Nursing
Diagnosis
and
Intervention
in Nursing Practice

Consulting Editors

For Part 2,
"Nursing Diagnoses"
MARY REARDON CASTLES, M.S.N., Ph.D.
Associate Professor
Wayne State University
College of Nursing

For Part 3,
"Nursing Interventions"
LORA B. ROACH, R.N., B.S., M.S.N.
Assistant Professor
The University of Texas at Arlington
School of Nursing

Nursing Diagnosis and Intervention in Nursing Practice

CLAIRE CAMPBELL, R.N., M.S.

Former Staff and Head Nurse, Medical-Surgical Nursing
Dallas County Hospital District
Parkland Memorial Hospital
and
Former Instructor
Texas Woman's University
Dallas Center

A Wiley Medical Publication
JOHN WILEY & SONS
New York   Chichester   Brisbane   Toronto

To
the Source of all our blessings
and to
Hugh, Clara, and loved ones
my devoted colleagues
and all those entrusted to our care

This book was set in Aster by Lexigraphics, Inc. It was printed and bound by Quinn & Boden Company, Inc. The designer was Suzanne Bennett. Margery Carazzone supervised copyediting and production.

Library of Congress Cataloging in Publication Data
Campbell, Claire.
    Nursing diagnosis and intervention in nursing practice.

    (A Wiley medical publication)
    Includes bibliographical references and indexes.
    1. Nursing. 2. Diagnosis. I. Castles, Mary Reardon. II. Roach, Lora B. III. Title.

RT41.C28   610.73   77-17095

ISBN 0-471-13307-8
Printed in the United States of America
10 9 8 7 6 5 4 3 2

Preface

This book is devoted to the nursing process and emphasizes the development and identification of nursing diagnoses and interventions. It is based on the concept that nursing diagnoses are determined from existing or potential health problems treated by professional nurses. These patient problems are identified in strictly nursing, rather than medical, terms. For years, nurses have been using medical diseases as the basis of nursing treatment. But today we are developing our own list of patient problems, which are not diseases, in an effort to establish a more precise nursing profession.

Nursing Diagnosis and Intervention in Nursing Practice is designed for professional registered nurses involved in clinical practice or in education and for students learning nursing care. It describes the step-by-step system of thought that nurses use in analyzing and solving patient problems in giving nursing care, in much the same way that physicians analyze diseases and treat them. The book is intended to be a quick, practical source from which patient care plans can be made and is applicable to the Problem Oriented Record System. Additionally, it provides a common basis of communication among nurse colleagues for the practice of nursing until a standard nomenclature of nursing diagnosis can be developed.

In Part 1, the theory that supports nursing diagnosis and intervention and its integration into the nursing process is discussed. In Chapter 4, the organization of the book, the interrelationship of its various parts, and how the book is intended to be used are described in detail. Also, since the concept of nursing diagnosis and the use of physical examination skills are both relatively new in nursing, a description is given of how nursing diagnoses can be arrived at through assessment by physical examination.

Part 2 lists 730 nursing diagnoses. For each diagnosis included, assessment data, possible etiology, the nursing diagnosis, a nursing plan, appropriate nursing interventions, and evaluation criteria are given. The nursing diagnosis list presented here is considered a beginning and is not a comprehensive, final list or an attempt to develop a taxonomy. The classification system is flexible enough so that new diagnoses can be added, and it is expected that this list will lend itself to refinement.

Part 3 lists all the nursing interventions found in Part 2, including for each a definition, a rationale, the human needs resolved by the intervention, and any contraindications for its use. These interventions are grouped into four categories: nursing treatments, nursing observations, health teaching, and medical treatments performed by nurses. Those nursing interventions that are performed by nurses as part of the expanded role in nursing are identified by a code (ExR), as are those that are performed by nurses in emergencies (ET). Although the nursing interventions have been stated specifically in an effort to clarify nursing functions, these interventions are not intended to initiate formula-type nursing. They are presented as alternatives from which the nurse can choose those interventions appropriate to the individual patient in a specific health-related situation.

Part 4 consists of references and indexes. The four indexes list the nursing diagnoses (alphabetically and by subject) and the nursing interventions (alphabetically and by subject) that are found in the book. Thus, they ease the finding of material within Parts 2 and 3 and provide a quick reference for nursing diagnosis and intervention labels.

Nursing diagnosis, as a step in the nursing process, is in its infancy. However, as the science of professional nursing continues to advance, the development of nursing diagnosis and intervention should progress rapidly. It is my hope that this book will further that development and promote greater freedom among professional nurses in making decisions as they plan and provide care.

C. C.

Acknowledgments

This book originally evolved from the association of the following registered nurses and the author, all of whom were involved together in the pursuit of graduate studies:

SUZANNE J. BEACH, R.N., M.S., Director of the Department of Nursing, Children's Medical Center of Dallas, Dallas, Texas

DOLORES CHUMCHAL BERKOVSKY, R.N., M.S., Community Nurse Practitioner, Catholic Social Services, former Associate Professor in Nursing, Texas Christian University, Fort Worth, Texas

CECILIA M. HOLLAND, R.N., M.S.N., Staff Nurse, Sam Rayburn Memorial Veterans Center, Bonham, Texas, former Instructor in Nursing, Paris Junior College, Paris, Texas

HAZEL M. JAY, R.N., M.Ed., M.S., Associate Professor, Graduate Advisor, The University of Texas at Arlington School of Nursing, former Director of Continuing Education, The University of Texas at Arlington School of Nursing, Arlington, Texas

CLAIRE JENKINS JOHNSON, R.N., M.S., Critical Care Nurse Consultant, Dallas, Texas, former Director, Critical-Care Nursing Course, School of Allied Health Sciences, University of Texas Health Science Center, Dallas, Texas

ANNE KUEMPEL, R.N., B.S.N., M.S., Director of Nurses, St. David's Hospital, former Assistant Executive Secretary, Board of Nurse Examiners for the State of Texas, Austin, Texas

SHIRLEY J. PINTERICH, R.N., M.S., Associate Professor of Nursing and Chairman, Southwestern Union College, Keene, Texas, former Instructor in Nursing, Union College, Denver, Colorado

MARY K. OLSON ROBITAILLE, R.N., M.S., Nephrology Nurse Clinician, Detroit, Michigan

WANDA J. THOMPSON, R.N., M.S., Assistant Professor of Nursing and Director of the Family Nurse Practitioner Program, The University of Texas at Arlington School of Nursing, Arlington, Texas, former Assistant Professor of Nursing, Dallas Baptist College, Dallas, Texas

LINDA S. WHITE, R.N., M.S., former Director, Accelerated Program in Nursing, University of Tennessee, College of Nursing, Memphis, Tennessee

KATHLEEN S. WINGER, R.N., M.S., former Associate Director of Nursing, St. Paul's Hospital, Dallas, Texas

As the study of nursing diagnoses and interventions progressed, other health professionals became involved. Without the expertise and outstanding generosity of the nursing colleagues and others listed below, this work could never have achieved completion:

PAULINE BAKER BOSWELL, R.N., Assistant Head Nurse, General Surgery, Presbyterian Hospital of Dallas, former Head Nurse, General Surgery, Dallas County Hospital District, Parkland Memorial Hospital, Dallas, Texas

JESSIE F. BEWLEY, R.N., M.S., former Assistant Professor, Texas Woman's University, College of Nursing, Dallas Center, and Instructor of Nursing, Parkland Hospital School of Nursing, Dallas, Texas

BERNADETTE CLAUS, R.N., Office Nursing, Southwest Clinic, former Staff Nurse, St. Paul's Hospital, Dallas, Texas

CHERYL CONATSER, R.N., M.S., Adolescent Clinical Nurse, Specialist in Hematology-Oncology, Children's Medical Center of Dallas, former Instructor, Pediatric Nursing, El Centro College, Dallas, Texas

MARGARET HARTY, B.S., M.A., Ed.D., Vice President of the Institute of Health Sciences, Texas Woman's University, College of Nursing, Denton, Texas

JUDITH HENLEY, R.N., M.S., Instructor in Nursing, Texas Woman's University, College of Nursing, Dallas Center, former Head Nurse and Inservice Instructor in Maternity Nursing, Dallas County Hospital District, Parkland Memorial Hospital, Dallas, Texas

TEDDY LANGFORD, M.S.N., Ph.D., Associate Dean for Education, University of Colorado School of Nursing, Denver, Colorado, former Vice President for Academic Affairs, University of Texas System School of Nursing, Austin, Texas

LOUISE LORRAINE LASTELICK, R.N., M.S., Assistant Professor of Nursing, University of Southwestern Louisiana, Lafayette, Louisiana, former Assistant Supervisor, Neurosurgery Division, Baylor University Medical Center, Dallas, Texas

MARGARET McCLUSKY McLEROY, R.N., M.S., Assistant Professor, Texas Woman's University, College of Nursing, Dallas Center, former Instructor, St. Paul's Hospital School of Nursing, Dallas, Texas

ANN RUTH ROBERSON, R.N., Industrial Nurse, Occupational Health Services, Otis Engineering Corporation, former Staff and Head Nurse of Surgical Specialties, Dallas County Hospital District, Parkland Memorial Hospital, Dallas, Texas

JOSEPHINE SIMONSON, M.A., Consultant in Speech, Texas Neurological Institute at Medical City of Dallas and Presbyterian Hospital of Dallas, Dallas, Texas

JUDY SPINELLA, R.N., M.S.N., Assistant Professor, University of Texas at Arlington School of Nursing, Arlington, Texas, former Staff Nurse, John Peter Smith Hospital, Fort Worth, Texas

MARY LOVATT SMITH TRAGUS, R.N., M.S.N., Rehabilitation Specialist, International Rehabilitation Associates, Inc., former Instructor of Nursing, Texas Woman's University, College of Nursing, Dallas Center, Dallas, Texas

NANCY J. VOLLMER, R.N., M.S., Assistant Director of Nursing, Dallas County Hospital District, Parkland Memorial Hospital, former Assistant Professor of Nursing, Texas Woman's University, College of Nursing, Dallas Center, Dallas, Texas

BETTY H. WADE, R.N., M.S.N., Associate Dean, College of Nursing, Texas Woman's University, College of Nursing, Dallas Center, Dallas, Texas, former Staff Nurse, Head Nurse, Supervisor, Medical Nursing and Clinical Research Center, University of Alabama Hospitals and Clinics Birmingham, Birmingham, Alabama

CAROL WARE, R.N., B.S.N., M.B.A., Programmer, Presbyterian Hospital of Dallas, Dallas, Texas

OPAL WHITE, R.N., M.P.H., D.N.S., former Professor, Texas Woman's University, College of Nursing, Dallas Center, Dallas, Texas, and Professor and Coordinator, University of Colorado School of Nursing, Denver, Colorado

FRANCES WHITED, R.N., B.S., Assistant Professor, Texas Woman's University, College of Nursing, Dallas Center, former Staff Nurse, Dallas City Health Department, Dallas, Texas

JULIA M. WILSON, M.D., Cardiologist, Ottawa, Canada

EVELYN B. WORMSER, R.N., M.S., Assistant Professor of Psychiatry-Mental Health, Family Nurse Practitioner Program, The University of Texas at Arlington School of Nursing, Arlington, Texas

Sincere appreciation is also extended to the 100 registered nurses and 233 senior and junior nursing students (1971–1972) who participated in this effort, to Lynda L. Kelly, Ph.D., to Martha Ann Edwards and Saundra G. Haun for their secretarial services, and to the entire staff of John Wiley & Sons, Inc., especially Nursing Editor Cathy Somer, former Editor Earl Shepherd, and Production Editor Margery Carazzone.

Contents

PART 2
NURSING DIAGNOSES

PART 3
NURSING INTERVENTIONS

PART 4
REFERENCES AND INDEXES

Part 1.

The Theory of Nursing Diagnosis and Intervention

1.
A Human Need Approach to Nursing Diagnosis

In 1939 the physiologist Cannon (82:24)* described homeostasis as an attempt by the body to maintain a state of constancy in its internal environment. Since that time, other physiologists have agreed with this theory. Guyton stated that "the term homeostasis is used by physiologists to mean maintenance of static, or constant, conditions in the internal environment. Essentially all the organs and tissues of the body perform functions that help to maintain these constant conditions" (180:3). Ganong concurred that "a large part of physiology is concerned with regulatory mechanisms which act to maintain the constancy of the internal environment" (160:18).

In 1954 Maslow (292:35–36) stated that each person has basic human needs that are vital to the integration of the homeostatic system. These needs are essential components, and they must be gratified if there is to be a healthy existence. He categorized them according to their priority, with the highest priority being assigned to those needs most important to maintaining life: the physiologic and safety needs. Maslow (292:37–47) believed that once these most basic needs were met, human beings could move forward to meet their needs for belonging, esteem, esteem from others, and self-actualization.

Maslow's categories (292:37–47) followed this sequence of priority, in descending order:

Physiologic needs
Safety needs
Belongingness needs
Esteem needs
Esteem from others needs
Self-actualization needs

Under each of these six categories he further identified specific needs appropriate to each category, but he did not list them in order of priority.

*See p. 51 for an explanation of the reference numbering system.

Maslow's theory (292:35–36) emphasized that when a human being undergoes intense stress, the normal integration of the organism is threatened. When the basic human needs are not met, the person is in a state of disequilibrium. He stated that since a human being is and behaves as a harmoniously coordinated organism, when one system is out of harmony the whole being is affected. When a person is hungry, not only is his nutritional balance disturbed, but his attitudes, tolerance for stress, and many other factors are temporarily in disharmony. When his hunger is satisfied, the normal state of homeostasis is regained. In order to maintain a state of harmony, a person receives signals from his body in the form of appetites or motivational drives toward those needs that are unmet within the organism. If the body is lacking in regard to a specific chemical component, the organism will move toward replacing that component so that equilibrium can be restored.

This attempt to maintain balance occurs on all levels of human existence, from the most basic physiologic need to the highest self-actualization need. The person, by attempting to restore harmony, achieves balance and regains a state of health. Maslow (292:29–33) stated that when human needs are gratified, health is improved, because the person once again becomes an integrated whole.

According to Maslow (292:57), basic need deprivation results in an unhealthy state in the individual. Since the person in an unhealthy state becomes the concern of the professional nurse, nurses must learn to recognize human needs. Beland stated that "in illness the capacity of the individual to cope with disturbances in his environment, in such a manner that his needs are satisfied, is reduced" (32:46). She further described the functions of the nurse in helping the patient maintain homeostasis as those of "modifying the external environment so the adaptations the patient is required to make are within his capacity to make, supporting the efforts of the patient to adapt or respond, and providing him with the materials required to maintain the constancy of his internal environment" (32:46). If homeostasis and need gratification are necessary for health, then nurses who help patients resolve need deprivations are simultaneously helping them resolve their health problems.

Nurses also must recognize that it is the patient's awareness that some of his needs are unmet that forces him to acknowledge the he has health problems and that compels him to attempt to solve them.

Professional nurses have long recognized that certain human needs take priority over others. Some needs must be met immediately, while others can be postponed, especially during an illness in which life itself is threatened.

The concept that need deprivation results in unhealthy states led to the development of nursing diagnoses, which imply human-need deprivation and nursing interventions that resolve, diminish, or prevent human needs.

2.
The Study of Nursing Diagnoses and Nursing Interventions

In order that Maslow's human need theory (292:37–47) might be applied to the nursing process, a list of nursing diagnoses was developed. Although professional nurses have for many years been making judgments about patient interaction with existing or potential health problems, the effort to formalize nursing diagnosis statements is in its infancy. A number of essential factors must be considered in the development of nursing diagnoses:

Health needs of the consumer
Legislation, as it affects nursing diagnoses in all areas of professional nursing, including practice at advanced and specialized levels
Realities of current nursing practice
Curricula in schools of nursing
Differentiation of nursing and medical interventions
Patient problems, as exemplified in the nursing literature
Definitions of nursing diagnosis, as exemplified in the nursing literature

HEALTH NEEDS OF THE CONSUMER

The health needs of the consumer, as he perceives them, have been greatly influenced by recent advances in scientific knowledge and technology. The consumer today enjoys a higher level of education and receives better information than he did just a few years ago. The consumer is now seeking more complete health care and health maintenance; he has an educated desire to know what the current health problems are and how they can be treated or prevented, as well as how the environment, lifestyles, and society in general influence health. The consumer seeks to be able to adapt to health problems in a manner compatible with a productive life and sound economics.

The emergence of an informed public and the recent advances in technology have helped to expand the number of health professions and the scope

5

of their activities in an effort to integrate health services for the increased benefit of the patient. This, in turn, increases the need for the nursing profession to state explicitly those nursing diagnoses of patient problems that are specific to nursing. Doing so will make it easier for nursing to integrate its services with those of other health professionals and, at the same time, remain accountable for activities specific to nursing.

LEGISLATION

As the consumer has become better informed, his quest for health has prompted new legislation and revision of existing laws and nursing practice acts designed to protect the consumer. Several states have rewritten their laws to meet consumer and practitioner demands, and others are in the process of doing so.

The question of whether nursing diagnosis should be defined by law has provoked considerable debate. Professional nurses have endeavored to avoid implying medical diagnoses in the terminology used in nursing diagnoses. To do so would not be permissible under the medical and nursing acts of most states, and it would serve no purpose to duplicate already existing health services.

If medical diagnoses are to be kept separate from nursing diagnoses, the differences between the two must be clearly defined.

The Division of Library and Archival Services of the American Medical Association has suggested that a generally accepted definition of medical diagnosis is to be found in the *Attorney's Dictionary of Medicine and Word Finder*. The definition states that a medical diagnosis is "the determination of what kind of a disease a patient is suffering from, especially the art of distinguishing between several possibilities" (376:27).

Murchison and Nichols stated that "almost all courts would agree that [medical] diagnosis is the determination of a disease from its symptoms" (321:95). They indicated that medical "diagnosis would be the selection of one disease from the possibility of diseases suggested by symptoms" (321:94). A Colorado statute refers to medical diagnosis as "the ascertaining of a disease or ailment by its symptoms" (321:94). Such statements clearly indicate that the diagnosis of disease is considered a medical responsibility. Such diagnosis is and always has been part of the practice of medicine.

Since medical diagnosis is clearly the identification of disease, what then is nursing diagnosis? Nursing today is involved in two areas of nursing activity that have an effect on the definition of nursing diagnosis. These activities are delivery of basic nursing care, and interventions associated with the expanded role of nursing.

Henderson described basic nursing care (193:16–17) as including those activities or providing those conditions under which the patient can, unaided, accomplish the following:

Breathe normally
Eat and drink normally
Eliminate body wastes

Move and maintain desirable positions
Sleep and rest
Select suitable clothes; dress and undress
Maintain body temperature within normal range by adjusting clo-
thing or modifying the environment
Keep the body clean and well groomed and protect the integument
Avoid dangers in the environment and avoid injuring others
Communicate with others in expressing emotions, needs, fears, or
opinions
Worship according to one's faith
Work in such a way that there is a sense of accomplishment
Play or participate in various forms of recreation
Learn, discover, or satisfy the curiosity that leads to normal develop-
ment and health and use the available health facilities.

These general components of basic nursing care may be categorized as
"hygienic, psychologic, environmental, safety, spiritual, social, rehabilitative, health instruction, prevention," (101:103) and comfort. They are compatible with the definitions of nursing that appear in most state nursing
practice acts, and they are patterned after the American Nurses Association
definition of nursing practice, which reads: "The practice of professional
nursing means the performance for compensation of any acts in the observation, care and counsel of the ill, injured or infirm or in the maintenance of
health or prevention of illness of others or in the supervision and teaching
of other personnel or in the administration of medications and treatments
prescribed by licensed physicians or dentists, requiring for all these functions substantial, specialized judgment and skill based on knowledge and
application of the principles of biological, physical and social sciences. The
foregoing shall not be deemed to include acts of diagnosis [implying medical diagnosis] or prescription of therapeutic or corrective measures" (616:2).
    These general components of nursing care provide areas for independent
nursing diagnosis and nursing intervention. However, in addition to basic
nursing care, the increased demands of the consumer for improved health
services have placed new responsibilities on the nurse. Many diverse factors
(isolated geographic areas, substandard communities, critical care units,
care specific to certain age groups) have contributed to the development of
new nursing activities that are either more comprehensive or more
specialized. These will be discussed in terms of the expanded role of nursing.
    The nurse in an expanded role performs physical examinations, identifies
normal and abnormal findings, orders drugs, and initiates therapy not previously associated with nursing (564:15–16). She treats uncomplicated and
chronic illnesses, common childhood conditions, and minor injuries; she
manages normal pregnancy, labor, and delivery and provides acute and
emergency care (228:507–510).
    In the 1970 U.S. Department of Health, Education and Welfare "Report on
Extending the Scope of Nursing Practice," it was stated that "the functions of
nurses are changing primarily because nurses have demonstrated their competence to perform a greater variety of functions" (614:12). These changing

functions tend to complicate the question of what the nurse can diagnose without infringing on the physician's medical diagnosis.

Some clarification of the term nursing diagnosis has been attempted. In 1973 the American Nurses Association, in its *Generic Standards of Practice*, referred to nursing diagnosis as "judgments about the health status of the patient which are distinct from diagnosis of other health professionals" (551:91).

Nursing practice acts generally restrict the professional nurse by incorporating statements such as "the foregoing shall not be deemed to include acts of [medical] diagnosis or prescription of therapeutic or corrective measures" (616:3). A "Position on Nursing Practice" published by the Michigan Nurses Association has stated that nurses assist the patient with health problems that include "existing or potential deficits in the ability to breathe, eat, drink, eliminate, maintain hygiene and comfort, exercise and rest, insure safety from environmental hazards, communicate, express emotional and spiritual needs and learn" (228:159). The California Nurses Association has indicated that the professional nurse identifies "each person's physical, psychologic and social needs, and assists the individual and his family to achieve an optimal health regime and dignified death" (228:160).

According to Mundinger and Jauron, the New York Nurse Practice Act describes nursing diagnosis as "human responses to actual or potential health problems" (536:94).

These definitions, which reflect the general professional and legislative approaches to nursing diagnosis, support the broad concept of a range of health care problems that can be treated independently by nurses. Because of this broad concept, the question has arisen whether nursing diagnosis, which does not include the identification of diseases, involves the identification of signs and symptoms of disease.

Lesnik and Anderson indicated that professional nurses have several areas of independent function. One of these is "the observation of symptoms and reactions including symptomatology of physical and mental conditions and needs, requiring evaluation or application of principles based upon the biologic, the physical, and social sciences" (259:259). Murchison and Nichols stated that "the nurse is properly allowed the responsibility of judging the gravity of symptoms without engaging in [medical] diagnosis" (321:95). They were of the opinion that in areas such as diagnosis of dysrhythmias, "when the nurse judges that the patient exhibits ventricular fibrillation she is merely observing a symptom, not diagnosing the disease suggested. In determining that the patient is suffering a true cardiac arrest, she is exercising judgment as to the seriousness of the symptom, but she is not ascertaining the nature of the disease" (321:94).

The foregoing statements support the concept that nurses should identify and evaluate signs and symptoms but they do not determine the disease possibilities represented. The physician "infers from signs and symptoms the abnormalities in function and structure" (316:20). The nurse infers from signs and symptoms their effects on the patient's capacity to function. The nurse may help the patient to cope with his signs and symptoms by suggesting a changed pattern of living; alternatively, if nursing intervention is appropriate, the nurse may relieve (261:119) the signs and symptoms so that the patient's living pattern remains unchanged but his life is no longer threatened. If certain nursing-related patient problems are themselves the signs and symptoms, they must be labeled as such in terms of a nursing diagnosis. It is essential that the scope and limits of nursing diagnosis be developed not in terms of the minimum legal requirements of nursing performance but in terms of the maximum legal extent of nursing practice. Even though this level is not presently encouraged in some states, the consumer's demand for maximum health care will support nursing practice designed to provide such care.

THE REALITIES OF CURRENT NURSING PRACTICE

In the process of developing a terminology for nursing diagnosis, the realities of current nursing practice must be considered. The nursing judgments that are being made and recorded in everyday contact with patients must be examined. In hospitals, community health agencies, or wherever the professional nurse may be, nursing judgments are being made and identified in nursing terms, even though such terms have not been compiled into a nomenclature of diagnoses. The realities of practice are a major source for a terminology of nursing diagnosis.

CURRICULA IN SCHOOLS OF NURSING

Prior and Silverstein suggested that "a nurse who meets the requirements for professional nursing practice . . . possesses a body of selective knowledge, relevant to the health sciences, drawn from the biologic, the physical and psychosocial basic sciences and selected medical science knowledge" (190:95). The basic knowledge of the professional nurse determines the kind and number of nursing diagnoses that can be made. The extent of this basic knowledge is determined primarily by the curriculum to which the nurse has been exposed. That curriculum, in addition to its determining effect on the nurse's level of knowledge, is also reflected in nursing practice.

DIFFERENTIATION OF NURSING AND MEDICAL INTERVENTIONS

In order to establish a terminology for nursing diagnosis, one must recognize that "nursing diagnoses are limited to areas of independent nursing action" (536:96). When the nurse recognizes a health problem but is not authorized to act independently to assist the patient in resolving that particular problem, she must work in conjunction with the physician. When a health problem is recognized by the nurse and she initiates treatment on the basis of standing medical orders or refers the patient to the physician, resolution of the problem is within the scope of medicine, not the scope of nursing, even though the nurse assists in resolving the problem.

Murchison and Nichols stated that "the differentiation of the doctor's diagnosis and a nursing diagnosis is based on the courses of action open to each professional after the decision from the observation is made" (321:97). The American Nurses Association Committee on Legislation (625:2) and Lesnik and Anderson (259:260) agree that one of the six independent areas of nursing is "the application and the execution of nursing procedures and techniques" (259:260).

If the nurse is to be able to determine which health problems nursing can resolve, diminish, or prevent, there must be a clear distinction between those interventions that are nursing treatments applicable to nursing diagnoses and those that are medical treatments carried out by the nurse. It must be recognized that today, as in the past, physicians direct many nursing procedures and techniques. Traditionally, "the medical components of nursing care have included those aspects of medical treatment delegated by the physician to the nurse" (101:103). This medical component has long been prevalent in nursing activities. The physician's direction of some nursing treatments and the frequency with which nurses carry out medical treatments have led to the misconception by patients, nurses, and physicians that all nursing interventions are medical treatments, when in fact they are nursing treatments. A statement of a health problem is not a nursing diagnosis unless the nurse can independently treat the health problem. Therefore nurses must clearly define what the nursing treatments are before they can determine which health problems fall within the nursing domain.

PATIENT PROBLEMS IN NURSING LITERATURE

Each patient has a number of patient problems that center around his attempt to maintain or regain health. The patient problems may be medical, nursing, sociologic, etc. (435:25–40). Nurses frequently make identifications of patient problems that are then referred to and treated by physicians, social workers, etc. However, only those identifications that describe "actual or potential health problems which nurses are capable [of treating] and licensed to treat" (611:9) are considered nursing diagnoses.

In any attempt to compile a list of nursing diagnoses, one of the most significant resources is the nursing literature. Nursing literature has been a consistent source of guidance for nurses in their efforts to solve health problems. Even though the health problems that have been recognized by nurses have not been stated in the form of nursing diagnoses, they have been expressed in such a way that they can be used as the basis for new efforts to identify nursing diagnoses. The nursing literature describes such patient problems as *wrist drop* (391:320), *indigestion* (4:459), *malnutrition* (325:73), and *increased cardiac work load* (71:269). Such problem identification can provide the basic terminology for nursing diagnoses.

DEFINITIONS OF NURSING DIAGNOSIS
IN NURSING LITERATURE

In addition to examples of the patient problems that can generate a terminology of nursing diagnosis, the literature contains statements of what professional nurses believe a nursing diagnosis to be. Gebbie and Lavin defined a nursing diagnosis as "the identification of those patient problems or concerns most frequently identified by nurses, problems which are usually identified by nurses before they are recognized by other health care workers, and problems which are amenable to some intervention which is available in the present or potential scope of nursing practice" (500:250). Komarita considered nursing diagnosis to be a "determination of the nature and extent of nursing problems presented by the individual patients or families receiving care" (517:91), and Marriner indicated that a "nursing diagnosis is a statement of a conclusion based on scientific principles and indicating the patient's need for nursing care" (289:32). Mundinger and Jauron stated that a diagnosis "is essentially an inference about a state that is undesirable. . . . As nurses, we are responsible for diagnosing and treating human responses to health problems" (536:96). At the 1976 American Nurses Association biennial convention, the House of Delegates in its Resolution on the Classification System of Nursing Diagnosis stated that "nursing diagnosis describes actual or potential health problems which nurses are capable [of treating] and licensed to treat" (611:9).

All these definitions reflect the basic concept of identifying patient problems and initiating independent nursing treatment. They contribute significantly to the effort to develop a standardized terminology for nursing diagnosis.

THE STUDY OF NURSING DIAGNOSES
AND NURSING INTERVENTIONS

Following a review of the literature, lists of possible nursing diagnoses and nursing interventions were compiled. Then 233 junior and senior nursing students in a large community hospital were asked to make nursing assessments of 550 patients over an 8½-month period. These students were providing care in the following clinical areas: general medicine; isolation; pediatrics; premature nursery; obstetrics; general chest; long-term chest diseases; eye, ear, nose, and throat diseases; general surgery; trauma; rehabilitation; neurology; neurosurgery; public health. Among the 550 patients there was a total of 344 different medical diagnoses.

The students were given the lists of possible nursing diagnoses and nursing interventions and were instructed to use them as references. They were asked to search for and add health problems and interventions appropriate to nursing that were not on the lists. They were also to determine whether the problems listed actually occurred in the clinical area and whether the nursing interventions were feasible.

The students wrote care plans for each of their patients. These care plans were reviewed by a nursing instructor and were thoroughly discussed with the students to confirm that all probable patient problems and appropriate nursing interventions had been included. New problems and interventions were added to the lists as they were identified.

The final list of patient problems was reevaluated by a panel of clinical judges, and criteria for the acceptance of a patient problem as a nursing diagnosis were developed. These criteria were accepted:

The diagnosis is a human response or resource limitation
The professional nurse can legally prescribe and carry out treatment independent of medical direction
The diagnosis occurs repeatedly in a significant number of patients
The diagnosis is a consequence of, contributing factor to, or potential danger leading to illness, injury, disease, or health maintenance
One or more human needs as identified by Maslow exist
The supporting data are such that they can be obtained and analyzed by the professional nurse in the light of nursing knowledge
The supporting data present two or more related facts
The patient problem is not a specific disease identified as such in the standard medical classification systems

In an effort to rule out patient problems that involved medical diagnoses, diagnostic statements were examined to determine whether they were listed in the *International Classification of Disease* (424) or *The Standard Nomenclature of Disease and Operations* (417).

The fact that diagnostic statements applicable to the areas of hygiene, assistance, comfort, prevention, education, and safety do not appear in listings of medical diagnoses confirms that these areas of health care are within the scope of nursing. However, the medical classifications consulted included not only medical diagnoses of disease but also signs, symptoms, and ill-defined conditions. Since professional nurses assume considerable responsibility for patient health from the standpoint of physiologic function, the question arose whether nurses could use already established medical terminology. It also became clear that it is important to distinguish between medical diagnosis of disease and generally used medical terminology.

In this study, medical diagnosis has been defined as "the determination of what kind of a disease a patient is suffering from, especially the art of distinguishing between several possibilities" (376:D27). Medical terminology, as used in this study, means those words used by an occupational group that become definite scientific terms and become a part of the language as a whole (101:103).

The American Medical Association has stated in *Current Medical Terminology* (16) that those who should use medical terminology to facilitate standardization in communication include "practitioners of medicine and the specialties, educators, investigators in fundamental and clinical medicine, medical students, interns, nurses, medical record librarians, etc." (16:iii).

Since almost all authorities and the courts agree that medical diagnosis is the determination of a disease from its symptoms (321:95), and since this is clearly the function of the physician, a nursing diagnosis cannot be a statement of disease. However, it has been determined that there are some common medical terms shared by all health professionals. Gebbie and Lavin stated that "there is no prohibition against using a label from another field if we [nurses] use it with the characteristics and accuracy usually expected and it says what we want it to say" (500:253). Murchison and Nichols suggested that in many aspects "nursing and medical practice are interrelated and undistinguishable from each other" (321:101). In the 1970 "American Medical Association Position Paper on Nursing" and in the "U.S. Department of Health, Education and Welfare Report on Extending the Scope of Nursing Practice," it was stated that an "identical act or procedure may be the practice of medicine when carried out by a physician and the practice of nursing when carried out by a nurse" (228:295).

The use of a common terminology to identify health problems results in what is essentially a system of *dual diagnosis*. Such diagnoses pertain to more than one professional domain. The diagnosis of disease is considered to be the exclusive prerogative of the physician, while the diagnosis of human responses and resource limitations is the exclusive prerogative of the nurse. There is, however, an area of dual responsibility and dual activity that may be found in the mutual diagnosis and treatment of the signs, symptoms, and ill-defined conditions identified in the medical classifications. This duality does not constitute an infringement of one profession on the other; rather, it is a cooperative effort between two professions seeking to provide health care.

An example of dual diagnosis is seen in *emergency-phase cardiac arrest*; the diagnosis can be arrived at by either the doctor or the nurse. Each practitioner can institute independent treatment procedures. *Malnutrition, indigestion,* and *muscle spasms* are other examples of conditions that may be identified and treated by either the doctor or the nurse.

Since the "nurse is able to recognize physical symptoms of illness commonly identified with organic changes, as well as manifestations of illness" (190:95), the medical terminology used for certain signs, symptoms, and processes may become nursing diagnostic statements. The list of nursing diagnoses established by this study consists of diagnoses related to human responses and resource limitations, some of which involve dual diagnosis, as described previously.

One area of concern that is not covered explicitly in this text involves the possible nursing diagnoses for which there are no independent nursing interventions. Examples of such possible nursing diagnoses are the dysrhythmias. These are diagnoses that are made by nurses in critical care units, and their identification is within the scope of nursing knowledge. However, there are no independent nursing interventions appropriate to these diagnoses, and all intervention is physician-directed. Since the dysrhythmias do not involve medical diagnoses of disease, there is the potential for them to fall into the sphere of nursing diagnosis. Their identification cannot presently be considered a nursing diagnosis, since there are no independent nursing interventions. Discussion of these conditions and others like them must be reserved until such time as nursing treatment may become expanded to the point that nurses can function independently in the treatment of such conditions.

The diagnoses meeting the criteria established by the panel of judges were reviewed and categorized as either human responses or resource limitations. A diagnosis was categorized as a *human response* if it was a reaction, effect, or behavior that could be interpreted as indicating existing or potential unwellness. A diagnosis was categorized as a *resource limitation* if it indicated a lack of ability, a lack of source of supply, or a lack of source of support that contributed to existing or potential unwellness.

Further examination of the diagnoses established that the general areas of human response generating nursing diagnoses were the following:

Discomfort, pain, or distress related to:
    diagnostic procedures
    environment
    health therapy
    imposed restrictions
    internal body sensations
    lifesaving devices
    prosthetic aids
    sleep and rest
    spiritual life
Difficult adaptation to:
    crisis situations
    life stages
    lifestyle interruptions
    role changes
Distressed human relationships
Difficulty in handling one's own emotional responses
Impairment of independent self-maintenance
Poor health practice despite adequate health knowledge
Signs and symptoms
Normal physiologic changes occurring in various life stages
Uncomplicated illnesses
Minor injuries
Acute and emergency conditions
Existing health states that must be maintained under health care supervision

Areas of resource limitation were found to include:

Health knowledge deficits involving:
    existing health hazards
    health examinations
    health therapy
    management of a specific health practice
    management of surgical body alterations
    nonrecognition of problems
    potential health hazards

problem solving
use of assistive communication devices
use of assistive health devices
Limitations related to:
environmental influences
preexisting (inherited, accidental) body disorders, deformities, or
nonhealth tendencies
sociocultural influences

These areas of human responses and resource limitations are included to provide examples of components of the health-life situation to which nursing interventions are appropriate.

Each diagnosis was then defined. The associated subjective (symptoms), objective (signs), and related data and etiology were established from the literature. Then, using Maslow's list of human needs (292:37–47), the human needs that could be inferred from the diagnosis were established on the basis of the definition, the subjective, objective, and related data, the etiology, and clinical judgment.

Maslow (292:37–47) ranked the broad categories of human needs in a hierarchy of descending priority from physiologic, safety, belongingness, self-esteem, esteem from others, self-actualization. However, he did not specify by priority the specific needs that he listed as subcategories under his main headings. In this study of nursing diagnosis and intervention, Maslow's subcategories of specific needs (292:37–47) were assigned priority rankings. One hundred registered nurses and 50 junior and 50 senior nursing students were asked to rank the subcategory needs from the most significant to the least significant according to their importance in nursing. Priorities were established as shown in Table 2-1.

Table 2-1
Priority Ranking of Maslow's Subcategories of Human Needs

PHYSIOLOGIC NEEDS
Oxygen, circulation
Water-salt balance
Food balance
Acid-base balance
Waste elimination
Normal temperature
Sleep, rest, relaxation
Activity, exercise
Energy
Comfort
Stimulation
Cleanliness
Sexuality

SAFETY NEEDS
Protection from physical harm

Table 2-1   continued

SAFETY NEEDS *continued*
Protection from psychologic threat
Freedom from pain
Stability
Dependence
Predictable, orderly world

BELONGINGNESS NEEDS
Love and affection
Acceptance
Warm, communicating relationships
Approval from others
Unity with loved ones
Group companionship

SELF-ESTEEM NEEDS
Sense of value, usefulness
High evaluation of self
Adequacy
Self-reliance
Goal achievement
Mastery and competence in skills
Independence
Endurance

ESTEEM FROM OTHERS NEEDS
Recognition
Dignity
Appreciation from others
Importance, influence
Reputation of good character
Attention
Status
Dominance over others

SELF-ACTUALIZATION NEEDS
Personal growth and maturity
Awareness of potential
Increased learning
Full development of potential
Improved values
Religious, philosophic satisfaction
Increased creativity
Increased reality perception and problem-solving abilities
Less rigid conventionality
Less of the familiar, more of the novel
Greater satisfaction in beauty
Increased pleasantness
Less of the simple, more of the complex

The list of nursing interventions that the students had been using was also reviewed by the panel of judges. It was recognized that a specific list of interventions might be interpreted by some as limiting the scope of nursing practice; however, for this study it was necessary that the interventions be identified so that nursing diagnoses could be determined. It was also recognized that additional nursing interventions could and should be added in the future and that the listing of specific interventions can be seen as an expanding rather than a limiting process in that it gives the nurse a clearer view of the vast scope of nursing practice.

Criteria for acceptance of a nursing intervention were determined:

The nursing action falls within the legal scope of nursing activity
The rationale and effects of the nursing action are within the scope of nursing knowledge and skills
The nursing action resolves, diminishes, or prevents one or more human needs.

Each nursing intervention statement was structured so as to involve only a single nursing action. The rationale for implementation and the contraindications were identified in the literature.

While the full range of health interventions available to the patient was being reviewed, the question of which health interventions are nursing interventions and which are medical interventions arose. The differentiation in Table 2-2 is based on extensive review of the relevant literature. Nursing interventions are single-action treatments that are ordered by a professional nurse and carried out by a professional nurse or by a nursing assistant under professional nursing supervision. They are listed in Table 2-2.

Table 2-2
Nursing Interventions

BASIC NURSING TREATMENTS
Airway patency maintenance (71:50)
Alignment, body (70:133)
Ambulation, patient (271:1742)
Ambulation with mechanical aids (71:29)
Aseptic technique, maintenance of (71:818)
Baths, emollient: starch, bran, oatmeal (271:1756)
Bath, sitz (271:1755)
Bathing (366:184)
Bathing, sponge (71:726)
Bed-making (271:1743)
Binder applications (366:175)
Bladder irrigations, management of (71:469)
Bladder training (71:36)
Blakemore tube inflation and deflation (71:441)
Blood transfusion, management of (71:199)
Bowel elimination (70:473)
Bowel training (71:38)
Breast pump, use of (461:636–637)
Catheterization, urinary (271:1748)

Table 2-2   continued

BASIC NURSING TREATMENTS *continued*

Catheter, management of urinary (71:467)
Chest drainage, management of (70:260)
CircOlectric frames, placing on (71:757)
Cold applications (271:1754)
Cold packs (271:1754)
Cold sponges (271:1755)
Cough exercises (70:234)
Deep breathing exercises (71:50)
Denture care (366:177)
Douche, vaginal (71:535)
Dressing and undressing, assistance with (454:163)
Dressings, nonmedicated wet (71:569)
Dressings, occlusive (71:571)
Dressings, wound (71:64)
Ear hygiene (70:745)
Eating assistance (271:1745)
Electrolytes, food and oral fluid replacement of (472:63)
Enemas (271:1747)
Environment, modification of (271:1742)
Expression of breast milk, manual (461:637)
Fluid replacement, oral (472:36)
Food appropriateness for eating, determining (242:104)
Food preference, assistance with (242:103)
Footboard, application of (70:168)
Gastric tube, management of (71:385)
Hair care (271:1744)
Heat applications, dry (271:1752
Heat applications, moist (271:1752)
Hot packs (271:1754)
Hyperalimentation, management of (71:1086)
Intravenous infusion, management of (70:85)
Irrigations, nonmedicated low-pressure: eye, ear, nose (271:1749); wound
    (71:908)
Isolation technique (271:1757)
Isometric exercises (71:7)
Massage, back (71:799)
Massage, uterine fundus (71:1001)
Nail care (271:1744)
Nursing-care-related referrals (71:38)
Nutrition, maintaining balanced (242:103)
Nutritional supplements, nonprescription (70:671)
Oral hygiene (271:1746)
Oxygen therapy, management of (71:131)
Perineal care (71:537)
Positioning of the body (71:5)
Postmortem care (366:293)
Postural drainage (271:1752)
Predeath care (70:40)
Range-of-motion exercises (70:161)
Restraints (271:1746)

Table 2 2   continued

BASIC NURSING TREATMENTS *continued*

Skin care (271:1744)
Steam inhalation, nonmedicated (271:1751)
Stryker frame, placing on (71:763)
Teaching, patient (71:25)
Tracheostomy, management of (71:99)
Traction, management of (70:852)
Trochanter roll, application of (71:19)
Tube feedings, management of (71:395)
Urine elimination (70:473)

EMERGENCY NURSING TREATMENTS

Bivalve cast (71:778)
Cardiac compression, external (71:901)
Defibrillation (70:418)
Gastric lavage (366:440)
Intravenous infusion, initiation of (71:905)
Nasogastric intubation (71:911)
Oxygen therapy, initiation of (71:909)
Positive pressure therapy, initiation of (71:902)
Pulmonary resuscitation (70:950)
Rotating tourniquets (71:283)
Splinting, fracture (71:916)
Tetanus prophylaxis (71:907)
Tracheostomy (71:933)

ADDITIONAL NURSING MEASURES PERFORMED BY NURSES IN THE EXPANDED
    ROLE

Anesthetics, application of local (562:16)
Drugs, nonprescription (562:16)
Immunization (228:288)
Incision and extension of wounds not involved with major blood vessels,
    nerves, or tendons (562:16)
Management of common childhood conditions (228:508)
Management of the healthy newborn (228:509)
Management of uncomplicated labor and delivery (228:509)
Management of uncomplicated postpartum period (228:508)
Management of uncomplicated pregnancy (228:508)
Suture removal (71:64)
Suturing (562:16)

Medical interventions are treatments that are ordered by the physician
and are carried out by the physician or by someone under the supervision of
the physician. They are listed in Table 2-3.

Since one of the six independent functions of nursing is "the application
and execution of nursing procedures and techniques" (259:260), professional nurses can initiate nursing interventions for the consumer's benefit
without physician direction. Independent intervention with nursing procedures and techniques does not imply that physicians should not order nursing treatments; in many instances the physician relies heavily on nursing

Table 2-3
Medical Interventions

Aerosol inhalation, medicated (271:1724)
Anesthesia, administration of (417:607–610)
Back exercises, prescribing (71:800)
Bed rest, prescribing (391:781)
Blakemore tube insertion (70:524)
Blood transfusion, prescribing (70:94)
Braces, prescribing (70:175)
Burger exercises, prescribing (71:320)
Burger-Allen postural exercises, prescribing (70:329)
Cardiac compression (417:1043)
Cast application (391:318)
Cauterization (391:902)
Chemotherapy perfusion, prescribing (70:185)
Chest drainage, water-sealed (391:249)
Colostomy irrigation (242:272)
Contact lens, prescribing (70:721)
Contrast baths, prescribing (70:329)
Crutches, prescribing (70:174)
Crutch gait, prescribing (70:174)
Cutdown, arterial (271:1731)
Defibrillation (70:418)
Diets specific to diseases (271:1770)
Dressings, medicated wet (242:232)
Drugs, prescribing nasal spray and sublingual (271:1724), intradermal
    (271:1725), subcutaneous (271:1727), intramuscular (271:1728), intracar-
    diac and intraarterial (271:1731), intrathecal (271:1732), rectal
    (271:1733), aerosol inhalation, and vaginal (271:1734)
Ear irrigations, medicated (71:685)
Eye irrigations, medicated (71:685)
Endotracheal intubation (71:105)
Eyeglasses, prescribing (70:721)
Fluid and electrolyte replacement (70:83)
Gastric cooling (70:462)
Gastric gavage (366:450)
Hearing aids, prescribing (70:756)
Hemodialysis (391:1102)
Hyperalimentation, prescribing (71:1086)
Hypodermoclysis, prescribing (271:1728)
Hypothermia (391:1086)
Incision and drainage (366:715)
Intraarterial infusion (70:186)
Intravenous infusion, prescribing (271:1729)
Nasogastric and intestinal intubation and aspiration (271:1738)
Nebulization, medicated (271:1724)
Nutritional supplements, prescribing (70:669)
Operative procedures (417:517–606)
Orthotist, prescribing (70:175)
Oxygen therapy, prescribing (271:1725)

Table 2-3   continued

Pacemaker insertion (391:1048)
Paracentesis (271:1735)
Pericardicentesis (271:1736)
Peritoneal dialysis (391:1106)
Phlebotomy (391:579)
Phototherapy treatment (71:1130)
Postmastectomy exercises, prescribing (391:935)
Prosthesis, prescribing (70:175)
Pulmonary resuscitation (242:346)
Radiation therapy (70:201)
Radioisotope therapy (70:202)
Reduction of fractures and dislocations (366:816)
Splinting, fracture (71:916)
Suture removal (71:64)
Suturing (391:220)
Thoracentesis (271:1736)
Tidal drainage (242:319)
Tube feedings, prescribing (71:395)
Rotating tourniquets (391:611)
Tracheal aspiration (271:1741)
Traction, prescribing (391:327)
Tracheostomy (70:222)
Urinary bladder installations, medicated (242:319)

interventions in his effort to cure the disease being treated. It does imply, however, that professional nurses are free to perform nursing procedures independent of physician direction when those nursing treatments apply to health problems that fall within the nursing domain.

Of the total number of nursing interventions that have been listed in this study, 99.98% can be performed independent of physician direction. Only 0.02% of these nursing interventions require direction from the physician.

Discussion by the judges also led to the conclusion that it is convenient to group nursing interventions in a few broad categories. The work of Matheney (293:99–100) and that of Maloney (282:63–66) were combined to produce the list of nursing intervention categories shown in Table 2-4.

An assistive nursing intervention is one in which the nurse helps carry out those normal daily activities that cannot be carried out by the patient.

A hygienic nursing intervention is one that is necessary for the maintenance of cleanliness.

A rehabilitative nursing intervention is one that supports improved or independent activity and function in one of the following areas: mobility; management of specific devices, supplies, and body alterations; retraining for bowel and bladder function; measures to ease work and conserve physical energy; clothing adjustments specific to health problems; budgeting; planning with the family and agencies; referral to resource persons; involvement of the patient in community and social affairs.

Table 2-4
Nursing Intervention Categories

Assistive nursing interventions
Hygienic nursing interventions
Rehabilitative nursing interventions
Supportive nursing interventions
Preventive nursing interventions
Observational nursing interventions
Educative nursing interventions

A supportive nursing intervention is one in which the nurse provides needed objects (oxygen, nutrition, fluids), facilitates processes or activities (elimination, body alignment, exercise, rest, sleep, entertainment), provides physical or psychologic comfort or healing measures, or simply maintains a healthy environment.

A preventive nursing intervention is one in which the nurse provides protective or precautionary measures to avert physical or behavioral illness, injury, disease, or threat or to prevent complications or recurrences of physical or behavioral disorders, malfunctioning of therapeutic devices, or noneffective treatments.

An observational nursing intervention is one in which the nurse examines, checks, inspects, and monitors behavioral and physical responses to illness, injury, and disease and their associated therapies.

An educative nursing intervention is one in which the nurse provides satisfactory and accurate health information and explanation of treatment.

In summary, during the first phase of the study three lists were developed: a list of nursing diagnoses, each with its definition, etiology, and supporting data; a list of nursing interventions, each with its definition and rationale; a list of human needs developed as subcategories under Maslow's six major needs categories and ranked by a panel of clinical nurses.

In the second phase the human needs assigned to each diagnosis were derived from the definition, etiology, supporting data, and clinical judgment. They were listed according to the priorities established by the panel of clinical nurses. Nursing interventions that specifically resolved, diminished, or prevented the human needs of each diagnosis were assigned to the nursing diagnosis.

As the study proceeded, it was determined that the goals appropriate to each nursing diagnosis should fit into a consistent and basic pattern.

Since Abdellah's "Twenty-One Nursing Problems" (2:280–281) lend themselves to goal statements and are familiar to most clinical nurses, they were used. With only minimal changes in wording, they served as a standard framework of expected outcomes, as shown in Table 2-5.

These nursing goals provide a statement of the expected outcome that will occur if the human needs are resolved, diminished, or prevented. They reflect those factors that must be changed if the patient is to regain or maintain health.

Table 2-5
Primary Nurse-Patient Goals (2:280–281)

To maintain
 oxygen to all cells
 nutrition to all cells
 elimination of wastes
 fluid and electrolyte balance
 regulating mechanisms and functions
 sensory function and stimulation

To achieve
 good hygiene
 comfort
 activity and exercise
 sleep, rest, and relaxation
 positive expressions, feelings, and reactions
 effective verbal and nonverbal communications
 productive interpersonal relationships
 spiritual goals
 a therapeutic environment
 awareness of needs and/or use of resources
 optimum function

To prevent
 accident, physical injury, deformity, infection, and hypersensitivity response
 emotional injury

In the process of determining which of Abdellah's goals were suitable to each of Maslow's needs, it became evident that in some cases several goals could be applied to one need. This led to confused and disorderly association between the two. Therefore it was decided that only the primary goal or most appropriate goal should be assigned to each of Maslow's needs. By using only one primary goal, the nursing process could be kept orderly. The goals are realistically attainable and are subject to evaluation. A primary nurse-patient goal was thus assigned to each human need as shown in Table 2-6.

Once the goals to be associated with the human needs of each nursing diagnosis were established, evaluation criteria were developed, as shown in Table 2-7.

Table 2-6
Primary Nurse-Patient Goals Associated With Maslow's Needs

MASLOW'S NEEDS (292:37–47)	PRIMARY NURSE-PATIENT GOALS (2:280–281)
PHYSIOLOGIC NEEDS	
Oxygen, circulation	To maintain oxygen to all cells

Table 2-6   continued

MASLOW'S NEEDS (292:37–47)	PRIMARY NURSE-PATIENT GOALS (2:280–281)

PHYSIOLOGIC NEEDS *continued*

Water-salt balance	To maintain fluid and electrolyte balance
Food balance	To maintain nutrition to all cells
Acid-base balance, waste elimination, normal temperature	To maintain regulating mechanisms and functions
Sleep, rest, relaxation	To achieve sleep, rest, and relaxation
Activity, exercise	To achieve activity and exercise
Energy	To maintain regulating mechanisms and functions
Comfort	To achieve comfort
Stimulation	To maintain sensory function and stimulation
Cleanliness	To achieve good hygiene
Sexuality	To achieve productive interpersonal relationships

SAFETY NEEDS

Protection from physical harm	To prevent accident, physical injury, deformity, infection, and hypersensitivity response
Protection from psychologic threat	To prevent emotional injury
Freedom from pain	To achieve comfort
Stability	To achieve a therapeutic environment
Dependence	To achieve comfort
Predictable, orderly world	To achieve a therapeutic environment

BELONGINGNESS NEEDS

Love and affection, acceptance	To achieve productive interpersonal relationships
Warm, communicating relationships	To achieve effective verbal and nonverbal communications
Approval from others, unity with loved ones, group compansionship	To achieve productive interpersonal relationships

ESTEEM NEEDS

Sense of value, usefulness, high evaluation of self, adequacy, self-reliance	To achieve positive expressions, feelings, and reactions
Goal achievement, mastery and competence in skills, independence	To achieve optimum function
Endurance	To achieve positive expressions, feelings, and reactions

Table 2-6 continued

MASLOW'S NEEDS (292:37–47)	PRIMARY NURSE-PATIENT GOALS (2:280–281)
ESTEEM FROM OTHERS NEEDS	
Recognition, dignity, appreciation from others, importance, influence, reputation of good character, attention, status, dominance over others	To achieve productive interpersonal relationships
SELF-ACTUALIZATION NEEDS	
Personal growth and maturity, awareness of potential	To achieve optimum function
Increased learning	To achieve awareness of needs and/or use of resources
Full development of potential	To achieve optimum function
Improved values	To achieve positive expressions, feelings, and reactions
Religious, philosophic satisfaction	To achieve spiritual goals
Increased creativity, increased reality perception and problem-solving abilities	To achieve optimum function
Less rigid conventionality, less of the familiar, more of the novel, greater satisfaction in beauty	To achieve a therapeutic environment
Increased pleasantness	To achieve positive expressions, feelings, and reactions
Less of the simple, more of the complex	To achieve optimum function

Table 2-7
Evaluation Guideline

CRITERIA[a]	DATA INDICATING THAT CRITERIA ARE MET[b]
GOAL: To maintain oxygen to all cells (includes oxygen absorption and circulation)	
Good skin and mucous membrane color	Obj. D: Warm, moist, natural color to skin, nails, lips, ear lobes
Vital signs within normal limits	Obj. D: Respiratory rate: 30–60 infant 20–30 child 15–24 adolescent

Table 2-7   continued

CRITERIA[a]	DATA INDICATING THAT CRITERIA ARE MET[b]
	16–20 adult
	Pulse Rate:
	120–160 fetal
	80–180 infant
	70–140 child
	50–110 adolescent
	70–82 adult
	BP: Infants 90/60
	3–6 years 110/70
	7–10 years 120/80
	11–17 years 130/80
	18–44 years 140/90
	45–64 years 150/95
	65 or older 160/95
Laboratory studies within normal limits	Obj. D: Blood:
	Hemoglobin:
	15–18 gm% infant
	14.5–16.5 gm% male
	13.0–15.5 gm% female
	Hematocrit:
	43–50% male
	40–45% female
	O_2 saturation: 95–97%
	CO_2:
	20–26 mEq/liter infant
	26–28 mEq/liter adult
	PO_2 (PaO_2): 80–110 mm Hg
	PCO_2 ($PaCO_2$): 35.45 mm Hg

GOAL: To maintain fluid-electrolyte balance (includes equal intake and output of fluid for body tissues and cells; includes balance of the body salts of sodium, potassium, chloride, calcium, and magnesium)

Normal body hydration	Obj. D: Good skin turgor
	Thin secretions
	Moist mucous membranes
	No edema, ascites, venous distention
	Sub. D: Absence of thirst
	Absence of irritability that accompanies fluid retention
Laboratory studies within normal limits	Obj. D: Blood sodium 136–145 mEq/liter

Table 2-7   continued

CRITERIA[a]	DATA INDICATING THAT CRITERIA ARE MET[b]
	potassium 3.5–5 mEq/liter chloride 100–106 mEq/liter magnesium 1.5–2.5 mEq/liter calcium 4.5–5.7 mEq/liter Urine specific gravity: 1.010–1.030

GOAL: To maintain nutrition to all cells (includes adequate protein, carbohydrate, fat, vitamin, and mineral intake and absorption)

Normal body composition	Obj. D: Good bone and tooth development Good posture, with head erect, chest out, abdomen less protruding than chest Good skin turgor Clear skin and eyes Firm muscles Shining hair Subcutaneous fat sufficient to pad bones and muscles, but no more than 1-inch fold
Normal body functioning	Obj. D: Adequate elimination Prompt healing Daily weight stabilized at normal level for body build Adequate growth of 3–5 inches/year in children Sub. D: Good digestion
Vitality	Obj. D: Mental alertness Good concentration and attentiveness Sub. D: Absence of malaise, fatigue, weakness
Daily intake of essential food groups	Obj. D: Include milk, meat, fruits, vegetables, breads, cereals in daily diet

GOAL: To maintain regulating mechanisms and functions (includes acid-base balance, waste elimination, body temperature, and energy)

ACID-BASE BALANCE

Laboratory studies within normal limits	Obj. D: Blood pH: 7.35–7.45 Urine pH: 4.8–8.5

Table 2-7 continued

CRITERIA[a]	DATA INDICATING THAT CRITERIA ARE MET[b]
WASTE ELIMINATION: GASTROINTESTINAL Bowel elimination normal for individual	Obj. D: Soft stools, soft nondistended abdomen Sub. D: No abdominal pressure or abdominal cramping
WASTE ELIMINATION: KIDNEY Daily fluid output equal to fluid intake	Obj. D: Urine output: 1500–3000 cc daily, or equivalent to intake
Laboratory studies within normal limits	Obj. D: Blood urea nitrogen: 10–20 mg/100 ml Serum creatinine: 0.7–1.4 mg/100 ml Urine specific gravity: 1.010–1.030 Urine protein: Combistix or Urostix: Negative 24-hour urine: less than 50 mg Urine creatinine: 1.0–1.5 gm/24 hr Creatinine clearance: 70–130 ml/min
WASTE ELIMINATION: RESPIRATORY Normal respirations	Obj. D: Respiratory rate: 30–60 infant 20–30 child 15–24 adolescent 16–20 adult Rhythm and depth Regular breathing pattern Sub. D: No respiratory distress
Laboratory studies within normal limits	Obj. D: Blood: O_2 saturation: 95–97% CO_2: 20–26 mEq/liter infant 26–28 mEq/liter adult
WASTE ELIMINATION: SKIN Normal perspiration	Obj. D: Warm, slightly moist skin when at rest Perspiration adequate during strenuous activity and environmental heat

Table 2-7   continued

CRITERIA[a]	DATA INDICATING THAT CRITERIA ARE MET[b]
NORMAL TEMPERATURE Normal body temperature	Obj. D: 96.8°F (36°C)–99.5°F (37.5°C) orally 99.1°F (37.2°C)–100.5°F (38°C) rectally 98.1°F (36.7°C) axillary Sub. D: Feels neither hot nor cold
ENERGY Vitality	Obj. D: Mental alertness Good concentration, attentiveness Sub. D: Absence of malaise, fatigue, weakness
Adequate performance of work and play	Obj. D: Able to maintain self-care Can perform household or work activities Can participate in recreation and sports in addition to required daily activities Sub. D: Satisfied with work and play performance

GOAL: To maintain sensory function and stimulation (includes sight, hearing, touch, taste, smell, and arousal to stimuli)

SIGHT Ease of ambulation	Obj. D: Avoids contact with stable and moving objects when ambulating
Correct identification of environment	Obj. D: Correctly identifies persons and common objects
Positive visual tests	Obj. D: Correct identification of letters on Snellen eye chart from distance of 20 feet Correct identification of number of fingers held up in extended-finger visual test from distance of 2 feet
HEARING Correct responses to verbal communication	Obj. D: In environment free from major noise distraction: Appropriate action responses to verbal directions Appropriate verbal

Table 2-7   continued

CRITERIA[a]	DATA INDICATING THAT CRITERIA ARE MET[b]
	responses to questions Does not ask for message repetition
Positive hearing tests	Obj. D: Hears whisper at 15 feet and voice at 20 feet in whispered and spoken voice tests Positive Rinne test Positive Weber test Audiometry within normal limits
TOUCH	
Correct responses to touch communication	Obj. D: Indicates awareness of stimuli when touched by person out of sight (turning, verbal response, etc.)
Positive touch test	Sub. D: Feels pinprick Feels heat Feels cold Feels touch
TASTE	
Positive attitude toward food	Obj. D: No excessive use of salts, spices, sugar Sub. D: Indicates that food tastes good
Positive taste test	Sub. D: Can differentiate bitterness and sweetness
SMELL	
Positive smell test	Obj. D: Correctly identifies various odors Sub. D: Ascribes meanings to odors associated with various activities (smoke, gas, popcorn, etc.)
STIMULATION	
Positive responses to environment	Obj. D: Interest in environment Self-motivated activities Alertness

GOAL: To achieve good hygiene (includes personal and therapeutic cleanliness)	
General body cleanliness	Obj. D: Clean hair, eyes, ears, nose, mouth, skin, nails, teeth, clothes, linen No unpleasant body odor Sub. D: Feels clean and refreshed

Table 2-7   continued

CRITERIA[a]	DATA INDICATING THAT CRITERIA ARE MET[b]
Clean body alterations ·	Obj. D: Clean colostomy or ileostomy stoma, amputation stump, etc. Sub. D: Feels clean
Clean therapeutic devices	Obj. D: Clean dressing, cast, drainage systems, etc. Sub. D: Feels clean

GOAL: To achieve comfort (includes feelings of satisfaction and contentment)

Physical appearance (nonverbal expression) of comfort	Obj. D: Calm, contented, relaxed facial expression Normal posture Freedom of body movement Relaxed muscles when resting and motionless
Verbal expression of comfort	Sub. D: Expresses comfort, satisfaction, confidence in care Cessation of previous complaining

GOAL: To achieve activity and exercise (includes physical body action or
movements used in activities, vigorous body exertion to improve
health)

ACTIVITY

Frequent position change and body movement	Obj. D: Walking Sitting Standing
Participation in variety of activities	Obj. D: Work Recreation Creative arts, etc.

EXERCISE

Participation in daily physical exercise	Obj. D: Bicycling Tennis Jogging Running, etc.
Participation in therapeutic exercise	Obj. D: Range-of-motion exercises Isometric exercises Mastectomy exercises, etc.

GOAL: To achieve sleep, rest, and relaxation (includes freedom from physical or psychologic disturbance in rest, temporary loss of conscious
life in sleep, and relief of tension through pleasurable activity in
relaxation)

Table 2-7   continued

CRITERIA [a]	DATA INDICATING THAT CRITERIA ARE MET [b]
SLEEP AND REST	
Adequate sleep in 24 hours	Obj. D: 18–20 hours infant 10–14 hours children 7–9 hours adults 5–7 hours aged
Physical appearance of sufficient rest	Obj. D: No dark circles under eyes No yawning Clear (not red) conjunctiva Wide-open eyelids Good concentration Good coordination Sub. D: Absence of fatigue
RELAXATION	
Relaxed state while resting	Obj. D: Calm, serene facial expression Regular breathing without intermittent sighing Flaccid, limp muscles when motionless Complete absence of body movement for short periods No startle response to normal stimuli (being approached unexpectedly, bells ringing, etc.) Sub. D: Feels relaxed
Relaxed state while active	Obj. D: Calm, serene facial expression Performs activities at leisurely, unrushed pace Regular breathing without intermittent sighing Calm speech with intermittent silence Nonrigid, smooth, loose body movements and postures No startle response to normal stimuli (being approached unexpectedly, bells ringing, etc.) Sub. D: Feels relaxed

GOAL: To achieve positive expressions, feelings, and reactions (includes positive self-image and positive approach to life as shown in expressions of certainty and confidence)

Table 2-7   continued

CRITERIA[a]	DATA INDICATING THAT CRITERIA ARE MET[b]
Positive disposition	Obj. D: Uses cheerful conversation Smiles appropriately Sub. D: Indicates internal harmony despite life's challenges
Responds positively to new ideas and experiences	Obj. D: Takes action to shape environment whenever possible Sub. D: Enjoys challenge of new experiences
Expresses confidence in future	Obj. D: Makes plans for and looks forward to future activities Sub. D: Perceives future with pleasant anticipation
Expresses acceptance of past and present when there is no future	Obj. D: Realistically prepares for approaching termination of life by putting business in order, etc. Sub. D: Expression of having lived as best he could

GOAL: To achieve effective verbal and nonverbal communication (includes communication by speaking and by body activity)

Adequate communication delivery	Obj. D: Adequate expression of messages Adequate use of means other than speech for communication, such as writing, gesturing, esophageal speech, etc. No evidence of frustration in communications, such as crying, irritation, aggression, etc.
Adequate communication reception and process	Obj. D: Good attention to messages being sent Appropriate action responses to messages being sent Sub. D: Correct feedback of messages received

GOAL: To achieve productive interpersonal relationships (includes interactions with persons and groups)

Relates confidently with others	Obj. D: Responds pleasantly to others Sub. D: Feels sure of receiving love

Table 2-7   continued

CRITERIA[a]	DATA INDICATING THAT CRITERIA ARE MET[b]
	and support from others Experiences mutual trust, respect, acceptance from some others Enjoys some deep relationships
Positive response to therapeutically structured nurse-patient relationship, if and when needed	Obj. D: Functions well in permissive atmosphere when appropriate Cooperative with set limits, when appropriate
	Sub. D: Expresses positive feelings about nurse-patient relationship
Well-defined sexuality	Obj. D: Male: Has masculine appearance Relates well to male peers In youth, relates well to male authority figures Female: Has feminine appearance Relates well to female peers
	Sub. D: Male: Youth identifies with his father Female: Youth identifies with her mother Marriage is based on growth by both partners Marriage is mutual (equal) relationship, with neither party marrying for purpose of being taken care of
Reasonable adherence to cultural expectations	Obj. D: Positive social interaction with individuals and groups Activity directed toward fulfilling role identity
	Sub. D: Recognizes own effect on others in social situations

GOAL: To achieve spiritual goals (includes satisfaction for the spirit or soul in regard to one's relationship with a Supreme Being)

Table 2-7 *continued*

CRITERIA[a]	DATA INDICATING THAT CRITERIA ARE MET[b]
Positive statements regarding existence of and relationship to Supreme Being	Obj. D: Expresses trust in God Sub. D: Feels loved by God and love for God
Adequate participation in spiritual rituals desired	Obj. D: Expresses satisfaction with supplied religious articles, such as reading material, crucifix, rosary, etc. Satisfied with religious diet Peaceful facial expression following clergy visits or participation in religious services Sub. F: Feeling of satisfaction following ritual participation

GOAL: To achieve a therapeutic environment (includes those conditions and surroundings that promote healing as well as maintenance, maximum efficiency, or improvement of physical or behavioral functioning)

Patient's surroundings are clean	Obj. D: Patient's surroundings are free from dust, dirt, etc. Lies on clean bed linens Uses clean bathroom facilities Sub. D: Expresses satisfaction with cleanliness
Patient's surroundings are safe	Obj. D: Uses safety precautions, such as siderails, low bed, etc. Occupies a room geographically appropriate to his situation Sub. D: Expresses feelings of safety Perceives environment as orderly
Patient's surroundings are comfortable	Obj. D: Is in a room where temperature is appropriate to his situation: 68–72°F (20–22°C) normal 75–78°F (23.8–25.5°C) warm 65°F (18.3°C) cool 80°F (25.5°C) for premature infant Is in a room where humidity level is appropriate to his situation:

Table 2-7   continued

CRITERIA[a]	DATA INDICATING THAT CRITERIA ARE MET[b]
	40–45% normal 45–65% for premature infant Is in well-ventilated room Patient's movement is not hampered by environmental barriers
	Sub. D: No complaints of irritating noise or odors Perceives surroundings as pleasant
Patient's schedule is satisfactory	Obj. D: Patient's established daily routine is minimally interrupted by health care.
	Sub. D: Expresses satisfaction with daily routine Comfortable with visitor permissions and restrictions

GOAL: To achieve awareness of needs and/or use of resources (includes receiving health information, learning new skills, and referral to other resources for health improvement)

Recognizes that health needs exist	Sub. D: Verbally acknowledges need for behavior change to reestablish or maintain health Verbally acknowledges need for health maintenance assistance
Has acquired knowledge of health, health problems, and health solutions	Obj. D: Adequate score when tested over health material taught Adequate verbal feedback or return demonstration of health material or skills taught Increased independent self-direction in health maintenance Improved health status resulting from practice of health knowledge gained Increased application of specific health knowledge to other health situations
	Sub. D: Controls unhealthy behavior that formerly resulted in adverse

Table 2-7   continued

CRITERIA[a]	DATA INDICATING THAT CRITERIA ARE MET[b]
	physiologic and psychologic responses
Positive attitude toward available resources	Obj. D: Acceptance of suggestion of referral
Follow through on referral made to physician, nurse specialist, health or community agencies	Obj. D: Actively seeks health maintenance assistance Sub. D: Expresses satisfaction

GOAL: To achieve optimum function (includes highest level of functioning expected of the patient in his particular situation)

Adequate performance in relation to specific situation	Obj. D: Patient performs at expected level in: independent self-maintenance independent work performance independent recreation independent health maintenance
Positive attitude toward self-performance	Sub. D: Satisfaction with accomplishment of goals despite limitations

GOAL: To prevent accident, physical injury, deformity, infection, and hypersensitivity response (includes prevention of harmful unexpected incidents, pain or harm to the body, distortion or disfigurement of the body, entrance of pathogenic organisms into the body, or unfavorable antigen-antibody reactions)

ACCIDENT

No evidence of accidents having occurred	Obj. D: No physical sign of accident Sub. D: No subjective evidence of accident

PHYSICAL INJURY

No evidence of physical injury	Obj. D: No evidence of complications arising from drugs, treatments, or nursing care

DEFORMITY

No evidence of deformity resulting from health treatment	Obj. D: Hands, feet, limbs, spine in good alignment Hands, feet, limbs, spine

Table 2-7   continued

CRITERIA[a]	DATA INDICATING THAT CRITERIA ARE MET[b]
	functional where there is no pathology
	Sub. D: Absent or minimal joint stiffness or pain

INFECTION

Adequate energy level	Sub. D: No malaise, fatigue, weakness
Absence of infection	Obj. D: No evidence of: inflammation purulent drainage purulent secretions pain or aching Oral temperature reading: 98.6°F (37°C)
Laboratory findings within normal limits	Obj. D: Blood leukocyte count: 5,000–10,000 No urine erythrocytes, leukocytes, hemoglobin, hyaline or tubular casts Negative bacterial culture

HYPERSENSITIVITY RESPONSE

Adequate energy level	Obj. D: No malaise or weakness
Absence of hypersensitivity response	Obj. D: No sneezing, tearing, watery nasal discharge, wheezing, dyspnea, rashes, vomiting, diarrhea
	Sub. D: No nausea or nasal congestion
Laboratory studies within normal limits	Obj. D: Blood: total protein: 100% albumin: 53% or 3.5–5.5 g/dl a-globulin: 14% or 0.2–0.9 gm% b-globulin: 12% or 0.6–1.9 gm% g-globulin: 20% or 0.7–1.6 gm% sedimentation rate: 0–9 mm/hour males 0–20 mm/hour females leukocyte count: 5,000–10,000 eosinophil count: 1–4%

Table 2-7   continued

CRITERIA[a]	DATA INDICATING THAT CRITERIA ARE MET[b]

GOAL: To prevent emotional injury (includes preventing feelings of worthlessness, fear, anxiety, loss of dignity, ridicule, criticism, alienation, rejection, frustration, aloneness, inadequacy, insecurity, guilt, shame, loss of dominance, loss of individuality, emotional fatigue, conflict, failure)

Feels comfortable about himself	Obj. D: Has maintained same apparent emotional stability as existed prior to seeking health assistance Has improved state of emotional stability
	Sub. D: Expresses feelings of safety by maintaining identity, independence, and self-respect
Feels comfortable about his situation	Sub. D: Expresses feelings of safety by being able to make decisions regarding events occurring to him
Uses healthy coping mechanisms	Obj. D: At times of problems or crisis, reaches out to appropriate support systems (family, friends, church); may seek support from nurse when family, etc., is not available
	Sub. D: Expresses feelings of safety by his ability to cope with situation Employs healthy coping mechanisms, such as identification with favorable role models, substitution with alternate but satisfactory goals, etc. (see complete list under Identify Appropriate Use of Defense Mechanisms, p. 1478)
No evidence of emotional distress mannerisms after receiving health care	Obj. D: Has not developed acute distress mannerisms, such as twitches, nail biting, constantly pushing his call light, etc.

[a] These criteria are appraised as follows:
Each criterion under a goal may have one of the following numerical values:

Table 2-7   continued

0 means the criterion is irrelevant.

+1 means the criterion has been met.

−1 means the criterion has not been met.

If each of the criteria assigned to the goal is either 0 or +1, the goal has been accomplished.

If any of the criteria assigned to the goal are −1, the goal has not been accomplished.

[b] Obj. D: objective data; Sub. D: subjective data.

3.
The Nursing Process and Maslow's Human Need Theory

Maslow (292:29–33) believed that the basic needs of a person must be met if that person is to enjoy a state of health. Professional nurses can assist patients to meet needs and regain health by integrating Maslow's theory (292:35–47) with the nursing process.

DESCRIPTION OF THE NURSING PROCESS

The professional nursing process involves a system of problem solving, a step-by-step activity designed to obtain an understanding of the relevant factors in the patient's situation (261:14–15, 459:116). The steps of the process (261:14–15, 459:116) can be subdivided as follows:

Assessment
    Subjective data (symptoms)
    Objective data (signs)
    Related data
Possible etiology
Nursing diagnosis
Nursing plan
    Patient needs
    Primary nurse-patient goals
Nursing interventions
    Nursing treatments
    Nursing observations
    Health teaching
    Medical treatments performed by nurses
Evaluation

The nursing process is the basis for professional practice. It is sufficiently flexible to serve as a framework for the vast scope of professional functions and responsibilities. The flow of the process is depicted in Figure 3-1 (261:14–15, 459:116).

Figure 3-1
The Professional Nursing Process

NURSE	PATIENT
	presents problem (s)

Assessment: Gathering information
by means of the nursing history, a
physical examination, and laboratory findings. Analyzing the subjective,
objective, and related data.
Identifying the patient's strengths
and weaknesses.

Possible etiology: Identifying
the possible causes of the prob-
lem(s).

Nursing diagnosis: Identifying the
patient's problem(s) that the
nurse will treat.

Nursing plan: Identifying the
patient's human needs. Identifying the nurse-patient goals associated with the human needs.

Nursing intervention: Determining
the nursing treatments, nursing
observations, and health teaching that
will resolve, diminish, or prevent
the patient's needs.

Evaluation: Determining and
describing criteria for goal
evaluation. Appraising the
degree to which the criteria were
met.

NURSING PROCESS COMPARED WITH MEDICAL PROCESS

Physicians have long employed a process by which a planned series of activities serves as a basis for medical diagnosis and treatment. The
similarities and differences of the nursing process (261:14–15, 459:116) and
the medical process (113:1–9, 225:11–33, 316:17) are presented in Figure
3-2.

Figure 3-2

The Nursing Process Compared With the Medical Process

NURSING PROCESS	MEDICAL PROCESS
Assessment: Gathering information by means of the nursing history, physical examination, and laboratory findings. Analyzing the subjective, objective, and related data. Identifying the patient's strengths and weaknesses.	*Assessment:* Gathering information by means of the medical history, physical examination, laboratory findings, x-ray findings, and other studies.
	Data analysis: Determining which signs and symptoms are abnormal. Eliminating those that are irrelevant. Analyzing the significance of the signs and symptoms for abnormal body functions.
Possible etiology: Identifying the possible causes of the problem(s).	*Possible etiology:* Identifying causes and placing them in etiologic categories.
	Hypothesis preparation: Considering the diseases compatible with the signs and symptoms. Narrowing the list to a few diseases.
	Verification: Obtaining more specific data through further examination, studies, tissue examination, autopsy, etc.
Nursing diagnosis: Identifying the patient's problem(s) that the nurse will treat.	*Medical diagnosis:* Identifying and labeling the precise pathologic disease. If the disease cannot be identified, signs and symptoms are often treated.
Nursing plan: Identifying the patient's human needs. Identifying the nurse-patient goals associated with the human needs.	*Prognosis:* Projecting the expected outcome.
Nursing intervention: Determining the nursing treatments, nursing observations, and health teaching that will resolve, diminish, or prevent the patient's needs.	*Medical treatment:* Determining and administering the course of treatment that will cure the specific disease(s).
Evaluation: Determining and describing criteria for goal evaluation. Appraising the degree to which the criteria were met	

ASSESSMENT

Comprehensive assessment carried out in a highly skilled manner is essential for determining the relevant factors in the patient's situation. Once the patient presents his problem(s), relevant information must be gathered about the patient and his situation in anticipation of making a nursing diagnosis. Assessment data consist of any relevant information about the patient that gives evidence of physiologic, behavioral, sociologic, spiritual, and environmental impairments and strengths. In order for the nurse to be able to formulate a diagnosis, there must be supporting data; those data must clearly reveal two or more facts that relate to one another. If a patient complains that he is hurting, that alone is not sufficient for a diagnosis. If he states that he hurts, that he experiences a pounding sensation, and that the hurt occurs with each pounding, then these facts are sufficient to determine a diagnosis of *throbbing pain.*

Assessment techniques include talking with and listening to the patient to obtain a nursing history. The patient communicates his chief complaint, his past health status, current data, and some information about how he perceives himself.

The patient is always the primary source of information. Even if he should be limited to nonverbal communication because of impaired cerebral function, his condition will be the primary source of information for the nurse. Secondary sources of information include the family, physicians, other nurses, and records (261:35–36).

During the physical examination the nurse gathers data through observation, percussion, palpation, and auscultation. Laboratory studies are used to develop a complete data base.

Along with the patient's limitations, the nurse must also consider his strengths, i.e., those qualities, resources, or conditions that work in his favor as he attempts to cope with his presenting problem(s). As Maslow (292:35–36) pointed out, although unwellness brings about disequilibrium, the person's strengths keep pulling him back into balance and integration. The organism constantly attempts to maintain its normal state of equilibrium. Human beings have certain needs, some of which are not met during periods of unwellness. When a person attempts to cope with those needs that are unmet, his needs that have been met are sources of strength that help him cope. If a person has fever and his need is for a normal temperature, his strength may lie in the fact that he is in water-salt balance and has a good energy resource. If a person is suffering from anxiety and his need is for protection from psychologic threat, his strength may lie in the fact that he experiences warm, communicating relationships, unity with loved ones, and a high evaluation of self.

It is advantageous for both the nurse and the patient to recognize the patient's strengths as positive health factors. If the patient fails to recognize his strengths, it is the nurse's responsibility to promote this awareness.

Every effort should be made to gather as much information as possible in order to obtain a clear view of the patient's situation.

ETIOLOGY

Etiology involves determination of the cause of the patient's problem. If assessment of the problem is to be accurate, its cause must be considered. The nurse may recognize that a patient has poor hygiene. If the cause is that the patient is apathetic toward hygiene, then the diagnosis would be *inade-*

quate general hygiene. If the cause is paralysis resulting from a stroke, then the diagnosis would be *dependence on general hygiene.*

Knowledge of the cause of a problem also influences the nursing intervention. If the patient with poor hygiene has not been educated about hygiene, then the nursing intervention would be teaching. If the cause is paralysis, then the nursing intervention would be care. Thus the statement of etiology is essential to nursing intervention as well as to diagnosis.

NURSING DIAGNOSIS

Nursing diagnosis involves recognition of those patient problem(s) that the nurse is capable of treating and is licensed to treat (611:9). Each patient problem must be identified as either a human response or a resource limitation. As defined earlier, a *human response* is a reaction, effect, or behavior indicating existing or potential unwellness. A *resource limitation* is a lack of ability, lack of source of supply, or lack of source of support that contributes to existing or potential unwellness.

A human response is a reaction, effect, or behavior, such as *inability to sleep, phantom pain,* or *impaired arterial peripheral circulation.*

A resource limitation is a lack of ability, lack of source of supply, or lack of source of support that interferes with wellness, such as *dependence on general hygiene, inability to obtain health care,* or *inadequate information related to the surgical procedure.*

The nursing diagnosis cannot be made on the nurse's assumption that a certain situation will create a problem for the patient. A situation that creates a problem for one person may have no effect on another. However, when a patient with limited health knowledge is not able to identify his problem, or when a patient has focused his attention on other problems that are less significant, the professional nurse should guide the patient in problem identification.

If a medical diagnosis has been determined by the physician, the nurse may use it as a reference point. However, a confirmed medical diagnosis of pathology is not a prerequisite for making a nursing diagnosis.

The physician, in making a medical diagnosis, recognizes pathologic processes and focuses primarily on pathophysiologic etiology and organic unwellness (113:8). Through evaluation of basic data, the patient's problem is identified and labeled in terms of a specific disease. The nursing diagnostic statement indicates problem(s) that are consequences of, contributing factors to, or potential dangers leading to illness, injury, or disease.

Whereas the physician diagnoses the medical condition (e.g., Parkinson's disease), the nurse diagnoses the problems that are consequences of the disease (e.g., *difficulty ambulating, dependence on feeding, poor oral secretion control*). If the physician diagnoses the disease pneumococcal pneumonia, the nurse may diagnose a contributing factor: *inadequate information related to environmental cleanliness.* She may also diagnose a condition that potentially can lead to the disease: *potential infection transmission.* However, if during assessment the nurse recognizes subjective or objective data that indicate a specific disease, she should refer the patient to the physician for medical diagnosis and medical treatment.

The medical diagnosis is made with the intention of prescribing treatment that will cure the disease or reduce the injury. The nursing diagnosis is made with the intention of performing nursing interventions that will alleviate, diminish, or prevent human needs, assist in restoring normally independent functions lost because of disease or illness, and maintain optimum health and independent patient functioning. Both the physician and the nurse take into consideration their professional diagnostic and treatment responsibilities to the patient. In the activities of patient care, a sharing of skill and knowledge between the physician and nurse is necessary as they work together to alleviate human distress.

NURSING PLAN

Once the nursing diagnosis is made, the nurse should utilize Maslow's concept (292:37–47) to identify the patient's human needs. The term human need implies the absence of an essential component that is vital to an integrated body system (292:35–38). Every person who is in a healthy state has human needs that he can fulfill. Even when some needs are unsatisfied, a state of homeostasis may exist. But in the unhealthy state, deficiencies or failure to resolve or diminish human needs can result in disequilibrium. It is essential that nurses recognize need deprivation when making plans to help the patient reestablish health.

By identifying the human needs that pose difficulties for the patient, the nurse perceives the problem itself and the significant factors involved in the problem. For instance, when a diagnosis of *elevated body temperature* is made, the patient's problem, as stated, is simply an overproduction of body heat. When the human needs of water-salt balance, normal temperature, sleep, rest, and comfort are recognized, the nurse has detailed information about the overall effects of the problem. Knowledge of the human needs involved can assist the nurse in determining those nursing interventions that will be most beneficial to the patient.

In the planning process, the primary nurse-patient goals identify those aims of nursing care that nursing intervention should bring about. Primary nurse-patient goals should be determined fairly early, although they may not be accomplished for some time. Goals are to be mutually determined by the nurse and the patient; because of this cooperative factor, they are more likely to be reached.

In planning, the professional nurse involves the patient and his family in the determination of specific nursing interventions appropriate to resolving the human needs and accomplishing the goals associated with the nursing diagnosis. Since no two patients require exactly the same intervention, it is the responsibility of the professional nurse to use her skill and expertise to develop an individualized plan of care.

NURSING INTERVENTIONS

Nursing interventions include several activities that reflect nursing responsibility in the performance of health treatment:

Nursing interventions
Nursing treatments
Nursing observations
Health teaching
Medical treatments performed by nurses

A nursing intervention is a single-action nursing measure designed to resolve, diminish, or prevent the needs that are inferred from the patient's problem. In order to determine and initiate nursing interventions, one must have a scientific background and extensive education in nursing. Such interventions may be carried out only by the professional nurse or by someone under direct supervision of the professional nurse. There are three categories of independently initiated nursing interventions: nursing treatments, nursing observations, and health teaching.

Nursing treatments consist of those single-action nursing measures that provide assistance, regulation of the internal or external environment, support in functioning, and comfort, as well as those that facilitate hygiene, improved or independent activity, and prevention of illness or injury through protective and precautionary measures. Nursing observations consist of the single-action nursing measures of examining, checking, inspecting, and monitoring. Health teaching consists of those nursing measures that provide health information and explanation.

Nursing interventions are designed for the purpose of resolving, diminishing, or preventing human needs. If the nursing diagnosis indicates water-salt imbalance, then the nursing intervention must be such that the need for water-salt balance is met, as seen in Figure 3-3, or else the intervention is not appropriate to the diagnosis.

The fourth kind of nursing intervention to be considered involves activities that are medically directed. These are medical treatments that have been delegated by the physician to the nurse and are supervised by the physician (101:103). They include such medical treatments as intravenous infusion, peritoneal dialysis, and gastrointestinal aspiration. These medical treatments, although under medical supervision, are as much the responsi-

Figure 3-3
Human Needs Resolved by Nursing Intervention

Nursing diagnosis: inadequate fluid intake	Nursing intervention: increase fluid intake to about 2000 cc daily
Human need: water-salt balance	Need resolved by the intervention: water-salt imbalance

bility of the nurse as are the nursing interventions ordered and directed by the professional nurse.

The professional nurse has sole responsibility for ordering and initiating the nursing treatments, nursing observations, and health teaching described previously. They are the nurse's avenue for assisting patients in solving their health problem(s) within the realm of nursing.

EVALUATION

Once nursing interventions have been performed for and with the patient, evaluation is essential. Nursing evaluation is an appraisal of the effectiveness of nursing actions. Once the nurse has selected and initiated appropriate nursing interventions, the human needs of the patient theoretically should be resolved, diminished, or prevented. However, it must be determined whether the expected and desired results (goals) or the nursing interventions have actually been accomplished.

According to Mager (280:44–53), standards for evaluating the accomplishment of nursing goals consist of:

Describing the goal
Selecting measurable criteria for goal evaluation
Appraising the degree to which the criteria were met

Goal description involves a statement of expected outcome. Only by knowing the specific changes that are expected to occur can it be determined whether those changes actually did occur.

Selecting criteria for goal evaluation includes determining those specific criteria that will be the standards for evaluating each goal. After criteria are selected, the degree to which the criteria are met is appraised. If all the criteria assigned to the goal have a 0 or +1 value (i.e., all criteria are either irrelevant or met), then the goal has been accomplished. If one of the criteria is assigned a score of −1, the goal has not been accomplished.

Evaluation provides the professional nurse with information on whether the desired changes in the patient's condition were realized. Table 3-1 shows the steps used in determining whether the nursing goals have been accomplished.

The preceding chapters have indicated how the nursing process can be interrelated with the hierarchy of needs as described in Maslow's theory of motivation (293:35–58) to develop a framework for generating nursing diagnoses and nursing interventions.

Table 3-1
Evaluation

Determining nursing goals before initiating nursing interventions

Selecting criteria for goal evaluation

Appraising the degree to which the goal was met

4.
How to Use
This Book

This text is expected to reinforce the concept of the nursing process. It is intended to provide a common framework among nurse colleagues for the practice of nursing until a standardized nomenclature of nursing diagnoses can be developed. Part 1 consists of four chapters and discusses the theory that supports nursing diagnosis and intervention and its integration into the nursing process. The remaining chapters are divided into Part 2, Nursing Diagnoses, and Part 3, Nursing Interventions. The final section consists of the References and Indexes. Each of these sections is described in detail below.

PART 2. NURSING DIAGNOSES

The chapter headings in this part describe the material covered. The nursing diagnoses appear under main headings that generally reflect the subject matter.

Each nursing diagnosis is treated separately according to the following common format:

Assessment
    Subjective data
    Objective data
    Related data
Possible etiology
Nursing diagnosis
Nursing plan
    Patient needs
    Primary nurse-patient goals
Nursing interventions
    Nursing treatments
    Nursing observations
    Health teaching
    Medical treatments performed by nurses
Evaluation

The section on nursing assessment provides the subjective data (symptoms), objective data (signs), and related data that constitute the supporting information specific to a nursing diagnosis. The related data contain additional information, especially the conditions and diseases commonly associated with the nursing diagnoses.

The section on etiology includes the possible causes of the condition diagnosed. The nursing diagnosis is defined to clarify its meaning and provide greater assurance of correct identification of the problem.

The section on the nursing plan lists those human needs that are inferred from the patient's diagnosis. An awareness of these needs serves as the basis for later determining those nursing interventions that will resolve, diminish, or prevent the needs. The nursing plan also includes the primary nurse-patient goals that are appropriate to the human needs.

The nursing interventions applicable to each diagnosis are assigned to that diagnosis. They include those nursing treatments, nursing observations, and health teaching that can be independently initiated and carried out by the nurse. They also include medical treatments that are initiated by the physician but carried out by the nurse. The use of nursing interventions is highly dependent on patient and nurse perception of the diagnosis. Several patients may have the same diagnosis; yet the selection of interventions for each of those assigned to that diagnosis depends on the severity of the situation, the variables surrounding the patient, and his distinct individuality. The choice is also affected by the attitude and experience of the professional nurse.

The evaluation section lists those criteria that must be met if the primary nurse-patient goals, as listed in the section on the nursing plan, are to be considered accomplished. It is suggested that the criteria under each goal be reviewed and that the appropriate numerical appraisal $(0, +1, or -1)$ be applied to each set of criteria. If all the criteria appropriate to the goal are appraised as having a 0 or $+1$ numerical value, the goal has been met. If one of the criteria has a -1 numerical value, the goal has not been met, and new nursing interventions should be employed.

PART 3. NURSING INTERVENTIONS

Part 3 consists of a complete list of all the nursing interventions found in the section on nursing diagnoses. The nursing interventions are compiled into four separate chapters on nursing treatments, nursing observations, health teaching, and medical treatments performed by nurses. The interventions are listed in alphabetical order, and the format is as follows:

Definition of the nursing intervention
Rationale for the nursing intervention
Human needs that the nursing intervention resolves, diminishes, or prevents
Contraindications to performing the nursing interventions, when such exist

The accepted approach to writing nursing interventions is to answer these questions: Who? What? Where? When? It is the intent of this text to answer only one of these: What? This will provide a basic intervention that may be used as it is stated or may be slightly altered to meet individual situations. The professional nurse may add the information on who should perform and receive the treatment and how, when, and where it should be carried out. For example, the basic intervention may read: Give carbonated beverages. The nurse may wish to state: Give 240cc carbonated beverage, now.

Those nursing interventions that are performed by nurses as part of the expanded role in nursing bear the code ExR (expanded role). Those that are perfromed by nurses in life-threatening or emergency situations are coded ET (emergency treatment). These codes are also present, when indicated, in the nursing intervention section of each nursing diagnosis format.

The nursing treatments coded ET could have been listed under nursing treatments or under medical treatments performed by nurses. To avoid duplication, they have been listed only once under nursing treatments.

PART 4. REFERENCES AND INDEXES

All references are compiled together at the back of the book. Each reference is numbered, and that number is used to designate that reference anywhere in the text. When several references are mentioned together, they are separated by commas: (19, 128, 241). When page numbers are appropriate to a reference, they are separated from the reference number by a colon: (7:23–24, 130:50–54).

There are four indexes in this text:

Nursing Diagnoses Alphabetical Index
Nursing Diagnoses Subject Index
Nursing Interventions Alphabetical Index
Nursing Interventions Subject Index

These indexes have been arranged to make it easy to find material in Part 2 and Part 3 of the text. They also provide the nurse with a quick reference for nursing diagnosis and intervention labels. In the Nursing Interventions Subject Index, the interventions that apply to behavioral nursing diagnoses are all listed under the main heading Behavior, followed by subheadings. Any intervention throughout this index that falls in the category of medical treatments performed by nurses is coded MDRx.

The four indexes do not refer to the material in Part 1. However, information on these chapters is readily available in the Contents preceding the text.

NURSING DIAGNOSIS BY PHYSICAL EXAMINATION

Since the concept of nursing diagnosis and the use of physical examination skills are both relatively new in nursing, a description is given of how nursing diagnosis can be arrived at through assessment by physical examination. Table 4-1 is in no way intended as a physical examination guideline, for there are many fine books on physical examination already available. It is a description of clinical findings that suggest nursing diagnoses. All the nursing diagnoses given in this text are not included in this guideline; it is an effort to help the nurse understand how the nursing diagnosis statements can be arrived at.

Table 4-1

Nursing Diagnoses Commonly Associated With Clinical Findings (113, 225, 316)

CLINICAL FINDINGS	NURSING DIAGNOSES SUGGESTED BY CLINICAL FINDINGS

Note: See page 101 for explanation of use of brackets and parentheses.

MENTAL STATUS

Level of Response

Nonresponsive or slightly responsive to external stimuli [comatose, semiconscious, stuporous, lethargic]	Dependence on general hygiene Dependence on dressing Dependence on feeding Dependence on maintenance of a healthy environment Increased physical stimulation requirement Potential decubitus ulcer Potential inadequate pulmonary ventilation Potential accidental falling

Perception Related to Cerebral Function

Disorderly arrangement of ideas [confusion]; unable to recognize persons, location, or time [disorientation]	Intolerance for environmental disorder Dependence on general hygiene assistance Dependence on dressing assistance Dependence on eating assistance Dependence on maintenance of a healthy environment Potential accidental falling

Perception Related to the Senses

Believes that certain ideas are factual, when in reality they are not, such as thinking his bones are made of glass [delusions]	Inability to define reality Inadequate information related to coping with the mentally ill
Perceives through his senses objects that don't exist, such as seeing people who aren't there [hallucinations]	Misperception of the environment Maladaptive coping related to anxiety Inadequate information related to coping with the mentally ill
Interprets objects to be other than what they are, such as thinking that lace curtains are spiders [illusions]	Misperception of the environment Inadequate information related to coping with the mentally ill

Table 4-1 continued

CLINICAL FINDINGS	NURSING DIAGNOSES SUGGESTED BY CLINICAL FINDINGS
MENTAL STATUS *continued*	
Thought Process and Progression	
Short-term concentration on an activity or idea [limited attention span]; total or partial inability to recall past experiences and ideas [memory impairment]; diminished ability to evaluate situations and solve problems [impaired judgment]; spontaneous, unthinking responses or activities [impaired thought organization]	Dependence on general hygiene assistance Dependence on dressing assistance Dependence on eating assistance Dependence on maintenance of a healthy environment
EMOTIONAL STATUS	
Predominant Emotion	
Seldom, if ever, has visitors; verbally expresses feelings of being unloved; seeks attention from health care personnel	Inadequate emotional support related to aloneness
Self-concept	
Refuses to take care of his amputation stump	Difficult adaptation to altered body image
Interpersonal Relationships	
Confides secretly to the nurse that other patients' visitors are noisy	Distress related to disturbing visitors
Coping Mechanisms	
States that the doctors have mixed up the diagnostic study reports and incorrectly diagnosed his illness	Temporary denial requirement
Adjustment	
States that everyone at the hospital is very nice; but now and then is found weeping because he is unable to go home	Distress related to environmental dependence
Insight	
Expresses an inability to understand his constant feelings of loneliness, since there are so many people in the hospital setting	Inadequate insight related to self
COMMUNICATION	
Communication Skills	
Unable to organize words, phrases, and sentences; unable to use connecting words (such as *and*	Dependence on communication assistance related to impaired speech delivery

Table 4-1   continued

CLINICAL FINDINGS	NURSING DIAGNOSES SUGGESTED BY CLINICAL FINDINGS
COMMUNICATION *continued* and *the*) to form words, to speak, to communicate the correct name of objects; speaks using jumbled unrecognizable words and stiff verbalization, or speaks with hoarseness; aphasic; labored, painstaking enunciation; repetitious echoing of words; jerky, tremorous speech; stuttering; incorrectly spoken speech sounds; poor speech control from abnormal mouth and tongue movements; lisps	
Spoken words from others are heard as jumbled messages; cannot identify objects or messages by sound	Dependence on communication assistance related to impaired hearing
Unable to determine the meanings of written or printed words, to differentiate similarly shaped letters, and to read and relate the meaning	Dependence on communication assistance related to impaired reading reception
Unable to express self through writing; writes meaningless phrases; illegible writing	Dependence on communication assistance related to impaired writing ability

CLINICAL FINDINGS	NURSING DIAGNOSES SUGGESTED BY CLINICAL FINDINGS
INTEGUMENT *Skin Eruptions*	
Moles, skin cancer, warts, tumors	Potential skin irritation
Boils, carbuncles	External abscess Potential skin irritation
Brownish pink, small, irregular, burning skin elevations	Maculopapular skin discomfort Potential skin irritation
Solid, cone-shaped skin elevations [papules]	Papular skin discomfort Inadequate skin care Malnutrition Potential skin irritation
Fluid-filled skin elevations [blisters]	Vesicular skin discomfort Potential infection transmission Potential skin irritation
Round, smooth, level, dark or white skin spots [macules]	Macular skin discomfort Intradermal bleeding Potential skin injury related to decreased pigmentation Potential skin injury related to increased pigmentation

Table 4-1   continued

CLINICAL FINDINGS	NURSING DIAGNOSES SUGGESTED BY CLINICAL FINDINGS
INTEGUMENT *continued*	
Small, round, protruding mass or white cystic mass [nodules]	Nodular skin discomfort Malnutrition
Petechiae, bruising, hematoma, purpura	Intradermal bleeding Predisposition to bleeding or hemorrhage
Round, swollen skin elevation with white or pink edges [wheals]	Urticaria skin discomfort Pruritus skin discomfort Emergency phase blood transfusion reaction Potential skin irritation Inadequate information related to food allergy Inadequate information related to drug allergy
Pus-filled skin elevation [pustules]	Pustular skin discomfort Potential skin irritation Potential infection transmission
Skin Intactness Raw, rough wound [abrasion]	Burning pain Dependence on wound care Potential wound infection
Clean cut wound [incision]; ragged, broken wound [laceration]; deep wound [puncture]	Stabbing pain Throbbing pain Dependence on wound care Potential tetanus Potential wound infection Potential incisional tension
Nonsutured tracheostomy or chest tube wound	Inadequate wound closure Dependence on wound care Potential wound infection
Skin Moisture Skin dryness and flaking	Inadequate skin care Malnutrition Inadequate fluid intake Inadequate information related to skin care
Skin oiliness	Inadequate skin care Inadequate information related to skin care
Cold, clammy skin	Impaired arterial peripheral circulation Emergency phase impending shock Emergency phase anaphylactic shock

Table 4-1   continued

CLINICAL FINDINGS	NURSING DIAGNOSES SUGGESTED BY CLINICAL FINDINGS
INTEGUMENT *continued*	Emergency phase bacteremic shock Emergency phase cardiogenic shock Emergency phase hemorrhagic shock Emergency phase insulin shock
Skin Temperature Cool or cold skin	Decreased body temperature Cold intolerance Impaired arterial peripheral circulation
Very warm or hot skin	Elevated body temperature Heat intolerance
Skin Texture Calloused skin	Inadequate skin care Inadequate information related to skin care
Coarse skin	Dermal coarseness Inadequate information related to skin care
Translucent skin	Dermal fragility
When pinched, the skin maintains its fold for some time [dehydration]	Inadequate fluid intake
Persistence of an indentation when the thumb is pressed into the skin [pitting edema]	Edema related to localized tissue injury Dependence on skin care Inadequate information related to skin care
Skin Irritation Skin covered with dirt; unclean skin	Inadequate general hygiene Inadequate skin care Potential wound infection Inadequate information related to skin care
Mild skin redness with burning	Burning pain Erythema skin discomfort
Skin itching	Pruritus skin discomfort Inadequate skin care Inadequate fluid intake Insect bite Urticaria skin discomfort Inadequate information related to food allergy

Table 4-1   continued

CLINICAL FINDINGS	NURSING DIAGNOSES SUGGESTED BY CLINICAL FINDINGS
INTEGUMENT *continued*	Inadequate information related to skin allergy
	Inadequate information related to drug allergy
Skin Color	
Rosy skin color	Emergency phase oxygen toxicity
Pallor	Impaired arterial peripheral circulation
	Malnutrition
	Increased nutritional requirement related to blood loss
	Insufficient sleep and rest
	Emergency phase oxygen insufficiency
	Emergency phase hemorrhage
Red-streaked skin	Limited cellulitis
Bluish red skin after exposure to cold	Emergency phase frostbite
Deep yellow or orange skin without sclera coloring [carotenemia]	Inadequate information related to carotene skin discoloration
	Difficult adaptation to altered body image
Yellow skin with sclera yellowing [jaundice]	Jaundice skin discomfort
	Difficult adaptation to altered body image
Freckles, butterfly marking, port-wine angioma; brown, brownish yellow, red brown, or blue gray skin	Potential skin injury related to increased pigmentation
	Difficult adaptation to altered body image
Localized milk-white skin spots [vitiligo]; generalized congenital milk-white skin [albinism]	Potential skin injury related to decreased pigmentation
	Difficult adaptation to altered body image
Skin Necrosis	
Small, reddish gonorrheal crusted lesions; sticky, painless gumma lesions	Potential infection transmission
	Potential skin irritation
Brown or white open chancre sores	Oral tenderness (if in the mouth)
	Potential infection transmission
	Potential skin irritation

Table 4-1 continued

CLINICAL FINDINGS	NURSING DIAGNOSES SUGGESTED BY CLINICAL FINDINGS
INTEGUMENT *continued*	
Round area of broken skin tissue	Decubitus ulcer
	Increased nutritional requirement related to tissue healing
	Predisposition to bleeding or hemorrhage
	Potential skin irritation
	Potential wound infection
Red, irritated skin area	Threatening decubitus ulcer
	Dependence on skin care
	Inadequate information related to skin care
Local skin cyanosis or blackness	Stasis ulcer
	Impaired arterial peripheral circulation
	Potential skin irritation
Open circular lesion or deep cavity on lower extremity	Stasis ulcer
	Potential skin irritation
Skin stretching in pregnancy, ascites, or obesity	Potential skin striae
Skin Scarring	
Granulation tissue; a healing scar	Immobility requirement related to healing
	Increased nutritional requirement related to tissue healing
	Potential skin irritation
Perspiration	
Sweat having a disagreeable odor	Inadequate general hygiene
Inability to sweat	Inability to control body temperature
Excessive perspiration	Emotional nervousness
	Physiologic nervousness
	Dependence on diaphoresis hygiene
	Electrolyte imbalance related to diaphoresis
	Potential electrolyte imbalance related to diaphoresis
Salty perspiration	Inadequate fluid intake
White perspiration	Uremic frost skin discomfort

Table 4-1   continued

CLINICAL FINDINGS	NURSING DIAGNOSES SUGGESTED BY CLINICAL FINDINGS
INTEGUMENT *continued* *Hair* Excessive hair growth [hirsutism]	Difficult adaptation to altered body image
Diffuse or localized hair loss	Inadequate hair care Malnutrition Difficult adaptation to altered body image
Brittle hair	Malnutrition Inadequate hair care
Dry scaling on scalp and hair [dandruff]	Dandruff Inadequate hair care
Yellowish, greasy scale on infant's scalp [cradle cap]	Cradle cap Inadequate hair care
Edema, crusting, redness of the scalp, with hair broken close to the scalp [tinea capitis, ringworm]	Inadequate hair care Potential infection transmission
Unclean, tangled, matted, or oily hair	Inadequate hair care Dependence on hair care
Small, gray white hair areas; visible nits [lice]	Parasite infestation Inadequate hair care Potential infestation transmission
Crusted blood on scalp and hair	Inadequate hair care Dependence on hair care Dependence on wound care Potential wound infection
Nails Ragged, dirty, excessively long nails	Inadequate nail care Dependence on nail care Inadequate information related to nail care
Frayed nail layers (protein deficiency)	Malnutrition Inadequate information related to balanced nutrition Inadequate nail care Inadequate information related to nail care
Nail presses into soft skin tissue [ingrown nail]	Ingrown nail Inadequate information related to nail care

Table 4-1   continued

CLINICAL FINDINGS	NURSING DIAGNOSES SUGGESTED BY CLINICAL FINDINGS
INTEGUMENT *continued*	
White patches on nail surface (fungus infection)	Potential infection transmission
Cranium	
Cranial bulge; delayed fontanel closure; fontanel bulging; gradually increasing head circumference	Minimal intracranial pressure requirement Potential headache Potential vomiting
Cranial crepitation; cranial friction rub (cranial bone fracture)	Minimal intracranial pressure requirement Potential tissue injury related to fracture (skull) Potential headache
Cranial bruit (arterial aneurysm)	Potential arterial rupture
Bogginess or bleeding in area of temples or behind ear [Battle's sign] (skull fracture)	Minimal intracranial pressure requirement Predisposition to shock Potential tissue injury related to fracture (skull)
Face	
Facial swelling (protein deficiency; allergy; drug intolerance)	Malnutrition Adrenal steroid intolerance Inadequate information related to food allergy Difficult adaptation to altered body image
Sinus tenderness	Sinus congestion
Parotid gland swelling (mumps); submaxillary gland swelling	Parotid gland pain Impaired swallowing Chewing difficulty Dependence on oral hygiene Poor oral secretion control Potential infection transmission
Neck	
Neck stiffness	Limited range of motion Painful joint motion Potential limited range of motion
Painful lymph node swelling with skin flushing (inflammation)	Throbbing pain Edema related to localized tissue injury

Table 4 1   continued

CLINICAL FINDINGS	NURSING DIAGNOSES SUGGESTED BY CLINICAL FINDINGS
INTEGUMENT *continued*	
Palpable and enlarged thyroid gland; thyroid bruit (hyperthyroidism)	Additional rest requirement Increased nutritional requirement related to metabolsim Intolerance to stress Dependence on cardiac work load reduction
Presence of laryngectomy	Dependence on airway patency maintenance Dependence on laryngectomy management Inadequate information related to laryngectomy management Inadequate information related to use of an artificial larnyx Inadequate information related to esophageal speech
Presence of tracheostomy	Dependence on airway patency maintenance Dependence on tracheostomy management Dependence on communication assistance related to impaired speech delivery Inadequate information related to tracheostomy management
Hyperalimentation therapy	Dependence on hyperalimentation management
EYES *Lacrimation* Increased tearing	Emergency phase eye foreign body Inadequate information related to respiratory allergy
Lack of tears	Potential vision loss related to eye exposure
Eyelids Unable to blink or infrequent blinking; eyelid eversion [ectropion]; widened eye fissure with incomplete eyelid closure [lid lag]	Potential vision loss related to eye exposure

Table 4-1   continued

CLINICAL FINDINGS	NURSING DIAGNOSES SUGGESTED BY CLINICAL FINDINGS
Eyes *continued*	
Upper eyelid drooping [ptosis]	Dependence related to partial vision loss
Eyelid redness; pustule on the margin [sty]	External abscess
Eyelid blackness (trauma to the eye, nasal or skull fracture)	Intradermal bleeding Potential tissue injury related to fracture (skull)
Eyelid inflammatory edema (local infection, allergy)	Edema related to localized tissue injury Dependence related to partial vision loss
Eyelid noninflammatory edema (protein deficiency, allergy, acute nephritis)	Inadequate information related to skin allergy Malnutrition Inadequate information related to food allergy Dependence related to partial vision loss
Eye Prominence	
Excessive eye prominence [exophthalmos]	Minimal intraocular pressure requirement Potential vision loss related to eye exposure
Recessed eye [enophthalmos] (dehydration)	Inadequate fluid intake
Area Surrounding Eyes	
Dark shadows under eyes	Insufficient sleep and rest
Intraocular Pressure	
Increased eyeball firmness or tension (increased intraocular pressure)	Minimal intraocular pressure requirement
Decreased eyeball tension; soft eyeballs (dehydration)	Inadequate fluid intake
Eye Movements	
Uncoordinated eye movements (crossed eyes); jerking eye movements [nystagmus]; ocular paralysis [strabismus]	Dependence related to partial vision loss
Conjunctiva	
Conjunctival hemorrhage; conjunctival edema	Minimal intraocular pressure requirement
Pink, swollen conjunctiva (conjunctivitis)	Light intolerance discomfort Dependence related to partial vision loss Potential infection transmission

Table 4-1   continued

CLINICAL FINDINGS	NURSING DIAGNOSES SUGGESTED BY CLINICAL FINDINGS
Eyes *continued*	
Cornea	
Open ulcer or sore on cornea	Light intolerance discomfort
	Dependence related to partial vision loss
Corneal haze	Dependence related to partial vision loss
Cornea exposure to light causes pain	Light intolerance discomfort
Sclera	
Yellow sclera [jaundice]	Potential infection transmission
Blue sclera (osteogenesis imperfecta)	Predisposition to bone fracture
Iris and Pupil	
One pupil responds more rapidly or more slowly to light than the other; less than normal reflex response of one or both pupils; one pupil is dilated more than the other, but both respond to light (increased intracranial pressure)	Minimal intracranial pressure requirement
One pupil is dilated and does not react to light, but the other reacts normally (increased intracranial pressure, skull fracture, aneurysm, intracranial hemorrhage)	Minimal intracranial pressure requirement Potential tissue injury related to fracture (skull) Potential arterial rupture
Dilatation of both pupils with no reaction to light (increased intracranial pressure, food or drug poisoning, cardiac arrest)	Emergency phase food poisoning Emergency phase cardiac arrest Emergency phase analgesic poisoning Minimal intracranial pressure requirement
Constriction of both pupils with no reaction to light by either (anoxia, mushroom poisoning, morphine reaction)	Emergency phase oxygen insufficiency Emergency phase food poisoning Analgesic intolerance
Vision	
Difficulty in seeing at a distance [nearsightedness]; after age 40, difficulty in seeing at a close distance [farsightedness]; after age 40, difficulty in focusing [impaired visual accommodation]; 20/70 to 20/200 acuity in the best eye with the	Dependence related to partial vision loss

Table 4-1   continued

CLINICAL FINDINGS	NURSING DIAGNOSES SUGGESTED BY CLINICAL FINDINGS
EYES *continued* help of visual aid as determined by Snellen test	
Cannot perceive light [blindness]	Dependence related to total vision loss
Sees two objects instead of one [diplopia] (increased intracranial pressure, hypertension, food poisoning)	Dependence related to partial vision loss Minimal intracranial pressure requirement Increased arterial blood pressure Emergency phase food poisoning
Loss of nighttime visual acuity	Dependence related to partial vision loss Potential accidental automobile injury
Objects appear hazy, dim, indistinct, and blurred (hypertension, eye fatigue)	Increased arterial blood pressure Potential vision loss related to eye abuse
Ophthalmoscopic Examination White disk with sharply defined borders accompanied by vision loss [primary optic atrophy]	Dependence related to partial vision loss
White disk with indistinct margins, obscured lamina, and invisible physiologic cup (increased intracranial pressure)	Minimal intracranial pressure requirement
Disk edema and blurred borders accompanied by vision loss [papillitis]	Dependence related to partial vision loss Minimal intraocular pressure requirement
Disk edema and blurred borders without vision loss [papilledema] (hypertension, salicylate poisoning, increased intracranial pressure)	Increased arterial blood pressure Emergency phase noncorrosive poisoning (salicylates) Minimal intracranial pressure requirement Minimal intraocular pressure requirement
Retinal hemorrhages (hypertension, diabetes)	Increased arterial blood pressure Minimal intraocular pressure requirement
Retinal artery occlusion (vascular disease)	Minimal intraocular pressure requirement
Retinal artery sclerosis (arteriosclerosis)	Increased arterial blood pressure Predisposition to cerebral vascular accident

Table 4-1   continued

CLINICAL FINDINGS	NURSING DIAGNOSES SUGGESTED BY CLINICAL FINDINGS
Eyes *continued*	
Graywhite retinal spots with fluffy borders (hypertension, papilledema)	Predisposition to cerebral vascular accident Increased arterial blood pressure Minimal intraocular pressure requirement
Spidery retinal pigmentation (night blindness progressing to vision loss)	Dependence related to partial vision loss
Visual Aids and Prostheses	
Wears contact lenses	Dependence on contact lens care Inadequate information related to contact lens use Potential vision loss related to trauma
Wears eyeglasses	Inadequate information related to eyeglass use Potential vision loss related to trauma
Has artificial eye	Inadequate information related to artificial-eye use Dependence on artificial-eye care
Habits Related to Vision Activities	
Working in a poorly lighted environment; watching television in a dark room	Potential vision loss related to eye abuse
Ears	
Ear Discharges	
Excessive wax in ear canal	Impacted cerumen Tinnitus discomfort
Bloody ear discharge (skull fracture, ruptured tympanic membrane)	Minimal intracranial pressure requirement Dependence on body drainage hygiene
Purulent ear discharge (infection, inflammation)	Earache Ear foreign body Dependence on body drainage hygiene
Serous ear discharge (infection, skull fracture)	Earache Minimal intracranial pressure requirement Dependence on body drainage hygiene

Table 4-1   continued

CLINICAL FINDINGS	NURSING DIAGNOSES SUGGESTED BY CLINICAL FINDINGS
EARS *continued*	
Middle Ear	
Amber, blue, yellow, or chalky white tympanic membrane; bulging of tympanic membrane; painful ear (infection)	Earache Additional rest requirement
Pinhole or larger punctures in tympanic membrane [perforated eardrum] with impaired hearing	Dependence on communication assistance related to impaired hearing
Hearing	
Cannot hear normal sounds at 20, 15, or 10 feet distance; can hear watch ticking only when it is less than 2 feet from ear; bone conduction is as long as or longer than air conduction; air conduction is not twice as long as bone conduction (partial or complete hearing loss)	Dependence on communication assistance related to impaired hearing
Buzzing sound in ear from ear disorders, drugs, or insect intrusion	Tinnitus discomfort Ear foreign body
Complains about minimum noise in the environment	Sound sensitivity Temporary minimal stress requirement
Is chronically exposed to loud noises; plays with ears; puts foreign objects into ears	Potential hearing loss related to trauma
Hearing Devices	
Has difficulty with hearing aid	Inadequate information related to hearing aid use
NOSE	
Nasal Discharge	
Cerebrospinal fluid nasal discharge [cerebral rhinorrhea] (head injury)	Dependence on body drainage hygiene Minimal intracranial pressure requirement
Watery nasal discharge (sinusitis, allergy)	Inadequate nasal hygiene Dependence on body drainage hygiene Inadequate information related to respiratory allergy
Mucoid nasal discharge (common cold)	Inadequate nasal hygiene Dependence on body drainage hygiene

Table 4-1   continued

CLINICAL FINDINGS	NURSING DIAGNOSES SUGGESTED BY CLINICAL FINDINGS
Nose *continued*	
	Tenacious airway secretions
	Inadequate information related to respiratory allergy
Bloody nasal discharge (epistaxis, hypertension, trauma, infection, blood dyscrasias)	Epistaxis
	Predisposition to bleeding
	Increased arterial blood pressure
Nasal secretions draining down back of throat	Postnasal drainage
	Inadequate information related to respiratory allergy
Purulent nasal discharge (infection)	Dependence on body drainage hygiene
	Potential infection transmission
External Nose	
Nasal crusting	Inadequate nasal hygiene
Periorbital edema (inflammation, abscess)	Edema related to localized tissue injury
	Dependence related to partial vision loss (if severe)
Internal Nose	
Nasal deviation; air will not pass through one or both nares; adenoid enlargement; nasal polyps; accumulated nasal secretions	Airway obstruction
	Potential airway obstruction
Red, boggy turbinates	Sinus congestion
Nose-Related Activity	
Putting foreign objects in nose	Airway obstruction
	Potential airway obstruction
Poor disposal of tissues used for nasal hygiene	Inadequate disposal of respiratory excreta
	Potential infection transmission
Therapy Related to Nose	
Presence of nasal packing	Nasal pack discomfort
	Impaired swallowing
Presence of nasogastric or intestinal tube	Dependence on nasogastric tube management
	Dependence on intestinal tube management
	Potential electrolyte imbalance related to gastric suction
Mouth	
Oral Discharge	
Mouth bleeding	Oral bleeding

Table 4-1   continued

CLINICAL FINDINGS	NURSING DIAGNOSES SUGGESTED BY CLINICAL FINDINGS
MOUTH *continued*	Chewing difficulty Inadequate oral hygiene Dependence on oral hygiene Potential malnutrition (if prolonged) Potential inadequate fluid intake (if prolonged)
External Mouth: Lips Splitting or parching of lip tissue	Inadequate fluid intake Inadequate information related to skin care
Cleft lip	Sucking difficulty
Tissue splitting at angles of mouth (vitamin B deficiency)	Malnutrition Burning pain
Internal Mouth: Teeth Decayed teeth; broken teeth; loose teeth; partial or total loss of teeth	Chewing difficulty Inadequate oral hygiene Potential malnutrition
Widely spaced teeth	Chewing difficulty
Crowded teeth	Predisposition to tooth decay
Accumulation of hard crusty tartar on teeth margins [plaque]	Inadequate oral hygiene Dependence on oral hygiene
Tooth pain on exposure to cold, heat, pressure, or sour food and drink	Sensitive teeth Chewing difficulty Potential malnutrition
Infant's incoming teeth	Teething pain
Presence of dentures	Dependence on denture care Difficult adaptation to altered body image Potential airway obstruction
Poorly fitting dentures	Chewing difficulty Oral mucosa irritation related to dentures Potential malnutrition Potential airway obstruction
Brown, yellow, orange, gray, or black teeth stains	Inadequate oral hygiene
Ingesting tea, coffee, or drugs or smoking	Potential teeth discoloration
Internal Mouth: Gums Bleeding gums (vitamin C deficiency, trauma, blood dyscrasias, dental plaque)	Gum bleeding Predisposition to bleeding Malnutrition Inadequate oral hygiene Dependence on oral hygiene

Table 4-1   continued

CLINICAL FINDINGS	NURSING DIAGNOSES SUGGESTED BY CLINICAL FINDINGS
MOUTH *continued*	
Gum inflammation; purulent gums (periodontitis)	Chewing difficulty Predisposition to bleeding Inadequate oral hygiene Dependence on oral hygiene Potential infection transmission
Gum hyperplasia (leukemia, Dilantin toxicity)	Drug toxicity (Dilantin) Chewing difficulty Dependence on oral hygiene
Receding gums (aging, periodontitis)	Inadequate oral hygiene Dependence on oral hygiene
Slightly red gums	Chewing difficulty Oral mucosa irritation related to dentures Inadequate oral hygiene Dependence on oral hygiene
Internal Mouth: Tongue	
Tongue vesicles; tongue splitting; denuded tongue	Oral tenderness Chewing difficulty Dependence on oral hygiene Inadequate oral hygiene Potential malnutrition (if prolonged) Potential inadequate fluid intake (if prolonged)
Ulcerated tongue (syphilis, tuberculosis, herpes simplex, niacin deficiency)	Oral tenderness Chewing difficulty Malnutrition Inadequate oral hygiene Dependence on oral hygiene Potential infection transmission Potential malnutrition (if prolonged) Potential inadequate fluid intake (if prolonged)
Bright red tongue (niacin deficiency)	Malnutrition
Longitudinally furrowed tongue (dehydration)	Inadequate fluid intake Dependence on oral hygiene
Large or swollen tongue	Airway obstruction Potential airway obstruction Chewing difficulty Dependence on oral hygiene Dependence on communication assistance related to impaired speech delivery
Poor tongue control; tongue deviates to paralyzed side; tongue quivering	Chewing difficulty Impaired swallowing Dependence on communication

Table 4-1   continued

CLINICAL FINDINGS	NURSING DIAGNOSES SUGGESTED BY CLINICAL FINDINGS
Mouth *continued*	assistance related to impaired speech delivery
Burning tongue (riboflavin deficiency)	Malnutrition Dependence on oral hygiene
Strawberry tongue, denuded and beefy red (scarlet fever)	Dependence on oral hygiene Potential infection transmission
Internal Mouth: Oral Mucosa	
Bright red, inflamed oral mucosa (thrush); white thickened mucosa plaques (Monilia)	Oral tenderness Chewing difficulty Inadequate oral hygiene Dependence on oral hygiene Potential infection transmission
Pale oral mucosa	Malnutrition Increased nutritional requirement related to blood loss
Blue oral mucosa (cyanosis)	Emergency phase oxygen insufficiency
Hemorrhagic spots on roof of mouth (infectious mononucleosis)	Oral tenderness Dependence on oral hygiene Predisposition to bleeding Potential infection transmission
Koplik spots (measles)	Dependence on oral hygiene Potential infection transmission
White precancerous spots or tumors on oral mucosa, especially tongue and cheeks (leukoplasia)	Chewing difficulty Inadequate oral hygiene Dependence on oral hygiene Predisposition to bleeding
Ulceration and/or tissue sloughing of oral mucosa (carcinoma, syphilis)	Chewing difficulty Oral tenderness Inadequate oral hygiene Dependence on oral hygiene Predisposition to bleeding
Internal Mouth: Oral Cavity	
Uvula deviates to nonparalyzed side; gagging is not stimulated (hemiplegia)	Chewing difficulty Impaired swallowing Dependence on communication assistance related to impaired speech delivery
Cleft palate	Sucking difficulty
Presence of surgical sutures in mouth	Chewing difficulty Oral tenderness Inadequate oral hygiene Dependence on oral hygiene Predisposition to bleeding

Table 4-1   continued

CLINICAL FINDINGS	NURSING DIAGNOSES SUGGESTED BY CLINICAL FINDINGS
Mouth *continued* Presence of endotracheal tube	Dependence on endotracheal tube management Dependence on airway patency maintenance Dependence on oral hygiene
Internal Mouth: Tonsils White or yellow tonsil ulceration and edema (tonsillitis)	Throat soreness Impaired swallowing Potential airway obstruction Dependence on oral hygiene
Internal Mouth: Throat Throat redness and swelling (inflammation, infection)	Throat soreness Impaired swallowing Dependence on oral hygiene Potential malnutrition (if prolonged) Potential inadequate fluid intake (if prolonged)
Hoarseness (infection, allergy, foreign body, inhalation of gas irritants)	Airway obstruction Emergency phase pulmonary irritant inhalation Inadequate information related to respiratory allergy Dependence on communication assistance related to impaired speech delivery
Salivary Gland Swollen salivary glands	Parotid gland pain Chewing difficulty Impaired swallowing Dependence on oral hygiene Potential infection transmission
Decreased salivation	Chewing difficulty Impaired swallowing Thirst discomfort Dependence on oral hygiene
Increased salivation	Poor oral secretion control Dependence on oral hygiene
Jaw Jaw stiffness	Chewing difficulty Poor oral secretion control Dependence on communication assistance related to impaired speech delivery Potential malnutrition (if prolonged) Potential airway obstruction

Table 4-1   continued

CLINICAL FINDINGS	NURSING DIAGNOSES SUGGESTED BY CLINICAL FINDINGS
Hᴇᴀʀᴛ *continued*	
Wired jaw	Poor oral secretion control
	Dependence on communication assistance related to impaired speech delivery
	Potential malnutrition
	Potential inadequate fluid intake
	Potential airway obstruction
Hᴇᴀʀᴛ	
Precordial (Anterior Chest) Inspection	
Visible apical impulse (left ventricular hypertrophy, valve stenosis and insufficiency, thyrotoxicosis)	Dependence on cardiac work load reduction
	Additional rest requirement
	Potential oxygen insufficiency
Visible right ventricular impulse (valve stenosis and insufficiency, right ventricular hypertrophy)	Dependence on cardiac work load reduction
	Additional rest requirement
	Potential oxygen insufficiency
Precordial bulge (cardiac hypertrophy, syphilitic aneurysm)	Dependence on cardiac work load reduction
	Potential arterial rupture
	Additional rest requirement
	Potential oxygen insufficiency
Precordial (Anterior Chest) Palpation	Dependence on cardiac work load reduction
Accentuated apical thrust [precordial thrust] (valve stenosis and insufficiency, thyrotoxicosis)	Increased arterial blood pressure
	Additional rest requirement
	Dependence on cardiac work load reduction
Base pulsation (valve stenosis, aortic aneurysm)	Potential arterial rupture
	Potential oxygen insufficiency
Accentuated right ventricular thrust [precordial heave] (thyrotoxicosis, valve stenosis and insufficiency); palpable sensation like a purring cat [precordial thrill] (valve stenosis); palpable rubbing-leather sensation [precordial friction rub] (pericarditis)	Dependence on cardiac work load reduction
	Additional rest requirement
	Potential oxygen insufficiency
Precordial Percussion	
Widened cardiac dullness (cardiac dilatation or pericardial effusion)	Dependence on cardiac work load reduction
	Additional rest requirement

Table 4-1   continued

CLINICAL FINDINGS	NURSING DIAGNOSES SUGGESTED BY CLINICAL FINDINGS

HEART *continued*
Auscultation of Irregular Heart Rate
  with Normal Rhythm
Rate below 60 (sinus bradycardia)
	Emergency phase oxygen
	  insufficiency (in OHD)
	Digitalis toxicity
	Minimum activity tolerance (in
	  OHD)
	Mild activity tolerance (in OHD)

Rate of 35–60 (second-degree heart
  block)
	Dependence on cardiac work load
	  reduction
	Digitalis toxicity
	Minimum activity tolerance
	Mild activity tolerance
	Moderate activity tolerance

Rate of 25–60, not accelerated by
  exertion (third-degree heart
  block)
	Digitalis toxicity
	Dependence on nursing supervision
	  of cardiac monitoring
	Dependence on cardiac pacemaker
	  management
	Predisposition to shock
	  (cardiogenic)
	Dependence on cardiac work load
	  reduction

Rate above 100 (sinus tachycardia);
  rate 140–240 (atrial tachycardia)
	Digitalis toxicity
	Excessive caffeine intake
	Potential dysrhythmia aggravation
	Dependence on cardiac work load
	  reduction
	Emergency phase oxygen
	  insufficiency
	Potential oxygen insufficiency
	Additional rest requirement
	Predisposition to shock
	  (cardiogenic)

Rate 75–180 (atrial flutter); rate
  80–160 with regular rhythm and
  then one irregular rhythm (atrial
  fibrillation); rate 150–250
  (ventricular tachycardia)
	Digitalis toxicity
	Emergency phase oxygen
	  insufficiency
	Dependence on nursing supervision
	  of cardiac monitoring
	Dependence on cardiac pacemaker
	  management
	Dependence on cardiac work load
	  reduction
	Minimum activity tolerance
	Mild activity tolerance
	Additional rest requirement

Table 4-1   continued

CLINICAL FINDINGS	NURSING DIAGNOSES SUGGESTED BY CLINICAL FINDINGS
HEART *continued*	Predisposition to shock (cardiogenic)
Auscultation of Irregular Rhythm Extra beats following normal beats [premature beats]	Digitalis toxicity Excessive caffeine intake Increased arterial blood pressure Potential dysrhythmia aggravation
Chaotic rhythm with rate above 400 (atrial fibrillation)	Digitalis toxicity Emergency phase oxygen insufficiency Increased arterial blood pressure Minimum activity tolerance Dependence on cardiac work load reduction Predisposition to shock (cardiogenic)
One normal beat followed by a second premature beat [bigeminy]; three normal beats followed by a pause, or two normal beats followed by a premature beat, or one normal beat followed by two premature beats [trigeminy]; two, three, or four beats followed by a pause [dropped beats]	Digitalis toxicity Excessive caffeine intake Epinephrine intolerance Potential oxygen insufficiency
Monitoring Irregular Rhythms Undefinable by Auscultation Premature (junctional) contraction	Digitalis toxicity Dependence on nursing supervision of cardiac monitoring Potential oxygen insufficiency
Bundle branch block	Digitalis toxicity Dependence on nursing supervision of cardiac monitoring Dependence on cardiac pacemaker management Predisposition to shock (cardiogenic) Emergency phase oxygen insufficiency (in OHD)
First-degree heart block	Drug toxicity (digitalis, atropine, Isuprel) Emergency phase oxygen insufficiency (in OHD)

Table 4-1   continued

CLINICAL FINDINGS	NURSING DIAGNOSES SUGGESTED BY CLINICAL FINDINGS
HEART *continued*	
	Minimum activity tolerance
	Mild activity tolerance
	Dependence on cardiac work load reduction
	Predisposition to shock (cardiogenic in OHD)
Atrial standstill	Digitalis toxicity
	Emergency phase cardiac arrest
	Emergency phase oxygen insufficiency
	Dependence on nursing supervision of cardiac monitoring
	Dependence on cardiac pacemaker management
	Predisposition to shock (cardiogenic)
Atrial tachycardia with block	Digitalis toxicity
	Emergency phase oxygen insufficiency
	Predisposition to shock (cardiogenic)
	Dependence on nursing supervision of cardiac monitoring
	Dependence on cardiac pacemaker management
	Dependence on cardiac work load reduction
Sinus arrest	Digitalis toxicity
	Emergency phase oxygen insufficiency
	Dependence on nursing supervision of cardiac monitoring
Ventricular flutter	Drug toxicity (digitalis, quinidine)
	Emergency phase cardiac arrest
	Emergency phase oxygen insufficiency
	Dependence on nursing supervision of cardiac monitoring
Ventricular fibrillation	Digitalis toxicity
	Emergency phase cardiac arrest
	Emergency phase oxygen insufficiency
	Dependence on nursing supervision of cardiac monitoring
Ventricular standstill	Digitalis toxicity
	Emergency phase cardiac arrest

Table 4-1   continued

CLINICAL FINDINGS	NURSING DIAGNOSES SUGGESTED BY CLINICAL FINDINGS
HEART *continued*	Dependence on nursing supervision of cardiac monitoring
Auscultation of Heart Sounds Loud first sounds (valve stenosis, thyrotoxicosis, fever, hypertension)	Increased arterial blood pressure Elevated body temperature Dependence on cardiac work load reduction Additional rest requirement Potential oxygen insufficiency
Faint first sounds (first-degree block, cardiac ischemia)	Emergency phase oxygen insufficiency (in OHD) Predisposition to shock (cardiogenic) Dependence on cardiac work load reduction Additional rest requirement
First sound splitting (bundle branch block)	Emergency phase oxygen insufficiency (in OHD) Predisposition to shock (cardiogenic) Dependence on nursing supervision of cardiac monitoring Dependence on cardiac pacemaker management
Loud aortic second sound (hypertension, valve stenosis or insufficiency, aortic aneurysm)	Increased arterial blood pressure Dependence on cardiac work load reduction Additional rest requirement Potential oxygen insufficiency Potential arterial rupture
Faint aortic second sound (valve stenosis)	Dependence on cardiac work load reduction Additional rest requirement Potential oxygen insufficiency
Loud pulmonic second sound (valve stenosis, ventricular failure, septal defect)	Emergency phase oxygen insufficiency Predisposition to shock (cardiogenic) Dependence on cardiac work load reduction Additional rest requirement Potential oxygen insufficiency Potential pulmonary edema

Table 4-1 continued

CLINICAL FINDINGS	NURSING DIAGNOSES SUGGESTED BY CLINICAL FINDINGS
HEART *continued*	
Faint pulmonic second sound (valve stenosis, septal defect)	Dependence on cardiac work load reduction Additional rest requirement Potential oxygen insufficiency
Inspiratory second sound splitting (valve stenosis or insufficiency, septal defect, bundle branch block); expiratory second sound splitting (valve stenosis, left bundle branch block)	Emergency phase oxygen insufficiency Dependence on cardiac work load reduction Additional rest requirement Potential oxygen insufficiency Potential dysrhythmia aggravation
Left ventricular gallop (valve insufficiency, cardiac failure); right ventricular gallop (cardiac failure)	Emergency phase oxygen insufficiency Emergency phase cardiogenic shock Predisposition to shock (cardiogenic) Dependence on cardiac work load reduction Additional rest requirement Potential oxygen insufficiency
Presystolic gallop (valve stenosis, hypertension, hyperthyroidism, anemia, heart disease)	Dependence on cardiac work load reduction Additional rest requirement Potential oxygen insufficiency
Diastolic or systolic ejection murmur (valve stenosis); diastolic or systolic regurgitant murmur (valve stenosis or insufficiency)	Dependence on cardiac work load reduction Additional rest requirement Potential oxygen insufficiency
Absence of heart sounds (ventricular standstill)	Emergency phase cardiac arrest
Cardiac Assistance or Surveillance Devices	
Patient being monitored	Distress related to cardiac monitoring Dependence on nursing supervision of cardiac monitoring
Presence of pacemaker	Dependence on cardiac pacemaker management Distress related to cardiac pacemaker Pacemaker failure Inadequate information related to portable pacemaker use

Table 4-1   continued

CLINICAL FINDINGS	NURSING DIAGNOSES SUGGESTED BY CLINICAL FINDINGS
BLOOD PRESSURE	
Systolic blood pressure between 140 and 150	Increased arterial blood pressure Epinephrine intolerance Predisposition to hypertension Inadequate information related to hypertension
Diastolic blood pressure between 90 and 100	Increased arterial blood pressure Predisposition to hypertension Inadequate information related to hypertension
Systolic pressure above 150; diastolic pressure above 100	Dependence on cardiac work load reduction Predisposition to cerebral vascular accident Lifestyle inappropriate to hypertension Epinephrine intolerance Inadequate information related to hypertension
Systolic pressure below 100; diastolic pressure below 60	Decreased arterial blood pressure Predisposition to shock Potential oxygen insufficiency Potential inadequate urinary output
Sudden drop in blood pressure when changing from lying to sitting or from sitting to standing position, or when a pregnant woman lies flat	Postural hypotension
Decreased pulse pressure with less than 30 points between systolic and diastolic pressures (valve stenosis, pericarditis)	Dependence on cardiac work load reduction Additional rest requirement Potential oxygen insufficiency
Increased pulse pressure with more than 50 points between systolic and diastolic pressures (hypertension, valve insufficiency, thyrotoxicosis)	Increased arterial blood pressure Inadequate information related to hypertension Dependence on cardiac work load reduction Additional rest requirement Potential oxygen insufficiency
Circulation	
Barely perceptible temporal, carotid, or subclavian pulse or no pulse	Impaired arterial peripheral circulation

Table 4-1 continued

CLINICAL FINDINGS	NURSING DIAGNOSES SUGGESTED BY CLINICAL FINDINGS
BLOOD PRESSURE *continued*	
Barely perceptible brachial, radial, ulnar, femoral, dorsal pedis, popliteal, or posterior tibial pulse or no pulse	Impaired arterial peripheral circulation Cold intolerance
Distended neck, arm, or leg veins (left ventricular failure, fluid overload)	Emergency phase circulatory overload Increased arterial blood pressure Dependence on cardiac work load reduction
Calf tenderness, positive Homan's sign (thrombophlebitis)	Potential thrombus displacement
Presence of petechiae, hematoma, bruising, purpura	Intradermal bleeding
Loss of 500 cc or more of blood	Emergency phase hemorrhage Predisposition to shock (hemorrhagic) Emergency phase impending shock
Circulation Related Therapy	
Intravenous therapy being given	Parenteral infusion discomfort Dependence on arteriovenous cutdown management Dependence on intravenous infusion management Dependence on umbilical infusion management
Blood transfusion being given	Dependence on blood transfusion management
Rash, fever, etc., developing during blood transfusion	Emergency phase blood transfusion reaction
Hypodermoclysis being given	Dependence on hypodermoclysis management
CHEST AND LUNGS	
Respirations	
Fewer than 12 respirations per minute [bradypnea]	Sedative intolerance Analgesic intolerance Inadequate pulmonary ventilation Potential oxygen insufficiency
More than 16 respirations per minute [tachypnea]	Hyperventilation Epinephrine intolerance Distressed respiratory effort Potential carbon dioxide insufficiency Potential alkalosis

Table 4-1   continued

CLINICAL FINDINGS	NURSING DIAGNOSES SUGGESTED BY CLINICAL FINDINGS
CHEST AND LUNGS *continued*	
Alternate breathing cessation and rapid breathing [Biot respirations] (meningitis)	Distressed respiratory effort Minimal intracranial pressure requirement
Painful breathing (inflammation, trauma)	Painful respirations Potential inadequate pulmonary ventilation
Dyspneic, deep, slow respirations [Kussmaul breathing] (diabetic acidosis, uremia, hemorrhage, pneumonia)	Emergency phase diabetic acidosis Distressed respiratory effort
Coughing up blood [hemoptysis] (tuberculosis, cancer, congestive heart failure, pulmonary embolism, hypertension, hemophilia, leukemia)	Potential infection transmission Predisposition to bleeding or hemorrhage Increased arterial blood pressure
Productive cough with sputum expectoration (inflammation, irritation)	Potential infection transmission
Thorax Inspection	
Thoracic deformity (barrel chest, pectus excavatum, pectus neonatum, kyphosis, lordosis, scoliosis)	Inadequate pulmonary ventilation Potential inadequate pulmonary ventilation Potential decubitus ulcer (with kyphosis)
Respiratory Movements	
Accessory muscle breathing (asthma, emphysema)	Excessive carbon dioxide retention Potential carbon dioxide toxicity
Abnormal bulging of interspaces during expiration and retraction during inspiration [flail chest] (rib fracture)	Distressed respiratory effort Painful respirations
Dyspnea at rest (cardiac and respiratory disorders)	Emergency phase oxygen insufficiency Distressed respiratory effort Minimum activity tolerance Potential oxygen insufficiency
Dyspnea on exertion (cardiac and respiratory disorders, hypertension, anemia)	Distressed respiratory effort Minimum activity tolerance Mild activity tolerance Potential oxygen insufficiency
Mouth breathing	Mouth breathing discomfort Airway obstruction Nasal congestion

Table 4-1   continued

CLINICAL FINDINGS	NURSING DIAGNOSES SUGGESTED BY CLINICAL FINDINGS
CHEST AND LUNGS *continued*	
Difficulty in breathing when lying down, relieved by sitting up or standing [orthopnea]	Emergency phase oxygen insufficiency Distressed respiratory effort Potential oxygen insufficiency
Noisy snoring [stertorous respirations]	Airway obstruction Potential airway obstruction
Cough	
Brassy, barking, nonproductive, wheezing, spasmodic, or hacking cough	Cough discomfort
Thorax Palpation and Percussion	
Thoracic tenderness or swelling (trauma)	Painful respirations Potential tissue injury related to fracture (rib)
Decreased diaphragmatic descent (pleural effusion, pulmonary atelectasis, diaphragmatic paralysis, pneumonia)	Inadequate pulmonary ventilation Potential infection transmission Potential inadequate pulmonary ventilation
Thoracic skin crepitation (pneumothorax, subcutaneous emphysema)	Inadequate pulmonary ventilation Potential inadequate pulmonary ventilation
Tracheal deviation (pulmonary atelectasis, pleural effusion, spontaneous pneumothorax)	Inadequate pulmonary ventilation Potential inadequate pulmonary ventilation
Percussion cracked-pot sounds (pulmonary cavity in advanced tuberculosis)	Potential infection transmission
Percussion dullness (pulmonary atelectasis, pulmonary consolidation, pulmonary congestion); percussion flatness (pulmonary consolidation, pleural effusion, pulmonary congestion)	Inadequate pulmonary ventilation Potential inadequate pulmonary ventilation
Percussion hyperresonance (emphysema, pleural effusion, pneumothorax); percussion tympany (pulmonary cavity, pneumothorax)	Inadequate pulmonary ventilation Excessive carbon dioxide retention Potential inadequate pulmonary ventilation
Thorax Auscultation	
Short inspiratory breathing; prolonged expiratory breathing; tubular sound over lung area [bronchial breathing]	Emergency phase pulmonary edema Distressed respiratory effort Excessive carbon dioxide retention Potential carbon dioxide toxicity

Table 4-1   continued

CLINICAL FINDINGS	NURSING DIAGNOSES SUGGESTED BY CLINICAL FINDINGS
CHEST AND LUNGS *continued*	
(emphysema, pulmonary consolidation, pulmonary edema)	Potential oxygen insufficiency Potential inadequate pulmonary ventilation
Equal inspiratory and expiratory breath sounds in lower lobes of lung [bronchovesicular breathing] (pulmonary consolidation)	Distressed respiratory effort Potential oxygen insufficiency Potential inadequate pulmonary ventilation
Amphoric breathing sound, like air being blown over a bottle (pneumothorax)	Emergency phase oxygen insufficiency Potential oxygen insufficiency
Wheezing breath sounds, hissing, whistling expiration (pulmonary atelectasis, airway obstruction, pulmonary edema, bronchitis)	Emergency phase oxygen insufficiency Emergency phase pulmonary edema Distressed respiratory effort Inadequate pulmonary ventilation Airway obstruction Potential oxygen insufficiency
No breath sounds (pleural effusion, emphysema, pulmonary atelectasis)	Emergency phase respiratory arrest Airway obstruction Distressed respiratory effort Excessive carbon dioxide retention Potential oxygen insufficiency Potential carbon dioxide toxicity
Decreased breath sounds (pulmonary atelectasis, pleural effusion, emphysema, airway obstruction, pulmonary infection, pneumothorax)	Emergency phase respiratory arrest Airway obstruction Inadequate pulmonary ventilation Excessive carbon dioxide retention Distressed respiratory effort Potential oxygen insufficiency Potential carbon dioxide toxicity
Bubbling rales (pulmonary edema, congestion, cavity infection, embolus)	Emergency phase oxygen insufficiency Emergency phase pulmonary edema Distressed respiratory effort Pulmonary secretion congestion Inadequate pulmonary ventilation Potential oxygen insufficiency
Crackling rales (pulmonary congestion, consolidation, embolus, infection, cardiac failure)	Emergency phase oxygen insufficiency Emergency phase cardiogenic shock Distressed respiratory effort Inadequate pulmonary ventilation Potential oxygen insufficiency Pulmonary secretion congestion

Table 4-1   continued

CLINICAL FINDINGS	NURSING DIAGNOSES SUGGESTED BY CLINICAL FINDINGS
CHEST AND LUNGS *continued*	
Gurgling rales (pulmonary edema, airway obstruction)	Emergency phase pulmonary edema Airway obstruction Inadequate pulmonary ventilation
Musical rales (pulmonary congestion, pulmonary edema); sonorous rhonchi (pulmonary edema, congestion)	Emergency phase pulmonary edema Pulmonary secretion congestion
Pleural friction rub (pulmonary embolus, pleurisy)	Emergency phase oxygen insufficiency Painful respirations Potential inadequate pulmonary ventilation
Crepitus rib sound (rib fracture)	Painful respirations Limited range of motion Potential inadequate pulmonary ventilation Potential tissue injury related to fracture (rib)
Decreased voice sounds (pulmonary atelectasis, congestion, emphysema, pneumothorax)	Emergency phase oxygen insufficiency Excessive carbon dioxide retention Inadequate pulmonary ventilation Pulmonary secretion congestion Distressed respiratory effort Potential oxygen insufficiency
Decreased vocal/tactile fremitus (pulmonary atelectasis, pleural effusion, emphysema, pneumothorax)	Inadequate pulmonary ventilation Excessive carbon dioxide retention Potential inadequate pulmonary ventilation Potential oxygen insufficiency
Increased vocal/tactile fremitus (pulmonary consolidation)	Potential oxygen insufficiency
Egophony (pulmonary consolidation, pleural effusion)	Potential inadequate pulmonary ventilation Potential oxygen insufficiency
Pectoriloquy (pulmonary consolidation, pulmonary embolus, pulmonary atelectasis)	Emergency phase oxygen insufficiency Inadequate pulmonary ventilation Potential oxygen insufficiency Potential inadequate pulmonary ventilation
Bronchophony (pulmonary consolidation)	Potential oxygen insufficiency

Table 4-1   continued

CLINICAL FINDINGS	NURSING DIAGNOSES SUGGESTED BY CLINICAL FINDINGS
CHEST AND LUNGS *continued* *Respiratory-Related Therapy* Difficulty with artificial ventilation therapy	Artificial ventilation discomfort
System for closed-chest drainage	Dependence on closed-chest drainage management
Nonfunctioning system for closed-chest drainage	Interrupted closed-chest drainage

CLINICAL FINDINGS	NURSING DIAGNOSES
ABDOMEN *Abdominal Inspection* Dilated abdominal veins (body thinness, inferior vena cava obstruction)	Malnutrition
Visible peristalsis (bowel obstruction)	Emergency phase acute gastric dilatation Cramping pain Potential vomiting
Visible pulsation over wide abdominal area (hypertension, aneurysm)	Increased arterial blood pressure Potential arterial rupture
Generalized uniform abdominal roundness, with umbilicus deep in abdomen	Obesity Flatulence
Single abdominal curve from xiphoid to pubis, everted umbilicus, bulging flanks (ascites); double abdominal curve, everted umbilicus, fluid wave (ovarian cyst)	Increased intraabdominal pressure discomfort
Enlarged upper abdominal half (abdominal distention)	Flatulence Increased intraabdominal pressure discomfort
Enlarged lower abdominal half or third (bladder distention)	Inadequate urinary output related to urine retention Increased intraabdominal pressure discomfort
Inward depression of abdominal wall	Malnutrition
Abdominal wall protrusion in inguinal and femoral areas (herniation)	Potential impaired intestinal circulation

Table 4-1   continued

CLINICAL FINDINGS	NURSING DIAGNOSES SUGGESTED BY CLINICAL FINDINGS
ABDOMEN *continued*	
Bursting of abdominal incision with protrusion of abdominal contents	Emergency phase abdominal evisceration Predisposition to shock Predisposition to bleeding or hemorrhage Potential wound infection
Healing newborn umbilical cord	Dependence on umbilical hygiene
Presence of colostomy	Dependence on colostomy management Inadequate information related to colostomy management Difficult adaptation to altered body image Unpleasant sensory stimulation Potential electrolyte imbalance related to colostomy drainage
Presence of ileostomy	Dependence on ileostomy management Inadequate information related to ileostomy care Difficult adaptation to altered body image Unpleasant sensory stimulation Potential electrolyte imbalance related to ileostomy drainage
Presence of T-tube for drainage	Dependence on local drainage tube hygiene Dependence on common-duct T-tube management Potential electrolyte imbalance related to T-tube drainage
Presence of gastrostomy	Dependence on gastrostomy feeding management Potential diarrhea
Presence of jejunostomy	Dependence on jejunostomy feeding management Potential diarrhea
Abdominal Auscultation	
Diminished bowel sounds or no sounds (peritonitis, intestinal obstruction, spinal cord injury)	Emergency phase acute gastric dilatation Predisposition to shock Peritoneal irritation pain Potential constipation

Table 4-1   continued

CLINICAL FINDINGS	NURSING DIAGNOSES SUGGESTED BY CLINICAL FINDINGS
ABDOMEN *continued*	
Gurgling bowel sounds (early intestinal obstruction, gastric inflammation)	Gastric irritation Diarrhea Cramping pain Biliary colic pain
Rushing bowel sounds (intestinal obstruction, intraabdominal mass, strangulated hernia)	Emergency phase acute gastric dilatation Predisposition to shock Increased intraabdominal pressure discomfort Cramping pain
Peritoneal friction rub (peritoneal inflammation)	Predisposition to shock Peritoneal irritation pain
Abdominal bruit (aneurysm)	Potential arterial rupture
Abdominal Palpation	
Localized tenderness (localized inflammation)	Tenderness Peritoneal irritation pain
Rebound tenderness (peritoneal inflammation); cutaneous hyperesthesia (inflammation)	Peritoneal irritation pain
Involuntary abdominal rigidity (abdominal infection or mass)	Peritoneal irritation pain Increased intraabdominal pressure discomfort
Abdominal mass	Increased intraabdominal pressure discomfort
Spleen enlargement (mononucleosis, endocarditis, etc.)	Predisposition to bleeding or hemorrhage Increased intraabdominal pressure discomfort Potential spleen rupture Potential infection transmission
Liver enlargement (hepatitis, cirrhosis)	Increased intraabdominal pressure discomfort Potential infection transmission
Palpable bladder	Inadequate urinary output related to urine retention
Abdominal Percussion	
Abdominal tympany (intestinal obstruction, ascites, gastric dilatation)	Emergency phase acute gastric dilatation Increased intraabdominal pressure discomfort Flatulence

Table 4-1 continued

CLINICAL FINDINGS	NURSING DIAGNOSES SUGGESTED BY CLINICAL FINDINGS
ABDOMEN *continued*	
Percussion dullness below 11th rib (spleen enlargement)	Predisposition to bleeding or hemorrhage Increased intraabdominal pressure discomfort Potential spleen rupture Potential infection transmission
Percussion resonance extending below costal margin (liver enlargement)	Increased intraabdominal pressure discomfort Potential infection transmission
Anal Inspection	
Anal redness	Painful defecation Potential painful defecation
Reddened masses protruding from rectum	Hemorrhoidal pain Painful defecation Potential painful defecation
Anal itching	Pruritus discomfort Inadequate information related to transmission of intestinal worms
Rectal Inspection and Palpation	
Narrowed rectal lumen; rectal polyps	Painful defecation Potential painful defecation
Hard stool in rectum	Fecal impaction Potential painful defecation
Dark, tarry stools	Emergency phase hemorrhage Predisposition to shock
Gastrointestinal-Related Discomforts	
Sense of epigastric fullness	Indigestion
Burning midsternal sensation	Heartburn
Feeling that vomiting is about to occur	Nausea
Ejection of stomach contents through mouth [vomiting]	Vomiting Hyperemesis Electrolyte imbalance related to vomiting Potential electrolyte imbalance related to vomiting Dependence on oral hygiene Inadequate information related to safe food handling Inadequate information related to foreign food hazards Minimal intracranial pressure requirement Additional rest requirement

Table 4-1   continued

CLINICAL FINDINGS	NURSING DIAGNOSES SUGGESTED BY CLINICAL FINDINGS

ABDOMEN *continued*

Vomiting bright red blood [hematemesis] (neoplasm, esophageal varices, gastric ulceration)	Emergency phase hemorrhage Predisposition to shock Dependence on oral hygiene
Passage of liquid stools at frequent intervals [diarrhea]	Diarrhea Electrolyte imbalance related to diarrhea Potential electrolyte imbalance related to diarrhea Gastric irritation Dependence on incontinence hygiene Inadequate information related to food allergy Inadequate information related to foreign food hazards Inadequate information related to safe food handling Additional rest requirement Dependence on convenient toilet facilities
Diarrhea occurring 30 minutes to 1 hour following meals	Post-meal diarrhea Electrolyte imbalance related to diarrhea Potential electrolyte imbalance related to diarrhea Dependence on convenient toilet facilities
No interest in food	Anorexia Potential malnutrition
Little interest in food	Blunted appetite Potential malnutrition
Insatiable appetite (hyperthyroidism)	Increased nutritional requirement related to metabolism Potential obesity
Failure of infant or child to gain normal weight and height [failure to thrive]	Sucking difficulty Inadequate information related to solid food feeding Inadequate information related to infant bottle feeding Chewing difficulty Malnutrition
Chronic rechewing of regurgitated food	Chronic rumination Inadequate oral hygiene Dependence on oral hygiene

Table 4-1   continued

CLINICAL FINDINGS	NURSING DIAGNOSES SUGGESTED BY CLINICAL FINDINGS
ABDOMEN *continued*	
Displeasure with available food	Food selection dissatisfaction Difficulty maintaining religious diet
Displeasure with prescribed diet	Therapeutic diet dissatisfaction Inadequate information related to prescribed diet Noncompliance to the therapeutic regime
Eating inconsistently, changing one's diet according to the latest fad	Inadequate information related to fad dieting Potential malnutrition

CLINICAL FINDINGS	NURSING DIAGNOSES SUGGESTED BY CLINICAL FINDINGS
FEMALE REPRODUCTIVE SYSTEM	
Breast Inspection	
Bloody nipple discharge, breast dimpling, breast asymmetry, breast peau d'orange, inverted breast nipple	Dependence on body drainage hygiene Dependence on skin care Inadequate information related to breast cancer Potential skin irritation
Open sore on breast nipple	Dependence on wound care Potential skin irritation
Inflammatory abscess of breast	External abscess Limited range of motion (arm) Potential skin irritation
Purulent nipple discharge	Dependence on body drainage hygiene Potential skin irritation Potential infection transmission
Split in breast nipple tissue	Cracked-nipple pain Potential skin irritation
Very large, heavy normal breasts	Pendulous breast discomfort
Breast soreness	Breast tenderness Inadequate information related to premenstrual tension
Breast fullness with milk	Breast engorgement Excessive lactation
Lack of breast milk	Lactation deficiency Lactation suppression
Breast Palpation	
Breast tumor	Dependence on skin care Pendulous breast discomfort Inadequate information related to breast cancer Inadequate information related to surgical procedure

Table 4-1   continued

CLINICAL FINDINGS	NURSING DIAGNOSES SUGGESTED BY CLINICAL FINDINGS

FEMALE REPRODUCTIVE SYSTEM *continued*
Breast Transillumination

| Stippled breast areas indicating mass | Inadequate information related to breast cancer |
| | Inadequate information related to the surgical procedure |

Breast Surgery

Recent breast amputation	Limited range of motion
	Difficult adaptation to altered body image
	Inadequate information related to postmastectomy management

Abdominal Inspection and Palpation
See Abdomen, p. 84

Inspection of External Female Genitalia

Vulva itching	Pruritus discomfort
	Inadequate feminine hygiene
	Dependence on feminine hygiene
	Potential skin irritation
Wartlike lesions on vulva (gonorrhea, syphilis)	Potential infection transmission
	Potential skin irritation
Vulva redness and edema	Edema related to localized tissue injury
	Burning pain
	Inadequate feminine hygiene
	Dependence on feminine hygiene
	Dependence on skin care
	Potential skin irritation
Healing episiotomy incision	Burning pain
	Dependence on episiotomy care
	Potential skin irritation
	Potential wound infection
Vaginal orifice reveals cheesy, creamy white, frothy white, or thick yellow vaginal discharge (inflammation)	Inadequate feminine hygiene
	Potential infection transmission
	Potential genitourinary infection
Vaginal orifice reveals foul odor, brown (chocolate) vaginal discharge; positive pap smear (malignancy)	Inadequate information related to uterine cancer
	Inadequate feminine hygiene
Irregular vaginal bleeding	Bleeding
	Emergency phase hemorrhage
	Inadequate information related to abnormal vaginal bleeding
	Inadequate information related to postsurgical vaginal bleeding

Table 4-1   continued

CLINICAL FINDINGS	NURSING DIAGNOSES SUGGESTED BY CLINICAL FINDINGS
FEMALE REPRODUCTIVE SYSTEM *continued* *Inspection and Palpation of Internal Female Organs* *Vagina*	
Vaginal wall redness (gonorrhea, *trichomonas* or other infection); vaginal wall tenderness or inflammation	Dependence on feminine hygiene Inadequate feminine hygiene Potential infection transmission
Vaginal wall blueness (pregnancy, tumor); vaginal wall tumor	Dependence on nursing supervision of normal pregnancy Inadequate information related to the surgical procedure
Cervical Os	
Purulent or mucopurulent cervical os discharge (gonorrhea, puerperal infection)	Inadequate feminine hygiene Dependence on feminine hygiene Potential infection transmission
Soft, bright red polyps	Inadequate information related to the surgical procedure
Cervix	
Cervical softness (pregnancy)	Dependence on nursing supervision of normal pregnancy
Cervical blueness (pregnancy, pelvic tumor)	Dependence on nursing supervision of normal pregnancy Inadequate information related to the surgical procedure
Cervical ulcer (foreign body irritation, syphilis, tuberculosis); if chronic with induration, it indicates carcinoma	Inadequate information related to the surgical procedure Potential infection transmission
Bartholin gland tenderness and inflammation (gonorrhea)	Throbbing pain Potential infection transmission
Pelvic Floor	
Vaginal fistula	Dependence on incontinence hygiene Electrolyte imbalance related to fistula drainage Potential electrolyte imbalance related to fistula drainage Dependence on convenient toilet facilities
Bladder prolapse into vagina [cystocele], with residual urine and urinary frequency	Inadequate urinary output related to urine retention Potential genitourinary infection Dependence on convenient toilet facilities

Table 4-1   continued

CLINICAL FINDINGS	NURSING DIAGNOSES SUGGESTED BY CLINICAL FINDINGS
FEMALE REPRODUCTIVE SYSTEM *continued*	
Rectal prolapse into vagina [rectocele]	Constipation Potential constipation
Uterine prolapse into vagina, with urinary frequency	Dependence on convenient toilet facilities
Uterine Palpation	
Uterine tenderness with discharge (infection)	Potential infection transmission Backache
Uterine enlargement (pregnancy, painless fibroid nodules)	Increased intraabdominal pressure discomfort Potential varicose veins Dependence on nursing supervision of normal pregnancy Inadequate information related to the surgical procedure
Uterine enlargement with bloody discharge (carcinoma)	Increased intraabdominal pressure discomfort Dependence on feminine hygiene Inadequate feminine hygiene Inadequate information related to uterine cancer Inadequate information related to the surgical procedure
MALE REPRODUCTIVE SYSTEM	
Inspection and Palpation of Penis	
Penis swelling (trauma, edema from any cause)	Edema related to localized tissue injury Potential skin irritation
Penis ulceration (gonorrhea, syphilis)	Dependence on wound care Inadequate information related to the surgical procedure Potential infection transmission
Painless ulceration, or wartlike growth on penis (carcinoma)	Dependence on wound care Inadequate information related to surgical procedure Potential skin irritation
Penis foreskin excision	Dependence on circumcision care
Urethral stricture evidenced by minimal force and size of urinary stream	Painful urination Dependence on convenient toilet facilities Inadequate urinary output related to urine retention

Table 4-1   continued

CLINICAL FINDINGS	NURSING DIAGNOSES SUGGESTED BY CLINICAL FINDINGS
MALE REPRODUCTIVE SYSTEM *continued*	
Purulent or nonpurulent urethral discharge (gonorrhea, genitourinary infection)	Painful urination Increased hydration requirement Potential infection transmission
Inspection and Palpation of the Testes	
Painful testicle swelling (mumps)	Edema related to localized tissue injury Throbbing pain Additional rest requirement Potential infection transmission
Inspection and Palpation of Epididymis	
Epididymis swelling and tenderness	Edema related to localized tissue injury
Palpation of Prostate Gland	
Benign prostate enlargement with residual urine, hesitancy, nocturia	Inadequate urinary output related to urine retention Potential genitourinary infection Dependence on convenient toilet facilities
Swollen, painful prostate with dysuria, frequency and nocturia, or inability to void	Inadequate urinary output related to urine retention Potential genitourinary infection Dependence on convenient toilet facilities Painful urination
Problems Related to Stages of Male Reproductive Cycle	
Onset of period when male becomes capable of reproduction (age 14–15)	Inadequate information related to male puberty
Period of lessening sexual activity in male (age 50–60)	Inadequate information related to male climacteric Difficult adaptation to altered body image
Therapy Related to Genitourinary System	
Presence of urinary catheter	Dependence on indwelling urinary catheter management Inadequate information related to urinary catheter care Inadequate urinary output related to urinary catheter obstruction Potential genitourinary infection
Presence of decompression urinary drainage system	Dependence on decompression urinary drainage management

Table 4-1 continued

CLINICAL FINDINGS	NURSING DIAGNOSES SUGGESTED BY CLINICAL FINDINGS
MALE REPRODUCTIVE SYSTEM *continued*	
Presence of tidal drainage system	Dependence on tidal drainage management
Presence of nephrostomy tube	Dependence on nephrostomy drainage management
Presence of suprapubic catheter	Dependence on suprapubic drainage management
Presence of ureteroileostomy	Dependence on ureteroileostomy management Potential skin irritation
Presence of ureterosigmoidostomy	Dependence on ureterosigmoidostomy management Potential genitourinary infection Potential skin irritation
Presence of cutaneous ureterostomy	Dependence on ureterostomy management Potential skin irritation
Peritoneal dialysis therapy	Dependence on peritoneal dialysis management Increased intraabdominal pressure discomfort Predisposition to shock
Hemodialysis therapy	Dependence on arteriovenous shunt management Dependence on hemodialysis management Inadequate information related to arteriovenous shunt management Inadequate information related to home dialysis management Nonacceptance of increased dependency

MUSCULOSKELETAL AND NEUROLOGIC SYSTEMS	
Inspection and Palpation of Bone	
Bone soreness when touched (infection, neoplasm, trauma, leukemia, anemia)	Bone pain Limited range of motion Difficulty ambulating Potential bone fracture
Bone crepitation; nonresistance to abnormal positioning; severe nonalignment; loss of movement [fracture]	Potential tissue injury related to fracture
Unequal lower limb bone length	Difficulty ambulating Potential accidental falling

Table 4-1   continued

CLINICAL FINDINGS	NURSING DIAGNOSES SUGGESTED BY CLINICAL FINDINGS

MUSCULOSKELETAL AND NEUROLOGIC SYSTEMS *continued*

Inspection and Palpation of Joints

Joint swelling	Edema related to localized tissue injury Limited range of motion Difficulty ambulating Painful joint motion Potential limited range of motion
Joint inflammation	Painful joint motion Throbbing pain Limited range of motion Difficulty ambulating Potential limited range of motion
Joint muscle appears shortened	Joint contracture Limited hand dexterity Difficulty ambulating
Inability to move joint [joint freezing]	Limited range of motion Limited hand dexterity Difficulty ambulating
Difficulty in moving joint in circular, forward, inward, outward, rotation, or straight position; feeling of stiffness	Limited range of motion Limited hand dexterity Potential limited range of motion Potential accidental falling
Limb nonalignment, either inward or outward from body	Irregular joint rotation Potential joint contracture

Inspection and Palpation of Ligaments

Torn, tender ligament; excessive joint motion; extreme joint pain	Sprain Limited range of motion Limited hand dexterity Difficulty ambulating
Ligament out of normal contour; bone separated from its normal joint position; nonaligned joint [bone dislocation]	Limited range of motion Limited hand dexterity Difficulty ambulating

Inspection and Palpation of Muscle

Difference in measured sizes of muscles reveals atrophy or hypertrophy; inability to move muscles against resistance exerted by examiner [muscle weakness]	Difficulty sitting up Difficulty standing up Difficulty turning self Difficulty ambulating
Continuous state of muscular contraction	Muscle spasm

Table 4-1   continued

CLINICAL FINDINGS	NURSING DIAGNOSES SUGGESTED BY CLINICAL FINDINGS

MUSCULOSKELETAL AND NEUROLOGIC SYSTEMS *continued*

Brief muscle contraction	Involuntary muscle twitching Restless leg discomfort
Involuntary action or nonaction tremors [chorea or athetoid movements]	Limited hand dexterity Dependence on general hygiene assistance Dependence on dressing assistance Dependence on eating assistance Dependence on feeding Embarrassment related to social exposure
Involuntary muscle contraction occurring with muscle stretching [muscle spasticity]	Muscle spasm Dependence on dressing assistance Dependence on general hygiene assistance Dependence on eating assistance Depending on feeding Difficulty ambulating Potential muscle spasm Potential joint contracture Potential accidental falling Potential limited range of motion
Intense muscle resistance to passive movement [muscle rigidity]	Limited hand dexterity Limited range of motion Difficulty ambulating Potential joint contracture Potential limited range of motion
Stiff extension position [decerebrate rigidity]; stiff flexion or extension position [decorticate rigidity]	Potential joint contracture Potential decubitus ulcer
Muscle contraction and relaxation at slower rate than normal; loss of tone [muscle hypertonia]	Potential footdrop Potential wristdrop
Inability to move muscles of half of body [hemiplegia]	Difficulty ambulating Difficulty standing up Difficulty sitting up Difficulty transferring Difficulty turning self Dependence on dressing assistance Dependence on general hygiene assistance Dependence on eating assistance Impaired swallowing Difficult adaptation to altered body image

Table 4-1   continued

CLINICAL FINDINGS	NURSING DIAGNOSES SUGGESTED BY CLINICAL FINDINGS
MUSCULOSKELETAL AND NEUROLOGIC SYSTEMS *continued*	Dependence on communication assistance related to impaired speech delivery Potential decubitus ulcer Potential accidental falling
Inability to move muscles in one limb [monoplegia]	Difficulty ambulating Difficulty standing up Difficulty transferring Dependence on dressing assistance Dependence on general hygiene assistance Dependence on eating assistance Difficult adaptation to altered body image Potential accidental falling
Inability to move muscles in both lower limbs [paraplegia]	Difficulty transferring Dependence on dressing assistance Dependence on general hygiene Difficult adaptation to altered body image Dependence on retraining for elimination control Potential decubitus ulcer Potential accidental falling
Inability to move muscles in all four extremities [quadriplegia]	Dependence on general hygiene Dependence on dressing Dependence on feeding Dependence on incontinence hygiene Nonacceptance of increased dependency Difficult adaptation to altered body image Dependence on retraining for elimination control Inadequate information related to hygienic care of the dependent person Potential decubitus ulcer Potential impaired pulmonary ventilation
Inspection and Palpation of Limbs and Appendices	
Absence of finger, toe, or limb since birth or from trauma or surgery	Limited hand dexterity Difficulty ambulating

Table 4-1   continued

CLINICAL FINDINGS	NURSING DIAGNOSES SUGGESTED BY CLINICAL FINDINGS
MUSCULOSKELETAL AND NEUROLOGIC SYSTEMS *continued*	
	Phantom pain
	Phantom-limb discomfort
	Dependence on amputation stump care
	Difficult adaptation to altered body image
Hand, finger, or wrist deformity; diminished or no grip	Limited hand dexterity
	Limited range of motion
	Dependence on eating assistance
	Dependence on feeding
	Dependence on general hygiene assistance
	Dependence on dressing assistance
Inspection and Palpation of Spine	
Abnormal curvature of spine, such as scoliosis, kyphosis, lordosis, or spinal indentation	Difficulty ambulating
	Muscle spasm
	Backache
	Potential decubitus ulcer
Spinal protrusions such as spina bifida or meningocele	Potential decubitus ulcer
	Difficulty turning self
Therapeutic or Ambulating Devices	
Presence of wet cast	Potential bone deformity
Cast fits too tightly or too loosely	Potential impaired arterial peripheral circulation
	Potential skin irritation
	Potential bone deformity
Difficult ambulation with cast, cane, crutches, walker, or brace	Inadequate information related to brace manipulation
	Inadequate information related to cane use
	Inadequate information related to crutch manipulation
	Inadequate information related to walker manipulation
	Potential accidental falling
Brace fits too tightly or too loosely; nonalignment of brace joints and limb joints	Potential skin irritation
	Potential accidental falling
Difficulty in using wheelchair	Inadequate information related to wheelchair manipulation
	Immobility related to architectural barriers
Presence of cervical collar	Cervical collar discomfort
Traction therapy	Dependence on traction management
Nonfunctioning traction therapy	Disrupted traction

Table 4-1   continued

CLINICAL FINDINGS	NURSING DIAGNOSES SUGGESTED BY CLINICAL FINDINGS

MUSCULOSKELETAL AND NEUROLOGIC SYSTEMS *continued*

Recent application of artificial limb	Inadequate information related to limb prosthesis

Cranial Nerves

Olfactory nerve: inability to correctly identify odors such as tobacco, coffee, etc.	Impaired ability to taste food Potential accidental burn Potential accidental suffocation
Optic nerve: any variation from 20/20 vision	Dependence related to total vision loss Dependence related to partial visual loss
Oculomotor nerve: cannot follow moving finger with smooth eye movements (intracranial pressure, aneurysm, subarachnoid hemorrhage)	Potential arterial rupture Minimal intracranial pressure requirement Dependence related to partial vision loss
Trochlear nerve: inability to look downward or laterally to the side, in addition to double vision	Dependence related to partial vision loss
Pupillary responses (see Eyes, p. 61)	
Trigeminal nerve: no response or dull response of cheek or jaw area when touched with cotton, pin, or cold or warm objects; tongue blade can be pulled out from between teeth when teeth are closed (mastication nerve paralysis)	Chewing difficulty Burning pain (facial)
Abducens nerve: inability to look to side (aneurysm, increased intracranial pressure)	Minimal intracranial pressure requirement Potential arterial rupture
Facial nerve: inability to wrinkle forehead, raise eyebrows, frown, or smile; inability to differentiate tastes such as sugar and salt; one-sided facial paralysis; inability to blink	Chewing difficulty Impaired ability to taste food Potential malnutrition Dependence on communication assistance related to impaired speech delivery Potential vision loss related to eye exposure
Acoustic nerve (see Hearing, under Ears, p. 66)	
Glossopharyngeal and vagus nerves: touching back of tongue with tongue blade fails to stimulate gag reflex; uvula fails to elevate	Impaired swallowing Chronic regurgitation

Table 4-1   continued

CLINICAL FINDINGS	NURSING DIAGNOSES SUGGESTED BY CLINICAL FINDINGS

MUSCULOSKELETAL AND NEUROLOGIC SYSTEMS *continued*

when patient says "Ah," which indicates bilateral paralysis; uvula elevates on only one side when patient says "Ah," which indicates unilateral paralysis

Accessory nerve: inability to raise shoulders or turn head against resistance exerted by examiner	Limited range of motion
Hypoglossal nerve: protruded tongue reveals tremors, involuntary movements, or deviation toward weak side	Chewing difficulty Impaired swallowing

Coordination

With eyes closed, patient cannot touch his finger to his nose; inability to pat the knees rapidly while alternating palms and backs of hands; inability to run one's heel down shin of opposite leg; inability to walk a straight line heel-to-toe	Difficulty ambulating Potential accidental falling
Environment seems to be swirling around [vertigo]	Vertigo Difficulty ambulating Potential accidental falling Potential nausea Potential vomiting
Whirling or swimming sensation in head (dizziness)	Drug toxicity Difficulty ambulating Increased arterial blood pressure Antihypertensive drug intolerance Postural hypotension Potential nausea Potential accidental falling

Sensory Responses

Inability to feel when touched with cotton, pin, or cold or warm objects [impaired tactile sense]	Potential accidental burn Potential decubitus ulcer
Inability to determine direction of positioned toes with eyes closed [impaired position sense]; inability to differentiate varied weights in palms of hands [impaired pressure sense]; inability to distinguish body parts and right from left [impaired position sense]	Difficulty ambulating Dependence on general hygiene assistance Dependence on eating assistance Potential accidental falling

Table 4-1   continued

CLINICAL FINDINGS	NURSING DIAGNOSES SUGGESTED BY CLINICAL FINDINGS
MUSCULOSKELETAL AND NEUROLOGIC SYSTEMS *continued*	
Poor sucking reflex	Diminished sucking Potential malnutrition
Hyperactive sucking reflex	Unsatisfied sucking
Deep Reflex Responses	
Diminished deep reflex responses or no responses, which indicates impaired motor function	Difficulty ambulating Potential accidental falling
Hyperactive deep reflex responses, which indicates clonus [spasm]	Potential muscle spasm

Note: Words in brackets [] are synonymous with clinical findings. Words in parentheses () are conditions associated with clinical findings.

Part 2.

Nursing Diagnoses

5.

NURSING DIAGNOSES RELATED TO
Acid-Base Balance

POTENTIAL ACID-BASE IMBALANCE

Predisposition to Acidosis (271,325)

ASSESSMENT

Objective Data
Fever
Prolonged use of weight reduction, crash, or fad diets
Prolonged intake of highly acid drugs such as ammonium chloride
Profuse and prolonged sweating
Impaired carbohydrate metabolism
Impaired kidney function

Related Data
Laboratory Findings:
Prolonged increased blood carbon dioxide

Commonly Related Conditions:
Starvation
Dehydration

Commonly Related Diseases:
Diabetes mellitus
Emphysema
Renal failure
Hepatitis

POSSIBLE ETIOLOGY

When carbohydrate reserves are depleted, the body obtains its energy through protein and fat metabolism which leads to acidosis. In fever, carbohydrate demands are increased while carbohydrate intake is usually decreased. In poor nutritional intake, the carbohydrate reserve is not adequate to meet body demands. Impaired carbohydrate metabolism, as in diabetes, fails to control the blood sugar which results in increased fat metabolism and the accumulation of blood ketones.

Adequate sodium is needed to combine with carbonic acid and maintain a normal pH. In profuse sweating and impaired kidney function, the loss of sodium reduces the amount available to combine with carbonic acid.

NURSING DIAGNOSIS

Predisposition to acidosis: a susceptibility to an imbalanced chemical state of decreased bicarbonate (alkali) and increased carbonic acid

PLANNING

Patient Needs	Primary Nurse-Patient Goals
Water-salt balance	To maintain fluid and electrolyte balance
Acid-base balance	To maintain regulating mechanisms and functions
Protection from physical harm	To prevent physical injury
Increased learning	To achieve awareness of needs

NURSING INTERVENTIONS

Nursing Treatments
Balance nutritional intake (if intake is poor)
Give high-sodium fluids orally
    AND
Encourage increased sodium-food intake (during prolonged, profuse sweating or impaired renal function where there is sodium loss)
Encourage increased calorie intake (during fever)

Nursing Observations
Monitor blood studies for abnormal acid-base
Monitor blood studies for abnormal gas exchange (if patient has emphysema)
Monitor blood studies for abnormal glucose (if patient has diabetes)
Test the urine for pH
Test the urine for sugar and acetone (if patient has diabetes)
Inspect for dehydration
Observe for complaints of dizziness
Observe for complaints of malaise
Observe for complaints of pain (abdominal)
Observe for complaints of thirst
Observe for complaints of weakness
Observe for restlessness
Observe for vomiting
Observe the breath for abnormal odors
Observe the level of consciousness

Health Teaching
Describe those symptoms which should be reported (weakness, malaise, nausea, vomiting, restlessness)

Explain the causes of the health problem
Explain the reason for and intended effect of the therapy
Teach the principles of good nutrition
Describe the manifestations of impending diabetic coma

EVALUATION

See the evaluation criteria for each specific goal in Chapter 2.

Predisposition to Alkalosis (271,325)

ASSESSMENT

Objective Data
Excessive ingestion of sodium bicarbonate and other alkalis
Severe, prolonged vomiting
Severe, prolonged diarrhea
Prolonged gastric suction therapy
Prolonged use of diuretics without potassium replacement
Rapid, deep breathing
Prolonged adrenocortical steroid therapy

Related Data
Laboratory Findings:
Low blood potassium
Commonly Related Conditions:
Infant diarrhea
Hyperemesis
Hyperventilation
Chronic indigestion
Commonly Related Diseases:
Cushing's syndrome

POSSIBLE ETIOLOGY

Excessive carbonic acid loss. Excessive bicarbonate intake. Incompatible nutritional intake and insulin dosage. The administration of adrenal cortical hormones.

NURSING DIAGNOSIS

Predisposition to alkalosis: a susceptibility to an imbalanced chemical state of increased bicarbonate (alkali) and decreased carbonic acid

PLANNING

Patient Needs	Primary Nurse-Patient Goals
Water-salt balance	To maintain fluid and electrolyte balance
Acid-base balance	To maintain regulating mechanisms and functions

Protection from physical harm   To prevent physical injury
Increased learning   To achieve awareness of needs

NURSING INTERVENTIONS

Nursing Treatments
Give citrus fruit juice (if tolerated during prolonged vomiting and diarrhea)
Give high potassim fluids orally
    AND
Encourage increased potassium-food intake (when on diuretics or adreno-
    corticosteroids and during vomiting and diarrhea)
Refrain from giving bicarbonates
Refrain from giving carbonated beverages
Irrigate the gastric tube with saline

Nursing Observations
Monitor blood studies for abnormal acid-base
Test the urine for pH
Inspect the hands for tremors
Inspect the chest for respiratory rate and rhythm
Observe for complaints of weakness
Observe for convulsions
Observe for irritability
Observe for restlessness
Observe for tetany
Observe for vomiting

Health Teaching
Describe those symptoms that should be reported (lethargy, tetany, tremor,
    convulsions, vomiting)
Explain the causes of the health problem
Explain the reason for and intended effect of the therapy
Recommend that alkalis be used conservatively
Teach how to do breath-holding (if inclined to hyperventilation)

Medical Treatments Performed by Nurses
Give the prescribed drugs

EVALUATION

See the evaluation criteria for each specific goal in Chapter 2.

EMERGENCY ACID IMBALANCE

Emergency Phase Acidosis
(192,271,325)

ASSESSMENT

Subjective Data
Weakness
Malaise
Dull headache

Abdominal pain
Nausea

Objective Data
Restlessness
Vomiting
Dehydration
Deep, rapid respirations
Edema, sometimes
Decreased temperature
Lethargy
Stupor
Coma
Shock
Acetone breath

Related Data
Laboratory Findings:
Acid urine with pH 4.6–5.2
Blood pH below 7.2
Increased blood carbon dioxide

Commonly Related Conditions:
Starvation
Dehydration

Commonly Related Diseases:
Emphysema
Renal failure
Hepatitis

POSSIBLE ETIOLOGY

Urea retention due to kidney impairment. Excessive ingestion of acid drugs
and foods. Loss of sodium through profuse sweating. Carbohydrate depletion through fever or poor nutrition.

NURSING DIAGNOSIS

Emergency phase acidosis: the need for immediate health care as a result of
an imbalanced chemical state of excess carbonic acid and decreased bicarbonate (alkali)

PLANNING

Patient Needs	**Primary Nurse-Patient Goals**
Water-salt balance	To maintain fluid and electrolyte balance
Acid-base balance	To maintain regulating mechanisms and functions
Rest	To achieve rest
Comfort	To achieve comfort

Protection from physical harm   To prevent physical injury

Increased learning   To achieve awareness of needs

NURSING INTERVENTIONS

Nursing Treatments

Administer intravenous fluids (ET) (1000 cc of 0.45% normal saline)
    OR
Give salt-soda solution orally (if intravenous fluids are not available)
Administer intermittent positive pressure breathing (ET) (for respiratory
    acidosis)
Place on complete bed rest
Cover with warm blankets
Attend the patient constantly
Consult with the physician (immediately)

Nursing Observations

Measure the intake
Measure the output
Monitor the blood pressure
Monitor blood studies for abnormal acid-base
Test the urine for pH
Inspect the chest for respiratory rate and rhythm
Palpate the pulse for rate, rhythm, and volume

Health Teaching

Explain the causes of the health problem
Explain the reason for and intended effect of the therapy

Medical Treatments Performed by Nurses

Give the prescribed drugs (sodium bicarbonate, sodium lactate, potassium)

EVALUATION

See evaluation criteria for each specific goal in Chapter 2.

Emergency Phase Diabetic Acidosis (192,271,325)

ASSESSMENT

Subjective Data

Early Stage:
Malaise
Excessive appetite

Midstage:
Dizziness
Nausea
Severe thirst

Objective Data

Early Stage:
Restlessness

Mental dullness
Fruity or acetone breath
Midstage:
Vomiting
Dehydration
Dry, flushed skin
Deep, rapid respirations
Polyuria

Related Data

Laboratory Findings (Early Stage):
Urine glucose and acetone

Laboratory Findings (Midstage):
Urine glucose and acetone
Acid urine with pH 4.6–5.2

Commonly Related Diseases:
Diabetes mellitus

POSSIBLE ETIOLOGY

Improper insulin dosage or administration in the treatment of impaired carbohydrate metabolism. Infection. Surgical or other stress.

NURSING DIAGNOSIS

Emergency phase diabetic acidosis: the need for immediate health care as a result of an imbalanced chemical state of excess carbonic acid and decreased bicarbonate related to impaired carbohydrate metabolism

PLANNING

Patient Needs	**Primary Nurse-Patient Goals**
Water-salt balance	To maintain fluid and electrolyte balance
Acid-base balance	To maintain regulating mechanisms and functions
Rest	To achieve rest
Comfort	To achieve comfort
Protection from physical harm	To prevent physical injury
Increased learning	To achieve awareness of needs

NURSING INTERVENTIONS

Nursing Treatments

Administer intravenous fluids (ET) (5% glucose in saline or Ringer's solution)
   OR
Give salt-soda solution orally (if insulin or intravenous fluids are not available)
Place on complete bed rest
Cover with warm blankets

Attend the patient constantly
Consult with the physician (immediately)
Catheterize with an indwelling urinary catheter (to facilitate urine testing)

Nursing Observations
Measure the intake
Measure the output
Monitor the blood pressure
Monitor blood studies for abnormal (increased) glucose (every 2 hours)
Monitor blood studies for abnormal acid-base
Test the urine for sugar and acetone (every 30 minutes)
Test the urine for pH
Inspect the abdomen for distention
Observe for complaints of pain (abdominal)
Inspect the chest for respiratory rate and rhythm
Palpate the pulse for rate, rhythm, and volume

Health Teaching
Explain the causes of the health problem
Explain the reason for and intended effect of the therapy

Medical Treatments Performed by Nurses
Give the prescribed drugs (fast-acting, crystalline, insulin 50 units every 1–2
    hours until urine glucose reaches normal)

EVALUATION

See the evaluation criteria for each specific goal in Chapter 2.

EMERGENCY ALKALI IMBALANCE

Emergency Phase Alkalosis (247,271)

ASSESSMENT

Subjective Data
Anxiety
Lethargy

Objective Data
Irritability
Restlessness
Tetany (despite normal blood calcium)
Tremor
Convulsions
Flaccid muscle weakness (when blood potassium low)
Shallow respirations (in alkali excess)
Vomiting
Irregular cardiac rhythm

Related Data

Laboratory Findings:
Increased blood bicarbonate and pH
Normal or decreased blood chloride
Alkaline urine

Commonly Related Conditions:
Infant diarrhea
Hyperemesis
Hyperventilation
Chronic indigestion

Commonly Related Diseases:
Cushing's syndrome

POSSIBLE ETIOLOGY

Excess sodium bicarbonate intake. Chloride loss through prolonged vomiting. Potassium loss through diuresis. Carbon loss though hyperventilation.

NURSING DIAGNOSIS

Emergency phase alkalosis: the need for immediate health care as a result of an imbalanced chemical state of excess bicarbonate and decreased carbonic acid

PLANNING

Patient Needs	**Primary Nurse-Patient Goals**
Water-salt balance	To maintain fluid and electrolyte balance
Acid-base balance	To maintain regulating mechanisms and functions
Rest	To achieve rest
Comfort	To achieve comfort
Protection from physical harm	To prevent physical injury
Increased learning	To achieve awareness of needs

NURSING INTERVENTIONS

Nursing Treatments
Give high-potassium fluids orally (if on diuretics, adrenocorticosteroids, or vomiting)
    OR
Give high-sodium fluids orally (if dehydrated)
    OR
Administer intravenous fluids (ET) (isotonic saline) (if dehydrated or vomiting)
Refrain from giving bicarbonates
Provide a paper bag for breathing (if hyperventilating)

Place on complete bed rest
Cover with warm blankets
Attend the patient constantly
Consult with the physician (immediately)

Nursing Observations
Monitor the blood pressure
Monitor blood studies for abnormal acid-base
Test the urine for pH
Inspect the chest for respiratory rate and rhythm
Palpate the pulse for rate, rhythm, and volume

Health Teaching
Explain the causes of the health problem
Explain the reason for and intended effect of the therapy
Teach how to do breath-holding (if hyperventilating)
Recommend that alkalis be used conservatively

Medical Treatments Performed by Nurses
Give the prescribed drugs (ammonium chloride, potassium, calcium gluco-
nate)

EVALUATION

See the evaluation criteria for each specific goal in Chapter 2.

6.

NURSING DIAGNOSES RELATED TO
Behavior

ANGER

Anger Related to Being Ill (299,420)

ASSESSMENT

Subjective Data
Feels bitter that the illness happened to him
Feels resentment and hostility toward those who are well
Wonders "Why me?" "What did I ever do to deserve this?"
Perceives that others are involved in life's trivia while he is struggling to
   function or survive

Objective Data
Uncooperative
Demanding
Verbalizes bitterness
Irritability

Related Data
Commonly Related Diseases:
Any disease or injury

POSSIBLE ETIOLOGY

Stress related to illness. An attempt to maintain self-esteem and reduce
anxiety in the presence of threat.

NURSING DIAGNOSIS

Anger related to being ill: feelings of intense emotional displeasure that one
is in poor or failing health

PLANNING

Patient Needs   **Primary Nurse-Patient Goals**
Comfort   To achieve comfort

Protection from psychologic threat

To prevent emotional injury

Acceptance

To achieve productive interpersonal relationships

Warm, communicating relationships

To achieve effective verbal and nonverbal communications

Adequacy

To achieve positive expressions, feelings, reactions

Increased learning

To achieve awareness of needs

NURSING INTERVENTIONS

Nursing Treatments

Approach unhurriedly
Provide an atmosphere of acceptance
Express empathy
Encourage the expression of feelings
Listen attentively

AND

Talk with the patient
Offer feedback of the patient's expressed feelings
Recognize the need for the use of appropriate defense mechanisms
Encourage the use of normal coping mechanisms
Explore with the patient his strengths and resources
Touch the patient judiciously
Refrain from negatively criticizing

Nursing Observations

Determine the degree of insight
Evaluate the significance of emotional distress mannerisms
Evaluate the significance of nonverbal communication
Observe for an excessive stress level
Observe for evidence that the patient is reaching out for emotional support
Observe for a favorable response to therapy

Health Teaching

Explain how to obtain release from emotional stress
Explain that the person's emotional response is appropriate and commonly experienced
Explain and offer hope that the emotional pain will decrease with time

EVALUATION

See the evaluation criteria for each specific goal in Chapter 2.

Anger Related to Desertion by a Departed Loved One

ASSESSMENT

Subjective Data

Feels bitter toward the person who is gone
Experiences resentment and hostility

Perceives that the departure of the loved one has left him alone and without the support he deserves

May experience guilt for feeling angry

Objective Data

Verbalizes bitterness

Fault-finding

Related Data

Commonly Related Conditions:

Separation anxiety

Commonly Related Diseases:

None

  OR

Depressive neurosis or reactive depression

POSSIBLE ETIOLOGY

An attempt to maintain self-esteem and reduce anxiety in the presence of threat. A normal part of the grief process.

NURSING DIAGNOSIS

Anger related to desertion by a departed loved one: feelings of intense emotional displeasure that one has been left by a significant other through death or an unresolvable life situation

PLANNING

Patient Needs	**Primary Nurse-Patient Goals**
Comfort	To achieve comfort
Protection from psychologic threat	To prevent emotional injury
Acceptance	To achieve productive interpersonal relationships
Warm, communicating relationships	To achieve effective verbal and nonverbal communications
Personal growth and maturity	To achieve optimum function
Increased learning	To achieve awareness of needs
Increased reality perception and problem-solving ability	To achieve optimum function

NURSING INTERVENTIONS

Nursing Treatments

Approach unhurriedly

Provide an atmosphere of acceptance

Express empathy

Encourage the expression of feelings

Listen attentively

  AND

Talk with the patient

Offer feedback of the patient's expressed feelings

Recognize the need for the use of appropriate defense mechanisms
Encourage the use of normal coping mechanisms
Encourage enhanced involvement in already established relationships
Explore with the patient his strengths and resources (especially his support system)
Recognize the need for unique personal adjustments to change
Touch the patient judiciously
Refrain from negatively criticizing

Nursing Observations
Determine the degree of insight
Evaluate the significance of emotional distress mannerisms
Evaluate the significance of nonverbal communication
Observe for an excessive stress level
Observe for evidence that the patient is reaching out for emotional support
Observe for a favorable response to therapy

Health Teaching
Explain how to obtain release from emotional stress
Explain that the person's emotional response is appropriate and commonly experienced
Explain and offer hope that the emotional pain will decrease with time

EVALUATION

See the evaluation criteria for each specific goal in Chapter 2.

Inability to Control Anger (299,420)

ASSESSMENT

Subjective Data
May fear his own anger and capacity for destructiveness
Unable to restrain angry impulses
Inadequacy feelings
Frustration
Anxiety

Objective Data
Anger is easily aroused
Violent angry outbursts
Temper tantrums
Throwing objects
Use of profanity
Quarrelsome
Demanding
Shouting and fist-pounding
Commanding voice tone
Uncooperative
Acts out before others

Related data
Commonly Related Diseases:
None

POSSIBLE ETIOLOGY

Lack of early training in self-discipline and social skills. Identification with adults poorly trained in social skills. Prolonged stress. An attempt to maintain self-esteem or reduce anxiety.

NURSING DIAGNOSIS

Inability to control anger: the inability to restrain angry impulses

PLANNING

Patient Needs	Primary Nurse-Patient Goals
Relaxation	To achieve relaxation
Protection from psychologic threat	To prevent emotional injury
Acceptance	To achieve productive interpersonal relationships
Warm, communicating relationships	To achieve effective verbal and nonverbal communications
High evaluation of self, adequacy	To achieve positive expressions, feelings, reactions
Personal growth and maturity	To achieve optimum function
Increased learning	To achieve awareness of needs
Increased reality perception and problem-solving ability	To achieve optimum function

NURSING INTERVENTIONS

Nursing Treatments
Approach unhurriedly
Demonstrate calmness
Provide an atmosphere of acceptance
Encourage the expression of feelings
Listen attentively
    AND
Talk with the patient
Offer feedback of the patient's expressed feelings
Encourage the use of normal coping mechanisms
Explore with the patient his strengths and resources
Explore with the patient reasons for recurring problems
Explore with the patient the effects of his behavior on others
Encourage respect for the rights of others
Encourage participation in therapeutic group interaction
Suggest more appropriate means of emotional expression
Ignore undesirable behavior
    OR
Set limits on unacceptable behavior
Remove the stimulus for the emotion
Provide seclusion (if needed)
    OR
Restrain the patient (if combative)
Reduce the demands placed upon the patient

Refrain from arguing
Refrain from negatively criticizing
Refrain from using punitive measures in exercising authority
Touch the patient judiciously
Provide emotional support for persons significant to the patient

Nursing Observations
Determine the degree of insight
Determine the precipitating factors (of the anger)
Evaluate the person's relatedness with others
Evaluate the significance of emotional distress mannerisms
Evaluate the significance of nonverbal communication
Identify disturbing conversation topics
Identify emotion-stimulating events
Identify potentially destructive behavior
Determine the extent of group pressure conformity (in relation to destruc-
     tive behavior)
Identify life values significant to the person
Identify appropriate use of defense mechanisms
Observe for an excessive stress level
Observe for evidence that the patient is reaching out for emotional support
Observe for behavior modification

Health Teaching
Explain the causes of the health problem
Advise against causing defensive responses in others
Explain what is considered justifiable aggression
Advise that highly emotional situations be avoided
Emphasize the importance of recognizing tension within oneself
Explain how to obtain release from emotional stress
Explain how to channel emotional energy into activity
Recommend methods for achieving total relaxation
Explain the importance of remaining calm
Explain why persons should maintain self-control
Explain the importance of maintaining a positive self-attitude
Recommend that behavioral limits be set (by the family)
Explain how to set behavioral limits

EVALUATION

See the evaluation criteria for each specific goal in Chapter 2.

Maladaptive Coping Related to Anger (299,420)

ASSESSMENT

Subjective Data
May outwardly appear to control anger
Once offended, seldom forgives or reconciliates
May harbor angry feelings for days or months

Perceives others as enemies
Perceives power over others as success

Objective Data
Belittles, ridicules, and criticizes others
Exploits, intimidates, teases, and bullies others
Deliberately seeks controversy
Makes sarcastic remarks
Sulking
Rejects the person who is the object of the anger
Exhibitionism
Burns, tears down, mutilates, injures, or dismantles objects or persons
Appears to enjoy destructiveness
Is unable to discuss his anger and resolve the problem with others

Related Data
Commonly Related Conditions:
Sexual deviance
Commonly Related Diseases:
None
  OR
Alcoholism psychosis
Paranoid schizophrenia
Paranoid involutional psychosis
Manic-depressive psychosis
Psychopathic personality
Sociopathic personality

POSSIBLE ETIOLOGY

Chronic, inappropriate use of defense mechanisms such as projection, repression, or symbolism. Inability to resolve frustration or threat. A real or supposed threat with a desire for retaliation. An attempt to protect oneself against future injury.

NURSING DIAGNOSIS

Maladaptive coping related to anger: the expression of intense emotional displeasure in an unhealthy, deceptive, or destructive manner

PLANNING

Patient Needs	Primary Nurse-Patient Goals
Comfort	To achieve comfort
Protection from psychologic threat	To prevent emotional injury
Acceptance	To achieve productive interpersonal relationships
Warm, communicating relationships	To achieve effective verbal and nonverbal communications
Personal growth and maturity	To achieve optimum function
Increased learning	To achieve awareness of needs

Increased reality perception and   To achieve optimum function
  problem-solving ability

NURSING INTERVENTIONS

Nursing Treatments
Approach unhurriedly
Provide an atmosphere of acceptance
Encourage the expression of feelings
Listen attentively
  AND
Talk with the patient
Offer feedback of the patient's expressed feelings
Encourage the use of normal coping mechanisms
Encourage mutual problem solving
Explore with the patient his strengths and resources
Explore with the patient reasons for criticism of others
Encourage realistic perception of others
Explore with the patient the effects of his behavior on others
Encourage respect for the rights of others
Encourage participation in therapeutic group interaction
Explore with the patient the need for dominance
Support a realistic assessment of the situation
Suggest more appropriate means of emotional expression
Set limits on unacceptable behavior
Provide seclusion (if needed)
Refrain from arguing
Refrain from negatively criticizing
Refrain from using punitive measures in exercising authority
Touch the patient judiciously

Nursing Observations
Determine the degree of insight
Determine the precipitating factors (of the anger)
Evaluate the person's relatedness with others
Evaluate the significance of emotional distress mannerisms
Evaluate the significance of nonverbal communication
Identify disturbing conversation topics
Identify emotion-stimulating events
Identify potentially destructive behavior
Identify life values significant to the person
Identify appropriate use of defense mechanisms
Identify inappropriate use of defense mechanisms
Observe for an excessive stress level
Observe for evidence that the patient is reaching out for emotional support
Observe for behavior modification

Health Teaching
Explain the causes of the health problem
Advise against causing defensive responses in others
Explain what is considered justifiable aggression

Advise that negative responses from others be regarded with minimum
   significance
Explain how to obtain release from emotional stress
Explain how to channel emotional energy into activity
Explain why persons should maintain self-control
Recommend that behavior limits be set (by the family)
Explain how to set behavioral limits

EVALUATION

See the evaluation criteria for each specific goal in Chapter 2.

POTENTIAL ANGER

Potential Active Aggression (299,420)

ASSESSMENT

Subjective Data
Feelings of low self-esteem and powerlessness
Has little or no fear of punishment
Perceives aggression as a normal response to threat
Tends to see other persons as a source of danger or threat, and himself as
   vulnerable even if such is not true
Believes that others exist to satisfy his needs

Objective Data
Poorly educated in social skills
Early exposure to parental rejection, threats, aggression, and inconsistent
   parental discipline
No external motivation toward standards of high performance
Seldom exposed to affection
Self-indulgent
Chronic loss of emotional control
Exploitive, manipulative behavior for self-satisfaction
Appears to gain pleasure from bullying others
Previous active aggression
Alcohol consumption reveals aggressiveness

Related Data
Commonly Related Diseases:
None
   OR
Alcoholism psychosis
Paranoid schizophrenia
Manic-depressive psychosis
Psychopathic personality

POSSIBLE ETIOLOGY

Frustration of a desired goal or goals. Lack of early training in self-
discipline and social skills. Prolonged stress.

NURSING DIAGNOSIS

Potential active aggression: the possibility that the person will become actively aggressive toward others

PLANNING

Patient Needs	**Primary Nurse-Patient Goals**
Comfort	To achieve comfort
Protection from psychologic threat	To prevent emotional injury
Acceptance	To achieve productive interpersonal relationships
Warm, communicating relationships	To achieve effective verbal and nonverbal communications
Sense of value, usefulness, high evaluation of self	To achieve positive expressions, feelings, reactions
Personal growth and maturity	To achieve optimum function
Increased learning	To achieve awareness of needs
Increased reality perception and problem-solving ability	To achieve optimum function

NURSING INTERVENTIONS

Nursing Treatments
Approach unhurriedly
Demonstrate calmness
Provide an atmosphere of acceptance
Express warmth and friendliness
Avoid causing intense emotional situations
Encourage the expression of feelings
Listen attentively
    AND
Talk with the patient
Encourage the use of normal coping mechanisms
Encourage mutual problem solving
Explore with the patient his strengths and resources
Encourage the substitution of undesirable habits with favorable habits
Explore with the patient the effects of his behavior on others
Encourage respect for the rights of others
Encourage role-playing to develop sensitivity
Encourage participation in therapeutic group interaction
Encourage acceptance of partial goal satisfaction (if frustration precipitates aggression)
Encourage noncompetitive activities (if competition precipitates aggression)
Support a realistic assessment of the situation (if misperception precipitates aggression)

Suggest more appropriate means of emotional expression
Suggest more appropriate means of need gratification (if pleasure is gained
    from hurting others)
Set limits on unacceptable behavior
Provide seclusion (if needed)
Reduce the demands placed upon the patient
Refrain from arguing
Refrain from negatively criticizing
Refrain from using punitive measures in exercising authority

Nursing Observations
Determine the degree of insight
Evaluate the person's relatedness with others
Evaluate the significance of emotional distress mannerisms
Evaluate the significance of nonverbal communication
Identify abnormal perceptions
Identify abnormal thought content
Identify disturbing conversation topics
Identify emotion-stimulating events
Identify inappropriate emotional responses
Identify potentially destructive behavior
Determine the extent of group pressure conformity (in relation to potential
    destructive behavior)
Identify life values significant to the person
Identify appropriate use of defense mechanisms
Identify inappropriate use of defense mechanisms
Observe for evidence that the patient is reaching out for emotional support
Observe for an excessive stress level

Health Teaching
Advise against causing defensive responses in others
Explain what is considered justifiable aggression
Advise that highly emotional situations be avoided
Advise that negative responses from others be regarded with minimum
    significance
Advise that significant persons express love for one another
Advise that discipline be consistent
Explain how to obtain release from emotional stress
Explain how to channel emotional energy into activity
Teach how to use the problem-solving method
Explain why persons should maintain self-control
Recommend that behavioral limits be set (by the family)
Explain how to set behavioral limits

EVALUATION

See the evaluation criteria for each specific goal in Chapter 2.

ANXIETY

Inadequate Emotional Support Related to Mild Anxiety (187,196,260,263, 295,298,344,399,492,508,530,538)

ASSESSMENT

Subjective Data

A painful, emotional uneasiness and feeling of dread that is mildly difficult to endure

A sudden momentary upsurge if acute

Constant and of indefinite duration if chronic

Sense of helplessness

Unsettled, vaguely confused feeling

Feeling of weakness

Wants to escape the situation

Minimum focus on himself

Perception is altered in that he sees, hears, and grasps more than when in a nonanxiety state

Unaccountable nervousness

Preoccupied with the anxiety

Objective Data

Appears forlorn and upset

At the time of need, the person has a limited, nonexistent, or temporarily absent support system of significant others

May reach out for help through crying, attention-seeking behavior, touching persons or objects, seeking someone to talk with, etc.

May appear withdrawn

Maintains some interest in the external environment

Restlessness

Talkative or verbally very quiet

Mood swings

Unusually sensitive

Related Data

Commonly Related Conditions:

Caffeine and epinephrine drug intolerance

Hypoglycemia

Anoxia

Premenstrual edema

Commonly Related Diseases:

None

  OR

Any disease or injury, especially:

Hypoparathyroidism

Myocardial infarction

Neurocirculatory asthenia

Thrombophlebitis

Mesenteric vascular occlusion
Anxiety neurosis

POSSIBLE ETIOLOGY

Lack of interest on the part of one's usually supportive world of family, friends, and church. The unavailability of persons who usually offer support. The presence of *anxiety from psychologic causes:* Situational inadequacy feelings; the absence of meaning in a situation that does not make sense. Disturbed interpersonal relationships. Inability to meet the expectations of significant others. Forced adaptation to change. Conflict between dependence and independence. Conflict between desires and moral standards. Poorly defined goals. Lack of fulfillment in life. Suppressed aggressive impulses. *Anxiety from physical causes:* Inadequate tissue oxygenation. Increased lactic acid blood levels binding calcium from nerve endings. Decreased blood glucose stimulates the adrenal gland to secrete epinephrine (adrenalin) for the purpose of elevating the blood sugar, and the increased epinephrine level results in anxiety. Drug side effects.

NURSING DIAGNOSIS

Inadequate emotional support related to mild anxiety: little or no comfort or sustaining measures received from others while one is enduring mild anxiety

PLANNING

Patient Needs	**Primary Nurse-Patient Goals**
Relaxation	To achieve relaxation
Comfort	To achieve comfort
Protection from psychologic threat	To prevent emotional injury
Predictable, orderly world	To achieve a therapeutic environment
Acceptance	To achieve productive interpersonal relationships
Warm, communicating relationships	To achieve effective verbal and nonverbal communications
High evaluation of self, adequacy	To achieve positive expressions, feelings, reactions
Personal growth and maturity	To achieve optimum function
Increased learning	To achieve awareness of needs
Increased reality perception and problem-solving ability	To achieve optimum function

NURSING INTERVENTIONS

Nursing Treatments
General Interventions:
Approach unhurriedly

Demonstrate calmness
Express empathy
Express warmth and friendliness
Provide an atmosphere of acceptance
Touch the patient judiciously
Reassure verbally
Attend the patient constantly (until the acute episode subsides)
    AND
Provide frequent patient contact (thereafter)
Arrange a structured environment (suitable to the patient)
Arrange situations which encourage patient autonomy
Encourage the expression of feelings
Listen attentively
    AND
Talk with the patient
Offer feedback of the patient's expressed feelings
Encourage patient questions (if such will relieve the distress)
Provide reliable information
Do not allow unpleasant surprise situations
Avoid causing painful emotional situations
Provide objects which symbolize safeness
Encourage mutual problem solving
Support a realistic assessment of the situation
Introduce to persons who have successfully undergone the same experience
Encourage the use of normal coping mechanisms
Explore with the patient his strengths and resources
Encourage the person to face the anxiety
Reduce the demands placed upon the patient
Refrain from performing nonessential procedures
Refrain from negatively criticizing

Call the patient's family to the
    bedside
    OR
Encourage telephone calls between
    significant persons

} (if the patient prefers or strongly needs significant others and if significant others are available as a support system)

Specific to Chronic Anxiety:
Explore with the patient reasons for recurring problems (precipitating the anxiety)
Encourage identification of specific life values (if poorly defined values are precipitating the anxiety)
Emphasize the person's normal characteristics (if there is self-condemnation for experiencing anxiety)
Encourage active diversional activities (to promote periods of rest from anxiety)

Nursing Observations
Determine the degree of insight
Determine the precipitating factors

Determine the relieving factors
Evaluate the significance of emotional distress mannerisms
Evaluate the significance of nonverbal communication
Identify disturbing conversation topics
Identify life values significant to the person
Identify appropriate use of defense mechanisms
Identify inappropriate use of defense mechanisms
Observe for drug reactions (to
   caffeine or epinephrine)
Monitor blood studies for abnormal
   (decreased) glucose
Monitor blood studies for abnormal
   (decreased) parathyroid function   (indicating the anxiety is of physical
Monitor blood studies for abnormal   origin)
   gas exchange (decreased O_2 level)
Monitor blood studies for abnormal
   (increased) adrenal function
Monitor blood studies for increased
   lactic acid
Observe for evidence of a favorable response to therapy

Health Teaching
Explain that the person's emotional response is appropriate and commonly
   experienced
Explain and offer hope that the emotional pain will decrease with time
Explain that some tension is normal
Explain how to obtain release from emotional stress
Advise against fighting anxiety
Explain how to channel emotional energy into activity
Teach how to use the problem-solving method
Describe those symptoms which should be reported (severe anxiety)

EVALUATION

See the evaluation criteria for each specific goal in Chapter 2.

Inadequate Emotional Support Related to Moderate Anxiety (187,196,260, 263,295,298,344,399,492,508,530,538)

ASSESSMENT

Subjective Data
A painful emotional uneasiness and feeling of dread that is very difficult to
   endure
A sudden momentary upsurge if acute
Constant and of indefinite duration if chronic
Sense of helplessness
Unsettled, vaguely confused feeling
Feeling of weakness

Wants to escape the situation
Narrowed sensory perception
Unaware of peripheral activities
Considerable fatigue
Internal shaking or trembling
Preoccupied with the anxiety

Objective Data
Appears forlorn and upset
At the time of need, the person has a limited, nonexistent, or temporarily
  absent support system of significant others
May reach out for help through crying, attention-seeking behavior, touching
  persons or objects, seeking someone to talk with, etc.
May appear withdrawn
Voice tremors
Sweating
Increased pulse rate
Increased respiratory rate
Increased blood pressure
Overeating or anorexia
Difficulty sleeping
Selective inattention
Difficulty performing poorly developed or recently acquired skills
Easily performs long-established skills
Uses safe, habitual behavioral responses

Related Data
Commonly Related Conditions:
Caffeine and epinephrine drug intolerance
Hypoglycemia
Anoxia
Commonly Related Diseases:
None
   OR
Any disease or injury, especially:
Hypoparathyroidism
Myocardial infarction
Neurocirculatory asthenia
Thrombophlebitis
Mesenteric vascular occlusion
Alzheimer's disease
Carcinoma
Anxiety psychoneurosis

POSSIBLE ETIOLOGY

Lack of interest on the part of one's usually supportive world of family,
friends, and church. The unavailability of persons who usually offer support. The presence of *anxiety from psychologic causes:* Situational inadequa-

cy feelings; the absence of meaning in a situation that does not make sense. Disturbed interpersonal relationships. Inability to meet the expectations of significant others. Forced adaptation to change. Conflict between dependence and independence. Conflict between desires and moral standards. Poorly defined goals. Lack of fulfillment in life. Suppressed aggressive impulses. *Anxiety from physical causes:* Inadequate tissue oxygenation. Increased lactic acid blood levels binding calcium from nerve endings. Decreased blood glucose stimulates the adrenal gland to secrete epinephrine (adrenalin) for the purpose of elevating the blood sugar, and the increased epinephrine level results in anxiety. Drug side effects.

NURSING DIAGNOSIS

Inadequate emotional support related to moderate anxiety: little or no comfort or sustaining measures received from others while enduring moderate anxiety.

PLANNING

Patient Needs	**Primary Nurse-Patient Goals**
Rest, relaxation	To achieve rest, relaxation
Comfort	To achieve comfort
Protection from physical harm	To prevent physical injury
Protection from psychologic threat	To prevent emotional injury
Predictable, orderly world	To achieve a therapeutic environment
Acceptance	To achieve productive interpersonal relationships
Warm, communicating relationships	To achieve effective verbal and nonverbal communications
High evaluation of self, adequacy	To achieve positive expressions, feelings, reactions
Personal growth and maturity	To achieve optimum function
Increased learning	To achieve awareness of needs
Religious-philosophic satisfaction	To achieve spiritual goals
Increased reality perception and problem-solving ability	To achieve optimum function
Increased pleasantness	To achieve positive expressions, feelings, reactions

NURSING INTERVENTIONS

Nursing Treatments

General Interventions:
Approach unhurriedly
Demonstrate calmness

Express empathy
Express warmth and friendliness
Provide an atmosphere of acceptance
Touch the patient judiciously
Reassure verbally
Attend the patient constantly (until the acute episode subsides)
    AND
Provide frequent patient contact (thereafter) ˙
Arrange a structured environment (suitable to the patient)
Arrange orderly surroundings
Establish routines familiar to the patient
Provide quiet
Arrange situations which encourage patient autonomy

Massage gently
    OR   } (for the relaxing effect)
Bathe in warm water

Encourage adequate rest
Avoid placing the patient on enforced inactivity
Encourage the expression of feelings
Listen attentively
    AND
Talk with the patient
Offer feedback of the patient's expressed feelings
Encourage patient questions (if such will relieve the distress)
Provide reliable information
Do not allow unpleasant surprise situations
Avoid causing painful emotional situations
Provide objects which symbolize safeness
Encourage mutual problem solving
Support a realistic assessment of the situation
Introduce to persons who have successfully undergone the same experience
Encourage the use of normal coping mechanisms
Encourage the use of spiritual resources
Explore with the patient his strengths and resources
Encourage the person to face the anxiety
Reduce the demands placed upon the patient
Refrain from performing nonessential procedures
Refrain from negatively criticizing

Call the patient's family to the
    bedside   (if the patient prefers or strongly
    OR   }   needs significant others and if the
Encourage telephone calls between   significant others are available as
    significant persons   a support system)
Restrict unwanted visitors

Specific to Chronic Anxiety:
Explore with the patient the reasons for recurring problems (of anxiety)

Encourage identification of specific life values (if poorly defined values are precipitating the anxiety)
Encourage active diversional activities (to promote periods of rest from anxiety)
Present change gradually
Encourage gradual mastery of a situation
Encourage planned one-day-at-a-time living
Encourage the sharing of common problems with others
Encourage habitual peaceful thinking

Nursing Observations
Determine the degree of insight
Determine the precipitating factors
Determine the relieving factors
Evaluate the signficance of emotional distress mannerisms
Evaluate the significance of nonverbal communication
Identify disturbing conversation topics
Identify life values significant to the person
Identify appropriate use of defense mechanisms
Identify inappropriate use of defense mechanisms
Observe for evidence of a favorable response to therapy

Observe for drug reactions (to caffeine or epinephrine)
Monitor blood studies for abnormal (decreased) glucose
Monitor blood studies for abnormal (decreased) parathyroid function
Monitor blood studies for abnormal gas exchange (decreased O_2 level)
Monitor blood studies for abnormal (increased) adrenal function
Monitor blood studies for increased lactic acid

} (indicating the anxiety is of physical origin)

Health Teaching
Explain that the person's emotional response is appropriate and commonly experienced
Explain and offer hope that the emotional pain will decrease with time
Explain the importance of recognizing tension within oneself
Explain that fatigue should be recognized as a stress factor
Explain the need to recognize highly stressful situations
Explain how to obtain release from emotional stress
Advise against fighting anxiety
Explain the difference between freedom from anxiety and freedom from problems
Explain the importance of offering emotional support to one another
Explain the importance of remaining calm

Explain how to channel emotional energy into activity
Explain how to reduce muscular tension
Recommend methods for reducing sensory stimulation
Recommend methods for achieving total relaxation
Recommend a habitual, positive mental attitude
Explain the need to predict and plan for change
Teach how to use the problem-solving method

Medical Treatments Performed by Nurses
Give the prescribed drug

EVALUATION

See the evaluation criteria for each specific goal in Chapter 2.

Inadequate Emotional Support Related to Severe Anxiety (187,196,260,263, 295,298,344,399,492,508,530,538)
ASSESSMENT

Subjective Data
An intensely painful emotional uneasiness or dread that is extremely difficult to endure
A sudden momentary upsurge if acute
Constant and of indefinite duration if chronic
Sense of helplessness
Unsettled, vaguely confused feeling
Feeling of weakness
Wants to escape the situation
Greatly narrowed perception
Focuses on details
Unable to distinguish between safe and harmful stimuli
Temporarily unable to learn
Preoccupied with the anxiety

Objective Data
Appears forlorn and upset
At the time of need, the person has a limited, nonexistent, or temporarily absent support system of significant others
May reach out for help through crying, attention-seeking behavior, touching persons or objects, seeking someone to talk with, etc.
May appear withdrawn
Increased pulse rate (tachycardia)
Increased respiratory rate
Increased blood pressure
Hyperventilation
Overeating or anorexia
Difficulty sleeping

Is easily distracted
Overtalkative
  OR
Verbally very quiet
Mental blocking
Irritability
Poorly organized behavior
May develop manifestations of hysteria such as paralysis, pain

Related Data

Commonly Related Conditions:
Caffeine and epinephrine drug intolerance when such drugs are adminis-
  tered
Hypoglycemia
Anoxia

Commonly Related Diseases:
None
  OR
Any disease or injury, especially:
Hypoparathyroidism
Myocardial infarction
Neurocirculatory asthenia
Thrombophlebitis
Mesenteric vascular occlusion
Alzheimer's disease
Anxiety psychoneurosis
Hysterical neurosis

POSSIBLE ETIOLOGY

Lack of interest on the part of one's usually supportive world of family,
friends, and church. The unavailability of persons who usually offer support. The presence of *anxiety from psychologic causes:* Situational inadequacy feelings; the absence of meaning in a situation that does not make sense.
Disturbed interpersonal relationships. Inability to meet the expectations of
significant others. Forced adaptation to change. Conflict between dependence and independence. Conflict between desires and moral standards.
Poorly defined goals. Lack of fulfillment in life. Suppressed aggressive impulses. *Anxiety from physical causes:* Inadequate tissue oxygenation. Increased blood lactic acid levels binding calcium from nerve endings. Decreased blood glucose stimulates the adrenal gland to secrete epinephrine
(adrenalin) for the purpose of elevating the blood sugar, and the increased
epinephrine level results in anxiety. Drug side effects.

NURSING DIAGNOSIS

Inadequate emotional support related to severe anxiety: little or no comfort
or sustaining measures received from others while enduring severe anxiety

PLANNING

Patient Needs	Primary Nurse-Patient Goals
Rest, relaxation	To achieve rest, relaxation
Comfort	To achieve comfort
Protection from psychologic threat	To prevent emotional injury
Predictable, orderly world	To achieve a therapeutic environment
Acceptance	To achieve productive interpersonal relationships
Warm, communicating relationships	To achieve effective verbal and nonverbal communications
High evaluation of self, adequacy	To achieve positive expressions, feelings, reactions
Personal growth and maturity	To achieve optimum function
Increased learning	To achieve awareness of needs and/or use of resources
Religious-philosophic satisfaction	To achieve spiritual goals
Increased reality perception and problem-solving ability	To achieve optimum function

NURSING INTERVENTIONS

Nursing Treatments

General Interventions:
Approach unhurriedly
Demonstrate calmness
Express empathy
Express warmth and friendliness
Provide an atmosphere of acceptance
Touch the patient judiciously
Reassure verbally
Attend the patient constantly (until the acute episode subsides)
   AND
Provide frequent patient contact (thereafter)
Arrange a structured environment (suitable to the patient)
Arrange orderly surroundings
Establish routines familiar to the patient
Provide quiet
Acknowledge dependency (if it is increased by the level of anxiety)
Massage gently
   OR   } (for the relaxation effect)
Bathe in warm water
Encourage adequate rest
Avoid placing the patient on enforced inactivity

Encourage the expression of feelings
Listen attentively
  AND
Talk with the patient
Offer feedback of the patient's expressed feelings
Encourage patient questions (if such will relieve the distress)
Provide reliable information
Give important messages only when the patient is receptive
Do not allow unpleasant surprise situations
Avoid causing painful emotional situations
Provide emotionally safe experiences
Provide objects which symbolize safeness
Encourage mutual problem solving
Support a realistic assessment of the situation
Introduce to persons who have successfully undergone the same experience
Encourage the use of normal coping mechanisms
Encourage the use of spiritual resources
Explore with the patient his strengths and resources
Encourage the person to face the anxiety
Reduce the demands placed upon the patient
Refrain from performing nonessential procedures
Refrain from negatively criticizing

Call the patient's family to the
  bedside   (if the patient prefers or strongly
  OR   needs significant others and if the
Encourage telephone calls between   significant others are available as
  significant persons   a support system)

Restrict unwanted visitors

Specific to Chronic Anxiety:
Explore with the patient the reasons for recurring problems (related to the
  anxiety)
Encourage identification of specific life values (if poorly defined values are
  precipitating the anxiety)
Encourage active diversional activities (to promote periods of rest from an-
  xiety)
Encourage gradual mastery of a situation
Encourage planned one-day-at-a-time living
Encourage the sharing of common problems with others

Nursing Observations
Determine the degree of insight
Determine the precipitating factors
Determine the relieving factors
Evaluate the significance of emotional distress mannerisms
Evaluate the significance of nonverbal communication
Identify disturbing conversation topics
Identify life values significant to the person

Identify appropriate use of defense mechanisms
Identify inappropriate use of defense mechanisms
Observe for drug reactions (to
    caffeine or epinephrine)
Monitor blood studies for abnormal
    (decreased) glucose
Monitor blood studies for abnormal
    (decreased) parathyroid function   (indicating the anxiety is of physical
Monitor blood studies for abnormal   origin)
    gas exchange (decreased O₂ level)
Monitor blood studies for abnormal
    (increased) adrenal function
Monitor blood studies for increased
    lactic acid
Observe for evidence of a favorable response to therapy

Health Teaching
Explain that the person's emotional response is appropriate (if it is) and
    commonly experienced
Explain and offer hope that the emotional pain will decrease with time
Explain the importance of recognizing tension within oneself
Explain that fatigue should be recognized as a stress factor
Explain the need to recognize highly stressful situations
Explain how to obtain release from emotional stress
Advise against fighting anxiety
Explain the difference between freedom from anxiety and freedom from
    problems
Explain the importance of offering emotional support to one another
Explain how to channel emotional energy into activity
Explain how to reduce muscular tension
Recommend methods for reducing sensory stimulation
Recommend methods for achieving total relaxation
Recommend a habitual, positive mental attitude
Teach how to use problem-solving method

Medical Treatments Performed by Nurses
Give the prescribed drug

EVALUATION

See the evaluation criteria for each specific goal in Chapter 2.

Maladaptive Coping Related to Anxiety
(260,263,295,298,344,399,492,530,538)

ASSESSMENT

Subjective Data
Experiences the feeling that something terrible is about to happen
Is unable to attribute the anxiety to a specific situation but associates it
    with multiple situations

Experiences anxiety when in a crowd
Feels intensely threatened if he loses control of the situation
Preoccupation with fantasized sickness
Unexplainable nervousness
Indulges in hallucinations and delusions

Objective Data
Blames the anxiety-producing situation on persons, objects, or events
Uses demanding behavior to regain control
Is awakened by nightmares
Refuses to discuss anxiety-provoking subjects
Displays prolonged, severely regressive behavior

Related Data
Commonly Related Diseases:
Anxiety psychoneurosis
Hysterical neurosis

POSSIBLE ETIOLOGY

Chronic use of inappropriate defense mechanisms such as repression, prolonged denial, projection, regression. The inability to channel anxiety into activity.

NURSING DIAGNOSIS

Maladaptive coping related to anxiety: attempts to reduce the painfulness of anxiety through unhealthy methods

PLANNING

Patient Needs	**Primary Nurse-Patient Goals**
Comfort	To achieve comfort
Protection from psychologic threat	To prevent emotional injury
Warm, communicating relationships	To achieve effective verbal and nonverbal communications
Personal growth and maturity	To achieve optimum function
Increased learning	To achieve awareness of needs
Increased reality perception and problem-solving ability	To achieve optimum function

NURSING INTERVENTIONS

Nursing Treatments
Approach unhurriedly
Provide an atmosphere of acceptance
Express warmth and friendliness
Provide frequent patient contact
Ask questions which encourage answers that reflect reality perception
Encourage the expression of feelings
Listen attentively
    AND
Talk with the patient

Offer feedback of the patient's expressed feelings
Encourage planned one-day-at-a-time living
Encourage identification of specific life values
Encourage the practical application of the accepted value system
Encourage mutual problem solving
Encourage patient questions
Encourage the sharing of common problems with others
Support a realistic assessment of the situation
Encourage the reduction of generalizations to specifics
Encourage the use of normal coping mechanisms
Explore superficial topics and reasons for avoiding in-depth feelings
Explore with the patient his strengths and resources
Encourage the person to face the anxiety
Explore with the patient reasons for criticism of others
Explore with the patient reasons for recurring problems (related to the anx-
    iety)
Explore with the patient the effects of his behavior on others
Explore with the patient the need for attention
Explore with the patient the need for dominance
Give important messages only when the patient is receptive
Introduce to persons who have successfully undergone the same experience
Provide emotionally safe experiences
Reduce the demands placed upon the patient
Refrain from performing nonessential procedures
Refrain from negatively criticizing
Set limits on unacceptable behavior
Touch the patient judiciously
Make a referral (to a psychiatric nurse specialist)

Nursing Observations
Determine the degree of insight
Estimate the degree of stress experienced
Evaluate the person's relatedness with others
Evaluate the significance of emotional distress mannerisms
Evaluate the significance of nonverbal communication
Identify abnormal perceptions
Identify abnormal thought content
Identify attention span abnormalities
Observe for impaired judgment
Identify disturbing conversation topics
Identify emotion-stimulating events
Identify inappropriate emotional responses
Identify life values significant to the person
Identify inappropriate use of defense mechanisms
Observe for an excessive stress level
Observe for evidence that the patient is reaching out for emotional support
Observe for evidence of a favorable response to therapy

Health Teaching
Advise against fighting anxiety

Describe those factors which intensify anxiety
Emphasize the importance of recognizing tension within oneself
Explain the need to recognize highly stressful situations
Explain how to obtain release from emotional stress
Explain that anxiety often disguises itself
Explain the difference between freedom from anxiety and freedom from
    problems
Explain how to channel emotional energy into activity
Explain how to reduce muscular tension
Recommend methods for achieving total relaxation
Teach how to use the problem-solving method
Describe the behavior pattern indicating emotional maturity

EVALUATION

See the evaluation criteria for each specific goal in Chapter 2.

ANXIETY, POTENTIAL

Potential Anxiety Related to Illness
(196,260,263,295,298,344,399,530,538)

ASSESSMENT

Subjective Data
Awareness of a potential threat of dependence, sickness, suffering, pain,
    death, or loss of integrity

Objective Data
Person is thrust into an unknown health care situation
Is awaiting or undergoing diagnostic examinations, surgery, anesthesia,
    pain, therapeutic procedures, or confirmation of a diagnosis
Is separated from significant others because of health care
Is being questioned about his health status in a manner which infringes on
    his privacy
Family and/or health personnel have communicated disbelief in the
    patient's symptoms
Is exposed to the illness or death of a loved one
Person has been prevented from practicing superstitious rituals regarding
    health
Person is physically restrained for health purposes

Related Data
Commonly Related Conditions:
Caffeine and epinephrine drug intolerance
Hypoglycemia
Anoxia
Premenstrual cerebral edema

Commonly Related Diseases:
None
> OR

Any disease or injury, especially:
Hypoparathyroidism
Myocardial infarction
Chorea
Glomerulonephritis
Thrombophlebitis
Mesenteric vascular occlusion
Acute intestinal obstruction

POSSIBLE ETIOLOGY

Anticipation of physical harm and/or psychologic threat. Forced adaptation to change because of the health status. Inability to use one's usual methods for coping with anxiety because of impaired health. Feelings of inadequacy.

NURSING DIAGNOSIS

Potential anxiety related to illness: the probability that anxiety will be aroused as a result of existing or suspected illness or association with ill persons

PLANNING

Patient Needs

Comfort

Protection from psychologic threat

Warm, communicating
  relationships

Increased learning

Increased reality perception and
  problem-solving ability

Primary Nurse-Patient Goals

To achieve comfort

To prevent emotional injury

To achieve effective verbal and
  nonverbal communications

To achieve awareness of needs

To achieve optimum function

NURSING INTERVENTIONS

Nursing Treatments
Approach unhurriedly
Reassure verbally
Demonstrate calmness
Express warmth and friendliness
Provide an atmosphere of acceptance
Attend the patient constantly (during potential anxiety-producing proce-
  dures, etc.)
> AND

Provide frequent patient contact (at other times)
Arrange situations which encourage patient autonomy
Avoid causing embarrassing situations
Avoid causing intense emotional situations

Do not allow unpleasant surprise situations
Establish routines familiar to the patient
Encourage the expression of feelings
Listen attentively
    AND
Talk with the patient
Encourage patient questions
Encourage gradual mastery of a situation
Encourage mutual problem solving
Encourage the use of normal coping mechanisms
Ensure the patient's feeling of safety before introducing unpleasantness
Introduce one anxiety situation at a time
Introduce to persons who have successfully undergone the same experience
Present change gradually
Provide objects which symbolize safeness
Provide reliable information
Recognize the need for the use of appropriate defense mechanisms
Recognize the need for superstition
Reduce the demands placed upon the patient
Refrain from performing nonessential procedures
Use a chest restraint (to allow freedom of movement which reduces anxiety)
Tour the patient through the health care facility
Touch the patient judiciously
Involve the family (as much as possible)

Nursing Observations
Evaluate the significance of emotional distress mannerisms
Evaluate the significance of nonverbal communication
Identify disturbing conversation topics
Observe for evidence that the patient is reaching out for emotional support
Observe for an excessive stress level

Health Teaching
Explain the importance of offering emotional support to one another (to
    prevent anxiety)
Explain the reason for and intended effect of the therapy

EVALUATION

See the evaluation criteria for each specific goal in Chapter 2.

CONFLICT

Conflict Related to a High-Risk Health Procedure (12,94,372)

ASSESSMENT

Subjective Data
Person is preoccupied with thoughts about potential high-risk surgery, drug
    therapy, diagnostic procedures, etc.

Perceives the choice as both acceptable and unacceptable
Desires the health effect of the procedure while fearing its unfavorable consequences

Objective Data
Appears frequently contemplative
Fails to take any decisive action
May initiate conversation regarding the procedure
May seek the advice of others

Related Data
Commonly Related Conditions:
Open-heart surgery
Kidney transplant surgery
Cancer chemotherapy
Brain surgery
Commonly Related Diseases:
Coronary artery disease
Renal failure
Cancer of the internal organs or tissue
    OR
Any potentially terminal illness

POSSIBLE ETIOLOGY

Fear that the procedure will be fatal. Concern that if the procedure is ineffective, present responsibilities could not be carried out because of its unfavorable consequences on the health.

NURSING DIAGNOSIS

Conflict related to a high-risk health procedure: an internal struggle in which the person cannot decide if he should take the risk of a dangerous but medically recommended therapeutic or diagnostic procedure

PLANNING

Patient Needs	**Primary Nurse-Patient Goals**
Comfort	To achieve comfort
Protection from psychologic threat	To prevent emotional injury
Warm, communicating relationships	To achieve effective verbal and nonverbal communications
Adequacy	To achieve positive expressions, feelings, reactions
Personal growth and maturity	To achieve optimum function
Increased learning	To achieve awareness of needs
Increased reality perception and problem-solving ability	To achieve optimum function

NURSING INTERVENTIONS

Nursing Treatments

Approach unhurriedly

Demonstrate calmness

Provide an atmosphere of acceptance

Ask questions which encourage answers that reflect reality perception

Assist the patient in defining consistent life standards

Encourage the expression of feelings

Listen attentively

    AND

Talk with the patient

Offer feedback of the patient's expressed feelings

Reveal the patient's ambivalent feelings

Encourage patient questions

Provide reliable information

Maintain honesty

Encourage decision-making

Encourage the sharing of common problems with others

Introduce to persons who have successfully undergone the same experience

Explore with the patient his strengths and resources

Support a realistic assessment of the situation

Involve the family (as much as possible)

Nursing Observations

Determine the degree of insight

Evaluate the significance of emotional distress mannerisms

Evaluate the significance of nonverbal communication

Identify life values significant to the person

Identify appropriate use of defense mechanisms

Identify inappropriate use of defense mechanisms

Observe for an excessive stress level

Observe for evidence that the patient is reaching out for emotional support

Observe for evidence of a favorable response to therapy

Health Teaching

Explain that some tension is normal

Teach how to use the problem-solving method

Explain the reason for and intended effect of the therapy

EVALUATION

See the evaluation criteria for each specific goal in Chapter 2.

Conflict Related to the Health Care of a Significant Other (12,94,372)

ASSESSMENT

Subjective Data

Person is preoccupied with thoughts about:

    whether certain treatments should be performed on a loved one

whether the loved one should be cared for at home or in a nursing home
whether the person should be committed to a mental institution or drug
or alcohol center
Person perceives the choice as both acceptable and unacceptable

Objective Data
Appears frequently contemplative
Fails to take any decisive action
May initiate conversation regarding the problem
May seek the advice of others

Related Data
Commonly Related Conditions:
Confusion
Aging
Commonly Related Diseases:
Cerebral vascular accident
Parkinson's disease
Multiple sclerosis
Spinal cord injury
Schizophrenia
Arteriosclerosis
Alcoholism
Drug addiction

POSSIBLE ETIOLOGY

Fear of making the wrong choice. Concern that the significant other would
not approve of the choice if it were his to make.

NURSING DIAGNOSIS

Conflict related to the health care of a significant other: an internal struggle
in which the person cannot decide what health care he should approve or
instigate for a loved one

PLANNING

Patient Needs	Primary Nurse-Patient Goals
Comfort	To achieve comfort
Protection from psychologic threat	To prevent emotional injury
Acceptance	To achieve productive interpersonal relationships
Warm, communicating relationships	To achieve effective verbal and nonverbal communications
Adequacy	To achieve positive expressions, feelings, reactions
Personal growth and maturity	To achieve optimum function

Increased learning

To achieve awareness of needs and/or use of resources

Increased reality perception and problem-solving ability

To achieve optimum function

NURSING INTERVENTIONS

Nursing Treatments
Approach unhurriedly
Demonstrate calmness
Provide an atmosphere of acceptance
Ask questions which encourage answers that reflect reality perception
Assist the patient in defining consistent life standards
Encourage the expression of feelings
Listen attentively
   AND
Talk with the patient (the family member experiencing conflict)
Offer feedback of the patient's expressed feelings
Reveal the patient's ambivalent feelings
Encourage patient questions
Provide reliable information
Maintain honesty
Encourage decision-making
Encourage the sharing of common problems with others
Introduce to persons who have successfully undergone the same experience
Explore with the patient his strengths and resources
Support a realistic assessment of the situation
Involve the family (as much as possible)

Nursing Observations
Determine the degree of insight
Evaluate the significance of emotional distress mannerisms
Evaluate the significance of nonverbal communication
Identify life values significant to the person
Identify appropriate use of defense mechanisms
Identify inappropriate use of defense mechanisms
Observe for an excessive stress level
Observe for evidence that the patient is reaching out for emotional support
Observe for evidence of a favorable response to therapy

Health Teaching
Explain that some tension is normal
Teach how to use the problem-solving method
Explain the reason for and intended effect of the therapy (intended for the loved one)

EVALUATION
See the evaluation criteria for each specific goal in Chapter 2.

Reluctance to Donate Blood

ASSESSMENT

Subjective Data

Person would like to donate a pint of his blood

Feels uncertain as to whether or not he should

Felt enthusiastic to give the blood during the acute emergency, with decreased motivation as the emergency subsides

Feels insecure as to what the giving of blood will do to his own health

Perceives the loss of a pint of blood as loss of part of himself

Finds it difficult to perceive the giving of blood as an extension of the self

Perceives the choice of giving blood as both acceptable and unacceptable

Objective Data

Person has a loved one or friend who received a blood transfusion

Person has been asked to donate a pint of blood

Friends or relatives may be heard both encouraging or discouraging the prospective donor from giving the blood

Related Data

Commonly Related Conditions:
Hemorrhage

Commonly Related Diseases:
Hemophilia
Aplastic anemia

POSSIBLE ETIOLOGY

A desire to fulfill one's humane ideals opposed by one's desire to feel safe. Lack of information. Fear of an unknown situation. Negative persuasion from external forces. Feelings of inadequacy.

NURSING DIAGNOSIS

Reluctance to donate blood: a hesitancy in which the person cannot decide whether or not to give blood as a replacement for blood transfused to a loved one or friend

PLANNING

Patient Needs	Primary Nurse-Patient Goals
Comfort	To achieve comfort
Protection from psychologic threat	To prevent emotional injury
Acceptance	To achieve productive interpersonal relationships
Warm, communicating relationships	To achieve effective verbal and nonverbal communications
Adequacy	To achieve positive expressions, feelings, reactions
Increased learning	To achieve awareness of needs

NURSING INTERVENTIONS

Nursing Treatments
Approach unhurriedly
Provide an atmosphere of acceptance
Reassure verbally
Encourage the expression of feelings
  AND
Listen attentively
Discuss the anticipated procedure (include the information that most adults
    have ten pints of blood in their body, that only one pint is donated, that
    it is done by needle puncture, that the body will replace the lost blood
    within several weeks, and that little or no discomfort will be experi-
    enced)
Explore with the patient (donor) how he would feel in situations experi-
    enced by others (if he needed blood and could not get it)
Introduce to persons (donors) who have successfully undergone the same
    experience
Make a referral (to the blood bank)

Nursing Observations
Determine the degree of insight
Observe for an excessive stress level
Observe for evidence that the person is reaching out for emotional support
Observe for evidence of a favorable response to therapy

Health Teaching
Explain that the person's emotional response is appropriate and commonly
    experienced by others
Explain that some tension is normal
Explain the importance of blood replacement after transfusion

EVALUATION

See the evaluation criteria for each specific goal in Chapter 2.

DEPENDENCE-INDEPENDENCE

Difficult Adaptation to Health Care Termination

ASSESSMENT

Subjective Data
Feels anxious or uneasy about no longer having supervised health care
May doubt his ability to maintain his health upon termination of care
Often perceives it as a permanent break with the health care worker
Feels that his invested trust and favorable relationship are lost
May experience anger
Sense of aloneness and threat

Objective Data

Verbalizes that he wishes the physician or nurse would continue to see him

May openly reject the idea of new health personnel taking the place of others

Frequently telephones about minor health problems

May ask permission at the time of termination to visit at a later date if he should later desire to

Related Data

Commonly Related Conditions:
Separation anxiety

Commonly Related Diseases:
Any disease or injury

POSSIBLE ETIOLOGY

Loss of dependence on a reliable person. Feelings of inadequacy to meet one's own health needs. A normal part of the grief process.

NURSING DIAGNOSIS

Difficult adaptation to health care termination: a period of difficult emotional adjustment in which the person attempts to adapt to the conclusion of a therapeutic relationship that has been perceived as highly favorable

PLANNING

Patient Needs	**Primary Nurse-Patient Goals**
Comfort	To achieve comfort
Protection from psychologic threat	To prevent emotional injury
Acceptance	To achieve productive interpersonal relationships
Warm, communicating relationships	To achieve effective verbal and nonverbal communications
Adequacy	To achieve positive expressions, feelings, reactions
Independence	To achieve optimum function
Increased learning	To achieve awareness of varying needs
Increased reality perception and problem-solving ability	To achieve optimum function

NURSING INTERVENTIONS

Nursing Treatments

Approach unhurriedly

Provide an atmosphere of acceptance

Reassure verbally

Encourage the expression of feelings

Listen attentively
   AND
Talk with the patient

Offer feedback of the patient's expressed feelings
Encourage patient questions
Encourage decision-making
Encourage the use of normal coping mechanisms
Explore with the patient his strengths and resources
Provide prior notification of an impending separation
Offer assurance that return visits are acceptable despite termination of the
    therapeutic relationship
Introduce the patient to replacement personnel before an impending sep-
    aration
Recognize the need for unique personal adjustments to change
Refrain from negatively criticizing
Support a realistic assessment of the situation
Involve the family (as a support system)

Nursing Observations
Determine the degree of insight
Evaluate the significance of emotional distress mannerisms
Evaluate the significance of nonverbal communication
Identify disturbing conversation topics
Identify appropriate use of defense mechanisms
Identify inappropriate use of defense mechanisms
Identify the current dominant emotion
Observe for an excessive stress level
Observe for evidence that the patient is reaching out for emotional support
Observe for evidence of a favorable response to therapy

Health Teaching
Explain that the person's emotional response is appropriate and commonly
    experienced
Explain the importance of maintaining a positive self-attitude (regarding
    one's ability to maintain his health)

EVALUATION

See the evaluation criteria for each specific goal in Chapter 2.

Difficult Adaptation to Illness
Dependency (511)

ASSESSMENT

Subjective Data
Anxiety, sometimes severe at the onset of dependence
Lessened self-esteem
Temporarily denies the illness causing the dependence

Objective Data
Attempts to maintain normal functioning ability even though the ability is
    lessened
At first, refuses help from others, but gradually accepts more and more help

Related Data

Commonly Related Diseases:
Any disease or injury

POSSIBLE ETIOLOGY

Man's adaptive mechanisms require time and insight to allow him to make transitions and still feel safe and comfortable

NURSING DIAGNOSIS

Difficult adaptation to illness dependency: a period of difficult emotional adjustment in which the person attempts to adapt to the realization of illness and the increased need to depend on others

PLANNING

Patient Needs	Primary Nurse-Patient Goals
Comfort	To achieve comfort
Protection from psychologic threat	To prevent emotional injury
Dependence	To achieve comfort
Acceptance	To achieve productive interpersonal relationships
Warm, communicating relationships	To achieve effective verbal and nonverbal communications
High evaluation of self	To achieve positive expressions, feelings, reactions
Independence	To achieve optimum function
Dignity	To achieve productive interpersonal relationships
Increased learning	To achieve awareness of needs
Increased reality perception and problem-solving ability	To achieve optimum function despite limitations

NURSING INTERVENTIONS

Nursing Treatments
Approach unhurriedly
Provide an atmosphere of acceptance
Acknowledge dependency
Arrange situations which encourage patient autonomy
Encourage the expression of feelings
Listen attentively
    AND
Talk with the patient
Offer feedback of the patient's expressed feelings
Encourage patient in illness adjustment
Explore with the patient his strengths and resources
Recognize the need for the use of appropriate defense mechanisms
Recognize the need for unique personal adjustments to change

Support a realistic assessment of the situation
Refrain from performing nonessential procedures
Refrain from negatively criticizing
Respond immediately to the patient's call

Nursing Observations
Determine the degree of insight
Evaluate the person's relatedness with others (in regard to dependence-independence)
Evaluate the significance of emotional distress mannerisms
Evaluate the significance of nonverbal communication
Identify disturbing conversation topics
Identify life values significant to the person
Identify appropriate use of defense mechanisms
Identify inappropriate use of defense mechanisms
Observe for an excessive stress level
Observe for impaired self-attitudes
Observe for evidence that the patient is reaching out for emotional support
Observe for evidence of a favorable response to therapy

Health Teaching
Explain that the person's emotional response (adjustment difficulty) is normal and commonly experienced by others
Explain that ill persons are often hypersensitive (about their dependence)
Explain that some tension is normal
Recommend a habitual, positive mental attitude

EVALUATION

See the evaluation criteria for each specific goal in Chapter 2.

Difficult Adaptation to Independence During Health Renewal (511)

ASSESSMENT

Subjective Data
As body health is gradually restored, the person becomes aware that he must begin to assume normal activities and responsibilities
When health is partially restored but not fully recovered, the person feels reluctant to give up his ego-centered concern for himself and the attention derived from others

Objective Data
Person is convalescing
Is gradually becoming more and more active
May attempt independent activity without success at first, but later with success

Related Data
Commonly Related Diseases:
Any disease or injury

POSSIBLE ETIOLOGY

Man's adaptive mechanisms require time and insight to allow him to make transitions and still feel safe and comfortable. Healing frequently requires considerable time.

NURSING DIAGNOSIS

Difficult adaptation to independence during health renewal: a period of difficult emotional adjustment during which the person attempts to adapt from the dependent state of illness to the independence of health

PLANNING

Patient Needs	Primary Nurse-Patient Goals
Comfort	To achieve comfort
Protection from psychologic threat	To prevent emotional injury
Dependence	To achieve comfort
Warm, commmunicating relationships	To achieve effective verbal and nonverbal communications
High evaluation of self	To achieve positive expressions, feelings, reactions
Independence	To achieve optimum function
Increased learning	To achieve awareness of needs and/or use of resources
Increased reality perception and problem-solving ability	To achieve optimum function

NURSING INTERVENTIONS

Nursing Treatments
Approach unhurriedly
Provide an atmosphere of acceptance
Arrange situations which encourage patient autonomy
Encourage acceptance of responsibility (a little at a time)
Encourage self-performance
Encourage the expression of feelings
Listen attentively
Talk with the patient
Encourage patience in illness adjustment
Explore with the patient his strengths and resources
Recognize the need for the use of appropriate defense mechanisms
Recognize the need for unique personal adjustments to change
Refrain from negatively criticizing

Nursing Observations
Determine the degree of insight
Evaluate the person's relatedness to others (in regard to dependence-independence)
Evaluate the significance of emotional distress mannerisms
Evaluate the significance of nonverbal communication

Identify disturbing conversation topics
Identify life values significant to the person (attitudes toward independence)
Identify appropriate use of defense mechanisms
Identify inappropriate use of defense mechanisms
Observe for an excessive stress level
Observe for fatigue (if independence is attempted too early)
Observe for evidence that the patient is reaching out for emotional support
Observe for evidence of a favorable response to therapy

Health Teaching
Recommend that independence be encouraged (at a comfortable level for
    the patient)
Recommend a habitual, positive mental attitude

EVALUATION

See the evaluation criteria for each specific goal in Chapter 2.

Difficult Withdrawal From Dependence on Life-Support Systems (391)

ASSESSMENT

Subjective Data
Intense awareness that one's existence has been maintained by a life-
    supporting device
Intense anxiety if the device is not readily available

Objective Data
Frequently calls for the therapeutic device even though it is not needed
Verbally resists removal of the device
Asks to have the device within sight

Related Data
Common among people with pacemakers, on prolonged oxygen or intermit-
    tent positive pressure therapy, or on respirators

Commonly Related Conditions:
Separation anxiety

Commonly Related Diseases:
Myasthenia gravis
Guillain Barre disease
Cervical spinal cord injury
Myocardial infarction
Poliomyelitis
Cerebral vascular accident

POSSIBLE ETIOLOGY

An earlier need for life-support systems that resulted in dependency feelings

NURSING DIAGNOSIS

Difficult withdrawal from dependence on life-support systems: a period of
difficult emotional adjustment during which the person relinquishes his re-

liance on life-support systems and reestablishes confidence in his body's ability to maintain life unaided

PLANNING

Patient Needs	Primary Nurse-Patient Goals
Comfort	To achieve comfort
Protection from psychologic threat	To prevent emotional injury
Adequacy	To achieve positive expressions, feelings, reactions
Independence	To achieve optimum function
Increased learning	To achieve awareness of needs

NURSING INTERVENTIONS

Nursing Treatments
Approach unhurriedly
Reassure verbally (that the person is safe without the life-support system)
Demonstrate calmness
Provide an atmosphere of acceptance
Attend the patient constantly (at the initial withdrawal)
    AND
Provide frequent patient contact (thereafter)
    AND
Respond immediately to the patient's call (especially during withdrawal periods)
Increase the weaning time off therapeutic devices gradually
Place equipment within sight (until the person feels more secure)
Encourage the expression of feelings
Listen attentively
    AND
Talk with the patient
Encourage gradual mastery of the situation
Encourage the use of normal coping mechanisms
Provide radio and television for diversion (during withdrawal periods)
Recognize the need for unique personal adjustments to change
Support a realistic assessment of the situation

Nursing Observations
Determine the degree of insight
Evaluate the significance of emotional distress mannerisms
Evaluate the significance of nonverbal communication
Identify disturbing conversation topics
Observe for an excessive stress level
Observe for evidence that the patient is reaching out for emotional support
Observe for evidence of a favorable response to therapy

Health Teaching
Describe those symptoms which should be reported (during the withdrawal)

Explain that the person's emotional response is appropriate and commonly
    experienced
Explain the importance of remaining calm
Recommend a habitual, positive mental attidude

EVALUATION

See the evaluation criteria for each specific goal in Chapter 2.

Distress Related to Potential
Unavailable Maintenance Drugs

ASSESSMENT

Subjective Data
Vividly perceives that his life is dependent on maintenance drugs
Quick to imagine what could happen if the drug were unavailable
Intense dependency feelings

Objective Data
Frequently checks to be sure he has his drugs
Displays anxiety if a scheduled dose is missed or late
Verbalizes anxiety if there is any problem with drug refills

Related Data
The person is taking drugs such as Prostigmin for myasthenia gravis, cor-
    tisone for Addison's disease, insulin for diabetes

Commonly Related Diseases:
Diabetes mellitus
Addison's disease
Myasthenia gravis
Asthma
Emphysema

POSSIBLE ETIOLOGY

The reality of the physical harm or death that could result if the therapeutic
drugs were not taken

NURSING DIAGNOSIS

Distress related to potential unavailable maintenance drugs: feelings of intense reliance on certain drugs essential to the support of life accompanied
by the worry that the drug might for some reason become unavailable

PLANNING

Patient Needs	Primary Nurse-Patient Goals
Comfort	To achieve comfort
Protection from psychologic threat	To prevent emotional injury
Dependence	To achieve comfort
Increased learning	To achieve awareness of needs and/or use of resources

Increased reality perception and   To achieve optimum function
    problem-solving ability

NURSING INTERVENTIONS

Nursing Treatments
Approach unhurriedly
Reassure verbally (that the drug is available)
Demonstrate calmness
Provide an atmosphere of acceptance
Encourage the expression of feelings
Listen attentively
    AND
Talk with the patient
Encourage early replacement of dwindling therapeutic supplies

Nursing Observations
Determine the degree of insight
Evaluate the significance of emotional distress mannerisms
Evaluate the significance of nonverbal communication
Identify disturbing conversation topics (about the drug)
Observe for evidence that the patient is reaching out for emotional support
Observe for an excessive stress level

Health Teaching
Explain that the person's emotional response is appropriate and commonly
    experienced
Explain how to obtain therapeutic supplies
Recommend that extra therapeutic supplies be carried (especially on trips,
    etc.)

Medical Treatments Performed by Nurses
Give the prescribed drugs (on time)

EVALUATION

See the evaluation criteria for each specific goal in Chapter 2.

Distress Related to Environmental Dependence (12,372)

ASSESSMENT

Subjective Data
Intense desire to return home or to familiar surroundings
Longingness
Melancholy
Grieving

Objective Data
Weeping
Verbal expression of wanting to go home

Related Data

Commonly Related Diseases:
Any disease or injury

POSSIBLE ETIOLOGY

Absence from the security of one's home. Dependence on the persons and environment within the home. A normal part of the grief process.

NURSING DIAGNOSIS

Distress related to environmental dependence: an intense desire to return to an environment perceived as familiar and safe.

PLANNING

Patient Needs	Primary Nurse-Patient Goals
Comfort	To achieve comfort
Protection from psychologic threat	To prevent emotional injury
Dependence	To achieve comfort
Predictable, orderly world	To achieve a therapeutic environment
Acceptance	To achieve productive interpersonal relationships
Warm, communicating relationships	To achieve effective verbal and nonverbal communications
Increased learning	To achieve awareness of needs

NURSING INTERVENTIONS

Nursing Treatments
Approach unhurriedly
Reassure verbally
Demonstrate calmness
Provide an atmosphere of acceptance
Arrange pleasant surroundings
Establish routines familiar to the patient
Encourage the expression of feelings
Listen attentively
    AND
Talk with the patient
Grant special requests
Provide objects which symbolize safeness (and are significant with the person's home)
Encourage visiting by significant others
Support a realistic assessment of the situation

Nursing Observations
Determine the extent of emotional flexibility
Determine the degree of insight
Evaluate the significance of emotional distress mannerisms

Evaluate the significance of nonverbal communication
Identify disturbing conversation topics
Observe for an excessive stress level
Observe for evidence that the patient is reaching out for emotional support
Observe for evidence of a favorable response to therapy

Health Teaching
Explain that the person's emotional response is appropriate and commonly experienced
Explain the reason for and intended effect of the therapy (which is detaining the person from going home)

EVALUATION

See the evaluation criteria for each specific goal in Chapter 2.

Excessive Compliance Related to Illness Dependency

ASSESSMENT

Subjective Data
Worries about displeasing others
Anxiety
Withholds information that may result in conflict

Objective Data
Seldom, if ever, complains
Agreeable at all times
Avoids unpleasantness
Gives gifts out of proportion to the relationship
Often labeled the "good patient"
Does not question that which affects him, but blindly accepts everything

Related Data
Commonly Related Diseases:
Any disease or injury

POSSIBLE ETIOLOGY

Inadequacy feelings. Poor self-esteem. Dependence needs. Poorly defined self-image. Emotional aging. Overprotection. Poorly developed abilities. A flight response to avoid conflict.

NURSING DIAGNOSIS

Excessive compliance related to illness dependency: a submissive, enduring attitude in which there is no resistance to direction from others regarding one's health care

PLANNING

Patient Needs	**Primary Nurse-Patient Goals**
Protection from psychologic threat	To prevent emotional injury

Warm, communicating relationships	To achieve effective verbal and nonverbal communications
High evaluation of self, adequacy, self-reliance	To achieve positive expressions, feelings, reactions
Personal growth and maturity	To achieve optimum function
Increased learning	To achieve awareness of needs
Increased reality perception and problem-solving ability	To achieve optimum function

NURSING INTERVENTIONS

Nursing Treatments
Approach unhurriedly
Express warmth and friendliness
Arrange situations which encourage patient autonomy
Encourage the expression of feelings
Listen attentively
    AND
Talk with the patient
Encourage patient questions
Encourage mutual problem solving
Encourage decision-making (about health care)
Support a realistic assessment of the situation
Provide frequent patient contact (to assure that his needs are met)
Arrange a predischarge planning conference (with patient participation)

Nursing Observations
Determine the degree of insight
Evaluate the significance of emotional distress mannerisms
Evaluate the significance of nonverbal communication
Identify disturbing conversation topics
Observe for an excessive stress level
Observe for evidence that the patient is reaching out for emotional support
Observe for behavior modification

Health Teaching
Describe those symptoms which should be reported
Explain the importance of maintaining a positive self-attitude

EVALUATION

See the evaluation criteria for each specific goal in Chapter 2.

Inability to Admit Dependency Habituation (198,251,266,385,330)

ASSESSMENT

Subjective Data
Anxiety over the possibility of being dependent, followed by quick dismissal of such thoughts
Anger at others who suggest that dependence exists

Objective Data

Insists that drinking, smoking or drug abuse can be stopped whenever the abuser desires to do so

States that he simply does not want to stop

Terminates the habit for a short period in order to establish self-assurance of nondependence, then returns to the habit because of the dependence

If the habituation is alcohol, there is failure to recognize that the gradual increase in the amount and frequency of alcohol use, the poor dietary intake, slackened personal appearance, and nonattendance to responsibilities are related to the alcohol dependence

If the habituation is smoking, there is failure to recognize that the breathlessness, chronic productive cough, elevated blood pressure, lessened sense of taste and smell, poor appetite, and tachycardia are related to the smoking dependence

If the habituation is narcotic or barbiturate drug abuse, there is failure to recognize that gradual increase in drug dosage, guarding of personal possessions, inability to complete goals, wearing of long-sleeved clothing and sunglasses, and painful body sensations if drug dosage is decreased are related to drug dependence

Related Data

Commonly Related Conditions:
Drug habituation
Smoking habituation

Commonly Related Diseases:
Alcoholism

POSSIBLE ETIOLOGY

A dependence need that is sufficiently strong to outweigh logic and reason. Feelings of shame or guilt if the need is admitted. Feelings of inadequacy to overcome the need.

NURSING DIAGNOSIS

Inability to admit dependency habituation: an inability to recognize in oneself a habitual need for the intake of chemical products as a source of pleasure and strength

PLANNING

Patient Needs	**Primary Nurse-Patient Goals**
Protection from psychologic threat	To prevent emotional injury
Acceptance	To achieve productive interpersonal relationships
Warm, communicating relationships	To achieve effective verbal and nonverbal communications
Adequacy	To achieve positive expressions, feelings, reactions
Personal growth and maturity	To achieve optimum function
Increased learning	To achieve awareness of needs

Increased reality perception and problem-solving ability

To achieve optimum function

NURSING INTERVENTIONS

Nursing Treatments
Acknowledge dependency
Approach unhurriedly
Provide an atmosphere of acceptance
Encourage acceptance of self-limitations
Encourage the expression of feelings
Listen attentively
  AND
Talk with the patient
Offer feedback of the patient's expressed feelings
Ask questions which encourage answers that reflect reality perception
Encourage the reduction of generalizations to specifics
Explore superficial topics and reasons for avoiding in-depth feelings
Explore with the patient his strengths and resources
Explore with the patient reasons for recurring problems (related to the habituation)
Explore with the patient the effects of his behavior on others
Encourage gradual mastery of a situation
Encourage mutual problem solving
Encourage participation in therapeutic group interaction
Encourage the substitution of undesirable habits with favorable habits
Encourage the use of normal coping mechanisms
Introduce to persons who have successfully undergone the same experience (of admitting dependency habituation)
Recognize the need for the use of appropriate defense mechanisms
Recognize the need for unique personal adjustments to change
Refrain from negatively criticizing
Suggest more appropriate means of need gratification
Support a realistic assessment of the situation

Nursing Observations
Determine the degree of insight
Determine the extent of group pressure conformity (on dependency habituation)
Evaluate the significance of emotional distress mannerisms
Evaluate the significance of nonverbal communication
Identify disturbing conversation topics
Identify life values significant to the person
Identify appropriate use of defense mechanisms
Identify inappropriate use of defense mechanisms
Observe for an excessive stress level
Observe for evidence that the patient is reaching out for emotional support
Observe for behavior modification

Health Teaching
Advise early correction of problems

Explain the importance of maintaining a positive self-attitude
Explain that ill persons are often hypersensitive (about the habituation)
Explain the causes of the health problem
Explain that the person's emotional response is appropriate and commonly
  experienced

EVALUATION

See the evaluation criteria for each specific goal in Chapter 2.

Inadequate Autonomy Related to Health Care (118,199)

ASSESSMENT

Subjective Data
Feels highly threatened by lack of control of the health care situation
Desires to be and is capable of being independent

Objective Data
Overprotective behavior displayed by significant others
Little opportunity for making his own decisions
Displays irritable and demanding behavior as a means of gaining control of
  the situation

Related Data
Commonly Related Diseases:
Any disease or injury

POSSIBLE ETIOLOGY

Previous painful dependence experiences. Fear and anxiousness that loss of
control will allow others to impose harm on him. Readiness to be more
independent as health is being regained.

NURSING DIAGNOSIS

Inadequate autonomy related to health care: a feeling that one does not
have adequate independence and control of his health care situation

PLANNING

Patient Needs	Primary Nurse-Patient Goals
Comfort	To achieve comfort
Protection from psychologic threat	To prevent emotional injury
Acceptance	To achieve productive interpersonal relationships
Warm, communicating relationships	To achieve effective verbal and nonverbal communications
Independence	To achieve optimum function
Increased learning	To achieve awareness of needs
Increased reality perception and problem-solving ability	To achieve optimum function

NURSING INTERVENTIONS

Nursing Treatments

Approach unhurriedly

Provide an atmosphere of acceptance

Arrange situations which encourage patient autonomy

Encourage self-performance (regarding health care)

Encourage decision-making (regarding health care)

Encourage the expression of feelings

Listen attentively
   AND
Talk with the patient

Encourage the use of normal coping mechanisms

Refrain from performing nonessential procedures

Arrange a predischarge planning conference (with patient participation)

Nursing Observations

Observe for evidence that the patient is reaching out for emotional support

Observe for evidence of a favorable response to therapy

Health Teaching

Recommend that independence be encouraged

EVALUATION

See the evaluation criteria for each specific goal in Chapter 2.

Inadequate Emotional Support Related to Drug Dependency Withdrawal (148,187,251,266,360,423,508)

ASSESSMENT

Subjective Data

Sense of helplessness

Unsettled, vaguely confused feeling

Feels that the withdrawal period is very difficult to endure

Feeling of weakness

Wants to escape the situation

Intense insecure feelings

Preoccupied with the dependence on drugs

Objective Data

Appears forlorn and upset

At the time of need, the person has a limited, nonexistent, or temporarily absent support system of significant others

May reach out for help through crying, attention-seeking behavior, touching persons or objects, seeking someone to talk with, etc.

May appear withdrawn

If the dependence is alcohol, the withdrawal signs are vomiting, insomnia, diarrhea, tachycardia, fever, tremors, poor memory, disorientation, and hallucinations

If the dependence is drugs, the withdrawal signs are tremor, vomiting, muscle twitching, diarrhea, profuse sweating, chills, seizures, delirium, hallucinations, delusions, and disorientation

If the dependence is smoking, the withdrawal signs are constipation or diarrhea, urinary frequency, coughing, dyspnea, sweating, tremors, and depression

Related Data

Commonly Related Conditions:
Drug habituation
Smoking habituation

Commonly Related Diseases:
Alcoholism
Sociopathic personality

POSSIBLE ETIOLOGY

Lack of interest on the part of one's usually supportive world of family, friends, and church. The unavailability of persons who usually offer support. Hopelessness on the part of significant others who have given up trying to help the person with a dependence habituation.

NURSING DIAGNOSIS

Inadequate emotional support related to drug dependency withdrawal: little or no comfort or sustaining measures received from others while enduring a period of withdrawal from chemical substances

PLANNING

Patient Needs	Primary Nurse-Patient Goals
Comfort	To achieve comfort
Protection from psychologic threat	To prevent emotional injury
Acceptance	To achieve productive interpersonal relationships
Warm, communicating relationships	To achieve effective verbal and nonverbal communications
Adequacy, endurance	To achieve positive expressions, feelings, reactions
Personal growth and maturity	To achieve optimum function
Increased learning	To achieve awareness of needs
Increased reality perception and problem-solving ability	To achieve optimum function

NURSING INTERVENTIONS

Nursing Treatments
Approach unhurriedly
Demonstrate calmness
Express empathy
Express warmth and friendliness
Provide an atmosphere of acceptance

Touch the patient judiciously
Reassure verbally (that the withdrawal pain will subside)
Attend the patient constantly (until the acute episode subsides)
> AND

Provide frequent patient contact (thereafter)
Arrange a structured environment (suitable to the patient)
Encourage the expression of feelings
Listen attentively
> AND

Talk with the patient
Offer feedback of the patient's expressed feelings
Encourage patient questions (if such will relieve the distress)
Do not allow unpleasant surprise situations
Provide objects which symbolize safeness
Encourage mutual problem solving
Support a realistic assessment of the situation
Introduce to persons who have successfully undergone the same experience
Encourage the use of normal coping mechanisms
Explore with the patient his strengths and resources
Reduce the demands placed upon the patient
Refrain from performing nonessential procedures
Refrain from negatively criticizing

Call the patient's family to the
    bedside
> OR

Encourage telephone calls between
    significant persons

} (if the patient prefers or strongly needs significant others and if the significant others are available as a support system)

Nursing Observations
Determine the degree of insight
Evaluate the significance of emotional distress mannerisms
Evaluate the significance of nonverbal communications
Identify disturbing conversation topics
Observe for an excessive stress level

Health Teaching
Describe those symptoms which should be reported (physical symptoms related to the withdrawal)
Explain that the person's emotional response is appropriate and commonly experienced

EVALUATION

See the evaluation criteria for each specific goal in Chapter 2.

Nonacceptance of Increased Dependency (511)

ASSESSMENT

Subjective Data
Severe anxiety especially at the onset of dependency

Diminished self-esteem

Frustration

Objective Data

Irritability

Refuses help from others

Deliberately attempts to exceed his limitations to prove his independence

May omit medications or treatments in an effort to prove independence from them

Aggressive toward persons who attempt to curtail his activities or offer help

Verbally assures others of his capabilities

Expresses pride in his independence

Frequently discusses future wellness and independence

Related Data

Common among persons on dialysis therapy, persons having cardiac pacemakers, persons on prolonged intermittent positive pressure treatments for chronic pulmonary disorders, and persons dependent on drugs, such as diabetics having to rely on insulin

Commonly Related Diseases:

Cervical or thoracic spinal cord injury

Carcinoma

Tuberculosis

Muscular dystrophy

Poliomyelitis

Glomerulonephritis

Multiple sclerosis

Cerebral vascular accident

POSSIBLE ETIOLOGY

The threat of diminished self-esteem when there is loss of or diminished physical or mental function

NURSING DIAGNOSIS

Nonacceptance of increased dependency: the inability to accept that one must be more reliant on others to meet one's needs that were independently met in the past

PLANNING

Patient Needs	Primary Nurse-Patient Goals
Comfort	To achieve comfort
Protection from psychologic threat	To prevent emotional injury
Dependence	To achieve comfort
Acceptance	To achieve productive interpersonal relationships
High evaluation of self	To achieve positive expressions, feelings, reactions

Independence | To achieve optimum function

Dignity | To achieve productive interpersonal relationships

Increased learning | To achieve awareness of needs

NURSING INTERVENTIONS

Nursing Treatments

Approach unhurriedly

Provide an atmosphere of acceptance

Arrange situations which encourage patient autonomy

Emphasize the person's value as an individual (despite the increased dependence)

Encourage the expression of feelings

Listen attentively
AND
Talk with the patient

Offer feedback of the patient's expressed feelings

Encourage acceptance of interdependency

Encourage acceptance of self-limitations

Explore with the patient his strengths and resources

Recognize the need for the use of appropriate defense mechanisms

Recognize the need for unique personal adjustments to change

Support a realistic assessment of the situation

Refrain from performing nonessential procedures

Refrain from negatively criticizing

Nursing Observations

Determine the degree of insight

Evaluate the person's relatedness with others (in regard to dependence-independence)

Evaluate the significance of emotional distress mannerisms

Evaluate the significance of nonverbal communication

Identify disturbing conversation topics

Identify life values significant to the person (regarding dependence)

Identify appropriate use of defense mechanisms

Identify inappropriate use of defense mechanisms

Observe for an excessive stress level

Observe for impaired self-attitudes

Observe for evidence that the patient is reaching out for emotional support

Observe for evidence of a favorable response to therapy

Health Teaching

Explain that the person's emotional response is appropriate and commonly experienced

Explain the importance of maintaining a positive self-attitude (despite the increased dependence)

EVALUATION

See the evaluation criteria for each specific goal in Chapter 2.

DEPRESSION

Inadequate Emotional Support Related to Mild Depression (80,118,148,187, 199,331,360,504,508)

ASSESSMENT

Subjective Data

Sense of helplessness
Unsettled, vaguely confused feeling
Feels that the depression is mildly difficult to endure
Feeling of weakness
Wants to escape the situation
Feels slightly let down, discouraged, or hopeless
Chronically worries
Prolonged self-analysis
Oversensitive
Fearful
Insecure
Chronically fatigued
Preoccupied with the depression

Objective Data

Appears forlorn and upset
At the time of need, the person has a limited, nonexistent, or temporarily
    absent support system of significant others
May reach out for help through crying, attention-seeking behavior, touching
    persons or objects, seeking someone to talk with, etc.
May appear withdrawn
Saddened facial expression
Decreased attendance to personal appearance
Decreased interest in food

Related Data

Commonly Related Conditions:
Hypoglycemia
Commonly Related Diseases:
Any disease or injury
    OR
Cushing's Disease
Thyrotoxicosis
Glomerulonephritis
Carcinoma
Depression neurosis

POSSIBLE ETIOLOGY

Psychologic causes: Lack of interest on the part of one's usually supportive
world of family, friends, and church. The unavailability of persons who
usually offer support. Depression resulting from a stressful life situation,

poor emotional adaptation, or feelings of failure, unworthiness, guilt or anger. Inability to fulfill expectations *Physical causes:* Decreased norepinephrine or blood glucose level.

NURSING DIAGNOSIS

Inadequate emotional support related to mild depression: little or no comfort or sustaining measures received from others while one is enduring mild depression

PLANNING

Patient Needs	**Primary Nurse-Patient Goals**
Comfort	To achieve comfort
Stimulation	To maintain stimulation
Protection from psychologic threat	To prevent emotional injury
Acceptance	To achieve productive interpersonal relationships
Warm, communicating relationships	To achieve effective verbal and nonverbal communications
Sense of value, usefulness, high evaluation of self, adequacy, endurance	To achieve positive expressions, feelings, reactions
Personal growth and maturity	To achieve optimum function
Increased learning	To achieve awareness of needs
Increased reality perception and problem-solving ability	To achieve optimum function
Increased pleasantness	To achieve positive expressions, feelings, reactions

NURSING INTERVENTIONS

Nursing Treatments
Approach unhurriedly
Demonstrate calmness
Express empathy
Express warmth and friendliness
Provide an atmosphere of acceptance
Touch the patient judiciously
Reassure verbally
Attend the patient constantly
   OR
Provide frequent patient contact
Arrange a structured environment (suitable to the patient)
Arrange pleasant surroundings
Encourage the expression of feelings
Listen attentively
   AND
Talk with the patient

Offer feedback of the patient's expressed feelings
Encourage patient questions (if such will relieve the distress)
Provide objects which symbolize safeness
Encourage mutual problem solving
   AND
Encourage the sharing of common problems with others
Encourage the reduction of generalizations to specifics
Encourage acceptance of self-limitations
Encourage awareness of positive responses from others
Explore with the patient reasons for self-criticism
Encourage identification of specific life values
Explore with the patient his strengths and resources
Support a realistic assessment of the situation
Encourage gradual mastery of a situation
Encourage the use of normal coping mechanisms
Encourage involvement in helping others
Encourage involvement in totally new interests
Encourage meaningful activity
Encourage a full day of activities
Encourage active diversional activities
Encourage balanced long- and short-range goals
Encourage planned one-day-at-a-time living
Encourage pride in appearance
Encourage the enjoyment of life's simple things
Offer hope
Introduce to persons who have successfully undergone the same experience
Recognize the need for unique personal adjustments to change
Reduce the demands placed upon the patient
Refrain from performing nonessential procedures
Refrain from negatively criticizing

Call the patient's family to the
   bedside
   OR
Encourage telephone calls between
   significant persons
} (if the patient prefers or strongly needs significant others and if the significant others are available as a support system)

Nursing Observations
Determine the degree of insight
Determine the precipitating factors
Determine the relieving factors
Evaluate the person's relatedness with others
Evaluate the significance of emotional distress mechanisms
Evaluate the significance of nonverbal communication
Identify disturbing conversation topics
Identify life values significant to the person
Identify appropriate use of defense mechanisms
Identify inappropriate use of defense mechanisms
Observe for an excessive stress level
Observe for impaired judgment

Observe for impaired self-attitudes

Monitor blood studies for abnormal (decreased) adrenal function

Monitor blood studies for abnormal (decreased) glucose

} (indicating the depression is of a physical origin)

Observe for a favorable response to therapy

Health Teaching

Advise that negative responses from others be regarded with minimum significance

Advise that significant persons express acceptance of one another

Advise that significant persons express love for one another

Explain the importance of offering emotional support to one another

Describe those symptoms which should be reported (severe depression)

Emphasize the importance of recognizing tension within oneself

Explain the need to recognize highly stressful situations

Explain the importance of maintaining a positive self-attitude

Explain that the person's emotional response is appropriate and commonly experienced

Teach how to use the problem-solving method

EVALUATION

See the evaluation criteria for each specific goal in Chapter 2.

Inadequate Emotional Support Related to Moderate Depression (80,118,148, 187,199,331,504,508)

ASSESSMENT

Subjective Data

Sense of helplessness

Unsettled, vaguely confused feeling

Feels that the depression is very difficult to endure

Feeling of weakness

Wants to escape the situation

Feels considerably let down, discouraged, or hopeless

May experience guilt feelings

Poverty of ideas

Impaired judgment

Disorientation, sometimes

Severe fatigue

Preoccupied with the depression

Objective Data

Appears forlorn and upset

At the time of need, the person has a limited, nonexistent, or temporarily absent support system of significant others

May reach out for help through excessive crying, touching persons or objects, seeking someone to talk with, withdrawal

Lowered eyelids
Drooping mouth and head
Shrinking body movements
Diminished activity
Low voice pitch
Slow speech
Considerable self-neglect
Little interest in food
Morbid, verbal self-criticism

Related Data

Commonly Related Conditions:
Hypoglycemia

Commonly Related Diseases:
Any disease
    OR
Cushing's disease
Thyrotoxicosis
Glomerulonephritis
Carcinoma
Melancholia involutional psychosis
Simple senile psychosis
Pellagra

POSSIBLE ETIOLOGY

Psychologic causes: Lack of interest on the part of one's usually supportive world of family, friends, and church. The unavailability of persons who usually offer support. Depression resulting from a stressful life situation, poor emotional adaptation, or feelings of failure, unworthiness, guilt, or anger. Inability to fulfill expectations. *Physical causes:* Decreased norephinephrine or blood glucose level.

NURSING DIAGNOSIS

Inadequate emotional support related to moderate depression: little or no comfort or sustaining measures received from others while one is enduring moderate depression

PLANNING

Patient Needs	Primary Nurse-Patient Goals
Rest	To achieve rest
Comfort	To achieve comfort
Stimulation	To maintain sensory function and stimulation
Protection from psychologic threat	To prevent emotional injury
Dependence	To achieve comfort
Acceptance	To achieve productive interpersonal relationships

Warm, communicating relationships

To achieve effective verbal and nonverbal communications

Sense of value, usefulness, high evaluation of self, adequacy, endurance

To achieve positive expressions, feelings, reactions

Personal growth and maturity

To achieve optimum function

Increased learning

To achieve awareness of needs

Increased reality perception and problem-solving ability

To achieve optimum function

Increased pleasantness

To achieve positive expressions, feelings, reactions

NURSING INTERVENTIONS

Nursing Treatments
Approach unhurriedly
Demonstrate calmness
Express empathy
Express warmth and friendliness
Provide an atmosphere of acceptance
Touch the patient judiciously
Reassure verbally
Attend the patient constantly
   OR
Provide frequent patient contact
Sit with the patient
Stimulate by movement, touch, sternal pressure, or speech
Arrange a structured environment (suitable to the patient)
Arrange pleasant surroundings
Acknowledge dependency
   BUT
Encourage self-performance
Encourage the expression of feelings
Listen attentively
   AND
Talk with the patient
Offer feedback of the patient's expressed feelings
Encourage patient questions (if such will relieve the distress)
Encourage attentive patient listening
Do not allow unpleasant surprise situations
Provide objects which symbolize safeness
Encourage mutual problem solving
   AND
Encourage the sharing of common problems with others
Encourage the reduction of generalizations to specifics
Encourage acceptance of self-limitations
Encourage awareness of positive responses from others
Explore with the patient reasons for self-criticism

Encourage identification of specific life values
Explore with the patient his strengths and resources
Support a realistic assessment of the situation
Encourage gradual mastery of a situation
Encourage the use of normal coping mechanisms
Encourage alternate rest and activity
Encourage meaningful activity
Encourage active diversional activities
Encourage balanced long- and short-range goals
Encourage planned one-day-at-a-time living
Encourage pride in appearance
Encourage the enjoyment of life's simple things
Offer hope
Use direct eye contact to terminate excessive crying
Introduce to persons who have successfully undergone the same experience
Recognize the need for unique personal adjustments to change
Reduce the demands placed upon the patient
Refrain from performing nonessential procedures
Refrain from negatively criticizing
Encourage patient to make a verbal no-suicide contract (there is always a
    suicide risk in depression)
Call the patient's family to the bedside ⎫ (if the patient prefers or strongly
    OR   ⎪ needs significant others and if the
Encourage telephone calls   ⎬ significant others are available as
    between significant persons   ⎭ a support system)

Nursing observations
Determine the degree of insight
Determine the precipitating factors
Determine the relieving factors
Evaluate the significance of emotional distress mannerisms
Evaluate the significance of nonverbal communication
Identify disturbing conversation topics
Identify life values significant to the person
Identify appropriate use of defense mechanisms
Identify inappropriate use of defense mechanisms
Observe for an excessive stress level
Observe for presuicide calmness
Monitor blood studies for abnormal ⎫
    (decreased) adrenal function   ⎪ (indicating the depression is of phys-
Monitor blood studies for abnormal   ⎬   ical origin)
    (decreased) glucose   ⎭

Observe for a favorable response to therapy

Health Teaching
Advise that negative responses from others be regarded with minimum
    significance
Advise that significant persons express acceptance of one another

Advise that significant persons express love for one another
Explain the importance of offering emotional support to one another
Emphasize the importance of recognizing tension within oneself
Explain the need to recognize highly stressful situations
Explain the importance of maintaining a positive self-attitude
Teach how to use the problem-solving method

EVALUATION

See the evaluation criteria for each specific goal in Chapter 2.

Inadequate Emotional Support Related to Severe Depression (80,118,148, 187,199,331,360,504,508)

ASSESSMENT

Subjective Data
Sense of helplessness
Unsettled, vaguely confused feeling
Feels that the depression is extremely difficult to endure
Feeling of weakness
Wants to escape the situation
Feels intensely let down, discouraged, or hopeless
Severe feelings of gloom
Preoccupied with the object of the depression
Impaired judgment

Objective Data
Appears forlorn and upset
At the time of need, the person has a limited, nonexistent, or temporarily
    absent support system of significant others
May reach out for help through excessive crying, touching persons or ob-
    jects, withdrawal
Slow thought response
Little or no activity
Stooped shoulders
Walks slowly
Does not speak unless spoken to
Severe self-neglect
Refusal to eat

Related Data
Commonly Related Diseases:
Any disease
    OR
Cushing's disease
Thyrotoxicosis
Glomerulonephritis
Carcinoma
Manic-depressive psychosis

Involutional melancholia
Pellagra

POSSIBLE ETIOLOGY

Psychologic causes: Lack of interest on the part of one's usually supportive world of family, friends, and church. The unavailability of persons who usually offer support. Depression resulting from a stressful life situation, poor emotional adaptation, or feelings of failure, unworthiness, guilt, or anger. Inability to fulfill expectations. *Physical causes:* Decreased norepinephrine or blood glucose level.

NURSING DIAGNOSIS

Inadequate emotional support related to severe depression: little or no comfort or sustaining measures received from others while one is enduring severe depression

PLANNING

Patient Needs	Primary Nurse-Patient Goals
Rest	To achieve rest
Comfort	To achieve comfort
Stimulation	To maintain sensory function and stimulation
Protection from psychologic threat	To prevent emotional injury
Acceptance	To achieve productive interpersonal relationships
Warm, communicating relationships	To achieve effective verbal and nonverbal communications
Sense of value, usefulness, high evaluation of self, adequacy, endurance	To achieve positive expressions, feelings, reactions
Personal growth and maturity	To achieve optimum function
Increased learning	To achieve awareness of needs
Increased reality perception and problem-solving ability	To achieve optimum function
Increased pleasantness	To achieve positive expressions, feelings, reactions

NURSING INTERVENTIONS

Nursing Treatments
Approach unhurriedly
Demonstrate calmness
Express empathy
Express warmth and friendliness
Provide an atmosphere of acceptance
Touch the patient judiciously
Reassure verbally

Attend the patient constantly
   OR
Provide frequent patient contact
Sit with the patient
Stimulate by movement, touch, sternal pressure, or verbally
Arrange a structured environment (suitable to the patient)
Arrange pleasant surroundings
Acknowledge dependency
   BUT
Encourage self-performance
Encourage the expression of feelings
Listen attentively
   AND
Talk with the patient
Offer feedback of the patient's expressed feelings
Encourage attentive patient listening
Do not allow unpleasant surprise situations
Provide objects which symbolize safeness
Encourage mutual problem solving
Encourage acceptance of self-limitations
Encourage awareness of positive responses from others
Explore with the patient reasons for self-criticism
Encourage identification of specific life values
Explore with the patient his strengths and resources
Support a realistic assessment of the situation
Encourage gradual mastery of a situation
Encourage the use of normal coping mechanisms
Encourage alternate rest and activity
Encourage meaningful activity
Encourage passive diversional activities (if response is very slow)
Encourage active diversional activities (whenever possible)
Encourage planned one-day-at-a-time living
Encourage pride in appearance
Encourage the enjoyment of life's simple things
Offer hope
Use direct eye contact to terminate excessive crying
Recognize the need for unique personal adjustments to change
Reduce the demands placed upon the patient
Refrain from performing nonessential procedures
Refrain from negatively criticizing
Encourage patient to make a verbal no-suicide contract (there is always a
   suicide risk in depression)
Call the patient's family to the bedside ⎫(if the patient prefers or strongly
   OR   ⎬ needs significant others and if the
Encourage telephone calls between ⎭ significant others are available as
   significant persons   a support system)

Nursing Observations
Determine the degree of insight

Determine the precipitating factors
Determine the relieving factors
Evaluate the person's relatedness with others
Evaluate the significance of emotional distress mannerisms
Evaluate the significance of nonverbal communication
Identify disturbing conversation topics
Identify life values significant to the person
Identify appropriate use of defense mechanisms
Identify inappropriate use of defense mechanisms
Observe for presuicide calmness
Monitor blood studies for abnormal
   (decreased) adrenal function $\Big\}$ (indicating the depression is of phys-
Monitor blood studies for abnormal   ical origin)
   (decreased) glucose
Observe for a favorable response to therapy

Health Teaching
Advise that negative responses from others be regarded with minimum
   significance
Advise that significant persons express acceptance of one another
Advise that significant persons express love for one another
Explain the importance of offering emotional support to one another
Emphasize the importance of recognizing tension within oneself
Explain the need to recognize highly stressful situations
Explain the importance of maintaining a positive self-attitude
Teach how to use the problem-solving method (if the person is responsive)

EVALUATION

See the evaluation criteria for each specific goal in Chapter 2.

DEPRESSION, POTENTIAL

Potential Depression (80,118,199,331)

ASSESSMENT

Subjective Data
Slight feeling of gloom
Perceives goals as vague
Nervousness
Inadequacy feelings

Objective Data
Restlessness
Spontaneous crying

Related Data
Commonly Related Conditions:
Childbirth and parenthood
Senility

Drug toxicity
Mental or physical fatigue
Altered body image
Loss of loved one or personal possessions
Surgical procedures
Commonly Related Diseases:
Any disease or injury
Myocardial infarction
Emphysema
Cerebral vascular accident
Spinal cord injury
Cancer

POSSIBLE ETIOLOGY

Severe stress. Lack of clearly defined goals. Toxic reactions. Endocrine imbalance. Severe situational change. Limitations imposed upon the person by illness.

NURSING DIAGNOSIS

Potential depression: the possibility that emotional depression could develop

PLANNING

Patient Needs	Primary Nurse-Patient Goals
Sleep, rest, relaxation	To achieve sleep, rest, relaxation
Comfort	To achieve comfort
Protection from psychologic threat	To prevent emotional injury
Acceptance	To achieve productive interpersonal relationships
Warm, communicating relationships	To achieve effective verbal and nonverbal communications
Sense of value, usefulness, high evaluation of self, adequacy	To achieve positive expressions, feelings, reactions
Awareness of potential	To achieve optimum function
Increased learning	To achieve awareness of needs and/or use of resources
Increased reality perception and problem-solving ability	To achieve optimum function

NURSING INTERVENTIONS

Nursing Treatments
Approach unhurriedly
Provide an atmosphere of acceptance
Avoid causing painful emotional situations
Encourage the expression of feelings
Listen attentively
AND
Talk with the patient

Offer feedback of the patient's expressed feelings
Encourage gradual mastery of a situation
Encourage planned one-day-at-a-time living (especially during severe stress)
Encourage acceptance of self-limitations
Introduce one anxiety situation at a time
Introduce to persons who have successfully undergone the same experience
Encourage identification of specific life values
Encourage the practical application of the accepted value system
Encourage the use of normal coping mechanisms
Support a realistic assessment of the situation
Encourage laughter
Encourage meaningful activity
Encourage mutual problem solving
Encourage new goals at past goal achievement
Encourage adequate rest
Encourage the enjoyment of life's simple things
Recognize the need for the use of appropriate defense mechanisms
Recognize the need for unique personal adjustments to change
Reduce the demands placed upon the patient
Refrain from performing nonessential procedures

Nursing Observations
Determine the degree of insight
Evaluate the person's relatedness with others
Evaluate the significance of emotional distress mannerisms
Evaluate the significance of nonverbal communication
Identify disturbing conversation topics
Identify inappropriate emotional responses
Identify life values significant to the person
Identify appropriate use of defense mechanisms
Identify inappropriate use of defense mechanisms
Observe for an excessive stress level
Observe for impaired self-attitudes
Observe for evidence that the patient is reaching out for emotional support
Observe for evidence of a favorable response to therapy

Health Teaching
Advise early correction of problems
Advise occasional respite from responsibility
Advise that negative responses from others be regarded with minimum significance
Advise that significant persons express acceptance of one another
Advise that significant persons express love for one another
Explain the importance of offering emotional support to one another
Emphasize the need for realistic expectation of others
Emphasize the importance of recognizing tension within oneself
Explain that fatigue should be recognized as a stress factor

Explain the need to recognize highly stressful situations
Explain the importance of maintaining a positive self-attitude
Explain how to obtain release from emotional stress
Explain that some tension is normal
Recommend methods for achieving total relaxation
Teach how to use the problem-solving method

EVALUATION

See the evaluation criteria for each specific goal in Chapter 2.

EMBARRASSMENT

Embarrassment Related to Body Exposure

ASSESSMENT

Subjective Data
Person is uncomfortable undressing or being undressed in front of others
Perceives his body as very private
Feels humiliated

Objective Data
Clings to clothing or sheets when undressed in front of another
Undresses only partially
Reluctant to assume positions necessary for examination or treatment
May object to being bathed or viewed by others, but especially members of
  the opposite sex

Related Data
Commonly Related Diseases:
Any disease or injury

POSSIBLE ETIOLOGY

Strong modesty values. Lack of consideration by health personnel.

NURSING DIAGNOSIS

Embarrassment related to body exposure: a sense of uneasiness and loss of
composure associated with exposure of the body while undergoing health
examinations or procedures

PLANNING

Patient Needs	**Primary Nurse-Patient Goals**
Comfort	To achieve comfort
Protection from psychologic threat	To prevent emotional injury
Warm, communicating relationships	To achieve effective verbal and nonverbal communications

Dignity

To achieve productive interpersonal relationships

Increased learning

To achieve awareness of needs

NURSING INTERVENTIONS

Nursing Treatments

Reassure verbally (that the person will be protected from unnecessary body exposure)

Encourage the expression of feelings

Listen attentively

Express empathy

Demonstrate calmness

Provide an atmosphere of acceptance

Avoid causing embarrassing situations

Drape modestly

Encourage self-performance (of bath, etc., if the person is able)

Talk with the patient (as a diversion during examinations or procedures)

Screen the patient for privacy

Keep the patient's door closed

Nursing Observations

Determine the precipitating factors

Determine the relieving factors

Evaluate the significance of emotional distress mannerisms

Evaluate the significance of nonverbal communications

Identify disturbing conversation topics

Observe for an excessive stress level

Observe for evidence that the patient is reaching out for emotional support

Observe for evidence of a favorable response to therapy

Health Teaching

Explain that the person's emotional response is appropriate and commonly experienced

Explain the reason for and intended effect of the therapy or examination

EVALUATION

See the evaluation criteria for each specific goal in Chapter 2.

Embarrassment Related to Social Exposure

ASSESSMENT

Subjective Data

Person feels that the health impairment has made him less socially acceptable

Sensitive to the comments of others

Feels humiliated

Objective Data
Prefers not to meet with other people
Pulls the bed curtain around himself
Keeps the door closed
Patient has any of the following, which are *visible* evidence of illness: drainage tubing and container (especially G. U. bags), nasogastric tubes, permanent tracheostomy and laryngectomy tubes, arteriovenous shunt, hand tremors, abnormal gait, incontinence, obesity, severe weight loss, hair loss from chemotherapy, jaundice, skin rash, use of a wheelchair, cane, crutch, or walker

Related Data
Commonly Related Conditions:
Cachexia
Commonly Related Diseases:
Parkinson's disease
Chorea
Laennec's cirrhosis
Cerebral vascular accident
Spinal cord injury
Trauma causing disfigurement such as severe burns or leg amputation

POSSIBLE ETIOLOGY

Fear of loss of esteem from others. Feelings of inadequacy. Low self-esteem.

NURSING DIAGNOSIS

Embarrassment related to social exposure: a sense of uneasiness and loss of composure when health impairment is visible and subject to the observation of others during social contacts

PLANNING

Patient Needs	**Primary Nurse-Patient Goals**
Comfort	To achieve comfort
Protection from psychologic threat	To prevent emotional injury
Warm, communicating relationships	To achieve effective verbal and nonverbal communications
High evaluation of self, adequacy	To achieve positive expressions, feelings, reactions
Dignity	To achieve productive interpersonal relationships
Increased learning	To achieve awareness of needs

NURSING INTERVENTIONS

Nursing Treatments
Approach unhurriedly
Reassure verbally (that the person will be protected from unnecessary social exposure)

Provide an atmosphere of acceptance
Avoid causing embarrassing situations
Encourage the expression of feelings
Listen attentively
   AND
Talk with the patient
Encourage acceptance of self-limitations
Screen the patient for privacy
Keep the patient's door closed
Restrict unwanted visitors
Keep treatment equipment
   (drainage systems, etc.) out of
   sight
Cover the head (with a wig or scarf
   if there is hair loss) } (when exposed to social contacts)
Sit the patient in an armchair
   (instead of a wheelchair)
Protect with plastic pants (if
   incontinent)
Introduce to persons who have successfully undergone the same
   experience
Recognize the need for the use of appropriate defense mechanisms
Recognize the need for unique personal adjustments to change
Socialize gradually

Nursing Observations
Determine the degree of insight
Evaluate the significance of emotional distress mannerisms
Evaluate the significance of nonverbal communication
Identify disturbing conversation topics
Identify life values significant to the person
Identify appropriate use of defense mechanisms
Identify inappropriate use of defense mechanisms
Observe for an excessive stress level
Observe for evidence that the patient is reaching out for emotional support
Observe for a favorable response to therapy

Health Teaching
Explain that the person's emotional response is appropriate and commonly
   experienced
Advise that negative responses from others be regarded with minimum
   significance
Explain the importance of maintaining a positive self-attitude
Explain how to adjust clothing to
   meet health needs } (which will reduce visiblity of im-
Teach how to use assistive eating   pairment during social exposure)
   devices

EVALUATION
See the evaluation criteria for each specific goal in Chapter 2.

FEAR

Inadequate Emotional Support Related to Fear (95,118,199,331)

ASSESSMENT

Subjective Data
Sense of helplessness
Unsettled, vaguely confused feeling
Feels that the fear is very difficult to endure
Feeling of weakness
Wants to escape the situation
Feels highly threatened
Profound feelings of fright and alarm
Often imagines the worst
Preoccupied with the fear

Objective Data
Appears forlorn and upset
At the time of need, the person has a limited, nonexistent, or temporarily
    absent support system of significant others
May reach out for help through crying, attention-seeking behavior, touching
    persons or objects, seeking someone to talk with, etc.
May appear withdrawn
Rapid respirations
Profuse sweating
Tachycardia
Increased blood pressure
Restlessness
Insomnia
Weeping
Uncooperative, sometimes
Clings to objects which symbolize security

Related Data
Commonly Related Diseases:
Any disease or injury

POSSIBLE ETIOLOGY

Lack of interest on the part of one's usually supportive world of family,
friends, and church. The unavailability of persons who usually offer support. Fear resulting from any of the following causes: feelings of inadequacy
to defend oneself, lack of knowledge and experience regarding a situation,
previous similar frightening experiences, poor early dependency relationships, vivid imagination, and the inability of a child to distinguish between
real and imaginary dangers.

NURSING DIAGNOSIS

Inadequate emotional support related to fear: little or no comfort or sustaining measures received from others while one is enduring fear

PLANNING

Patient Needs	**Primary Nurse-Patient Goals**
Relaxation	To achieve relaxation
Comfort	To achieve comfort
Protection from psychologic threat	To prevent emotional injury
Warm, communicating relationships	To achieve effective verbal and nonverbal communications
Adequacy	To achieve positive expressions, feelings, reactions
Increased learning	To achieve awareness of needs

NURSING INTERVENTIONS

Nursing Treatments

Approach unhurriedly
Demonstrate calmness
Express empathy
Express warmth and friendliness
Provide an atmosphere of acceptance
Touch the patient judiciously
Reassure verbally
Attend the patient constantly (until the acute episode subsides)
    AND
Provide frequent patient contact (thereafter)
Arrange a structured environment (suitable to the patient)
Arrange orderly surroundings
Establish routines familiar to the patient
Provide quiet
Arrange situations which encourage patient autonomy (if the fear is based on dependency)
Massage gently
    OR   } (for the relaxing effect)
Bathe in warm water
Encourage the expression of feelings
Listen attentively
    AND
Talk with the patient
Offer feedback of the patient's expressed feelings
Encourage patient questions (if such will relieve the distress)
Provide reliable information
Do not allow unpleasant surprise situations
Avoid causing painful emotional situations
Provide objects which symbolize safeness
Encourage mutual problem solving
Support a realistic assessment of the situation
Introduce to persons who have successfully undergone the same experience
Encourage the use of normal coping mechanisms

Explore with the patient his strengths and resources
Encourage the person to face the fear
Reduce the demands placed upon the patient
Refrain from performing nonessential procedures
Refrain from negatively criticizing
Call the patient's family to the
    bedside   } (if the patient prefers or strongly
    OR   needs significant others and if the
Encourage telephone calls between   significant others are available as
    significant persons   a support system)
Explore with the patient reasons for recurring problems (related to the fear)
Encourage active diversional activities (to promote periods of rest from
    fear)
Present change gradually
Encourage gradual mastery of a situation
Encourage planned one-day-at-a-time living
Encourage the sharing of common problems with others
Recognize the need for unique personal adjustments to change
Encourage exploration of the dark when fearful of the dark
    AND
Provide a nightlight

Nursing Observations
Determine the degree of insight
Determine the precipitating factors
Determine the relieving factors
Evaluate the significance of emotional distress mannerisms
Evaluate the significance of nonverbal communication
Evaluate disturbing conversation topics
Identify life values significant to the person
Identify appropriate use of defense mechanisms
Identify inappropriate use of defense mechanisms
Observe for an excessive stress level
Observe for evidence of a favorable response to therapy

Health Teaching
Explain that the person's emotional response is appropriate and commonly
    experienced
Explain and offer hope that the emotional pain will decrease with time
Emphasize the importance of recognizing tension within oneself
Explain that fatigue should be recognized as a stress factor
Explain the need to recognize highly stressful situations
Explain how to obtain release from emotional stress
Advise against fighting fear
Explain that fear often disguises itself
Explain the causes of fear of death

Explain the difference between freedom from fear and freedom from prob-
lems
Explain the importance of offering emotional support to one another
Explain the importance of remaining calm
Explain how to channel emotional energy into activity
Explain how to reduce muscular tension
Recommend methods for reducing sensory stimulation
Recommend methods for achieving total relaxation
Recommend a habitual, positive mental attitude
Explain the need to predict and plan for change
Teach how to use the problem-solving method

Medical Treatments Performed by Nurses
Give the prescribed drug

EVALUATION

See the evaluation criteria for each specific goal in Chapter 2.

Maladaptive Coping Related to Fear
(95,118,199,331)

ASSESSMENT

Subjective Data
Fear is magnified out of proportion to reality
Has an exaggerated fear of things and situations one normally fears
Fears things and situations one normally does not fear
Experiences fright and even terror
Experiences hallucinations or delusions

Objective Data
May go to extremes to avoid the feared object
Blames others for the situation
Profuse sweating
Poor motor control
Tachycardia
Increased blood pressure

Related Data
Commonly Related Diseases:
Phobic neurosis

POSSIBLE ETIOLOGY

Chronic, inappropriate use of defense mechanisms such as repression,
reaction formation, displacement, and symbolism. Displacement of fear
from its real source to objects or events. Conflict arising in the phallic stage
of development. An inability to defend oneself against threat. Conditioned
learning in situations eliciting a strong fear response. Overpowering feelings of inadequacy. Forced adaptation to change.

NURSING DIAGNOSIS

Maladaptive coping related to fear: an unhealthy attempt to cope with feelings of fright and alarm

PLANNING

Patient Needs	**Primary Nurse-Patient Goals**
Relaxation	To achieve relaxation
Comfort	To achieve comfort
Protection from psychologic threat	To prevent emotional injury
Predictable, orderly world	To achieve a therapeutic environment
Warm, communicating relationships	To achieve effective verbal and nonverbal communications
Adequacy	To achieve positive expressions, feelings, reactions
Personal growth and maturity	To achieve optimum function
Increased learning	To achieve awareness of needs
Increased reality perception and problem-solving ability	To achieve optimum function

NURSING INTERVENTIONS

Nursing Treatments
Approach unhurriedly
Provide an atmosphere of acceptance
Express warmth and friendliness
Provide frequent patient contact
Ask questions which encourage answers that reflect reality perception
Encourage the expression of feelings
Listen attentively
    AND
Talk with the patient
Offer feedback of the patient's expressed feelings
Encourage patient questions
Encourage gradual mastery of a situation
Encourage planned one-day-at-a-time living
Encourage the sharing of common problems with others
Support a realistic assessment of the situation
Encourage the reduction of generalizations to specifics
Encourage the use of normal coping mechanisms
Explore superficial topics and reasons for avoiding in-depth feelings
Explore with the patient his strengths and resources
Encourage the person to face the fear
Explore with the patient reasons for criticism of others
Explore with the patient reasons for recurring problems (related to the fear)
Explore with the patient the effects of his behavior on others
Give important messages only when the patient is receptive
Introduce to persons who have successfully undergone the same experience
Provide emotionally safe experiences
Reduce the demands placed upon the patient
Refrain from performing nonessential procedures
Refrain from negatively criticizing

Touch the patient judiciously
Make a referral (to a psychiatric nurse specialist)

Nursing Observations
Determine the degree of insight
Estimate the degree of stress experienced
Evaluate the person's relatedness with others
Evaluate the significance of emotional distress mannerisms
Evaluate the significance of nonverbal communications
Identify abnormal perceptions
Identify abnormal thought content
Identify attention span abnormalities
Observe for impaired judgment
Identify disturbing conversation topics
Identify emotion-stimulating events
Identify inappropriate emotional responses
Identify life values significant to the person
Identify inappropriate use of defense mechanisms
Observe for an excessive stress level
Observe for evidence that the patient is reaching out for emotional support
Observe for evidence of a favorable response to therapy

Health Teaching
Advise against fighting fear
Describe those factors which intensify fear
Emphasize the importance of recognizing tension within oneself
Explain the importance of maintaining a positive self-attitude
Explain how to obtain release from emotional stress
Explain that fear often disguises itself
Explain the difference between freedom from fear and freedom from
    problems
Explain how to channel emotional energy into activity
Explain how to reduce muscular tension
Recommend methods for achieving total relaxation
Teach how to use the problem-solving method
Describe the behavior pattern indicating emotional maturity

EVALUATION

See the evaluation criteria for each specific goal in Chapter 2.

FRUSTRATION

Frustration Related to Slow Cure Progression (281,440)

ASSESSMENT

Subjective Data
Irritability
Experiences internal tension

Is less and less able to tolerate stress and pain

Objective Data
Nervous mannerisms
Verbally strikes out at others
Throws or slams down the object of frustration, such as a cane or crutch
May outwardly attempt to establish a wellness routine on his own but discovers he cannot maintain it
Moodiness

Related Data
Commonly Related Diseases:
Alcoholism
Spinal cord injury
Myocardial infarction
Carcinoma
Third-degree burn
Bone fracture

POSSIBLE ETIOLOGY

Chronic blocking of a desired goal. Long-term illness. The body's adaptation to wellness reaches a plateau, and from that point, progress toward health is very slow. Unforeseen health complications.

NURSING DIAGNOSIS

Frustration related to slow cure progression: emotional irritation and aggressive impulses resulting from a slow recovery that extends over a prolonged period and thwarts the goal of regaining health immediately

PLANNING

Patient Needs	Primary Nurse-Patient Goals
Comfort	To achieve comfort
Protection from psychologic threat	To prevent emotional injury
Warm, communicating relationships	To achieve effective verbal and nonverbal communications
Adequacy	To achieve positive expressions, feelings, reactions
Goal achievement	To achieve optimum function
Endurance	To achieve positive expressions, feelings, reactions
Personal growth and maturity	To achieve optimum function
Increased learning	To achieve awareness of needs and/or use of resources
Increased reality perception and problem-solving ability	To achieve optimum function

NURSING INTERVENTIONS

Nursing Treatments
Approach unhurriedly

Demonstrate calmness
Provide an atmosphere of acceptance
Reassure verbally
Express empathy
Discourage the setting of time limits
Encourage acceptance of partial goal satisfaction
Encourage single goal seeking
Encourage balanced long- and short-range goals
Encourage strivings toward realistic goals
Suggest substitute means of goal attainment
Encourage gradual mastery of a situation
Encourage the expression of feelings
Listen attentively
    AND
Talk with the patient
Offer feedback of the patient's expressed feelings
Encourage laughter
Encourage patience in illness adjustment
Encourage planned one-day-at-a-time living
Encourage the sharing of common problems with others
Encourage the use of normal coping mechanisms
Explore with the patient his strengths and resources
Verbalize daily the patient's successful progress
Support a realistic assessment of the situation
Offer praise
Introduce to persons who have successfully undergone the same experience
Reduce the demands placed upon the patient
Refrain from performing nonessential procedures
Refrain from negatively criticizing
Refrain from teasing

Nursing Observations
Determine the degree of insight
Determine the precipitating factors
Determine the relieving factors
Evaluate the person's relatedness with others
Evaluate the significance of emotional distress mannerisms
Evaluate the significance of nonverbal communication
Identify disturbing conversation topics
Observe for an excessive stress level
Observe for evidence that the patient is reaching out for emotional support
Observe for evidence of a favorable response to therapy

Health Teaching
Explain that the person's emotional response is appropriate and commonly
    experienced
Explain the importance of offering emotional support to one another
Emphasize the importance of recognizing tension within oneself
Explain that fatigue should be recognized as a stress factor
Explain how to obtain release from emotional stress

Explain the importance of maintaining a positive self-attitude
Explain that ill persons are often hypersensitive (to frustration)

EVALUATION

See the evaluation criteria for each specific goal in Chapter 2.

GRIEF

Failure to Grieve (264,494)

ASSESSMENT

Subjective Data
Sense of emotional numbness
No feeling
Loss of self-esteem
Guilt
Severe depression
Ambivalence
Anger

Objective Data
Remains emotionally composed
Does not weep
Does not discuss or seldom discusses the loss
Behavior changes begin to occur sometime after the loss, especially around
  anniversaries

Related Data
Commonly Related Conditions:
Any significant loss
Commonly Related Diseases:
Any disease or injury

POSSIBLE ETIOLOGY

The absence of family members with whom one can grieve. A desire to remain strong in the face of crisis.

NURSING DIAGNOSIS

Failure to grieve: failure to express sorrow and deep inner turmoil at the
time of a significant loss

PLANNING

Patient Needs	**Primary Nurse-Patient Goals**
Comfort	To achieve comfort
Protection from psychologic threat	To prevent emotional injury
Warm, communicating relationships	To achieve effective verbal and nonverbal communications

Personal growth and maturity To achieve optimum function
Increased learning To achieve awareness of needs

NURSING INTERVENTIONS

Nursing Treatments

Approach unhurriedly
Provide an atmosphere of acceptance
Express empathy
Reassure verbally
Communicate that the nurse feels comfortable with the patient's discussions of death (in relation to a departed loved one)
Encourage acceptance of self-limitations (to endure the repressed grief)
Encourage crying
Encourage the expression of feelings
Listen attentively
    AND
Talk with the patient
Offer feedback of the patient's expressed feelings
Encourage the sharing of common problems with others
Encourage the person to face grief
Encourage the use of normal coping mechanisms
Explore superficial topics and reasons for avoiding in-depth feelings
Explore with the patient his strengths and resources
Explore with the patient reasons for self-criticism (about his wanting to grieve)
Support a realistic assessment of the situation
Recognize the need for the use of appropriate defense mechanisms
Recognize the need for unique personal adjustments to change
Refrain from negatively criticizing

Nursing Observations

Determine the degree of insight
Estimate the degree of stress experienced
Evaluate the person's relatedness with others
Evaluate the significance of emotional distress mannerisms
Evaluate the significance of nonverbal communication
Identify disturbing conversation topics
Identify emotion-stimulating events
Observe for an excessive stress level
Observe for impaired self-attitudes
Observe for evidence that the patient is reaching out for emotional support
Observe for evidence of a favorable response to therapy

Health Teaching

Explain that the person's emotional response is appropriate and commonly experienced
Explain and offer hope that the emotional pain will decrease with time
Advise that negative responses from others be regarded with minimum significance (regarding grieving)

Advise that significant persons express acceptance of one another
Explain the importance of offering emotional support to one another
Describe the normal stages of grief
Emphasize the importance of recognizing tension within oneself
Explain how to obtain release from emotional stress
Explain that undesirable thoughts and feelings are normal
Advise that children participate in grief-related activities

EVALUATION

See the evaluation criteria for each specific goal in Chapter 2.

Inability to Control Grief (264,494)

ASSESSMENT

Subjective Data
Overwhelming grief
Exhaustion

Objective Data
Sobbing
Hysterical behavior
Loss of emotional control
Inability to function

Related Data
Commonly Related Diseases:
Any disease or injury

POSSIBLE ETIOLOGY

An attempt to relieve emotional tension or hurt and to restore inner equilibrium. Severe depression.

NURSING DIAGNOSIS

Inability to control grief: excessive audible lamenting as an expression of sorrow over one's loss

PLANNING

Patient Needs	Primary Nurse-Patient Goals
Comfort	To achieve comfort
Protection from psychologic threat	To prevent emotional injury
Warm, communicating relationships	To achieve effective verbal and nonverbal communications
Adequacy	To achieve positive expressions, feelings, reactions
Personal growth and maturity	To achieve optimum function
Increased learning	To achieve awareness of needs
Religious-philosophic satisfaction	To achieve spiritual goals

Increased reality perception and   To achieve optimum function
   problem-solving ability

NURSING INTERVENTIONS

Nursing Treatments
Approach unhurriedly
Express empathy
Demonstrate calmness
Avoid causing painful emotional situations
Use direct eye contact to terminate excessive crying
Encourage the expression of feelings
Listen attentively
    AND
Talk with the patient
Encourage the use of normal coping mechanisms
Encourage the use of spiritual resources
Explore with the patient his strengths and resources
Explore with the patient previous displays of courage
Explore with the patient the effects of his behavior on others
Give drugs judiciously for emotional repression
Provide seclusion (if needed)
Reduce the demands placed upon the patient
Refrain from performing nonessential procedures
Refrain from negatively criticizing
Set limits on unacceptable behavior
Suggest more appropriate means of emotional expression

Nursing Observations
Determine the degree of insight
Evaluate the person's relatedness with others
Evaluate the significance of emotional distress mannerisms
Evaluate the significance of nonverbal communication
Evaluate the significance of spirituality in the patient's life
Identify disturbing conversation topics
Identify emotion-stimulating events
Observe for evidence that the patient is reaching out for emotional support
Observe for behavior modification

Health Teaching
Explain and offer hope that the emotional pain will decrease with time
Advise that highly emotional situations be avoided
Advise that significant persons express love for one another
Explain the importance of offering emotional support to one another
Describe those symptoms which should be reported (personality disorders)
Explain how to obtain release from emotional stress
Explain why persons should maintain self-control
Explain how to channel emotional energy into activity

Recommend a habitual, positive mental attitude
Describe the behavior pattern indicating emotional maturity

Medical Treatments Performed by Nurses
Give the prescribed drug

EVALUATION

See the evaluation criteria for each specific goal in Chapter 2.

Inability to Resolve Grief (264,494)

ASSESSMENT

Subjective Data
Considerable thought is directed toward the deceased
Thoughts of the loved one remain painful and are not pleasurable even occasionally

Objective Data
Cannot renew old, external interests
Cannot find new persons with whom love can be shared and received
Continues to weep openly

Related Data
Grieving has lasted considerably longer than a year from the time of loss
Commonly Related Diseases:
None

POSSIBLE ETIOLOGY

Inability to cope with a serious loss. An inability to restructure life into a stable, meaningful situation.

NURSING DIAGNOSIS

Inability to resolve grief: the inability to work through and set aside one's loss and begin a new life

PLANNING

Patient Needs	Primary Nurse-Patient Goals
Comfort	To achieve comfort
Protection from psychologic threat	To prevent emotional injury
Warm, communicating relationships	To achieve effective verbal and nonverbal communications
Sense of value, usefulness, adequacy	To achieve positive expressions, feelings, reactions
Personal growth and maturity	To achieve optimum function
Increased learning	To achieve awareness of needs
Increased reality perception and problem-solving ability	To achieve optimum function

Increased pleasantness

To achieve positive expressions, feelings, reactions

NURSING INTERVENTIONS

Nursing Treatments

Approach unhurriedly
Provide an atmosphere of acceptance
Reassure verbally
Express empathy
Encourage the expression of feelings
Listen attentively
    AND
Talk with the patient
Offer feedback of the patient's expressed feelings
Explore superficial topics and reasons for avoiding in-depth feelings
Explore with the patient his strengths and resources
Explore with the patient the effects of his behavior on others
Support a realistic assessment of the situation
Assist the patient in restructuring his lifestyle
Assist the patient in setting standards of a meaningful existence
Emphasize the person's value as an individual
Encourage acceptance of the right to pleasure
Encourage a full day of activities
Encourage enhanced involvement in already established relationships
Encourage meaningful activity
Encourage renewal of former interests
Encourage planned one-day-at-a-time living
Encourage social activities
Encourage the use of normal coping mechanisms
Introduce to persons who have successfully undergone the same experience
Recognize the need for unique personal adjustments to change
Refrain from negatively criticizing
Encourage involvement in helping others

Nursing Observations

Determine the degree of insight
Estimate the degree of stress experienced
Evaluate the person's relatedness with others
Evaluate the significance of emotional distress mannerisms
Evaluate the significance of nonverbal communication
Identify disturbing conversation topics
Identify life values significant to the person
Identify appropriate use of defense mechanisms
Identify inappropriate use of defense mechanisms
Identify the current dominant emotion
Observe for an excessive stress level
Observe for impaired self-attitudes

Observe for evidence that the patient is reaching out for emotional support
Observe for evidence of a favorable response to therapy

Health Teaching
Explain and offer hope that the emotional pain will decrease with time
Advise that significant persons express love for one another
Explain the importance of offering emotional support to one another
Describe the normal stages of grief
Explain how to obtain release from emotional stress
Explain how to channel emotional energy into activity
Recommend a habitual, positive mental attitude

EVALUATION

See the evaluation criteria for each specific goal in Chapter 2.

Inadequate Emotional Support Related to Anticipatory Grieving (148,187,264, 360,494,502,508)

ASSESSMENT

Subjective Data
Awareness of an impending loss
Intense sadness and torment
Sense of helplessness
Unsettled, vaguely confused feeling
Feels that the grief is very difficult to endure
Feeling of weakness
Wants to escape the situation
Preoccupied with the anticipated loss

Objective Data
Appears forlorn and upset
At the time of need, the person has a limited, nonexistent, or temporarily
    absent support system of significant others
May reach out for help through crying, attention-seeking behavior, touching
    persons or objects, seeking someone to talk with, etc.
May appear withdrawn
Impending loss may be so intolerable that the person leaves the scene

Related Data
Commonly Related Diseases:
Any disease or injury

POSSIBLE ETIOLOGY

Lack of interest on the part of one's usually supportive world of family,
friends, and church. The unavailability of persons who usually offer support. The preoccupation of significant others with their own grieving so that

they are unable to be supportive. Undeniable awareness that the loss of a significant person or situation is about to occur.

NURSING DIAGNOSIS

Inadequate emotional support related to anticipatory grieving: little or no comfort or sustaining measures received from others while one is suffering the inner turmoil of grief and sorrow during the period prior to the death or loss of a significant person or factor in one's life

PLANNING

Patient Needs	Primary Nurse-Patient Goals
Comfort	To achieve comfort
Protection from psychologic threat	To prevent emotional injury
Warm, communicating relationships	To achieve effective verbal and nonverbal communications
Unity with loved ones	To achieve productive interpersonal relationships
Personal growth and maturity	To achieve optimum function
Increased learning	To achieve awareness of needs
Religious-philosophic satisfaction	To achieve spiritual goals

NURSING INTERVENTIONS

Nursing Treatments
Approach unhurriedly
Demonstrate calmness
Express empathy
Provide an atmosphere of acceptance
Touch the patient judiciously
Reassure verbally
Attend the patient constantly
    OR
Provide frequent patient contact
Encourage the expression of feelings
Listen attentively
    AND
Talk with the patient
Offer feedback of the patient's expressed feelings
Provide objects which symbolize safeness
Support a realistic assessment of the situation
Encourage the use of normal coping mechanisms
Explore with the patient his strengths and resources
Reduce the demands placed upon the patient
Refrain from performing nonessential procedures
Refrain from negatively criticizing

Call the patient's family to the bedside

OR

Encourage telephone calls between significant persons

} (if the patient prefers or strongly needs significant others and if the significant others are available as a support system)

Assist the family to prepare for life changes which will occur after the loved one's death

Encourage gradual mastery of a situation

Encourage planned one-day-at-a-time living

Encourage the use of spiritual resources

Recognize the need for unique personal adjustments to change

Nursing Observations

Determine the degree of insight

Estimate the degree of stress experienced

Evaluate the person's relatedness with others

Evaluate the significance of emotional distress mechanisms

Evaluate the significance of nonverbal communication

Identify disturbing conversation topics

Identify appropriate use of defense mechanisms

Identify inappropriate use of defense mechanisms

Observe for an excessive stress level

Observe for evidence of a favorable response to therapy

Health Teaching

Explain that the person's emotional response is appropriate and commonly experienced

Explain and offer hope that the emotional pain will decrease with time

Advise that significant persons express love for one another

Explain the importance of offering emotional support to one another

EVALUATION

See the evaluation criteria for each specific goal in Chapter 2.

Inadequate Emotional Support Related to Dying (148,187,264,360,494,502, 508)

ASSESSMENT

Subjective Data

An awareness that one's health condition is rapidly worsening

Sense of helplessness

Unsettled, vaguely confused feeling

No longer denies the approaching death, but feels that the thought of dying is very difficult to endure

Feeling of weakness

Wants to escape the situation

Preoccupied with his inner turmoil

In the predeath anger phase, the person experiences bitterness and resentment

In the predeath bargaining phase, the person secretly bargains with God for health and time

May perceive the illness as punishment, which increases guilt feelings

In the predeath depression phase, the person perceives with great sadness his loss of past and future meaningful persons, objects, and situations

Objective Data

Appears forlorn and upset

At the time of need, the person has a limited, nonexistent, or temporarily absent support system of significant others

May reach out for help through crying, attention-seeking behavior, touching persons or objects, seeking someone to talk with, etc.

May appear withdrawn

In the predeath anger phase, the person is quick to blame others

Complains chronically

Invokes negative responses from others through demanding behavior

In the predeath bargaining phase, the person may impose self-punishment

In the predeath depression phase, the person does not respond with hope to treatments

Related Data

Commonly Related Diseases:
Any fatal disease or injury
Depressive neurosis

POSSIBLE ETIOLOGY

Lack of interest on the part of one's usually supportive world of family, friends, and church. The unavailability of persons who usually offer support. The preoccupation of significant others with anticipatory grieving for the dying person, so that they are unable to be supportive. A need to adapt emotionally to the truth of approaching death.

NURSING DIAGNOSIS

Inadequate emotional support related to dying: little or no comfort or sustaining measures received from others while one is suffering the inner turmoil that results from awareness that one's life is soon to come to an end

PLANNING

Patient Needs	**Primary Nurse-Patient Goals**
Comfort	To achieve comfort
Protection from psychologic threat	To prevent emotional injury
Acceptance	To achieve productive interpersonal relationships
Warm, communicating relationships	To achieve effective verbal and nonverbal communications

Unity with loved ones	To achieve productive interpersonal relationships
High evaluation of self, adequacy, endurance	To achieve positive expressions, feelings, reactions
Dignity	To achieve productive interpersonal relationships
Personal growth and maturity	To achieve optimum function
Increased learning	To achieve awareness of needs
Religious-philosophic satisfaction	To achieve spiritual goals

NURSING INTERVENTIONS

Nursing Treatments
Approach unhurriedly
Demonstrate calmness
Express empathy
Express warmth and friendliness
Provide an atmosphere of acceptance
Touch the patient judiciously
Reassure verbally
Attend the patient constantly
    OR
Provide frequent patient contact
Encourage the expression of feelings
Listen attentively
Talk with the patient
    BUT
Terminate emotionally threatening conversation immediately
Communicate that the nurse feels comfortable with the patient's discussions of death
Offer feedback of the patient's expressed feelings
Encourage patient questions (if such will relieve the distress)
Provide objects which symbolize safeness
Encourage mutual problem solving
Support a realistic assessment of the situation
Encourage gradual mastery of a situation
Encourage planned one-day-at-a-time living } (during the early stages of dying)
Encourage meaningful activity
Recognize the need for the use of appropriate defense mechanisms
Encourage the use of normal coping mechanisms
Encourage the use of spiritual resources
Explore with the patient his strengths and resources
Reduce the demands placed upon the patient
Refrain from performing nonessential procedures

Refrain from negatively criticizing

Call the patient's family to the
bedside

OR

Encourage telephone calls between
significant persons

} (if the patient prefers or strongly
needs significant others and if the
significant others are available as
a support system)

Involve the family (as much as possible)

Provide emotional support for persons significant to the patient (so they can
more adequately support the dying person)

Suggest that one relative remain with the dying person

Place in a room with a patient having a favorable prognosis

Provide conditions which the patient desires for peaceful dying

Refrain from making a specific length-of-life estimate

Reinforce concern throughout the entire illness

Assist the dying person with detachment from life

Assist the dying person with unfinished business

Nursing Observations

Determine the degree of insight

Estimate the degree of stress experienced

Evaluate the person's relatedness with others

Evaluate the significance of emotional distress mannerisms

Evaluate the significance of nonverbal communication

Evaluate the significance of spirituality in the patient's life

Identify disturbing conversation topics

Identify emotion-stimulating events

Identify life values significant to the person

Identify appropriate use of defense mechanisms

Identify inappropriate use of defense mechanisms

Observe for an excessive stress level

Observe for impaired self-attitudes

Determine the extent of the child's comprehension of death

Observe for evidence of a favorable response to therapy

Health Teaching

Explain that the person's emotional response is appropriate and commonly
experienced

Explain and offer hope that the emotional pain will decrease with time

Advise that significant persons express acceptance of one another

Advise that significant persons express love for one another

Explain the importance of offering emotional support to one another

Explain the importance of maintaining a positive self-attitude

Explain the causes of fear of death

EVALUATION

See the evaluation criteria for each specific goal in Chapter 2.

Inadequate Emotional Support Related to Grieving (148,187,264,360,494, 502,508)

ASSESSMENT

Subjective Data

Sense of helplessness
Unsettled, vaguely confused feeling
Feels that the grief is very difficult to endure
Feeling of weakness
Wants to escape the situation
Preoccupied with his loss
May wonder if his grieving is normal, since he receives little response from
    others
During the initial grief phase, the person:
    feels intensely sad
    feels lessened self-esteem
    feels a sense of unreality
    resists attempts by others to turn his thoughts away from the loss
Ambivalence
Guilt
Anger
Throat tightness
Intense threat
Panic, sometimes
Cannot accept that he could love another with the same depth
During the grief work phase, the person:
    perceives the deceased's personal belongings as symbolic of him
    dwells on memories of the deceased until each memory has been
      thoroughly worked over
    wonders if he will ever stop grieving
During the resolving grief phase, the person:
    dwells less and less on thoughts directed toward the deceased
    finds that thoughts of the loved one become less painful, even pleasur-
      able at times, and he feels he needs less emotional support

Objective Data

Appears forlorn and upset
At the time of need, the person has a limited, nonexistent, or temporarily
    absent support system of significant others
May reach out for help through crying, attention-seeking behavior, touching
    persons or objects, seeking someone to talk with, etc.
May appear withdrawn
During the initial grief phase, the person:
    displays disinterest in the environment
    displays periodic weeping

displays restlessness
displays aimlessness
is emotionally distant from others
displays slowed motor and speech activity
spends considerable time talking about the deceased
displays loss of appetite
displays insomnia
makes self-accusations for past unkindnesses shown the deceased
displays excessive activity until the emotional pain is tolerable
usually clings to favorite possessions (as a child to a toy)
During the grief work phase, the person:
unknowingly assumes some mannerisms or behavioral characteristics of the deceased
verbally idealizes the deceased, with concentration on good qualities and inability to remember faults
makes endowments or memorials in an attempt to symbolize the deceased
During the resolving grief phase, the person:
begins to renew old, external interests
attempts to find new persons with whom love can be shared and received and feels he needs less emotional support

Related Data

Children respond to loved one's death differently at various ages. Prior to age 3 years, there is little or no understanding of death; the primary concern is separation from the mother. At age 5 years, death is perceived as an end that can be reversed; children recognize that the dead cannot move; their reaction is unemotional. The child of 6 years is aware of death, responds emotionally, relates death to illness, and fears that his parents may die and leave him; he does not believe he will ever die. At age 7 years, the cause of death and burial rites are an interest; the child suspects he may die, but denies it. At age 8 years, interest centers on the hereafter and there is acceptance that everyone dies. The child of 9 years accepts the inevitability of his death but is too preoccupied to be interested.

Commonly Related Conditions:
Death
Job loss
Retirement
Divorce
Geographic changes
Isolation
Loneliness

Commonly Related Diseases:
Any disease or injury, especially those causing paralysis of the body or body parts or loss of body function

POSSIBLE ETIOLOGY

Lack of interest on the part of one's usually supportive world of family, friends, and church. The unavailability of persons who usually offer support. The preoccupation of significant others with their own grieving, so that they are unable to be supportive. The need to grieve when a love, identity, and dependence relationship is interrupted and the consciousness gradually attempts to detach itself from the loss, reestablish emotional stability, and restructure life into a stable, meaningful situation.

NURSING DIAGNOSIS

Inadequate emotional support related to grieving: little or no comfort or sustaining measures received from others while one is suffering the inner turmoil that results when one loses a loved one, a body part, or a meaningful situation or object

PLANNING

Patient Needs	Primary Nurse-Patient Goals
Comfort	To achieve comfort
Protection from psychologic threat	To prevent emotional injury
Acceptance	To achieve productive interpersonal relationship
Warm, communicating relationships	To achieve effective verbal and nonverbal communications
Unity with loved ones	To achieve effective verbal and nonverbal communications
Adequacy, endurance	To achieve positive expressions, feelings, reactions
Personal growth and maturity	To achieve optimum function
Increased learning	To achieve awareness of needs
Religious-philosophic satisfaction	To achieve spiritual goals

NURSING INTERVENTIONS

Nursing Treatments
Approach unhurriedly
Demonstrate calmness
Express empathy
Express warmth and friendliness
Provide an atmosphere of acceptance
Touch the patient judiciously
Reassure verbally
Attend the patient constantly
    OR
Provide frequent patient contact

Encourage the expression of feelings
Listen attentively
AND
Talk with the patient
Offer feedback of the patient's expressed feelings
Provide objects which symbolize safeness
Support a realistic assessment of the situation
Introduce to persons who have successfully undergone the same experience
Recognize the need for the use of appropriate defense mechanisms
Encourage the use of normal coping mechanisms
Explore with the patient his strengths and resources
Reduce the demands placed upon the patient
Refrain from performing nonessential procedures
Refrain from negatively criticizing
Call the patient's family to
  the bedside
OR
Encourage telephone calls
  between significant persons
} (if the patient prefers or strongly needs significant others and if the significant others are available as a support system)

Avoid causing painful emotional situations
Discourage decision-making when one is under severe stress
Encourage gradual mastery of a situation
Encourage planned one-day-at-a-time living
Encourage the use of normal coping mechanisms
Encourage the use of spiritual resources
Recognize the need for unique personal adjustments to change

Nursing Observations
Determine the degree of insight
Estimate the degree of stress experienced
Evaluate the person's relatedness with others
Evaluate the significance of emotional distress mannerisms
Evaluate the significance of nonverbal communication
Identify disturbing conversation topics
Identify appropriate use of defense mechanisms
Identify inappropriate use of defense mechanisms
Observe for an excessive stress level
Determine the extent of the child's comprehension of death
Observe for evidence of a favorable response to therapy

Health Teaching
Explain that the person's emotional response is appropriate and commonly experienced
Explain and offer hope that the emotional pain will decrease with time
Advise that significant persons express love for one another
Explain the importance of offering emotional support to one another
Describe the normal stages of grief
Advise against correlating God's love and death to children
Advise that children participate in grief-related activities

EVALUATION

See the evaluation criteria for each specific goal in Chapter 2.

Inadequate Emotional Support Related to Poor Prognosis (140,148,173,187, 248,504,508)

ASSESSMENT

Subjective Data

Sense of helplessness

Unsettled, vaguely confused feeling

Feels that the poor prognosis is difficult to endure

Feeling of weakness

Wants to escape the situation

Preoccupied much of the time with thoughts of the poor prognosis

Is struggling internally to cope with the reality of the situation

Feels overwhelmed for some time following the revelation of the poor prognosis

Objective Data

Appears forlorn and upset after recently being told of the prognosis

At the time of need, the person has a limited, nonexistent, or temporarily absent support system of significant others

May reach out for help through crying, attention-seeking behavior, touching persons or objects, seeking someone to talk with, etc.

Related Data

Commonly Related Diseases:

Carcinoma

Glomerulonephritis

Parkinson's disease

Cerebral vascular accident

Leukemia

Aplastic anemia

POSSIBLE ETIOLOGY

Lack of interest on the part of one's usually supportive world of family, friends, and church. The unavailability of persons who usually offer support. The preoccupation of significant others who are trying to cope with their own reaction to the poor prognosis of their loved one, so that they are unable to be supportive.

NURSING DIAGNOSIS

Inadequate emotional support related to poor prognosis: little or no comfort or sustaining measures received from others during the period when one is trying to adjust emotionally to the reality of an unfavorable outlook regarding disease progression

PLANNING

Patient Needs	**Primary Nurse-Patient Goals**
Comfort	To achieve comfort
Protection from psychologic threat	To prevent emotional injury
Warm, communicating relationships	To achieve effective verbal and nonverbal communications
Adequacy, endurance	To achieve positive expressions, feelings, reactions
Personal growth and maturity	To achieve optimum function
Increased learning	To achieve awareness of needs
Religious-philosophic satisfaction	To achieve spiritual goals
Increased reality perception and problem-solving ability	To achieve optimum function

NURSING INTERVENTIONS

Nursing Treatments
Approach unhurriedly
Demonstrate calmness
Express empathy
Express warmth and friendliness
Provide an atmosphere of acceptance
Touch the patient judiciously
Reassure verbally
Offer hope
Attend the patient constantly
   OR
Provide frequent patient contact
Encourage the expression of feelings
Listen attentively
Talk with the patient
   BUT
Terminate emotionally threatening conversation immediately
Offer feedback of the patient's expressed feelings
Encourage patient questions (if such will relieve the distress)
Provide reliable information
Do not allow unpleasant surprise situations
Provide objects which symbolize safeness
Encourage mutual problem solving
Support a realistic assessment of the situation
Introduce to persons who have successfully undergone the same experience
Recognize the need for the use of appropriate defense mechanisms
Encourage the use of normal coping mechanisms
Encourage the use of spiritual resources
Explore with the patient his strengths and resources

Reduce the demands placed upon the patient
Refrain from performing nonessential procedures
Refrain from negatively criticizing
Call the patient's family to the
  bedside
  OR
Encourage telephone calls
  between significant persons
} (if the patient prefers or strongly needs significant others and if the significant others are available as a support system)
Assist the patient in setting standards of a meaningful existence
Encourage meaningful activity
Emphasize the person's value as an individual
Encourage gradual mastery of a situation
Encourage planned one-day-at-a-time living
Explore with the patient previous displays of courage
Recognize the need for unique personal adjustments to change

Nursing Observations
Determine the degree of insight
Determine the extent of the comprehension of a poor prognosis
Estimate the degree of stress experienced
Evaluate the person's relatedness with others
Evaluate the significance of emotional distress mannerisms
Evaluate the significance of nonverbal communication
Evaluate the significance of spirituality in the patient's life
Identify disturbing conversation topics
Identify inappropriate emotional responses
Identify reality-acceptance clues
Identify life values significant to the person
Identify appropriate use of defense mechanisms
Identify inappropriate use of defense mechanisms
Identify the current dominant emotion
Observe for an excessive stress level
Observe for impaired self-attitudes
Observe for evidence of a favorable response to therapy

Health Teaching
Explain that the person's emotional response is appropriate and commonly
  experienced
Explain and offer hope that the emotional pain will decrease with time
Advise that a poor prognosis be shared with significant others
Advise that significant persons express love for one another
Explain the importance of offering emotional support to one another
Explain how to obtain release from emotional stress
Recommend a habitual, positive mental attitude

EVALUATION

See the evaluation criteria for each specific goal in Chapter 2.

Inadequate Family Support Related to Predeath Acceptance (140,148,173, 187,248,504,508)

ASSESSMENT

Subjective Data

Person is aware that his family cannot yet accept losing him

Person does not want life prolonged, but struggles to stay alive for his family

Wishes to die in peace

Perceives that death would be a relief

Objective Data

Person who is dying gives evidence of having accepted the approaching death by:

being passive

frequently sleeping

narrowing interests

preferring not to be bothered but being left alone

not talking much to visitors

The family gives evidence of not having accepted the approaching death by:

refusing to discuss the possibility of death with the person

discussing what they will do when the patient gets well

verbalizing that he cannot die because they cannot go on without him

Related Data

Commonly Related Diseases:

Any fatal disease

POSSIBLE ETIOLOGY

The existence of sufficient time and emotional maturity on the part of the ill person to relinquish the struggle for life, accompanied by an inability or lack of time for the family to have coped with the reality of his approaching death.

NURSING DIAGNOSIS

Inadequate family support related to predeath acceptance: a lack of family acceptance of a loved one's approaching death that exists after the ill loved one has accepted and is resigned to the reality of his own nearness to death

PLANNING

Patient Needs	Primary Nurse-Patient Goals
Comfort	To achieve comfort
Protection from psychologic threat	To prevent emotional injury
Warm, communicating relationships	To achieve effective verbal and nonverbal communications
Unity with loved ones	To achieve productive interpersonal relationships

Dignity	To achieve productive interpersonal relationships
Increased learning (by the family)	To achieve awareness of needs
Religious-philosophic satisfaction	To achieve spiritual goals

NURSING INTERVENTIONS

Nursing Treatments
Approach unhurriedly
Demonstrate calmness
Express empathy
Express warmth and friendliness
Provide an atmosphere of acceptance
Tough the patient judiciously
Reassure verbally
Avoid reinforcing hope after predeath acceptance
Attend the patient constantly
    OR
Provide frequent patient contact
Encourage the expression of feelings (by both the patient and the family)
Ask questions (of family members) which encourage answers that reflect reality perception
Explore superficial topics and reasons for avoiding in-depth feelings
Listen attentively
    AND
Talk with the patient (and the family)
Offer feedback of the patient's expressed feelings
Encourage patient questions (if such will relieve the distress)
Encourage mutual problem solving
Support a realistic assessment of the situation (by the family, and by the patient, as regards the loved one's emotions)
Encourage the use of normal coping mechanisms
Encourage the use of spiritual resources (by the family)
Recognize the need for unique personal adjustments to change
Refrain from negatively criticizing (the family)
Involve the family (as much as possible)
Encourage family support of the patient's acceptance of death
Assist the family to prepare for life changes which will occur after the loved one's death
Provide emotional support for persons significant to the patient

Nursing Observations
Determine the degree of insight (by both the patient and the family)
Evaluate the significance of emotional distress mannerisms
Evaluate the significance of nonverbal communication
Identify disturbing conversation topics
Observe for behavior modification (by the family)

Health Teaching
Advise that significant persons express love for one another

Explain the importance of offering emotional support to one another

EVALUATION

See the evaluation criteria for each specific goal in Chapter 2.

LOVE AND AFFECTION

Impaired Ability to Express Love (156,157)

ASSESSMENT

Subjective Data
Embarrassment
Strong feelings of love

Objective Data
Slow in leading up to verbal expressions of love
Avoids verbal expressions of love, but performs activities which are hoped
   will be interpreted as expressions of love

Related Data
Commonly Related Diseases:
None

POSSIBLE ETIOLOGY

Poor social skills. Lack of self-confidence. Fear of rejection. The person did
not experience the feeling of love in the oral stage, and not having felt love,
does not know how to give love. The person never learned to trust, so he
mistrusts.

NURSING DIAGNOSIS

Inability to express love: difficulty in outwardly demonstrating to others
love that is felt for them

PLANNING

Patient Needs	Primary Nurse-Patient Goals
Comfort	To achieve comfort
Protection from psychologic threat	To prevent emotional injury
Acceptance	To achieve productive interpersonal relationships
Warm, communicating relationships	To achieve effective verbal and nonverbal communications
Adequacy	To achieve positive expressions, feelings, reactions
Personal growth and maturity	To achieve optimum function
Increased learning	To achieve awareness of needs

NURSING INTERVENTIONS

Nursing Treatments

Approach unhurriedly
Provide an atmosphere of acceptance
Reassure verbally
Encourage the expression of feelings
Listen attentively
   AND
Talk with the patient
Offer feedback of the patient's expressed feelings
Create giving situations
Provide emotionally safe experiences
Encourage awareness of positive responses from others
Explore superficial topics and reasons for avoiding in-depth feelings
Explore with the patient his strength and resources
Explore with the patient how he would feel in situations experienced by
   others (if love was not expressed)
Explore with the patient reasons for recurring problems (related to the ina-
   bility to express love)
Explore with the patient the effects of his behavior on others
Recognize the need for the use of appropriate defense mechanisms
Refrain from negatively criticizing

Nursing Observations

Determine the degree of insight
Evaluate the person's relatedness with others
Evaluate the significance of nonverbal communication
Identify disturbing conversation topics
Identify life values significant to the person
Identify appropriate use of defense mechanisms
Identify inappropriate use of defense mechanisms
Observe for an excessive stress level
Observe for impaired self-attitudes
Observe for evidence that the patient is reaching out for emotional support
Observe for a favorable response to therapy

Health Teaching

Advise that negative responses from others be regarded with minimum
   significance
Advise that significant persons express acceptance of one another
Advise that significant persons express love for one another
Explain the importance of offering emotional support to one another
Explain the importance of maintaining a positive self-attitude
Explain the causes of the health problem

EVALUATION

See the evaluation criteria for each specific goal in Chapter 2.

Impaired Ability to Receive Love (156,157)

ASSESSMENT

Subjective Data
Internal uneasiness
Rejects the possibility that he is loved for what he is
Thinks that love given to him is based on ulterior motives
Fears loss of individuality if he allows others to love him

Objective Data
Gruff attitude
Pushes the loving person away
Fails to return love gestures

Related Data
Commonly Related Diseases:
None

POSSIBLE ETIOLOGY

Past unpleasant love experiences. An attempt to protect oneself against emotional hurt. The person did not experience the feeling of love in the oral stage, and not having felt love, does not know how to give love. The person never learned to trust, so he mistrusts.

NURSING DIAGNOSIS

Imparied ability to receive: discomfort when accepting love from others

PLANNING

Patient Needs	Primary Nurse-Patient Goals
Comfort	To achieve comfort
Protection from psychologic threat	To prevent emotional injury
Acceptance	To achieve productive interpersonal relationships
Warm, communicating relationships	To achieve effective verbal and nonverbal communications
Adequacy	To achieve positive expressions, feelings, reactions
Personal growth and maturity	To achieve optimum function
Increased learning	To achieve awareness of needs

NURSING INTERVENTIONS

Nursing Treatments
Approach unhurriedly
Provide an atmosphere of acceptance
Encourage the expression of feelings
Listen attentively
AND
Talk with the patient

Offer feedback of the patient's expressed feelings
Provide receiving situations
Provide emotionally safe experiences
Encourage awareness of positive responses from others
Explore superficial topics and reasons for avoiding in-depth feelings
Explore with the patient his strengths and resources
Explore with the patient how he would feel in situations experienced by others (if his love was not accepted)
Explore with the patient reasons for recurring problems (related to the inability to receive love)
Explore with the patient the effects of his behavior on others
Recognize the need for the use of appropriate defense mechanisms
Refrain from negatively criticizing

Nursing Observations
Determine the degree of insight
Evaluate the person's relatedness with others
Evaluate the significance of emotional distress mannerisms
Evaluate the significance of nonverbal communication
Identify disturbing conversation topics
Identify life values significant to the person
Identify appropriate use of defense mechanisms
Identify inappropriate use of defense mechanisms
Observe for impaired self-attitude
Observe for evidence that the patient is reaching out for emotional support
Observe for a favorable response to therapy

Health Teaching
Advise that negative responses from others be regarded with minimum significance
Advise that significant persons express acceptance of one another
Advise that significant persons express love for one another
Explain the importance of offering emotional support to one another
Explain the importance of maintaining a positive self-attitude
Explain the causes of the health problem

EVALUATION

See the evaluation criteria for each specific goal in Chapter 2.

Inadequate Parent-Child Bonding

ASSESSMENT

Subjective Data
Parent feels little or no attachment to his or her child
May feel angry about the responsibility the child has brought
Does not perceive herself or himself as a parent

Objective Data
Parent does not hold the baby
Does not make eye contact with the baby

Leaves the baby unattended on the bed

Does not talk to the baby

OR

May talk to the baby at length about the pain and suffering it caused the mother during birth

Refers to the child as it, he, or she rather than calling the infant by name

If the child is a girl, the parent may refer to her as him, especially if the parent wanted a boy

Displays little or no interest in the child

May be neglectful in failing to feed, clothe, bathe, or supervise the child

May be abusive in that the parent inflicts physical or mental harm on the child

Related Data

Commonly Related Conditions:

Failure to thrive

Commonly Related Diseases:

None

POSSIBLE ETIOLOGY

Childhood rejection of the adult by his own parents. Hostility toward the child. Parental emotional instability. Parental inability to assume responsibility. Feelings of parental inadequacy. A very young mother may be unable to assume the parent role since she has not completed her own childhood developmental stage.

NURSING DIAGNOSIS

Inadequate parent-child bonding: lack of a parent's feeling of union or love for and responsibility to his or her child.

PLANNING

Patient Needs	**Primary Nurse-Patient Goals**
Protection from psychologic threat	To prevent emotional injury
Acceptance	To achieve productive interpersonal relationships
Warm, communicating relationships	To achieve effective verbal and nonverbal communications
Adequacy	To achieve positive expressions, feelings, reactions
Personal growth and maturity	To achieve optimum function
Increased learning	To achieve awareness of needs and/or use of resources
Increased reality perception	To achieve optimum function

NURSING INTERVENTIONS

Nursing Treatments

Provide an atmosphere of acceptance

Express warmth and friendliness
Touch the patient judiciously
Encourage acceptance of responsibility (for the child)
Encourage awareness of positive responses from others (the child)
Encourage the expression of feelings
Listen attentively
    AND
Talk with the patient
Offer feedback of the patient's expressed feelings
Create giving situations
Provide emotionally safe experiences
Encourage participation in therapeutic group interaction
Encourage recognition of one's various roles in life
Encourage role-playing to develop sensitivity
Encourage the use of normal coping mechanisms
Explore superficial topics and reasons for avoiding in-depth feelings
Explore with the patient his strengths and resources
Explore with the patient reasons for recurring problems
Explore with the patient the effects of his behavior on others
Introduce to persons who have successfully undergone the same experience
Recognize the need for appropriate defense mechanisms
Recognize the need for unique personal adjustments to change
Refrain from negatively criticizing
Support a realistic assessment of the situation

Nursing Observations
Determine the degree of insight
Evaluate the person's relatedness with others
Evaluate the significance of nonverbal communication
Identify disturbing conversation topics
Identify inappropriate emotional responses
Identify life values significant to the person
Identify appropriate use of defense mechanisms
Identify inappropriate use of defense mechanisms
Identify the current dominant emotion
Observe for an excessive stress level
Observe for evidence that the patient is reaching out for emotional support
Observe for behavior modification

Health Teaching
Advise early correction of problems
Emphasize the importance of recognizing tension within oneself
Explain the importance of maintaining a positive self-attitude
Explain that parental attitudes affect child development
Explain that undesirable thoughts and feelings are normal
Explain the causes of the health problem

EVALUATION

See the evaluation criteria for each specific goal in Chapter 2.

Intimacy Avoidance (156,157)

ASSESSMENT

Subjective Data

Feels uncomfortable when there is a possibility of intimacy with others

Objective Data

Avoids activities that require involvement with others
An aloof manner
Does not give affection responses or encourage them from others
Indulges in work almost to the exclusion of all else

Related Data

Commonly Related Diseases:
None
   OR
Schizophrenia

POSSIBLE ETIOLOGY

Parental discouragement of closeness during childhood. Fear of emotional hurt.

NURSING DIAGNOSIS

Intimacy avoidance: an attempt to delay or avoid having emotional feelings or involvement with a person or situation

PLANNING

Patient Needs	Primary Nurse-Patient Goals
Comfort	To achieve comfort
Protection from psychologic threat	To prevent emotional injury
Acceptance	To achieve productive interpersonal relationships
Warm, communicating relationships	To achieve effective verbal and nonverbal communications
Adequacy	To achieve positive expressions, feelings, reactions
Personal growth and maturity	To achieve optimum function
Increased learning	To achieve awareness of needs

NURSING INTERVENTIONS

Nursing Treatments

Approach unhurriedly
Provide an atmosphere of acceptance
Reassure verbally
Encourage the expression of feelings
Listen attentively
   AND
Talk with the patient
Offer feedback of the patient's expressed feelings
Create giving situations

Provide receiving situations
Provide emotionally safe experiences
Encourage awareness of positive responses from others
Explore superficial topics and reasons for avoiding in-depth feelings
Explore with the patient his strengths and resources
Explore with the patient how he would feel in situations experienced by others (if others avoided intimacy with him)
Explore with the patient reasons for recurring problems (related to the intimacy avoidance)
Explore with the patient the effects of his behavior on others
Recognize the need for the use of appropriate defense mechanisms
Refrain from negatively criticizing

Nursing Observations
Determine the degree of insight
Evaluate the person's relatedness with others
Evaluate the significance of emotional distress mannerisms
Evaluate the significance of nonverbal communication
Identify disturbing conversation topics
Identify life values significant to the person
Identify appropriate use of defense mechanisms
Identify inappropriate use of defense mechanisms
Observe for an excessive stress level
Observe for impaired self-attitudes
Observe for evidence that the patient is reaching out for emotional support
Observe for a favorable response to therapy

Health Teaching
Advise that negative responses from others be regarded with minimum significance
Advise that significant persons express acceptance of one another
Advise that significant persons express love for one another
Explain the importance of offering emotional support to one another
Explain the importance of maintaining a positive self-attitude
Explain the causes of the health problem

EVALUATION

See the evaluation criteria for each specific goal in Chapter 2.

Maladaptive Love Response (156,157)

ASSESSMENT

Subjective Data
Perceives the giving of love to another as a loss of one's self

Objective Data
Gives love only on the condition that the person meet standards set up by the lover
Withholds love from persons to whom giving love is appropriate
Limits one's love relationship to only one person in an exclusive love relationship

Protects the loved person to the point of denying that person the opportunity for self-actualization

Total submission of oneself to another person

Related Data

Commonly Related Diseases:
None
> OR

Psychoneurosis

POSSIBLE ETIOLOGY

A desire to control the recipient of love to satisfy one's own needs. Inability to give love because of painful past love experiences. Early feelings of rejection because of parents' constant messages of disapproval. Poor development of the skills of loving. Hostility toward the loved one. Love needs were unmet in the oral stage causing a sense of separateness and isolation. Lack of understanding regarding the qualities of mature love and trust. Strong dependency needs. Feelings of low self-esteem or inadequacy.

NURSING DIAGNOSIS

Maladaptive love responses: the inability to exchange mature love between persons, wherein growth and development are fostered in one party by the other

PLANNING

Patient Needs	**Primary Nurse-Patient Goals**
Protection from psychologic threat	To prevent emotional injury
Acceptance	To achieve productive interpersonal relationships
Warm, communicating relationships	To achieve effective verbal and nonverbal communications
High evaluation of self, adequacy	To achieve positive expressions, feelings, reactions
Independence	To achieve optimum function
Personal growth and maturity	To achieve optimum function
Increased learning	To achieve awareness of needs

NURSING INTERVENTIONS

Nursing Treatments
Approach unhurriedly
Provide an atmosphere of acceptance
Reassure verbally
Encourage the expression of feelings
Listen attentively
> AND

Talk with the patient
Offer feedback of the patient's expressed feelings
Provide emotionally safe experiences

Explore superficial topics and reasons for avoiding in-depth feelings
Explore with the patient his strengths and resources
Explore with the patient how he would feel in situations experienced by
  others
Explore with the patient reasons for recurring problems
Explore with the patient the effects of his behavior on others
Recognize the need for the use of appropriate defense mechanisms
Refrain from negatively criticizing
Make a referral (to a psychiatric nurse specialist)

Nursing Observations
Determine the degree of insight
Evaluate the person's relatedness with others
Evaluate the significance of emotional distress mannerisms
Evaluate the significance of nonverbal communication
Identify disturbing conversation topics
Identify life values significant to the person
Identify appropriate use of defense mechanisms
Identify inappropriate use of defense mechanisms
Observe for an excessive stress level
Observe for impaired self-attitudes
Observe for evidence that the patient is reaching out for emotional support
Observe for behavior modification

Health Teaching
Advise against causing defensive responses in others
Advise against communicating double-meaning messages
Explain the importance of offering emotional support to one another
Explain the importance of maintaining a positive self-attitude
Recommend that independence be encouraged (in a love relationship)
Recommend that behavioral limits be set
Explain how to set behavioral limits

EVALUATION

See the evaluation criteria for each specific goal in Chapter 2.

Maladaptive Response to Adequate Loving (156,157)

ASSESSMENT

Subjective Data
Fails to perceive his love relationship as inadequate

Objective Data
Expects others to be exceptionally thoughtful
Finds fault with others who fail to meet his excessive need for love
Wants love on his terms only
Wants many frequent attentions
Wants constant evidence that the lover still loves and approves of him

Related Data

Commonly Related Diseases:
None
   OR
Psychoneurosis

POSSIBLE ETIOLOGY

Feelings of low self-esteem or inadequacy. Need to dominate the love relationship. Never developed basic trust in the oral stage of development.

NURSING DIAGNOSIS

Maladaptive response to adequate loving: a demand for more love than is being given even though the love being given is adequate

PLANNING

Patient Needs	**Primary Nurse-Patient Goals**
Comfort	To achieve comfort
Protection from psychologic threat	To prevent emotional injury
Acceptance	To achieve productive interpersonal relationships
Warm, communicating relationships	To achieve effective verbal and nonverbal communications
High evaluation of self, adequacy	To achieve positive expressions, feelings, reactions
Personal growth and maturity	To achieve optimum function
Increased learning	To achieve awareness of needs
Increased reality perception and problem-solving ability	To achieve optimum function

NURSING INTERVENTIONS

Nursing Treatments
Approach unhurriedly
Provide an atmosphere of acceptance
Reassure verbally
Encourage the expression of feelings
Listen attentively
   AND
Talk with the patient
Offer feedback of the patient's expressed feelings
Explore superficial topics and reasons for avoiding in-depth feelings
Explore with the patient reasons for recurring problems
Explore with the patient the effects of his behavior on others
Explore with the patient the need for approval
Explore with the patient the need for attention
Explore with the patient the need for dominance
Recognize the need for the use of appropriate defense mechanisms
Refrain from negatively criticizing
Make a referral (to a psychiatric nurse specialist)

Nursing Observations

Determine the degree of insight
Evaluate the person's relatedness with others
Evaluate the significance of emotional distress mannerisms
Evaluate the significance of nonverbal communication
Identify disturbing conversation topics
Observe for an excessive stress level
Observe for impaired self-attitudes
Observe for evidence that the patient is reaching out for emotional support
Observe for behavior modification

Health Teaching

Advise that negative responses from others be regarded with minimum
    significance
Emphasize the need for realistic expectations of others
Explain the causes of the health problem
Recommend that behavioral limits be set
Explain how to set behavioral limits

EVALUATION

See the evaluation criteria for each specific goal in Chapter 2.

GUILT

Guilt Related to Genetic Imperfections of Offspring (33,239,403)

ASSESSMENT

Subjective Data

Feelings of remorse or regret
Repeated self-accusation and self-condemnation
Feelings of disgrace and dishonor
Cannot forgive himself
Expects reproach from others, usually close relatives
Preoccupied with the situation

Objective Data

Person has parented a child with some physical or mental defect
May behave in a manner that forces punishment on himself

Related Data

Commonly Related Conditions:
Mental retardation
Deafness
Blindness
Prematurity

Commonly Related Diseases:
Mongolism
Hydrocephalus
Cerebral palsy

POSSIBLE ETIOLOGY

The perception that the child's weakness is a result of hereditary factors. The interpretation of one's own behavior as being at variance with or contrary to the standards one has set for oneself.

NURSING DIAGNOSIS

Guilt related to genetic imperfections of offspring: feelings of guilt about having transmitted to a child defective hereditary characteristics resulting in the child's physical or mental weakness

PLANNING

Patient Needs	Primary Nurse-Patient Goals
Comfort	To achieve comfort
Protection from psychologic threat	To prevent emotional injury
Acceptance	To achieve productive interpersonal relationships
Warm, communicating relationships	To achieve effective verbal and nonverbal communications
Personal growth and maturity	To achieve optimum function
Increased learning	To achieve awareness of needs
Increased reality perception and problem-solving ability	To achieve optimum function

NURSING INTERVENTIONS

Nursing Treatments
Approach unhurriedly
Provide an atmosphere of acceptance
Express empathy
Reassure verbally
Provide frequent patient contact
Encourage acceptance of forgiveness offered by others
Encourage the expression of feelings
Listen attentively
  AND
Talk with the patient
Offer feedback of the patient's expressed feelings
Provide reliable information
Encourage the sharing of common problems with others
Encourage strivings toward realistic goals (of helping the child overcome his weakness)
Encourage the use of normal coping mechanisms
Explore with the patient his strengths and resources (and those of the child)
Explore with the patient reasons for self-criticism
Explore with the patient the effects of his behavior on others (how one's guilt affects the child's self-perception)
Introduce to persons who have successfully undergone the same experience
Involve the family (as much as possible)

Recognize the need for the use of appropriate defense mechanisms
Divert attention from preoccupation with guilt
Support a realistic assessment of the situation

Nursing Observations
Determine the extent of behavioral suggestibility (guilt implied by others)
Determine the degree of insight
Evaluate the person's relatedness with others
Evaluate the significance of emotional distress mannerisms
Evaluate the significance of nonverbal communication
Identify disturbing conversation topics
Identify life values significant to the person
Identify appropriate use of defense mechanisms
Identify inappropriate use of defense mechanisms
Observe for an excessive stress level
Observe for impaired self-attitudes
Observe for evidence that the patient is reaching out for emotional support
Observe for evidence of a favorable response to therapy

Health Teaching
Explain that the person's emotional response is appropriate and commonly
    experienced
Explain and offer hope that the emotional pain will decrease with time
Advise that negative responses from others be regarded with minimum
    significance
Advise that significant persons express acceptance of one another
Advise that significant persons express love for one another
Explain the importance of offering emotional support to one another
Explain the importance of maintaing a positive self-attitude
Explain how to obtain release from emotional stress
Explain the difference between a mature and a rigid conscience
Explain the difference between real and neurotic guilt
Explain the genetic factors involved in the disease

EVALUATION

See the evaluation criteria for each specific goal in Chapter 2.

Guilt Related to Injury Inflicted on Others (33,239,403)

ASSESSMENT

Subjective Data
Feelings of remorse or regret
Repeated self-accusation and self-condemnation
Feelings of disgrace and dishonor
Cannot forgive himself
Expects reproach from others
Preoccupation with the situation

Objective Data

Person has injured or killed someone in an automobile accident, fire, etc.

Person did not take proper precautionary measures, which led someone (often a child) to accidental drowning, poisoning, etc.

Person has physically abused someone else

Related Data

Commonly Related Conditions:

Poisoning

Drowning

Commonly Related Diseases:

First-, second-, or third-degree burns

Bone fracture

Cerebral concussion

POSSIBLE ETIOLOGY

The interpretation of one's own behavior as being at variance with or contrary to the standards one has set for oneself

NURSING DIAGNOSIS

Guilt related to injury inflicted on others: feelings of guilt about having caused injury to another through commission or omission

PLANNING

Patient Needs	Primary Nurse-Patient Goals
Comfort	To achieve comfort
Protection from psychologic threat	To prevent emotional injury
Acceptance	To achieve productive interpersonal relationships
Warm, communicating relationships	To achieve effective verbal and nonverbal communications
Personal growth and maturity	To achieve optimum function
Increased learning	To achieve awareness of needs
Increased reality perception and problem-solving ability	To achieve optimum function

NURSING INTERVENTIONS

Nursing Treatments

Approach unhurriedly

Provide an atmosphere of acceptance

Express empathy

Reassure verbally

Provide frequent patient contact

Divert attention from preoccupation with guilt

Encourage acceptance of forgiveness offered by others

Encourage admission of wrongdoing

Encourage the expression of feelings

Listen attentively
  AND
Talk with the patient
Offer feedback of the patient's expressed feelings
Encourage mutual problem solving
Recognize the need for the use of appropriate defense mechanisms
Encourage the use of normal coping mechanisms
Explore with the patient his strengths and resources
Explore with the patient reasons for self-criticism
Explore with the patient the effects of his behavior on others (when guilt
    affects his ability to function)
Suggest that reparation will diminish guilt
Support a realistic assessment of the situation
Introduce to persons who have successfully undergone the same experience
Refrain from negatively criticizing
Make a referral (to a psychiatric nurse specialist if the injury was from
    abuse)

Nursing Observations
Determine the degree of insight
Evaluate the person's relatedness with others
Evaluate the significance of emotional distress mannerisms
Evaluate the significance of nonverbal communication
Identify disturbing conversation topics
Identify life values significant to the person
Identify appropriate use of defense mechanisms
Identify inappropriate use of defense mechanisms
Observe for excessive talking
Observe for impaired self-attitudes
Observe for evidence that the patient is reaching out for emotional support
Observe for evidence of a favorable response to therapy

Health Teaching
Explain that the person's emotional response is appropriate and commonly
    experienced
Explain and offer hope that the emotional pain will decrease with time
Advise that negative responses from others be regarded with minimum
    significance
Advise that significant persons express acceptance of one another
Advise that significant persons express love for one another
Explain the importance of offering emotional support to one another
Explain the importance of maintaining a positive self-attitude
Explain how to obtain release from emotional stress
Explain the causes of the health problem

EVALUATION
See the evaluation criteria for each specific goal in Chapter 2.

Guilt Related to Moral Conflict
With Medical Ethics (33,239,403)

ASSESSMENT

Subjective Data

Feelings of remorse or regret

Repeated self-accusation and self-condemnation

Feelings of disgrace and dishonor

Cannot forgive himself

Preoccupation with the situation

If the treatment was unsuccessful, the person feels the lack of success is a
form of punishment

Objective Data

Person has:

agreed to allow a loved one to die

received a blood transfusion

taken medication that is morally objectionable to him

had an abortion because of pressure from others

had a sterilization procedure

Related Data

Commonly Related Diseases:

Any disease or injury

POSSIBLE ETIOLOGY

Differences in established moral and medical ethics. A tendency to revert to
long-established moral codes even after contrary moral decisions have been
made and put into effect. The interpretation of one's own behavior as being
at variance with or contrary to the standards one has set for oneself.

NURSING DIAGNOSIS

Guilt related to moral conflict with medical ethics: feelings of guilt about
having made a choice of and accepted health treatment that is contrary to
one's moral code but is acceptable to the medical community

PLANNING

Patient Needs	Primary Nurse-Patient Goals
Comfort	To achieve comfort
Protection from psychologic threat	To prevent emotional injury
Acceptance	To achieve productive interpersonal relationships
Warm, communicating relationships	To achieve effective verbal and nonverbal communications
Increased learning	To achieve awareness of needs
Religious-philosophic satisfaction	To achieve spiritual goals
Increased reality perception and problem-solving ability	To achieve optimum function

NURSING INTERVENTIONS

Nursing Treatments

Approach unhurriedly
Provide an atmosphere of acceptance
Express empathy
Reassure verbally
Provide frequent patient contact
Divert attention from preoccupation with guilt
Encourage acceptance of forgiveness offered by others
Encourage the expression of feelings
Listen attentively
    AND
Talk with the patient
Offer feedback of the patient's expressed feelings
Encourage identification of specific life values
Encourage the practical application of the accepted value system
Encourage the sharing of common problems with others
Encourage the use of normal coping mechanisms
Encourage the use of spiritual resources
Support a realistic assessment of the situation
Refrain from negatively criticizing
Make a referral (to a psychiatric nurse specialist and/or a chaplin)

Nursing Observations

Determine the degree of insight
Determine the extent of group pressure conformity
Evaluate the person's relatedness with others
Evaluate the significance of emotional distress mannerisms
Evaluate the significance of nonverbal communication
Identify disturbing conversation topics
Identify life values significant to the person
Identify appropriate use of defense mechanisms
Identify inappropriate use of defense mechanisms
Observe for an excessive stress level
Observe for impaired self-attitudes
Observe for evidence that the patient is reaching out for emotional support
Observe for evidence of a favorable response to therapy

Health Teaching

Explain that the person's emotional response is appropriate and commonly
    experienced
Advise that negative responses from others be regarded with minimum
    significance
Advise that significant persons express acceptance of one another
Advise that significant persons express love for one another
Explain the importance of offering emotional support to one another
Explain the importance of maintaining a positive self-attitude

Explain how to obtain release from emotional stress
Explain the difference between a mature and a rigid conscience

EVALUATION

See the evaluation criteria for each specific goal in Chapter 2.

Guilt Related to Irrevocable Past Behavior (33,239,403)

ASSESSMENT

Subjective Data

Feelings of remorse or regret
Repeated self-accusation and self-condemnation
Feeling of disgrace and dishonor
Cannot forgive himself
Expects reproach from others
Preoccupation with the situation
Contemplates what he could have done or should be doing for his loved one
Realizes that the opportunity to express feeling to the significant other is lost forever

Objective Data

Significant other is dying or has died
A person is dying and realizes that he has not done all he wanted to for those he is leaving behind

Related Data

Commonly Related Diseases:
Any disease or injury resulting in death

POSSIBLE ETIOLOGY

An awareness of the effect of one's behavior on others. The realization that the past cannot be changed once one of the persons involved has died. The interpretation of one's own behavior as being at variance with or contrary to the standards one has set for oneself.

NURSING DIAGNOSIS

Guilt related to irrevocable past behavior: feelings of guilt about not having performed kindnesses or about having indulged in unkindness toward a significant other to whom amends can no longer be made

PLANNING

Patient Needs	**Primary Nurse-Patient Goals**
Comfort	To achieve comfort
Protection from psychologic threat	To prevent emotional injury
Acceptance	To achieve productive interpersonal relationships
Warm, communicating relationships	To achieve effective verbal and nonverbal communications

Personal growth and maturity

Increased learning

Increased reality perception and problem-solving ability

To achieve optimum function

To achieve awareness of needs

To achieve optimum function

NURSING INTERVENTIONS

Nursing Treatments

Approach unhurriedly

Provide an atmosphere of acceptance

Express empathy

Reassure verbally

Provide frequent patient contact

Divert attention from preoccupation with guilt

Encourage acceptance of forgiveness offered by others

Encourage acceptance of self-limitations

Encourage admission of wrongdoing

Encourage the expression of feelings

Listen attentively
    AND
Talk with the patient

Offer feedback of the patient's expressed feelings

Encourage the sharing of common problems with others

Encourage the use of normal coping mechanisms

Explore with the patient reasons for self-criticism

Support a realistic assessment of the situation

Refrain from negatively criticizing

Nursing Observations

Determine the degree of insight

Evaluate the person's relatedness with others

Evaluate the significance of emotional distress mannerisms

Evaluate the significance of nonverbal communication

Identify disturbing conversation topics

Identify life values significant to the person

Identify appropriate use of defense mechanisms

Observe for an excessive stress level

Observe for impaired self-attitudes

Observe for evidence that the patient is reaching out for emotional support

Observe for evidence of a favorable response to therapy

Health Teaching

Explain that the person's emotional response is appropriate and commonly experienced

Advise that negative responses from others be regarded with minimum significance

Advise that significant persons express acceptance of one another

Advise that significant persons express love for one another

Explain the importance of offering emotional support to one another

Explain the importance of maintaining a positive self-attitude

Explain how to obtain release from emotional stress
Explain the difference between a mature and a rigid conscience
Explain the difference between real and neurotic guilt

EVALUATION

See the evaluation critièria for each specific goal in Chapter 2.

Guilt Related to the Burden of Illness on Others (33,239,403)

ASSESSMENT

Subjective Data

Feelings of remorse or regret
Repeated self-accusation and self-condemnation
Feelings of disgrace and dishonor
Person perceives that his illness has brought hardship and sorrow to others
Is preoccupied with the effect of his illness on others and how things might
  have been had he not become ill
Wonders about his loveworthiness
Wonders if the family feels unexpressed anger toward him
Senses the weariness of others who wait on him and their decreased resis-
  tance to exposure to illness
Feels that he deserves some reproach for having become a burden on others

Objective Data

Apologizes for being ill
Verbalizes comments indicating diminished self-esteem

Related Data

The more serious the illness and the resulting hardship on others, the greater the feeling of guilt

Commonly Related Diseases:

Any disease or injury

POSSIBLE ETIOLOGY

Feelings of inadequacy that one has not lived up to one's responsibilities or
self-established standards. The fact that illness does actually put a burden
on others.

NURSING DIAGNOSIS

Guilt related to the burden of illness on others: feelings of guilt regarding
the hardships and suffering that one's illness places on significant others

PLANNING

Patient Needs	Primary Nurse-Patient Goals
Comfort	To achieve comfort
Protection from psychologic threat	To prevent emotional injury
Acceptance	To achieve productive interpersonal relationships

Warm, communicating relationships

Unity with loved ones

High evaluation of self

Increased learning

To achieve effective verbal and nonverbal communications

To achieve productive interpersonal relationships

To achieve positive expressions, feelings, reactions

To achieve awareness of needs

NURSING INTERVENTIONS

Nursing Treatments
Approach unhurriedly
Provide an atmosphere of acceptance
Express empathy
Reassure verbally
Provide frequent patient contact
Divert attention from preoccupation with guilt
Encourage acceptance of forgiveness offered by others
Encourage acceptance of self-limitations
Encourage acceptance of responsibility (as much as possible)
Encourage the expression of feelings
Listen attentively
    AND
Talk with the patient
Offer feedback of the patient's expressed feelings
Encourage the sharing of common problems with others
Encourage the use of normal coping mechanisms
Explore with the patient reasons for self-criticism
Support a realistic assessment of the situation
Refrain from negatively criticizing

Nursing Observations
Determine the degree of insight
Evaluate the person's relatedness with others
Evaluate the significance of emotional distress mannerisms
Evaluate the significance of nonverbal communication
Identify disturbing conversation topics
Identify life values significant to the person
Identify appropriate use of defense mechanisms
Identify inappropriate use of defense mechanisms
Observe for an excessive stress level
Observe for impaired self-attitudes
Observe for evidence that the patient is reaching out for emotional support
Observe for evidence of a favorable response to therapy

Health Teaching
Explain that the person's emotional response is appropriate and commonly experienced
Advise that negative responses from others be regarded with minimum significance

Advise that significant persons express acceptance of one another
Advise that significant persons express love for one another
Explain the importance of offering emotional support to one another
Explain the importance of maintaining a positive self-attitude
Explain how to obtain release from emotional stress

EVALUATION

See the evaluation criteria for each specific goal in Chapter 2.

Guilt Related to the Perception of Illness as Punishment

ASSESSMENT

Subjective Data

Feelings of remorse or regret
Repeated self-accusation and self-condemnation
Feelings of disgrace and dishonor
Preoccupied with thoughts of past behavior that he perceives deserves
  punishment

Objective Data

Verbalizes comments indicating that he deserves the illness or that the illness is his own fault

Related Data

Commonly Related Diseases:
Any disease or injury

POSSIBLE ETIOLOGY

The interpretation of one's own behavior as being at variance with or contrary to the standards one has set for oneself

NURSING DIAGNOSIS

Guilt related to the perception of illness as punishment: feelings of guilt
evolving from interpreting one's illness as a punishment for past unacceptable behavior

PLANNING

Patient Needs	**Primary Nurse-Patient Goals**
Comfort	To achieve comfort
Protection from psychologic threat	To prevent emotional injury
Acceptance	To achieve productive interpersonal relationships
Warm, communicating relationships	To achieve effective verbal and nonverbal communications
Personal growth and maturity	To achieve optimum function
Increased learning	To achieve awareness of needs

Increased reality perception and   To achieve optimum function
   problem-solving ability

NURSING INTERVENTIONS

Nursing Treatments

Approach unhurriedly
Provide an atmosphere of acceptance
Express empathy
Reassure verbally
Provide frequent patient contact
Divert attention from preoccupation with guilt
Encourage the expression of feelings
Listen attentively
   AND
Talk with the patient
Offer feedback of the patient's expressed feelings
Encourage the sharing of common problems with others
Encourage the use of normal coping mechanisms
Explore with the patient reasons for self-criticism
Support a realistic assessment of the situation
Refrain from negatively criticizing

Nursing Observations

Determine the degree of insight
Evaluate the significance of emotional distress mannerisms
Evaluate the significance of nonverbal communication
Identify disturbing conversation topics
Identify life values significant to the person
Identify appropriate use of defense mechanisms
Identify inappropriate use of defense mechanisms
Observe for an excessive stress level
Observe for impaired self-attitudes
Observe for evidence that the patient is reaching out for emotional support
Observe for evidence of a favorable response to therapy

Health Teaching

Explain that the person's emotional response is appropriate and commonly
   experienced
Advise that negative responses from others be regarded with minimum
   significance
Advise that significant persons express acceptance of one another
Advise that significant persons express love for one another
Explain the importance of offering emotional support to one another
Explain the importance of maintaining a positive self-attitude
Explain how to obtain release from emotional stress
Explain the difference between a mature and a rigid conscience
Explain the difference between real and neurotic guilt

EVALUATION

See the evaluation criteria for each specific goal in Chapter 2.

LONELINESS

Inadequate Emotional Support Related to Aloneness (148,187,360,502,508)

ASSESSMENT

Subjective Data
Sense of helplessness
Unsettled, vaguely confused feeling
Feels that the aloneness is intensely difficult to endure
Feeling of weakness
Feels forsaken by others
Sense of isolation and emptiness
Feels there is no one to share his suffering with
Feels desolate, deserted, and all by himself
Watches people go by and is inwardly crying out to them
Wants to escape the situation
Preoccupation with the aloneness

Objective Data
Appears forlorn and upset
At the time of need, the person has a limited, nonexistent, or temporarily absent support system of significant others
May reach out for help through crying, attention-seeking behavior, touching persons or objects, seeking someone to talk with, etc.
Detains health personnel whenever possible
Starts conversations with strangers
May appear withdrawn

Related Data
Commonly Related Diseases:
Any disease or injury

POSSIBLE ETIOLOGY

Lack of interest on the part of one's usually supportive world of family, friends, and church. The unavailability of persons who usually offer support. Being alone for a prolonged period. Physical limitations. Health restrictions due to communicable disease. Long-term illness in one environmental setting.

PLANNING

Patient Needs	Primary Nurse-Patient Goals
Comfort	To achieve comfort
Protection from psychologic threat	To prevent emotional injury
Warm, communicating relationships	To achieve effective verbal and nonverbal communications
Group companionship	To achieve productive interpersonal relationships
Attention	To achieve productive interpersonal relationships

Increased learning

Increased problem-solving ability

To achieve awareness of needs

To achieve optimum function

NURSING INTERVENTIONS

Nursing Treatments

Approach unhurriedly

Express empathy

Express warmth and friendliness

Provide an atmosphere of acceptance

Touch the patient judiciously

Reassure verbally

Attend the patient constantly (until the acute episode subsides)
    AND

Provide frequent patient contact (thereafter)

Arrange a structured environment (suitable to the patient)

Arrange geographic placement (so the patient can see the nurse and other
    people)

Keep the patient's door open

Provide a compatible room companion

Encourage the expression of feelings

Listen attentively
    AND

Talk with the patient

Offer feedback of the patient's expressed feelings

Provide objects which symbolize safeness

Encourage mutual problem solving

Support a realistic assessment of the situation

Call the patient's family to the
    bedside

    OR

Encourage telephone calls between
    significant persons

(if the patient prefers or strongly needs significant others and if the significant others are available as a support system)

Allow unlimited visiting

Encourage awareness of positive responses from others

Specific to Independent, Ambulatory Persons:

Encourage visits with friends when lonely

Encourage involvement in helping others

Encourage meaningful activity

Encourage relationships between persons with common interests
    and goals

Nursing Observations

Determine the degree of insight

Evaluate the person's relatedness with others

Evaluate the significance of emotional distress mannerisms

Evaluate the significance of nonverbal communication

Identify disturbing conversation topics

Identify emotion-stimulating events

Observe for an excessive stress level
Observe for impaired self-attitudes
Observe for evidence of a favorable response to therapy

Health Teaching

Explain that the person's emotional response is appropriate and commonly
  experienced
Advise that significant persons express acceptance of one another
Advise that significant persons express love for one another
Explain the importance of offering emotional support to one another
Explain that ill persons are often hypersensitive

EVALUATION

See the evaluation criteria for each specific goal in Chapter 2.

REJECTION

Rejection Related to Anticipatory Loss by Others

ASSESSMENT

Subjective Data

Person feels suddenly left out from contact with a family member or friend
Sadness
Feels the person does not care about him
Is keenly aware of the changed relationship
May wonder what he has done to cause loss of the significant person

Objective Data

Significant person has stopped or greatly reduced his usual visits or telephone
  calls
Significant person may send cards or flowers to reduce his own guilt but
  avoids personal contact with the patient
If the significant person continues his contact with the patient, he assumes an
  aloof, noncaring, or hostile attitude toward him

Related Data

Commonly Related Diseases:
Any disease or injury having a poor prognosis

POSSIBLE ETIOLOGY

Early emotional withdrawal on the part of persons significant to the patient in
order that they might reduce or prevent their own pain of loss

NURSING DIAGNOSIS

Rejection related to anticipatory loss by others: feelings of being emotionally
slighted or cut off from significant persons once those persons learn of the
patient's poor prognosis

PLANNING

Patient Needs	**Primary Nurse-Patient Goals**
Comfort	To achieve comfort
Protection from psychologic threat	To prevent emotional injury
Warm, communicating relationships	To achieve effective verbal and nonverbal communications
Unity with loved ones	To achieve productive interpersonal relationships
Increased learning	To achieve awareness of needs

NURSING INTERVENTIONS

Nursing Treatments

Approach unhurriedly
Express empathy
Reassure verbally
Provide an atmosphere of acceptance
Touch the patient judiciously
Encourage acceptance of limitations in others
Encourage awareness of positive responses from others
Encourage the expression of feelings
Listen attentively
　　AND
Talk with the patient
Offer feedback of the patient's expressed feelings
Support a realistic assessment of the situation
Encourage realistic perception of others
Encourage the use of normal coping mechanisms
Explore with the patient his strengths and resources (in other significant persons)
Provide emotional support for persons significant to the patient (so they can support the patient)
Encourage visiting by significant others

Nursing Observations

Determine the degree of insight
Evaluate the person's relatedness with others
Evaluate the significance of emotional distress mannerisms
Evaluate the significance of nonverbal communication
Identify disturbing conversation topics
Observe for an excessive stress level
Observe for impaired self-attitudes
Observe for evidence that the patient is reaching out for emotional support
Observe for evidence of a favorable response to therapy

Health Teaching

Explain the causes of the health problem
Advise that negative responses from others be regarded with minimum significance

Advise that significant persons express acceptance of one another
Advise that significant persons express love for one another
Explain the importance of offering emotional support to one another
Emphasize the need for realistic expectations of others
Explain the importance of maintaining a positive self-attitude

EVALUATION

See the evaluation criteria for each specific goal in Chapter 2.

SENSITIVITY

Excessive Sensitivity Response (392)

ASSESSMENT

Subjective Data
Highly imaginative
High self-esteem
Concerned about other person's attitude toward him
Feels a deep sense of social responsibility
Becomes so involved with others that he feels their hurt, or is hurt by them

Objective Data
Outgoing, warm, and emotional
Unaggressive
Tolerant
Intelligent
Considerate
Independent
Highly motivated and open to new experiences
Curious about and deeply involved with people
Nondefensive in interpersonal relationships

Related Data
Commonly Related Diseases:
None

POSSIBLE ETIOLOGY

Satisfactory emotional relationships that cause an individual to move toward other persons

NURSING DIAGNOSIS

Excessive sensitivity response: intense involvement with other persons and the needs of other persons, which causes great emotional pain

PLANNING

Patient Needs	Primary Nurse-Patient Goals
Comfort	To achieve comfort
Protection from psychologic threat	To prevent emotional injury

Increased learning   To achieve awareness of needs

NURSING INTERVENTIONS

Nursing Treatments
Approach unhurriedly
Reassure verbally
Touch the patient judiciously
Encourage the expression of feelings
Listen attentively
   AND
Talk with the patient
Offer feedback of the patient's expressed feelings
Encourage acceptance of unpleasantness
Encourage realistic perception of others
Support a realistic assessment of the situation
Encourage the use of normal coping mechanisms

Nursing Observations
Determine the degree of insight
Evaluate the person's relatedness with others
Evaluate the significance of emotional distress mannerisms
Evaluate the significance of nonverbal communication
Identify disturbing conversation topics
Identify emotion-stimulating events
Observe for an excessive stress level
Observe for a favorable response to therapy

Health Teaching
Explain that the person's emotional response is appropriate and commonly
   experienced
Advise that negative responses from others be regarded with minimum
   significance
Explain the need for realistic expectations of others
Explain the importance of maintaining a positive self-attitude

EVALUATION

See the evaluation criteria for each specific goal in Chapter 2.

Impaired Sensitivity Response (392)

ASSESSMENT

Subjective Data
Feels no strong ties to other people
Low self-esteem
Little empathy for the misfortune of others
Seldom considers that his actions might bring suffering or misfortune to
   others

Objective Data
Rigid personality
Introverted

Distrustful
Aloofness
Aggressive
Independent
Dominating

Related Data

Commonly Related Diseases:
None
   OR
Sociopathic or schizoid personality

POSSIBLE ETIOLOGY

Almost total preoccupation with one's own problems. Limited suffering within one's own life. Lack of experience and training in feelings appropriate to different situations. Early emotional relationships were unsatisfying; so the person feels he cannot invest love but must keep it to himself. Poor perception of what is required in one's social role.

NURSING DIAGNOSIS

Impaired sensitivity response: a decreased ability to perceive emotional responses and needs in other persons

PLANNING

Patient Needs	**Primary Nurse-Patient Goals**
Acceptance	To achieve productive interpersonal relationships
Warm, communicating relationships	To achieve effective verbal and nonverbal communications
Personal growth and maturity	To achieve optimum function
Increased learning	To achieve awareness of needs
Increased reality perception and problem-solving ability	To achieve optimum function

NURSING INTERVENTIONS

Nursing Treatments

Approach unhurriedly
Provide an atmosphere of acceptance
Encourage the expression of feelings
Listen attentively
   AND
Talk with the patient
Offer feedback of the patient's expressed feelings
Encourage identification of specific life values
Encourage the practical application of the accepted value system
Encourage involvement in helping others
Encourage respect for the rights of others
Encourage role-playing to develop sensitivity

Encourage the sharing of common problems with others
Explore superficial topics and reasons for avoiding in-depth feelings
Explore with the patient how he would feel in situations experienced by others
Explore with the patient reasons for recurring problems
Explore with the patient the effects of his behavior on others
Refrain from negatively criticizing
Set limits on unacceptable behavior (if the insensitivity is severe)

Nursing Observations
Determine the degree of insight
Evaluate the person's relatedness with others
Identify inappropriate emotional responses
Identify life values significant to the person
Identify appropriate use of defense mechanisms
Identify the current dominant emotion
Observe for evidence of a favorable response to therapy

Health Teaching
Explain the causes of the health problem
Advise against causing defensive responses in others
Explain the importance of offering emotional support to one another
Recommend that behavioral limits be set (if the insensitivity is severe)
Explain how to set behavioral limits

EVALUATION

See the evaluation criteria for each specific goal in Chapter 2.

SHAME

Shame Related to Being Ill
(12,94,372)

ASSESSMENT

Subjective Data
Feelings of unworthiness
Humiliation
Mortification

Objective Data
Openly blames himself for his illness or injury
Attempts to keep the illness from others
Family or friends may make derogatory remarks about the illness or how it could have been prevented

Related Data
Commonly Related Diseases:
Any disease or injury, but especially such diseases as syphilis, gonorrhea, leprosy, epilepsy, and tuberculosis

POSSIBLE ETIOLOGY

Sociocultural attitudes toward illness, especially certain illnesses that have for generations had evil connotations. Feelings of inadequacy. Activities that caused the illness or injury. Fear of loss of employment.

NURSING DIAGNOSIS

Shame related to being ill: a feeling of disgrace or shortcoming for having become ill or contracted some disease

PLANNING

Patient Needs	Primary Nurse-Patient Goals
Comfort	To achieve comfort
Protection from psychologic threat	To prevent emotional injury
Acceptance	To achieve productive interpersonal relationships
Warm, communicating relationships	To achieve effective verbal and nonverbal communications
Adequacy	To achieve positive expressions, feelings, reactions
Increased learning	To achieve awareness of needs

NURSING INTERVENTIONS

Nursing Treatments
Approach unhurriedly
Provide an atmosphere of acceptance
Reassure verbally
Touch the patient judiciously
Avoid causing painful emotional situations
Empahsize the person's value as an individual
Encourage acceptance of self-limitations
Encourage awareness of positive responses from others
Encourage the expression of feelings
Listen attentively
    AND
Talk with the patient
Offer feedback of the patient's expressed feelings
Encourage patient questions (about the illness)
Provide reliable information
Support a realistic assessment of the situation
Encourage the use of normal coping mechanisms
Explore with the patient reasons for criticisms by others
Explore with the patient reasons for self-criticism
Introduce to persons who have successfully undergone the same experience
Refrain from negatively criticizing

Nursing Observations
Determine the degree of insight

Evaluate the person's relatedness with others
Evaluate the significance of emotional distress mannerisms
Evaluate the significance of nonverbal communication
Identify disturbing conversation topics
Observe for an excessive stress level
Observe for evidence that the patient is reaching out for emotional support
Observe for impaired self-attitudes
Observe for evidence of a favorable response to therapy

Health Teaching
Explain that the person's emotional response is appropriate and commonly
 experienced
Advise that negative responses from others be regarded with minimum
 significance
Advise that significant persons express acceptance of one another
Advise that significant persons express love for one another
Explain the importance of offering emotional support to one another
Explain the importance of maintaining a positive self-attitude

EVALUATION

See the evaluation criteria for each specific goal in Chapter 2.

Shame Related to Changed Behavior During Illness (12,94,372)

ASSESSMENT

Subjective Data
Feeling of unworthiness
Humiliation
Mortification
Feels he should be reproached

Objective Data
Person has openly cried
Displayed demanding or angry behavior
Called out for help
Indulged in self-pity
Given less time and concern to significant others

Related Data
Commonly Related Diseases:
Any disease or injury

POSSIBLE ETIOLOGY

Stress caused by illness that results in reduced emotional control. The struggle to cope simultaneously with the illness, treatments, and other life problems.

NURSING DIAGNOSIS

Shame related to changed behavior during illness: a feeling of disgrace or shortcoming for having displayed behavior during illness that one would, under normal circumstances, consider unacceptable behavior for oneself

PLANNING

Patient Needs	**Primary Nurse-Patient Goals**
Comfort	To achieve comfort
Protection from psychologic threat	To prevent emotional injury
Acceptance	To achieve productive interpersonal relationships
Warm, communicating relationships	To achieve effective verbal and nonverbal communications
Increased learning	To achieve awareness of needs

NURSING INTERVENTIONS

Nursing Treatments
Approach unhurriedly
Express empathy
Provide an atmosphere of acceptance
Reassure verbally
Touch the patient judiciously
Avoid causing painful emotional situations
Emphasize the person's value as an individual
Encourage acceptance of self-limitations
Encourage awareness of positive responses from others
Encourage the expression of feelings
Listen attentively
   AND
Talk with the patient
Offer feedback of the patient's expressed feelings
Explore with the patient the reasons for self-criticism
Encourage the use of normal coping mechanisms
Recognize the need for the use of appropriate defense mechanisms
Refrain from negatively criticizing

Nursing Observations
Determine the degree of insight
Evaluate the significance of emotional distress mannerisms
Evaluate the significance of nonverbal communication
Identify disturbing conversation topics
Identify life values significant to the person
Observe for an excessive stress level
Observe for impaired self-attitudes
Observe for evidence that the patient is reaching out for emotional support
Observe for evidence of a favorable response to therapy

Health Teaching
Explain that the person's emotional response is appropriate and commonly experienced

Advise that significant persons express acceptance of one another
Advise that significant persons express love for one another
Explain the importance of offering emotional support to one another
Explain the importance of maintaining a positive self-attitude

EVALUATION

See the evaluation criteria for each specific goal in Chapter 2.

SUFFERING

Inadequate Emotional Support Related to the Endurance of Pain (148,187, 360,502,508)

ASSESSMENT

Subjective Data
Sense of helplessness
Unsettled, vaguely confused feeling
Feeling of weakness
Feels that his pain is very difficult to endure
Wants to escape the situation
Is experiencing severe pain
Preoccupation with the pain

Objective Data
Appears forlorn and upset
At the time of need, the person has a limited, nonexistent, or temporarily absent support system of significant others
May reach out for help through crying, attention-seeking behavior, touching persons or objects, seeking someone to talk with, etc.
May display quiet endurance, emotional excitement, or sometimes personality disorganization

Related Data
Commonly Related Diseases:
Any painful disease or injury

POSSIBLE ETIOLOGY

Lack of interest on the part of one's usually supportive world of family, friends, and church. The unavailability of persons who usually offer support. Long-term pain that decreases the ability to endure it. Intense pain that quickly depletes one's strength.

NURSING DIAGNOSIS

Inadequate emotional support related to the endurance of pain: little or no comfort or sustaining measures received from others while enduring severe pain .

PLANNING

Patient Needs	**Primary Nurse-Patient Goals**
Comfort	To achieve comfort
Protection from psychologic threat	To prevent emotional injury
Warm, communicating relationships	To achieve effective verbal and nonverbal communications
Adequacy, endurance	To achieve positive expressions, feelings, reactions
Increased learning	To achieve awareness of needs

NURSING INTERVENTIONS

Nursing Treatments
Approach unhurriedly
Demonstrate calmness
Express empathy
Communicate nurse sensitivity to the person's pain
Express warmth and friendliness
Provide an atmosphere of acceptance
Touch the patient judiciously
Reassure verbally
Attend the patient constantly (until the acute episode subsides)
    AND
Provide frequent patient contact (thereafter)
Sit with the patient
Encourage the expression of feelings
Listen attentively
    AND
Talk with the patient
Offer feedback of the patient's expressed feelings
Encourage patient questions (if such will relieve the distress)
Provide objects which symbolize safeness
Encourage mutual problem solving
Introduce to persons who have successfully undergone the same experience
Encourage the use of normal coping mechanisms
Explore with the patient his strengths and resources
Reduce the demands placed upon the patient
Refrain from performing nonessential procedures
Refrain from negatively criticizing
Call the patient's family to the bedside
    OR
Encourage telephone calls between significant persons
} (if the patient prefers or strongly needs significant others and if the significant others are available as a support system)
Ask the patient what makes him comfortable
Discuss possible pain-reducing measures
Explain that there are nondrug measures available for pain relief
Provide a pain-relief measure of the patient's choice

Offer assurance of other measures if the pain-relief method fails
Reassure that the pain will subside
Reduce the demands placed upon the patient
Respond immediately to the patient's call
Use positive suggestion in pain relief
Encourage active diversional
   activities
   OR   } (for prolonged pain)
Encourage passive diversional
   activities

Nursing Observations
Estimate the degree of pain experienced
Evaluate the pain for intensity and quality
Observe for nonverbal communication of pain
Observe for an excessive stress level
Evaluate the effectiveness of the pain-relief measures
Observe for evidence of a favorable response to therapy

Health Teaching
Explain that it is acceptable to admit the existence of pain (if the patient is
   quietly enduring the pain)
Explain the causes of fear of pain
Explain how to describe pain
Explain the reason for delay in giving a pain-relief drug

EVALUATION

See the evaluation criteria for each specific goal in Chapter 2.

Inadequate Emotional Support Related to Progressive Illness (148,187,360, 502, 508)

ASSESSMENT

Subjective Data
Person perceives that the illness is gradually worsening
Person feels that this awareness is very difficult to endure
Sense of helplessness
Unsettled, vaguely confused feeling
Feeling of weakness
Wants to escape the situation
Preoccupied with the progressive illness

Objective Data
Appears forlorn and upset
At the time of need, the person has a limited, nonexistent, or temporarily
   absent support system of significant others
May reach out for help through crying, attention-seeking behavior, touching
   persons or objects, seeking someone to talk with, etc.
May appear withdrawn

Makes comments such as these: "I'm not getting any better, and no one will help me." "I feel sicker and sicker, and no one can do anything for me." "The sicker I get, the harder it is to bear it alone."

Related Data

Commonly Related Conditions:
Gradual hearing or vision loss

Commonly Related Diseases:
Glomerulonephritis
Multiple Sclerosis
Carcinoma
Cardiac failure
Parkinson's disease
Myasthenia gravis

POSSIBLE ETIOLOGY

Lack of interest on the part of one's usually supportive world of family, friends, and church. The unavailability of persons who usually offer support. Prolonged disease progression that exhausts the supportive capacity of significant others.

NURSING DIAGNOSIS

Inadequate emotional support related to progressive illness: little or no comfort or sustaining measures received from others as one's disease progressively worsens

PLANNING

Patient Needs	**Primary Nurse-Patient Goals**
Comfort	To achieve comfort
Protection from psychologic threat	To prevent emotional injury
Warm, communicating relationships	To achieve effective verbal and nonverbal communications
Adequacy, endurance	To achieve positive expressions, feelings, reactions
Personal growth and maturity	To achieve optimum function
Increased learning	To achieve awareness of needs
Religious-philosophic satisfaction	To achieve spiritual goals

NURSING INTERVENTIONS

Nursing Treatments
Approach unhurriedly
Demonstrate calmness
Express empathy
Express warmth and friendliness
Provide an atmosphere of acceptance
Touch the patient judiciously
Reassure verbally

Offer hope
Attend the patient constantly (until the acute episode subsides)
AND
Provide frequent patient contact (thereafter)
Arrange a structured environment (suitable to the patient)
Encourage the expression of feelings
Listen attentively
AND
Talk with the patient
Offer feedback of the patient's expressed feelings
Encourage patient questions (if such will relieve the distress)
Provide objects which symbolize safeness
Encourage mutual problem solving
Encourage the use of normal coping mechanisms
Explore with the patient his strengths and resources
Reduce the demands placed upon the patient
Refrain from performing nonessential procedures
Refrain from negatively criticizing
Call the patient's family to the
  bedside
OR
Encourage telephone calls between
  significant persons
} (if the patient prefers or strongly needs significant others and if the significant others are available as a support system)

Assist the patient in setting standards of a meaningful existence
Encourage meaningful activity (if possible)
Emphasize the person's value as an individual
Encourage awareness of positive responses from others
Explore with the patient previous displays of courage
Reinforce concern throughout the entire illness

Nursing Observations
Determine the degree of insight
Evaluate the significance of emotional distress mannerisms
Evaluate the significance of nonverbal communication
Identify disturbing conversation topics
Observe for an excessive stress level
Observe for impaired self-attitudes
Observe for evidence of a favorable response to therapy

Health Teaching
Explain that the person's emotional response is appropriate and commonly
  experienced
Advise that significant persons express acceptance of one another
Advise that significant persons express love for one another
Explain the importance of offering emotional support to one another
Recommend a habitual, positive mental attitude

EVALUATION

See the evaluation criteria for each specific goal in Chapter 2.

Inadequate Emotional Support Related to the Endurance of Diagnostic Studies (148,187,360,502,508)

ASSESSMENT

Subjective Data

Sense of helplessness

Unsettled, vaguely confused feeling

Feels that the diagnostic studies are difficult to endure

Experiences pain, discomfort, or weakness resulting from the studies

Feels that the invasive studies are an intrusion on his very personal and private body

May feel that his body is being mutilated with probes, tubes, needles, etc.

Experiences a loss of dignity

Feels that he cannot take much more

Wants to escape from the studies

Preoccupied with the studies

Objective Data

Person is undergoing a series of diagnostic studies

Studies are over a prolonged period of time (more than 2–3 days)

Studies are done day after day with little or no rest in between

Diagnostic conclusion may be difficult to determine

Appears forlorn and upset

At the time of need, the person has a limited, nonexistent, or temporarily absent support system of significant others

May reach out for help through crying, attention-seeking behavior, touching persons or objects, seeking someone to talk with, etc.

May appear withdrawn

Related Data

Commonly Related Diseases:
Any disease or injury

POSSIBLE ETIOLOGY

Lack of interest on the part of one's usually supportive world of family, friends, and church. The unavailability of persons who usually offer support. The need to perform diagnostic studies in order to reach a medical diagnosis.

NURSING DIAGNOSIS

Inadequate emotional support related to the endurance of diagnostic studies: little or no comfort or sustaining measures received from others while one is enduring diagnostic studies

PLANNING

Patient Needs	Primary Nurse-Patient Goals
Rest	To achieve rest
Comfort	To achieve comfort

Protection from psychologic threat	To prevent emotional injury
Acceptance	To achieve productive interpersonal relationships
Warm, communicating relationships	To achieve effective verbal and nonverbal communications
Adequacy, endurance	To achieve positive expressions, feelings, reactions
Increased learning	To achieve awareness of needs

NURSING INTERVENTIONS

Nursing Treatments
Approach unhurriedly
Demonstrate calmness
Express empathy
Express warmth and friendliness
Provide an atmosphere of acceptance
Touch the patient judiciously
Reassure verbally
Attend the patient constantly (until the acute episode subsides)
    AND
Provide frequent patient contact (thereafter)
Arrange a structured environment (suitable to the patient)
Encourage adequate rest
Encourage the expression of feelings
Listen attentively
    AND
Talk with the patient
Offer feedback of the patient's expressed feelings
Encourage patient questions (if such will relieve the distress)
Arrange situations which encourage patient autonomy
Do not allow unpleasant surprise situations
Ensure the patient's feeling of safety before introducing unpleasantness
Introduce one anxiety situation at a time
Ask the patient what makes him/her comfortable
Grant special requests
Provide objects which symbolize safeness
Encourage mutual problem solving
Introduce to persons who have successfully undergone the same experience
Encourage the use of normal coping mechanisms
Explore with the patient his strengths and resources
Reduce the demands placed upon the patient
Refrain from performing nonessential procedures
Refrain from negatively criticizing
Call the patient's family to the
    bedside
    OR
Encourage telephone calls between
    significant persons

} (if the patient prefers or strongly needs significant others and if the significant others are available as a support system)

Nursing Observations

Evaluate the significance of emotional distress mannerisms

Evaluate the significance of nonverbal communication

Identify disturbing conversation topics

Observe for an excessive stress level

Observe for a favorable response to therapy

Health Teaching

Explain that the person's emotional response is appropriate and commonly
experienced

Explain the importance of offering emotional support to one another

Explain the reason for and intended effect of the study or examination

EVALUATION

See the evaluation criteria for each specific goal in Chapter 2.

Inadequate Emotional Support Related to the Endurance of Health Treatment (148,187,360,502,508)

ASSESSMENT

Subjective Data

Sense of helplessness

Unsettled, vaguely confused feeling

Feels that the treatment is difficult to endure

Experiences pain, discomfort, or weakness resulting from the treatment

May feel that being cured is not worth what must be endured during treatment

Feels that he cannot take much more

Wants to escape from the treatment

Preoccupied with the treatment

Objective Data

Person is undergoing a series of treatments

Treatment occurs over a prolonged period of time

Treatment occurs quite often (once or several times a week, or daily)

Person is having treatments such as burn wound dressing changes, cobalt
therapy or chemotherapy, dialysis, frequent injections or intravenous
therapy, shock treatments, painful exercise, etc.

Appears forlorn and upset

At the time of need, the person has a limited, nonexistent, or temporarily
absent support system of significant others

May reach out for help through crying, attention-seeking behavior, touching
persons or objects, seeking someone to talk with, etc.

May appear withdrawn

Related Data

Commonly Related Diseases:

Any disease or injury

POSSIBLE ETIOLOGY

Lack of interest on the part of one's usually supportive world of family, friends, and church. The unavailability of persons who usually offer support. The need to perform treatments for their curative effect.

NURSING DIAGNOSIS

Inadequate emotional support related to the endurance of health treatment: little or no comfort or sustaining measures received from others while one is enduring health treatment

PLANNING

Patient Needs	Primary Nurse-Patient Goals
Rest	To achieve rest
Protection from psychologic threat	To prevent emotional injury
Acceptance	To achieve productive interpersonal relationships
Warm, communicating relationships	To achieve effective verbal and nonverbal communications
Adequacy, endurance	To achieve positive expressions, feelings, reactions
Increased learning	To achieve awareness of needs

NURSING INTERVENTIONS

Nursing Treatments
Approach unhurriedly
Demonstrate calmness
Express empathy
Express warmth and friendliness
Provide an atmosphere of acceptance
Touch the patient judiciously
Reassure verbally
Attend the patient constantly (until the acute episode subsides)
    AND
Provide frequent patient contact (thereafter)
Arrange a structured environment (suitable to the patient)
Encourage adequate rest
Encourage the expression of feelings
Listen attentively
    AND
Talk with the patient
Offer feedback of the patient's expressed feelings
Encourage patient questions (if such will relieve the distress)
Arrange situations which encourage patient autonomy
Do not allow unpleasant surprise situations
Ensure the patient's feeling of safety before introducing unpleasantness
Ask the patient what makes him/her comfortable

Grant special requests
Provide objects which symbolize safeness
Encourage mutual problem solving
Introduce to persons who have successfully undergone the same experience
Encourage the use of normal coping mechanisms
Explore with the patient his strengths and resources
Reduce the demands placed upon the patient
Refrain from performing nonessential procedures
Refrain from negatively criticizing
Call the patient's family to the
   bedside
   OR
Encourage telephone calls between
   significant persons
} (if the patient prefers or strongly needs significant others and if the significant others are available as a support system)

Nursing Observations
Evaluate the significance of emotional distress mannerisms
Evaluate the significance of nonverbal communication
Identify disturbing conversation topics
Observe for an excessive stress level
Observe for evidence of a favorable response to therapy

Health Teaching
Explain that the person's emotional response is appropriate and commonly experienced
Explain the importance of offering emotional support to one another
Explain the reason for and intended effect of the therapy

EVALUATION
See the evaluation criteria for each specific goal in Chapter 2.

TRUST

Inability to Trust (118,199,331)
ASSESSMENT
Subjective Data
Feels doubtful about the competence of others
Feels suspicious about the integrity of another's relationship with him
Fears that the effects of the actions of others may prove harmful to him

Objective Data
Questions health personnel regarding every detail of treatment
Frequently uncooperative
Unable to establish close interpersonal relationships
Checks and rechecks all interactions with others to be sure he has not been taken advantage of

Prone to displays of jealousy
May accuse persons of causing him injury when such was neither intended
   nor inflicted

Related Data
Commonly Related Diseases:
None
   OR
Paranoid schizophrenia or involutional psychosis
Psychoneurosis
Organic brain syndrome

POSSIBLE ETIOLOGY

Negative past experiences. Imagined injury. Inadequate or incorrect information. An unstable self-image. Unsuccessful oral stage development.

NURSING DIAGNOSIS

Inability to trust: the inability to feel confident regarding the competence and reliability of other persons

PLANNING

Patient Needs	Primary Nurse-Patient Goals
Comfort	To achieve comfort
Protection from psychologic threat	To prevent emotional injury
Stability, predictable, orderly world	To achieve a therapeutic environment
Acceptance	To achieve productive interpersonal relationships
Warm, communicating relationships	To achieve effective verbal and nonverbal communications
High evaluation of self	To achieve positive expressions, feelings, reactions
Personal growth and maturity	To achieve optimum function
Increased learning	To achieve awareness of needs
Increased reality perception and problem-solving ability	To achieve optimum function

NURSING INTERVENTIONS

Nursing Treatments
Approach unhurriedly
Provide an atmosphere of acceptance
Demonstrate calmness
Arrange situations which encourage patient autonomy
Avoid causing intense emotional situations
Encourage the expression of feelings
Listen attentively
   AND

Talk with the patient
    BUT
Terminate emotionally threatening conversation immediately
Offer feedback of the patient's expressed feelings
Support a realistic assessment of the situation
Encourage the reduction of generalizations to specifics (regarding who or what is distrusted)
Explore with the patient reasons for recurring problems
Explore with the patient the effects of his behavior on others
Ensure the patient's feeling of safety before introducing unpleasantness
Introduce one anxiety situation at a time
Provide emotionally safe experiences
Provide objects which symbolize safeness
Limit touching of suspicious persons
Maintain consistent staff behavior
Maintain honesty
Maintain social formality   } (whichever is most suitable to the
    OR   patient)
Maintain social informality
Follow through on promises
    OR
Refrain from making promises
Provide reliable information
Refrain from arguing
Refrain from teasing
Refrain from negatively criticizing
Refrain from performing nonessential procedures
Set limits on unacceptable behavior

Nursing Observations
Determine the degree of insight
Determine the precipitating factors
Determine the relieving factors
Evaluate the person's relatedness with others
Evaluate the significance of emotional distress mannerisms
Evaluate the significance of nonverbal communications
Identify abnormal perceptions
Identify abnormal thought content
Identify disturbing conversation topics
Identify emotion-stimulating events
Identify inappropriate emotional responses
Identify potentially destructive behavior
Observe for an excessive stress level
Observe for impaired judgment
Observe for impaired self-attitudes
Observe for incoherent thinking
Observe for evidence of a favorable response to therapy

Health Teaching

Advise that negative responses from others be regarded with minimum significance

Advise that significant persons express acceptance of one another

Advise that significant persons express love for one another

Explain the importance of offering emotional support to one another

Explain the need for realistic expectations of others

Explain the causes of the health problem

Describe those symptoms which should be reported (paranoia)

Explain that ill persons are often hypersensitive

Recommend that behavioral limits be set (for excessive distrust)

Explain how to set behavioral limits

EVALUATION

See the evaluation criteria for each specific goal in Chapter 2.

TRUST, POTENTIAL LACK OF

Potential Distrust Related to Health Care

ASSESSMENT

Subjective Data

A trusting patient wonders if health personnel are reliable or competent

A distrusting patient looks for lack of integrity in his health care

Objective Data

Person's health problems are incorrectly diagnosed

Treatments which should be started are delayed or changed

Person discovers that family members received different information about his health care and status than he did

Person is given false hopes regarding health improvement or cure

Person is receiving placebos

Related Data

Commonly Related Diseases:

Any disease or injury

POSSIBLE ETIOLOGY

The well-meaning actions of persons who feel that deception will benefit the patient

NURSING DIAGNOSIS

Potential distrust related to health care: the possibility that a trusting person will recognize deceptive practices in his health care and will develop a sense of distrust regarding such care

PLANNING

Patient Needs	**Primary Nurse-Patient Goals**
Comfort	To achieve comfort
Protection from psychologic threat	To prevent emotional injury
Acceptance	To achieve productive interpersonal relationships
Warm, communicating relationships	To achieve effective verbal and nonverbal communications
Dignity	To achieve productive interpersonal relationships
Increased learning	To achieve awareness of needs

NURSING INTERVENTIONS

Nursing Treatments
Approach unhurriedly
Provide an atmosphere of acceptance
Demonstrate calmness
Express warmth and friendliness
Touch the patient judiciously
Arrange situations which encourage patient autonomy
Avoid causing painful emotional situations
Ensure the patient's feeling of safety before introducing unpleasantness
Maintain consistent staff behavior
Maintain honesty
Follow through on promises
    OR
Refrain from making promises
Maintain social formality
    OR   } (whichever is most suitable to the patient)
Maintain social informality
Provide emotionally safe experiences
Talk with the patient
Encourage patient questions
Listen attentively
Provide reliable information
Provide frequent patient contact
Refrain from negatively criticizing
Refrain from performing nonessential procedures
Involve the family (as much as possible)

Nursing Observations
Evaluate the significance of emotional distress mannerisms
Evaluate the significance of nonverbal communication
Identify disturbing conversation topics
Observe for an excessive stress level

Health Teaching
Explain the reason for and intended effect of the therapy

EVALUATION

See the evaluation criteria for each specific goal in Chapter 2.

EMOTIONAL EXPRESSION

Inadequate Emotional Expression
(118,199,264,331)

ASSESSMENT

Subjective Data
Keeps emotions pent up inside
Experiences deep feelings

Objective Data
Appears unemotional externally
An aloof mannerism
Seclusiveness
Physically removes himself from others when emotions cannot be concealed
Avoids touching others
Appears to use logic, not emotion, in all relationships

Related Data
Commonly Related Diseases:
None
    OR
Anxiety neurosis

POSSIBLE ETIOLOGY

Poor social skills. Lack of self-confidence. Fear of rejection or punishment.
An attempt to protect oneself against emotional hurt. Unpleasant past emotional experiences. Culturally restricted emotional expression. Repressive overcontrol by parents. Intellectualizes as a defense against feelings.

NURSING DIAGNOSIS

Inadequate emotional expression: the inability to externally express one's feelings as such feelings are experienced internally

PLANNING

Patient Needs	**Primary Nurse-Patient Goals**
Comfort	To achieve comfort
Protection from psychologic threat	To prevent emotional injury
Acceptance	To achieve productive interpersonal relationships
Warm, communicating relationships	To achieve effective verbal and nonverbal communications
Adequacy	To achieve positive expressions, feelings, reactions
Personal growth and maturity	To achieve optimum function
Increased learning	To achieve awareness of needs

NURSING INTERVENTIONS

Nursing Treatments

Approach unhurriedly

Provide an atmosphere of acceptance (for the expression of feelings)

Reassure verbally

Touch the patient judiciously

Acknowledge emotional concealment

Encourage the expression of feelings

Listen attentively

    AND

Talk with the patient

Offer feedback of the patient's expressed feelings

Explore superficial topics and reasons for avoiding in-depth feelings

    BUT

Terminate emotionally threatening conversation immediately

Encourage patient questions

Encourage crying (when appropriate)

Encourage laughter

Encourage participation in therapeutic group interaction

Encourage the sharing of common problems with others

Refrain from negatively criticizing

Nursing Observations

Determine the degree of insight

Identify inappropriate use of defense mechanisms (intellectualization)

Evaluate the significance of emotional distress mannerisms

Evaluate the significance of nonverbal communication

Identify disturbing conversation topics

Observe for an excessive stress level

Observe for evidence that the person is reaching out for emotional support

Observe for evidence of a favorable response to therapy

Health Teaching

Explain the causes of the health problem

Explain how to obtain release from emotional stress

Explain the importance of maintaining a positive self-attitude

EVALUATION

See the evaluation criteria for each specific goal in Chapter 2.

INAPPROPRIATE NEED GRATIFICATION

Need Gratification Through Diagnosed Illness

ASSESSMENT

Subjective Data

Person experiences pleasure in being ill

Feels a sense of importance not experienced in everyday living

Objective Data
Person has received a medical diagnosis of illness
Frequently complains of the illness or pain, which focuses attention on him
Prolongs the illness as much as possible
Encourages others to wait on him

Related Data
Commonly Related Diseases:
Psychoneurosis
Psychophysiologic illness (peptic ulcers, asthma, etc.)
Any illness or disease

POSSIBLE ETIOLOGY

The absence of life experiences that gratify the need for attention and affection from others

NURSING DIAGNOSIS

Need gratification through diagnosed illness: the consistent use of acutal illness as a means of meeting one's needs for attention and affection

PLANNING

Patient Needs	Primary Nurse-Patient Goals
Comfort	To achieve comfort
Protection from psychologic threat	To prevent emotional injury
Love and affection, acceptance	To achieve productive interpersonal relationships
Warm, communicating relationships	To achieve effective verbal and nonverbal communications
Attention	To achieve productive interpersonal relationships
Personal growth and maturity	To achieve optimum function
Increased learning	To achieve awareness of needs
Increased reality perception and problem-solving ability	To achieve optimum function

NURSING INTERVENTIONS

Nursing Treatments
Approach unhurriedly
Provide an atmosphere of acceptance
Encourage the expression of feelings
Listen attentively
    AND
Talk with the patient
Suggest more appropriate means of need gratification
Explore with the patient reasons for recurring problems
Explore with the patient the effects of his behavior on others
Explore with the patient the need for attention
Encourage self-performance
Refrain from negatively criticizing

Assist the patient in setting standards of a meaningful existence
Encourage meaningful activity

Nursing Observations
Determine the degree of insight
Evaluate the person's relatedness with others
Evaluate the significance of emotional distress mannerisms
Evaluate the significance of nonverbal communications
Identify disturbing conversation topics
Observe for an excessive stress level
Observe for evidence that the patient is reaching out for emotional support
Observe for evidence of a favorable response to therapy

Health Teaching
Advise that significant persons express love for one another
Explain the importance of offering emotional support to one another
Explain the importance of maintaining a positive self-attitude
Explain the causes of the health problem

EVALUATION

See the evaluation criteria for each specific goal in Chapter 2.

Need Gratification Through Fantasized Illness (12,13,94,372)

ASSESSMENT

Subjective Data
Person perceives his body as vulnerable and sickly
Has strange inner sensations directed toward different organs
Worries excessively about his own health

Objective Data
Develops an illness following exposure to conversation about that illness
Endless verbal descriptions of ailments
Warns others about germs and infection

Related Data
Commonly Related Diseases:
None
  OR
Hypochondriasis
Psychoneurosis

POSSIBLE ETIOLOGY

Perception of the self as ill to meet the needs for dependency, attention, or love gratification. Displaced anxiety. Insecurity feelings.

NURSING DIAGNOSIS

Need gratification through fantasized illness: preoccupation with fantasized illness as a means of meeting one's needs for attention and affection

PLANNING

Patient Needs	Primary Nurse-Patient
Comfort	To achieve comfort
Protection from psychologic threat	To prevent emotional injury
Acceptance	To achieve productive interpersonal relationships
Warm, communicating relationships	To achieve effective verbal and nonverbal communications
Adequacy	To achieve positive expressions, feelings, reactions
Attention	To achieve productive interpersonal relationships
Personal growth and maturity	To achieve optimum function
Increased learning	To achieve awareness of needs
Increased reality perception and problem-solving ability	To achieve optimum function
Increased pleasantness	To achieve positive expressions, feelings, reactions

NURSING INTERVENTIONS

Nursing Treatments
Approach unhurriedly
Provide an atmosphere of acceptance
Emphasize the person's normal characteristics
Encourage the expression of feelings (about his body)
Listen attentively
    AND
Talk with the patient
Suggest more appropriate means of need gratification
Provide reliable information (about the health status)
Explore with the patient reasons for recurring problems
Explore with the patient the effects of his behavior on others
Explore with the patient the need for attention
Support a realistic assessment of the situation
Refrain from negatively criticizing
Assist the patient in setting standards of a meaningful existence
Encourage meaningful activity

Nursing Observations
Determine the extent of behavioral suggestibility
Determine the degree of insight
Determine the precipitating factors
Determine the relieving factors
Evaluate the person's relatedness with others
Evaluate the significance of emotional distress mannerisms
Evaluate the significance of nonverbal communication

Identify disturbing conversation topics
Observe for emotional instability
Observe for an excessive stress level
Observe for evidence that the patient is reaching out for emotional support
Observe for evidence of a favorable response to therapy

Health Teaching
Advise that significant persons express love for one another
Explain the importance of offering emotional support to one another
Explain the importance of maintaining a positive self-attitude
Explain the causes of the health problem

EVALUATION

See the evaluation criteria for each specific goal in Chapter 2.

DEFENSE RESPONSES

Emotional Shock (12,13,94,372)

ASSESSMENT

Subjective Data
Intense anxiety
Poor concentration ability
Thought disorganization
Nightmares

Objective Data
Wide-eyed facial expression
Activity is temporarily limited
Dazed appearance
Unable to sleep
Nervous behavior

Related Data
Commonly Related Diseases:
None
   OR
Any very serious disease or injury

POSSIBLE ETIOLOGY

An adaptation response to extreme surprise or danger

NURSING DIAGNOSIS

Emotional shock: a temporary period of being emotionally overpowered or insensible

PLANNING

Patient Needs	Primary Nurse-Patient Goals
Sleep, rest, relaxation	To achieve sleep, rest, relaxation
Comfort	To achieve comfort

Protection from physical harm	To prevent physical injury
Protection from psychologic threat	To prevent emotional injury
Dependence	To achieve comfort
Acceptance	To achieve productive interpersonal relationships
Warm, communicating relationships	To achieve effective verbal and nonverbal communications
Adequacy	To achieve positive expressions, feelings, reactions
Personal growth and maturity	To achieve optimum function
Increased learning	To achieve awareness of needs
Religious-philosophic satisfaction	To achieve spiritual goals

NURSING INTERVENTIONS

Nursing Treatments
Approach unhurriedly
Acknowledge dependency
Provide an atmosphere of acceptance
Demonstrate calmness
Reassure verbally
Attend the patient constantly
    OR
Provide frequent patient contact
Encourage adequate rest
Provide quiet
Restrict unwanted visitors
Involve the family (as much as possible)
Establish routines familiar to the patient
Avoid causing painful emotional situations
Discourage decision-making when one is under severe stress
Do not allow unpleasant surprise situations
Encourage the expression of feelings
Listen attentively
    AND
Talk with the patient
Encourage crying
Recognize the need for the use of appropriate defense mechanisms
Encourage the use of normal coping mechanisms
Encourage the use of spiritual resources
Explore with the patient his strengths and resources
Ensure the patient's feeling of safety before introducing unpleasantness
Provide emotionally safe experiences
Provide emotional support for persons significant to the patient
Provide objects which symbolize safeness
Reduce the demands placed upon the patient
Refrain from performing nonessential procedures

Nursing Observations

Determine the degree of insight

Determine the precipitating factors

Determine the relieving factors

Estimate the degree of stress experienced

Evaluate the person's relatedness with others

Evaluate the significance of emotional distress mannerisms

Evaluate the significance of nonverbal communication

Identify disturbing conversation topics

Identify inappropriate emotional responses

Identify reality-acceptance clues

Identify appropriate use of defense mechanisms

Identify inappropriate use of defense mechanisms

Identify the current dominant emotion

Observe for evidence that the patient is reaching out for emotional support

Observe for evidence of a favorable response to therapy

Health teaching

Explain that the person's emotional response is appropriate and commonly
    experienced

Explain the importance of offering emotional support to one another

Explain how to obtain release from emotional stress

Explain the causes of the health problem

Medical Treatments Performed by Nurses

Give the prescribed drugs

EVALUATION

See the evaluation criteria for each specific goal in Chapter 2.

Temporary Emotional Privacy Requirement

ASSESSMENT

Subjective Data

Desires emotional release without social stigma

Desires decreased external stess in order to reestablish internal equilibrium

Objective Data

Asks to be left alone

Sits facing away from others

Related Data

Commonly Related Diseases:

None

    OR

Any disease or injury

POSSIBLE ETIOLOGY

The need to reestablish emotional equilibrium

NURSING DIAGNOSIS

Temporary emotional privacy requirement: the need to temporarily be by oneself in a place of solitude during a period of intense emotional feeling

PLANNING

Patient Needs	Primary Nurse-Patient Goals
Comfort	To achieve comfort
Protection from psychologic threat	To prevent emotional injury
Acceptance	To achieve productive interpersonal relationships
Personal growth and maturity	To achieve optimum function
Increased learning	To achieve awareness of needs

NURSING INTERVENTIONS

Nursing Treatments
Approach unhurriedly
Provide an atmosphere of acceptance
Express empathy
Reassure verbally (that the nurse is available whenever needed)
Place in a private room
   OR
Provide seclusion
Keep the patient's door closed
Provide quiet
Restrict unwanted visitors
Recognize the need for the use of appropriate defense mechanism
Encourage the use of normal coping mechanisms
Reduce the demands placed upon the patient
Refrain from performing nonessential procedures

Nursing Observations
Determine the degree of insight
Evaluate the significance of emotional distress mannerisms
Evaluate the significance of nonverbal communication
Identify disturbing conversation topics
Identify appropriate use of defense mechanisms
Identify inappropriate use of defense mechanisms
Observe for an excessive stress level
Observe for evidence that the patient is reaching out for emotional support

Health Teaching
Advise that significant persons express acceptance of one another
Explain the importance of offering emotional support to one another

EVALUATION

See the evaluation criteria for each specific goal in Chapter 2.

Temporary Partial Denial Requirement
(12,13,94,372)

ASSESSMENT

Subjective Data

Feels highly threatened

Feels bitterness, anger, depression

May bargain with God to change the situation

Internal struggling to recognize the truth

Objective Data

Can occasionally discuss the painful experience

Indicates a desire to discuss it, but only when feeling strong

Discussion begins regarding the painful experience, then suddenly changes
to a more pleasant topic

Related Data

Commonly Related Diseases:

Any fatal or severe disease or injury

POSSIBLE ETIOLOGY

Inability to adapt to the full realization of the painful experience. The setting aside of painful thoughts in order to live normally.

NURSING DIAGNOSIS

Temporary partial-denial requirement: a temporary need to partially deny
a painful reality

PLANNING

Patient Needs	Primary Nurse-Patient Goals
Comfort	To achieve comfort
Protection from psychologic threat	To prevent emotional injury
Acceptance	To achieve productive interpersonal relationships
Warm, communicating relationships	To achieve effective verbal and nonverbal communications
Adequacy	To achieve positive expressions, feeling, reactions
Personal growth and maturity	To achieve optimum function
Increased learning	To achieve awareness of needs
Increased reality perception and problem-solving ability	To achieve optimum function

NURSING INTERVENTIONS

Nursing Treatments

Approach unhurriedly

Provide an atmosphere of acceptance

Recognize the need for the use of appropriate defense mechanisms (by sup-
porting the denial)
Encourage the use of normal coping mechanisms
Recognize the need for unique personal adjustments to change
Encourage the expression of feelings
Listen attentively
    AND
Talk with the patient
Offer feedback of the patient's expressed feelings
Ask questions which encourage answers that reflect reality perception
    AND
Explore superficial topics and reasons for avoiding in-depth feelings
    BUT
Terminate emotionally threatening conversation immediately
Ensure the patient's feeling of safety before introducing unpleasantness
Provide emotionally safe experiences
Provide objects which symbolize safeness
Support a realistic assessment of the situation
Encourage mutual problem solving
Explore with the patient his strengths and resources

Nursing Observations
Determine the degree of insight
Evaluate the person's relatedness with others
Evaluate the significance of emotional distress mannerisms
Evaluate the significance of nonverbal communications
Identify disturbing conversation topics
Identify emotion-stimulating events
Identify reality-acceptance clues
Identify appropriate use of defense mechanisms
Identify inappropriate use of defense mechanisms
Identify the current dominant emotion
Observe for an excessive stress level
Observe for evidence that the patient is reaching out for emotional support
Observe for evidence of a favorable response to therapy

Health Teaching
Explain that the person's emotional response is appropriate and commonly
experienced
Explain and offer hope that the emotional pain will decrease with time
Advise that significant persons express acceptance of one another
Explain the importance of offering emotional support to one another
Explain that persons making emotional adjustments prefer doing so at their
own pace

EVALUATION

See the evaluation criteria for each specific goal in Chapter 2.

Temporary Total Denial Requirement (12,13,94,372)

ASSESSMENT

Subjective Data
Sense of unreality
Feels highly threatened

Objective Data
Exclaims "No, it can't be. It isn't true."
Claims that x-rays or test results are incorrect
Travels from doctor to doctor seeking to refute the truth
Resorts to faith healers, sometimes
Still seeks treatment, despite the denial

Related Data
Occurs in family members as well as in the sick person
Commonly Related Diseases:
Any fatal or severe disease or injury

POSSIBLE ETIOLOGY

Inability of man to immediately adapt to the full realization of mortality or vulnerability. An attempt to allow time for adaptation so that less radical defenses can be used at a later time. Permits the person to set aside thoughts of the painful experience so that he can lead a normal life.

NURSING DIAGNOSIS

Temporary total denial requirement: a temporary, immediate response of nonacceptance occurring when a person is informed of a very painful reality

PLANNING

Patient Needs	Primary Nurse-Patient Goals
Comfort	To achieve comfort
Protection from psychologic threat	To prevent emotional injury
Acceptance	To achieve productive interpersonal relationships
Warm, communicating relationships	To achieve effective verbal and nonverbal communications
Adequacy	To achieve positive expressions, feelings, reactions
Personal growth and maturity	To achieve optimum function
Increased learning	To achieve awareness of needs

NURSING INTERVENTIONS

Nursing Treatments
Approach unhurriedly
Provide an atmosphere of acceptance
Reassure verbally (that the nurse is available to discuss the problem)
Recognize the need for the use of appropriate defense mechanisms (by supporting the denial)

Encourage the use of normal coping mechanisms
Recognize the need for unique personal adjustments to change
Encourage the expression of feelings
Listen attentively
  AND
Talk with the patient
Offer feedback of the patient's expressed feelings
Ensure the patient's feelings of safety before introducing unpleasantness
Provide emotionally safe experiences
Provide objects which symbolize safeness
Encourage mutual problem solving
Explore with the patient his strengths and resources

Nursing Observations
Determine the degree of insight
Evaluate the person's relatedness with others
Evaluate the significance of emotional distress mannerisms
Evaluate the significance of nonverbal communication
Identify disturbing conversation topics
Identify emotion-stimulating events
Identify reality-acceptance clues
Identify appropriate use of defense mechanisms
Identify inappropriate use of defense mechanisms
Identify the current dominant emotion
Observe for an excessive stress level
Observe for evidence that the patient is reaching out for emotional support
Observe for evidence of a favorable response to therapy

Health Teaching
Explain that the person's emotional response is appropriate and commonly
    experienced
Explain and offer hope that the emotional pain will decrease with time
Advise that significant persons express acceptance of one another
Explain the importance of offering emotional support to one another

EVALUATION

See the evaluation criteria for each specific goal in Chapter 2.

SELF-CONCEPT

Altered Self-concept Related to Illness Reinforcement by Others (12,94,98, 118)

ASSESSMENT

Subjective Data
Patient perceives himself as too ill to continue activities he has been per-
    forming
Heightened anxiety

Objective Data

Verbal confirmation and overemphasis of the seriousness of the illness by
   the reinforcing party
Reinforcer pampers the patient
Patient responds by prolonging his illness
Diminished ability to function

Related Data

Commonly Related Diseases:
None
   OR
Any disease

POSSIBLE ETIOLOGY

Overprotectiveness. Displaced hostility on the part of the reinforcer. An inadequate attempt at social activity by the reinforcer.

NURSING DIAGNOSIS

Altered self-concept related to illness reinforcement by others: external and
unwarranted enhancement of the seriousness of a person's illness by
another person

PLANNING

Patient Needs	**Primary Nurse-Patient Goals**
Protection from psychologic threat	To prevent emotional injury
Warm, communicating relationships	To achieve effective verbal and nonverbal communications
Adequacy	To achieve positive expressions, feelings, reactions
Increased learning	To achieve awareness of needs
Increased reality perception and problem-solving ability	To achieve optimum function

NURSING INTERVENTIONS

Nursing Treatments

Approach unhurriedly
Reassure verbally
Emphasize the person's normal characteristics
Encourage self-performance
Encourage maintenance of an established favorable reputation
Encourage awareness of positive responses from others
Encourage the expression of feelings (by both the patient and the visitor)
Listen attentively
   AND
Talk with the patient (and visitor)
Provide reliable information (about the patient's health status)
Support a realistic assessment of the situation

Explore with the patient his strengths and resources
Explore with the patient the effects of his behavior on others
Refrain from negatively criticizing
Restrict unwanted visitors

Nursing Observations
Determine the extent of behavioral suggestibility
Determine the degree of insight
Determine the precipitating factors
Evaluate the person's relatedness with others
Evaluate the significance of emotional distress mannerisms
Evaluate the significance of nonverbal communication
Identify disturbing conversation topics
Observe for an excessive stress level
Observe for impaired self-attitudes
Observe for evidence of a favorable response to therapy

Health Teaching
Advise that negative responses from others be regarded with minimum
    significance
Explain the importance of offering emotional support to one another
Explain the importance of maintaining a positive self-attitude
Explain the causes of the health problem

EVALUATION

See the evaluation criteria for each specific goal in Chapter 2.

Difficult Adaptation to Altered Body Image (118,199,331,540,552,558)

ASSESSMENT

Subjective Data
Self-displeasure
Sadness
Despair
Grief
Worries about physical changes
Finds the thought of physical or mental limitations intolerable

Objective Data
Verbalizes discontent with the present body
Weeping
Irritability
Refuses to admit that he cannot work as hard or as long, that he is unable
    to perform strenuous physical activity, that his responses are slower,
    that he has difficulty learning new things, or that his memory is less
    reliable
Attempts difficult physical or mental tasks despite limitations
Resorts to considerable reminiscing about his stronger, healthier days

Related Data

Commonly Related Conditions:
Aging
Radical mastectomy
Colostomy, ileostomy, or ureteroileostomy

Commonly Related Diseases:
Bone or skin cancer
Limb amputation
Knife wounds of the face or arm
Second- or third-degree burns
Addison's disease
Acromegaly
   OR
Any disease that changes bodily appearance or function

POSSIBLE ETIOLOGY

Loss of a body part. Impaired body function. Body disfigurement. The threat of diminished self-esteem.

NURSING DIAGNOSIS

Difficult adaptation to altered body image: a period of difficult emotional adjustment in which one attempts to adapt to the perception of one's body as different from the original and acceptable body that previously represented oneself

PLANNING

Patient Needs	Primary Nurse-Patient Goals
Comfort	To achieve comfort
Protection from psychologic threat	To prevent emotional injury
Acceptance	To achieve productive interpersonal relationships
Warm, communicating relationships	To achieve effective verbal and nonverbal communications
High evaluation of self, adequacy	To achieve positive expressions, feelings, reactions
Dignity	To achieve productive interpersonal relationships
Personal growth and maturity	To achieve optimum function
Increased learning	To achieve awareness of needs
Increased reality perception and problem-solving ability	To achieve optimum function

NURSING INTERVENTIONS

Nursing Treatments
Approach unhurriedly
Provide an atmosphere of acceptance
Express empathy

Reassure verbally
Provide frequent patient contact
Avoid causing painful emotional situations
Emphasize the person's value as an individual
Emphasize the person's normal characteristics
Encourage acceptance of self-limitations
Encourage awareness of positive responses from others
Encourage the expression of feelings
Listen attentively
    AND
Talk with the patient
Offer feedback of the patient's expressed feelings
Encourage patient questions
Encourage patience in illness adjustment
Encourage the sharing of common problems with others
Recognize the need for the use of appropriate defense mechanisms
Encourage the use of normal coping mechanisms
Recognize the need for unique personal adjustments to change
Explore with the patient his strengths and resources
Introduce to persons who have successfully undergone the same experience
Reduce the demands placed upon the patient
Refrain from negatively criticizing

Nursing Observations
Determine the degree of insight
Evaluate the significance of emotional distress mannerisms
Evaluate the significance of nonverbal communication
Identify disturbing conversation topics
Identify life values significant to the person
Identify appropriate use of defense mechanisms
Identify inappropriate use of defense mechanisms
Identify the current dominant emotion
Observe for evidence that the patient is reaching out for emotional support
Observe for evidence of a favorable response to therapy

Health Teaching
Explain that the person's emotional response is appropriate and commonly
    experienced
Explain and offer hope that the emotional pain will decrease with time
Advise that negative responses from others be regarded with minimum
    significance
Advise that significant persons express acceptance of one another
Explain the importance of offering emotional support to one another
Explain the importance of maintaining a positive self-attitude
Explain how to obtain release from emotional stress
Explain that ill persons are often hypersensitive

EVALUATION

See the evaluation criteria for each specific goal in Chapter 2.

Difficult Adaptation to Childlessness
(12,13,94,118,372)

ASSESSMENT

Subjective Data

Anxiety regarding diminished self-concept, social acceptance, and social roles
Guilt
Depression

Objective Data

Couple has been married several years
Have unsuccessfully attempted to have children
Verbalize frequently how much they want a child

Related Data

Commonly Related Diseases:
Cervicitis
Vaginitis
Salpingitis
Endometritis
Hypothyroidism
Ovarian cyst
Uterine retroversion
Seminal duct obstruction
Cryptorchidism

POSSIBLE ETIOLOGY

Feelings of inadequacy. Unfulfilled need gratification. Reproductive organ disorders.

NURSING DIAGNOSIS

Difficult adaptation to childlessness: a period of difficult emotional adjustment in which the persons attempt to adapt to the realization that they are unable to conceive human life

PLANNING

Patient Needs	**Primary Nurse-Patient Goals**
Comfort	To achieve comfort
Protection from psycholgic threat	To prevent emotional injury
Acceptance	To achieve productive interpersonal relationships
Warm, communicating relationships	To achieve effective verbal and nonverbal communications
Adequacy	To achieve positive expressions, feelings, reactions
Personal growth and maturity	To achieve optimum function
Increased learning	To achieve awareness of needs and/or use of resources

Increased reality perception and   To achieve optimum function
   problem-solving ability

NURSING INTERVENTIONS

Nursing Treatments
Approach unhurriedly
Provide an atmosphere of acceptance
Express empathy
Reassure verbally
Emphasize the person's value as an individual
Emphasize the person's normal characteristics
Encourage acceptance of self-limitations
Encourage the expression of feelings
Listen attentively
   AND
Talk with the patient
Offer feedback of the patient's expressed feelings
Assist the patient in setting standards of a meaningful existence
Encourage meaningful activity
Recognize the need for the use of appropriate defense mechanisms
Encourage the use of normal coping mechanisms
Suggest possible child adoption
Make a referral (to a physician if the couple has not seen a physician)

Nursing Observations
Determine the extent of behavioral suggestibility
Determine the degree of insight
Determine the extent of group pressure conformity
Evaluate the significance of emotional distress mannerisms
Evaluate the significance of nonverbal communication
Identify disturbing conversation topics
Identify life values significant to the person
Identify appropriate use of defense mechanisms
Identify inappropriate use of defense mechanisms
Observe for an excessive stress level
Observe for impaired self-attitudes
Observe for evidence that the patient is reaching out for emotional support
Observe for evidence of a favorable response to therapy

Health Teaching
Explain that the person's emotional response is appropriate and commonly
   experienced
Advise that negative responses from others be regarded with minimum
   significance
Advise that significant persons express acceptance of one another
Explain the importance of offering emotional support to one another
Explain the importance of maintaining a positive self-attitude

EVALUATION
See the evaluation criteria for each specific goal in Chapter 2.

Difficult Adaptation to Retirement (73,115)

ASSESSMENT

Subjective Data
Feels unneeded
Especially lonely from 9 A.M. to 5 P.M.
Worries about growing old
Lonesome for the social contacts enjoyed through previous work environment

Objective Data
Irritability
Verbal preoccupation with the good old days
Spends considerably more time sleeping
Fills leisure time with meaningless activity
Manifests evidence of increased illness

Related Data
Commonly Related Diseases:
None
   OR
Any disease that forces early retirement or occurs after retirement

POSSIBLE ETIOLOGY

Negative attitudes toward retirement. Dependence on work for need satisfaction. Interruption of the normal pattern of a meaningful life. Retirement required because of age.

NURSING DIAGNOSIS

Difficult adaptation to retirement: a period of difficult emotional adjustment in which the person attempts to adapt to loss of identity and established daily routine following withdrawal from employment

PLANNING

Patient Needs	Primary Nurse-Patient Goals
Activity	To achieve activity
Comfort	To achieve comfort
Protection from psychologic threat	To prevent emotional injury
Acceptance	To achieve productive interpersonal relationships
Warm, communicating relationships	To achieve effective verbal and nonverbal communications
Sense of value, usefulness	To achieve positive expressions, feelings, reactions
Recognition, dignity	To achieve productive interpersonal relationships
Personal growth and maturity	To achieve optimum function

Increased learning

Full development of potential

Increased reality perception and
problem-solving ability

To achieve awareness of needs

To achieve optimum function

To achieve optimum function

NURSING INTERVENTIONS

Nursing Treatments

Approach unhurriedly

Provide an atmosphere of acceptance

Express empathy

Express warmth and friendliness

Reassure verbally

Encourage the expression of feelings

Listen attentively

AND

Talk with the patient

Offer feedback of the patient's expressed feelings

Emphasize the person's value as an individual

Assist the patient in restructuring his lifestyle

Assist the patient in setting standards of a meaningful existence

Encourage meaningful activity

Encourage involvement in community affairs

Encourage involvement in helping others

Encourage involvement in totally new interests

Encourage renewal of former interests

Encourage part-time employment

Encourage planned one-day-at-a-time living

Encourage visits with friends when lonely

Encourage mutual problem solving

Recognize the need for the use of appropriate defense mechanisms

Encourage the use of normal coping mechanisms

Recognize the need for unique personal adjustments to change

Explore with the patient his strengths and resources

Nursing Observations

Determine the degree of insight

Estimate the degree of stress experienced

Evaluate the person's relatedness with others

Evaluate the significance of emotional distress mannerisms

Evaluate the significance of nonverbal communication

Identify disturbing conversation topics

Identify life values significant to the person

Identify appropriate use of defense mechanisms

Identify inappropriate use of defense mechanisms

Observe for an excessive stress level

Observe for impaired self-attitudes

Observe for evidence that the patient is reaching out for emotional support

Observe for evidence of a favorable response to therapy

Health Teaching

Explain that the person's emotional response is appropriate and commonly experienced

Explain that positive retirement goals are essential to health

Explain the importance of offering emotional support to one another

Explain the importance of maintaining a positive self-attitude

Emphasize the importance of planning and anticipating future activities

Explain that persons making emotional adjustments prefer doing so at their own pace

EVALUATION

See the evaluation criteria for each specific goal in Chapter 2.

Diminished Self-esteem Related to Illness (12,13,94,118,372)

ASSESSMENT

Subjective Data

Intense feeling of humiliation

Perceives that his sick body no longer measures up to the standards by which it can be considered an object of value

Perceives that since his body is part of what makes up his total being, then he is a person of less value than he was before the illness

Feels that others perceive him with less respect because of his illness

Sensitive to comments by others about the illness

Quick to perceive the strengths of others

Preoccupied with his own weakness

Objective Data

May blame others for the illness

Withdrawn from social contacts

Personal appearance is not attended to as well as in the past

Related Data

Commonly Related Conditions:
Aging

Commonly Related Diseases:
Parkinson's disease
Multiple Sclerosis
Rheumatoid arthiritis
Cerebral vascular accident
Cervical, thoracic, or lumbar spinal injury
Myocardial infarction
Limb amputation

POSSIBLE ETIOLOGY

Poorly defined self-image. The loss of a life situation through illness that in the past maintained self-esteem.

NURSING DIAGNOSIS

Diminished self-esteem related to illness: the perception of oneself as of less value than others as a result of being ill

PLANNING

Patient Needs	Primary Nurse-Patient Goals
Comfort	To achieve comfort
Protection from psychologic threat	To prevent emotional injury
Acceptance	To achieve productive interpersonal relationships
Warm, communicating relationships	To achieve effective verbal and nonverbal communications
High evaluation of self, adequacy	To achieve positive expressions, feelings, reactions
Personal growth and maturity	To achieve optimum function
Increased learning	To achieve awareness of needs
Increased reality perception and problem-solving ability	To achieve optimum function

NURSING INTERVENTIONS

Nursing Treatments
Approach unhurriedly
Provide an atmosphere of acceptance
Express empathy
Reassure verbally
Express warmth and friendliness
Emphasize the person's value as an individual
Emphasize the person's normal characteristics
Encourage acceptance of self-limitations
Encourage awareness of positive responses from others
Encourage the expression of feelings
Listen attentively
    AND
Talk with the patient
Offer feedback of the patient's expressed feelings
Encourage the sharing of common problems with others
Recognize the need for the use of appropriate defense mechanisms
Encourage the use of normal coping mechanisms
Recognize the need for unique personal adjustments to change
Explore wtith the patient his strengths and resources
Explore with the patient reasons for self-criticism
Introduce to persons who have successfully undergone the same experience
Support a realistic assessment of the situation

Nursing Observations
Determine the degree of insight
Evaluate the person's relatedness with others
Evaluate the significance of emotional distress mannerisms

Evaluate the significance of nonverbal communication
Identify disturbing conversation topics
Identify life values significant to the person
Identify appropriate use of defense mechanisms
Identify inappropriate use of defense mechanisms
Observe for an excessive stress level
Observe for impaired self-attitudes
Observe for evidence that the patient is reaching out for emotional support
Observe for evidence of a favorable response to therapy

Health Teaching

Explain that the person's emotional response is appropriate and commonly
  experienced
Advise that negative responses from others be regarded with minimum
  significance
Advise that significant persons express acceptance of one another
Explain the importance of offering emotional support to one another
Explain the importance of maintaining a positive self-attitude
Explain that ill persons are often hypersensitive
Explain the causes of the health problem

EVALUATION

See the evaluation criteria for each specific goal in Chapter 2.

Inadequate Self-concept (98,115,372)

ASSESSMENT

Subjective Data

Person feels that he is not sure who he is
Experiences a sense of vague self-identity
Is intensely aware of trying to mentally clarify who he is

Objective Data

Displays a variety of behaviors in an effort to find one suitable to his identity

Related Data

Commonly Related Diseases:
None
  OR
Any disease or injury

POSSIBLE ETIOLOGY

Lack of direction toward the future. A sudden life change that has altered
one's self-concept. The person cannot mentally or emotionally determine a
total identity and is not mature enough to establish an identity.

NURSING DIAGNOSIS

Inadequate self-concept: the inability of the person to clearly define who he
is in relation to being a separate person with distinct qualities from others

PLANNING

Patient Needs	**Primary Nurse-Patient Goals**
Comfort	To achieve comfort
Protection from psychologic threat	To prevent emotional injury
Acceptance	To achieve productive interpersonal relationships
Sense of value, usefulness, high evaluation of self, adequacy	To achieve positive expressions, feelings, reactions
Personal growth and maturity	To achieve optimum function
Increased learning	To achieve awareness of needs

NURSING INTERVENTIONS

Nursing Treatments

Approach unhurriedly
Provide an atmosphere of acceptance
Express empathy
Reassure verbally
Emphasize the person's value as an individual
Encourage awareness of positive responses from others
Encourage differentiation between self ideal and actual self
Encourage the expression of feelings
Listen attentively
    AND
Talk with the patient
Offer feedback of the patient's expressed feelings
Encourage honesty in presenting oneself to others
Encourage identification of specific life values
Encourage identification of success standards
Encourage identification of values acquired from one's own culture
Encourage identification of values in common with the values of others
Encourage the practical application of the accepted value system
Encourage recognition of one's various roles in life
Encourage the substitution of real-life endeavors for fantasized endeavors
Encourage participation in therapeutic group interaction
Encourage the use of normal coping mechanisms
Refrain from negatively criticizing
Refrain from personality comparisons

Nursing Observations

Determine the degree of insight
Evaluate the person's relatedness with others
Evaluate the significance of emotional distress mannerisms
Evaluate the significance of nonverbal communication
Identify disturbing conversation topics
Identify life values significant to the person
Observe for an excessive stress level
Observe for impaired self-attitudes

Observe for evidence that the patient is reaching out for emotional support
Observe for evidence of a favorable response to therapy

Health Teaching
Advise against verbally comparing significant persons
Advise that negative responses from others be regarded with minimum significance
Advise that significant persons express acceptance of one another
Explain the importance of offering emotional support to one another
Explain the importance of maintaining a positive self-attitude
Explain that persons making emotional adjustments prefer doing so at their own pace
Teach how to use the problem-solving method

EVALUATION

See the evaluation criteria for each specific goal in Chapter 2.

Loss of Individuality Related to Institutionalization

ASSESSMENT

Subjective Data
Low self-esteem
Feels he is just one of many

Objective Data
Conforms to established routines as expected
Finds his identity listed by number, not name
Unable to obtain special consideration
Suddenly demands individual attention

Related Data
Has been institutionalized for some time
Commonly Related Diseases:
None
    OR
Any disease or injury

POSSIBLE ETIOLOGY

Lack of concern for persons as individuals. Imposed stress and time limitations when the needs of large numbers of people must be met.

NURSING DIAGNOSIS

Loss of individuality related to institutionalization: lack of regard for the person's separateness, distinct characteristics, and needs, as distinguished from those of another

PLANNING

Patient Needs	**Primary Nurse-Patient Goals**
Comfort	To achieve comfort
Protection from psychologic threat	To prevent emotional injury

High evaluation of self

Recognition, dignity, importance, attention

To achieve positive expressions, feelings, reactions

To achieve productive interpersonal relationships

NURSING INTERVENTIONS

Nursing Treatments
Approach unhurriedly
Express empathy
Touch the patient judiciously
Provide frequent patient contact
Sit with the patient (whenever possible)
Grant special requests
Emphasize the person's value as an individual
Encourage the expression of feelings
Listen attentively
    AND
Talk with the patient
Offer feedback of the patient's expressed feelings
Use the patient's name frequently

Nursing Observations
Determine the degree of insight
Evaluate the significance of emotional distress mannerisms
Evaluate the significance of nonverbal communication
Identify disturbing conversation topics
Observe for an excessive stress level
Observe for impaired self-attitudes
Observe for evidence of a favorable response to therapy

Health Teaching
Explain that the person's emotional response is appropriate and commonly experienced
Explain the importance of maintaining a positive self-attitude
Explain the causes of the health problem

EVALUATION

See the evaluation criteria for each specific goal in Chapter 2.

Self-dissatisfaction Related to an Unfulfilled Life Cycle (173,248)

ASSESSMENT

Subjective Data
Dwells on dreams of new endeavors that can never be completed because of age
Envious of the young
Despair

Objective Data
Verbalizes about what he would do if life could only be lived over again
Displays antagonism toward the young

Related Data

Commonly Related Diseases:
None
    OR
Any disease during mature adulthood

POSSIBLE ETIOLOGY

Dissatisfaction with what one's life has been. Desire to live life over again.

NURSING DIAGNOSIS

Self-dissatisfaction related to an unfulfilled life cycle: dissatisfaction with the fact that one has only a single life cycle, that it is about to end, and that everything intended was not accomplished

PLANNING

Patient Needs	Primary Nurse-Patient Goals
Comfort	To achieve comfort
Protection from psychologic threat	To prevent emotional injury
Acceptance	To achieve productive interpersonal relationships
Warm, communicating relationships	To achieve effective verbal and nonverbal communications
High evaluation of self	To achieve positive expressions, feelings, reactions
Independence	To achieve optimum function
Dignity	To achieve productive interpersonal relationships
Personal growth and maturity	To achieve optimum function
Increased learning	To achieve awareness of needs
Increased reality perception and problem-solving ability	To achieve optimum function

NURSING INTERVENTIONS

Nursing Treatments
Approach unhurriedly
Provide an atmosphere of acceptance
Express empathy
Encourage the expression of feelings
Listen attentively
    AND
Talk with the patient
Offer feedback of the patient's expressed feelings
Emphasize the person's value as an individual
Encourage acceptance of partial goal satisfaction
Encourage awareness of positive responses from others (regarding accomplishments)

Encourage strivings toward realistic goals
Encourage the substitution of real-life endeavors for fantisized endeavors
Encourage the use of normal coping mechanisms
Explore with the patient previous achievements of success
Explore with the patient his strength and resources
Support a realistic assessment of the situation

Nursing Observations
Determine the degree of insight
Evaluate the significance of emotional distress mannerisms
Evaluate the significance of nonverbal communication
Identify disturbing conversation topics
Identify life values significant to the person
Identify appropriate use of defense mechanisms
Identify inappropriate use of defense mechanisms
Observe for an excessive stress level
Observe for impaired self-attitudes
Observe for evidence that the patient is reaching out for emotional support
Observe for evidence of a favorable response to therapy

Health Teaching
Explain that the person's emotional response is appropriate and commonly
     experienced
Emphasize the importance of planning and anticipating future activities
     (realistically)
Explain the importance of maintaining a positive self-attitude
Explain the causes of the health problem

EVALUATION

See the evaluation criteria for each specific goal in Chapter 2.

Self-dissatisfaction Related to the Developing Body (12,94,372)

ASSESSMENT

Subjective Data
The young child perceives his body as less than that of other children
May perceive deformed body parts as related to, but as separate from, the
     whole body
Perceives body changes during growth as threatening

Objective Data
Poor coordination
Small body
Poor body posture
Deformed body
Withdraws from participation in childhood competition
Verbally expresses dissatisfaction with his limitations
Attempts to excel in mental activities

Related Data

Commonly Related Diseases:
None
  OR
Muscular dystrophy
Cerebral palsy

POSSIBLE ETIOLOGY

Inability to perform motor skills as well as other children. Presence of deformities or unsightly scars. Unpleasant facial features. Inherited frail body.

NURSING DIAGNOSIS

Self-dissatisfaction related to the developing body: the gradual perception of a child that his body is not as acceptable or as competent as those of other children

PLANNING

Patient Needs	**Primary Nurse-Patient Goals**
Comfort	To achieve comfort
Protection from psychologic threat	To prevent emotional injury
Acceptance	To achieve productive interpersonal relationships
Warm, communicating relationships	To achieve effective verbal and nonverbal communications
High evaluation of self, adequacy	To achieve positive expressions, feelings, and reactions
Increased learning	To achieve awareness of needs

NURSING INTERVENTIONS

Nursing Treatments
Approach unhurriedly
Provide an atmosphere of acceptance
Express empathy
Reassure verbally
Touch the patient judiciously
Express warmth and friendliness
Listen attentively
  AND
Talk with the patient
Offer feedback of the patient's expressed feelings
Avoid causing embarrassing situations
Avoid causing painful emotional situations
Provide emotionally safe experiences
Emphasize the person's value as an individual
Emphasize the person's normal characteristics
Encourage acceptance of self-limitations
Assist the patient in setting standards of a meaningful existence
Encourage meaningful activity

Encourage realistic perception of others
Encourage the sharing of common problems with others
Recognize the need for the use of appropriate defense mechanisms
Encourage the use of normal coping mechanisms
Explore with the patient his strengths and resources
Explore with the patient reasons for self-criticism
Support a realistic assessment of the situation
Introduce to persons who have successfully undergone the same experience

Nursing Observations
Determine the degree of insight
Determine the extent of group pressure conformity
Evaluate the person's relatedness with others
Evaluate the significance of emotional distress mannerisms
Evaluate the significance of nonverbal communication
Identify disturbing conversation topics
Identify emotion-stimulating events
Identify life values significant to the person
Identify appropriate use of defense mechanisms
Identify inappropriate use of defense mechanisms
Observe for evidence that the person is reaching out for emotional support
Observe for evidence of a favorable response to therapy

Health Teaching
Explain that the person's emotional response is appropriate and commonly
    experienced
Advise against verbally comparing significant persons
Advise that negative responses from others be regarded with minimum
    significance
Advise that significant persons express acceptance of one another
Advise that significant persons express love for one another
Explain the importance of offering emotional support to one another
Explain the importance of maintaining a positive self-attitude
Explain that parental attitudes affect child development
Teach how to use the problem-solving method

EVALUATION

See the evaluation criteria for each specific goal in Chapter 2.

Sense of Inadequacy (12,13,94,372)

ASSESSMENT

Subjective Data
Perceives himself as inadequate and worthless in the eyes of others
Perceives failure on starting any activity
Experiences discomforting emptiness, hopelessness, threat, and fearfulness
Indulges in considerable fantasy

Objective Data
Easily discouraged
Intolerance to minor rebuffs

Easily embarrassed
Timid
Lacks openness to new ideas and thoughts
Poorly motivated, not attempting new experiences
Habitual procrastination
Malingering, irresponsible behavior
Envious of others
Overrates the virtues of superiors and persons in high positions
Underrates the virtues of persons in a status beneath him
Does not make friends easily
Indulges in extreme egotism by relating everything to himself
Pushes his children to achieve great things
Lies to protect himself
Habitually participates in highly dangerous activities to prove his adequacy
Quick to resist change
Excessively dominant over things

Related Data

Commonly Related Diseases:
None
  OR
Any disease or injury

POSSIBLE ETIOLOGY

Feelings of inadequacy. The inability to try one's abilities because of overprotective authority figures. Parental establishment of goals too high for a
child to reach. Anxiety and disapproval of failure expressed by significant
persons. The person was dominated into submissiveness as a child by one or
both parents and as an adult dominates others to reduce his sense of inadequacy.

NURSING DIAGNOSIS

Sense of inadequacy: a feeling that one is not adequate and capable in a
situation

PLANNING

Patient Needs	**Primary Nurse-Patient Goals**
Comfort	To achieve comfort
Protection from psychologic threat	To prevent emotional injury
Acceptance	To achieve productive interpersonal relationships
Warm, communicating relationships	To achieve effective verbal and nonverbal communications
High evaluation of self, adequacy, self-reliance	To achieve positive expressions, feeling, reactions
Goal achievement	To achieve optimum function

Personal growth and maturity	To achieve optimum function
Increased learning	To achieve awareness of needs
Full development of potential	To achieve optimum function
Increased reality perception and problem-solving ability	To achieve optimum function

NURSING INTERVENTIONS

Nursing Treatments
Approach unhurriedly
Provide an atmosphere of acceptance
Demonstrate calmness
Express empathy
Reassure verbally
Provide frequent patient contact
Encourage the expression of feelings
Listen attentively
    AND
Talk with the patient
Offer feedback of the patient's expressed feelings
Emphasize the person's value as an individual
Emphasize the person's normal characteristics
Encourage awareness of positive responses from others
Encourage identification of specific life values
Encourage identification of success standards
Encourage realistic perception of others
Encourage self-performance
Encourage the sharing of common problems with others
Encourage single goal seeking
Encourage strivings toward realistic goals
Explore with the patient his strengths and resources
Explore with the patient previous achievements of success
Explore with the patient previous displays of courage
Explore with the patient reasons for recurring problems
Explore with the patient the effects of his behavior on others
Introduce to persons who have successfully undergone the same experience
Support a realistic assessment of the situation
Reduce the demands placed upon the patient
Refrain from negatively criticizing

Nursing Observations
Determine the degree of insight
Determine the precipitating factors
Determine the relieving factors
Evaluate the person's relatedness with others
Evaluate the significance of emotional distress mannerisms
Evaluate the significance of nonverbal communication
Identify disturbing conversation topics
Identify inappropriate emotional responses

Identify life values significant to the person
Identify appropriate use of defense mechanisms
Identify inappropriate use of defense mechanisms
Observe for an excessive stress level
Observe for evidence that the patient is reaching out for emotional support
Observe for evidence of a favorable response to therapy

Health Teaching
Advise that negative responses from others be regarded with minimum
    significance
Advise that significant persons express acceptance of one another
Advise that significant persons express love for one another
Explain the importance of offering emotional support to one another
Explain the need for realistic expectations of others
Emphasize the need to develop self-reliance
Teach how to use the problem-solving method
Explain the causes of the health problem

EVALUATION

See the evaluation criteria for each specific goal in Chapter 2.

Sense of Meaninglessness
(12,13,94,372)

ASSESSMENT

Subjective Data
Feelings of alienation, emptiness, and worthlessness
Unable to perceive the situation and himself as having a meaningful rela-
    tionship
Feels he has little or no effect on persons or situations, that he does not
    matter
Feels unneeded by family and friends

Objective Data
Verbalizes his unimportance in the scheme of things
Lacks specific goals

Related Data
Commonly Related Conditions:
Retirement
Children leaving home
Commonly Related Diseases:
None
    OR
Any disease that limits one from participation in meaningful activity, such
    as cerebral vascular accident, myocardial infarction. Parkinson's disease,
    or cervical, thoracic, or lumbar spinal injury, psychotic depression

POSSIBLE ETIOLOGY

Negative self-esteem. Inability to identify with and accept cultural goals
and values. Lack of creative functioning and goal striving. Forced removal
from meaningful employment or activities.

NURSING DIAGNOSIS

Sense of meaninglessness: a feeling that one's life has no purpose or significance

PLANNING

Patient Needs	Primary Nurse-Patient Goals
Comfort	To achieve comfort
Protection from psychologic threat	To prevent emotional injury
Acceptance	To achieve productive interpersonal relationships
Warm, communicating relationships	To achieve effective verbal and nonverbal communications
Sense of value, usefulness, high evaluation of self	To achieve positive expressions, feelings, reactions
Goal achievement	To achieve optimum function
Personal growth and maturity	To achieve optimum function
Increased learning	To achieve awareness of needs
Full development of potentialities	To achieve optimum function
Religious-philosophic satisfaction	To achieve spiritual goals
Increased pleasantness	To achieve positive expressions, feelings, reactions

NURSING INTERVENTIONS

Nursing Treatments
Approach unhurriedly
Provide an atmosphere of acceptance
Express empathy
Reassure verbally
Encourage the expression of feelings
Listen attentively
   AND
Talk with the patient
Offer feedback of the patient's expressed feelings
Assist the patient in setting standards of a meaningful existence
Encourage meaningful activity
Encourage involvement in community affairs
Encourage involvement in helping others
Emphasize the person's value as an individual
Encourage awareness of positive responses from others
Encourage family-shared pleasures
Encourage family-shared responsibility
Encourage families to seek the opinions of elders
Encourage planned one-day-at-a-time living
Encourage relationships between persons with common interests and goals
Explore with the patient his strengths and resources
Support a realistic assessment of the situation

Introduce to persons who have successfully undergone the same experience
Refrain from negativly criticizing

Nursing Observations
Determine the degree of insight
Determine the precipitating factors
Determine the relieving factors
Evaluate the person's relatedness with others
Evaluate the significance of emotional distress mannerisms
Evaluate the significance of nonverbal communication
Identify disturbing conversation topics
Observe for an excessive stress level
Observe for impaired self-attitudes
Observe for evidence that the patient is reaching out for emotional support
Observe for evidence of a favorable response to therapy

Health Teaching
Explain that the person's emotional response is appropriate and commonly experienced
Advise that significant persons express acceptance of one another
Advise that significant persons express love for one another
Explain the importance of offering emotional support to one another
Explain the importance of maintaining a positive self-attitude
Emphasize the importance of planning and anticipating future activities
Recommend that passive activities be avoided

EVALUATION

See the evaluation criteria for each specific goal in Chapter 2.

SEXUALITY

Difficult Adaptation to Role Reversal
(45,115,118,415)

ASSESSMENT
Subjective Data
Humiliation
Fears rejection
Decreased self-esteem
Considerable anxiety

Objective Data
Woman financially supports the family, although her husband had done so previously
Man assumes household chores, which his wife previously did
Can no longer assume previous responsibilities, which remain unattended to or are divided or assigned to others

Related Data
Commonly Related Conditions:
Aging

Commonly Related Diseases:
None
OR
Any disease or injury

POSSIBLE ETIOLOGY

Illness forced changes in social codes related to one's sex. Health problems that alter one's physical capacity. Different life stages that alter the person's role.

NURSING DIAGNOSIS

Difficult adaptation to role reversal: a period of difficult emotional adjustment in which the person attempts to adapt to the loss of some of the social components that make up the total personality structure of being a whole man or woman

PLANNING

Patient Needs	Primary Nurse-Patient Goals
Comfort	To achieve comfort
Protection from psychologic threat	To prevent emotional injury
Acceptance	To achieve productive interpersonal relationships
Warm, communicating relationships	To achieve effective verbal and nonverbal communications
High evaluation of self	To achieve positive expressions, feelings, reactions
Independence	To achieve optimum function
Dignity	To achieve productive interpersonal relationships
Personal growth and maturity	To achieve optimum function
Increased learning	To achieve awareness of needs
Increased reality perception and problem-solving ability	To achieve optimum function

NURSING INTERVENTIONS

Nursing Treatments
Approach unhurriedly
Provide an atmosphere of acceptance
Express empathy
Express warmth and friendliness
Arrange situations which encourage patient autonomy
Assist the patient in restructuring his lifestyle
Emphasize the person's value as an individual
Encourage acceptance of interdependency
Encourage acceptance of self-limitations
Encourage the expression of feelings

Listen attentively
    AND
Talk with the patient
Offer feedback of the patient's expressed feelings
Encourage the sharing of common problems with others
Encourage strivings toward realistic goals
Recognize the need for the use of appropriate defense mechanisms
Encourage the use of normal coping mechanisms
Recognize the need for unique personal adjustments to change
Explore with the patient his strengths and resources
Explore with the patient reasons for self-criticism
Support a realistic assessment of the situation
Introduce to persons who have successfully undergone the same experience
Provide objects which symbolize sex identity

Nursing Observations
Determine the degree of insight
Evaluate the person's relatedness with others
Evaluate the significance of emotional distress mannerisms
Evaluate the significance of nonverbal communication
Identify disturbing conversation topics
Identify life values significant to the person
Identify appropriate use of defense mechanisms
Identify inappropriate use of defense mechanisms
Observe for an excessive stress level
Observe for impaired self-attitudes
Observe for evidence that the patient is reaching out for emotional support
Observe for evidence of a favorable response to therapy

Health Teaching
Explain that the person's emotional response is appropriate and commonly
    experienced
Advise that significant persons express acceptance of one another
Advise that significant persons express love for one another
Explain the importance of offering emotional support to one another
Explain the importance of maintaining a positive self-attitude
Explain that ill persons are often hypersensitive
Explain that persons making emotional adjustments prefer doing so at their
    own pace

EVALUATION

See the evaluation criteria for each specific goal in Chapter 2.

Reduced Female Sexual Response (65,415)

ASSESSMENT

Subjective Data
Decreased sexual desire and responsiveness
Perceives sexual activities as undesirable

Female perceives herself as merely an instrument of male gratification, not a love object

Guilt

Anxiety and frustration of the partner

Objective Data

Blames reduced response on natural or surgical menopause or hormonal deficiency

Complains of changed attitudes in the partner

Previous aggressive personality becomes passive

Related Data

Commonly Related Diseases:

None
  OR
Hypopituitarism

POSSIBLE ETIOLOGY

Lack of sexual experience. Surgical removal of the pituitary gland. Recent emotional trauma, especially from the spouse. Lack of social motivation. Preoccupation with stressful problems or responsibilities.

NURSING DIAGNOSIS

Reduced female sexual response: diminished ability of the female to respond to sexual activity

PLANNING

Patient Needs	**Primary Nurse-Patient**
Relaxation	To achieve relaxation
Comfort	To achieve comfort
Sexuality	To achieve productive interpersonal relationships
Protection from psychologic threat	To prevent emotional injury
Love and affection, acceptance	To achieve productive interpersonal relationships
Warm, communicating relationships	To achieve effective verbal and nonverbal communications
High evaluation of self, adequacy	To achieve positive expressions, feelings, reactions
Personal growth and maturity	To achieve optimum function
Increased learning	To achieve awareness of needs
Increased reality perception and problem-solving ability	To achieve optimum function

NURSING INTERVENTIONS

Nursing Treatments

Approach unhurriedly

Provide an atmosphere of acceptance

Express empathy
Reassure verbally
Encourage awareness of positive responses from others (the partner)
Encourage the expression of feelings
Listen attentively
  AND
Talk with the patient
Offer feedback of the patient's expressed feelings
Recognize the need for the use of appropriate defense mechanisms
Encourage the use of normal coping mechanisms
Explore superficial topics and reasons for voiding in-depth feelings
Explore with the patient his strengths and resources
Explore with the patient reasons for recurring problems
Explore with the patient the effects of his behavior on others (the partner)
Provide emotional support for persons significant to the patient
Refrain from negatively criticizing
Support a realistic assessment of the situation

Nursing Observations
Determine the degree of insight
Evaluate the person's relatedness with others
Evaluate the significance of emotional distress mannerisms
Evaluate the significance of nonverbal communication
Identify disturbing conversation topics
Identify life values significant to the person
Identify appropriate use of defense mechanisms
Identify inappropriate use of defense mechanisms
Observe for an excessive stress level
Observe for evidence that the patient is reaching out for emotional support
Observe for evidence of a favorable response to therapy

Health Teaching
Advise against causing defensive responses in others
Advise that significant persons express acceptance of one another
Advise that significant persons express love for one another
Explain the importance of offering emotional support to one another
Explain the importance of recognizing tension within oneself
Explain the need for realistic expectations of others
Explain that fatigue should be recognized as a stress factor
Explain the importance of maintaining a positive self-attitude
Explain that relaxation is essential for successful sexual response
Explain that sexual response normally varies
Explain the emotional causes of reduced sexual response
Explain the physical causes of reduced sexual response
Relate the criteria for successful sexual response

EVALUATION

See the evaluation criteria for each specific goal in Chapter 2.

Reduced Male Sexual Response
(65,415)

ASSESSMENT

Subjective Data
Diminished sexual satisfaction
Grief
Anxiety
Depression
Worries about mate's reaction
Male perceives himself as less of a man

Objective Data
Partially or totally unable to perform sexual activities
Focuses more on preintercourse sexual activity

Related Data
Commonly Related Conditions:
Aging
Commonly Related Diseases:
Syphilis
Multiple sclerosis
Cerebral vascular accident
Cervical or thoracic spinal cord injury
Renal failure

POSSIBLE ETIOLOGY

Congenital abnormality. Fear of causing pregnancy or acquiring venereal disease. Religious beliefs. Emotional immaturity. Inability to give love to others. Alcohol or drug abuse. Spinal cord nerve damage. Chemical imbalance resulting from dialysis.

NURSING DIAGNOSIS

Reduced male sexual response: inability of the male to perform the sex act satisfactorily

PLANNING

Patient Needs	Primary Nurse-Patient Goals
Relaxation	To achieve relaxation
Comfort	To achieve comfort
Sexuality	To achieve productive interpersonal relationships
Protection from psychologic threat	To prevent emotional injury
Love and affection, acceptance	To achieve productive interpersonal relationships
Warm, communicating relationships	To achieve effective verbal and nonverbal communications

High evaluation of self, adequacy	To achieve positive expressions, feelings, reactions
Personal growth and maturity	To achieve optimum function
Increased learning	To achieve awareness of needs
Increased reality perception and problem-solving ability	To achieve optimum function
Increased pleasantness	To achieve positive expressions, feelings, reactions

NURSING INTERVENTIONS

Nursing Treatments
Approach unhurriedly
Provide an atmosphere of acceptance
Express empathy
Reassure verbally
Encourage awareness of positive responses from others (the partner)
Encourage the expression of feelings
Listen attentively
    AND
Talk with the patient
Offer feedback of the patient's expressed feelings
Recognize the need for the use of appropriate defense mechanisms
Encourage the use of normal coping mechanisms
Explore superficial topics and reasons for avoiding in-depth feelings
Explore with the patient his strengths and resources
Explore with the patient reasons for recurring problems
Explore with the patient the effects of his behavior on others (the partner)
Provide emotional support for persons significant to the patient
Refrain from negatively criticizing
Support a realistic assessment of the situation

Nursing Observations
Determine the degree of insight
Evaluate the person's relatedness with others
Evaluate the significance of emotional distress mannerisms
Evaluate the significance of nonverbal communication
Identify disturbing conversation topics
Identify life values significant to the person
Identify appropriate use of defense mechanisms
Identify inappropriate use of defense mechanisms
Observe for an excessive stress level
Observe for evidence that the patient is reaching out for emotional support
Observe for evidence of a favorable response to therapy

Health Teaching
Advise against causing defensive responses in others
Advise that significant persons express acceptance of one another
Advise that significant persons express love for one another
Explain the importance of offering emotional support to one another

Emphasize the importance of recognizing tension within oneself
Explain the need for realistic expectations of others
Explain that fatigue should be recognized as a stress factor
Explain the importance of maintaining a positive self-attitude
Explain that relaxation is essential for successful sexual response
Explain that sexual response normally varies
Explain the physical causes of reduced sexual response
Relate the criteria for successful sexual response

EVALUATION

See the evaluation criteria for each specific goal in Chapter 2.

Rejection Related to Sex Misidentification (12,372,471)

ASSESSMENT

Subjective Data
Cannot accept himself as a man or herself as a woman
Desires to be a person of the opposite sex
Person feels that he is not acceptable to others
Feels that he does not receive the care and attention he deserves because of his variance from social standards of the majority

Objective Data
Female:
Displays generally accepted male behavior and dress
Prefers to work in male-identified occupations
Is competitive
Is aggressive
Has coarse body movements
Male:
Displays generally accepted female behavior and dress
Is preoccupied with domestic affairs
Prefers female-identified occupations and working with women rather than men
Prefers sentimental and romantic movies and literature
Has feminine body movements

Related Data
Commonly Related Condtions:
Transsexualism

POSSIBLE ETIOLOGY

Conflict over gender identity. The child's inability to find warm, affectionate, rewarding relationships with the parent of the same sex causes the child to identify with the parent of the opposite sex. If, in the child's early years, one parent is not available to assume his or her role, the child may be forced to assume that parent's role indirectly. Early childhood reward for behavior usually reserved for the opposite sex. Fear or hate of the parent of the same sex.

NURSING DIAGNOSIS

Rejection related to sex misidentification: feeling of being rebuffed by others because one assumes social characteristics usually reserved for the opposite sex

PLANNING

Patient Needs	Primary Nurse-Patient Goals
Comfort	To achieve comfort
Sexuality	To achieve productive interpersonal relationships
Protection from psychologic threat	To prevent emotional injury
Acceptance	To achieve productive interpersonal relationships
Warm, communicating relationships	To achieve effective verbal and nonverbal communications
High evaluation of self	To achieve positive expressions, feelings, reactions
Personal growth and maturity	To achieve optimum function
Increased learning	To achieve awareness of needs
Increased reality perception and problem-solving ability	To achieve optimum function

NURSING INTERVENTIONS

Nursing Treatments
Approach unhurriedly
Provide an atmosphere of acceptance
Reassure verbally
Provide frequent patient contact
Avoid causing painful emotional situations
Emphasize the person's value as an individual
Encourage awareness of positive responses from others
Encourage the expression of feelings
Listen attentively
　　AND
Talk with the patient
Offer feedback of the patient's expressed feelings
Explore superficial topics and reasons for avoiding in-depth feelings
Explore with the patient his strengths and resources
Explore with the patient reasons for criticism by others
Explore with the patient reasons for criticism of others
Explore with the patient reasons for recurring problems
Recognize the need for the use of appropriate defense mechanisms
Encourage the use of normal coping mechanisms
Refrain from negatively criticizing

Nursing Observations
Determine the degree of insight
Evaluate the person's relatedness with others

Evaluate the significance of emotional distress mannerisms
Evaluate the significance of nonverbal communication
Identify disturbing conversation topics
Identify life values significant to the person
Identify appropriate use of defense mechanisms
Identify inappropriate use of defense mechanisms
Observe for an excessive stress level
Observe for evidence that the patient is reaching out for emotional support
Observe for evidence of a favorable response to therapy

Health Teaching
Advise that negative responses from others be regarded with minimum
     significance
Advise that significant persons express acceptance of one another
Explain the importance of offering emotional support to one another
Explain the need for realistic expectations of others
Explain the importance of maintaining a positive self-attitude

EVALUATION

See the evaluation criteria for each specific goal in Chapter 2.

Rejection Related to Variant Sexual Preferences (48,372,415)

ASSESSMENT

Subjective Data
Person feels that he is not acceptable to others
Feels that he does not receive the care and attention he deserves because of
     his variance from social standards of the majority
Fantasizes that his spouse is of the same sex
Derives strong emotional satisfaction from members of the same sex

Objective Data
Sometimes there is a partnership in which one member assumes an active
     male role and the other a passive female role, although both are of the
     same sex
Married to a member of the opposite sex, but would rather be married to a
     member of the same sex

Related Data
Commonly Related Conditions:
Homosexuality

POSSIBLE ETIOLOGY

Fear of being overwhelmed or exploited by members of the opposite sex.
Lack of affection from the parent of the opposite sex during childhood.

NURSING DIAGNOSIS

Rejection related to variant sexual preferences: feelings of being rebuffed by
others because of one's preference for having sexual relationships with
members of the same sex, rather than with members of the opposite sex

PLANNING

Patient Needs	**Primary Nurse-Patient Goals**
Sexuality	To achieve productive interpersonal relationships
Protection from psychologic threat	To prevent emotional injury
Acceptance	To achieve productive interpersonal relationships
Warm, communicating relationships	To achieve effective verbal and nonverbal communication
High evaluation of self	To achieve positive expressions, feelings, reactions
Personal growth and maturity	To achieve optimum function
Increased learning	To achieve awareness of needs
Increased reality perception and problem-solving ability	To achieve optimum function

NURSING INTERVENTIONS

Nursing Treatments

Approach unhurriedly
Provide an atmosphere of acceptance
Reassure verbally
Provide frequent patient contact
Avoid causing painful emotional situations
Emphasize the person's value as an individual
Encourage awareness of positive responses from others
Encourage the expression of feelings
Listen attentively
    AND
Talk with the patient
Offer feedback of the patient's expressed feelings
Explore superficial topics and reasons for avoiding in-depth feelings
Explore with the patient his strengths and resources
Explore with the patient reasons for criticism by others
Explore with the patient reasons for criticism of others
Explore with the patient reasons for recurring problems
Recognize the need for the use of appropriate defense mechanisms
Encourage the use of normal coping mechanisms
Refrain from negatively criticizing

Nursing Observations

Determine the degree of insight
Evaluate the person's relatedness with others
Evaluate the significance of emotional distress mannerisms
Evaluate the significance of nonverbal communication
Identify disturbing conversation topics
Identify life values significant to the person
Identify appropriate use of defense mechanisms

Identify inappropriate use of defense mechanisms
Observe for an excessive stress level
Observe for evidence that the patient is reaching out for emotional support
Observe for evidence of a favorable response to therapy

Health Teaching
Advise that negative responses from others be regarded with minimum
    significance
Advise that significant persons express acceptance of one another
Explain the importance of offering emotional support to one another
Explain the need for realistic expectations of others
Explain the importance of maintaining a positive self-attitude

EVALUATION

See the evaluation critieria for each specific goal in Chapter 2.

Self-dissatisfaction Related to Sex Misidentification (12,372,471)

ASSESSMENT

Subjective Data
Cannot accept himself as a man or herself as a woman
Desires to be a person of the opposite sex
Dislikes himself for wanting to be of the opposite sex
Feels he is not an acceptable person
Desires to change his behavior

Objective Data
Female:
Displays generally accepted male behavior and dress
Prefers to work in male-identified occupations
Is competitive
Is aggressive
Has coarse body movements

Male:
Displays generally accepted female behavior and dress
Is preoccupied with domestic affairs
Prefers female-identified occupations and working with women rather than
    men
Prefers sentimental and romantic movies and literature
Has feminine body movements

Related Data
Commonly Related Conditions:
Transsexualism

POSSIBLE ETIOLOGY

Conflict over gender identity. The child's inability to find warm, affectionate, rewarding relationships with the parent of the same sex causes the
child to identify with the parent of the opposite sex. If, in the child's early

years, one parent is not available to assume his or her role, the child may be forced to indirectly assume that parent's role. Early childhood reward for behavior usually reserved for the opposite sex. Fear or hate of the parent of the same sex.

NURSING DIAGNOSIS

Self-dissatisfaction related to sex misidentification: unhappiness with oneself for having assumed social characteristics usually reserved for the opposite sex

PLANNING

Patient Needs	Primary Nurse-Patient Goals
Comfort	To achieve comfort
Sexuality	To achieve productive interpersonal relationships
Protection from psychologic threat	To prevent emotional injury
Acceptance	To achieve productive interpersonal relationships
Warm, communicating relationships	To achieve effective verbal and nonverbal communication
High evaluation of self	To achieve positive expressions, feelings, reactions
Personal growth and maturity	To achieve optimum function
Increased learning	To achieve awareness of needs
Increased reality perception and problem-solving ability	To achieve optimum function

NURSING INTERVENTIONS

Nursing Treatments
Approach unhurriedly
Provide an atmosphere of acceptance
Reassure verbally
Emphasize the person's value as an individual
Encourage the expression of feelings
Listen attentively
    AND
Talk with the patient
Offer feedback of the patient's expressed feelings
Explore with the patient reasons for self-criticism
Explore with the patient his strengths and resources
Assist the patient in defining consistent life standards
Encourage the practical application of the accepted value system
Assist the patient in restructuring his lifestyle
Introduce to persons who have successfully undergone the same experience
Provide objects which symbolize sex identity
Recognize the need for the use of appropriate defense mechanisms
Encourage the use of normal coping mechanisms
Refrain from negatively criticizing

Nursing Observations
Determine the degree of insight
Evaluate the person's relatedness with others
Evaluate the significance of emotional distress mannerisms
Evaluate the significance of nonverbal communication
Identify disturbing conversation topics
Identify life values significant to the person
Identify appropriate use of defense mechanisms
Identify inappropriate use of defense mechanisms
Observe for an excessive stress level
Observe for evidence that the patient is reaching out for emotional support
Observe for behavior modification

Health Teaching
Advise that negative responses from others be regarded with minimum
   significance
Advise that significant persons express acceptance of one another
Explain the importance of offering emotional support to one another
Explain the importance of maintaining a positive self-attitude
Explain the causes of the health problem
Teach how to use the problem-solving method

EVALUATION

See the evaluation criteria for each specific goal in Chapter 2.

STRESS, EXTERNAL

Distress Related to an Incompatible Room Companion (141,380,487)

ASSESSMENT

Subjective Data
Greatly annoyed with the other person
Preoccupation with the other's undesirable qualities

Objective Data
Emotional upset over small problems (such as when to close or open a win-
   dow, when to turn the TV on or off)
One person screens himself from, or constantly turns away from, the other
Difficulty sharing the bathroom
One confidentially reports the other to the nursing staff
One remains out of the room most of the time

Related Data
Commonly Related Diseases:
Any disease

POSSIBLE ETIOLOGY

Frame of reference discrepancy between persons. Varying social and moral
standards. Lack of common interests. Susceptibility to irritation as a result
of illness.

NURSING DIAGNOSIS

Distress related to an incompatible room companion: a state of emotional or mental suffering brought about by the inability to coexist in harmony with the person with whom one is sharing a room during an illness

PLANNING

Patient Needs

Comfort

Protection from psychologic threat

Acceptance

Warm, communicating
  relationships

Increased learning

Primary Nurse-Patient Goals

To achieve comfort

To prevent emotional injury

To achieve productive interpersonal
  relationships

To achieve effective verbal and
  nonverbal communications

To achieve awareness of needs

NURSING INTERVENTIONS

Nursing Treatments

Approach unhurriedly
Provide an atmosphere of acceptance
Reassure verbally
Demonstrate calmness
Encourage the expression of feelings
Listen attentively
  AND
Talk with the patient
Encourage mutual problem solving
Provide a compatible room companion
  OR
Place in a private room

Nursing Observations

Determine the precipitating factors
Determine the relieving factors
Evaluate the person's relatedness with others
Evaluate the significance of emotional distress mannerisms
Evaluate the significance of nonverbal communication
Identify disturbing conversation topics
Observe for an excessive stress level
Observe for evidence of a favorable response to therapy

Health Teaching

Advise that negative responses from others be regarded with minimum
  significance
Explain the need for realistic expectations of others

EVALUATION

See the evaluation criteria for each specific goal in Chapter 2.

Distress Related to an Unwelcomed Hospital Discharge (141,380,487)

ASSESSMENT

Subjective Data
Insecurity related to being alone at home

Objective Data
Verbalizes a preference for not being discharged
Comments on the pleasant hospital environment, if it is superior to the home environment
Actively socializes with staff and other patients
Develops illness complaints a day or two prior to discharge

Related Data
Commonly Related Diseases:
Any disease or injury

POSSIBLE ETIOLOGY

Inadequacy feelings. Poor need gratification outside the hospital setting. May actually not feel well enough to go home.

NURSING DIAGNOSIS

Distress related to an unwelcomed hospital discharge: a state of emotional or mental suffering brought about by a negative attitude toward the termination of hospitalization

PLANNING

Patient Needs	Primary Nurse-Patient Goals
Comfort	To achieve comfort
Protection from psychologic threat	To prevent emotional injury
Acceptance	To achieve productive interpersonal relationships
Warm, communicating relationships	To achieve effective verbal and nonverbal communications
Adequacy	To achieve positive expressions, feelings, reactions
Increased learning	To achieve awareness of needs
Increased reality perception and problem-solving ability	To achieve optimum function

NURSING OBSERVATIONS

Nursing Treatments
Approach unhurriedly
Provide an atmosphere of acceptance
Reassure verbally
Express empathy

Touch the patient judiciously
Encourage the expression of feelings
Listen attentively
   AND
Talk with the patient
Offer feedback of the patient's expressed feelings
Encourage mutual problem solving
Arrange a predischarge planning conference
Explore with the patient his strengths and resources
Present change gradually
Offer assurance that return visits are acceptable despite termination of the
   therapeutic relationship
Recognize the need for unique personal adjustments to change
Encourage the use of normal coping mechanisms
Support a realistic assessment of the situation
Involve the family (as much as possible)

Nursing Observations
Determine the degree of insight
Evaluate the person's relatedness with others
Evaluate the significance of emotional distress mannerisms
Evaluate the significance of nonverbal communications
Identify disturbing conversation topics
Observe for an excessive stress level
Observe for evidence that the patient is reaching out for emotional support
Observe for evidence of a favorable response to therapy

Health Teaching
Explain the importance of offering emotional support to one another
Teach how to use the problem-solving method

EVALUATION

See the evaluation criteria for each specific goal in Chapter 2.

Distress Related to Chronic Family Discord (141,282,380,487)

ASSESSMENT

Subjective Data
Highly suspicious
Intense competition between family members
Defense-oriented, not task-oriented, family
Love does not prevail in the family climate

Objective Data
Dissension
Yelling, shouting
Quarreling
Verbalized negative, destructive inferences
Physically harm each other

Related Data

Commonly Related Conditions:
Emotional immaturity

POSSIBLE ETIOLOGY

Incompatible frames of reference between family members. Opposing need satisfaction. Inadequate problem-solving abilities. Interference from relatives or outside sources. Unrealistic perception of problems due to emotional involvement or fatigue.

NURSING DIAGNOSIS

Chronic family discord: a state of emotional or mental suffering brought about by a persistent lack of agreement and peaceful coexistence between family members

PLANNING

Patient Needs	Primary Nurse-Patient Goals
Rest, relaxation	To achieve rest, relaxation
Comfort	To achieve comfort
Protection from physical harm	To prevent physical injury
Protection from psychologic threat	To prevent emotional injury
Love and affection, acceptance	To achieve productive interpersonal relationships
Warm, communicating relationships	To achieve effective verbal and nonverbal communications
Personal growth and maturity	To achieve optimum function
Increased learning	To achieve awareness of needs
Increased reality perception and problem-solving ability	To achieve optimum function
Increased pleasantness	To achieve positive expressions, feelings, reactions

NURSING INTERVENTIONS

Nursing Treatments
Approach unhurriedly
Provide an atmosphere of acceptance
Demonstrate calmness
Encourage the expression of feelings
Listen attentively
   AND
Talk with the patient
Offer feedback of the patient's expressed feelings
Encourage acceptance of interdependency
Encourage acceptance of limitations in others
Encourage acceptance of self-limitations
Encourage awareness of positive responses from others
Encourage family-shared pleasures

Encourage family-shared responsibility
Encourage mutual problem solving
Encourage participation in therapeutic group interaction
Encourage realistic perception of others
Encourage respect for the rights of others
Encourage the reduction of generalizations to specifics
Explore superficial topics and reasons for avoiding in-depth feelings
Explore with the patient his strengths and resources
Explore with the patient reasons for criticism by others
Explore with the patient reasons for criticism of others
Explore with the patient reasons for likes and dislikes
Explore with the patient reasons for recurring problems
Explore with the patient the effects of his behavior on others
Provide emotionally safe experiences
Recognize the need for the use of appropriate defense mechanisms
Encourage the use of normal coping mechanisms
Refrain from arguing
Refrain from negatively criticizing
Set limits on unacceptable behavior
Suggest more appropriate means of emotional expression
Suggest more appropriate means of need gratification
Support a realistic assessment of the situation

Nursing Observations
Determine the degree of insight
Determine the precipitating factors
Determine the relieving factors
Evaluate the person's relatedness with others
Evaluate the significance of emotional distress mannerisms
Evaluate the significance of nonverbal communication
Identify disturbing conversation topics
Identify emotion-stimulating events
Identify inappropriate emotional responses
Identify life values significant to the person
Identify appropriate use of defense mechanisms
Identify inappropriate use of defense mechanisms
Identify the current dominant emotion
Observe for emotional instability
Observe for an excessive stress level
Observe for impaired self-attitudes
Observe for evidence that the patient is reaching out for emotional support
Observe for evidence of a favorable response to therapy

Health Teaching
Advise against causing defensive responses in others
Advise against communicating double-meaning messages
Advise against emphasizing past problems caused by another
Advise against verbally comparing significant persons
Advise early correction of problems
Advise that highly emotional situations be avoided

Advise that negative responses from others be regarded with minimum significance
Advise that significant persons express acceptance of one another
Advise that significant persons express love for one another
Explain the importance of offering emotional support to one another
Emphasize the importance of recognizing tension within oneself
Explain the need for realistic expectations of others
Explain that fatigue should be recognized as a stress factor·
Explain the need to recognize highly stressful situations
Explain the importance of maintaining a positive self-attitude
Explain how to obtain release from emotional stress
Explain that undesirable thoughts and feelings are normal
Explain that unpleasant conversation increases stress
Explain the importance of correct message interpretation
Explain the importance of remaining calm
Explain why persons should maintain self-control
Explain how to channel emotional energy into activity
Recommend methods for achieving total relaxation
Recommend that behavioral limits be set
Explain how to set behavioral limits
Teach how to use the problem-solving method

EVALUATION

See the evaluation criteria for each specific goal in Chapter 2.

Distress Related to Disturbing Visitors (141,380,487)

ASSESSMENT

Subjective Data

Fatigue when visitors stay too long or come in large numbers
Embarrassment when visitors become demanding or arrive at moments when privacy is essential

Objective Data

Emotionally upset when visitors bring bad news or the burden of their own problems
Unable to rest when visitors arrive at all hours

Related Data

Commonly Related Diseases:
Any disease or injury

POSSIBLE ETIOLOGY

Lack of knowledge or sensitivity to the needs of ill persons. Visitors' preoccupation with meeting their own needs.

NURSING DIAGNOSIS

Distress related to disturbing visitors: a state of emotional or mental suffering brought about when persons who visit an ill patient cause weariness, confusion, disturbance, or aggravation for the patient

PLANNING

Patient Needs

Comfort

Protection from physical harm

Protection from psychologic threat

Increased learning

Primary Nurse-Patient Goals

To achieve comfort

To prevent physical injury

To prevent emotional injury

To achieve awareness of needs

NURSING INTERVENTIONS

Nursing Treatments

Approach unhurriedly

Express empathy

Demonstrate calmness

Encourage the expression of feelings

Listen attentively

  AND

Talk with the patient (and visitor)

Limit excessive demands (by the visitor)

Restrict unwanted visitors

Nursing Observations

Evaluate the significance of emotional distress mannerisms (manifested by the patient)

Evaluate the significance of nonverbal communication

Identify disturbing conversation topics

Observe for an excessive stress level

Observe for evidence that the patient is reaching out for emotional support

Observe for behavior modification (by the visitor)

Observe for evidence of a favorable response to therapy (by the patient)

Health Teaching

Explain that ill persons are often hypersensitive

Explain that socialization depletes the ill patient's energy

Explain that unpleasant conversation increases stress

EVALUATION

See the evaluation criteria for each specific goal in Chapter 2.

Distress Related to Temporary Family Disorganization (141,380,487)

ASSESSMENT

Subjective Data

Family members feel lonely and experience increased tension

Hope that things will soon be back to normal

Objective Data

Temporary loss of one family member from the family scene

Routine family life is disrupted

May be daily, time-consuming trips to the hospital
Family members are temporarily assuming new roles
Children may be temporarily parentless
Family frequently asks when the ill person can come home
May insist that the physician discharge the patient

Related Data

Commonly Related Diseases:
None
   OR
Any disease

POSSIBLE ETIOLOGY

Temporary separation of family members by illness

NURSING DIAGNOSIS

Distress related to temporary family disorganization: a state of emotional or mental suffering occurring when the basic family structure is temporarily altered, even though in time the previous living pattern will be reestablished

PLANNING

Patient Needs	**Primary Nurse-Patient Goals**
Comfort	To achieve comfort
Protection from psychologic threat	To prevent emotional injury
Predictable, orderly world	To achieve a therapeutic environment
Warm, communicating relationships	To achieve effective verbal and nonverbal communications
High evaluation of self, adequacy, self-reliance, endurance	To achieve positive expressions, feelings, reactions
Increased learning	To achieve awareness of needs
Increased reality perception and problem-solving ability	To achieve optimum function

NURSING INTERVENTIONS

Nursing Treatments
Approach unhurriedly
Provide an atmosphere of acceptance
Express empathy
Reassure verbally
Demonstrate calmness
Provide frequent patient contact
Encourage the expression of feelings
Listen attentively
   AND
Talk with the patient
Offer feedback of the patient's expressed feelings

Avoid causing intense emotional situations
Do not allow unpleasant surprise situations
Encourage balanced long- and short-range goals
Encourage strivings toward realistic goals
Encourage family-shared responsibilities
Encourage gradual mastery of a situation
Encourage mutual problem solving
Encourage planned one-day-at-a-time living
Encourage the sharing of common problems with others
Establish routines familiar to the patient
Explore with the patient his strengths and resources
Explore with the patient previous achievements of success
Explore with the patient previous displays of courage
Ensure the patient's feeling of safety before introducing unpleasantness
Provide emotionally safe experiences
Recognize the need for the use of appropriate defense mechanisms
Encourage the use of normal coping mechanisms
Recognize the need for unique personal adjustments to change
Present change gradually
Reduce demands placed upon the patient
Support a realistic assessment of the situation
Introduce to persons who have successfully undergone the same experience

Nursing Observations
Determine the degree of insight
Estimate the degree of stress experienced
Evaluate the person's relatedness with others
Evaluate the significance of emotional distress mannerisms
Evaluate the significance of nonverbal communication
Identify disturbing conversation topics
Identify life values significant to the person
Identify appropriate use of defense mechanisms
Identify inappropriate use of defense mechanisms
Observe for an excessive stress level
Observe for evidence that the patient is reaching out for emotional support
Observe for evidence of a favorable response to therapy

Health Teaching
Explain that the person's emotional response is appropriate and commonly
    experienced
Advise that highly emotional situations be avoided
Advise that significant persons express acceptance of one another
Advise that significant persons express love for one another
Explain the importance of offering emotional support to one another
Explain how to obtain release from emotional stress
Explain the need to predict and plan for change
Teach how to use the problem-solving method

EVALUATION
See the evaluation criteria for each specific goal in Chapter 2.

Distress Related to Family Reorganization (141,380,487)

ASSESSMENT

Subjective Data
Anxiety
Insecurity feelings until new patterns are well established

Objective Data
Adjustment to new family additions (new baby, grandparents coming to live with the family)
Adjustment to a new location and new friends when the family moves
Altered family responsibilities when the mother starts working
Relearning social skills when moving to a new social status
In death and divorce, substitute persons are sought to replace the lost person

Related Data
Commonly Related Diseases:
None
   OR
Any disease

POSSIBLE ETIOLOGY

The need for time to adjust to new patterns of living

NURSING DIAGNOSIS

Distress related to family reorganization: a state of emotional or mental suffering when the basic structure of family membership or routine has been permanently changed and the family reorganizes its living pattern into a new, permanent stable structure

PLANNING

Patient Needs	Primary Nurse-Patient Goals
Comfort	To achieve comfort
Protection from psychologic threat	To prevent emotional injury
Predictable, orderly world	To achieve a therapeutic environment
Acceptance	To achieve productive interpersonal relationships
Warm, communicating relationships	To achieve effective verbal and nonverbal communications
Unity with loved ones	To achieve productive interpersonal relationships
High evaluation of self, adequacy	To achieve positive expressions, feelings, reactions
Personal growth and maturity	To achieve optimum function
Increased learning	To achieve awareness of needs

Increased reality perception and problem-solving ability

To achieve optimum function

NURSING INTERVENTIONS

Nursing Treatments
Approach unhurriedly
Provide an atmosphere of acceptance
Express empathy
Reassure verbally
Demonstrate calmness
Provide frequent patient contact
Encourage the expression of feelings
Listen attentively
    AND
Talk with the patient
Offer feedback of the patient's expressed feelings
Assist the patient in restructuring his lifestyle
Avoid causing intense emotional situations
Do not allow unpleasant surprise situations
Encourage balanced long- and short-range goals
Encourage strivings toward realistic goals
Encourage family-shared pleasures
Encourage family-shared responsibilities
Encourage gradual mastery of a situation
Encourage mutual problem solving
Encourage planned one-day-at-a-time living
Encourage the sharing of common problems with others
Establish routines familiar to the patient
Explore with the patient his strengths and resources
Explore with the patient previous achievements of success
Explore with the patient previous displays of courage
Ensure the patient's feeling of safety before introducing unpleasantness
Provide emotionally safe experiences
Recognize the need for the use of appropriate defense mechanisms
Encourage the use of normal coping mechanisms
Recognize the need for unique personal adjustments to change
Present change gradually
Reduce demands placed upon the patient
Support a realistic assessment of the situation
Introduce to persons who have successfully undergone the same experience

Nursing Observations
Determine the degree of insight
Estimate the degree of stress experienced
Evaluate the person's relatedness with others
Evaluate the significance of emotional distress mannerisms
Evaluate the significance of nonverbal communication
Identify disturbing conversation topics
Identify life values significant to the person

Identify appropriate use of defense mechanisms
Identify inappropriate use of defense mechanisms
Observe for an excessive stress level
Observe for evidence that the patient is reaching out for emotional support
Observe for evidence of a favorable response to therapy

Health Teaching
Explain that the person's emotional response is appropriate and commonly
  experienced
Advise that highly emotional situations be avoided
Advise that significant persons express acceptance of one another
Advise that significant persons express love for one another
Explain the importance of offering emotional support to one another
Explain how to obtain release from emotional stress
Explain the need to predict and plan for change
Recommend a habitual, positive mental attitude
Teach how to use the problem-solving method

EVALUATION

See the evaluation criteria for each specific goal in Chapter 2.

Distress Related to Home-Pass Intolerance (141,380,487)

ASSESSMENT

Subjective Data
Anxiety
Anger
Weeping

Objective Data
Reluctance to go home on a pass
Gives many reasons for not going home
May become ill at the time of the scheduled pass
If forced to go home, the return to the hospital occurs long before the
  scheduled time of return

Related Data
Commonly Related Diseases:
Any disease or injury, especially: cerebral vascular accident or cervical,
  thoracic, or spinal cord injury

POSSIBLE ETIOLOGY

Unstable family situation. Inadequate home facilities from the standpoint
of the patient's disability. Inadequacy feelings when in the world of well
persons. Patient perception of lack of family interest. Prolonged hospitalization lasting for months or years.

NURSING DIAGNOSIS

Distress related to home-pass intolerance: a state of emotional or mental
suffering brought about by the inability to comfortably tolerate leaving the
hospital for a short period and adapting to the world of well people

PLANNING

Patient Needs	**Primary Nurse-Patient Goals**
Comfort	To achieve comfort
Protection from psychologic threat	To prevent emotional injury
Acceptance	To achieve productive interpersonal relationships
Adequacy	To achieve positive expressions, feelings, reactions
Independence	To achieve optimum function
Increased learning	To achieve awareness of needs
Increased reality perception and problem-solving ability	To achieve optimum function

NURSING INTERVENTIONS

Nursing Treatments

Approach unhurriedly
Provide an atmosphere of acceptance
Reassure verbally
Express empathy
Touch the patient judiciously
Encourage the expression of feelings
Listen attentively
　AND
Talk with the patient (and the family)
Offer feedback of the patient's expressed feelings
Encourage mutual problem solving
Encourage gradual mastery of a situation (by going home for a few hours at a time)
Explore with the patient his strengths and resources
Explore with the patient previous achievements of success
Explore with the patient previous displays of courage
Recognize the need for the use of appropriate defense mechanisms
Encourage the use of normal coping mechanisms
Recognize the need for unique personal adjustments to change
Support a realistic assessment of the situation
Involve the family (as much as possible)
Provide a home visit (to evaluate the patient's problem)

Nursing Observations

Determine the extent of emotional flexibility
Determine the degree of insight
Determine the precipitating factors
Determine the relieving factors
Evaluate the person's relatedness with others
Evaluate the safety of the environment (at home)
Evaluate the significance of emotional distress mannerisms
Evaluate the significance of nonverbal communication

Identify disturbing conversation topics
Observe for an excessive stress level
Observe for evidence that the patient is reaching out for emotional support
Observe for evidence of a favorable response to therapy

Health Teaching
Explain that the person's emotional response is appropriate and commonly
    experienced
Advise that significant persons express acceptance of one another
Advise that significant persons express love for one another
Explain the importance of offering emotional support to one another
Explain the importance of maintaining a positive self-attitude
Explain the causes of the health problem
Explain the need to predict and plan for change
Teach how to use the problem-solving method

EVALUATION

See the evaluation criteria for each specific goal in Chapter 2.

Distress Related to Illness-Imposed Family Hardship (141,380,487)

ASSESSMENT

Subjective Data
Family feels some anger about the imposed hardships
Feels obligated to care for the ill person

Objective Data
Family no longer indulges in life's extras
Are barely able to make ends meet
Children complain about doing without
Someone must remain at home to care for the ill person
Social activities are curtailed, both in the home and away from home

Related Data
Commonly Related Diseases:
Any disease or injury

POSSIBLE ETIOLOGY

Illness that restricts family income and activity and depletes resources

NURSING DIAGNOSIS

Distress related to illness-imposed family hardship: a state of emotional or
mental suffering brought about by hardships imposed on a family because
of illness of one member

PLANNING

Patient Needs	**Primary Nurse-Patient Goals**
Comfort	To achieve comfort
Protection from psychologic threat	To prevent emotional injury

Acceptance	To achieve productive interpersonal relationships
Adequacy	To achieve positive expressions, feelings reactions
Increased learning	To achieve awareness of needs and/or use of resources
Increased reality perception and problem-solving ability	To achieve optimum function

NURSING INTERVENTIONS

Nursing Treatments
Approach unhurriedly
Provide an atmosphere of acceptance
Express empathy
Express warmth and friendliness
Reassure verbally
Encourage the expression of feelings
Listen attentively
    AND
Talk with the patient
Offer feedback of the patient's expressed feelings
Reveal the patient's ambivalent feelings
Offer hope
Offer praise
Encourage balanced long- and short-range goals
Encourage family-shared pleasures
Encourage family-shared responsibility
Encourage gradual mastery of a situation
Encourage planned one-day-at-a-time living
Encourage mutual problem solving
Encourage the sharing of common problems with others
Encourage strivings toward realistic goals
Explore with the patient his strengths and resources
Explore with the patient previous achievements of success
Explore with the patient previous displays of courage
Provide emotional support for persons significant to the patient
Encourage the use of normal coping mechanisms
Recognize the need for unique personal adjustments to change
Suggest that volunteers might offer assistance with home care
Support a realistic assessment of the situation
Introduce to persons who have successfully undergone the same experience
Make a referral (to the appropriate social agencies)

Nursing Observations
Determine the degree of insight
Estimate the degree of stress experienced
Evaluate the significance of emotional distress mannerisms
Evaluate the significance of nonverbal communication

Identify disturbing conversation topics
Observe for an excessive stress level
Observe for evidence that the family is reaching out for emotional support
Observe for evidence of a favorable response to therapy

Health Teaching
Explain that the person's emotional response is appropriate and commonly
    experienced
Advise occasional respite from responsibility (for family members)
Advise that significant persons express acceptance of one another
Advise that significant persons express love for one another
Explain the importance of offering emotional support to one another
Explain that fatigue should be recognized as a stress factor
Explain how to obtain release from emotional stress
Recommend methods for achieving total relaxation
Recommend a habitual, positive mental attitude
Teach how to use the problem-solving method

EVALUATION

See the evaluation criteria for each specific goal in Chapter 2.

Distress Related to Restricted Visitors
(141,380,487)

ASSESSMENT

Subjective Data
Loneliness because of visitor limitations

Objective Data
Requests special visitor permission for loved ones
Working visitors complain of being unable to visit because of restrictions
Visitors often disregard the institutional restrictions and visit anyway

Related Data
Commonly Related Diseases:
Any disease or injury

POSSIBLE ETIOLOGY

Institutional rules designed to meet the needs of the majority

NURSING DIAGNOSIS

Distress related to restricted visitors: a state of emotional or mental suffering brought about by restrictions placed on the time of day during which
visiting the ill is permitted

PLANNING

Patient Needs	**Primary Nurse-Patient Goals**
Comfort	To achieve comfort
Protection from psychologic threat	To prevent emotional injury
Acceptance	To achieve productive interpersonal relationships

Warm, communicating relationships — To achieve effective verbal and nonverbal communications

NURSING INTERVENTIONS

Nursing Treatments
Approach unhurriedly
Provide an atmosphere of acceptance
Express empathy
Encourage the expression of feelings
Listen attentively
   AND
Talk with the patient
Arrange situations which encourage patient autonomy
Grant special requests
Allow unlimited visiting

Nursing Observations
Observe for evidence of a favorable response to therapy

Health Teaching
Explain that the person's emotional response is appropriate and commonly experienced
Explain the reason for and intended effect of the therapy (visitor restrictions)

EVALUATION
See the evaluation criteria for each specific goal in Chapter 2.

Intolerance to Stress (141,380,487)

ASSESSMENT

Subjective Data
Keenly perceives the environment
Perceives dangers and problems often overlooked by others
Dislikes multiple, simultaneous changes
Easily frustrated
Anxious under minor stress

Objective Data
Startled by slight sound
Cries easily
Irritability
Appears nervous and high-strung
Has more than normal difficulty in maintaining healthy development at different age levels
Overly responsive to other persons' needs
Avoids tension-producing situations

Related Data
Commonly Related Diseases:
None
   OR

Any physical disease
   OR
Simple senile psychosis
Alcoholism
Conversion hysteria psychoneurosis
Neurasthenia psychoneurosis
Anxiety psychoneurosis
Thyrotoxicosis
Addison's disease
Simmonds' disease
Multiple sclerosis

POSSIBLE ETIOLOGY

Constitutional weaknesses. Decreased self-confidence. Lack of previous success in meeting psychologic and biologic needs. Poor intellectual competence. Endocrine imbalance. Neurologic disorders. Prolonged stress.

NURSING DIAGNOSIS

Intolerance to stress: the inability to endure high levels of pressure without physiologic and/or psychologic impairment

PLANNING

Patient Needs

Sleep, rest, relaxation

Comfort

Protection from physical harm

Protection from psychologic threat

Predictable, orderly world

Acceptance

Warm, communicating
   relationships

Increased learning

Increased reality perception and
   problem-solving ability

Primary Nurse-Patient Goals

To achieve sleep, rest, relaxation

To achieve comfort

To prevent physical harm

To prevent emotional injury

To achieve a therapeutic
   environment

To achieve productive interpersonal
   relationships

To achieve effective verbal and
   nonverbal communications

To achieve awareness of needs

To achieve optimum function

NURSING INTERVENTIONS

Nursing Treatments

Approach unhurriedly
Provide an atmosphere of acceptance
Express empathy
Demonstrate calmness
Arrange orderly surroundings
Arrange pleasant surroundings
Arrange a structured environment
Establish routines familiar to the patient
Provide quiet

Place in a private room
Recognize the need for unique personal adjustments to change
Present change gradually
Discourage decision-making when one is under severe stress
Encourage single goal seeking
Ensure the patient's feeling of safety before introducing unpleasantness
Introduce one anxiety situation at a time
Provide emotionally safe experiences
Provide objects which symbolize safeness
Recognize the need for the use of appropriate defense mechanisms
Encourage the use of normal coping mechanisms
Reduce the demands placed upon the patient
Refrain from performing nonessential procedures

Nursing Observations
Estimate the degree of stress experienced
Observe for an excessive stress level

Health Teaching
Advise occasional respite from responsibility
Advise that highly emotional situations be avoided
Emphasize the importance of recognizing tension within oneself
Explain that fatigue should be recognized as a stress factor
Explain the need to recognize highly stressful situations
Explain how to obtain release from emotional stress
Explain that unpleasant conversation increases stress
Explain the need to predict and plan for change
Recommend methods for reducing sensory stimulation
Recommend methods for noise reduction
Recommend methods for achieving total relaxation

EVALUATION

See the evaluation criteria for each specific goal in Chapter 2.

STRESS, POTENTIAL EXTERNAL

Potential Encounter With Multiple Situational Stressors (141,380,487)

ASSESSMENT

Subjective Data
Anticipatory tension

Objective Data
Pressured into making numerous decisions within a short time
Multiple life changes are about to occur simultaneously, such as having to have surgery shortly after the death of a loved one and while adjusting to a new job

Related Data

Commonly Related Diseases:
None
   OR
Any disease

POSSIBLE ETIOLOGY

Changes and problems evolving from a life situation

NURSING DIAGNOSIS

Potential encounter with multiple situational stressors: the likelihood that one will be simultaneously confronted with numerous tension-producing situations that require maximum adaptation

PLANNING

Patient Needs	**Primary Nurse-Patient Goals**
Rest, relaxation	To achieve rest and relaxation
Protection from psychologic threat	To prevent emotional injury
Predictable, orderly world	To achieve a therapeutic environment
Warm, communicating relationships	To achieve effective verbal and nonverbal communications
Increased learning	To achieve awareness of needs
Increased reality perception and problem-solving ability	To achieve optimum function

NURSING INTERVENTIONS

Nursing Treatments
Approach unhurriedly
Arrange orderly surroundings
Arrange pleasant surroundings
Arrange a structured environment
Establish routines familiar to the patient
Provide quiet
Provide frequent patient contact
Recognize the need for unique personal adjustments to change
Present change gradually
Discourage decision-making when one is under severe stress
Explore with the patient his strengths and resources
Ensure the patient's feeling of safety before introducing unpleasantness
Introduce one anxiety situation at a time
Provide emotionally safe experiences
Provide objects which symbolize safeness
Recognize the need for the use of appropriate defense mechanisms
Encourage the use of normal coping mechanisms
Reduce the demands placed upon the patient
Refrain from performing nonessential procedures

Nursing Observations
Estimate the degree of stress experienced
Observe for evidence that the patient is reaching out for emotional support
Observe for an excessive stress level

Health Teaching
Explain the importance of offering emotional support to one another
Explain the need to recognize highly stressful situations
Explain how to obtain release from emotional stress
Explain that unpleasant conversation increases stress
Explain the need to predict and plan for change
Recommend methods for reducing sensory stimulation
Recommend methods for noise reduction
Recommend methods for achieving total relaxation

EVALUATION

See the evaluation criteria for each specific goal in Chapter 2.

STRESS, INTERNAL

Emotional Irritability (12,94,118,199, 331,372)

ASSESSMENT

Subjective Data
Easily angered
Fatigued

Objective Data
Uncooperative
Antagonistic
Sour, cynical
Critical of others
Bitter toward others
Fretful
Quarrelsome
Nonconforming

Related Data
Commonly Related Diseases:
Any disease or injury
     OR
Manic-depressive psychosis
Melancholia involutional psychosis
Epidemic encephalitis psychosis
General paresis psychosis
Simple senile psychosis
Anxiety psychoneurosis

POSSIBLE ETIOLOGY

Lack of comfort and satisfaction with oneself. Emotional disequilibrium. Prolonged frustration and stress. Perception of threat.

NURSING DIAGNOSIS

Emotional irritability: a quick, impatient, emotional excitement response to annoyance

PLANNING

Patient Needs	**Primary Nurse-Patient Goals**
Comfort	To achieve comfort
Protection from psychologic threat	To prevent emotional injury
Acceptance	To achieve productive interpersonal relationships
Warm, communicating relationships	To achieve effective verbal and nonverbal communications
High evaluation of self	To achieve positive expressions, feelings, reactions
Personal growth and maturity	To achieve optimum function
Increased learning	To achieve awareness of needs
Increased reality perception and problem-solving ability	To achieve optimum function

NURSING INTERVENTIONS

Nursing Treatments
Approach unhurriedly
Provide an atmosphere of acceptance
Express empathy
Reassure verbally
Demonstrate calmness
Arrange orderly surroundings
Arrange pleasant surroundings
Arrange a structured environment
Establish routines familiar to the patient
Provide quiet
Provide frequent patient contact
Avoid causing intense emotional situations
Encourage the expression of feelings
Listen attentively
    AND
Talk with the patient
Offer feedback of the patient's expressed feelings
Encourage laughter
Encourage mutual problem solving
Encourage single goal seeking
Encourage strivings toward realistic goals

Explore with the patient his strengths and resources
Ensure the patient's feeling of safety before introducing unpleasantness
Introduce one anxiety situation at a time
Provide emotionally safe experiences
Recognize the need for the use of appropriate defense mechanisms
Encourage the use of normal coping mechanisms
Reduce the demands placed upon the patient
Refrain from performing nonessential procedures
Refrain from negatively criticizing
Refrain from arguing
Refrain from teasing
Set limits on unacceptable behavior (if the irritability is severe)
Encourage adequate rest
Massage gently
   OR   } (for the relaxing effect)
Bathe in warm water
Give drugs judiciously for emotional repression

Nursing Observations

Determine the extent of emotional flexibility
Determine the degree of insight
Determine the precipitating factors
Evaluate the person's relatedness with others
Evaluate the significance of emotional distress mannerisms
Evaluate the significance of nonverbal communication
Identify disturbing conversation topics
Identify emotion-stimulating events
Identify inappropriate emotional responses
Identify potentially destructive behavior
Identify appropriate use of defense mechanisms
Identify inappropriate use of defense mechanisms
Identify the current dominant emotion
Observe for emotional instability
Observe for an excessive stress level
Observe for impaired self-attitudes
Observe for evidence that the patient is reaching out for emotional support
Observe for evidence of a favorable response to therapy

Health Teaching

Explain that the person's emotional response is appropriate and commonly
   experienced
Advise that highly emotional situations be avoided
Advise that negative responses from others be regarded with minimum
   significance
Advise that significant persons express acceptance of one another
Explain the importance of offering emotional support to one another
Emphasize the importance of recognizing tension within oneself
Explain the need for realistic expectations of others
Explain that fatigue should be recognized as a stress factor
Explain the need to recognize highly stressful situations

Explain the importance of maintaining a positive self-attitude
Explain how to obtain release from emotional stress
Explain that ill persons are often hypersensitive
Explain that unpleasant conversation increases stress
Explain the causes of the health problem
Explain why persons should maintain self-control
Recommend methods for achieving total relaxation
Recommend that behavioral limits be set (if the irritability is severe)
Explain how to set behavioral limits
Teach how to use the problem-solving method

Medical Treatments Performed by Nurses
Give the prescribed drugs

EVALUATION

See the evaluation criteria for each specific goal in Chapter 2.

Emotional Nervousness (12,94,118, 199,331,372)

ASSESSMENT

Subjective Data
Fatigue
Fearful
Apprehensive
Headache or peculiar head sensations

Objective Data
Insomnia
Forgetfulness
Weeps easily
Giddiness
Anorexia
Urinary frequency
Nail-biting
Habitual gesturing or fidgeting
Cigarette puffing
Habitually pushes eyeglasses in place
Habitually clears the throat or coughs
Tugs at the ear

Related Data
Commonly Related Diseases:
None
   OR
Anxiety psychoneurosis

POSSIBLE ETIOLOGY

Prolonged emotional stress. Overload of the central nervous system with tension.

NURSING DIAGNOSIS

Emotional nervousness: an unnatural, uncomfortable feeling of internal tension evident in emotional expression

PLANNING

Patient Needs	**Primary Nurse-Patient Goals**
Sleep, rest, relaxation	To achieve sleep, rest, relaxation
Comfort	To achieve comfort
Protection from psychologic threat	To prevent emotional injury
Acceptance	To achieve productive interpersonal relationships
Warm, communicating relationships	To achieve effective verbal and nonverbal communications
High evaluation of self, adequacy	To achieve positive expressions, feelings, reactions
Personal growth and maturity	To achieve optimum function
Increased learning	To achieve awareness of needs
Increased reality perception and problem-solving ability	To achieve optimum function

NURSING INTERVENTIONS

Nursing Treatments
Approach unhurriedly
Provide an atmosphere of acceptance
Express empathy
Reassure verbally
Demonstrate calmness
Arrange orderly surroundings
Arrange pleasant surroundings
Arrange a structured environment
Establish routines familiar to the patient
Provide quiet
Provide frequent patient contact
Avoid causing intense emotional situations
Encourage the expression of feelings
Listen attentively
    AND
Talk with the patient
Offer feedback of the patient's expressed feelings
Encourage laughter
Encourage mutual problem solving
Encourage single goal seeking
Encourage strivings toward realistic goals
Explore with the patient his strengths and resources
Ensure the patient's feeling of safety before introducing unpleasantness
Introduce one anxiety situation at a time
Provide emotionally safe experiences
Recognize the need for the use of appropriate defense mechanisms

Encourage the use of normal coping mechanisms
Reduce the demands placed upon the patient
Refrain from performing nonessential procedures
Refrain from negatively criticizing
Refrain from arguing
Refrain from teasing
Encourage adequate rest
Massage gently
  OR   } (for the relaxing effect)
Bathe in warm water

Nursing Observations
Determine the degree of insight
Determine the precipitating factors
Determine the relieving factors
Evaluate the person's relatedness with others
Evaluate the significance of emotional distress mannerisms
Evaluate the significance of nonverbal communication
Identify disturbing conversation topics
Observe for an excessive stress level
Observe for evidence that the patient is reaching out for emotional support
Observe for evidence of a favorable response to therapy

Health Teaching
Explain that the person's emotional response is appropriate and commonly
    experienced
Advise that highly emotional situations be avoided
Advise that significant persons express acceptance of one another
Explain the importance of offering emotional support to one another
Describe the behavior pattern indicating overstimulation
Emphasize the importance of recognizing tension within oneself
Explain that fatigue should be recognized as a stress factor
Explain the need to recognize highly stressful situations
Explain how to obtain release from emotional stress
Explain that unpleasant conversation increases stress
Explain the causes of the health problem
Recommend methods for reducing sensory stimulation
Recommend methods for achieving total relaxation
Teach how to use the problem-solving method

Medical Treatments Performed by Nurses
Give the prescribed drugs

EVALUATION

See the evaluation criteria for each specific goal in Chapter 2.

Physical Irritability (32,247,372,453)

ASSESSMENT

Subjective Data
Sudden angry responses
Fatigue

Objective Data
Startle reaction to minor stimuli
Cries easily
Irritability
Overactivity

Related Data
Manifestations are of recent origin

Commonly Related Conditions:
Cardiac arrhythmias
Diplopia
Farsightedness
Nearsightedness
Indigestion
Puberty changes
Fever
Hepatic coma
Impending respiratory arrest
Menses
Menopause
Edema
Electrolyte and acid-base imbalance

Commonly Related Diseases:
Asthma
Hypertension
Eczema
Hay fever
Beriberi
Epilepsy
Milk alkali syndrome
Scurvy
Sydenham's chorea
Kwashiorkor
Rocky Mountain spotted fever
Tuberculous
Meningitis
Brucellosis
Thyrotoxicosis
Addison's disease

POSSIBLE ETIOLOGY

Prolonged nerve stimulation. Sensitive nerve fibers. Endocrine hyperactivity. Increased internal body pressures. Chronic skin or respiratory irritations. Hormonal changes.

NURSING DIAGNOSIS

Physical irritabiltiy: excessive response to external stimuli as a result of physical imbalance

PLANNING

Patient Needs	**Primary Nurse-Patient Goals**
Sleep, rest, relaxation	To achieve sleep, rest, relaxation
Comfort	To achieve comfort
Protection from physical harm	To prevent physical injury
Acceptance	To achieve productive interpersonal relationships
Warm, communicating relationships	To achieve effective verbal and nonverbal communications
Increased learning	To achieve awareness of needs

NURSING INTERVENTIONS

Nursing Treatments

Approach unhurriedly
Provide an atmosphere of acceptance
Express empathy
Reassure verbally
Demonstrate calmness
Arrange orderly surroundings
Arrange pleasant surroundings
Arrange a structured environment
Establish routines familiar to the patient
Provide quiet
Provide frequent patient contact
Avoid causing intense emotional situations
Encourage the expression of feelings
Listen attentively
    AND
Talk with the patient
Ensure the patient's feeling of safety before introducing unpleasantness
Introduce one anxiety situation at a time
Provide emotionally safe experiences
Reduce the demands placed upon the patient
Refrain from performing nonessential procedures
Encourage adequate rest
Massage gently
    OR   } (for the relaxing effect)
Bathe in warm water

Nursing Observations

Determine the precipitating factors
Monitor blood studies for abnormal acid-base
Monitor blood studies for abnormal adrenal function
Monitor blood studies for abnormal electrolytes
Monitor blood studies for abnormal gas exchange
Monitor blood studies for abnormal thyroid function
Auscultate the apical heartbeat for rate and rhythm

Inspect the chest for respiratory rate and rhythm
Palpate the pulse for rate, rhythm, and volume
Monitor the oral temperature (for fever)
Inspect for edema
Test the eyes for impaired vision
Determine the relieving factors
Observe for an excessive stress level
Observe for evidence that the patient is reaching out for emotional support
Observe for evidence of a favorable response to therapy

Health Teaching
Advise that highly emotional situations be avoided
Explain the importance of offering emotional support to one another
Describe the behavior pattern indicating overstimulation
Explain that fatigue should be recognized as a stress factor
Recommend methods for reducing sensory stimulation
Recommend methods for achieving total relaxation
Explain the causes of the health problem

Medical Treatments Performed by Nurses
Give the prescribed drugs

EVALUATION

See the evaluation criteria for each specific goal in Chapter 2.

Physical Nervousness (32,247,372, 453)

ASSESSMENT

Subjective Data
Anger
Fatigue
Moodiness
Internal shakiness

Objective Data
Restlessness
Weeping
Overactivity or underactivity

Related Data
Manifestations are of recent origin
Commonly Related Conditions:
Tachycardia
Drug toxicity
Insulin shock
Tetany
Adolescence
Menses
Menopause
Hypoglycemia

Commonly Related Diseases:
Hyperthyroidism
Pheochromocytoma
Hypertension
Cushing's disease

POSSIBLE ETIOLOGY

Hypersensitivity of neuron fibers. Metabolic dysfunction. Hormonal imbalance.

NURSING DIAGNOSIS

Physical nervousness: an unnatural, uncomfortable feeling of internal tension as a result of physical imbalance

PLANNING

Patient Needs	Primary Nurse-Patient Goals
Sleep, rest, relaxation	To achieve sleep, rest, relaxation
Comfort	To achieve comfort
Protection from physical harm	To prevent physical injury
Acceptance	To achieve productive interpersonal relationships
Warm, communicating relationships	To achieve effective verbal and nonverbal communications
Increased learning	To achieve awareness of needs

NURSING INTERVENTIONS

Nursing Treatments
Approach unhurriedly
Provide an atmosphere of acceptance
Express empathy
Reasssure verbally
Demonstrate calmness
Arrange orderly surroundings
Arrange pleasant surroundings
Arrange a structured environment
Establish routines familiar to the patient
Provide quiet
Provide frequent patient contact
Avoid causing intense emotional situations
Encourage the expression of feelings
Listen attentively
    AND
Talk with the patient
Ensure the patient's feeling of safety before introducing unpleasantness
Introduce one anxiety situation at a time
Provide emotionally safe experiences
Reduce the demands placed upon the patient

Refrain from performing nonessential procedures
Encourage adequate rest
Massage gently
   OR   } (for the relaxing effect)
Bathe in warm water

Nursing Observations
Determine the precipitating factors
Monitor blood studies for abnormal glucose
Monitor blood studies for abnormal adrenal function
Monitor blood studies for abnormal thyroid function
Observe for drug reactions
Observe for shock
Monitor the blood pressure (for increase)
Determine the relieving factors
Observe for an excessive stress level
Observe for evidence that the patient is reaching out for emotional support
Observe for evidence of a favorable response to therapy

Health Teaching
Advise that highly emotional situations be avoided
Explain the importance of offering emotional support to one another
Explain that fatigue should be recognized as a stress factor
Recommend methods for reducing sensory stimulation
Recommend methods for achieving total relaxation
Explain the causes of the health problem

Medical Treatments Performed by Nurses
Give the prescribed drugs

EVALUATION

See the evaluation criteria for each specific goal in Chapter 2.

INSIGHT AND PROBLEM SOLVING

Inability to Define Reality (12,94,118, 199,372)

ASSESSMENT

Subjective Data
May be preoccupied with delusions or hallucinations
Unable to perceive danger
Tendency toward fantasy

Objective Data
Displays little interest in the real world
Unable to function effectively

Related Data

Commonly Related Diseases:
Any severe disease
   OR
Melancholia involutional psychosis
Schizophrenia
Cerebral arteriosclerosis
Senile psychosis
Chronic brain syndrome
Manic-depressive psychosis

POSSIBLE ETIOLOGY

Excessive stress. Organic or functional disorders. Inadequacy feelings in dealing with the real world.

NURSING DIAGNOSIS

Inability to define reality: inability to distinguish between what is real and what is unreal

PLANNING

Patient Needs	**Primary Nurse-Patient Goals**
Comfort	To achieve comfort
Protection from physical harm	To prevent physical injury
Protection from psychologic threat	To prevent emotional injury
Dependence	To achieve comfort
Warm, communicating relationships	To achieve effective verbal and nonverbal communications
High evaluation of self, adequacy	To achieve positive expressions, feelings reactions
Dignity	To achieve productive interpersonal relationships
Personal growth and maturity	To achieve optimum function
Increased learning	To achieve awareness of needs
Increased reality perception and problem-solving ability	To achieve optimum function

NURSING INTERVENTIONS

Nursing Treatments
Approach unhurriedly
Acknowledge dependency
Provide an atmosphere of acceptance
Reassure verbally
Demonstrate calmness
Provide frequent patient contact
Arrange a structured environment
Provide quiet

Avoid causing intense emotional situations
Encourage the expression of feelings
Listen attentively
  AND
Talk with the patient
Offer feedback of the patient's expressed feelings
Ask questions which encourage answers that reflect reality perception
Explore superficial topics and reasons for avoiding in-depth feelings
  BUT
Terminate emotionally threatening conversation immediately
Encourage realistic perception of others
Encourage the reduction of generalizations to specifics
Encourage the substitution of real-life endeavors for fantasized endeavors
Explore with the patient his strengths and resources
Ensure the patient's feeling of safety before introducing unpleasantness
Introduce one anxiety situation at a time
Limit conversation to short discussions
Encourage active diversional activities (if possible)
Refrain from entering into delusions, hallucinations, or illusions
Encourage the use of normal coping mechanisms
Reduce the demands placed upon the patient
Refrain from performing nonessential procedures
Use the patient's name frequently
Provide emotional support for persons significant to the patient

Nursing Observations
Determine the degree of insight
Evaluate the safety of the environment
Evaluate the significance of emotional distress mannerisms
Evaluate the significance of nonverbal communication
Identify abnormal perceptions
Identify abnormal throught content
Identify disturbing conversation topics
Identify reality-acceptance clues
Identify life values significant to the person
Identify appropriate use of defense mechanisms
Identify inappropriate use of defense mechanisms
Observe for an excessive stress level
Observe for evidence that the patient is reaching out for emotional support
Observe for behavior modification

Health Teaching
Recommend more effective methods of coping
Advise against denouncing erroneous perceptions
Advise that highly emotional situations be avoided
Advise that significant persons express acceptance of one another
Advise that significant persons express love for one another
Explain the importance of offering emotional support to one another
Explain the need for realistic expectations of others

Explain the importance of maintaining a positive self-attitude
Explain the causes of the health problem
Recommend methods for reducing sensory stimulation
Recommend methods for achieving total relaxation

EVALUATION

See the evaluation criteria for each specific goal in Chapter 2.

Inadequate Insight Related to Interpersonal Relationships (35,282,372)

ASSESSMENT

Subjective Data
Unaware of his negative or positive stimulus value to other persons
Perceives himself with more abilities than he actually has
Fails to recognize his true motives in a relationship
Changes his perception of himself to fit the situation

Objective Data
Blames others for his difficulties
Verbally expresses an inability to understand why other people react to him
as they do

Related Data
Commonly Related Diseases:
None

POSSIBLE ETIOLOGY

Lack of education. Inconsistent values or standards.

NURSING DIAGNOSIS

Inadequate insight related to interpersonal relationships: the inability to recognize that how others react to one is the result of how one acts toward others

PLANNING

Patient Needs	Primary Nurse-Patient Goals
Protection for psychologic threat	To prevent emotional injury
Acceptance	To achieve productive interpersonal relationships
Warm, communicating relationships	To achieve effective verbal and non-verbal communications
High evaluation of self	To achieve positive expressions, feelings, reactions
Personal growth and maturity	To achieve optimum function
Increased learning	To achieve awareness of needs
Increased reality perception and problem-solving ability	To achieve optimum function

NURSING INTERVENTIONS

Nursing Treatments
Approach unhurriedly
Provide an atmosphere of acceptance
Reassure verbally
Provide frequent patient contact
Encourage the expression of feelings
Listen attentively
    AND
Talk with the patient
Offer feedback of the patient's expressed feelings
Ask questions which encourage answers that reflect reality perception
Explore superficial topics and reasons for avoiding in-depth feelings
Encourage acceptance of limitations in others
Encourage acceptance of self-limitations
Ecnourage honesty in presenting oneself
Encourage awareness of positive responses from others
Encourage enhanced involvement in already-established relationships
Encourage participation in therapeutic group interaction
Encourage role-playing to develop sensitivity
Encourage realistic perception of others
Encourage respect for the rights of others
Encourage the reduction of generalizations to specifics
Explore with the patient his strengths and resources
Explore with the patient reasons for criticism by others
Explore with the patient reasons for criticism of others
Explore with the patient reasons for likes and dislikes
Explore with the patient the effects of his behavior on others
Recognize the need for the use of appropriate defense mechanisms
Encourage the use of normal coping mechanisms
Refrain from negatively criticizing
Support a realistic assessment of the situation

Nursing Observations
Determine the degree of insight
Evaluate the person's relatedness with others
Evaluate the significance of emotional distresss mannerisms
Evaluate the significance of nonverbal communication
Identify disturbing conversation topics
Identify appropriate use of defense mechanisms
Identify inappropriate use of defense mechanisms
Observe for an excessive stress level
Observe for evidence of a favorable response to therapy

Health Teaching
Recommend more effective methods of coping
Advise that negative responses from others be regarded with minimum
    significance

Advise that significant persons express acceptance of one another
Explain the importance of offering emotional support to one another
Describe the behavior pattern indicating emotional maturity
Explain the need for realistic expectation of others
Recommend a habitual, positive mental attitude
Teach how to use the problem-solving method

EVALUATION

See the evaluation criteria for each specific goal in Chapter 2.

Inadequate Insight Related to Self (35,94,372)

ASSESSMENT

Subjective Data
Worries about his emotional responses
Either does not perceive his behavior as abnormal or perceives his behavior
   as abnormal but fails to recognize the severity of the abnormality

Objective Data
Blames others for his difficulties

Related Data
Commonly Related Diseases:
None
   OR
Psychoneurosis
Schizophrenia

POSSIBLE ETIOLOGY

Lack of education. Unfamiliarity with norms.

NURSING DIAGNOSIS

Inadequate insight related to self: the inability to identify one's own behavioral responses or to understand their cause

PLANNING

Patient Needs	Primary Nurse-Patient Goals
Protection from psychologic threat	To prevent emotional injury
Acceptance	To achieve productive interpersonal relationships
Warm, communicatiing relationships	To achieve effective verbal and nonverbal communications
Personal growth and maturity	To achieve optimum function
Increased learning	To achieve awareness of needs
Increased reality perception and problem-solving ability	To achieve optimum function

NURSING INTERVENTIONS

Nursing Treatments
Approach unhurriedly
Provide an atmosphere of acceptance
Reassure verbally
Provide frequent patient contact
Encourage the expression of feelings
Listen attentively
    AND
Talk with the patient
Offer feedback of the patient's expressed feelings
Ask questions which encourage answers that reflect reality perception
Explore superficial topics and reasons for avoiding in-depth feelings
Encourage acceptance of self-limitations
Encourage honesty in presenting oneself
Encourage participation in therapeutic group interaction
Explore with the patient his strengths and resources
Explore with the patient reasons for criticism by others
Explore with the patient reasons for criticism of others
Explore with the patient reasons for likes and dislikes
Explore with the patient reasons for recurring problems
Explore with the patient reasons for self-criticism
Explore with the patient the effects of his behavior on others
Recognize the need for the use of appropriate defense mechanisms
Encourage the use of normal coping mechanisms
Refrain from negatively criticizing
Support a realistic assessment of the situation

Nursing Observations
Determine the degree of insight
Evaluate the significance of emotional distress mannerisms
Evaluate the significance of nonverbal communication
Identify disturbing conversation topics
Identify appropriate use of defense mechanisms
Identify inappropriate use of defense mechanisms
Observe for an excessive stress level
Observe for evidence of a favorable response to therapy

Health Teaching
Recommend more effective methods of coping
Advise that negative responses from others be regarded with minimum
    significance
Describe the behavior pattern indicating emotional maturity
Explain the importance of maintaining a positive self-attitude
Explain that undesirable thoughts and feelings are normal
Teach how to use the problem-solving method

EVALUATION

See the evaluation criteria for each specific goal in Chapter 2.

Poor Problem-Solving Ability (543)

ASSESSMENT

Subjective Data
Helplessness
Anxiety

Objective Data
Does not recognize that there is a problem
Recognizes that there is a problem but is unable to identify it
Unable to determine a solution to the problem
Knows of multiple solutions but is unable to decide on one and act
Preoccupied with the problem rather than the solution

Related Data
Commonly Related Conditions:
Emotional distress
Commonly Related Diseases:
None
  OR
Any disease or injury

POSSIBLE ETIOLOGY

Inability to accept one's own judgments and decisions. Dealing with internal stress, which decreases the ability to deal with external stress. Poor problem-solving techniques. Habitual negative thinking. Inability to anticipate a situation's outcome. Situational inadequacy feelings.

NURSING DIAGNOSIS

Poor problem-solving ability: difficulty evaluating, determining solutions to, and acting to realize problems

PLANNING

Patient Needs	Primary Nurse-Patient Goals
Comfort	To achieve comfort
Protection from psychologic threat	To prevent emotional injury
Acceptance	To achieve productive interpersonal relationships
Warm, communicating relationships	To achieve effective verbal and nonverbal communications
Adequacy	To achieve positive expressions, feelings, reactions
Increased learning	To achieve awareness of needs and/or use of resources
Increased problem-solving ability	To achieve optimum function

NURSING INTERVENTIONS

Nursing Treatments
Approach unhurriedly
Provide an atmosphere of acceptance

Reassure verbally
Demonstrate calmness
Avoid causing embarrassing situations
Encourage the expression of feelings
Listen attentively
  AND
Talk with the patient
Encourage patient questions
Provide reliable information
Discourage decision-making when one is under severe stress
Encourage acceptance of unpleasantness
Encourage balanced long- and short-range goals
Encourage gradual mastery of a situation
Encourage mutual problem solving
Encourage the sharing of common problems with others
Explore with the patient his strengths and resources
Explore with the patient reasons for recurring problems
Support a realistic assessment of the situation

Nursing Observations
Determine the degree of insight
Identify disturbing conversation topics
Identify appropriate use of defense mechanisms
Identify inappropriate use of defense mechanisms
Observe for impaired judgment
Observe for evidence of a favorable response to therapy

Health Teaching
Advise early correction of problems
Explain the causes of the health problem
Teach how to use the problem-solving method

EVALUATION

See the evaluation criteria for each specific goal in Chapter 2.

THERAPEUTIC RELATIONSHIP

Inadequate Therapeutic Relationship (118,199,331,537)

ASSESSMENT

Subjective Data
Intense emotional involvement with the patient
Lack of nonjudgmental acceptance by the therapist
Deliberate dishonesty on the part of either party

Objective Data
Poor identification of patient problems and goals
Lack of responsibility between the patient and therapist

Poor communication between parties
Insufficient time spent in developing the relationship
Disrespect for one another

Related Data

Commonly Related Diseases:
None
   OR
Any disease

POSSIBLE ETIOLOGY

Lack of definition in terms of limits, roles, and relationship with the patient. The therapist's attempt to meet his own needs rather than those of the patient.

NURSING DIAGNOSIS

Inadequate therapeutic relationship: a nurse-patient relationship that does not contribute to the patient's well-being or personal growth

PLANNING

Patient Needs	**Primary Nurse-Patient Goals**
Comfort	To achieve comfort
Protection from psychologic threat	To prevent emotional injury
Acceptance	To achieve productive interpersonal relationships
Warm, communicating relationships	To achieve effective verbal and nonverbal communications
Personal growth and maturity	To achieve optimum function
Increased learning	To achieve awareness of needs
Increased reality perception and problem-solving ability	To achieve optimum function

NURSING INTERVENTIONS

Nursing Treatments
Approach unhurriedly
Provide an atmosphere of acceptance
Express empathy
Express warmth and friendliness
Demonstrate calmness
Provide frequent patient contact
Encourage acceptance of responsibility (by both the patient and therapist)
Encourage balanced long- and short-range goals
Encourage honesty in presenting oneself to others (by the patient)
Maintain honesty (with the patient)
Encourage mutual problem solving
Encourage patient questions
Provide reliable information
Encourage respect for the rights of others.

Maintain consistent staff behavior

Maintain social formality ⎫
    OR   ⎬ (whichever is most suitable to the
Maintain social informality ⎭   patient)

Nursing Observations
Determine the degree of insight
Evaluate the significance of emotional distress mannerisms
Evaluate the significance of nonverbal communication
Observe for a favorable response to therapy

Health Teaching
Teach how to use the problem-solving method
Explain the reason for and intended effect of the therapy

EVALUATION

See the evaluation criteria for each specific goal in Chapter 2.

GENERAL INFORMATION RELATED TO BEHAVIOR

Inadequate Information Related to Child Growth and Development (135,208)

ASSESSMENT

Subjective Data
Person confirms a lack of information

Objective Data
Person's actions indicate a lack of information regarding the fact:

that each child's growth and development occur at a consistent but often a more rapid or slower rate than others

that each phase of development has specific characteristic traits

that the factors which influence growth and development include intelligence, sex, nutrition, presence or absence of injury or disease, endocrine gland function, race, and the position of the child in the family

that the developmental stages include:

the prenatal period from conception to birth during which there is intrauterine physiologic growth

the infancy period from birth to 14 days of life during which there is a period of adjustment to the environment with little or no physical growth. The infant can perform simple reflex activities such as sucking, yawning, grunting, stretching, etc.

the babyhood period from 14 days (2 weeks) to 3 years during which body control is learned. Skills are developed in feeding and dressing oneself, walking, talking, and playing. The child learns to trust and gradually develops some independence. The first physical growth cycle occurs.

the childhood period from age 3 years to puberty (age 11–13 years) during which the child learns to control the environment and make social adjustments. He begins to develop a conscience and becomes involved in the industry of accomplishing work activities. The second physical growth cycle occurs.

the adolescent period from puberty (age 11–13 years) to maturity (21 years) during which a sense of identity is developed. The third growth cycle occurs in which there is rapid physiologic development of secondary sex characteristics. The person gains independence from adults and becomes ready for the intimacy of marriage and work responsibilities.

Related Data

Commonly Related Diseases:
None
   OR
Any disease or injury

POSSIBLE ETIOLOGY

Lack of instruction. Little or no contact with small children during the growth and development years.

NURSING DIAGNOSIS

Inadequate information related to child growth and development: lack of information regarding the orderly progression of life stages which occur in a child from conception to maturity

PLANNING

Patient Needs	Primary Nurse-Patient Goals
Comfort	To achieve comfort
Independence	To achieve positive expressions, feelings, reactions
Increased learning	To achieve awareness of needs
Increased reality perception and problem-solving ability	To achieve optimum function

NURSING INTERVENTIONS

Nursing Treatments
Approach unhurriedly
Encourage patient questions
Provide reliable information (about child growth and development)

Nursing Observations
Evaluate the response to teaching

Health Teaching
Explain that parental attitudes affect child development
Emphasize that children need guidance
Advise early correction of problems (during growth and development)

Inform of the resources available for health care (when growth and development are not normal)

EVALUATION

See the evaluation criteria for each specific goal in Chapter 2.

Inadequate Information Related to Child Socialization

ASSESSMENT

Subjective Data

Person confirms a lack of information

Conflict when hearing the opinions of others regarding child socialization

Objective Data

Person's actions indicate a lack of information regarding:

how to raise a child

how to correctly provide discipline

how to cope with a child who responds differently than most children

Related Data

Commonly Related Diseases:

None

POSSIBLE ETIOLOGY

Lack of instruction

NURSING DIAGNOSIS

Inadequate information related to child socialization: a lack of information regarding the correct methods to use in providing for the social development of a young person

PLANNING

Patient Needs	Primary Nurse-Patient Goals
Comfort	To achieve comfort
Warm, communicating relationships	To achieve effective verbal and nonverbal communications
Adequacy	To achieve positive expressions, feelings, reactions
Increased learning	To achieve awareness of needs and/or use of resources

NURSING INTERVENTIONS

Nursing Treatments

Approach unhurriedly

Reassure verbally

Encourage patient questions

Provide reliable information

Nursing Observations
Evaluate the response to teaching

Health Teaching
Advise early correction of problems
Advise against verbally comparing significant persons
Emphasize that children need guidance
Explain that parental attitudes affect child development
Advise that discipline be consistent
Inform that bribing and threatening are ineffective child discipline methods
Inform that isolation, loss of treat, and restriction are effective child discipline methods
Recommend that independence be encouraged
Emphasize the need to develop self-reliance

EVALUATION

See the evaluation criteria for each specific goal in Chapter 2.

Inadequate Information Related to Coping With the Mentally III (46,118,199,586,594)

ASSESSMENT

Subjective Data
Person confirms a lack of information

Objective Data
Person's actions indicate a lack of information regarding:
    how to help the mentally ill person
    where to obtain health assistance for the mentally ill

Related Data
Commonly Related Diseases:
Psychoneurosis
Schizophrenia

POSSIBLE ETIOLOGY

Lack of instruction. No previous experience with the mentally ill.

NURSING DIAGNOSIS

Inadequate information related to coping with the mentally ill: lack of information regarding how to approach and help persons who are mentally ill

PLANNING

Patient Needs	**Primary Nurse-Patient Goals**
Comfort	To achieve comfort
Protection from psychologic threat	To prevent emotional injury
Warm, communicating relationships	To achieve effective verbal and nonverbal communications

Adequacy	To achieve positive expressions, feelings, reactions
Increased learning	To achieve awareness of needs and/or use of resources

NURSING INTERVENTIONS

Nursing Treatments
Approach unhurriedly
Reassure verbally
Encourage patient questions
Provide reliable information
Make a referral (to the appropriate agency)

Nursing Observations
Determine the degree of insight
Identify disturbing conversation topics
Observe for an excessive stress level
Evaluate the response to teaching

Health Teaching
Advise early correction of problems
Advise against causing defensive responses in others
Advise against communicating double-meaning messages
Advise against emphasizing past problems caused by another
Advise against verbally comparing significant persons
Advise that highly emotional situations be avoided
Advise that significant persons express acceptance of one another
Advise that significant persons express love for one another
Explain the importance of offering emotional support to one another
Describe those symptoms which should be reported (combative behavior, loss of emotional control)
Explain that ill persons are often hypersensitive
Explain that the behavior of one family member is not a reflection on other family members
Explain that undesirable thoughts and feelings are normal
Explain the importance of remaining calm
Explain that persons making emotional adjustments prefer doing so at their own pace
Recommend that behavioral limits be set
Explain how to set behavioral limits
Relate the criteria for determining mental illness
Relate the accepted criteria for commitment of the mentally ill

EVALUATION
See the evaluation criteria for each specific goal in Chapter 2.

Inadequate Information Related to Mental Health Principles (52,118,372,405,587)

ASSESSMENT

Subjective Data
Person confirms a lack of information

Objective Data
Person's actions indicate a lack of information regarding:
the signs of good mental health
how to improve a basically healthy mental status
how to foster mental health in others

Related Data
Commonly Related Diseases:
None
OR
Any behavior disorder

POSSIBLE ETIOLOGY

Lack of instruction

NURSING DIAGNOSIS

Inadequate information related to mental health principles: lack of information regarding sound principles and their appropriate use in maintaining mental health

PLANNING

Patient Needs	Primary Nurse-Patient Goals
Comfort	To achieve comfort
Protection from psychologic threat	To prevent emotional injury
Warm, communicating relationships	To achieve effective verbal and nonverbal communications
Adequacy	To achieve positive expressions, feelings, reactions
Increased learning	To achieve awareness of needs

NURSING INTERVENTIONS

Nursing Treatments
Approach unhurriedly
Reassure verbally
Encourage patient questions
Provide reliable information

Nursing Observations
Evaluate the response to teaching

Health Teaching
Advise early correction of problems
Advise against causing defensive responses in others
Advise against communicating double-meaning messages
Advise against emphasizing past problems caused by another
Advise against verbally comparing significant persons
Advise occasional respite from responsibility
Advise that highly emotional situations be avoided
Advise that negative responses from others be regarded with minimum
    significance
Advise that significant persons express acceptance of one another
Advise that significant persons express love for one another
Explain the importance of offering emotional support to one another
Describe the behavior pattern indicating emotional maturity
Emphasize the importance of recognizing tension within oneself
Explain the need for realistic expectations of others
Explain that fatigue should be recognized as a stress factor
Explain the need to recognize highly stressful situations
Explain the importance of maintaining a positive self-attitude
Explain how to obtain release from emotional stress
Explain that ill persons are often hypersensitive
Explain that parental attitudes affect child development
Explain that recreation aids total heath
Explain that recreation supports personal growth and is not an escape
    mechanism
Explain that undesirable thoughts and feelings are normal
Emphasize the importance of planning and anticipating future activities
Explain the importance of remaining calm
Explain the need to predict and plan for change
Explain how to channel emotional energy into activity
Emphasize the need to develop self-reliance
Recommend methods for achieving total relaxation
Recommend that independence be encouraged
Recommend that passive activities be avoided
Recommend a habitual, positive mental attitude
Teach how to use the problem-solving method

EVALUATION

See the evaluation criteria for each specific goal in Chapter 2.

7.

NURSING DIAGNOSES RELATED TO
Body Fluids

ALTERED FLUID INTAKE

Inadequate Fluid Intake (32,325,391)

ASSESSMENT

Subjective Data
Thirst
Generalized weakness
Burning on urination

Objective Data
Daily fluid intake of less than 800 cc
Dry skin and mucous membranes
Poor skin turgor
Weight loss
Salty perspiration
Decreased urinary output

Related Data

Laboratory Findings:
Increased urine specific gravity
Increased hematocrit and red blood count

Commonly Related Conditions:
Dehydration
Disorientation
Comatose states

Commonly Related Diseases:
None
    OR
Esophageal stricture
Oral carcinoma
Cerebral vascular accident

POSSIBLE ETIOLOGY

Fluid inaccessibility. Refusal to take fluids. Inability to drink fluids.

NURSING DIAGNOSIS

Inadequate fluid intake: a daily intake of fluids below the normally required level

PLANNING

Patient Needs	**Primary Nurse-Patient Goals**
Water-salt balance	To maintain fluid and electrolyte balance
Comfort	To achieve comfort
Protection from physical harm	To prevent physical injury
Increased learning	To achieve awareness of needs

NURSING INTERVENTIONS

Nursing Treatments
Increase fluid intake to about 2000 cc daily
Provide fresh drinking water
Provide fluid selection
Give small, frequent drinks

Nursing Observations
Measure the intake
Measure the output

Health Teaching
Explain the reason for and intended effect of the therapy
Instruct to increase fluid intake

Medical Treatments Performed by Nurses
Administer fluids by hypodermoclysis
Administer intravenous fluids

EVALUATION

See the evaluation criteria for each specific goal in Chapter 2.

Increased Hydration Requirement (32,325)

ASSESSMENT

Subjective Data
Thirst

Objective Data
Elevated body temperature
Diarrhea
Vomiting
Profuse perspiration

Hemorrhage
Genitourinary infection
Renal calculi

Related Data

Commonly Related Conditions:
Fever

Commonly Related Diseases:
Gastritis
Pyelonephritis
Cystitis
Dysentery

POSSIBLE ETIOLOGY

Need to remove bacteria or undesirable waste products from the body. Excessive fluid loss.

NURSING DIAGNOSIS

Increased hydration requirement: an above-normal need for the intake of large amounts of fluid

PLANNING

Patient Needs	**Primary Nurse-Patient Goals**
Water-salt balance	To maintain fluid and electrolyte balance
Waste elimination	To maintain regulating mechanisms and functions
Protection from physical harm	To prevent physical injury, infection
Increased learning	To achieve awareness of needs

NURSING INTERVENTIONS

Nursing Treatments
Increase fluid intake to about 3000 cc daily
Provide fresh drinking water
Provide fluid selection
Give small, frequent drinks

Nursing Observations
Measure the intake
Measure the output

Health Teaching
Explain the causes of the health problem
Explain the reason for and intended effect of the therapy
Instruct to increase fluid intake

Medical Treatments Performed by Nurses
Administer fluids by hypodermoclysis
Administer intravenous fluids

EVALUATION

See the evaluation criteria for each specific goal in Chapter 2.

POTENTIAL ALTERED FLUID INTAKE

Potential Inadequate Fluid Intake (32,325,391)

ASSESSMENT

Subjective Data
Mouth tenderness
Generalized weakness

Objective Data
Difficulty swallowing
Wired or stiff jaw
Confusion

Related Data
Commonly Related Conditions:
Depression
Senility
Oral surgery

Commonly Related Diseases:
Cerebral vascular accident
Laryngeal carcinoma

POSSIBLE ETIOLOGY

Unavailability of fluids. Lack of interest in or ability to take fluids.

NURSING DIAGNOSIS

Potential inadequate fluid intake: the possibility that a sufficient amount of fluid will not be taken

PLANNING

Patient Needs	**Primary Nurse-Patient Goals**
Protection from physical harm	To prevent physical injury
Increased learning	To achieve awareness of needs

NURSING INTERVENTIONS

Nursing Treatments
Balance fluid intake to equal output
Provide fresh drinking water
Provide fluid selection
Give small, frequent drinks

Nursing Observations
Measure the intake
Measure the output

Health Teaching
Explain the reason for and intended effect of the therapy
Instruct to increase fluid intake

Medical Treatments Performed by Nurses
Administer fluids by hypodermoclysis
Administer intravenous fluids

EVALUATION

See the evaluation criteria for each specific goal in Chapter 2.

FLUID RETENTION

Edema Related to Localized Tissue Injury (271,325,453)

ASSESSMENT

Subjective Data
Skin tightness and heaviness
Pain
Sensory loss in severely edematous tissue

Objective Data
Localized swelling
Glossy skin
Heat and redness
Impaired mobility

Related Data
Recent tissue injury such as trauma, surgery, allergic response
Commonly Related Conditions:
Mastectomy
Cellulitis
Bruise
Abscess
Sprain
Eye contusion
Commonly Related Diseases:
Bone fracture
Thrombophlebitis
Rheumatoid arthritis
First-, second-, or third-degree burns

POSSIBLE ETIOLOGY

Lymphatic obstruction. Inflammation which dilates blood vessels and increases blood flow to the area, increasing capillary pressure which causes the escape of fluid into tissues. Trauma from blunt objects, burns, wounds, etc. The presence of histamines in an allergic response.

NURSING DIAGNOSIS

Edema related to localized tissue injury: fluid accumulation within body tissues as a result of direct injury to the tissue

PLANNING

Patient Needs	**Primary Nurse-Patient Goals**
Circulation	To maintain oxygen to all cells
Rest	To achieve rest
Comfort	To achieve comfort
Protection from physical harm	To prevent physical injury
Increased learning	To achieve awareness of needs

NURSING INTERVENTIONS

Nursing Treatments
Apply heat by a gooseneck lamp
    OR
Apply a heat cradle
    OR
Apply a hot water bottle
    OR
Apply a warm, moist compress
Elevate the affected body part
Apply an elastic bandage
Massage gently
    AND
Exercise in range of motion (for lymph obstruction)
Remove constrictive clothing
Give nonprescription drugs (ExR) (antihistamines for allergic response)
Handle gently
Lubricate the skin with cocoa butter, glycerine, lanolin, mineral oil, or olive
    oil (if the skin is intact)

Nursing Observations
Observe for complaints of pain
Observe for evidence of a favorable response to therapy

Health Teaching
Describe those symptoms which should be reported (increased edema, pain)
Explain the causes of the health problem
Explain the reason for and intended effect of the therapy
Instruct to elevate the body part
Advise against wearing constrictive clothing
Teach how to apply heat therapy

EVALUATION

See the evaluation criteria for each specific goal in Chapter 2.

POTENTIAL FLUID RETENTION

Potential Edema Related to Localized Tissue Injury (271,325,453)

ASSESSMENT

Objective Data
Interrupted tissue intactness
Bruising
Redness and/or heat

Related Data
Commonly Related Conditions:
Mastectomy
Cellulitis
Bruise
Abscess

Commonly Related Diseases:
Bone fracture
Rheumatoid arthritis
First-, second-, or third-degree burns

POSSIBLE ETIOLOGY

Lymphatic obstruction. Inflammation. Trauma from blunt objects, burns, wounds, insect bites, bone fracture, etc. An allergic response.

NURSING DIAGNOSIS

Potential edema related to localized tissue injury: the possibility that fluid accumulation will occur within body tissues as a result of direct injury to the tissue

PLANNING

Patient Needs
Protection from physical harm
Increased learning

Primary Nurse-Patient Goals
To prevent accident, physical injury
To achieve awareness of needs

NURSING INTERVENTIONS

Nursing Treatments
Apply a cold, moist compress
   OR
Apply an ice bag (immediately to the injured site)
Elevate the affected body part
Apply an elastic bandage
Give nonprescription drugs (ExR) (antihistamines for allergic response)
Massage gently
   AND
Exercise in range of motion (for lymph obstruction)
Remove constrictive clothing

Nursing Observations
Inspect for edema
Observe for complaints of pain

Health Teaching
Describe those symptoms which should be reported (skin tightness, pain)
Explain the causes of the health problem
Explain the reason for and intended effect of the therapy
Instruct to elevate the body part
Advise against wearing constrictive clothing

EVALUATION

See the evaluation criteria for each specific goal in Chapter 2.

FLUID RELATED DISCOMFORTS

Fluid Restriction Discomfort

ASSESSMENT

Subjective Data
Thirst
Preoccupation with fluid restriction

Objective Data
Patient has been put on a fluid restriction regime
Irritability
Frequently asks for fluids

Related Data
Commonly Related Conditions:
Ascites
Edema
Commonly Related Diseases:
Nephrosis
Glomerulonephritis
Laennec's cirrhosis
Congestive heart failure

POSSIBLE ETIOLOGY

Fluids are restricted as a therapeutic measure. The patient drinks the daily allotted fluid amount at one time or within a few hours, having little or nothing else to drink the remainder of the 24 hours.

NURSING DIAGNOSIS

Fluid restriction discomfort: a dryness discomfort resulting from a therapeutically imposed limit on the amount of fluid that can be taken in a 24-hour period

PLANNING

Patient Needs	**Primary Nurse-Patient Goals**
Comfort	To achieve comfort
Protection from physical harm	To prevent physical injury
Increased learning	To achieve awareness of needs

NURSING INTERVENTIONS

Nursing Treatments
Distribute the fluid intake over 24 hours
Give small, frequent drinks
Provide fluid selection
Provide cold water for mouth rinsing but not swallowing (between drinks)
Refresh with a mouthwash (between drinks)
Give hard candy (to suck on)

Nursing Observations
Observe for an excessive stress level

Health Teaching
Explain the reason for and intended effect of the therapy

EVALUATION

See the evaluation criteria for each specific goal in Chapter 2.

Thirst Discomfort (453)

ASSESSMENT

Subjective Data
Feeling of cotton in the mouth
Tongue thickness sensation
Desire to drink fluid

Objective Data
Parched lips
Little saliva

Related Data

Commonly Related Conditions:
Fever
Hemorrhage or chronic bleeding

Commonly Related Diseases:
Hyperparathyroidism
Dysentery
Diabetes mellitus or insipidus
Primary aldosteronism

POSSIBLE ETIOLOGY

Increased sodium retention. Excessive fluid loss through hemorrhage, vomiting, diarrhea, or polyuria.

NURSING DIAGNOSIS

Thirst discomfort: a dryness discomfort within the mouth and pharynx related to physiologic body changes

PLANNING

Patient Needs	Primary Nurse-Patient Goals
Water-salt balance	To maintain fluid and electrolyte balance
Comfort	To achieve comfort
Protection from physical harm	To prevent physical injury
Increased learning	To achieve awareness of needs

NURSING INTERVENTIONS

Nursing Treatments
Balance fluid intake to equal output
Provide fresh drinking water
Provide fluid selection
Moisten the mouth with cracked ice
Refrain from restricting fluids (in polyuria)

Nursing Observations
Measure the intake
Measure the output
Monitor blood studies for abnormal electrolytes (increased sodium)

Health Teaching
Explain the causes of the health problem

Medical Treatments Performed by Nurses
Administer intravenous fluids (for hemorrhage)

EVALUATION

See the evaluation criteria for each specific goal in Chapter 2.

FLUID THERAPY DEPENDENCE

Dependence on Arteriovenous Cutdown Management (70,71,391)

ASSESSMENT

Subjective Data
Person relies on nurses for:
cutdown patency
prevention of infection and embolus
correct fluid administration
dressing changes
supervision of flow rate
correct medication administration

Objective Data

Person has a venous cutdown

Related Data

Commonly Related Conditions:
Shock

Commonly Related Diseases:
Any disease or injury causing circulatory collapse

POSSIBLE ETIOLOGY

Need for fluids or fluid replacement. Inability to maintain fluid therapy by usual needle puncture. Prolonged intravenous therapy.

NURSING DIAGNOSIS

Dependence on arteriovenous cutdown management: reliance on nursing for the proper care and functioning of an arteriovenous cutdown

PLANNING

Patient Needs	**Primary Nurse-Patient Goals**
Comfort	To achieve comfort
Cleanliness	To achieve good hygiene
Protection from physical harm	To prevent physical injury, infection
Increased learning	To achieve awareness of needs

NURSING INTERVENTIONS

Nursing Treatments
Apply an antibiotic ointment (to the sutures)
Apply a sterile dressing (over the injection site)
Change the dressing frequently
Position (the arm) comfortably
Anchor the tubing securely
Provide sufficiently long tubing to allow freedom of movement

Nursing Observations
Check the tube (cutdown catheter) for patency
Check the solution (intravenous) for flow rate
Check for infiltration of the solution
Measure the intake
Measure the output
Observe for water intoxication

Health Teaching
Describe those symptoms which should be reported (burning pain at the cutdown site, tachycardia)
Explain the reason for and intended effect of the therapy

Medical Treatments Performed by Nurses
Administer intravenous fluids
Give the prescribed drugs (intravenously)

EVALUATION

See the evaluation criteria for each specific goal in Chapter 2.

Dependence on Blood Transfusion Management (70,391)

ASSESSMENT

Subjective Data

Person relies on nurses for:
   receiving the correct blood and at the proper flow rate
   observation for transfusion reaction signs
   infection prevention
Anxiety regarding blood transfusion safety
May fear dying because of blood transfusion implications

Objective Data

Person is receiving a blood transfusion

Related Data

Commonly Related Diseases:
Any disease or injury requiring blood replacement

POSSIBLE ETIOLOGY

Need to replace decreased blood volume or specific blood components

NURSING DIAGNOSIS

Dependence on blood transfusion management: reliance on nurses for the proper administration of a blood transfusion

PLANNING

Patient Needs	**Primary Nurse-Patient Goals**
Comfort	To achieve comfort
Cleanliness	To achieve good hygiene
Protection from physical harm	To prevent physical injury, infection
Increased learning	To achieve awareness of needs

NURSING INTERVENTIONS

Nursing Treatments

Attend the patient constantly (while the first 50 cc of blood is being administered)
Do not give blood unrefrigerated for more than one hour
Do not give blood which is over three weeks old
Administer isotonic saline intravenous fluid between the blood transfusion and glucose infusion
Do not inject drugs into a blood transfusion
Provide frequent patient contact
Restrict the blood transfusion rate to 500 cc every two to four hours
Apply a sterile dressing (over the injection site)
Anchor the tubing securely

Provide sufficiently long tubing to allow freedom of movement
Position (the arm) comfortably

Nursing Observations
Check the label on the blood container for correct patient identification
Check the tube (blood transfusion) for patency
Check the solution (blood) for flow rate
Check for infiltration of the solution
Measure the intake
Measure the output
Monitor the blood pressure
Monitor the oral temperature (for fever)
Observe for a blood transfusion reaction
Palpate the pulse for rate, rhythm (tachycardia), and volume

Health Teaching
Describe those symptoms which should be reported (chills, itching, rash, dyspnea)
Explain the reason for and intended effect of the therapy
Explain the importance of blood replacement after transfusion (to family)

Medical Treatments Performed by Nurses
Administer a blood transfusion

EVALUATION

See the evaluation criteria for each specific goal in Chapter 2.

Dependence on Hypodermoclysis Management (391)

ASSESSMENT

Subjective Data
Person relies on nurses for:
    infection prevention
    supervision of flow rate
    patency maintenance
    minimum tissue swelling
    correct fluid administration

Objective Data
Person is receiving hypodermoclysis

Related Data
Commonly Related Diseases:
Any disease or injury requiring fluid therapy

POSSIBLE ETIOLOGY

Inability to obtain adequate fluids by mouth or to receive fluids by venipuncture

NURSING DIAGNOSIS

Dependence on hypodermoclysis management: reliance on nurses for the administration of a hypodermoclysis

PLANNING

Patient Needs	**Primary Nurse-Patient Goals**
Water-salt balance	To maintain fluid and electrolyte balance
Comfort	To achieve comfort
Cleanliness	To achieve good hygiene
Protection from physical harm	To prevent physical injury, infection
Freedom from pain	To achieve comfort
Increased learning	To achieve awareness of needs

NURSING INTERVENTIONS

Nursing Treatments
Do not give electrolyte-free solutions by hypodermoclysis
Give only physiologic electrolyte fluids by hypodermoclysis
Do not add potassium to fluids given by hypodermoclysis
Regulate the hypodermoclysis rate to prevent painful swelling
Provide frequent patient contact
Position comfortably
Anchor the tubing securely
Provide sufficiently long tubing to allow freedom of movement
Apply a sterile dressing (following hypodermoclysis)

Nursing Observations
Check the tube (hypodermoclysis) for patency
Check the solution (hypodermoclysis) for flow rate
Measure the intake
Measure the output
Observe for complaints of pain

Health Teaching
Describe those symptoms which should be reported (pain)
Explain the reason for and intended effect of the therapy

Medical Treatments Performed by Nurses
Administer fluids by hypodermoclysis

EVALUATION

See the evaluation criteria for each specific goal in Chapter 2.

Dependence on Intravenous Infusion Management (70,391)

ASSESSMENT

Subjective Data
Person relies on nurses for:
    infusion patency
    prevention of infection and embolus
    correct fluid administration
    dressing changes

supervision of flow rate
correct medication administration
Anxiety regarding the safety of the intravenous infusions

Objective Data
Person is receiving an intravenous infusion

Related Data
Commonly Related Diseases:
Any disease or injury requiring intravenous fluid therapy

POSSIBLE ETIOLOGY

Need for fluids or fluid replacement

NURSING DIAGNOSIS

Dependence on intravenous infusion management: reliance on nurses for
the administration and functioning of intravenous fluids

PLANNING

Patient Needs	**Primary Nurse-Patient Goals**
Water-salt balance	To maintain fluid and electrolyte balance
Comfort	To achieve comfort
Cleanliness	To achieve good hygiene
Protection from physical harm	To prevent physical injury, infection
Increased learning	To achieve awareness of needs

NURSING INTERVENTIONS

Nursing Treatments
Distribute the intravenous fluid infusion over 12 to 24 hours
Do not allow foreign objects into the intravenous solution
Restrict the glucose intravenous solution rate according to the weight
Restrict the hypertonic intravenous solution rate to 200 cc per hour
Restrict the isotonic intravenous solution rate to 600 cc per hour
Position (the arm) comfortably
Anchor the tubing securely
Provide sufficiently long tubing to allow freedom of movement
Apply a sterile dressing (over the injection site)

Nursing Observations
Check the tube (intravenous) for patency
Check the solution (intravenous) for flow rate
Check for infiltration of the solution
Measure the intake
Measure the output
Monitor the blood pressure
Observe for water intoxication
Palpate the pulse for rate, rhythm, and volume

Health Teaching
Describe those symptoms which should be reported (dyspnea, orthopnea)
Explain the reason for and intended effect of the therapy

Medical Treatments Performed by Nurses
Administer intravenous fluids
Give the prescribed drugs (intravenously)

EVALUATION

See the evaluation criteria for each specific goal in Chapter 2.

Dependence on Umbilical Infusion Management

ASSESSMENT

Subjective Data
Infant relies on nurses for:
    infuson patency
    prevention of infection and embolus
    correct fluid administration
    dressing changes
    supervision of flow rate
    correct medication administration

Objective Data
Infant is receiving an umbilical vein infusion

Related Data
Commonly Related Conditions:
Prematurity
Commonly Related Diseases:
Any disease or injury requiring intravenous fluid therapy for newborns

POSSIBLE ETIOLOGY

The umbilical vein is more easily accessible for infusion than skin surface veins on newborn infants.

NURSING DIAGNOSIS

Dependence on umbilical infusion management: reliance on nurses for the administration of intravenous fluids through the infant's umbilical vein

PLANNING

Patient Needs	Primary Nurse-Patient Goals
Water-salt balance	To maintain fluid and electrolyte balance
Comfort	To achieve comfort
Cleanliness	To achieve good hygiene
Protection from physical harm	To prevent physical injury, infection
Increased learning	To achieve awareness of needs

NURSING INTERVENTIONS

Nursing Treatments
Clean with surgical soap (around the umbilicus)
Apply a sterile dressing
Provide frequent patient contact
Position comfortably
Anchor the tubing securely
Provide sufficiently long tubing to allow freedom of movement

Nursing Observations
Check the tube (umbilical infusion) for patency
Check the solution for flow rate
Check for infiltration of the solution

Health Teaching
Explain (to the parents) the reason for and intended effect of the therapy

Medical Treatments Performed by Nurses
Administer intravenous fluids
Give the prescribed drugs (intravenously)

EVALUATION

See the evaluation criteria for each specific goal in Chapter 2.

FLUID THERAPY DISCOMFORTS

Parenteral Infusion Discomfort

ASSESSMENT

Subjective Data
Cramping of the restricted limb
Soreness from the I.V. board
Painful tissue swelling, especially with hypodermoclysis
Anxiety regarding the infusion

Objective Data
Curtailed mobility
Limb restraint
Visible impatience with infusion slowness, speeding up or pulling out of the
    infusion
Requests to terminate the infusion

Related Data
Commonly Related Diseases:
Any disease or injury requiring fluid therapy

POSSIBLE ETIOLOGY

Need for intravenous infusion therapy

NURSING DIAGNOSIS

Parenteral infusion discomfort: annoyance or mild pain resulting from the infusion of fluid into tissues or veins

PLANNING

Patient Needs   **Primary Nurse-Patient Goals**

Comfort   To achieve comfort

Protection from physical harm   To prevent physical injury

Freedom from pain   To achieve comfort

Increased learning   To achieve awareness of needs

NURSING INTERVENTIONS

Nursing Treatments
Approach unhurriedly
Anticipate needs
Position comfortably
Change the patient's position frequently
Elevate the affected body part
Massage gently (around the infusion site)
Pad the bony prominences (if the limb is on an I.V. board)
Provide sufficiently long tubing to allow freedom of movement
Provide frequent patient contact
Sit with the patient (during the infusion)
Provide radio and television for diversion

Nursing Observations
Observe for complaints of pain

Health Teaching
Explain the reason for and intended effect of the therapy
Emphasize the danger of self-regulation of intravenous fluids

EVALUATION

See the evaluation criteria for each specific goal in Chapter 2.

EMERGENCY FLUID VOLUME EXCESS

Emergency Phase
Circulatory Overload (71)

ASSESSMENT

Subjective Data
Pounding headache
Back pain
Chills
Severe anxiety
Dyspnea

Objective Data
Coughing
Subcutaneous edema
Rapid pulse
Vein distention
Cyanosis
Shock
Urine output exceeds 50 cc per hour
Increased venous pressure above 10 cm

Related Data
Laboratory Findings:
Decreased blood sodium
Decreased urine specific gravity
Commonly Related Conditions:
Cardiac failure
Commonly Related Diseases:
Any disease or injury requiring intravenous fluid therapy or blood transfusion

POSSIBLE ETIOLOGY

Too rapid an administration of intravenous fluids or blood

NURSING DIAGNOSIS

Emergency phase circulatory overload: the need for immediate care as a result of excessive fluid within tissues, cells, and circulation

PLANNING

Patient Needs	**Primary Nurse-Patient Goals**
Oxygen, circulation	To maintain oxygen to all cells
Water-salt balance	To maintain fluid and electrolyte balance
Rest	To achieve rest
Comfort	To achieve comfort
Protection from physical harm	To prevent physical injury
Increased learning	To achieve awareness of needs

NURSING INTERVENTIONS

Nursing Treatments
Attend the patient constantly
Discontinue the intravenous infusion
    OR
Slow the intravenous infusion flow rate
Place on complete bed rest
Elevate the head
Place in the sitting position

Nursing Observations
Measure the intake

Measure the urine output hourly
Monitor the blood pressure
Monitor the central venous pressure
Palpate the pulse for rate, rhythm, and volume

Health Teaching
Explain the causes of the health problem
Explain the reason for and intended effect of the therapy

EVALUATION

See the evaluation criteria for each specific goal in Chapter 2.

8.
NURSING DIAGNOSES RELATED TO
Body Temperature

IRREGULAR BODY TEMPERATURE

Elevated Body Temperature (32,70)

ASSESSMENT

Subjective Data
Malaise
Headache
Internal feeling of warmth

Objective Data
Body temperature above 99.5° F (37.5° C) orally or 100.5° F (38.0° C) rectally
Rapid pulse
Increased respirations
Restlessness
Irritability
Chills, sometimes
Increased skin warmth and perspiration

Related Data
Commonly Related Conditions:
Dehydration
Blood transfusion reaction
Food allergy
Commonly Related Diseases:
Yellow fever
Typhoid fever
Rheumatic fever
Bacterial endocarditis
Pericarditis
Myocarditis
Myocardial infarction

Tuberculosis
Actinomycosis
Ulcerative colitis
Diverticulitis
Dysentery
Encephalitis
Endometritis
Gastritis
Gout
Hepatitis
Herpes zoster
Malaria
Pneumonia
Measles
Mumps
Rheumatoid arthritis
Parathyroid fever
Brucellosis
Mammary abscess
Pheochromocytoma
Thyrotoxicosis
Leukemia
Hodgkins's disease
Meningitis
Rat-bite fever
Tularemia
Rocky Mountain spotted fever
Metastatic carcinoma
Lupus erythematosus
Chickenpox
Smallpox
Roseola infantum
Infectious mononucleosis
Pertussus
Diptheria
Undulent fever
Influenza
Rabies
Tetanus
Anthrax
Bubonic plague
Dengue fever
Weil's disease
Kala-azar
Salmonella gastroentiritis
Photodermatitis
Exfoliative dermatitis
Dermatitis medicamentosa

Milaria
Otitis media
Mastoiditis
Bronchiectasis
Epididymitis
Mediastinitis
Lymphadenitis
Amyloidosis
Poliomyelitis
Colorado tick fever
Rickettsialpox
Epidemic louse-borne typhus
Histoplasmosis
Polyarteritis nodosa
Polymyositis
Acute pyogenic osteomyelitis
Glomerulonephritis
Renal calculi
Streptococcus throat

POSSIBLE ETIOLOGY

Hypothalmic disturbance. Infection. Increased metabolic rate. Impaired circulation. Central nervous system depression or damage. Emotional excitement. Drug reactions. High environmental temperature and humidity. Absence of sweat glands. Conditions of tissue destruction. Fluid imbalance. Antigen-antibody reaction.

NURSING DIAGNOSIS

Elevated body temperature: increased body heat production exceeding the amount of heat lost from the body

PLANNING

Patient Needs	Primary Nurse-Patient Goals
Water-salt balance	To maintain fluid and electrolyte balance
Normal temperature	To maintain regulating mechanisms and functions
Sleep, rest	To achieve sleep, rest
Comfort	To achieve comfort
Protection from physical harm	To prevent physical injury
Increased learning	To achieve awareness of needs

NURSING INTERVENTIONS

Nursing Treatments
Apply a cool, damp cloth to the face
Bathe in cool water
OR

Apply an ice bag (to the head and torso in very high fever)
    OR
Apply alcohol to the skin
Cover with lightweight blankets
Dress in lightweight clothing
Dress in minimum clothing
Maintain a cool room temperature
Increase drafts
Encourage adequate rest
Give nonprescription drugs (ExR) (antipyretics)
Increase fluid intake to about 2000 cc daily
Give iced liquids
Discourage oral stimulants
Refrain from giving hot liquids
Refrain from giving local heat applications

Nursing Observations
Measure the intake
Measure the output
Monitor the oral temperature
    OR
Monitor the rectal temperature
Obtain a bacterial culture (of blood, urine, sputum, stools)

Health Teaching
Explain the causes of the health problem
Explain the reason for and intended effect of the therapy
Teach how to clean a thermometer
Teach how to take a temperature
Explain how to estimate temperature by touch

Medical Treatments Performed by Nurses
Give the prescribed drugs
Place on a hypothermia blanket

EVALUATION

See the evaluation criteria for each specific goal in Chapter 2.

Decreased Body Temperature (32,70)

ASSESSMENT

Subjective Data
Chilliness
Numbness

Objective Data
Body temperature below 96° F (35.5° C) orally or 97° F (36.1° C) rectally
Pallor
Rapid or slow pulse
Slow respirations

Gooseflesh
Cool skin
Shivering

Related Data

Commonly Related Conditions:
Shock

Commonly Related Diseases:
Diabetes mellitus
Hypothyroidism
Arteriosclerosis
Simmond's disease
Pheochromocytoma

POSSIBLE ETIOLOGY

Increased heat loss. Impaired circulation. Lowered metabolic rate. Inadequate nutrition. Decreased body fat associated with aging.

NURSING DIAGNOSIS

Decreased body temperature: decreased body heat production below the normal amount of body heat

PLANNING

Patient Needs	**Primary Nurse-Patient Goals**
Circulation	To maintain oxygen to all cells
Food balance	To maintain nutrition to all cells
Normal temperature	To maintain regulating mechanisms and functions
Sleep, rest	To achieve sleep, rest
Comfort	To achieve comfort
Protection from physical harm	To prevent physical injury
Increased learning	To achieve awareness of needs

NURSING INTERVENTIONS

Nursing Treatments
Cover with warm blankets
Dress in warm clothing
Decrease drafts
Maintain a warm room temperature
Apply a heat cradle
Give warm liquids
Refrain from giving iced liquids
Encourage increased protein-food intake (if the problem is chronic)
Encourage moderate physical exercise
Encourage adequate rest
Refrain from giving local cold applications
Place only warm hands and objects on the patient

Nursing Observations
Monitor the oral temperature

Health Teaching
Explain the causes of the health problem
Explain the reason for and intended effect of therapy
Advise against exposure to inclement weather
Recommend the use of warm clothing

EVALUATION

See the evaluation criteria for each specific goal in Chapter 2.

Inability to Control Body Temperature (32,71)

ASSESSMENT

Subjective Data
Feelings of excessive warmth or coolness

Objective Data
Fluctuating body temperature
Fever precipitated by mild environmental heat
Hypothermia precipitated by mild environmental cold
Absence of sweating

Related Data
Commonly Related Conditions:
Heat stroke
Prematurity
Aging
Spinal shock following spinal cord injury
Commonly Related Diseases:
Cerebral vascular accident
Subdural hematoma
First-, second-, or third-degree burns
Addison's disease

POSSIBLE ETIOLOGY

Biochemical and metabolic imbalance. Nerve center damage at the base of the brain. Lack of subcutaneous body fat for insulation. Undeveloped temperature regulating mechanism. Loss of skin tissue through burns which reduces the capacity to regulate body temperature.

NURSING DIAGNOSIS

Inability to control body temperature: an impaired ability of the body's regulating mechanisms to maintain a normal temperature

PLANNING

Patient Needs
Normal temperature

Primary Nurse-Patient Goals
To maintain regulating mechanisms and functions

Comfort	To achieve comfort
Protection from physical harm	To prevent physical injury
Increased learning	To achieve awareness of needs

NURSING INTERVENTIONS

Nursing Treatments
Dress in lightweight clothing (in a warm environment)
Dress in warm clothing (in a cool environment)
Maintain a normal room temperature
Apply a heat cradle (if cold)
Place the newborn in an incubator
Refrain from giving hot liquids
Refrain from giving iced liquids
Refrain from giving oral stimulants
Delay bathing (until normal temperature is established)

Nursing Observations
Monitor the oral temperature
   OR
Monitor the rectal temperature
Check the environmental controls on the incubator periodically

Health Teaching
Advise against exposure to inclement weather
Advise against exposure to intense heat
Describe those symptoms which should be reported (fever or hypothermia)
Explain the causes of the health problem
Explain the reason for and intended effect of the therapy

EVALUATION

See the evaluation criteria for each specific goal in Chapter 2.

POTENTIAL IRREGULAR BODY TEMPERATURE

Potential Elevated Body Temperature (32,70)

ASSESSMENT

Objective Data
Recent fever
Poor fluid intake
Excessive fluid loss

Related Data
More likely to have fever following surgery and childbirth or when on vasodilating drugs such as epinephrine
Commonly Related Conditions:
Menopause
Dehydration

Commonly Related Diseases:
Thryotoxicosis
Herpes zoster
Leukemia
Hodgkin's disease

POSSIBLE ETIOLOGY

Infection. Increased metabolic rate. Impaired circulation. Central nervous system depression or damage. Drug reactions. High environmental temperature and humidity. Inadequate fluid intake.

NURSING DIAGNOSIS

Potential elevated body temperature: the possibility that a body temperature above 99.5° F orally or 100.5° F rectally will occur

PLANNING

Patient Needs	**Primary Nurse-Patient Goals**
Water-salt balance	To maintain fluid and electrolyte balance
Normal temperature	To maintain regulating mechanisms and functions
Protection from physical harm	To prevent physical injury
Increased learning	To achieve awareness of needs

NURSING INTERVENTIONS

Nursing Treatments
Balance fluid intake to equal output
Discourage oral stimulants
Cover with lightweight blankets
Dress in lightweight clothing
Maintain a cool room temperature
Refrain from giving hot liquids
Refrain from giving local heat applications

Nursing Observations
Monitor the oral temperature

Health Teaching
Describe those symptoms which should be reported (fever)
Explain the causes of the health problem
Explain the reason for and intended effect of the therapy

EVALUATION

See the evaluation criteria for each specific goal in Chapter 2.

Potential Decreased Body Temperature (32,70)

ASSESSMENT

Subjective Data
Chronic complaints of feeling cool

Objective Data
Prolonged bed rest
Poor nutrition
Impaired circulation

Related Data
Commonly Related Conditions:
Hemiplegia
Paraplegia
Commonly Related Diseases:
Myxedema
Arteriosclerosis
Diabetes mellitus

POSSIBLE ETIOLOGY

Decreased metabolic rate. Inadequate nutrition. Impaired peripheral nerve function. Poor tissue oxygenation.

NURSING DIAGNOSIS

Potential decreased body temperature: the probability that a body temperature below 96° F orally or 97° F rectally will occur

PLANNING

Patient Needs
Protection from physical harm
Increased learning

Primary Nurse-Patient Goals
To prevent physical injury
To achieve awareness of needs

NURSING INTERVENTIONS

Nursing Treatments
Decrease drafts
Drape for warmth
Dress in warm clothing
Maintain a warm room temperature
Refrain from giving iced liquids
Refrain from giving local cold applications
Encourage increased protein-food intake (if the problem is chronic)
Encourage moderate physical exercise

Nursing Observations
Monitor the oral temperature

Health Teaching
Describe those symptoms which should be reported (chills, low temperature)
Explain the causes of the health problem
Explain the reason for and intended effect of the therapy
Advise against exposure to inclement weather
Recommend the use of warm clothing

EVALUATION

See the evaluation criteria for each specific goal in Chapter 2.

EMERGENCY IRREGULAR BODY TEMPERATURE

Emergency Phase Heat Exhaustion (192,271)

ASSESSMENT

Subjective Data
Extreme fatigue
Headache
Nausea
Weakness
Abdominal or limb cramps, sometimes

Objective Data
Pallor
Profuse perspiration
Normal body temperature
Vomiting, sometimes

POSSIBLE ETIOLOGY

Vasodilatation occurs in response to intense environmental heat, and simultaneously there is an absence of increased blood volume which results in circulatory collapse.

NURSING DIAGNOSIS

Emergency phase heat exhaustion: the need for immediate health care as a result of the collapse of the peripheral circulatory system in response to exposure to intense environmental heat

PLANNING

Patient Needs	Primary Nurse-Patient Goals
Water-salt balance	To maintain fluid and electrolyte balance
Normal temperature	To maintain regulating mechanisms and functions
Sleep, rest	To achieve sleep, rest
Comfort	To achieve comfort
Protection from physical harm	To prevent physical injury
Increased learning	To achieve awareness of needs

NURSING INTERVENTIONS

Nursing Treatments
Give salt solution orally (one-half glass every 15 minutes for 1 hour)
    OR
Administer intravenous fluids (ET) (isotonic saline solution)
Bathe in cool water
Give iced liquids (iced coffee is preferable as a stimulant)
Place in the flat position (initially)

Place in the foot-elevated head-lowered (Trendelenburg) position (if the patient fails to respond)
Increase drafts (with an electric fan)
Maintain a cool room temperature
Refrain from giving hot liquids
Refrain from giving local heat applications

Nursing Observations
Monitor the blood pressure
Monitor the rectal temperature (every 15 minutes)

Health Teaching
Explain the reason for and intended effect of the therapy

EVALUATION

See the evaluation criteria for each specific goal in Chapter 2.

Emergency Phase Heat Stroke (71,192,271)

ASSESSMENT

Subjective Data
Headache
Dizziness
Nausea
Abdominal or extremity cramping

Objective Data
Tachycardia
Skin dryness
Flushed, hot skin
Temperature elevation to or above 106° F (41.1° C)
Unconsciousness, sometimes

Related Data
Persons aged 40 and over are most susceptible

POSSIBLE ETIOLOGY

A combined high or low environmental humidity, poor air circulation, and excessively high environmental temperature traumatize the body's heat-regulating mechanism.

NURSING DIAGNOSIS

Emergency phase heat stroke: the need for immediate health care as a result of impaired functioning of the body's heat-regulating mechanism in response to exposure to intense environmental heat

PLANNING

Patient Needs	Primary Nurse-Patient Goals
Water-salt balance	To maintain fluid and electrolyte balance
Normal temperature	To maintain regulating mechanisms and functions

Sleep, rest	To achieve sleep, rest
Comfort	To achieve comfort
Protection from physical harm	To prevent physical injury
Increased learning	To achieve awareness of needs

NURSING INTERVENTIONS

Nursing Treatments

Apply alcohol to the skin
   OR
Bathe in cool water   (until the temperature reaches
   OR   102° F, 38.8° C)
Apply an ice bag (around the torso)

Administer an enema (cold, saline if temperature remains elevated)
Massage gently (the entire body)
Administer intermittent positive pressure breathing (ET) (if cyanotic)
Administer intravenous fluids (ET) (isotonic solution only after temperature
   is below 102° F; give slowly)
Increase drafts (with an electric fan)
Maintain a cool room temperature
Refrain from giving hot liquids
Refrain from giving oral stimulants
Place on complete bed rest
Withhold the drugs (sedatives)

Nursing Observations

Monitor the blood pressure
Monitor the rectal temperature (every 15 minutes)
Measure the output

Health Teaching

Explain the reason for and intended effect of the therapy

Medical Treatments Performed by Nurses

Place on a hypothermia blanket

EVALUATION

See the evaluation criteria for each specific goal in Chapter 2.

INADEQUATE INFORMATION RELATED TO BODY TEMPERATURE

Inadequate Information Related to Heat Stroke

ASSESSMENT

Subjective Data

Person confirms a lack of information

Objective Data
Person's actions indicate a lack of information regarding:
   the dangers of intense environmental heat
   the need to stay out of midafternoon heat
   that the living pace must be slowed during intense heat
   that fluid and salt intake must be increased
   that heavy work and active sports should be postponed

POSSIBLE ETIOLOGY

Lack of instruction. No previous experience with intense environmental heat.

NURSING DIAGNOSIS

Inadequate information related to heat stroke: lack of information regarding the cause and prevention of heat stroke

PLANNING

Patient Needs

Protection from physical harm

Increased learning

Primary Nurse-Patient Goals

To prevent physical injury

To achieve awareness of needs

NURSING INTERVENTIONS

Nursing Treatments
Approach unhurriedly
Encourage patient questions
Encourage increased sodium-food intake

Nursing Observations
Evaluate the response to teaching

Health Teaching
Advise against exposure to intense heat
Instruct to increase fluid intake (when exposed to heat)
Recommend adherence to a moderate pace of living (especially during the hot months of the year)
Describe those symptoms which should be reported (tachycardia, skin flushing, headache, dizziness, nausea, high fever)
Explain the causes of the health problem

EVALUATION

See the evaluation criteria for each specific goal in Chapter 2.

9.

NURSING DIAGNOSES RELATED TO
The Cardiovascular
System

BLOOD CIRCULATION, ALTERED

Impaired Arterial Peripheral
Circulation (32,113)

ASSESSMENT

Objective Data
When the legs are dependent, the feet are blue or purple and the skin is cold
When the legs are elevated, the feet are pale and when the leg is lowered,
the normal color does not return within 20 seconds
Diminished arterial pulsations
Shiny skin appearance
Skin wrinkles when pinched
Lack of lango hair on the back of the hands, feet, fingers, and toes
Round scars covered with atrophied skin
Ulceration or gangrene
Slow-growing, dry, brittle thick nails

Related Data
Commonly Related Conditions:
Hemorrhage
Commonly Related Diseases:
Atherosclerosis
Buerger's disease
Arteriosclerosis
Myocardial infarction
Mitral or pulmonary stenosis

POSSIBLE ETIOLOGY

Reduced cardiac output. Vascular occlusion or constriction. Excessive
blood or fluid loss resulting in reduced blood volume to the skin surface.

NURSING DIAGNOSIS

Impaired arterial peripheral circulation: an inadequate supply of blood to extremity tissues

PLANNING

Patient Needs	Primary Nurse-Patient Goals
Oxygen, circulation	To maintain oxygen to all cells
Rest	To achieve rest
Exercise	To achieve exercise
Comfort	To achieve comfort
Protection from physical harm	To prevent physical injury
Increased learning	To achieve awareness of needs

NURSING INTERVENTIONS

Nursing Treatments

Place on complete bed rest
Place in the slight sitting (semi-Fowler's) position (with the legs at the heart level)
Maintain a warm room temperature
Dress in warm clothing (that fits loosely)
Bathe in warm water (never hot water)
Exercise in range of motion (passive)
Discourage smoking
Refrain from giving local heat applications
Refrain from giving local cold applications
Refrain from elevating the bed at the knee gatch
Refrain from placing a pillow under the knee
Refrain from tight bandaging
Remove constrictive clothing

Nursing Observations

Inspect the extremity for adequate circulation (periodically)
Palpate for arterial pulsations (periodically)
Monitor blood studies for abnormal gas exchange
Monitor blood studies for abnormal hematology

Health Teaching

Explain the causes of the health problem
Advise against wearing constrictive clothing
Explain the need to avoid mechanical trauma (to the affected area)
Inform that the extremities should be kept warm when the circulation is impaired (with loose clothing)
Instruct not to dangle the legs
Teach how to do isometric exercises
Explain the reason for and intended effect of the therapy

Medical Treatments Performed by Nurses

Give the prescribed exercises (Buerger-Allen exercises)

EVALUATION

See the evaluation criteria for each specific goal in Chapter 2.

Impaired Venous Peripheral Circulation (32,391)

ASSESSMENT

Subjective Data
Numbness and tingling
Extremity coldness

Objective Data
Mottled skin
Cyanosis or pallor
Swelling

Related Data
Commonly Related Diseases:
Thrombophlebitis
Phlebothrombosis

POSSIBLE ETIOLOGY

Valve incompetency of the veins. Loss of venous tone which results in blood pooling. Sluggish blood flow through the veins. Lack of exercise. Circulatory constriction from casts, etc.

NURSING DIAGNOSIS

Impaired venous peripheral circulation: a diminished ability of the blood circulating in the peripheral veins to maintain an adequate venous return of blood to the ventricles

PLANNING

Patient Needs	**Primary Nurse-Patient Goals**
Oxygen, circulation	To maintain oxygen to all cells
Activity, exercise	To achieve activity and exercise
Comfort	To achieve comfort
Protection from physical harm	To prevent physical injury
Increased learning	To achieve awareness of needs

NURSING INTERVENTIONS

Nursing Treatments
Ambulate the patient (as much as possible)
Apply elastic stockings
Bivalve and spread the cast to relieve pressure (ET)
Change the patient's position frequently
Discourage smoking
Elevate the extremity
Exercise in range of motion

Limit blood pressure cuff inflation to a few moments
Maintain a warm room temperature
Refrain from giving iced liquids
Refrain from elevating the bed at the knee gatch
Refrain from placing a pillow under the knee
Refrain from giving local cold applications
Refrain from tight bandaging
Remove constrictive clothing

Nursing Observations
Inspect the extremity for adequate circulation (periodically)
Monitor blood studies for abnormal hematology
Palpate for arterial pulsations (periodically)

Health Teaching
Explain the causes of the health problem
Advise against wearing constrictive clothing
Advise not to stand for prolonged periods
Advise that positions which impair circulation be avoided
Emphasize the danger of excessive body weight
Inform that the extremities should be kept warm when the circulation is
    impaired
Instruct not to dangle the legs
Instruct to change position frequently
Recommend activities which improve circulation
Teach how to do isometric exercises
Explain the reason for and intended effect of the therapy

Medical Treatments Performed by Nurses
Give the prescribed drugs

EVALUATION

See the evaluation criteria for each specific goal in Chapter 2.

Syncope (70,247)

ASSESSMENT

Subjective Data
Dizziness

Objective Data
Pallor
Temporary loss of consciousness
Sweating
Rapid pulse
Low blood pressure
Consciousness regained upon assuming the supine (flat on back) position

Related Data
Commonly Related Conditions:
Hypoglycemia
Pregnancy

Stokes-Adams syndrome
Heat prostration
Commonly Related Diseases:
Anemia
Rheumatic heart disease
Vasovagal syncope
Carotid sinus syncope
Aortic stenosis

POSSIBLE ETIOLOGY

Drug depression. Fear and anxiety. Decreased blood volume. Inadequate cardiac output.

NURSING DIAGNOSIS

Syncope (fainting) (impaired cerebral circulation) (neurogenic shock): loss of consciousness as a result of inadequate blood circulation to brain tissue

PLANNING

Patient Needs	**Primary Nurse-Patient Goals**
Oxygen, circulation	To maintain oxygen to all cells
Rest	To achieve rest
Comfort	To achieve comfort
Stimulation	To maintain sensory function and stimulation
Protection from physical harm	To prevent physical injury
Increased learning	To achieve awareness of needs

NURSING INTERVENTIONS

Nursing Treatments
Apply a cool, damp cloth to the face
Attend the patient constantly
Change the patient's position gradually
Cover with warm blankets
Discourage smoking (for some time after the episode)
Give hot coffee
    OR   } (if conscious)
Give hot tea
Give nonprescription drugs (ExR) (ammonia spirits)
Place in the flat position
    OR
Place in the foot-elevated head-lowered (Trendelenburg) position
Place on complete bed rest (until the episode subsides)
Refrain from giving iced liquids
Remove constrictive clothing

Nursing Observations
Auscultate the apical heartbeat for rate and rhythm
Inspect for hemorrhage
Monitor the blood pressure

Monitor blood studies for abnormal glucose
Monitor blood studies for abnormal hematology
Monitor the cardiogram (if there is evidence of impaired cardiac output)
Monitor the positional blood pressure
Observe for an excessive stress level
Observe for shock

Health Teaching
Describe the manifestations of circulatory impairment
Explain the causes of the health problem
Advise against exposure to intense heat
Advise against wearing constrictive clothing
Advise not to stand for prolonged periods
Advise that highly emotional situations be avoided
Advise that positions which impair circulation be avoided
Explain how to apply elastic stockings or an elastic bandage (to legs if the
    episode is recurrent)
Instruct to change position gradually (if the episode is recurrent)
Instruct to lower the head (until the episode subsides)
Explain the reason for and intended effect of the therapy

Medical Treatments Performed by Nurses
Give the prescribed drugs

EVALUATION

See the evaluation criteria for each specific goal in Chapter 2.

BLOOD CIRCULATION, POTENTiAL ALTERATION IN

Potential Arterial Rupture (247,453)

ASSESSMENT

Subjective Data
Awareness of a pulsating mass

Objective Data
Expanded arterial pulsation
Arterial bruit

Related Data
Commonly Related Diseases:
Syphilis
Cerebral, aortic, thoracic, or abdominal aneurysm

POSSIBLE ETIOLOGY

Arterial weakening from syphilis. Injury to the artery by bacterial infection
or trauma. Congenital weakness.

NURSING DIAGNOSIS

Potential arterial rupture: the strong possibility that an artery will rupture resulting in lethal hemorrhage

PLANNING

Patient Needs

Rest

Protection from physical harm

Increased learning

Primary Nurse-Patient Goals

To achieve rest

To prevent physical injury

To achieve awareness of needs

NURSING INTERVENTIONS

Nursing Treatments

Change the patient's position gradually
Discourage oral stimulants
Encourage adequate rest
Refrain from giving hot liquids
Refrain from giving iced liquids
Refrain from jarring the bed
Remove constrictive clothing

Nursing Observations

Monitor the blood pressure
Observe for shock (sudden)

Health Teaching

Explain the causes of the health problem
Advise against wearing constrictive clothing
Advise that highly emotional situations be avoided
Explain the need to avoid mechanical trauma (to the area of the aneurysm)
Explain the need to avoid overexertion
Inform that coughing should be avoided
Inform that elimination straining should be avoided
Inform that heavy lifting should be avoided
Instruct to change position gradually
Explain the reason for and intended effect of the therapy

EVALUATION

See the evaluation criteria for each specific goal in Chapter 2.

Potential Impaired Intestinal Circulation (247,453)

ASSESSMENT

Subjective Data

Nausea

Objective Data

Abdominal hernia
Chronic coughing, straining
Frequent heavy lifting

Related Data

Commonly Related Diseases:
Incisional hernia
Femoral hernia
Umbilical hernia
Inguinal hernia
Scrotal hernia

POSSIBLE ETIOLOGY

Pressure on the abdominal musculature will prevent adequate intestinal circulation

NURSING DIAGNOSIS

Potential impaired intestinal circulation: the possibility that circulation to the intestines will become impaired

PLANNING

Patient Needs
Protection from physical harm
Increased learning

Primary Nurse-Patient Goals
To prevent physical injury
To achieve awareness of needs

NURSING INTERVENTIONS

Nursing Treatments
Make a referral (to a physician if the patient has not seen a physician)

Nursing Observations
Auscultate the abdomen for abnormal bowel sounds (absent, diminished, or gurgling)
Observe for complaints of pain
Palpate for arterial pulsations (in the hernia area)

Health Teaching
Describe those symptoms which should be reported (tender mass, pain, vomiting)
Advise against wearing constrictive clothing
Inform that coughing should be avoided
Inform that elimination straining should be avoided
Inform that heavy lifting should be avoided
Recommend the use of a hernia support

EVALUATION

See the evaluation criteria for each specific goal in Chapter 2.

Potential Thrombus Displacement (71,391)

ASSESSMENT

Subjective Data
Person disregards aching, throbbing, upper calf pain

Objective Data

Person walks on a thrombosed leg, places a pilllow under, or massages a hot, tender, reddened calf area

Related Data

Commonly Related Diseases:
Thrombophlebitis
Phlebitis
Phlebothrombosis

POSSIBLE ETIOLOGY

A mass of fat, amniotic fluid, or air in a vein. The adherence of platelets to blood vessel endothelium until a mass is formed.

NURSING DIAGNOSIS

Potential thrombus displacement: the possibility that an existing thrombus will be dislodged from its position

PLANNING

Patient Needs	Primary Nurse-Patient Goals
Rest	To achieve rest
Protection form physical harm	To prevent physical injury
Increased learning	To achieve awareness of needs

NURSING INTERVENTIONS

Nursing Treatments

Do not massage (the leg)
Elevate the extremity
Elevate the foot of the bed (on 6-inch blocks)
Encourage adequate rest (of the limb)
Handle gently
Place on complete bed rest
Refrain from elevating the bed at the knee gatch
Refrain from placing a pillow under the knee

Nursing Observations

Inspect the extremity for adequate circulation (periodically)
Observe for complaints of pain (chest)
Observe for coughing
Observe for cyanosis
Observe for dyspnea
Observe for hemoptosis
Observe for shock

Health Teaching

Explain the causes of the health problem
Explain the reason for and intended effect of the therapy
Emphasize the danger of massaging a painful calf
Instruct not to dangle the legs

EVALUATION

See the evaluation criteria for each specific goal in Chapter 2.

Potential Varicose Veins (391)

ASSESSMENT

Subjective Data
Leg heaviness
Leg aching
Prolonged standing or sitting

Objective Data
Wears constrictive garments (girdles, garters, etc.)
Slight leg vein distention
Excess body weight

Related Data
History of family tendency toward varicose veins
Commonly Related Conditions:
Pregnancy
Obesity
Commonly Related Diseases:
Arteriosclerosis

POSSIBLE ETIOLOGY

Increased venous pressure. Weakened vein-wall elasticity.

NURSING DIAGNOSIS

Potential varicose veins: the probability that leg vein swelling will occur

PLANNING

Patient Needs
Circulation
Exercise
Protection from physical harm
Increased learning

Primary Nurse-Patient Goals
To maintain oxygen to all cells
To achieve exercise
To prevent physical injury
To achieve awareness of needs

NURSING INTERVENTIONS

Nursing Treatments
Apply an elastic bandage ⎫
    OR   ⎬ (to the legs)
Apply elastic stockings ⎭
Encourage moderate physical exercise (vigorous walking)
Refrain from tight bandaging
Remove constrictive clothing

Nursing Observations
Inspect the extremity for adequate circulation (periodically)

Health Teaching
Explain the causes of the health problem
Describe the manifestations of circulatory impairment
Advise against wearing constrictive clothing
Advise not to stand for prolonged periods
Emphasize the danger of excessive body weight
Instruct not to dangle the legs
Instruct to elevate the body part (the extremities whenever possible)
Recommend activities which improve circulation
Advise that positions which impair circulation be avoided
Explain how to apply elastic stockings or an elastic bandage (to the legs)
Explain the reason for and intended effect of the therapy

EVALUATION

See the evaluation criteria for each specific goal in Chapter 2.

Potential Impaired Peripheral Circulation (71,326,391)

ASSESSMENT

Objective Data
Prolonged sitting, standing, or bed rest
Crosses the legs at the thigh when sitting
Sits with the edge of the chair seat against the posterior knee
Pillows or blanket rolls are placed under the knee when in bed
Infrequent position change
Wears constrictive clothing
Excess weight in obesity or pregnancy
Restricted mobility

Related Data
Commonly Related Conditions:
Paralysis
Commonly Related Diseases:
Congestive heart failure
Cerebral vascular accident
Bone fracture
Arteriosclerosis

POSSIBLE ETIOLOGY

Immobility or insufficient exercise preventing normal blood flow with resulting blood pooling and/or clot formation. Weakened vein wall elasticity. Inadequate venous return to the heart during heart failure. Pressure on veins and arteries in the legs or pelvic area.

NURSING DIAGNOSIS

Potential impaired peripheral circulation (potential venous stasis) (potential blood pooling) (potential thrombus formation): the probability that blood will flow sluggishly through the circulatory system predisposing to inadequate tissue oxygenation or clot formation

PLANNING

Patient Needs	Primary Nurse-Patient Goals
Exercise	To achieve exercise
Protection from physical harm	To prevent physical injury
Increased learning	To achieve awareness of needs

NURSING INTERVENTIONS

Nursing Treatments

Ambulate the patient (as much as possible)

Apply an elastic bandage
   OR   } (to the legs)
Apply elastic stockings

Change the patient's position frequently

Elevate the foot of the bed (on 6-inch blocks)

Encourage deep breathing

Exercise in range of motion

Increase fluid intake to about 2000 cc daily (during periods of immobility)

Refrain from elevating the bed at the knee gatch

Refrain from placing a pillow under the knee

Refrain from tight bandaging

Remove constrictive clothing

Discourage smoking

Nursing Observations

Inspect the extremity for adequate circulation (periodically)

Observe for complaints of itching

Inspect for edema

Inspect the skin for discoloration (redness)

Palpate for arterial pulsations (periodically)

Health Teaching

Explain the causes of the health problem

Describe the manifestations of circulatory impairment

Advise that positions which impair circulation be avoided

Describe those symptoms which should be reported (skin coldness, blueness, pallor, swelling, numbness and tingling, ulceration, slow nail growth)

Advise against wearing constrictive clothing

Advise not to stand for prolonged periods

Emphasize the danger of excessive body weight

Instruct not to dangle the legs

Instruct to change position frequently

Instruct that pillows (blankets or trochanter rolls) not be placed under the knee

Recommend activities which improve circulation

Teach how to do isometric exercises
Explain how to apply elastic stockings or an elastic bandage (to the legs)
Explain the reason for and intended effect of the therapy

EVALUATION

See the evaluation criteria for each specific goal in Chapter 2.

BLOOD EMISSION

Bleeding (71,326,391)

ASSESSMENT

Subjective Data
Weakness

Objective Data
Blood oozing is visible from the body surface
Blood loss is minimal, slow, of short duration
Warm skin
Blood pressure normal or slightly hypotensive

Related Data
Commonly Related Diseases:
Minor trauma

POSSIBLE ETIOLOGY

Spontaneous blood vessel rupture. Platelet deficiency. Blood clotting defect or trauma.

NURSING DIAGNOSIS

Bleeding: slow loss of small amounts of blood

PLANNING

Patient Needs	Primary Nurse-Patient Goals
Water-salt balance	To maintain fluid and electrolyte balance
Rest	To achieve rest
Comfort	To achieve comfort
Cleanliness	To achieve good hygiene
Protection from physical harm	To prevent physical injury
Increased learning	To achieve awareness of needs

NURSING INTERVENTIONS

Nursing Treatments
Apply an ice bag
    OR
Apply manual pressure over the bleeding area
    OR

Apply a pressure dressing
Clean with surgical soap
Apply a sterile dressing
Elevate the affected body part
Immobilize the affected body part
Handle gently
Refrain from dislodging blood clots
Refrain from giving local heat applications
Encourage adequate rest
Discourage smoking (until the episode subsides)
Discourage oral stimulants (until the episode subsides)

Nursing Observations
Estimate the blood volume loss
Monitor the blood pressure
Monitor blood studies for abnormal hematology
Palpate the pulse for rate, rhythm, and volume

Health Teaching
Explain the causes of the health problem
Explain the need to avoid mechanical trauma (to the injured area)
Instruct to carefully move the injured body part
Instruct to increase fluid intake (in proportion to the amount of bleeding)
Explain the reason for and intended effect of the therapy

EVALUATION

See the evaluation criteria for each specific goal in Chapter 2.

Predisposition to Bleeding or Hemorrhage (71,271,326,391,453)

ASSESSMENT

Subjective Data
Recent bleeding or hemorrhage from or trauma to internal organs

Objective Data
Bruises easily
Frequent nose bleeds
Bleeding gums
Healing external wound or ulcer

Related Data
Laboratory Findings:
Increased bleeding time, clotting time, prothrombin time, partial thromboplastin time
Decreased blood antihemophiliac factor, fibrinogen, hematocrit, hemoglobin, or platelet count
Commonly Related Conditions:
Decubitus ulcers
Childbirth

Any form of surgery
Recent hemodialysis therapy
Diagnostic arteriogram or renal, liver, lung, or intestinal biopsy

Commonly Related Diseases:
Christmas disease
Glomerulonephritis
Laennec's cirrhosis
Leukemia
Scurvy
Cushing's syndrome
Hypothryoidism
Hemophilia
Gastric ulcer
Esophageal varices
Carcinoma
Bone fracture
Hypertension

POSSIBLE ETIOLOGY

Blood dyscrasias. Endocrine disorders. Blood coagulation defect in liver disorders. Inadequate Vitamin B or C intake. Drug formation of an antithrombin that prevents blood coagulation by inhibiting prothrombin conversion to thrombin. Pressure from tumors. Malignant cell invasion of tissue and arteries. Tender tissue not completely covered by healed integument.

NURSING DIAGNOSIS

Predisposition to bleeding or hemorrhage: a greater than normal inclination to bleed or hemorrhage

PLANNING

Patient Needs	Primary Nurse-Patient Goals
Rest	To achieve rest
Protection from physical harm	To prevent physical injury
Increased learning	To achieve awareness of needs

NURSING INTERVENTIONS

Nursing Treatments
Change the patient's position gradually
Handle gently
Place on complete bed rest (for possible internal bleeding)
Refrain from jarring the bed
Refrain from dislodging blood clots
Refrain from tight bandaging (for possible intradermal bleeding)
Refrain from pulling the patient across the sheets (if there is dermal fragility or open sores)
Brush the teeth with a soft toothbrush (for possible gum or oral bleeding)
Use small-gauge injection needles (for blood dyscrasias or impaired blood clotting)

Refrain from giving hot liquids
Refrain from giving oral stimulants
Withhold the drugs (salicylates)

Nursing Observations
Inspect for bleeding
Inspect for hemorrhage
Monitor blood studies for abnormal clotting mechanism
Monitor blood studies for abnormal hematology

Health Teaching
Explain the causes of the health problem
Describe those symptoms which should be reported (bleeding)
Advise against pulling off scabs
Inform that coughing should be avoided (for internal bleeding)
Advise not to stand for prolonged periods (for possible bleeding following
    childbirth, excessive menstrual flow, or rectal bleeding)
Instruct to change position gradually
Explain the need to avoid mechanical trauma
Instruct to carefully move the injured body part
Advise gentle nose blowing (for possible epistaxis)
    AND
Instruct not to pick the nose
Instruct to use a soft, new toothbrush and to apply only mild toothbrush
    pressure (for possible gum or oral bleeding)
Explain the reason for and intended effect of the therapy

Medical Treatments Performed by Nurses
Give the prescribed diet
Give the prescribed drugs

EVALUATION

See the evaluation criteria for each specific goal in Chapter 2.

BLOOD EMISSION
AT SPECIFIC SITES

Epistaxis (247)

ASSESSMENT

Subjective Data
Feels blood trickling down the back of the throat
Swallows blood

Objective Data
Blood oozing from the nose
Intermittent or continuous
Scant or profuse

Related Data

Commonly Related Conditions:
Pregnancy
Menstruation

Commonly Related Diseases:
Nasal fracture
Rhinitis
Measles
Sinusitis
Typhoid fever
Rheumatic fever
Scarlet fever
Hypertension
Sickle cell anemia
Chronic glomerulonephritis
Aortic coartation
Arteriosclerosis
Hemophilia
Syphilis
Diptheria
Leukemia
Scurvy
Laennec's cirrhosis
Tuberculosis
Thrombocytopenia purpura
Rendu-Osler Weber disease
von Willebrand's disease
Wegener's granulomatosis
Yellow fever

POSSIBLE ETIOLOGY

Blood clotting disorders. Nasal trauma. Atmospheric changes. Anticoagulant therapy.

NURSING DIAGNOSIS

Epistaxis: blood oozing or flowing from the nose

PLANNING

Patient Needs	**Primary Nurse-Patient Goals**
Rest	To achieve rest
Comfort	To achieve comfort
Protection from physical harm	To prevent physical injury
Increased learning	To achieve awareness of needs

NURSING INTERVENTIONS

Nursing Treatments
Apply an ice bag (to the back of the neck, under the upper lip and bridge of
the nose)

Apply manual pressure over the bleeding area (over the bridge of the nose and nostrils)
Change the patient's position gradually
Do not place in the flat position
Elevate the head
Encourage adequate rest
Withhold the drugs (if blood studies indicate anticoagulants are the cause and epistaxis is serious)

Nursing Observations
Estimate the blood volume loss
Monitor the blood pressure (if the bleeding is severe)
Monitor blood studies for abnormal clotting mechanism
Monitor blood studies for abnormal hemorrhage

Health Teaching
Explain the causes of the health problem
Explain how to prevent sneezing (temporarily)
Inform that coughing should be avoided (temporarily)
Inform that elimination straining should be avoided (temporarily)
Instruct not to blow the nose (temporarily)
Instruct not to pick the nose
Instruct not to swallow blood during epistaxis
Instruct to change position gradually
Explain the reason for and intended effect of the therapy

Medical Treatments Performed by Nurses
Give the prescribed drugs

EVALUATION

See the evaluation criteria for each specific goal in Chapter 2.

Gum Bleeding (70,391)

ASSESSMENT

Subjective Data
Unpleasant taste
Bleeding on gum stimulation

Objective Data
Blood oozing from the gum surface
Clot formation around the teeth

Related Data
Commonly Related Conditions:
Lead, arsenic, phosphorous, or mercury poisoning
Commonly Related Diseases:
Aplastic anemia
Monocytic and myelocytic leukemia
Scurvy

Pellegra
Trench mouth
Syphilis
Thrombocytopenia
Hodgkin's disease
Hemophilia
Yellow fever
Peridontal disease

POSSIBLE ETIOLOGY

Blood clotting disorders. Chemical or mechanical trauma. Infection. Tartar accumulation on the teeth.

NURSING DIAGNOSIS

Gum bleeding: blood oozing or flowing from the gums

PLANNING

Patient Needs	**Primary Nurse-Patient Goals**
Comfort	To achieve comfort
Cleanliness	To achieve good hygiene
Protection from physical harm	To prevent physical injury
Increased learning	To achieve awareness of needs

NURSING INTERVENTIONS

Nursing Treatments
Brush the teeth with a soft toothbrush
Give iced liquids
Refrain from giving hot liquids
Give soft foods
Refresh with a mouthwash
Swab the mouth with diluted glycerine
Make a referral (to a dentist if there is excessive plaque)

Nursing Observations
Estimate the blood volume loss (if bleeding is severe)
Inspect the gums for abnormalities
Inspect for renewed bleeding
Monitor blood studies for abnormal clotting mechanism
Monitor blood studies for abnormal hematology
Monitor blood studies for positive VDRL

Health Teaching
Explain the causes of the health problem
Instruct to use a soft, new toothbrush and to apply only mild toothbrush pressure
Explain the reason for and intended effect of the therapy

Medical Treatments Performed by Nurses
Give the prescribed drugs

EVALUATION

See the evaluation criteria for each specific goal in Chapter 2.

Intradermal Bleeding (113)

ASSESSMENT

Subjective Data

Pain associated with a bruise or hematoma

Objective Data

Purpura
Petechiae
Bruises
Hematomas

Related Data

Commonly Related Conditions:
Malnutrition
Premenopause

Commonly Related Diseases:
Cerebral concussion
Skin contusion
von Willebrand's disease
Typhus fever
Bubonic plague
Meningococcal meningitis
Allergic purpura
Chronic glomerulonephritis
Scurvy
Laennec's cirrhosis
Polycythemia vera
Subacute bacterial endocarditis
Rheumatic fever
Scarlet fever
Diptheria
Smallpox
Measles
Aplastic anemia

POSSIBLE ETIOLOGY

Bleeding from traumatized blood vessels under the skin. Capillary rupture.
Blood coagulation defect in liver disorders. Blood vessel or platelet abnormality. Vitamin C deficiency. Increased platelet destruction by an autoimmune process. Prolonged use of salicylates, bismuth, mercury, penicillin, atropine, or belladona.

NURSING DIAGNOSIS

Intradermal bleeding: loss of blood occurring under the skin

PLANNING

Patient Needs	Primary Nurse-Patient Goals
Comfort	To achieve comfort
Protection from physical harm	To prevent physical injury
Increased learning	To achieve awareness of needs

NURSING INTERVENTIONS

Nursing Treatments
Apply an ice bag
   OR
Apply manual pressure over the bleeding area (for a hematoma)
Handle gently

Nursing Observations
Monitor blood studies for abnormal clotting mechanism
Monitor blood studies for abnormal hematology

Health Teaching
Explain the causes of the health problem
Explain the need to avoid mechanical trauma

Medical Treatments Performed by Nurses
Give the prescribed drugs

EVALUATION

See the evaluation criteria for each specific goal in Chapter 2.

Oral Cavity Bleeding

ASSESSMENT

Subjective Data
Unpleasant taste
Spitting blood

Objective Data
Mild or profuse bleeding in the mouth
Blood clots in the mouth
Oral petechiae
Brownish-coated mucous membrane

Related Data
Commonly Related Diseases:
Leukemia
Thrombocytopenia
Hemophilia
Infectious mononucleosis

POSSIBLE ETIOLOGY

Accidental trauma. Blood clotting disorders. Surgery. Radium therapy.

NURSING DIAGNOSIS
Oral cavity bleeding: blood oozing or flowing from the mouth

PLANNING

Patient Needs	Primary Nurse-Patient Goals
Comfort	To achieve comfort
Cleanliness	To achieve good hygiene
Protection from physical harm	To prevent physical injury, infection
Increased learning	To achieve awareness of needs

NURSING INTERVENTIONS

Nursing Treatments
Apply an ice bag (to the external cheek for inner cheek bleeding)
Moisten the mouth with cracked ice
Give iced liquids
Refrain from giving hot liquids
Give pureed foods
   OR
Give soft foods
Discourage smoking
Refrain from dislodging blood clots
Brush the teeth with a soft toothbrush
Remove the dentures (if they irritate the mouth)
Refresh with a mouthwash (applied with a padded tongue blade)

Nursing Observations
Estimate the blood volume loss
Inspect for renewed bleeding
Monitor the blood pressure
Monitor blood studies for abnormal clotting mechanism
Monitor blood studies for abnormal hematology

Health Teaching
Explain the causes of the health problem
Explain the need to avoid mechanical trauma
Instruct not to vigorously rinse the mouth (if clots exist)
Instruct not to use a drinking straw
Instruct to use a soft, new toothbrush and to apply only mild toothbrush
   pressure (if bleeding is in the area of the teeth)
Explain the reason for and intended effect of the therapy

Medical Treatments Performed by Nurses
Give the prescribed drugs

EVALUATION
See the evaluation criteria for each specific goal in Chapter 2.

Rectal Bleeding (70,247)

ASSESSMENT

Subjective Data
Weakness
Pain

Objective Data
Bright blood in or on the stools
Rectal bleeding not associated with stools
Rapid pulse
Pallor

Related Data
Commonly Related Conditions:
Rectal polyps
Fecal impaction
Commonly Related Diseases:
Internal hemorrhoids
External hemorrhoids
Anal fissure
Anal fistula
Carcinoma of the rectum
Ulcerative proctitis

POSSIBLE ETIOLOGY

Injury to the rectal tissue. Intraabdominal pressure. Use of harsh purgatives.

NURSING DIAGNOSIS

Rectal bleeding: blood originating in and oozing from the rectum

PLANNING

Patient Needs	Primary Nurse-Patient Goals
Rest	To achieve rest
Comfort	To achieve comfort
Protection from physical harm	To prevent physical injury
Increased learning	To achieve awareness of needs

NURSING INTERVENTIONS

Nursing Treatments
Apply an ice bag (to the rectal area)
Change the patient's position gradually
Cover with warm blankets
Place on complete bed rest (if bleeding is severe)
Elevate the foot of the bed
Refrain from giving enemas
Refrain from giving laxatives

Refrain from inserting a rectal tube
Refrain from taking rectal temperatures

Nursing Observations
Estimate the blood volume loss
Inspect for renewed bleeding
Monitor the blood pressure
Monitor blood studies for abnormal hematology

Health Teaching
Explain the causes of the health problem
Advise not to stand for prolonged periods
Inform that coughing should be avoided
Inform that elimination straining should be avoided
Explain the reason for and intended effect of the therapy

EVALUATION

See the evaluation criteria for each specific goal in Chapter 2.

BLOOD PRESSURE, ALTERED ARTERIAL

Decreased Arterial Blood Pressure (32,71)

ASSESSMENT

Subjective Data
Weakness
Dizziness
Fatigue

Objective Data
Note: Although averages have been set for normal blood pressure, conclusions should be based on the person's baseline reading.
A blood pressure below 90/60 in adults
Faint pulse
Tachycardia

Related Data
Commonly Related Conditions:
Shock
Syncope
Cachexia
Hypoxia
Metabolic acidosis
Hyperventilation
Commonly Related Diseases:
Addison's disease
Myocardial infarction

Carcinoma
Neurasthenia
Simmonds' disease
Anemia
Mitral stenosis

POSSIBLE ETIOLOGY

Decreased cardiac output. Severe blood loss. Blood flow obstruction. Endocrine imbalance. Drug side effects. Intense emotion.

NURSING DIAGNOSIS

Decreased arterial blood pressure: systolic and diastolic blood pressure readings below normal limits

PLANNING

Patient Needs	Primary Nurse-Patient Goals
Oxygen, circulation	To maintain oxygen to all cells
Rest	To achieve rest
Comfort	To achieve comfort
Protection from physical harm	To prevent physical injury
Increased learning	To achieve awareness of needs

NURSING INTERVENTIONS

Nursing Treatments
Administer intravenous fluids (ET) (Ringer's lactate)
    OR
Increase the intravenous infusion flow rate
Give hot coffee
    OR
Give hot tea
Place in the foot-elevated head-lowered (Trendelenburg) position
Place on complete bed rest (if severely hypotensive)
Change the patient's position gradually
Cover with warm blankets
Maintain a warm room temperature
Apply an elastic bandage ⎫
    OR   ⎬ (to the legs)
Apply elastic stockings ⎭
Withhold the drugs (if they precipitate the episode)

Nursing Observations
Inspect for hemorrhage
Monitor the blood pressure
Observe for shock

Health Teaching
Explain the causes of the health problem
Instruct to change position gradually

Explain how to apply elastic stockings or an elastic bandage
Explain the reason for and intended effect of the therapy

Medical Treatments Performed by Nurses
Administer intravenous fluids
Give the prescribed drugs

EVALUATION

See the evaluation criteria for each specific goal in Chapter 2.

Increased Arterial Blood Pressure (32,247,453,603)

ASSESSMENT

Subjective Data
Weakness
Dizziness
Fatigue
Headache

Objective Data
Note: Although averages have been set for normal blood pressure, conclusions should be based on the person's baseline reading.
Blood pressure readings above:

3–6 years	110/70	18–44 years	140/90
7–10 years	120/80	45–64 years	150/95
11–17 years	130/80	65 or older	160/95

Flushed face
Epistaxis

Related Data

Commonly Related Conditions:
Edema
Obesity
Pregnancy toxemia
Carbon dioxide retention

Commonly Related Diseases:
Arteriovenous fistula
Thyrotoxicosis
Cerebral tumor
Patent ductus arteriosus
Pheochromocytoma
Glomerulonephritis
Aortic coarctation
Polyarteritis nodosa
Primary hyperaldosteronism
Cushing's syndrome
Acromegaly

Hypertensive encephalopathy
Arteriosclerosis
Chronic pyelonephritis
Cerebral vascular accident
Essential or malignant hypertension
Polycystic kidney disease
Anemia
Congestive heart failure
Aortic stenosis
Aortic regurgitation

POSSIBLE ETIOLOGY

Changes in arterial elasticity. Increased resistance by the arterial wall. Increased force in ventricular contraction. Drug side effects. Increased fluid volume within the arteries. Increased metabolic rate. Highly emotional situations. Fluid overload.

NURSING DIAGNOSIS

Increased arterial blood pressure: systolic and diastolic blood pressure readings above normal limits

PLANNING

Patient Needs	Primary Nurse-Patient Goals
Food balance	To maintain nutrition to all cells
Rest, relaxation	To achieve rest and relaxation
Comfort	To achieve comfort
Protection from physical harm	To prevent physical injury
Increased learning	To achieve awareness of needs

NURSING INTERVENTIONS

Nursing Treatments

Change the patient's position gradually
Elevate the head
Do not place in the flat position
Provide quiet
Encourage adequate rest
Massage gently (for a relaxing effect)
Maintain a normal room temperature
Discourage oral stimulants
Substitute caffeine-free coffee
Avoid causing intense emotional situations
Discourage smoking
Slow the intravenous infusion flow rate
Make a referral (to a physician if the condition is recurrent)

Nursing Observations
Monitor the blood pressure

Health Teaching
Explain the causes of the health problem
Advise that highly emotional situations be avoided
Emphasize the danger of excessive body weight
Inform that (intense) coughing should be avoided
Inform that elimination straining should be avoided
Instruct to change position gradually (to lie down slowly)
Explain the reason for and intended effect of the therapy

Medical Treatments Performed by Nurses
Give the prescribed diet
Give the prescribed drugs

EVALUATION

See the evaluation criteria for each specific goal in Chapter 2.

Postural Hypotension (247,453)

ASSESSMENT

Subjective Data
Dizziness
Lightheadedness
Faintness

Objective Data
Below-normal systolic and diastolic blood pressure readings
Tachycardia
Pallor

Related Data
Onset during sudden change from a lying to a sitting or a sitting to a standing position, or when lying flat on the back during pregnancy

Commonly Related Conditions:
Pregnancy
Commonly Related Diseases:
None
  OR
Peripheral neuropathy
Primary autonomic insufficiency
Simmonds' disease

POSSIBLE ETIOLOGY

Blood pooling in the extremities. Drug side effects.

NURSING DIAGNOSIS

Postural hypotension: decreased blood pressure readings occurring with a
sudden position change

PLANNING

Patient Needs

Oxygen, circulation

Comfort

Protection from physical harm

Increased learning

Primary Nurse-Patient Goals

To maintain oxygen to all cells

To achieve comfort

To prevent physical injury

To achieve awareness of needs

NURSING INTERVENTIONS

Nursing Treatments

Apply an elastic bandage ⎫
   OR   ⎬ (to the legs while in bed)
Apply elastic stockings ⎭

Change the patient's position gradually

Do not place in the flat position (during pregnancy)

Place in the side-lying position (during pregnancy)

Give hot coffee ⎫
   OR   ⎬ (while in bed)
Give hot tea ⎭

Remove constrictive clothing

Nursing Observations

Monitor the blood pressure

Observe for syncope

Health Teaching

Explain the causes of the health problem

Instruct to change position gradually

Advise against wearing constrictive clothing

Explain how to apply elastic stockings or an elastic bandage (to the legs)

Teach how to take a blood pressure

Explain the reason for and intended effect of the therapy

Medical Treatments Performed by Nurses

Give the prescribed drugs (ephedrine sulfate)

EVALUATION

See the evaluation criteria for each specific goal in Chapter 2.

BLOOD PRESSURE, HYPERTENSIVE ALTERATION IN

Dependence on Nursing Supervision of Controlled Hypertension (247,453)

ASSESSMENT

Subjective Data

Person relies on nurses for: ·

   periodic blood pressure readings

observation for antihypertensive drug intolerance
observation for adherence to and success of the diet
observation for complications related to hypertension

Objective Data
Blood pressure readings are lowered and stable with medical treatment

Related Data
Commonly Related Diseases:
Essential or malignant hypertension

POSSIBLE ETIOLOGY

Confirmed medical diagnosis of hypertension. On antihypertensive therapy regime.

NURSING DIAGNOSIS

Dependence on nursing supervision of controlled hypertension: reliance on nurses to periodically evaluate the health status of the patient whose hypertensive condition is relatively stabilized by medication and diet

PLANNING

Patient Needs	**Primary Nurse-Patient Goals**
Comfort	To achieve comfort
Protection from physical harm	To prevent physical injury
Dependence	To achieve comfort
Increased learning	To achieve awareness of needs

NURSING INTERVENTIONS

Nursing Treatments
Approach unhurriedly
Encourage patient questions

Nursing Observations
Inspect the neck veins for distention
Inspect the skin for discoloration (flushing)
Measure the body weight
Monitor the blood pressure (for a diastolic above 90 mm Hg)
Monitor the positional blood pressure
Observe for complaints of dizziness
Observe for complaints of headache
Observe for complaints of tinnitus
Observe for drug reactions
Observe for fatigue
Review the dietary intake with the patient to determine adherence to the prescribed diet

Health Teaching
Explain the causes of the health problem
Advise against exposure to intense heat ⎫
Advise not to take hot baths ⎭ (when on antihypertensive drugs)

Advise that highly emotional situations be avoided
Explain that fatigue should be recognized as a stress factor
Emphasize the danger of excessive body weight
Recommend eating and drinking in moderation
Recommend adherence to a moderate pace of living
Recommend methods for achieving total relaxation
Teach how to take a blood pressure
Inform that a predisposition to the illness exists (in all family members)
Explain the reason for and intended effect of the therapy

EVALUATION

See the evaluation criteria for each specific goal in Chapter 2.

BLOOD PRESSURE, POTENTIAL HYPERTENSIVE ALTERATION IN

Lifestyle Inappropriate to Hypertension (59,159)

ASSESSMENT

Subjective Data
Intensely competitive in work and at home
Narrow range of interest
Overcontrolled, rigid social relationships
Frequent geographic changes through traveling or moving
Irregular daily schedule
Irregular and inadequate sleep pattern
Chronic overexertion
Chronic overeating, smoking, or drinking
Frequently emotionally upset

Objective Data
Confirmed medical diagnosis of hypertension

Related Data
Commonly Related Diseases:
Essential or malignant hypertension

POSSIBLE ETIOLOGY

Habitual stressful work and home behaviors. Lack of instruction as to how to adjust one's lifestyle appropriately.

NURSING DIAGNOSIS

Lifestyle inappropriate to hypertension: the existence of a daily life routine that antagonizes the hypertensive state

PLANNING

Patient Needs	**Primary Nurse-Patient Goals**
Sleep, rest, relaxation	To achieve sleep, rest, relaxation

Protection from physical harm   To prevent physical injury
Increased learning   To achieve awareness of needs

NURSING INTERVENTIONS

Nursing Treatments
Assist the patient in restructuring his lifestyle
Discourage oral stimulants
Discourage smoking
Encourage adequate rest
Encourage moderate physical exercise
Discourage strenuous activities

Nursing Observations
Monitor the blood pressure (periodically)
Observe for behavior modification

Health Teaching
Recommend a regular sleeping schedule
Advise that highly emotional situations be avoided
Explain that fatigue should be recognized as a stress factor
Recommend adherence to a moderate pace of living
Recommend eating and drinking in moderation
Recommend methods for achieving total relaxation
Explain the reason for and intended effect of the therapy

EVALUATION

See the evaluation criteria for each specific goal in Chapter 2.

Predisposition to Hypertension (59,159,247,453)

ASSESSMENT

Subjective Data
Smokes more than five cigarettes a day
Sedentary life with little or no physical activity
Had an emotionally stormy childhood in which behavior became submissive and compliant or excessively aggressive
Quick to perceive hostility in others and overresponds with quick retaliation, irritability, and aggression

Objective Data
Excessive body weight
Chronically high salt and fat intake
Gradual blood pressure rise with age

Related Data
History of urinary tract infection
Race:
Greatest predisposition in the Negro race
One or both parents had hypertension

Sex:
More common in women than in men

Commonly Related Conditions:
Pregnancy
Obesity

Commonly Related Diseases:
Essential or malignant hypertension
Cushing's syndrome

POSSIBLE ETIOLOGY

Physical status. Lifestyle. Familiar tendency.

NURSING DIAGNOSIS

Predisposition to hypertension: a high probability of developing hypertension

PLANNING

Patient Needs	**Primary Nurse-Patient Goals**
Protection from physical harm	To prevent physical injury
Increased learning	To achieve awareness of needs

NURSING INTERVENTIONS

Nursing Treatments
Discourage oral stimulants
Discourage smoking
Encourage moderate physical exercise
Discourage strenuous activities
Encourage adequate rest
Encourage decreased fatty-food intake
Encourage decreased sodium-food intake

Nursing Observations
Inspect the eyes for papilledema
Measure the body weight (periodically)
Monitor the blood pressure (for diastolic above 90)
Monitor the positional blood pressure
Observe for complaints of dizziness
Observe for complaints of headache
Observe for complaints of tinnitus
Observe for fatigue

Health Teaching
Explain the causes of the health problem
Advise that highly emotional situations be avoided
Explain that fatigue should be recognized as a stress factor
Recommend adherence to a moderate pace of living
Recommend eating and drinking in moderation
Emphasize the danger of excessive body weight
Advise periodic examinations for known hereditary predispositions

Describe those symptoms which should be reported (dizziness, headache, tinnitus, fatigue)

Explain the reason for and intended effect of the therapy

Medical Treatments Performed by Nurses
Give the prescribed diet (for weight reduction)

EVALUATION

See the evaluation criteria for each specific goal in Chapter 2.

CARDIAC FUNCTION, ALTERED

Dependence on Cardiac Workload Reduction (58,71,307,453)

ASSESSMENT

Subjective Data
Dyspnea
Easily fatigued
Weakness
Person relies on nurses for:
    physical care
    a controlled environment

Objective Data
Tachycardia
Bounding pulse
Apical-radial pulse deficit
Increased blood pressure
Edema

Related Data

Commonly Related Conditions:
Cardiac dysrhythmias
Commonly Related Diseases:
Myocardial infarction
Myocarditis
Bacterial endocarditis
Congestive heart failure
Coronary thrombosis
Severe anemia
Patent ductus arteriosus
Aortic stenosis or insufficiency

POSSIBLE ETIOLOGY

An increase in the blood volume the heart must pump, the amount of pressure the heart muscle must exert when contracting, and an accelerated need of the myocardium for oxygen. An increased metabolic rate. Obesity which increases the amount of tissue the heart must oxygenate. Increased vagal stimulation of the heart's activity. Pulmonary congestion. Reduced oxygen carrying capacity of the blood.

NURSING DIAGNOSIS

Dependence on cardiac workload reduction: reliance on nurses to provide care that supports a decreased consumption of oxygen by body tissues so the heart is allowed to rest and heal

PLANNING

Patient Needs	Primary Nurse-Patient Goals
Oxygen, circulation	To maintain oxygen to all cells
Normal temperature	To maintain regulating mechanisms and functions
Sleep, rest, relaxation	To achieve sleep, rest, relaxation
Exercise	To achieve exercise
Comfort	To achieve comfort
Protection from physical harm	To prevent physical injury
Dependence	To achieve comfort
Increased learning	To achieve awareness of needs

NURSING INTERVENTIONS

Nursing Treatments

Acknowledge dependency
Approach unhurriedly
Anticipate needs
Grant special requests
Provide quiet
Encourage adequate rest
Refrain from performing nonessential procedures
Maintain adequate atmospheric humidity
Maintain adequate room ventilation
Maintain a normal room temperature
Change the patient's position gradually
Elevate the head
Bathe in bed
Feed the patient
Give small, frequent feedings
Refrain from giving hot liquids
Refrain from giving iced liquids
Refrain from giving oral stimulants
Provide a bedpan
   OR
Provide a bedside commode
Exercise in range of motion (passive)
Discourage smoking
Massage gently (for the relaxing effect)
Limit visitors

Nursing Observations
Auscultate the apical heartbeat for rate and rhythm (periodically)
Auscultate the chest for abnormal heart sounds
Measure the intake
Measure the output
Monitor the blood pressure (for an increase)
Observe for complaints of pain (chest)
Observe for dyspnea
Observe for fatigue
Observe for complaints of weakness
Palpate the pulse for rate, rhythm, and volume (tachycardia or bounding
   pulse)

Health Teaching
Explain the causes of the health problem
Explain the need to avoid overexertion
Describe the cardiac signs of physical overactivity
Advise that highly emotional situations be avoided
Explain that fatigue should be recognized as a stress factor
Inform that coughing should be avoided
Inform that elimination straining should be avoided
Instruct to immediately report serious symptoms (pain, dyspnea, fatigue)
Explain the reason for and intended effect of the therapy

Medical Treatments Performed by Nurses
Administer humidified oxygen
Give the prescribed drugs

EVALUATION

See the evaluation criteria for each specific goal in Chapter 2.

CARDIAC FUNCTION, POTENTIAL ALTERATION IN

Potential Dysrhythmia Aggravation (300,306,382,408)

ASSESSMENT

Subjective Data
Fatigue

Objective Data
Presence of dysrhythmias
Overactivity
Use of stimulants

Related Data
Receiving drug therapy

Commonly Related Conditions:
Fever
Inflammation
Excitement
Exhaustion
Menopause
Hypoglycemia
Commonly Related Diseases:
Thyrotoxicosis
Myocardial infarction
Anemia

POSSIBLE ETIOLOGY

Existing but drug-controlled dysrhythmias. Metabolic changes. Drug side effects. Impaired myocardial nutrition.

NURSING DIAGNOSIS

Potential dysrhythmia aggravation: the possibility that a dysrhythmia will occur as a result of irritating factors

PLANNING

Patient Needs	**Primary Nurse-Patient Goals**
Protection from physical harm	To prevent physical injury
Increased learning	To achieve awareness of needs

NURSING INTERVENTIONS

Nursing Treatments
Encourage adequate rest
Discourage strenuous activities
Discourage oral stimulants
Refrain from giving oral stimulants
Substitute caffeine-free coffee
Discourage smoking
Withhold the drugs (such as epinephrine, atropine, thyroxine, aminophyl-
line)

Nursing Observations
Auscultate the apical heartbeat for rate and rhythm
Monitor the blood pressure
Monitor blood studies for abnormal cardiac enzymes
Monitor blood studies for abnormal electrolytes
Monitor blood studies for abnormal gas exchange
Monitor the cardiogram (periodically)
Palpate the pulse for rate, rhythm, and volume

Health Teaching
Explain the causes of the health problem
Advise that highly emotional situations be avoided

Explain the need to avoid overexertion
Instruct to use vagal stimulation methods to terminate dysrhythmias
Instruct to immediately report serious symptoms (pain, dyspnea)
Explain the reason for and intended effect of the therapy

Medical Treatments Performed by Nurses
Give the prescribed drugs

EVALUATION

See the evaluation criteria for each specific goal in Chapter 2.

CARDIOVASCULAR INJURY, POTENTIAL

Lifestyle Inappropriate to Cardiac Pathology (132,306)

ASSESSMENT

Subjective Data
Lives under a sense of time urgency
Persistent aggressive patterns of living
Experiences restlessness during leisure hours
Narrowed interests
Seeks refuge in work

Objective Data
Irregular daily schedule
Frequent geographic changes through traveling and moving
Multiple jobs
Crowded living conditions
Uses leisure time to fulfill civic, social, and educational obligations
Rarely, if ever, takes vacations
Chronically attempting to meet deadlines

Related Data
Commonly Related Diseases:
Myocardial infarction

POSSIBLE ETIOLOGY

Habitual stressful work and home behavior. Lack of information related to the cardiac condition.

NURSING DIAGNOSIS

Lifestyle inappropriate to cardiac pathology: a daily life routine that aggravates an existing cardiac condition

PLANNING

Patient Needs
Protection from physical harm
Increased learning

Primary Nurse-Patient Goals
To prevent physical injury
To achieve awareness of needs

NURSING INTERVENTIONS

Nursing Treatments
Assist the patient in restructuring his lifestyle
Encourage moderate physical exercise
Discourage strenuous activities
Encourage adequate rest
Encourage vacationing (as often as possible)
Discourage oral stimulants
Discourage smoking

Nursing Observations
Observe for behavior modification

Health Teaching
Recommend a regular sleeping schedule
Recommend a regular meal schedule
Advise that highly emotional situations be avoided
Explain that fatigue should be recognized as a stress factor
Recommend adherence to a moderate pace of living
Recommend methods for achieving total relaxation
Recommend the pursuit of only one activity at a time
Explain the reason for and intended effect of the therapy

EVALUATION

See the evaluation criteria for each specific goal in Chapter 2.

Potential Cardiac Overload
(58,71,306,453)

ASSESSMENT

Objective Data
Occasional excessive exercise
Overexertion
Overeating at a single meal
Increased metabolic rate
Emotional excitement
Intense environmental heat or severe cold
High environmental humidity
High altitudes

Related Data

Laboratory Findings:
Low blood hemoglobin

Commonly Related Conditions:
Pregnancy

Commonly Related Diseases:
Thyrotoxicosis

POSSIBLE ETIOLOGY

A heightened metabolic rate which increases energy requirements. Excessive exercise increasing the need for muscle oxygenation. Overeating which diverts blood from the heart to the stomach to produce gastric juices. Emotional excitement in which adrenalin stimulates rapid cardiac contractions. Adaptation to environmental heat in which the heart pumps more blood to the skin to provide perspiration for cooling. Environmental cold in which muscle contractions which warm the body require additional blood supply. High altitudes in which less oxygen is available to the body. Low hemoglobin which reduces the oxygen carrying capacity of the blood.

NURSING DIAGNOSIS

Potential cardiac overload: the possibility that the amount of work the heart must put forth in order to maintain tissue oxygenation will exceed the capacity of the heart to adapt

PLANNING

Patient Needs

Protection from physical harm

Increased learning

Primary Nurse-Patient Goals

To prevent physical injury

To achieve awareness of needs

NURSING INTERVENTIONS

Nursing Treatments
Discourage oral stimulants (in excess)
Discourage smoking
Discourage strenuous activities (if any discomforting symptoms occur)
Encourage adequate rest
Encourage moderate physical exercise

Nursing Observations
Monitor the blood pressure
Observe for complaints of pain (chest)
Observe for complaints of weakness
Observe for dyspnea
Observe for fatigue

Health Teaching
Advise against exposure to inclement weather (extreme cold)
Advise against exposure to intense heat
Advise that highly emotional situations be avoided
Describe the cardiac signs of physical overactivity
Explain the need to avoid overexertion
Recommend eating and drinking in moderation
Recommend that high altitudes be avoided after cardiac damage

EVALUATION

See the evaluation criteria for each specific goal in Chapter 2.

Predisposition to Cardiovascular Pathology (132,306)

ASSESSMENT

Subjective Data
Prolonged fatigue
Gains little satisfaction from accomplishments

Fails to enjoy life in general
Smokes over five cigarettes a day
Sense of time urgency

Objective Data
Excessive weight
Elevated blood pressure
Diet high in polysaturated fats, salt, and carbohydrates in the presence of
    increased blood cholesterol and high blood pressure
Fad dieting in which there is fluctuating excessive weight and weight loss
Lack of regular exercise
Frequent geographic movement
Frequent changes in modes of living
Frequent occupational change or change of position within an occupation
Little success in attaining life goals
Simultaneously working at two or more jobs
Takes only rare vacations
Lives in crowded conditions

Related Data
Family history of heart disease, cerebral vascular accident or diabetes
Commonly Related Diseases:
Atherosclerosis
Arteriosclerosis
Diabetes mellitus
Hypertension
Cushing's syndrome

ETIOLOGY

Genetic weakness. Prolonged physical and emotional stress.

NURSING DIAGNOSIS

Predisposition to cardiovascular pathology: a susceptibility to developing
cardiovascular abnormalities

PLANNING

Patient Needs	**Primary Nurse-Patient Goals**
Sleep, rest, relaxation	To achieve sleep, rest, relaxation
Activity, exercise	To achieve activity and exercise
Protection from physical harm	To prevent physical injury
Increased learning	To achieve awareness of needs

NURSING INTERVENTIONS

Nursing Treatments
Assist the patient in restructuring his lifestyle
Discourage oral stimulants
Discourage smoking
Encourage adequate rest
Encourage decreased carbohydrate intake
Encourage decreased fatty-food intake

Encourage decreased sodium-food intake
Encourage moderate physical exercise

Nursing Observations
Auscultate the apical heartbeat for rate and rhythm (periodically)
Monitor the blood pressure
Monitor blood studies for abnormal cardiac enzymes
Monitor blood studies for abnormal hematology
Monitor the cardiogram (periodically)
Observe for complaints of pain
Observe for dyspnea
Observe for fatigue
Observe for complaints of weakness
Palpate the pulse for rate, rhythm, and volume

Health Teaching
Explain the causes of the health problem
Advise that highly emotional situations be avoided
Emphasize the need to recognize fatigue as a stress factor
Explain the reason for and intended effect of the therapy
Emphasize the danger of crash-dieting
Emphasize the danger of excessive body weight
Recommend adherence to a moderate pace of living
Recommend methods for achieving total relaxation
Recommend the pursuit of only one activity (job) at a time
Inform that a predisposition to the illness exists
Describe those symptoms which should be reported (chest pain, dyspnea, weakness)

EVALUATION

See the evaluation criteria for each specific goal in Chapter 2.

Predisposition to Cerebral Vascular Accident (338)

ASSESSMENT

Subjective Data
Frequent headaches
Recurrent dizziness and lightheadedness
Intermittent facial or extremity numbness, prickling, or burning lasting only a few minutes

Objective Data
Elevated blood pressure
Obesity
Heavy smoking
Unexplainable memory lapses
Intermittent confusion, slurred speech, or facial or extremity coldness lasting only a few minutes

Related Data
Family history of cerebral vascular accidents

Sex:
More prevalent in females than in males

Commonly Related Diseases:
Hypertension
Aneurysm
Arteriosclerosis
Atherosclerosis
Arteritis

POSSIBLE ETIOLOGY

Excessive arterial pressure. Weakened arterial walls. Narrowing or inflammation of arteries. Intermittent short periods of decreased cerebral arterial blood flow without complete arterial obstruction. The release of adrenalin, precipitated by cigarette smoking, causes faster blood clotting which increases the danger of arterial thrombus.

NURSING DIAGNOSIS

Predisposition to cerebral vascular accident: a susceptibility toward diminished blood supply to the brain as a result of the rupture, clotting, or sclerosis of a cerebral vessel

PLANNING

Patient Needs	**Primary Nurse-Patient Goals**
Sleep, rest, relaxation	To achieve sleep, rest, relaxation
Activity, exercise	To achieve activity and exercise
Protection from physical harm	To prevent physical injury
Increased learning	To achieve awareness of needs

NURSING INTERVENTIONS

Nursing Treatments
Encourage adequate rest
Encourage moderate physical exercise
Discourage oral stimulants
Discourage smoking
Encourage decreased cholesterol-food intake
Encourage decreased sodium-food intake

Nursing Observations
Monitor the blood pressure (periodically)

Health Teaching
Explain the causes of the health problem
Advise that highly emotional situations be avoided
Explain that fatigue should be recognized as a stress factor
Emphasize the danger of excessive body weight
Inform that coughing should be avoided
Inform that elimination straining should be avoided

Recommend adherence to a moderate pace of living
Recommend methods for achieving total relaxation
Inform that a predisposition to the illness exists
Describe those symptoms which should be reported (dizziness, numbness, and tingling)
Explain the reason for and intended effect of the therapy

Medical Treatments Performed by Nurses
Give the prescribed drugs

EVALUATION

See the evaluation criteria for each specific goal in Chapter 2.

CARDIAC THERAPY DEPENDENCE

Dependence on Nursing Supervision of Cardiac Monitoring (234,382,408)

ASSESSMENT

Subjective Data
Person relies on nurses for:
    surveillance for abnormal heart patterns
    interpretation of abnormal heart patterns
    recognition of mechanical failure of the monitoring system

Objective Data
Person is being monitored for cardiac irregularities

Related Data
Commonly Related Diseases:
Myocardial infarction
Congestive heart failure

POSSIBLE ETIOLOGY

Need for accurate diagnosis and early detection of abnormal heart rates and rhythms

NURSING DIAGNOSIS

Dependence on nursing supervision of cardiac monitoring: reliance on nurses to read and interpret heart rate and rhythm recordings

PLANNING

Patient Needs	**Primary Nurse-Patient Goals**
Comfort	To achieve comfort
Protection from physical harm	To prevent physical injury

Dependence

Increased learning

To achieve comfort

To achieve awareness of needs

NURSING INTERVENTIONS

Nursing Treatments
Reassure verbally
Provide frequent patient contact
Provide standby emergency equipment and drugs (oxygen, defibrillator)
Unplug the electrical monitor during a bath
Consult with the physician (as needed)

Nursing Observations
Check the monitor electrodes for placement periodically
Monitor the cardiogram

Health Teaching
Monitor blood studies for abnormal cardiac enzymes
Monitor blood studies for abnormal electrolytes
Monitor blood studies for abnormal gas exchange
Explain the reason for and intended effect of the therapy

EVALUATION

See the evaluation criteria for each specific goal in Chapter 2.

Dependence on Cardiac-Pacemaker Management
(234,382,408,475,498)

ASSESSMENT

Subjective Data
Person relies on nurses for:
pacemaker stimulation when the heartbeat exceeds or goes below the
desired level
maintenance of the pacemaker device and electrodes
protection from the danger of pacemaker-related electrical shock

Objective Data
Person is attached to a pacemaker

Related Data
Commonly Related Conditions:
Atrial fibrillation
Ventricular fibrillation
A-V heart block with digitalis toxicity
Commonly Related Diseases:
Rheumatic heart disease
Myocardial infarction

POSSIBLE ETIOLOGY

Inability of the human cardiac pacemaker to fire adequate or normal stimulus for the maintenance of regular heartbeat

NURSING DIAGNOSIS

Dependence on cardiac-pacemaker management: reliance on nurses to maintain the functioning of an electrical device that supports rhythmic heartbeats through regular electrical stimulation of the cardiac muscle

PLANNING

Patient Needs	Primary Nurse-Patient Goals
Comfort	To achieve comfort
Protection from physical harm	To prevent physical injury
Dependence	To achieve comfort
Increased learning	To achieve awareness of needs

NURSING INTERVENTIONS

Nursing Treatments
Reassure verbally
Provide frequent patient contact
Defibrillate the heart muscle (ET) (as needed)
Apply an antibiotic ointment (on the skin around the pacemaker wires)
Clean with surgical soap (around the pacemaker wires)
Apply a sterile dressing (at the site of surgically implanted electrodes)
Tape the pacemaker wire to the patient
Avoid simultaneously touching electrical equipment and a patient with a
    pacemaker
Avoid simultaneous use of multiple electrical machines around pacemakers
Avoid using extension cords around pacemakers
Avoid using worn electrical cords, plugs, or outlets around pacemakers
Disconnect unused electrical equipment around pacemakers
Insulate exposed pacemaker electrodes
Use only three-prong electrical plugs in the patient area
Place on a nonelectric bed if wearing a pacemaker
Position the pacemaker generator box comfortably

Nursing Observations
Auscultate the apical heartbeat for rate and rhythm
Check the pacemaker for pacing rate

Health Teaching
Describe those symptoms which should be reported (pain, dyspnea)
Explain the reason for and intended effect of the therapy

EVALUATION

See the evaluation criteria for each specific goal in Chapter 2.

CARDIAC THERAPY DISCOMFORTS

Distress Related to Cardiac Monitoring

ASSESSMENT

Subjective Data

Anxious regarding the danger of electrical currents, blinking lights, and sudden alarms

Fears being alone

Distressed if electrodes come loose

Distressed if normal monitor patterns become irregular from loose electrodes or activity

Alarm disturbs sleep

Objective Data

Spends a considerable amount of time looking at the monitor

Moves very little in bed

Related Data

Commonly Related Conditions:

Cardiac dysrhythmias

Commonly Related Conditions:

Myocardial infarction

Congestive heart failure

POSSIBLE ETIOLOGY

Inadequate knowledge regarding the cardiac monitor

NURSING DIAGNOSIS

Distress related to cardiac monitoring (distress related to cardiac telemetry): excessive worry and concern regarding the application of a transmitting device which records the heart rate and rhythm

PLANNING

Patient Needs

Comfort

Protection from psychologic threat

Increased learning

Primary Nurse-Patient Goals

To achieve comfort

To prevent emotional injury

To achieve awareness of needs

NURSING INTERVENTIONS

·Nursing Treatments

Approach unhurriedly

Attend the patient constantly

OR

Provide frequent patient contact

Demonstrate calmness

Reassure verbally (frequently)
Encourage patient questions

Nursing Observations
Check the monitor electrodes for placement periodically
Observe for an excessive stress level

Health Teaching
Explain that monitors are safe
Explain how the equipment works
Explain the reason for and intended effect of the therapy

EVALUATION

See the evaluation criteria for each specific goal in Chapter 2.

Distress Related to Cardiac Pacemaker

ASSESSMENT

Subjective Data
Fears the electrical jolt will be fatal or perceives it as pain
Curious about pacemaker function

Objective Data
Little movement in bed
Self-restriction of activities when ambulatory
Removes external electrodes sometimes
May refuse to bathe when the pacemaker is attached

Related Data
Commonly Related Conditions:
Atrial fibrillation
Ventricular fibrillation
A-V heart block with digitalis toxicity
Commonly Related Diseases:
Rheumatic heart disease
Myocardial infarction

POSSIBLE ETIOLOGY

Lack of instruction in machine operation and reason for treatment

NURSING DIAGNOSIS

Distress related to cardiac pacemaker: worry and concern regarding the use on oneself of an electrical device that supports rhythmic heartbeats through regular electrical stimulation of the cardiac muscle

PLANNING

Patient Needs
Comfort
Protection from psychologic threat
Increased learning

Primary Nurse-Patient Goals
To achieve comfort
To prevent emotional injury
To achieve awareness of needs

NURSING INTERVENTIONS

Nursing Treatments
Approach unhurriedly
Demonstrate calmness
Reassure verbally (frequently)
Provide frequent patient contact
Encourage patient questions .

Nursing Observations
Observe for an excessive stress level

Health Teaching
Explain that pacemakers are safe
Explain how the equipment works
Explain the effects of the specific type pacemaker
Explain the reason for and intended effect of the therapy

EVALUATION

See the evaluation criteria for each specific goal in Chapter 2.

NONFUNCTIONING CARDIAC THERAPY DEVICES

Pacemaker Failure (475,498)

ASSESSMENT

Subjective Data
Dizziness
Chest pain

Objective Data
Generator light fails to flash
Dial needle fails to move immediately prior to a pulse beat
Electrical stimulus is not simultaneous with each heartbeat; may occur between heartbeats, or more than one stimulus to one heartbeat
Artifact fails to appear on the EKG strip prior to each QRS complex
Battery change is overdue
Increased or decreased pulse rate
Loss of consciousness

POSSIBLE ETIOLOGY

Mechanical insufficiency

NURSING DIAGNOSIS

Pacemaker failure: nonfunctioning of the cardiac electrical device that supports rhythmic heartbeats through regular electrical stimulation of the cardiac muscle

PLANNING

Patient Needs
Protection from physical harm
Increased learning

Primary Nurse-Patient Goals
To prevent physical injury
To achieve awareness of needs

NURSING INTERVENTIONS

Nursing Treatments
Attend the patient constantly (until the pacemaker is functioning)
Provide standby emergency equipment
Reassure verbally
Replace the pacemaker batteries

Nursing Observations
Auscultate the apical heartbeat for rate and rhythm
Monitor the cardiogram (as needed)

Health Teaching
Explain the causes of the health problem
Instruct to check the pulse daily when wearing a pacemaker

EVALUATION

See the evaluation criteria for each specific goal in Chapter 2.

LYMPH CIRCULATION, ALTERED

Impaired Lymph Circulation (71,247)

ASSESSMENT

Subjective Data
Pain

Objective Data
Extreme swelling of the extremities
Nonpitting edema
Coarse skin

Related Data
Commonly Related Conditions:
Radical mastectomy
Commonly Related Diseases:
Lymphangitis
Lymphadenitis
Elephantiasis
Milroy's disease
Carcinoma
Filariasis

POSSIBLE ETIOLOGY

Obstructed lymph flow to a body area. Inflammation of subcutaneous lymph vessels. Bacterial infection.

NURSING DIAGNOSIS

Impaired lymph circulation: lack of adequate lymph circulation through body tissues

PLANNING

Patient Needs	**Primary Nurse-Patient Goals**
Water-salt balance	To maintain fluid and electrolyte balance
Sleep, rest	To achieve sleep, rest
Comfort	To achieve comfort
Protection from physical harm	To prevent physical injury
Increased learning	To achieve awareness of needs

NURSING INTERVENTIONS

Nursing Treatments
Apply an elastic bandage
Refrain from tight bandaging
Change the patient's position frequently
Do not place in the flat position
Elevate the extremity
Handle gently
Massage gently
Do not start I.V.'s or draw blood in the affected extremity
Lubricate the skin with cocoa butter, glycerine, lanolin, mineral oil, or olive oil

Nursing Observations
Monitor the blood pressure (but avoid using the affected limb)
Inspect the extremity for adequate circulation
Observe for complaints of pain

Health Teaching
Explain the causes of the health problem
Explain the reason for and intended effect of the therapy
Explain how to apply an elastic bandage

Medical Treatments Performed by Nurses
Give the prescribed drugs (diuretics and antibiotics)

EVALUATION

See the evaluation criteria for each specific goal in Chapter 2.

LYMPH CIRCULATION, POTENTIAL ALTERATION IN

Potential Impaired Lymph Circulation (71,326,453)

ASSESSMENT

Objective Data
Generalized bacterial infection in a limb
Surgical removal of lymph nodes
Neoplasm within the lymph node area

Related Data

Commonly Related Conditions:
Radical mastectomy

Commonly Related Diseases:
Milroy's disease
Filariasis
Chronic lymphedema

POSSIBLE ETIOLOGY

Surgical procedures. Tissue inflammation. Lymph node obstruction by growths.

NURSING DIAGNOSIS

Potential impaired lymph circulation: the possibility that impairment of lymph circulation will occur

PLANNING

Patient Needs

Protection from physical harm

Increased learning

Primary Nurse-Patient Goals

To prevent physical injury

To achieve awareness of needs

NURSING INTERVENTIONS

Nursing Treatments

Apply an elastic bandage
Refrain from tight bandaging
Elevate the extremity
Massage gently
Exercise in range of motion
Refrain from giving intravenous or intramuscular injections (in the susceptible limb)
Remove constrictive clothing
Lubricate the skin with cocoa butter, glycerine, lanolin, mineral oil, or olive oil (several times daily)

Nursing Observations

Monitor the blood pressure (but avoid using the susceptible limb)
Inspect for edema
Inspect the skin for discoloration (redness)

Health Teaching

Advise not to stand for prolonged periods (if the legs are affected)
Explain the causes of the health problem
Explain the reason for and intended effect of the therapy
Explain how to apply an elastic bandage

EVALUATION

See the evaluation criteria for each specific goal in Chapter 2.

EMERGENCY BLOOD LOSS

Emergency Phase Hemorrhage
(71,247)

ASSESSMENT

Subjective Data
Generalized weakness
Anxiety

Objective Data
Decreased blood pressure
Rapid pulse
Rapid respirations
Extreme restlessness
Pallor
Cold skin
Confusion
Loss of consciousness

External Hemorrhage:
Bright red blood from surface wounds

Internal Hemorrhage:
Hematemesis—dark red, black, or brown vomitus
Tarry stools—black, sticky stools
Severe hemoptysis—bright red, frothy sputum
Severe hematuria—bright, red blood in the urine
Postpartum hemorrhage—bright, red blood from the vagina within 48
    hours following delivery

Related Data
Commonly Related Conditions:
Pregnancy
Commonly Related Diseases:
Gastric or peptic ulcer
Esophageal varices
Hemophilia
Trauma wound
Tuberculosis
Carcinoma

POSSIBLE ETIOLOGY

Spontaneous blood vessel rupture. Platelet deficiency. Blood clotting defect.
Trauma. Hemodialysis. Radiation therapy. Surgical procedure.

NURSING DIAGNOSIS

Emergency phase hemorrhage: the immediate loss of 500 cc or more of
blood from the body

PLANNING

Patient Needs	**Primary Nurse-Patient Goals**
Oxygen, circulation	To maintain oxygen to all cells
Water-salt balance	To maintain fluid and electrolyte balance
Sleep, rest	To achieve sleep, rest
Comfort	To achieve comfort
Protection from physical harm	To prevent physical injury
Increased learning	To achieve awareness of needs

NURSING INTERVENTIONS

Nursing Treatments

General Treatments:

Administer humidified oxygen (ET)

Administer intravenous fluids (ET) *(immediately)*

Give water orally (if able to drink and not receiving intravenous fluids, give as much as the patient can comfortably tolerate)

Attend the patient constantly

Cover with lightweight blankets

Handle gently

Maintain a warm room temperature

Place on complete bed rest

Position comfortably

Refrain from giving hot liquids

Refrain from giving oral stimulants

Refrain from local heat applications

Treatments Specific to External Hemorrhage:

Apply an ice bag (to the bleeding area)

Apply manual pressure over the bleeding area

Apply a pressure dressing

Apply a tourniquet between the extremity wound and the body (only if other methods fail)

Elevate the extremity

Immobilize the affected body part

Treatments Specific to Internal Hemorrhage:

Hematemesis or tarry stools—

    Restrict the intake to nothing by mouth

    Place in the flat position

    Refrain from inserting objects into a bleeding orifice

Hematuria—

    Place in the flat position

    Refrain from inserting objects into a bleeding orifice

Severe hemoptysis—

    Apply an ice bag (to the affected chest side)

    Place in the slight sitting (semi-Fowler's, semirecumbent) position

    Place on the affected side

Position with sandbags (to immobilize the chest)
Provide standby emergency equipment (airway suction machine)
Refrain from giving positive pressure breathing
Postpartum hemorrhage—
Elevate the foot of the bed
Massage the uterine fundus

Nursing Observations (Postemergency)
Estimate the blood volume loss
Inspect the chest for respiratory rate and rhythm
Measure the intake
Measure the output
Monitor the blood pressure (frequently)
Monitor blood studies for abnormal hematology
Observe for complaints of pain
Observe for dyspnea
Observe for shock
Palpate the pulse for rate, rhythm, and volume

Health Teaching
Explain the causes of the health problem
Explain the reason for and intended effect of the therapy

Medical Treatments Performed by Nurses
Administer a blood transfusion
Give the prescribed drugs (sedatives)

EVALUATION

See the evaluation criteria for each specific goal in Chapter 2.

EMERGENCY CIRCULATORY AND CARDIAC RESPONSES

Emergency Phase Acute Cardiac Episode (71,271,391)

ASSESSMENT

Subjective Data
Dyspnea
Severe precordial or substernal chest pain
Crushing chest sensation
Pain sometimes radiates to the left arm, shoulder, throat, jaw, or teeth
Nausea
Weakness

Objective Data
Pallor
Cold, clammy skin

Tachycardia
Decreased blood pressure
Vomiting
Loss of consciousness

Related Data
Commonly Related Diseases:
Myocardial infarction
Coronary thrombosis

POSSIBLE ETIOLOGY

Presence of a thrombus in a coronary artery. Arteriosclerotic closure of a
coronary artery.

NURSING DIAGNOSIS

Emergency phase acute cardiac episode: a need for immediate health care
resulting from a disruption of the blood supply to cardiac tissue

PLANNING

Patient Needs	Primary Nurse-Patient Goals
Oxygen, circulation	To maintain oxygen to all cells
Rest	To achieve rest
Comfort	To achieve comfort
Protection from physical harm	To prevent physical injury
Freedom from pain	To achieve comfort
Increased learning	To achieve awareness of needs

NURSING INTERVENTIONS

Nursing Treatments
Administer humidified oxygen (ET)
Elevate the head (unless in shock)
Place on complete bed rest
Cover with warm blankets
Refrain from giving oral stimulants
Attend the patient constantly
Reassure verbally
Consult with the physician (*immediately* if in an institution)
Make a referral (to the local emergency room if in the community)

Nursing Observations
Auscultate the chest for abnormal heart sounds
Auscultate the chest for rales (moist, crackling)
Inspect the chest for respiratory rate and rhythm
Monitor the blood pressure
Palpate the pulse for rate, rhythm, and volume

Health Teaching
Explain the reason for and intended effect of the therapy

Medical Treatments Performed by Nurses
Give the prescribed drugs (nitroglycerine if prescribed from previous cardiac episodes, analgesics)

EVALUATION

See the evaluation criteria for each specific goal in Chapter 2.

Emergency Phase Cardiac Arrest
(71,247,391)

ASSESSMENT

Objective Data
Sudden onset
No audible heartbeat
No audible blood pressure
No palpable pulse
Apnea
Dilated pupils
Cyanosis
Unconsciousness
Death within a few minutes if untreated

Related Data
Commonly Related Diseases:
Ventricular standstill
Commonly Related Diseases:
Myocardial infarction

POSSIBLE ETIOLOGY

Inadequate oxygenation of cardiac muscle fibers which prevents electrical maintenance of normal rhythms. Depressing effects of drugs.

NURSING DIAGNOSIS

Emergency phase cardiac arrest: a need for immediate health care upon the cessation of myocardial contraction and blood circulation

PLANNING

Patient Needs	Primary Nurse-Patient Goals
Oxygen, circulation	To maintain oxygen to all cells
Water-salt balance	To maintain fluid and electrolyte balance
Stimulation	To maintain stimulation
Protection from physical harm	To prevent physical injury
Increased learning	To achieve awareness of needs

NURSING INTERVENTIONS

Nursing Treatments
Insert an oral airway
Resuscitate breathing (ET) (until spontaneous respirations return)

Apply a precordial blow (ET) (if there is no carotid or femoral pulse or respiratons)

Initiate external cardiac massage (ET) (until spontaneous pulsations return and dilated pupils become normal)

Defibrillate the heart muscle (ET) (if cardiac massage is ineffective)

Administer intravenous fluids (ET)

Administer intermittent positive pressure breathing (ET) (after respirations are reestablished)

Elevate the extremities (the legs)

Place on complete bed rest

Attend the patient constantly

Nursing Observations (Postemergency)
Auscultate the apical heartbeat for rate and rhythm
Inspect the chest for respiratory rate and rhythm
Measure the intake
Measure the urine output hourly
Monitor the blood pressure
Monitor the cardiogram (if available)
Palpate for arterial pulsations (the carotid arteries, every 5 minutes)

Health Teaching
Explain the causes of the health problem (after the episode)
Explain the reason for and intended effect of the therapy (after the episode)

Medical Treatments Performed by Nurses
Give the prescribed drugs (epinephrine, sodium bicarbonate)

EVALUATION

See the evaluation criteria for each specific goal in Chapter 2.

Emergency Phase Anaphylactic Shock (19,54,192,247,271)

ASSESSMENT

Subjective Data
Anxiety
Dyspnea
Choking sensation

Objective Data
Edema
Cyanosis
Paresthesia
Coughing
Incontinence
Pupil dilatation
Decreased blood pressure
Unconsciousness
Onset within seconds of drug injection or insect bite, or within 30 minutes

POSSIBLE ETIOLOGY

Foreign protein in the blood produces an antigen-antibody reaction that results in blood vessel constriction

NURSING DIAGNOSIS

Emergency phase anaphylactic shock (emergency phase allergic shock): a need for immediate health care resulting from a sudden circulatory collapse resulting from foreign protein entering the blood

PLANNING

Patient Needs	Primary Nurse-Patient Goals
Oxygen, circulation	To maintain oxygen to all cells
Water-salt balance	To maintain fluid and electrolyte balance
Rest	To achieve rest
Comfort	To achieve comfort
Protection from physical harm	To prevent physical injury
Increased learning	To achieve awareness of needs

NURSING INTERVENTIONS

Nursing Treatments

Insert an oral airway (if needed)

Resuscitate breathing (ET)

Perform a tracheostomy (ET) (only if other respiratory resuscitation methods fail)

Administer humidified oxygen (ET) (if needed)

Administer intermittent positive pressure breathing (ET) (as needed)

Administer intravenous fluids (ET) (electrolyte solutions *immediately*)
    OR

Give salt-soda solution orally (1/2 tsp. baking soda and 1 tsp. salt in one quart water)
    OR

Give water orally (as much as the patient can tolerate up to one quart)

Give nonprescription drugs (ExR) (an antihistamine, use epinephrine in cold compounds or by inhaler if epinephrine is not available for subcutaneous administration)

Apply a tourniquet between the extremity wound and the body (if shock is due to an insect bite)

Place in the slight foot-elevated head-lowered (semi-Trendelenburg) position

Place on complete bed rest

Cover with lightweight blankets

Catheterize with an indwelling urinary catheter (for measuring output)

Maintain a warm room temperature

Provide standby emergency equipment (oxygen, tracheostomy tray)

Attend the patient constantly

Position comfortably

Nursing Observations (Postemergency)
Auscultate the apical heartbeat for rate and rhythm
Inspect the chest for respiratory rate and rhythm
Measure the intake
Measure the urine output hourly
Monitor the blood pressure
Palpate the pulse for rate, rhythm, and volume

Health Teaching
Explain the causes of the health problem (after the episode)
Explain the reason for and intended effect of the therapy (after the episode)

Medical Treatments Performed by Nurses
Give the prescribed drugs (epinephrine 1:1000 subcutaneously)

EVALUATION

See the evaluation criteria for each specific goal in Chapter 2.

Emergency Phase Bacteremic Shock (54,247,300,301,453)

ASSESSMENT

Objective Data
Decreased blood pressure
Fever
Chills
Initially, warm, flushed dry skin
Later, cold, clammy skin
Bounding pulse (early)

Related Data
Age:
Most frequently occurs in very young or very old persons
Commonly Related Diseases:
Diabetes mellitus
Cirrhosis
Carcinoma
Leukemia
Lymphoma
Gastritis
Pyleonephritis
Glomerulonephritis

POSSIBLE ETIOLOGY

The release of bacterial toxins affecting vascular quality

NURSING DIAGNOSIS

Emergency phase bacteremic shock (emergency phase septic shock) (emergency phase endotoxic shock) (emergency phase exotoxic shock): the need for immediate health care due to circulatory collapse resulting from bacterial invasion into the bloodstream

PLANNING

Patient Needs	Primary Nurse-Patient Goals
Oxygen, circulation	To maintain oxygen to all cells
Water-salt balance	To maintain fluid and electrolyte balance
Rest	To achieve rest
Comfort	To achieve comfort
Protection from physical harm	To prevent physical injury
Increased learning	To achieve awareness of needs

NURSING INTERVENTIONS

Nursing Treatments

Administer intravenous fluids (ET) (electrolyte solutions *immediately*)
   OR
Give salt-soda solution orally (1/2 tsp. baking soda and 1 tsp. salt in one quart water)
   OR
Give water orally (as much as the patient can tolerate up to one quart)
Administer humidified oxygen (ET) (if needed)
Place in the flat position
   OR
Place in the slight foot-elevated head-lowered (semi-Trendelenburg) position
Place on complete bed rest
Cover with lightweight blankets
Catheterize with an indwelling urinary catheter (for measuring output)
Maintain a warm room temperature
Provide standby emergency equipment (oxygen, airway suction machine)
Refrain from giving oral stimulants
Position comfortably

Nursing Observations (Postemergency)

Auscultate the apical heartbeat for rate and rhythm
Inspect the chest for respiratory rate and rhythm
Measure the intake
Measure the urine output hourly
Monitor the blood pressure (frequently)
Palpate the pulse for rate, rhythm, and volume

Health Teaching

Explain the causes of the health problem (after the episode)
Explain the reason and intended effect of the therapy (after the episode)

EVALUATION

See the evaluation criteria for each specific goal in Chapter 2.

Emergency Phase Cardiogenic Shock (54,247,300,301)

ASSESSMENT

Subjective Data
Dyspnea
Sudden, severe substernal and abdominal pain
Weakness

Objective Data
Pallor
Cyanosis
Semiconsciousness or unconsciousness
Confusion
Increased respirations
Decreased urinary output
Rapid, irregular, weak pulse
Decreased blood pressure
Crackling rales

Related Data
Commonly Related Diseases:
Cardiac arrhythmias
Commonly Related Diseases:
Myocardial infarction
Coronary thrombosis
Cardiac tamponade
Pulmonary embolism
Congestive heart failure

POSSIBLE ETIOLOGY

Inability of the heart to pump sufficient blood to all body parts, despite normal blood volume, resulting in inadequate circulation

NURSING DIAGNOSIS

Emergency phase cardiogenic shock (emergency phase cardiac failure): the need for immediate health care resulting from circulatory failure with insufficient blood movement through the body for adequate tissue oxygenation

PLANNING

Patient Needs	Primary Nurse-Patient Goals
Oxygen, circulation	To maintain oxygen to all cells
Water-salt balance	To maintain fluid and electrolyte balance
Rest	To achieve rest
Comfort	To achieve comfort
Protection from physical harm	To prevent physical injury
Increased learning	To achieve awareness of needs

NURSING INTERVENTIONS

Nursing Treatments

Administer intravenous fluids (ET) (electrolyte solutions *immediately*)

OR

Give salt-soda solution orally (1/2 tsp. baking soda and 1 tsp. salt in one quart water)

OR

Give water orally (as much as the patient can tolerate up to one quart)

Administer humidified oxygen (ET) (if needed)

Place in the flat position

OR

Place in the slight foot-elevated head-lowered (semi-Trendelenburg) position

Place on complete bed rest

Cover with lightweight blankets

Catheterize with an indwelling urinary catheter (for measuring output)

Maintain a warm room temperature

Provide standby emergency equipment (oxygen, airway suction machine)

Refrain from giving oral stimulants

Nursing Observations (Postemergency)

Auscultate the apical heartbeat for rate and rhythm

Inspect the chest for respiratory rate and rhythm

Measure the intake

Measure the urine output hourly

Monitor the blood pressure

Monitor blood studies for abnormal gas exchange

Monitor the central venous pressure

Palpate the pulse for rate, rhythm, and volume

Health Teaching

Explain the causes of the health problem (after the episode)

Explain the reason for and intended effect of the therapy (after the episode)

Medical Treatments Performed by Nurses

Give the prescribed drugs (antiarrhythmia, vasodilating, or constricting drugs)

EVALUATION

See the evaluation criteria for each specific goal in Chapter 2.

Emergency Phase Electrical Shock (271,453)

ASSESSMENT

Subjective Data

Disoriented

Objective Data

Person is frozen to an electrical source in a rigid position, and is unconscious

Respiratory paralysis

Ventricular fibrillation
Severe burns

POSSIBLE ETIOLOGY

The simultaneous touching of ungrounded electrical wires, tools, or appliances with wet skin or surfaces and the touching of metal objects such as rings, keys, pipes, etc. causes the person to ground himself to the earth. When a person accidentally grounds himself to an electrical current, the full charge of the electrical current is conducted into the person's body, and he becomes part of the electrical circuit.

NURSING DIAGNOSIS

Emergency phase electrical shock: the need for immediate health care as a result of accidental passage of an electric current through the body

PLANNING

Patient Needs	Primary Nurse-Patient Goals
Oxygen, circulation	To maintain oxygen to all cells
Rest	To achieve rest
Comfort	To achieve comfort
Protection from physical harm	To prevent physical injury
Increased learning	To achieve awareness of needs

NURSING INTERVENTIONS

Nursing Treatments
Cut off the electrical power source causing the injury
Remove the person from the electrocuting source with a nonconducting
     material
Resuscitate breathing (ET)
Initiate external cardiac massage (ET)
Defibrillate the heart muscle (ET) (if available)
Administer humidified oxygen (ET) (if available)
Place in the flat position
Cover with lightweight blankets
Give warm liquids (when conscious)
Refrain from giving oral stimulants
Place on complete bed rest
Attend the patient constantly
Make a referral (to a physician)

Nursing Observations (Postemergency)
Auscultate the apical heartbeat for rate and rhythm
Inspect the chest for respiratory rate and rhythm
Measure the intake
Measure the urine output hourly
Monitor the blood pressure
Observe for cyanosis
Palpate the pulse for rate, rhythm, and volume

Health Teaching
Explain the causes of the health problem (after the episode)

Explain the importance of standing on dry surfaces and wearing insulated rubber gloves and rubber soled shoes when working with electricity

Explain the importance of using grounded electrical equipment and appliances

Explain the reason for and intended effect of the therapy

EVALUATION

See the evaluation criteria for each specific goal in Chapter 2.

Emergency Phase Hemorrhagic Shock (54,247,271,300,391)

ASSESSMENT

Subjective Data
Anxiety
Thirst
Dizziness
Weakness
Pain, from injury

Objective Data
Restlessness
Rapid, weak, irregular pulse
Pallor
Cold, wet skin
Decreased blood pressure
Rapid respirations
Cyanosis
Decreased urinary output
Unconsciousness

Related Data
Commonly Related Diseases:
Any disease or injury involving severe hemorrhage

POSSIBLE ETIOLOGY

Excessive blood loss

NURSING DIAGNOSIS

Emergency phase hemorrhagic shock (emergency phase hypovolemic shock) (emergency phase hematogenic shock) (emergency phase surgical shock) (emergency phase traumatic shock) (emergency phase oligemic shock): the need for immediate health care due to circulatory collapse resulting from blood loss causing an inadequate circulating blood volume with impaired tissue oxygenation

PLANNING

Patient Needs
Oxygen, circulation

Primary Nurse-Patient Goals
To maintain oxygen to all cells

Water-salt balance   To maintain fluid and electrolyte balance

Rest   To achieve rest

Comfort   To achieve comfort

Protection from physical harm   To prevent physical injury

Increased learning   To achieve awareness of needs

NURSING INTERVENTIONS

Nursing Treatments

Administer intravenous fluids (ET) (electrolyte solutions *immediately*)

    OR

Give salt-soda solution orally (1/2 tsp. baking soda and 1 tsp. salt in one quart water)

    OR

Give water orally (as much as the patient can tolerate up to one quart)

Administer humidified oxygen (ET) (if needed)

Place in the flat position

    OR

Place in the slight foot-elevated head-lowered (semi-Trendelenburg position)

Place on complete bed rest

Cover with lightweight blankets

Catheterize with an indwelling urinary catheter (for measuring output)

Maintain a warm room temperature

Provide standby emergency equipment (oxygen, suction machine)

Refrain from giving oral stimulants

Nursing Observations (Postemergency)

Auscultate the apical heartbeat for rate and rhythm

Inspect the chest for respiratory rate and rhythm

Measure the intake

Measure the urine output hourly

Monitor the blood pressure

Monitor blood studies for abnormal gas exchange

Monitor the central venous pressure (if available)

Palpate the pulse for rate, rhythm, and volume

Health Teaching

Explain the causes of the health problem (after the episode)

Explain the reason for and intended effect of the therapy (after the episode)

Medical Treatments Performed by Nurses

Administer a blood transfusion

Give the prescribed drugs (sedatives)

EVALUATION

See the evaluation criteria for each specific goal in Chapter 2.

EMERGENCY CIRCULATORY AND CARDIAC RESPONSES, POTENTIAL

Emergency Phase Impending Shock (70,192,391)

ASSESSMENT

Subjective Data
Intense anxiety
Nervousness

Objective Data
Cool, moist skin
Pallor
Lip cyanosis
Rapid, thready pulse
Rapid, shallow respirations
Consistent decreasing blood pressure with a systolic less than 90 mm Hg
Restlessness
Irritability

Related Data
Commonly Related Diseases:
Myocardial infarction
Skull fracture
Trauma wound

POSSIBLE ETIOLOGY

Circulatory failure. Slow, but consistent, blood loss.

NURSING DIAGNOSIS

Emergency phase impending shock: the presence of signs and symptoms indicating that shock is imminent

PLANNING

Patient Needs	**Primary Nurse-Patient Goals**
Oxygen, circulation	To maintain oxygen to all cells
Water-salt balance	To maintain fluid and electrolyte balance
Sleep, rest	To achieve sleep, rest
Comfort	To achieve comfort
Protection from physical harm	To prevent physical injury
Increased learning	To achieve awareness of needs

NURSING INTERVENTIONS

Nursing Treatments
Administer intravenous fluids (ET) (electrolyte solutions)
   OR

Give salt-soda solution orally (1/2 tsp. baking soda and 1 tsp. salt in one
   quart water)
   OR
Give water orally (as much as the patient can tolerate up to one quart)
Cover with lightweight blankets
Place in the slight foot-elevated head-lowered (Semi-Trendelenburg) posi-
   tion
Place on complete bed rest
Refrain from giving iced liquids
Refrain from giving oral stimulants
Catheterize with an indwelling urinary catheter (to measure output)
Provide standby emergency equipment (oxygen)
Attend the patient constantly
Consult with the physician (*immediately* after the emergency treatment
   given)

Nursing Observations
Auscultate the apical heartbeat for rate and rhythm
Inspect the chest for respiratory rate and rhythm
Measure the intake
Measure the urine output hourly
Monitor the blood pressure
Palpate the pulse for rate, rhythm, and volume

Health Teaching
Explain the causes of the health problem
Explain the reason for and intended effect of the therapy

EVALUATION

See the evaluation criteria for each specific goal in Chapter 2.

Predisposition to Shock (70,247)

ASSESSMENT

Subjective Data
Emotional instability
Experiencing severe pain

Objective Data
Malnutrition
Senility or debility
Receiving immunosuppressive therapy
Receiving radiation therapy
Receiving corticosteroid or antihypertensive drugs
Recent local or general anesthesia
Evidence of bleeding

Related Data
Commonly Related Diseases:
Diabetes mellitus
Addison's disease
Hay fever or asthma
Glomerulonephritis

POSSIBLE ETIOLOGY

Decreased physiologic and biologic resistance to stress

NURSING DIAGNOSIS

Predisposition to shock: a susceptibility toward developing shock

PLANNING

Patient Needs

Protection from physical harm

Increased learning

Primary Nurse-Patient Goals

To prevent physical injury

To achieve awareness of needs

NURSING INTERVENTIONS

Nursing Treatments

Place on complete bed rest (if under severe stress)
   OR
Encourage adequate rest
Provide quiet
Cover with lightweight blankets
Handle gently
Maintain a warm room temperature
Reassure verbally
Give nonprescription drugs (ExR) (for pain)

Nursing Observations

Inspect the chest for respiratory rate and rhythm
Monitor the blood pressure
Palpate the pulse for rate, rhythm, and volume

Health Teaching

Explain the causes of the health problem
Explain the reason for and intended effect of the therapy

Medical Treatments Performed by Nurses

Administer a blood transfusion
Administer humidified oxygen
Administer intravenous fluids
Give the prescribed drugs (for pain)

EVALUATION

See the evaluation criteria for each specific goal in Chapter 2.

INADEQUATE HYPERTENSION MANAGEMENT

Inadequate Information Related to Hypertension (59,71,142,247,453)

ASSESSMENT

Subjective Data

Person confirms a lack of information

Objective Data

Person's actions indicate a lack of information regarding:
    what hypertension is
    the signs and symptoms of hypertension
    the causes of hypertension
    those precautions that can be taken to control the disease
    the reason for and effects of treatment

Related Data

Commonly Related Diseases:
Essential or malignant hypertension

POSSIBLE ETIOLOGY

No previous experience with the condition. Lack of instruction.

NURSING DIAGNOSIS

Inadequate information related to hypertension: lack of health information regarding the causes, effects, and therapeutic plan associated with hypertension

PLANNING

Patient Needs	**Primary Nurse-Patient Goals**
Comfort	To achieve comfort
Protection from physical harm	To prevent physical injury
Increased learning	To achieve awareness of needs

NURSING INTERVENTIONS

Nursing Treatments

Approach unhurriedly
Encourage patient questions
Discourage oral stimulants
Discourage smoking
Encourage moderate physical exercise
Discourage strenuous activities
Encourage adequate rest
Encourage decreased fatty-food intake
Encourage decreased sodium-food intake

Nursing Observations

Evaluate the response to teaching

Health Teaching

Explain the causes of the health problem
Advise against exposure to intense heat ⎱ (when on antihypertensive drugs)
Advise not to take hot baths ⎰
Advise that highly emotional situations be avoided
Explain that fatigue should be recognized as a stress factor
Emphasize the danger of excessive body weight
Recommend eating and drinking in moderation
Recommend adherence to a moderate pace of living

Recommend methods for achieving total relaxation
Teach how to take a blood pressure
Inform that a predisposition to the illness exists (in all family members)
Explain the reason for and intended effect of the therapy

EVALUATION

See the evaluation criteria for each specific goal in Chapter 2.

INADEQUATE CARDIAC-DEVICE MANAGEMENT

Inadequate Information Related to Portable Pacemaker Use (391,469,498)

ASSESSMENT

Subjective Data
Person confirms a lack of information

Objective Data
Person's actions indicate a lack of information regarding:
   how the pacemaker functions
   how or when it is worn
   the dangers associated with a pacemaker
   how to care for it

Related Data
Commonly Related Diseases:
Atrial fibrillation
Ventricular fibrillation
A-V heart block with digitalis toxicity
Commonly Related Diseases:
Rheumatic heart disease
Myocardial infarction

POSSIBLE ETIOLOGY

No previous experience with a pacemaker. Lack of instruction.

NURSING DIAGNOSIS

Inadequate information related to portable pacemaker use: lack of knowledge as to how one uses a portable cardiac pacemaker

PLANNING

Patient Needs	**Primary Nurse-Patient Goals**
Comfort	To achieve comfort
Protection from physical harm	To prevent physical injury
Mastery and competence in skills	To achieve optimum function
Increased learning	To achieve awareness of needs

NURSING INTERVENTIONS

Nursing Treatments
Approach unhurriedly
Encourage patient questions
Discourage oral stimulants

Nursing Observations
Check the pacemaker for pacing rate
Evaluate the response to teaching

Health Teaching
Explain that pacemakers are safe
Explain the effects of the specific type pacemaker
Explain how to detect pacemaker failure
Inform that bathing is permitted when wearing a pacemaker
Recommend the use of a pacemaker shirt
Inform that high-frequency signals should be avoided when wearing a pacemaker
Inform that battery-operated objects should be used when wearing a pacemaker (if the pacemaker is temporary [external])
Instruct not to use ungrounded electrical equipment when wearing a pacemaker
Instruct to check the pulse daily when wearing a pacemaker
Teach how to count a pulse
Explain the importance of wearing a Medic Alert tag (if the pacemaker is permanent [implanted])
Explain the reason for and intended effect of the therapy

EVALUATION

See the evaluation criteria for each specific goal in Chapter 2.

10.

NURSING DIAGNOSES RELATED TO
Communication

IMPAIRED COMMUNICATION DELIVERY

Dependence on Communication Assistance Related to Impaired Speech Delivery
(67,188,223,388,437,442,443,490,556)

ASSESSMENT

Subjective Data
Intense frustration
Sense of isolation
Anxiety
May perceive his speech to be logical and clear
Person relies on nurses for:
  assistance through appropriate communication methods
  assistance through appropriate communication devices
  an environment conducive to improved communication

Objective Data
Any of the Following:
The inability to form words or bring forth voice sounds
Maybe able only to blink his eyelids or shake his head for yes and no answers
Unable to organize words into phrases and sentences
Unable to select the correct words to describe what he wants to say
Spoken words are jumbled and unrecognizable
Simply repeats what has just been said
Weak voice sounds
Tremulous, jerky speech
Lisping
Slow, one-syllable-at-a-time speech

Sing-song, writhing up and down speech
Thick, slurred speech
Choppy, stuttering speech
Uncoordinated speech with involuntary disorganized mouth and tongue movements
Spastic, hesitant speech
Uses considerable gesturing

Related Data

Commonly Related Conditions:
Aging
Respiratory distress
Dysarthria
Tracheostomy
Hemiplegia
Deafness
Jargon aphasia
Motor aphasia

Commonly Related Diseases:
Harelip
Cleft palate
Multiple sclerosis
Cerebral vascular accident
Cerebral concussion
Friedreich's ataxia
Chorea
Cerebral tumor
Laryngeal carcinoma
Parkinson's disease
Laryngitis

POSSIBLE ETIOLOGY

Sensory or motor lesions. Congenital malformation of the speech organs. Hearing loss. Nervous system or cerebral disease or injury. Increased intracranial pressure. Vocal cord infection or inflammation. Pressure on the vocal cord from gland enlargement or tumor. Surgical airway. Surgical removal of the larynx. Lack of nerve impulses to the speech organs or cerebral speech center.

NURSING DIAGNOSIS

Dependence on communication assistance related to impaired speech delivery: reliance on nurses to offer assistance in communicating with others when there is an impaired ability to communicate by speech

PLANNING

Patient Needs	**Primary Nurse-Patient Goals**
Comfort	To achieve comfort

Protection from psychologic threat	To prevent emotional injury
Dependence	To achieve comfort
Acceptance	To achieve productive interpersonal relationships
Warm, communicating relationships	To achieve effective verbal and nonverbal communications
Mastery and competence in skills	To achieve optimum function
Increased learning	To achieve awareness of needs and/or use of resources

NURSING INTERVENTIONS

Nursing Treatments
Anticipate needs
Approach unhurriedly
Demonstrate calmness
Reassure verbally
Listen attentively
Provide an atmosphere of acceptance
Provide frequent patient contact
Arrange geographic placement (so the patient can see the nurses)
Provide quiet
Ask simple, direct questions
Encourage simple signal language during impaired communication
Limit communication to one person at a time
Limit patient use of the telephone
Provide picture cards of objects
    OR
Provide words-and-phrases cards
    OR
Provide writing pad and pencil
Refrain from asking the patient to repeat the message too often
Solicit the family's assistance in understanding the patient's speech
Talk with the patient
Touch the patient judiciously

Nursing Observations
Observe for an excessive stress level

Health Teaching
Advise that communication be delayed during fatigue
Describe those behaviors which usually occur in communication impairment
Explain that communication should be encouraged despite impairment
Explain that ill persons are often hypersensitive
Explain that questions need to be phrased for yes and no answers when there is impaired speech delivery
Explain that the tracheostomy must be covered in order to speak
Explain the causes of the health problem

Explain the importance of wearing a Medic Alert tag
Make a referral (to a speech therapist)

EVALUATION

See the evaluation criteria for each specific goal in Chapter 2.

Dependence on Communication Assistance Related to Impaired Writing Ability (437,443,490,556)

ASSESSMENT

Subjective Data
Intense frustration
Embarrassment
Person relies on nurses for:
    assistance through appropriate communication devices
    assistance by writing for the patient

Objective Data
Previously able to write

Any of the Following:
Unable to write sentences that express a meaningful idea
Unable to write or illegible writing

Related Data

Commonly Related Conditions:
Motor agraphia

Commonly Related Diseases:
Parkinson's disease
Cerebral vascular accident
Multiple sclerosis

POSSIBLE ETIOLOGY

Central nervous system lesions affecting the basal ganglion. Muscular incoordination. Injury to the brain's speech and writing center.

NURSING DIAGNOSIS

Dependence on communication assistance related to impaired writing ability: reliance on nurses to offer assistance in communicating with others when there is an impaired ability to communicate by writing

PLANNING

Patient Needs	Primary Nurse-Patient Goals
Protection from psychologic threat	To prevent emotional injury
Dependence	To achieve comfort
Acceptance	To achieve productive interpersonal relationships

Warm, communicating relationships

Mastery and competence in skills

Increased learning

To achieve effective verbal and nonverbal communications

To achieve optimum function

To achieve awareness of needs

NURSING INTERVENTIONS

Nursing Treatments
Approach unhurriedly
Provide an atmosphere of acceptance
Write messages (for the patient)
  OR
Avoid written communication (if it disturbs the person)
Provide alphabet letters for word composition

Nursing Observations
Observe for an excessive stress level

Health Teaching
Explain the causes of the health problem
Explain that ill persons are often hypersensitive
Recommend the use of a typewriter when unable to write

EVALUATION

See the evaluation criteria for each specific goal in Chapter 2.

IMPAIRED COMMUNICATION DELIVERY, POTENTIAL

Impending Speech Loss

ASSESSMENT

Subjective Data
Intense anxiety

Objective Data
Scheduled laryngectomy
Scheduled tracheostomy
Scheduled surgical removal of the tongue

Related Data
Commonly Related Conditions:
Airway obstruction
Commonly Related Diseases:
Laryngeal or tongue carcinoma

POSSIBLE ETIOLOGY

Surgical intervention

NURSING DIAGNOSIS

Impending speech loss: the existence of a situation that indicates that the person will be unable to communicate by speech within the near future

PLANNING

Patient Needs

Comfort

Warm, communicating
   relationships

Increased learning

Primary Nurse-Patient Goals

To achieve comfort

To achieve effective verbal and
   nonverbal communications

To achieve awareness of needs

NURSING INTERVENTIONS

Nursing Treatments
Approach unhurriedly
Arrange geographic placement (so patient can see the nurses)
Demonstrate calmness
Encourage patient questions
Make a referral (to a speech therapist)
Provide frequent patient contact
Provide reliable information
Reassure verbally

Nursing Observations
Observe for an excessive stress level

Health Teaching
Explain that questions need to be phrased for yes and no answers when
   there is impaired speech delivery
Inform that the tracheostomy must be covered in order to speak
Inform that artificial larynxes are available
Inform that esophageal speech therapy is available .

EVALUATION

See the evaluation criteria for each specific goal in Chapter 2.

IMPAIRED COMMUNICATION
RECEPTION

Dependence on Communication
Assistance Related to
Impaired Reading Reception
(67,114,188,368,419,437,442,443,490,556)

ASSESSMENT

Subjective Data
Intense frustration
Person relies on nurses for assistance through appropriate communication
   methods

Objective Data
No visual impairment

Any of the Following:
Unable to determine the meaning of written or printed words when the
   word is seen as a whole
Unable to differentiate similarly shaped letters in a word
Can visualize an object on paper but is unable to determine what it is
Holds books and papers upside down or sideways
May refuse to attempt to read

Related Data
Commonly Related Conditions:
Alexia aphasia
Dyslexia
Agnosia
Commonly Related Diseases:
Cerebral vascular accident
Cerebral tumor

POSSIBLE ETIOLOGY

Cerebral cortex lesions. Bilateral cerebral dominance.

NURSING DIAGNOSIS

Dependence on communication assistance related to impaired reading reception: reliance on nurses to offer assistance in communicating with
others when there is an inability to understand written or printed messages

PLANNING

Patient Needs	**Primary Nurse-Patient Goals**
Comfort	To achieve comfort
Protection from psychologic threat	To prevent emotional injury
Dependence	To achieve comfort
Acceptance	To achieve productive interpersonal relationships
Warm, communicating relationships	To achieve effective verbal and nonverbal communications
Increased learning	To achieve awareness of needs and/or use of resources

NURSING INTERVENTIONS

Nursing Treatments
Approach unhurriedly
Provide an atmosphere of acceptance
Avoid written communications
Offer reading material with familiar content (if the patient wants to read)
Provide objects related to the message (if the patient wants to read)
Read to the patient
Correct misinterpreted messages immediately
Obtain feedback of the communicated message
Make a referral (to a speech therapist)

Nursing Observations
Observe for an excessive stress level

Health Teaching
Advise that communication be delayed during fatigue
Describe those behaviors which usually occur in communication impairment
Explain that ill persons are often hypersensitive
Explain the importance of correct message interpretation
Explain the causes of the health problem

EVALUATION

See the evaluation criteria for each specific goal in Chapter 2.

Dependence on Communication Assistance Related to Impaired Hearing (67,188,388,437,442,443,490,556)

ASSESSMENT

Subjective Data
Intense frustration
Confusion
Person relies on nurses for:
   assistance through appropriate communication methods
   assistance through appropriate communication devices
   an environment conducive to improved communication

Objective Data
Any of the Following:
Cannot hear at all
Can hear only with difficulty
Can hear the spoken words of others clearly, but they are received as jumbled messages having no meaning
Cannot hear messages sent from a close distance but hears distant messages well
Cannot understand the language of the sender of the message

Related Data
Commonly Related Conditions:
Aging
Auditory agnosia
Commonly Related Diseases:
Otitis media
Cerebral vascular accident
Skull fracture
Meniere's disease

POSSIBLE ETIOLOGY

Cerebral cortex lesion. Hearing loss. Different cultural language.

NURSING DIAGNOSIS

Dependence on communication assistance related to impaired hearing: reliance on nurses to offer assistance in communicating with others when there is an inability to clearly understand verbal messages

PLANNING

Patient Needs	Primary Nurse-Patient Goals
Comfort	To achieve comfort
Protection from psychologic threat	To prevent emotional injury
Dependence	To achieve comfort
Acceptance	To achieve productive interpersonal relationships
Warm, communicating relationships	To achieve effective verbal and nonverbal communications
Increased learning	To achieve awareness of needs and/or use of resources

NURSING INTERVENTIONS

Nursing Treatments
Anticipate needs
Approach unhurriedly
Demonstrate calmness
Provide frequent patient contact
Avoid verbal communication (unless the patient can lip read or has partial hearing)
Write messages
    OR
Communicate by gesture
    OR
Provide picture cards of objects
    OR
Provide words-and-phrases cards
    OR
Encourage simple signal language during impaired communication
    OR
Provide a language interpreter
Give one direction at a time
Limit communication to one person at a time
Limit conversation to short discussions
Use simple words and short sentences
Use single-word communication
Provide objects related to the message
Give important messages only when the patient is receptive
Refrain from shouting at persons with communication disorders
Allow time for thought comprehension
Wait for a response to one message before delivering another
Obtain feedback of the communicated message

Correct misinterpreted messages immediately
Repeat the message until it is understood
Touch the patient judiciously

Nursing Observations
Observe for an excessive stress level

Health Teaching
Advise that communication be delayed during fatigue
Describe those behaviors which usually occur in communication impairment
Explain that communication should be encouraged despite impairment
Explain that ill persons are often hypersensitive
Explain that one's face should be kept visible when speaking to a deaf person
Instruct to use simple words when speaking with persons having impaired communication reception
Recommend the use of slow, distinct speech with persons having impaired communication reception
Explain the importance of correct message interpretation
Explain the causes of the health problem
Explain the importance of wearing a Medic Alert tag
Make a referral (to a speech therapist)

EVALUATION

See the evaluation criteria for each specific goal in Chapter 2.

IMPAIRED INTERPERSONAL COMMUNICATION

Difficulty Communicating With the Nurse (Physician)

ASSESSMENT

Subjective Data
Feels threatened or intimidated by the nurse (physician)
Perceives the nurse (physician) with awe
Wants to ask questions or make suggestions but fears a negative response
Is not sure he has a right to active participation in his health care
Does not understand medical terminology used by health personnel

Objective Data
Communication skills are intact
Appears tense
May start to ask a question or make a suggestion, but changes his mind
After the meeting with the nurse (or physician), the patient will then openly communicate to another health person (nursing assistant, etc.) what he would like to have discussed with the nurse (or physician)

Related Data

Commonly Related Diseases.
Any disease or injury

POSSIBLE ETIOLOGY

Patient feelings of inadequacy. Poorly defined role for the patient. Previous unsuccessful nurse (physician)-patient relationships. A busy, uninvolved attitude on the part of health personnel.

NURSING DIAGNOSIS

Difficulty communicating with the nurse (physician): an impaired ability to relate and exchange information, ideas, or suggestions with the nurse (or physician) regarding one's health status and care

PLANNING

Patient Needs	Primary Nurse-Patient Goals
Comfort	To achieve comfort
Protection from psychologic threat	To prevent emotional injury
Acceptance	To achieve productive interpersonal relationships
Warm, communicating relationships	To achieve effective verbal and nonverbal communications
Adequacy	To achieve positive expressions, feelings, reactions
Increased learning	To achieve awareness of needs

NURSING INTERVENTIONS

Nursing Treatments
Approach unhurriedly
Sit with the patient (rather than talking in a standing position)
Reassure verbally (that the patient should take an active role in his care)
Express warmth and friendliness
Express empathy
Use the patient's name frequently
Touch the patient judiciously
Encourage the expression of feelings
Encourage patient (or family) questions
Listen attentively
Provide reliable information
Provide an atmosphere of acceptance
Refrain from negatively criticizing
Consult with the physician (if the person's communication difficulty is with the doctor)

Nursing Observations
Evaluate the significance of emotional distress mannerisms
Evaluate the significance of nonverbal communication

Observe for an excessive stress level

Observe for evidence of a favorable response to therapy (improved communication)

Health Teaching

Explain that the person's emotional response is appropriate and commonly experienced

EVALUATION

See the evaluation criteria for each specific goal in Chapter 2.

INADEQUATE COMMUNICATION ASSISTANCE DEVICE MANAGEMENT

Inadequate Information Related to Use of an Artificial Larynx (573,574)

ASSESSMENT

Subjective Data

Person confirms a lack of information

Objective Data

Person's actions indicate a lack of information regarding:
   the availability of an artificial larynx
   how to place the larynx vibrator either externally against the side of the neck or internally toward the side and back of the mouth in order to produce sound

Related Data

Commonly Related Diseases:

Laryngeal carcinoma

POSSIBLE ETIOLOGY

No previous experience with an artificial larynx. Lack of instruction.

NURSING DIAGNOSIS

Inadequate information related to use of an artificial larynx: lack of information regarding how to use an artificial larynx

PLANNING

Patient Needs	**Primary Nurse-Patient Goals**
Comfort	To achieve comfort
Mastery and competence in skills	To achieve optimum function
Increased learning	To achieve awareness of needs and/or use of resources

NURSING INTERVENTIONS

Nursing Treatments

Approach unhurriedly

Reassure verbally

Encourage patient questions
Make a referral (to a speech therapist)
Encourage the use of an artificial larynx as directed by the speech therapist

Nursing Observations
Evaluate the response to teaching

Health Teaching
Explain that communication should be encouraged despite impairment
Explain that ill persons are often hypersensitive
Inform that artificial larynxes are available

EVALUATION

See the evaluation criteria for each specific goal in Chapter 2.

INADEQUATE COMMUNICATION ASSISTANCE METHOD MANAGEMENT

Inadequate Information Related to Esophageal Speech (573,574)

ASSESSMENT

Subjective Data
Person confirms a lack of information

Objective Data
Person's actions indicate a lack of information regarding:
    the availability of esophageal speech
    the proper technique for esophageal speech

Related Data

Commonly Related Diseases:
Laryngeal carcinoma

POSSIBLE ETIOLOGY

No previous experience with esophageal speech. Lack of information.

NURSING DIAGNOSIS

Inadequate information related to esophageal speech: lack of information regarding how to correctly use esophageal speech

PLANNING

Patient Needs	**Primary Nurse-Patient Goals**
Comfort	To achieve comfort
Mastery and competence in skills	To achieve optimum function
Increased learning	To achieve awareness of needs and/or use of resources

NURSING INTERVENTIONS

Nursing Treatments

Approach unhurriedly

Reassure verbally

Encourage patient questions

Limit conversation to short discussions (when esophageal speech is being learned)

Make a referral (to a speech therapist)

Encourage the use of esophageal speech as directed by the speech therapist

Nursing Observations

Evaluate the response to teaching

Health Teaching

Explain that communication should be encouraged despite impairment

Explain that ill persons are often hypersensitive

Inform that esophageal speech therapy is available

EVALUATION

See the evaluation criteria for each specific goal in Chapter 2.

INADEQUATE COMMUNICATION INFORMATION

Inadequate Information Related to Communication Impairment (388,556)

ASSESSMENT

Subjective Data

Person confirms a lack of information

Objective Data

Person's actions indicate a lack of information regarding:

the best methods to use when communicating with a person having impaired communication

the use of assistive communication devices

the most effective psychologic approach to use with persons having impaired communication

resources available, such as speech therapists

Related Data

Commonly Related Conditions:

Dysarthria

Jargon aphasia

Motor aphasia

Motor agraphia

Auditory agnosia

Commonly Related Diseases:
Cerebral vascular accident
Friedreich's ataxia
Chorea
Parkinson's disease
Multiple sclerosis

POSSIBLE ETIOLOGY

No previous experience with communication impairment. Lack of instruction.

NURSING DIAGNOSIS

Inadequate information related to communication impairment: lack of information regarding how to communicate with the person having impaired communication ability

PLANNING

Patient Needs	**Primary Nurse-Patient Goals**
Comfort	To achieve comfort
Warm, communicating relationships	To achieve effective verbal and nonverbal communications
Mastery and competence in skills	To achieve optimum function
Increased learning	To achieve awareness of needs and/or use of resources

NURSING INTERVENTIONS

Nursing Treatments
Approach unhurriedly
Reassure verbally
Encourage patient questions
Encourage simple signal language during impaired communication

Nursing Observations
Evaluate the response to teaching

Health Teaching
Advise against whispering around ill persons
Advise that communication be delayed during fatigue
Describe those behaviors which usually occur in communication impairment
Explain that communication should be encouraged despite impairment
Explain that poor speech is not outgrown
Explain that questions need to be phrased for yes and no answers when there is impaired speech delivery
Explain the importance of correct message interpretation
Instruct to use simple words when speaking with persons having impaired communication reception
Recommend communication by gesture

Recommend the use of slow, distinct speech with persons having impaired communication reception

EVALUATION

See the evaluation criteria for each specific goal in Chapter 2.

Inadequate Information Related to Delayed Speech Delivery (25,45,337,427)

ASSESSMENT

Subjective Data

Person confirms a lack of information

Objective Data

Person's actions indicate a lack of information regarding how to cope with a child, age 1–3, who freely uses gesture speech rather than verbalize, whose speech cannot be understood by strangers, who is slow in saying single words and sentences, who understands the spoken word, and is a poor listener

POSSIBLE ETIOLOGY

No previous experience with the problem. Lack of instruction.

NURSING DIAGNOSIS

Inadequate information related to delayed speech delivery: lack of information regarding how to cope with a child's failure to acquire understandable speech by the age of three

PLANNING

Patient Needs	Primary Nurse-Patient Goals
Comfort	To achieve comfort
Protection from psychologic threat	To prevent emotional injury
Warm, communicating relationships	To achieve effective verbal and nonverbal communications
Increased learning	To achieve awareness of needs and/or use of resources

NURSING INTERVENTIONS

Nursing Treatments
Approach unhurriedly
Reassure verbally
Encourage parent questions
Make a referral (to a speech therapist)

Nursing Observations
Evaluate the response to teaching

Health Teaching
Advise against responding to gesture speech

Advise early correction of problems
Explain that parental attitudes affect child development
Explain that poor speech is not outgrown
Explain the causes of the health problem (neurologic incoordination, family conflict during the speech learning period from the first to the third birthday)

EVALUATION

See the evaluation criteria for each specific goal in Chapter 2.

11.

NURSING DIAGNOSES RELATED TO
Drug Use

DRUG SIDE EFFECTS: DRUG ACCUMULATION

Drug Toxicity (246)

ASSESSMENT

Subjective Data
Nausea
Euphoria or mental depression
Confusion
Visual disturbances

Objective Data
Drowsiness
Vomiting
Irritability
Poor emotional control
Speech thickness
Involuntary eye movements
Pupillary changes
Respiratory depression
Irregular gait
Lack of coordination
Depressed reflexes

Related Data

Commonly Related Diseases:
Renal insufficiency or failure
Myocardial infarction

POSSIBLE ETIOLOGY

Cumulative effect of certain drugs. Impaired excretion of the drug.

NURSING DIAGNOSIS

Drug toxicity (drug intoxication): a cumulative drug reaction having a poisonous effect

PLANNING

Patient Needs

Waste elimination

Protection from physical harm

Increased learning

Primary Nurse-Patient Goals

To maintain regulating mechanisms and functions

To prevent physical injury

To achieve awareness of needs

NURSING INTERVENTIONS

Nursing Treatments

Attend the patient constantly (until the episode subsides)
Give water orally (as much as the patient can comfortably tolerate)
Withhold the drug

Nursing Observations

Observe the level of consciousness
Inspect the eyes for pupil equality and response changes
Monitor the blood pressure
Inspect the chest for respiratory rate and rhythm
Palpate the pulse for rate, rhythm, and volume

Health Teaching

Explain the causes of the health problem
Explain the reason for and intended effect of the therapy

EVALUATION

See the evaluation criteria for each specific goal in Chapter 2.

DRUG SIDE EFFECTS: SPECIFIC DRUG ACCUMULATION

Digitalis Toxicity (32,247,271,453)

ASSESSMENT

Subjective Data
Nausea
Malaise
Disorientation
Depression
Yellow vision
Blurred vision

Objective Data
Anorexia
Vomiting
Diarrhea sometimes

Dysrhythmias
Confusion

Related Data

Includes such drugs as Digitalis leaf, digoxin, digitoxin, Getalin, Lanatoside C, Quabain, Straphanthin

Persons who are aging, have myocardial infarction, renal insufficiency, hypothryoidism, infants and children are most susceptible

Commonly Related Diseases:
Any disease requiring digitalis therapy

POSSIBLE ETIOLOGY

A cumulative reaction of body cells to digitalis

NURSING DIAGNOSIS

Digitalis toxicity (digitalis intoxication): a cumulative reaction of digitalis preparations causing a poisonous effect

PLANNING

Patient Needs

Protection from physical harm

Increased learning

Primary Nurse-Patient Goals

To prevent physical injury

To achieve awareness of needs

NURSING INTERVENTIONS

Nursing Treatments
Consult with the physician (for drug dosage change)
Withhold the drug (digitalis)

Nursing Observations
Auscultate the apical heartbeat for rate and rhythm
Palpate the pulse for rate, rhythm, and volume

Health Teaching
Explain the causes of the health problem

Medical Treatments Performed by Nurses
Give the prescribed drugs (lidocaine or diphenylhydantoin)

EVALUATION

See the evaluation criteria for each specific goal in Chapter 2.

DRUG SIDE EFFECTS: DRUG ACCUMULATION, POTENTIAL

Potential Drug Toxicity

ASSESSMENT

Objective Data
Renal insufficiency
Dehydration
Debilitation

Related Data

Commonly Related Diseases:
Any disease requiring prolonged drug therapy

POSSIBLE ETIOLOGY

Incorrect drug dosage. Long-term drug therapy. Impaired excretion.

NURSING DIAGNOSIS

Potential drug toxicity (potential drug intoxication): the possibility that a cumulative drug reaction will have a poisonous effect

PLANNING

Patient Needs

Waste elimination

Protection from physical harm

Increased learning

Primary Nurse-Patient Goals

To maintain regulating mechanisms and functions

To prevent physical injury

To achieve awareness of needs

NURSING INTERVENTIONS

Nursing Treatments
Balance fluid intake to equal output

Nursing Observations
Inspect the chest for respiratory rate and rhythm (depression)
Inspect the eyes for pupil equality and response changes
Monitor blood studies for increased digitalis level
Monitor blood studies for increased quinidine level
Observe for complaints of headache
Observe for complaints of malaise
Observe for complaints of nausea
Observe for complaints of pain (abdominal or neuralgic)
Observe for complaints of weakness
Observe for confusion
Observe for emotional instability
Observe for euphoria
Observe for fatigue
Observe for impaired judgment
Observe for irritability
Observe for lethargy
Observe for vomiting
Palpate the pulse for rate (bradycardia), rhythm, and volume

Health Teaching
Describe those symptoms which should be reported (headache, weakness, fatigue, vomiting)
Teach how to count a pulse (if taking digitalis)
Teach how to administer medications

EVALUATION

See the evaluation criteria for each specific goal in Chapter 2.

DRUG SIDE EFFECTS: EXAGGERATED REACTION TO DRUGS

Adrenal-Steroid Intolerance (28,246)

ASSESSMENT

Subjective Data
Generalized weakness
Euphoria or depression

Objective Data
Increased urine output
Moon-faced edema
Restlessness
Increased blood pressure
Excessive weight gain

Related Data
Person is receiving such drugs as cortisone, hydrocortisone, prednisolone, and prednisone

Laboratory Findings:
Increased blood glucose, sodium, erythrocytes
Decreased blood potassium, calcium, phosphorous
Increased urine glucose and uric acid

Commonly Related Diseases:
Addison's disease
Multiple sclerosis

POSSIBLE ETIOLOGY

A therapeutic attempt to offset hyposecretion of adrenal gland hormones. Use of adrenal hormones to treat various diseases.

NURSING DIAGNOSIS

Adrenal-steroid intolerance: an exaggerated reaction to the chemical actions of adrenal hormones which, if given in smaller than normal doses, produces no unusual reaction

PLANNING

Patient Needs	**Primary Nurse-Patient Goals**
Water-salt balance	To maintain fluid and electrolyte balance
Comfort	To achieve comfort
Protection from physical harm	To prevent physical injury
Increased learning	To achieve awareness of needs

NURSING INTERVENTIONS

Nursing Treatments
Consult with the physician (regarding drug dosage change)

Encourage decreased sodium-food intake
Encourage increased potassium-food intake
Encourage increased protein-food intake
Give high-potassium fluids orally
Give low-sodium fluids orally
Refrain from giving enemas (which will further deplete the potassium)
Refrain from giving laxatives
Refrain from giving table salt
Restrict the fluid intake according to the weight gain
Substitute artificial salt

Nursing Observations
Measure the body weight (daily)
Measure the intake
Measure the output
Monitor the blood pressure
Monitor blood studies for abnormal electrolytes

Health Teaching
Explain the causes of the health problem
Explain the reason for and intended effect of the therapy

Medical Treatments Performed by Nurses
Give the prescribed diet (low sodium)
Give the prescribed drugs (diuretics)

EVALUATION

See the evaluation criteria for each specific goal in Chapter 2.

Alcohol Intolerance (246)

ASSESSMENT

Subjective Data
Very severe headache
Nausea

Objective Data
Facial flushing
Inability to stay awake
Poor coordination
Vomiting
Onset following one full drink or less

POSSIBLE ETIOLOGY

More rapid than normal metabolic processes quickly oxidize and hastily release alcohol into the blood and tissue. The person may be allergic to the alcohol itself, the aromatics which flavor the drink, or the cereals used to produce the alcohol. Consumption of champagne and sparkling wines produces quick effects since they contain carbonated beverages in which the absorption rate is increased by the carbon dioxide factor. Consumption of beer produces the slowest effect since it contains proteins and carbohydrates which are slowly absorbed.

NURSING DIAGNOSIS

Alcohol intolerance: an exaggerated reaction to the chemical actions of alcohol which, if given in smaller than normal doses, produces no unusual effect

PLANNING

Patient Needs

Waste elimination

Protection from physical harm

Increased learning

Primary Nurse-Patient Goals

To maintain regulating mechanisms and functions

To prevent physical injury

To achieve awareness of needs

NURSING INTERVENTIONS

Nursing Treatments
Attend the patient constantly (until the episode subsides)
Give hot coffee
   OR
Give hot tea
Give nonprescription drugs (ExR) (sodium bicarbonate)
Give water orally (as much as the patient can comfortably tolerate)
Withhold the drug (alcohol)

Nursing Observations
Inspect the chest for respiratory rate and rhythm
Monitor the blood pressure
Palpate the pulse for rate, rhythm, and volume
Determine the precipitating factors (the specific type alcohol)

Health Teaching
Advice that the precipitating factor (alcohol) be avoided
Explain the causes of the health problem

EVALUATION

See the evaluation criteria for each specific goal in Chapter 2.

Analgesic Intolerance (28,246)

ASSESSMENT

Subjective Data
Anxiety
Impaired concentration
Nausea

Objective Data
Respiratory depression
Stuporousness
Decreased pulse rate
Pupillary constriction
Vomiting

Related Data
Receiving such drugs as morphine, codeine, papaverine, Demerol

POSSIBLE ETIOLOGY

Central nervous system depression

NURSING DIAGNOSIS

Analgesic intolerance: an exaggerated reaction to the chemical actions of pain-relieving drugs which, if given in smaller than normal doses, produces no unusual reaction

PLANNING

Patient Needs

Waste elimination

Protection from physical harm

Increased learning

Primary Nurse-Patient Goals

To maintain regulating mechanisms and functions

To prevent physical injury

To achieve awareness of needs

NURSING INTERVENTIONS

Nursing Treatments

Attend the patient constantly (until the episode subsides)
Consult with the physician (regarding drug dosage change)
Give water orally (as much as the patient can comfortably tolerate)
Withhold the drug (analgesic)

Nursing Observations

Inspect the chest for respiratory rate and rhythm
Monitor the blood pressure
Observe the level of consciousness
Palpate the pulse for rate, rhythm, and volume

Health Teaching

Advise that the precipitating factor (the analgesic drug) be avoided
Explain the causes of the health problem
Explain the importance of wearing a Medic Alert tag

EVALUATION

See the evaluation criteria for each specific goal in Chapter 2.

Antibiotic Intolerance (28,246)

ASSESSMENT

Subjective Data

Numbness and tingling
Gastric irritation
Nausea

Objective Data

Fever
Reduced urine output
Vomiting
Loose stools

Related Data
Person is receiving such drugs as penicillin, erythromycin, Aureomycin, neomycin, Terramycin

Commonly Related Diseases:
Any disease or injury requiring antibiotic therapy

POSSIBLE ETIOLOGY

A chemical reaction of the specific drug

NURSING DIAGNOSIS

Antibiotic intolerance: an exaggerated reaction to the chemical actions of antibiotics which, if given in smaller than normal doses, produces no unusual reaction

PLANNING

Patient Needs

Waste elimination

Protection from physical harm

Increased learning

Primary Nurse-Patient Goals

To maintain regulating mechanisms and functions

To prevent physical injury

To achieve awareness of needs

NURSING INTERVENTIONS

Nursing Treatments
Attend the patient constantly (until the episode subsides)
Consult with the physician (regarding drug dosage changes)
Give water orally (as much as the patient can comfortably tolerate)
Withhold the drug

Nursing Observations
Monitor the blood pressure
Palpate the pulse for rate (tachycardia), rhythm, and volume
Observe for shock

Health Teaching
Advise that the precipitating factor (penicillin) be avoided
Explain the causes of the health problem
Explain the importance of wearing a Medic Alert tag
Explain the reason for and intended effect of the therapy

EVALUATION

See the evaluation criteria for each specific goal in Chapter 2.

Antihypertensive Drug Intolerance (28,32,142,159,453)

ASSESSMENT

Alpha-Methyldopa (Aldomet)

Subjective Data
Drowsiness
Mouth dryness

Malaise
Mental depression

Objective Data
Fever
Bradycardia
Postural hypotension

Guanethidine (Ismelin)

Subjective Data
Dizziness
Faintness

Objective Data
Edema
Postural hypotension

Hydralazine (Apresoline)

Subjective Data
Headache
Weakness
Palpitations
Nausea
Angina type chest pain
Muscle pain

Objective Data
Edema
Skin eruptions

Reserpine

Subjective Data
Nightmares
Mental depression

Objective Data
Nasal stuffiness
Lethargy

Thiazides and Diuretics

Subjective Data
Gastrointestinal irritation
Weakness
Muscle cramps
Headache
Nausea

Objective Data
Hypotension
Skin eruption
Male mammary gland enlargement

Related Data

Laboratory Findings:
Decreased blood potassium

Commonly Related Diseases:
Essential or malignant hypertension

POSSIBLE ETIOLOGY

Chemical reaction of the specific drug

NURSING DIAGNOSIS

Antihypertensive drug intolerance: an exaggerated reaction to the chemical effects of antihypertensive drugs which, if given in smaller than normal doses, produce no unusual reaction.

PLANNING

Patient Needs	**Primary Nurse-Patient Goals**
Protection from physical harm	To prevent physical injury
Increased learning	To achieve awareness of needs

NURSING INTERVENTIONS

Nursing Treatments

Encourage decreased sodium-food intake
Encourage increased potassium-food intake
Give high-potassium fluids orally
} (for muscle weakness, gastric irritation, low blood potassium)

Encourage decreased sodium-fluid intake
Restrict the fluid intake according to the weight gain
} (for edema)

Reassure verbally (that symptoms will subside in a few weeks)
} (for drowsiness, nasal stuffiness, or mouth dryness)

Withhold the drug
Consult with the physician (regarding drug dosage change)
} (for angina type chest pain, bradycardia, fever and malaise, headache, lethargy, male mammary gland enlargement, muscle pain, nightmares, palpitations, severe hypotension, skin eruptions, mental depression lasting more than a few days)

AND
Consult with the physician (regarding any side effects which persist)

Nursing Observations

Monitor the blood pressure
Monitor blood studies for abnormal electrolytes (increased sodium, decreased potassium)

Measure the body weight
Palpate the pulse for rate, rhythm, and volume

Health Teaching
Advise against exposure to intense heat
Advise not to stand for prolonged periods
Explain the need to avoid overexertion (especially strenuous exercise)
Explain how to apply elastic stockings or an elastic bandage (to the legs for
  dizziness, faintness, postural hypotension)
Instruct to change position gradually
Instruct to take medications immediately after meals (for nausea)
Explain the causes of the health problem
Explain the reason for and intended effect of the therapy

Medical Treatments Performed by Nurses
Give the prescribed drugs

EVALUATION

See the evaluation criteria for each specific goal in Chapter 2.

Caffeine Intolerance (28,246)

ASSESSMENT

Subjective Data
Palpitations
Nervousness
Anxiety
Headache
Nausea
Numbness and tingling
Itching

Objective Data
Facial flushing
Tachycardia
Trembling
Irritability
Insomnia
Vomiting
Muscle twitching

Related Data

Commonly Related Diseases:
Hyperthyroidism
Gastric or duodenal ulcer

POSSIBLE ETIOLOGY

In hyperthyroidism, the metabolic rate is so high that the stimulant effect
of caffeine further heightens the already overstimulated cardiac and respiratory systems and produces undesirable effects. Caffeine stimulates
hydrochloric acid in gastric juices.

NURSING DIAGNOSIS

Caffeine intolerance: an exaggerated reaction to the chemical actions of caffeine which, if given in smaller than normal doses, produces no unusual reaction

PLANNING

Patient Needs

Waste elimination

Protection from physical harm

Increased learning

Primary Nurse-Patient Goals

To maintain regulating mechanisms and functions

To prevent physical injury

To achieve awareness of needs

NURSING INTERVENTIONS

Nursing Treatments
Attend the patient constantly (until the episode subsides)
Consult with the physician (regarding drug dosage changes)
Discourage oral stimulants
Discourage smoking
Encourage adequate rest
Give water orally (as much as the patient can comfortably tolerate)
Maintain a cool room temperature
Refrain from giving oral stimulants
Withhold the drug

Nursing Observations
Auscultate the apical heartbeat for rate and rhythm
Monitor the blood pressure
Palpate the pulse for rate (tachycardia), rhythm, and volume

Health Teaching
Advise that the precipitating factor (caffeine) be avoided
Explain the causes of the health problem
Explain the importance of wearing a Medic Alert tag
Explain the reason for and intended effect of the therapy

Medical Treatments Performed by Nurses
Give the prescribed drugs (sedatives)

EVALUATION

See the evaluation criteria for each specific goal in Chapter 2.

Epinephrine Intolerance (28,246)

ASSESSMENT

Subjective Data
Anxiety
Palpitations

Headache
Precordial pain

Objective Data
Pallor
Tremor
Tachycardia
Dyspnea
Rapid respirations
Increased blood pressure
Pulmonary edema

Related Data
Taking such drugs as vasoconstrictors, cardiac stimulants, bronchiole relaxants.

Commonly Related Conditions:
Ventricular fibrillation

Commonly Related Diseases:
Thyrotoxicosis

POSSIBLE ETIOLOGY

Increased metabolic rate due to hyperthryoidism. Increased heart rate from excessive thryoid output is further increased by the epinephrine drug. Epinephrine acts as a vasoconstrictor and increases blood pressure. Allergic response.

NURSING DIAGNOSIS

Epinephrine intolerance: an exaggerated reaction to the chemical actions of epinephrine (adrenalin) which, if given in smaller than normal doses, produces no unusual reaction

PLANNING

Patient Needs
Waste elimination

Protection from physical harm
Increased learning

Primary Nurse-Patient Goals
To maintain regulating mechanisms and functions
To prevent physical injury
To achieve awareness of needs

NURSING INTERVENTIONS

Nursing Treatments
Attend the patient constantly (until the episode subsides)
Consult with the physician (regarding drug dosage change)
Discourage oral stimulants
Discourage smoking
Encourage adequate rest
Give water orally (as much as the patient can comfortably tolerate)
Maintain a cool room temperature
Refrain from giving oral stimulants
Withhold the drug

Nursing Observations
Auscultate the apical heartbeat for rate and rhythm
Monitor the blood pressure
Palpate the pulse for rate (tachycardia), rhythm, and volume

Health Teaching
Advise that the precipitating factor (epinephrine) be avoided
Explain the causes of the health problem
Explain the importance of wearing a Medic Alert tag
Explain the reason for and intended effect of the therapy

Medical Treatments Performed by Nurses
Give the prescribed drugs (sedatives)

EVALUATION

See the evaluation criteria for each specific goal in Chapter 2.

Estrogen-Steroid Intolerance (28,246)

ASSESSMENT

Subjective Data
Nausea
Abdominal cramping
Migraine headache

Objective Data
Vaginal bleeding or spotting
Breast soreness
Vomiting
Abdominal distention

Related Data
Receiving such drugs as diethylstilbestrol, estrone, estradiol
Commonly Related Conditions:
Menopause

POSSIBLE ETIOLOGY

Estrogen drug therapy given to relieve the estrogen deficiency of menopause

NURSING DIAGNOSIS

Estrogen-steroid intolerance: an exaggerated reaction to the chemical actions of estrogen hormones which, if given in smaller than normal doses, produces no unusual reaction

PLANNING

Patient Needs	**Primary Nurse-Patient Goals**
Comfort	To achieve comfort
Protection from physical harm	To prevent physical injury
Increased learning	To achieve awareness of needs

NURSING INTERVENTIONS

Nursing Treatments
Consult with the physician (regarding drug dosage change)
Withhold the drug

Health Teaching
Explain the causes of the health problem

EVALUATION

See the evaluation criteria for each specific goal in Chapter 2.

Insulin Intolerance (70,246)

ASSESSMENT

Subjective Data
Generalized weakness

Related Data
Laboratory Findings:
Decreased blood glucose
Decreased blood sodium
Commonly Related Conditions:
Hypoglycemia
Commonly Related Diseases:
Addison's disease

POSSIBLE ETIOLOGY

In Addison's disease, the lack of adrenalin prevents the adequate conversion of protein into glucose, causing periodic hypoglycemia. If the patient were to receive insulin, the glucose level would decrease even further.

NURSING DIAGNOSIS

Insulin intolerance: an exaggerated reaction to the chemical actions of insulin

PLANNING

Patient Needs
Protection from physical harm
Increased learning

Primary Nurse-Patient Goals
To prevent physical injury
To achieve awareness of needs

NURSING INTERVENTIONS

Nursing Treatments
Administer intravenous fluids (ET) (10% dextrose in water)
Attend the patient constantly (until the episode subsides)
Give high-glucose fluids orally (immediately)
Give high-sodium fluids orally
Withhold the drug (insulin)

Nursing Observations
Monitor the blood pressure
Monitor blood studies for abnormal electrolytes (decreased sodium)

Monitor blood studies for abnormal (decreased) glucose
Palpate the pulse for rate, rhythm, and volume

Health Teaching
Explain the causes of the health problem
Explain the importance of wearing a Medic Alert tag

EVALUATION

See the evaluation criteria for each specific goal in Chapter 2.

Salicylate Intolerance (28,246)

ASSESSMENT

Subjective Data
Nausea
Tinnitus
Dizziness

Objective Data
Increased respirations

POSSIBLE ETIOLOGY

Adverse drug effects on the central nervous system.

NURSING DIAGNOSIS

Salicylate intolerance: an exaggerated reaction to the chemical actions of salicylates which, if given in smaller than normal doses, produce no reaction

PLANNING

Patient Needs	**Primary Nurse-Patient Goals**
Waste elimination	To maintain regulating mechanisms and functions
Protection from physical harm	To prevent physical injury
Increased learning	To achieve awareness of needs

NURSING INTERVENTIONS

Nursing Treatments
Attend the patient constantly (until the episode subsides)
Consult with the physician (regarding drug dosage change)
Give water orally (as much as the patient can comfortably tolerate)
Withhold the drug

Nursing Observations
Inspect the chest for respiratory rate and rhythm (until the episode subsides)

Health Teaching
Advise that the precipitating factor (salicylates) be avoided
Explain the causes of the health problem
Explain the importance of wearing a Medic Alert tag
Explain the reason for and intended effect of the therapy

EVALUATION

See the evaluation criteria for each specific goal in Chapter 2.

Sedative Intolerance (28,246)

ASSESSMENT

Subjective Data
Prolonged depression
Unpleasant dreams

Objective Data
Respiratory depression or failure
Bradycardia
Severe listlessness
Restlessness
Delirium
Stupor
Coma

Related Data
Is receiving such drugs as chloral hydrate, paraldehyde, bromides, barbiturates (Seconal, Nembutal, Phenobarbital, Dilantin)
Commonly Related Diseases:
Cretinism

POSSIBLE ETIOLOGY

In hypothyroidism, the basal metabolic rate is below normal. Sedative drugs reduce this level even further and depress smooth muscle action. The low metabolic rate in hypothyroidism increases the time needed for excretion and prolongs drug effects on the body.

NURSING DIAGNOSIS

Sedative intolerance: an exaggerated reaction to the chemical actions of sedatives which, if given in smaller than normal doses, produce no unusual reaction

PLANNING

Patient Needs	**Primary Nurse-Patient Goals**
Waste elimination	To maintain regulating mechanisms and functions
Stimulation	To maintain sensory function and stimulation
Protection from physical harm	To prevent physical injury
Increased learning	To achieve awareness of needs

NURSING INTERVENTIONS

Nursing Treatments
Administer humidified oxygen (ET) (for severe respiratory distress)
Ambulate the patient (if possible)

Attend the patient constantly (until the episode subsides)
Give hot coffee
   OR
Give hot tea
Increase fluid intake to about 2000 cc daily (until the episode subsides)
Stimulate by movement, touch, sternal pressure, or speech
Withhold the drug

Nursing Observations
Monitor the blood pressure
Inspect the chest for respiratory rate and rhythm
Palpate the pulse for rate, rhythm, and volume

Health Teaching
Advise that the precipitating factor (sedative) be avoided
Explain the causes of the health problem
Explain the importance of wearing a Medic Alert tag
Explain the reason for and intended effect of the therapy

Medical Treatments Performed by Nurses
Give the prescribed drugs (caffeine or epinephrine)

EVALUATION

See the evaluation criteria for each specific goal in Chapter 2.

DRUG SIDE EFFECTS: EXAGGERATED REACTION TO DRUGS, POTENTIAL

Potential Drug Intolerance

ASSESSMENT

Objective data
Underweight
Debilitated
Increased metabolic rate
Decreased metabolic rate
Known intolerances to specific substances

Related Data

Commonly Related Conditions:
Cachexia

Commonly Related Diseases:
Thyrotoxicosis
Cretinism
Addison's disease

POSSIBLE ETIOLOGY

Excessively rapid drug absorption. Too large a drug dose for the debilitated body.

NURSING DIAGNOSIS

Potential drug intolerance: the probability that an exaggerated reaction to a drug will occur

PLANNING

Patient Needs

Protection from physical harm

Increased learning

Primary Nurse-Patient Goals

To prevent physical injury

To achieve awareness of needs

NURSING INTERVENTIONS

Nursing Treatments

Administer a drug sensitivity test

Withhold the drug (if the intolerance known)

Nursing Observations

Inspect the chest for respiratory rate and rhythm (depressed or rapid)

Inspect the eyes for pupil equality and response changes

Inspect for edema

Inspect the hands for tremors

Inspect the skin for discoloration (flushing)

Inspect the skin for pallor

Monitor the blood pressure

Observe for complaints of dizziness

Observe for complaints of headache

Observe for complaints of itching

Observe for complaints of nausea

Observe for complaints of numbness and tingling

Observe for complaints of pain

Observe for complaints of tinnitus

Observe for complaints of weakness

Observe for confusion

Observe for diarrhea

Observe for dyspnea

Observe for emotional instability

Observe for euphoria

Observe for irritability

Observe for lethargy

Observe for nasal congestion

Observe for nervousness

Observe for restlessness

Observe for tetany

Observe for vomiting

Palpate the pulse for rate, rhythm, and volume

Health Teaching

Describe those symptoms which should be reported (dizziness, itching, weakness, vomiting, etc.)

Explain the importance of wearing a Medic Alert tag (if the intolerance is known)

Recommend that self-medication be avoided

EVALUATION

See the evaluation criteria for each specific goal in Chapter 2.

DRUG SIDE EFFECTS: SPECIFIC EXAGGERATED REACTIONS TO DRUGS, POTENTIAL

Impending Drug Deafness

ASSESSMENT

Subjective Data
Complaints of hearing difficulty

Objective Data
Failure to respond to verbal communications as well as previously
Prolonged streptomycin therapy

Related Data
Commonly Related Diseases:
Tuberculosis

POSSIBLE ETIOLOGY

Damaging effect of drugs on the auditory nerves and tissue

NURSING DIAGNOSIS

Impending drug deafness: deafness which is threatening to occur as a result
of drug therapy

PLANNING

Patient Needs
Protection from physical harm

Increased learning

Primary Nurse-Patient Goals
To prevent phyical injury

To achieve awareness of needs

NURSING INTERVENTIONS

Nursing Treatments
Consult with the physician (regarding drug dosage change)
Withhold the drug

Nursing Observations
Test the ears for impaired hearing

Health Teaching
Explain the causes of the health problem

EVALUATION

See the evaluation criteria for each specific goal in Chapter 2.

Potential Flora Suppression

ASSESSMENT

Objective Data
Prolonged antibiotic therapy
High doses of antibiotics
Debilitation

Related Data
Taking such drugs as penicillin, chloramphenicol, Aureomycin, and Terramycin
Increased susceptibility during pregnancy and in diabetics
Commonly Related Diseases:
Monilia vaginal infection
Pulmonary moniliasis

POSSIBLE ETIOLOGY

When antibiotics destroy the bacteria for which they are intended, they also destroy normal bacteria. This allows organisms unaffected by the drug, which are no longer held in check by normal bacteria, to flourish and infect other body sites.

NURSING DIAGNOSIS

Potential flora suppression: the possibility that antibiotics may destroy the body's normal bacteria flora and cause infections in the intestines, respiratory tract, or vagina

PLANNING

Patient Needs	**Primary Nurse-Patient Goals**
Protection from physical harm	To prevent physical injury
Increased learning	To achieve awareness of needs

NURSING INTERVENTIONS

Nursing Treatments
Give buttermilk or yogurt (daily until drug therapy is terminated)
Give nonprescription drugs (ExR) (Lactinex)

Nursing Observations
Inspect the mucous membranes for abnormalities (white oral patches)
Inspect the nails for abnormalities (brownish color)
Monitor the oral temperature (for fever)
Observe for complaints of malaise
Observe for complaints of itching (vaginal or anal)
Observe for coughing

EVALUATION

See the evaluation criteria for each specific goal in Chapter 2.

DRUG ABUSE, POTENTIAL

Potential Drug Dependence
(17,32,88,501)

ASSESSMENT

Subjective Data
Enjoys the pleasurable effects of drugs

Objective Data
Intake of alcohol, drugs, or tobacco for anxiety, pain, or problem relief
Gradually increases the amount and/or frequency of drug or alcohol intake
Complaints of illness-related pain long after pain normally should have
   subsided
Children observing adults using drugs or alcohol excessively
Drug addiction by a pregnant mother
Emotional instability

Related Data
Commonly Related Conditions:
Tobacco habituation
Commonly Related Diseases:
Alcoholism
Drug addiction

POSSIBLE ETIOLOGY

Poor problem-solving ability. Prolonged drug use for therapeutic reasons.
Easy accessibility to the purchase of drugs.

NURSING DIAGNOSIS

Potential drug dependence: the possibility that dependency on drugs could
occur

PLANNING

Patient Needs	**Primary Nurse-Patient Goals**
Protection from physical harm	To prevent physical injury
Protection from psychologic threat	To prevent emotional injury
Increased learning	To achieve awareness of needs

NURSING INTERVENTIONS

Nursing Treatments
Accept and attempt to relieve unexplainable body complaints (with
   methods other than drugs)
Approach unhurriedly
Give drugs judiciously for emotional repression
Give nonprescription drugs (ExR) (that do not support dependence)
Make a referral (to the psychiatric nurse specialist)

Nursing Observations
Observe for euphoria (following drug administration)
Observe for an excessive stress level
Observe for requests for increased drug dosage
Observe the newborn for drug withdrawal

Health Teaching
Advise early correction of problems
Explain how to obtain release from emotional stress
Explain that drug dependence is an illness
Explain that drug use is not socially essential
Explain that it is essential to foster healthy drinking attitudes
Explain that long-term drug abuse reduces the pleasures derived from drug abuse
Explain that the use of drugs to solve problems is dangerous
Explain the importance of setting an example through abstinence from drug use
Explain the importance of staying well informed on drug abuse
Explain the psychologic cause of organic pain
Explain why persons resort to drug abuse
Recommend that self-medication be avoided
Teach how to use the problem-solving method

EVALUATION

See the evaluation criteria for each specific goal in Chapter 2.

DRUG THERAPY DEPENDENCE

Dependence on Drug Therapy Management

ASSESSMENT

Subjective Data
Person relies on nurses for:
    the administration of drug(s) in correct doses and at appropriate times
    observation and prevention of drug side effects

Objective Data
Person is receiving drug therapy

Related Data
Commonly Related Diseases:
Any disease requiring drug therapy

POSSIBLE ETIOLGGY

Lack of skill in drug administration. Impaired cerebral function.

NURSING DIAGNOSIS

Dependence on drug therapy management: reliance on nurses to provide the correct drugs, in appropriate doses at specific times

PLANNING

Patient Needs

Protection from physical harm

Dependence

Increased learning

Primary Nurse-Patient Goals

To prevent physical injury

To achieve comfort

To achieve awareness of needs

NURSING INTERVENTIONS

Nursing Treatments
Acknowledge dependence

Nursing Observations
Observe for drug reactions

Health Teaching
Describe those symptoms which should be reported (specific to the side effect of the drug)
Explain the reason for and intended effect of the (drug) therapy

Medical Treatment Performed by Nurses
Give the prescribed drugs

EVALUATION

See the evaluation criteria for each specific goal in Chapter 2.

Dependence on Nursing Supervision of Prescribed Drug Therapy

ASSESSMENT

Subjective Data
Person relies on nurses for:
    observation for drug side effects
    evaluation of the body's response in relation to the intended effect of the
        drug

Objective Data
Person is receiving prolonged drug therapy
Person is taking drugs prescribed by a physician

Related Data
Commonly Related Diseases:
Hypertension
Rheumatoid arthritis
Influenza

POSSIBLE ETIOLOGY

Taking drugs in the home situation. Unavailability of frequent medical attention.

NURSING DIAGNOSIS

Dependence on nursing supervision of prescribed drug therapy: reliance on nurses to intermittently evaluate the safety and effectiveness of prolonged drug therapy

PLANNING

Patient Needs
Protection from physical harm
Increased learning

Primary Nurse-Patient Goals
To prevent physical injury
To achieve awareness of needs

NURSING INTERVENTIONS

Nursing Treatments
Consult with the physician (when necessary)

Nursing Observatons
Observe for drug reactions
Observe for evidence of a favorable response to therapy

Health Teaching
Explain the reason for and intended effect of the therapy

EVALUATION

See the evaluation criteria for each specific goal in Chapter 2.

DRUG THERAPY DISCOMFORTS

Difficulty Ingesting Distasteful Drug(s)

ASSESSMENT

Subjective Data
Bitter, sour, or undesirable taste

Objective Data
Taking liquid or powdered drugs
Displeased facial expression
Refusal to take the drug after the first taste
Unfavorable appearance of the drug

Related Data

Commonly Related Diseases:
Any disease requiring drug therapy

POSSIBLE ETIOLOGY

The unfavorable taste of the chemicals from which drugs are made

NURSING DIAGNOSIS

Difficulty ingesting distasteful drug(s): the discomfort of having to take an unfavorable-tasting drug for health purposes

PLANNING

Patient Needs
Comfort
Protection from physical harm
Increased learning

Primary Nurse-Patient Goals
To achieve comfort
To prevent physical injury
To achieve awareness of needs

NURSING INTERVENTIONS

Nursing Treatments
Approach unhurriedly
Dilute the medication
Disguise drugs with fruit-flavored syrup
Do not disguise drugs in food
Follow distasteful drugs with fruit juice
Refrain from forcing distasteful drugs

Health Teaching
Explain the reason for and intended effect of the therapy

EVALUATION

See the evaluation criteria for each specific goal in Chapter 2.

DRUG THERAPY INACCURACY

Drug Duplication

ASSESSMENT

Subjective Data
Person mistakingly believes he is taking two or more different drugs
Conscienciously adheres to the prescribed dosages of each prescription
May or may not complain of toxic effects depending upon drug dosages and
   the length of time the duplication has occurred

Objective Data
Drugs were obtained by prescription
Each drug container is labeled correctly but one with the chemical name
   and the other with the generic name or with two different chemical or
   generic names for the same chemical compound
Each prescription appears to be a different drug, being of different color
   and pill or capsule size

Related Data

Commonly Related Diseases:
Any disease requiring drug therapy

POSSIBLE ETIOLOGY

Failure of the patient to inform the physician of his current drug therapy.
The person goes to several physicians, each of whom arrives at the same
diagnosis and prescribes the same drug therapy, being unaware that the
patient is seeking other medical advice. The existence of different generic
and chemical names for the same drug. The manufacture of the same drug
in different colors and sizes under different names.

NURSING DIAGNOSIS

Drug duplication: the simultaneous intake of multiple prescriptions of a
single drug that the patient believes to be several different drugs because of
drug labeling and appearances

PLANNING

Patient Needs

Protection from physical harm

Increased learning

Primary Nurse-Patient Goals

To prevent physical injury

To achieve awareness of needs

NURSING INTERVENTIONS

Nursing Treatments

Withhold the drug(s)

Increase the fluid intake to about 2000 cc daily (for several days)

Provide reliable information (regarding generic and chemical drug names)

Consult with the physician(s) (who prescribed the drugs)

Nursing Observations

Observe for drug reactions (specific to the drug)

Auscultate the apical heartbeat for rate and rhythm

Palpate the pulse for rate, rhythm, and volume

Inspect the chest for respiratory rate and rhythm

Health Teaching

Describe the manifestations of a drug reaction

Describe those symptoms which should be reported

Explain the reason for and intended effect of the therapy

EVALUATION

See the evaluation criteria for each specific goal in Chapter 2.

Inaccurate Therapeutic Drug Management

ASSESSMENT

Subjective Data

Person knows how to correctly take his medications

Objective Data

Medications are being taken at the wrong time of day

Drug dosages are incorrect

Drug preparation may be incorrect

Person may be taking the correct or incorrect drug

There is no drug duplication

Related Data

Commonly Related Diseases:

Any disease requiring drug therapy

POSSIBLE ETIOLOGY

Apathy. Determining one's own drug dosage according to how one feels. Suggestions from friends or relatives that the drugs be taken in a way not consistent with the prescription instructions.

NURSING DIAGNOSIS

Inaccurate therapeutic drug management: failure to give oneself the proper dosage of medication as prescribed by health personnel

PLANNING

Patient Needs

Protection from physical harm

Independence

Increased learning

Primary Nurse-Patient Goals

To prevent physical injury

To achieve optimum function

To achieve awareness of needs

NURSING INTERVENTIONS

Nursing Treatments

Give explicit directions (as to how and when the medications should be taken)

Provide frequent patient contact

Refrain from negatively criticizing

Explore with the patient reasons for recurring problems

Involve the family

Withhold the drug(s) (if the inaccuracy is chronic and potentially dangerous)

Consult with the physician (so he knows that the wrong dosages are being taken)

Nursing Observations

Observe for drug reactions

Observe for impaired judgment

Observe for impaired learning ability

Health Teaching

Explain the reason for and intended effect of the therapy (drug)

Describe the manifestations of a drug reaction

Describe the specific dangerous effects of poor health practices (regarding drugs)

Recommend that self-medication be avoided

EVALUATION

See the evaluation criteria for each specific goal in Chapter 2.

EMERGENCY DRUG SITUATIONS: POISONING

Emergency Phase Analgesic Poisoning (70,271,602)

ASSESSMENT

Note: Each analgesic has specific signs and symptoms for poisoning. Those presented here are *generally* applicable to analgesic poisoning.

Subjective Data

Mouth and throat dryness

Headache

Nausea

Blurred vision, sometimes

Objective Data
Pupil constriction followed by dilatation
Giddiness or euphoria
Slow, shallow, depressed respirations
Hypertension or hypotension
Tachycardia or bradycardia
Hot, dry or cold, clammy skin
Vomiting, sometimes
Convulsions
Progressive drowsiness, stupor, and unconsciousness

Related Data
Has ingested such drugs as opium (morphine, codeine), Demerol, etc.

Commonly Related Diseases:
None
   OR
Any disease or injury

POSSIBLE ETIOLOGY

Accidental or intentional drug ingestion

NURSING DIAGNOSIS

Emergency phase analgesic poisoning: the need for immediate health care upon the intake of excessive pain-relief medication

PLANNING

Patient Needs	**Primary Nurse-Patient Goals**
Oxygen, circulation	To maintain oxygen to all cells
Waste elimination	To maintain regulating mechanisms and functions
Stimulation	To maintain sensory function and stimulation
Protection from physical harm	To prevent physical injury
Increased learning	To achieve awareness of needs

NURSING INTERVENTIONS

Nursing Treatments
Resuscitate breathing (ET) (if necessary)
Administer humidified oxygen (ET)
Stimulate by movement, touch, sternal pressure, or speech
Give the universal antidote orally
   OR
Give hot coffee
   OR
Give hot tea
   OR
Give milk
   OR

Give magnesium sulfate solution orally
Lavage the stomach (ET)
Administer intravenous fluids (ET)
   OR
Give water orally (age 1–5 years, give 1–2 cups; over 5 years, give up to 1
   quart)
Attend the patient constantly (until the episode subsides)
Save the poison container for content analysis
Make a referral (to a physician, emergency room, or poison control center)

Nursing Observations
Inspect the chest for respiratory rate and rhythm
Measure the intake
Measure the output (for reduced urine output)
Monitor the blood pressure
Observe for shock
Palpate the pulse for rate, rhythm, and volume

Health Teaching
Emphasize that medicine cabinets should be locked
Recommend that self-medication be avoided
Explain the reason for and intended effect of the therapy

Medical Treatments Performed by Nurses
Give the prescribed drugs

EVALUATION

See the evaluation criteria for each specific goal in Chapter 2.

Emergency Phase Corrosive Poisoning (70,247,271,602)

ASSESSMENT

Note: Each caustic poison has specific signs and symptoms. Those presented here are *generally* applicable to corrosive poisons.

Subjective Data
Burning mouth, throat, esophageal, or abdominal pain
Nausea
Headache
Intense thirst

Objective Data
Corrosion or necrosis of lip, mouth, or throat mucous membranes
Restlessness
Vomiting
Diarrhea
Cold, clammy or dry, moist skin
Tremors
Weak, rapid, or slow pulse
Respiratory distress

Convulsions
Unconsciousness
Decreased temperature
Decreased blood pressure

Related Data
Person has ingested:
  a corrosive acid: iodine, sulfuric, Nitric, hydrochloric, or acetic acid,
    phenol (carbolic acid)
  a corrosive alkali: lye (sodium hydroxide), ammonia, washing soda
    (sodium carbonate), household bleach (sodium hypochlorite), potas-
    sium hydroxide (potash)

POSSIBLE ETIOLOGY

Accidental or intentional ingestion

NURSING DIAGNOSIS

Emergency phase corrosive poisoning: the need for immediate health care
upon the ingestion of poisonous products that have a necrotic effect on tissue

PLANNING

Patient Needs	**Primary Nurse-Patient Goals**
Waste elimination	To maintain regulating mechanisms and functions
Rest	To achieve rest
Comfort	To achieve comfort
Protection from physical harm	To prevent physical injury
Increased learning	To achieve awareness of needs and/or use of resources

NURSING INTERVENTIONS

Nursing Treatments
Give an antidote as recommended ⎫
  on the poison-container label   ⎪
  OR   ⎪
Give the universal antidote orally ⎬ (for any corrosive poison)
  OR   ⎪
Give charcoal solution orally   ⎪
  OR   ⎪
Give milk   ⎭
Give citrus fruit juice (for corrosive alkalis)
Give olive oil orally   ⎫
  OR   ⎬ (for ammonia, lye, washing soda,
Give raw egg white orally ⎭ phenol)
Give vinegar solution orally (for ammonia, lye, washing soda)
Give hot coffee (for phenol)
Give starch paste orally (for iodine)

Administer intravenous fluids (ET)
   OR
Give water orally (age 1–5 years, give 1–2 cups; over 5 years, give up to 1
   quart)
Refrain from gastric lavage
Do not induce vomiting (for corrosive poisons)
Refrain from giving bicarbonates (for acid corrosives)
Refrain from giving laxatives
Cover with warm blankets
Encourage adequate rest
Attend the patient constantly
Save the poison container for content analysis
Make a referral (to a physician, emergency room, or poison control center)

Nursing Observations
Inspect the chest for respiratory rate and rhythm
Inspect for hemorrhage (gastrointestinal)
Measure the intake
Measure the output (for reduced urine output)
Monitor the blood pressure
Observe for complaints of pain (abdominal or esophageal)
Observe for convulsions
Observe the level of consciousness
Palpate the pulse for rate, rhythm, and volume

Health Teaching
Emphasize that dangerous products should be stored out of reach

Medical Treatments Performed by Nurses
Give the prescribed drugs

EVALUATION

See the evaluation criteria for each specific goal in Chapter 2.

Emergency Phase Noncorrosive
Poisoning (70,247,271,602)

ASSESSMENT

Note: Each noncaustic poison has specific signs and symptoms. Those presented here are *generally* applicable to noncorrosive poisons.

Subjective Data
Burning mouth, throat, esophageal, or abdominal pain
Colicky abdominal pain
Nausea
Hallucinations or delirium
Headache
Thirst

Objective Data
Mental excitement or depression
Restlessness

Muscle twitching
Vomiting
Diarrhea
Cold, clammy skin
Weak, rapid pulse
Respiratory distress
Convulsions
Skin eruptions
Decreased blood pressure

Related Data

Person has ingested arsenic, aspirin, benzene (gasoline, kerosene, naphtha lighter or cleaning fluid), bichloride of mercury, bromides, camphor, cold or headache compounds, DDT, isopropyl (rubbing) alcohol, napthalene (moth balls), oil of wintergreen, pep pills, phosphorous, sodium fluoride, strychnine, turpentine, pine oil

POSSIBLE ETIOLOGY

Accidental or intentional ingestion

NURSING DIAGNOSIS

Emergency phase noncorrosive poisoning: the need for immediate health care upon the ingestion of poisonous products that do not necrose tissue

PLANNING

Patient Needs	Primary Nurse-Patient Goals
Waste elimination	To maintain regulating mechanisms and functions
Rest	To achieve rest
Comfort	To achieve comfort
Protection from physical harm	To prevent physical injury
Increased learning	To achieve awareness of needs and/or use of resources

NURSING INTERVENTIONS

Nursing Treatments

Induce vomiting *immediately* (except for petroleum products such as napthalene, benzene, or unless stuporous, unconscious, or convulsing)
Give an antidote as recommended on the poison container label
    OR
Give the universal antidote orally (for any noncorrosive poison)
    OR
Give milk (except for DDT, napthalene, bromides, phosphorus)
Give hot coffee (for napthalene and camphor)
Give hot tea (for napthalene)
Give magnesium sulfate solution orally (for DDT, bromides, bichloride or mercury)
Give raw egg white orally (for mercury)

Give sodium bicarbonate solution orally (for iron compounds, oil of winter-
  green, rubbing alcohol, cold or headache compounds, and phosphorus)
Give vegetable oil orally (for gasoline, pine oil, kerosene, turpentine)
Refrain from giving animal or vegetable oil orally (for DDT or phosphorus)
Lavage the stomach (ET)
Administer intravenous fluids (ET)
  OR
Give water orally (age 1–5 years, give 1–2 cups; over 5 years, give up to 1
  quart)
Cover with warm blankets
Encourage adequate rest
Attend the patient constantly (until the episode subsides)
Save the poison container for content analysis
Make a referral (to a physician, emergency room, or poison control center)

Nursing Observations
Inspect the chest for respiratory rate and rhythm
Inspect for hemorrhage (gastrointestinal)
Measure the intake
Measure the output (for reduced urine output)
Monitor the blood pressure
Observe for complaints of pain (abdominal)
Observe for convulsions
Observe the level of consciousness
Palpate the pulse for rate, rhythm, and volume

Health Teaching
Emphasize that dangerous products should be stored out of reach
Emphasize that medicine cabinets should be locked

Medical Treatments Performed by Nurses
Give the prescribed drugs

EVALUATION

See the evaluation criteria for each specific goal in Chapter 2.

Emergency Phase Sedative Poisoning (70,271)

ASSESSMENT

Note: Each sedative has specific signs and symptoms for poisoning. Those
presented here are *generally* applicable to sedative poisoning.

Subjective Data
Headache
Confusion

Objective Data
Pupil constriction or dilatation
Respiratory depression
Depressed or absent corneal and deep reflexes

Decreased urine output, sometimes
Progressive drowsiness, stupor, and unconsciousness

Related Data

Person has ingested Seconal, Nembutal, phenobarbital, Doriden, or other
sedatives

POSSIBLE ETIOLOGY

Accidental or intentional intake

NURSING DIAGNOSIS

Emergency phase sedative poisoning: the need for immediate health care
upon the intake of excessive sleep-inducing medication

PLANNING

Patient Needs	Primary Nurse-Patient Goals
Oxygen, circulation	To maintain oxygen to all cells
Waste elimination	To maintain regulating mechanisms and functions
Stimulation	To maintain sensory function and stimulation
Protection from physical harm	To prevent physical injury
Increased learning	To achieve awareness of needs and/or use of resources

NURSING INTERVENTIONS

Nursing Treatments

Resuscitate breathing (ET) (if necessary)
Administer humidified oxygen (ET) (for respiratory distress)
Stimulate by movement, touch, sternal pressure, or speech
Induce vomiting *immediately* (unless stuporous, unconscious, or convulsing)
Give the universal antidote orally
   OR
Give hot coffee
   OR
Give hot tea
   OR
Give magnesium sulfate solution orally
Lavage the stomach (ET)
Administer intravenous fluids (ET)
   OR
Give water orally (age 1–5 years, give 1–2 cups; over 5 years, give up to 1
   quart)
Attend the patient constantly (until the episode subsides)
Save the poison container for content analysis
Make a referral (to a physician, emergency room, or poison control center)

Nursing Observations

Inspect the chest for respiratory rate and rhythm
Measure the intake

Measure the output (for reduced urine output)
Monitor the blood pressure
Observe for complaints of pain (abdominal)
Observe for convulsions
Observe for dyspnea
Observe for shock
Observe the level of consciousness
Palpate the pulse for rate, rhythm, and volume

Health Teaching
Emphasize that medicine cabinets should be locked
Recommend that self-medication be avoided
Explain the reason for and intended effect of the therapy

Medical Treatments Performed by Nurses
Give the prescribed drugs

EVALUATION

See the evaluation criteria for each specific goal in Chapter 2.

Emergency Phase Tranquilizer Poisoning (70)

ASSESSMENT

Subjective Data
Confusion
Mental depression

Objective Data
Restlessness
Decreased blood pressure
Insomnia
Convulsions
Coma

Related Data
Person has ingested Compazine, Librium, Mellaril, Meprobamate, Prolixin,
Thorazine, Trilafon, Valium

POSSIBLE ETIOLOGY

Accidental or intentional drug ingestion

NURSING DIAGNOSIS

Emergency phase tranquilizer poisoning: the need for immediate health
care upon the intake of excessive amounts of tranquilizer medication

PLANNING

Patient Needs
Oxygen, circulation
Waste elimination

Primary Nurse-Patient Goals
To maintain oxygen to all cells
To maintain regulating mechanisms
and functions

Stimulation	To maintain sensory function and stimulation
Protection from physical harm	To prevent physical injury
Increased learning	To achieve awareness of needs and/or use of resources

NURSING INTERVENTIONS

Nursing Treatments

Induce vomiting *immediately* (unless stuporous, unconscious, or convulsing)
Give hot coffee
    OR
Give hot tea
    OR
Give the universal antidote orally
Lavage the stomach (ET)
Administer intravenous fluids (ET)
    OR
Give water orally (age 1–5 years, give 1–2 cups; over 5 years, give up to 1 quart)
Stimulate by movement, touch, sternal pressure, or speech
Attend the patient constantly (until the episode subsides)
Save the poison container for content analysis
Make a referral (to a physician, emergency room, or poison control center)

Nursing Observations

Inspect the chest for respiratory rate and rhythm
Measure the intake
Measure the output
Monitor the blood pressure
Observe for dyspnea
Observe for shock
Observe the level of consciousness
Palpate the pulse for rate, rhythm, and volume

Health Teaching

Emphasize that medicine cabinets should be locked
Recommend that self-medication be avoided
Explain the reason for and intended effect of the therapy

Medical Treatments Performed by Nurses

Give the prescribed drugs

EVALUATION

See the evaluation criteria for each specific goal in Chapter 2.

Emergency Phase Unknown-Agent Poisoning (414)

ASSESSMENT

Subjective Data
Dizziness
Nausea

Objective Data

Progressive drowsiness, stupor, and unconsciousness

Particles of poison on and in the mouth

Poison odor evident

Absence of the poison container

Unlabeled poison container

POSSIBLE ETIOLOGY

Accidental or intentional ingestion. Inability of the person to communicate what was ingested.

NURSING DIAGNOSIS

Emergency phase unknown-agent poisoning: the need for immediate health care upon the ingestion of a poison that cannot be immediately identified

PLANNING

Patient Needs	**Primary Nurse-Patient Goals**
Oxygen, circulation	To maintain oxygen to all cells
Waste elimination	To maintain regulating mechanisms and functions
Rest	To achieve rest
Comfort	To achieve comfort
Stimulation	To maintain sensory function and stimulation
Protection from physical harm	To prevent physical injury
Increased learning	To achieve awareness of needs and/or use of resources

NURSING INTERVENTIONS

Nursing Treatments

Administer humidified oxygen (ET) (for respiratory distress)

Stimulate by movement, touch, sternal pressure, or speech

Give the universal antidote orally

    OR

Give charcoal solution orally

    OR

Give hot coffee (if drowsy)

    OR

Give milk

Administer intravenous fluids (ET)

    OR

Give water orally (age 1–5 years, give 1–2 cups; over 5 years, give up to 1 quart)

Cover with warm blankets

Refrain from gastric lavage

Do not induce vomiting

Encourage adequate rest

Attend the patient constantly

Save the poison container for content analysis

Make a referral (to a physician, emergency room, or poison control center)

Nursing Observations

Inspect the chest for respiratory rate and rhythm

Inspect for hemorrhage (gastrointestinal)

Measure the intake

Measure the output (for reduced urine output)

Monitor the blood pressure

Observe for complaints of pain (abdominal)

Observe for convulsions

Observe for shock

Observe the level of consciousness

Palpate the pulse for rate, rhythm, and volume

Health Teaching

Emphasize that dangerous products should be stored out of reach

Emphasize that medicine cabinets should be locked

Explain the reason for and intended effect of the therapy

Medical Treatments Performed by Nurses

Give the prescribed drugs

EVALUATION

See the evaluation criteria for each specific goal in Chapter 2.

INADEQUATE INFORMATION RELATED TO DRUG USE

Inadequate Information Related to Alcohol Abuse (49,198,385,394,589)

ASSESSMENT

Subjective Data

Person confirms a lack of information

Objective Data

Person's actions indicate a lack of information regarding:

the signs and symptoms of alcohol abuse

the physiologic effects of alcohol consumption

the reasons why people drink alcohol

where to obtain help for alcoholism

Related Data

Commonly Related Diseases:

None

OR

Alcoholism

Laennec's cirrhosis
Pancreatitis

POSSIBLE ETIOLOGY

Lack of instruction. No previous experience with alcohol.

NURSING DIAGNOSIS

Inadequate information related to alcohol abuse: lack of information regarding the frequent use of alcoholic beverages

PLANNING

Patient Needs

Protection from physical harm
Protection from psychologic threat
Increased learning

Primary Nurse-Patient Goals

To prevent physical injury
To prevent emotional injury
To achieve awareness of needs
and/or use of resources

NURSING INTERVENTIONS

Nursing Treatments
Approach unhurriedly
Encourage patient questions

Nursing Observations
Evaluate the response to teaching

Health Teaching
Advise early correction of problems
Describe the behavior pattern indicating early-, intermediate-, and late-stage alcohol abuse
Describe the specific dangerous effects of poor health practices
Explain that drug (alcohol) dependence is an illness
Explain that drug (alcohol) use is not socially essential
Explain that long-term drug (alcohol) abuse reduces the pleasures derived from drug abuse
Explain that the use of drugs (alcohol) to solve problems is dangerous
Explain the importance of staying well informed on drug (alcohol) abuse
Explain why persons resort to drug (alcohol) abuse
Explain why persons should maintain self-control
Relate the accepted criteria for commitment of drug (alcohol) abusers

EVALUATION

See the evaluation criteria for each specific goal in Chapter 2.

Inadequate Information Related to Coping With the Alcohol Abuser (49,198,385,394,589)

ASSESSMENT

Subjective Data
Anxiety
Hopelessness

Guilt, sometimes
Person confirms a lack of information

Objective Data
Person's actions indicate a lack of information regarding:
    how to help an alcoholic loved one
    how to prevent a loved one from becoming an alcoholic
    where to seek help

Related Data
Commonly Related Diseases:
Alcoholism
Laennec's cirrhosis
Pancreatitis

POSSIBLE ETIOLOGY

Lack of instruction

NURSING DIAGNOSIS

Inadequate information related to coping with the alcohol abuser: lack of information regarding how one can help an alcoholic

PLANNING

Patient Needs

Comfort

Warm, communicating
    relationships

Increased learning

Primary Nurse-Patient Goals

To achieve comfort

To achieve effective verbal and
    nonverbal communications

To achieve awareness of needs
    and/or use of resources

NURSING INTERVENTIONS

Nursing Treatments
Approach unhurriedly
Reassure verbally
Encourage patient questions
Make a referral (to Al Anon)

Nursing Observations
Evaluate the response to teaching

Health Teaching
Advise against committing alcoholics to promises of sobriety
Advise against making emotional appeals to the alcoholic
Advise against emphasizing past problems caused by another
Advise against making excuses for the alcoholic
Advise against questioning the alcoholic about drinking
Advise against removing the alcoholic's liquor supply
Advise against threatening the alcoholic
Advise early correction of problems
Advise that others should not assume the alcoholic's responsibilities

Advise that the alcoholic's illness be discussed only during sobriety
Describe the behavior pattern indicating drug (alcohol) abuse
Explain that drug (alcohol) dependence is an illness
Explain the importance of setting an example through abstinence from drug (alcohol) use
Explain why persons resort to drug (alcohol) abuse
Relate the accepted criteria for commitment of drug (alcohol) users

EVALUATION

See the evaluation criteria for each specific goal in Chapter 2.

Inadequate Information Related to Narcotic-Barbiturate Drug Abuse (17,88,92,119,257,266,267,349,501)

ASSESSMENT

Subjective Data
Anxiety
Dependence
Person confirms a lack of information

Objective Data
Person's actions indicate a lack of information regarding:
    the signs and symptoms of narcotic abuse
    the physiologic effects of narcotic abuse
    the reasons why people turn to narcotic abuse
    where to obtain help

Related Data
Commonly Related Diseases:
None
    OR
Any long-term, painful disease or injury

POSSIBLE ETIOLOGY

Lack of instruction

NURSING DIAGNOSIS

Inadequate information related to narcotic-barbiturate drug abuse: lack of information regarding the excessive use of narcotics or barbiturate drugs

PLANNING

Patient Needs	Primary Nurse-Patient Goals
Protection from physical harm	To prevent physical injury
Protection from psychologic threat	To prevent emotional injury
Increased learning	To achieve awareness of needs and/or use of resources

NURSING INTERVENTIONS

Nursing Treatments
Approach unhurriedly
Reassure verbally
Encourage patient questions
Make a referral (to local drug clinics)

Nursing Observations
Evaluate the response to teaching

Health Teaching
Advise early correction of problems
Describe the behavior pattern indicating drug abuse
Describe the specific dangerous effects of poor health practices
Explain that drug dependence is an illness
Explain that drug use is not socially essential
Explain that long-term drug abuse reduces the pleasures derived from drug
    abuse
Explain that the use of drugs to solve problems is dangerous
Explain the importance of staying well informed on drug abuse
Explain why persons resort to drug abuse
Explain why persons should maintain self-control

EVALUATION

See the evaluation criteria for each specific goal in Chapter 2.

Inadequate Information Related to Coping With the Drug Abuser
(17,88,92,119,257,266,267,349,501)

ASSESSMENT

Subjective Data
Anxiety
Hopelessness
Guilt, sometimes
Person confirms a lack of information

Objective Data
Person's actions indicate a lack of information regarding:
    how to help the drug abuser
    how to prevent a loved one from becoming a drug abuser
    where to seek help

Related Data
Commonly Related Conditions:
Drug addiction

POSSIBLE ETIOLOGY

Lack of instruction. No previous experience with drug abuse.

NURSiNG DIAGNOSIS

Inadequate information related to coping with the drug abuser: lack of in
formation regarding how one can help a drug abuser

PLANNING

Patient Needs

Comfort

Warm, communicating
   relationships

Increased learning

Primary Nurse-Patient Goals

To achieve comfort

To achieve effective verbal and
   nonverbal communications

To achieve awareness of needs
   and/or use of resources

NURSING INTERVENTIONS

Nursing Treatments
Approach unhurriedly
Reassure verbally
Encourage patient questions
Make a referral (to local drug clinic)

Nursing Observations
Evaluate the response to teaching

Health Teaching
Advise acceptance of the drug user's return home
Advise against emphasizing past problems caused by another
Advise against intense surveillance of the drug user
Advise early correction of problems
Explain how to counteract the theories of drug users
Advise that the responsibility for drug abuse be placed on the abuser, not on
   other persons
Describe the behavior pattern indicating drug abuse
Explain that drug dependence is an illness
Explain that the use of drugs to solve problems is dangerous
Explain the importance of setting an example through abstinence from
   drug use
Explain the importance of staying well informed on drug abuse
Explain why persons resort to drug abuse
Recommend financial nonsupport of the drug user's habit
Relate the accepted criteria for commitment of drug users
Relate the accepted criteria for notifying authorities of drug abuse

EVALUATION

See the evaluation criteria for each specific goal in Chapter 2.

Inadequate Information Related to
Patent-Drug Abuse

ASSESSMENT

Subjective Data
Dependence
Person confirms a lack of information

Objective Data
Person's actions indicate a lack of information regarding:
   the unsafeness of chronically taking aspirin, laxatives, tonics, etc.
   the fact that even though there is no desire to increase the drug dosage, it
      is a form of habituation
   the fact that there are alternate methods for meeting physiologic needs

Related Data
Commonly Related Diseases:
None
   OR
Any disease or injury

POSSIBLE ETIOLOGY

Lack of instruction. Desire to relieve some health disequilibrium or discomfort. Learned habits from elders. The convincing effect of patent-drug advertisements.

NURSING DIAGNOSIS

Inadequate information related to patent-drug abuse: lack of information regarding the chronic use of patent drugs

PLANNING

Patient Needs

Comfort

Protection from physical harm

Increased learning

Primary Nurse-Patient Goals

To achieve comfort

To prevent physical injury

To achieve awareness of needs

NURSING INTERVENTIONS

Nursing Treatments
Approach unhurriedly
Encourage patient questions

Health Teaching
Advise early correction of problems (under medical direction)
Describe the specific dangerous effects of health practices (laxatives cause
   loss of intestinal tone, aspirin causes bleeding, etc.)
Explain the causes of the health problem
Recommend that self-medication be avoided

EVALUATION

See the evaluation criteria for each specific goal in Chapter 2.

Inadequate Information Related to Prescribed Self-medication

ASSESSMENT

Subjective Data
Anxiety, sometimes
Person confirms a lack of information

Objective Data

Person's actions indicate a lack of information regarding:
> the skill involved in administering a prescribed medication (injections, etc.)
> how to measure a medication
> how to mix a medication
> the time of day to take each dose
> the side effects to look for
> the purpose of the medication

Related Data

Commonly Related Diseases:
Any disease or injury requiring medication

POSSIBLE ETIOLOGY

First introduction to the specific medication. Lack of instruction.

NURSING DIAGNOSIS

Inadequate information related to prescribed self-medication: lack of information regarding how to give oneself medications prescribed by health personnel

PLANNING

Patient Needs	**Primary Nurse-Patient Goals**
Protection from physical harm	To prevent physical injury
Mastery and competence in skills, independence	To achieve optimum function
Increased learning	To achieve awareness of needs and/or use of resources

NURSING INTERVENTIONS

Nursing Treatments
Approach unhurriedly
Encourage patient questions

Nursing Observations
Evaluate the response to teaching

Health Teaching
Describe those symptoms which should be reported (specific to the drugs)
Explain how to give medications to children
Explain the reason for and intended effect of the therapy
Explain how to obtain therapeutic supplies (drugs, syringes, etc.)
Teach how to administer medications

EVALUATION

See the evaluation criteria for each specific goal in Chapter 2.

Inadequate Information Related to Tobacco Habituation (70,327)

ASSESSMENT

Subjective Data

Anxiety, sometimes

Person confirms a lack of information

Objective Data

Person's actions indicate a lack of information regarding:
    the signs and symptoms of tobacco habituation
    the physiologic effects of tobacco habituation
    the reasons why people chronically smoke
    where to obtain help for tobacco habituation
    methods used to stop smoking

Related Data

Commonly Related Conditions:

Chronic cough

Commonly Related Diseases:

Chronic bronchitis

Myocardial infarction

Laryngeal, pharyngeal, oral, and pulmonary carcinoma

Emphysema

Peptic ulcer

Hypertension

Buerger's disease

Arteriosclerosis

Atherosclerosis

POSSIBLE ETIOLOGY

Lack of instruction. No previous experience with the use of tobacco.

NURSING DIAGNOSIS

Inadequate information related to tobacco habituation: lack of information regarding the chronic use of tobacco

PLANNING

Patient Needs	**Primary Nurse-Patient Goals**
Protection from physical harm	To prevent physical injury
Increased learning	To achieve awareness of needs and/or use of resources

NURSING INTERVENTIONS

Nursing Treatments

Approach unhurriedly

Encourage patient questions

Make a referral (to programs for curing tobacco habituation)

Nursing Observations

Evaluate the response to teaching

Health Teaching

Describe the behavior pattern indicating drug (tobacco) abuse

Describe the specific dangerous effects of poor health practices

Describe those symptoms which should be reported (coughing, bloody or purulent sputum, mouth lesions)

Explain that drug (tobacco) use is not socially essential

Explain the causes of the health problem

Recommend methods used to stop smoking

EVALUATION

See the evaluation criteria for each specific goal in Chapter 2.

12.
NURSING DIAGNOSES RELATED TO
Electrolyte Imbalance

HYPONATREMIA DISORDERS

Electrolyte Imbalance Related to Fistula Drainage (300,301,326)

ASSESSMENT

Subjective Data
Abdominal and muscle cramping
Fatigue
Headache
Vertigo

Objective Data
Decreased blood pressure
Muscle weakness
Poor skin turgor

Related Data
History of prolonged fistula drainage

Laboratory Findings:
Decreased blood sodium

Commonly Related Diseases:
Rectal, vaginal, or colon fistula

POSSIBLE ETIOLOGY

Sodium is lost through excessive fistula drainage.

NURSING DIAGNOSIS

Electrolyte imbalance related to fistula drainage: a decreased blood sodium as a consequence of drainage loss through a fistula

PLANNING

Patient Needs	**Primary Nurse-Patient Goals**
Water-salt balance	To maintain fluid and electrolyte balance
Protection from physical harm	To prevent physical injury
Increased learning	To achieve awareness of needs

NURSING INTERVENTIONS

Nursing Treatments
Encourage increased sodium-food intake
Give high-sodium fluids orally

Nursing Observations
Monitor blood studies for abnormal electrolytes

Health Teaching
Explain the causes of the health problem
Explain the reason for and intended effect of the therapy

EVALUATION

See the evaluation criteria for each specific goal in Chapter 2.

Electrolyte Imbalance Related to Diaphoresis

ASSESSMENT

Subjective Data
Chilling

Objective Data
Very wet skin
Soaked clothing
Wet bed clothes

Related Data

Laboratory Findings:
Decreased blood sodium

Commonly Related Conditions:
Fever
Shock
Hypoglycemia

Commonly Related Diseases:
Malaria
Pneumonia

POSSIBLE ETIOLOGY

Profuse perspiration. Night sweats.

NURSING DIAGNOSIS

Electrolyte imbalance related to diaphoresis: the loss of large amounts of sodium from profuse perspiration

PLANNING

Patient Needs

Water-salt balance

Protection from physical harm

Increased learning

Primary Nurse-Patient Goals

To maintain fluid and electrolyte
balance

To prevent physical injury

To achieve awareness of needs

NURSING INTERVENTIONS

Nursing Treatments

Encourage increased sodium-food intake
Give high-sodium fluids orally

Nursing Observations

Monitor blood studies for abnormal electrolytes
Monitor the oral temperature

Health Teaching

Explain the causes of the health problem
Explain the reason for and intended effect of the therapy

EVALUATION

See the evaluation criteria for each specific goal in Chapter 2.

HYPONATREMIA DISORDERS, POTENTIAL

Potential Electrolyte Imbalance Related to Gastric Suction (71,391)

ASSESSMENT

Objective Data

Prolonged gastric suction
Failure to irrigate the gastric tube with saline

Related Data

Commonly Related Diseases:
Volvulus
Intussusception
Carcinoma
Pancreatitis

POSSIBLE ETIOLOGY

The loss of electrolytes through the suctioned gastric juices

NURSING DIAGNOSIS

Potential electrolyte imbalance related to gastric suction: the possibility that an unstable chemical body state of decreased salt will occur as a result of the drainage of gastric secretions

PLANNING

Patient Needs	**Primary Nurse-Patient Goals**
Water-salt balance	To maintain fluid and electrolyte balance
Protection from physical harm	To prevent physical injury
Increased learning	To achieve awareness of needs

NURSING INTERVENTIONS

Nursing Treatments
Irrigate the gastric tube with saline

Nursing Observations
Monitor the blood pressure (for decrease)
Monitor blood studies for abnormal electrolytes (decreased sodium)
Observe for complaints of headache
Observe for complaints of pain (abdominal or muscular cramps)
Observe for fatigue
Observe for complaints of weakness

Health Teaching
Explain the causes of the health problem
Explain the reason for and intended effect of the therapy

EVALUATION

See the evaluation criteria for each specific goal in Chapter 2.

Potential Electrolyte Imbalance Related to Paracentesis (300,326,391)

ASSESSMENT

Subjective Data
Weakness

Objective Data
Large volume of paracentesis fluid withdrawn
Frequent paracentesis

Related Data
Commonly Related Diseases:
Laennec's cirrhosis

POSSIBLE ETIOLOGY

Excessive loss of electrolyte containing fluid through paracentesis drainage

NURSING DIAGNOSIS

Potential electrolyte imbalance related to paracentesis: the possibility that an unstable chemical body state will exist in which a decrease of salts, resulting from the drainage of abdominal or thoracic fluid by syringe, will change the electrolyte composition of body fluid so it is not in the normal proportion seen in a healthy state

PLANNING

Patient Needs	**Primary Nurse-Patient Goals**
Water-salt balance	To maintain fluid and electrolyte balance
Protection from physical harm	To prevent physical injury
Increased learning	To achieve awareness of needs

NURSING INTERVENTIONS

Nursing Treatments
Encourage increased sodium-food intake
Give high-sodium fluids orally

Nursing Observations
Measure the output (paracentesis fluid)
Monitor the blood pressure (for decrease)
Monitor blood studies for abnormal electrolytes (decreased sodium)
Observe for complaints of headache
Observe for complaints of pain (abdominal or muscular cramps)
Observe for complaints of weakness
Observe for fatigue

Health Teaching
Explain the causes of the health problem
Explain the reason for and intended effect of the therapy

EVALUATION

See the evaluation criteria for each specific goal in Chapter 2.

Potential Electrolyte Imbalance Related to Inadaquate Salt Ingestion (300,301,326)

ASSESSMENT

Subjective Data
Weakness

Objective Data
On low-salt diet therapy
Prolonged therapy

Related Data
Commonly Related Diseases:
Myocardial infarction

Hypertension
Any disease requiring a low-salt diet

POSSIBLE ETIOLOGY

The unavailability of normal salts for absorption by the body prevents electrolyte compounds from chemically combining positive and negative electrical charges with water molecules in normal concentration

NURSING DIAGNOSIS

Potential electrolyte imbalance related to inadequate salt ingestion: the possibility that an unstable chemical body state will exist in which a decrease in salt intake will change the electrolyte composition of body fluid so it is not in the normal proportion seen in a healthy state

PLANNING

Patient Needs	Primary Nurse-Patient Goals
Water-salt balance	To maintain fluid and electrolyte balance
Protection from physical harm	To prevent physical injury
Increased learning	To achieve awareness of needs

NURSING INTERVENTIONS

Nursing Treatments
Encourage increased sodium-food intake

Nursing Observations
Monitor the blood pressure (for decrease)
Monitor blood studies for abnormal electrolytes (decreased sodium)
Observe for complaints of pain (cramping)
Observe for complaints of headache
Observe for complaints of weakness
Observe for fatigue

Health Teaching
Explain the causes of the health problem
Explain the reason for and intended effect of the therapy

EVALUATION

See the evaluation criteria for each specific goal in Chapter 2.

Potential Electrolyte Imbalance Related to Fistula Drainage (300,301,391)

ASSESSMENT

Objective Data
Profuse fistula drainage
Prolonged drainage

Related Data
Commonly Related Diseases:
Rectal, vaginal, or colon fistula

POSSIBLE ETIOLOGY

Excessive loss of electrolyte containing fluid through drainage

NURSING DIAGNOSIS

Potential electrolyte imbalance related to fistula drainage: the possibility that an unstable chemical body state will exist in which a decrease of salts through external fistula drainage will change the electrolyte composition of body fluid so it is not in the normal proportion seen in a healthy state

PLANNING

Patient Needs	Primary Nurse-Patient Goals
Water-salt balance	To maintain fluid and electrolyte balance
Protection from physical harm	To prevent physical injury
Increased learning	To achieve awareness of needs

NURSING INTERVENTIONS

Nursing Treatments
Encourage increased sodium-food intake
Give high-sodium fluids orally

Nursing Observations
Measure the intake
Measure the output
Monitor blood studies for abnormal electrolytes (decreased sodium)
Observe for complaints of headache
Observe for complaints of pain (abdominal or muscular cramps)
Observe for complaints of weakness
Observe for fatigue

Health Teaching
Explain the causes of the health problem
Explain the reason for and intended effect of the therapy

EVALUATION

See the evaluation criteria for each specific goal in Chapter 2.

HYPERNATREMIA DISORDERS, POTENTIAL

Potential Electrolyte Imbalance Related to Excessive Salt Ingestion (70)

ASSESSMENT

Objective Data
Chronic use of saline laxatives
Excessive use of table salt
Edema may exist

Related Data

Commonly Related Diseases:
Addison's disease

POSSIBLE ETIOLOGY

The excessive availability of normal salts for absorption by the body prevents normal electrolyte concentration

NURSING DIAGNOSIS

Potential electrolyte imbalance related to excessive salt ingestion: the possibility that an unstable chemical body state will exist, in which an increase in salt intake changes the electrolyte composition of body fluid so it is not in the normal proportion seen in a healthy state

PLANNING

Patient Needs	**Primary Nurse-Patient Goals**
Water-salt balance	To maintain fluid and electrolyte balance
Protection from physical harm	To prevent physical injury
Increased learning	To achieve awareness of needs

NURSING INTERVENTIONS

Nursing Treatments
Encourage decreased sodium-food intake
Give low-sodium fluids orally
Refrain from giving saline laxatives
Refrain from giving table salt
Substitute artificial salt

Nursing Observations
Measure the intake
Measure the output (for oliguria or anuria)
Inspect the mucous membranes for abnormalities (dryness)
Inspect the skin for discoloration (flushing)
Monitor blood studies for abnormal electrolytes (increased sodium)
Monitor the oral temperature (for elevation)
Observe for complaints of thirst

Health Teaching
Explain the causes of the health problem
Explain the reason for and intended effect of the therapy

EVALUATION

See the evaluation criteria for each specific goal in Chapter 2.

HYPOKALEMIA DISORDERS

Electrolyte Imbalance Related to Diuresis (300,326)

ASSESSMENT

Subjective Data
Weakness
Apathy
Confusion

Objective Data
Abdominal distention
Soft, flabby muscles
Cardiac arrhythmias

Related Data
History of prolonged diuretic therapy without potassium replacement

Laboratory Findings:
Decreased blood potassium

Commonly Related Diseases:
Congestive heart failure
Pulmonary edema
Glomerulonephritis
Myocardial infarction
Laennec's cirrhosis
Hypertension
Alcoholism

POSSIBLE ETIOLOGY

Diuretics cause sodium and potassium loss through urine excretion. This loss usually brings sodium levels to normal concentrations but results in potassium depletion.

NURSING DIAGNOSIS

Electrolyte imbalance related to diuresis: a decreased blood potassium resulting from drug-related increased urine output

PLANNING

Patient Needs	Primary Nurse-Patient Goals
Water-salt balance	To maintain fluid and electrolyte balance
Protection from physical harm	To prevent physical injury
Increased learning	To achieve awareness of needs

NURSING INTERVENTIONS

Nursing Treatments
Encourage increased potassium-food intake
Give high-potassium fluids orally
Refrain from giving enemas (which further deplete potassium)

Nursing Observations
Monitor blood studies for abnormal electrolytes

Health Teaching
Explain the causes of the health problem
Explain the reason for and intended effect of the therapy

EVALUATION

See the evaluation criteria for each specific goal in Chapter 2.

Electrolyte Imbalance Related to Malnutrition (300,326)

ASSESSMENT

Subjective Data
Weakness
Apathy
Confusion

Objective Data
Abdominal distention
Soft, flabby muscles

Related Data
History of inadequate dietary intake
Laboratory Findings:
Decreased blood potassium

POSSIBLE ETIOLOGY

An inadequate intake of potassium reduces the normal blood potassium level

NURSING DIAGNOSIS

Electrolyte imbalance related to malnutrition: a decreased blood potassium as a consequence of inadequate dietary intake of potassium

PLANNING

Patient Needs	**Primary Nurse-Patient Goals**
Water-salt balance	To maintain fluid and electrolyte balance
Protection from physical harm	To prevent physical injury
Increased learning	To achieve awareness of needs

NURSING INTERVENTIONS

Nursing Treatments
Encourage increased potassium-food intake
Give high-potassium fluids orally

Nursing Observations
Monitor blood studies for abnormal electrolytes

Health Teaching
Explain the causes of the health problem
Explain the reason for and intended effect of the therapy

EVALUATION

See the evaluation criteria for each specific goal in Chapter 2.

HYPOKALEMIA DISORDERS, POTENTIAL

Potential Electrolyte Imbalance Related to Diuresis (300,301,326,391)

ASSESSMENT

Objective Data
Receiving diuretic therapy daily
Prolonged therapy
Less than 30 mEq of potassium is being replaced daily

Related Data
Commonly Related Diseases:
Myocardial infarction
Laennec's cirrhosis
Hypertension
Alcoholism
Congestive heart failure
Pulmonary edema
Glomerulonephritis

POSSIBLE ETIOLOGY

In diuresis, fluid reabsorption from the renal tubules is prevented with a loss of sodium and potassium in the urine. This diuresis may bring sodium levels to a normal state but causes potassium depletion. If diuresis continues after a normal blood sodium level has been reached, sodium depletion in addition to potassium depletion will occur.

NURSING DIAGNOSIS

Potential electrolyte imbalance related to diuresis: the possibility that an unstable chemical body state will exist in which drug-related increased urine excretion will change the electrolyte composition of body fluid so it is not in the normal proportion seen in a healthy state

PLANNING

Patient Needs	Primary Nurse-Patient Goals
Water-salt balance	To maintain fluid and electrolyte balance

Protection from physical harm	To prevent physical injury
Increased learning	To achieve awareness of needs

NURSING INTERVENTIONS

Nursing Treatments

Encourage increased potassium-food intake

Give high-potassium fluids orally

Encourage increased sodium-food intake } (only if the sodium blood level has reached normal and diuresis is continued)

Give high-sodium fluids orally

Refrain from giving enemas (which further deplete potassium)

Nursing Observations

Measure the intake

Measure the output

Monitor the blood pressure (for decrease)

Monitor blood studies for abnormal electrolytes (decreased potassium and sodium)

Observe for complaints of headache

Observe for complaints of pain (abdominal cramping)

Observe for complaints of weakness

Observe for fatigue

Observe for confusion

Health Teaching

Explain the causes of the health problem

Explain the reason for and intended effect of the therapy

EVALUATION

See the evaluation criteria for each specific goal in Chapter 2.

HYPERKALEMIA DISORDERS, POTENTIAL

Potential Electrolyte Imbalance Related to Potassium Infusion (271,300,301,326)

ASSESSMENT

Objective Data

Receiving slow, prolonged intravenous therapy with large doses of potassium added

Receiving rapid infusion of normal doses of potassium intravenously

Related Data

Commonly Related Diseases:

Any disease or injury requiring intravenous fluid therapy

POSSIBLE ETIOLOGY

Blood saturation with potassium prevents the electrolyte compounds from chemically combining positive and negative electrical charges with water molecules in normal concentration.

NURSING DIAGNOSIS

Potential electrolyte imbalance related to potassium infusion: the possibility that an unstable chemical body state will exist in which the intravenous infusion of potassium will change the electrolyte composition of body fluid so it is not in the normal proportion seen in a healthy state

PLANNING

Patient Needs

Water-salt balance

Protection from physical harm

Increased learning

Primary Nurse-Patient Goals

To maintain fluid and electrolyte balance

To prevent physical injury

To achieve awareness of needs

NURSING INTERVENTIONS

Nursing Treatments
Give low-potassium fluids orally
Refrain from giving potassium-containing drugs and solutions
Restrict the intravenous potassium to 20 mEq per hour or 200 mEq per 24 hours

Nursing Observations
Monitor blood studies for abnormal electrolytes (increased potassium)
Observe for complaints of numbness and tingling
Observe for complaints of weakness
Observe for confusion

Health Teaching
Explain the causes of the health problem
Explain the reason for and intended effect of the therapy

EVALUATION

See the evaluation criteria for each specific goal in Chapter 2.

HYPOCALCEMIA DISORDERS

Electrolyte Imbalance Related to Inadequate Calcium Intake (300,301,326)

ASSESSMENT

Subjective Data
Numbness and tingling of the extremities
Muscle twitching

Muscle cramping
Palpitations

Objective Data
Positive Chvostek's sign
Irritability
Rough, dry skin and sparse hair (if the condition is chronic)

Related Data
History of inadequate dietary intake under normal circumstances or during
  pregnancy, lactation, or rapid childhood growth

Laboratory Findings:
Decreased blood calcium, increased blood phosphate

Commonly Related Conditions:
Pregnancy
Lactation
Normal growth

POSSIBLE ETIOLOGY

An inadequate intake of calcium reduces the normal blood calcium level.
When the body requires additional calcium, if the intake is not adequate,
the blood level will decrease below normal.

NURSING DIAGNOSIS

Electrolyte imbalance related to inadequate calcium intake: a decreased
blood calcium as a consequence of inadequate dietary intake of calcium to
meet body needs

PLANNING

Patient Needs	**Primary Nurse-Patient Goals**
Water-salt balance	To maintain fluid and electrolyte balance
Protection from physical harm	To prevent physical injury
Increased learning	To achieve awareness of needs

NURSING INTERVENTIONS

Nursing Treatments
Encourage increased calcium-food intake
Give high-calcium fluids orally

Nursing Observations
Monitor blood studies for abnormal electrolytes

Health Teaching
Explain the causes of the health problem
Explain the reason for and intended effect of the therapy

EVALUATION

See the evaluation criteria for each specific goal in Chapter 2.

HYPOCALCEMIA DISORDERS, POTENTIAL

Potential Electrolyte Imbalance Related to Blood Transfusion (326)

ASSESSMENT

Objective Data
Receiving intensive blood transfusion therapy
Blood has citric acid added

Related Data
Commonly Related Diseases:
Hemophilia
Peptic ulcer
Accidental trauma

POSSIBLE ETIOLOGY

Citric acid in citrated blood binds the calcium within the circulatory system and reduces the blood calcium level.

NURSING DIAGNOSIS

Potential electrolyte imbalance related to blood transfusion: the possibility that an unstable chemical body state will exist in which a large volume of transfused blood will change the electrolyte composition of body fluid so it is not in the normal proportion seen in a healthy state

PLANNING

Patient Needs	**Primary Nurse-Patient Goals**
Water-salt balance	To maintain fluid and electrolyte balance
Protection from physical harm	To prevent physical injury
Increased learning	To achieve awareness of needs

NURSING INTERVENTIONS

Nursing Treatments
Give high-calcium fluids orally

Nursing Observations
Monitor the blood pressure (for decrease)
Monitor blood studies for abnormal electrolytes (decreased calcium)
Observe for complaints of numbness and tingling
Observe for complaints of pain (muscle cramps)
Observe for fatigue
Observe for irritability
Observe for muscle twitching

Health Teaching
Explain the causes of the health problem
Explain the reason for and intended effect of the therapy

EVALUATION

See the evaluation criteria for each specific goal in Chapter 2.

HYPERCALCEMIA DISORDERS

Electrolyte Imbalance Related to Excessive Calcium Intake (300,326)

ASSESSMENT

Subjective Data
Muscle weakness
Localized or generalized bone pain
Headache
Polyuria
Excessive thirst
Nausea
Fatigue

Objective Data
Anorexia
Constipation
Stuporous
Coma, sometimes

Related Data
History of excessive and prolonged milk, alkali, vitamin D, or calcium intake

Laboratory Findings:
Increased blood calcium
Decreased blood phosphate

Commonly Related Conditions:
Chronic indigestion

Commonly Related Diseases:
Peptic or duodenal ulcer

POSSIBLE ETIOLOGY

An excessive intake of calcium elevates the normal blood calcium level

NURSING DIAGNOSIS

Electrolyte imbalance related to excessive calcium intake: an increased blood calcium as a consequence of excessive drug or dietary intake of calcium

PLANNING

Patient Needs	**Primary Nurse-Patient Goals**
Water-salt balance	To maintain fluid and electrolyte balance
Protection from physical harm	To prevent physical injury
Increased learning	To achieve awareness of needs

NURSING INTERVENTIONS

Nursing Treatments
Encourage decreased calcium-food intake
Give low-calcium fluids orally
Increase fluid intake to about 2000 cc daily
Withhold the drug (calcium, alkalis)

Nursing Observations
Monitor blood studies for abnormal electrolytes

Health Teaching
Explain the causes of the health problem
Explain the reason for and intended effect of the therapy
Recommend that alkalis be used conservatively

EVALUATION

See the evaluation criteria for each specific goal in Chapter 2.

HYPERCALCEMIA DISORDERS, POTENTIAL

Potential Electrolyte Imbalance Related to Excessive Alkali Ingestion (271,326)

ASSESSMENT

Objective Data
Receiving prolonged antacid therapy
Prolonged milk-ulcer regime

Related Data
Commonly Related Diseases:
Gastric or peptic ulcer

POSSIBLE ETIOLOGY

Excessive alkali intake inhibits renal excretion of calcium. Blood saturation with calcium cations contained in milk and alkalis prevents electrolyte compounds from chemically combining positive and negative electrical charges with water molecules in normal concentration.

NURSING DIAGNOSIS

Potential electrolyte imbalance related to excessive alkali ingestion: the possibility that an unstable chemical body state will exist in which an increase in neutralizing acids will change the electrolyte composition of body fluids so it is not in the normal proportion seen in a healthy state

PLANNING

Patient Needs	Primary Nurse-Patient Goals
Water-salt balance	To maintain fluid and electrolyte balance
Acid-base balance	To maintain regulating mechanisms and functions
Protection from physical harm	To prevent physical injury
Increased learning	To achieve awareness of needs

NURSING INTERVENTIONS

Nursing Treatments
Encourage decreased calcium-food intake
Give low-calcium fluids orally

Nursing Observations
Measure the body weight (for weight loss)
Monitor blood studies for abnormal electrolytes (increased calcium)
Observe for complaints of constipation
Observe for complaints of headache
Observe for complaints of nausea
Observe for complaints of thirst
Observe for complaints of weakness
Observe for complaints of pain (bone)
Observe for fatigue

Health Teaching
Explain the causes of the health problem
Explain the reason for and intended effect of the therapy

EVALUATION

See the evaluation criteria for each specific goal in Chapter 2.

HYPONATREMIA-HYPOKALEMIA DISORDERS

Electrolyte Imbalance Related to Vomiting (300,301,326)

ASSESSMENT

Subjective Data
Weakness (K)
Apathy (K)

Confusion (K)
Headache (Na)
Vertigo (Na)
Fatigue (Na)
Abdominal and muscle cramps (Na)

Objective Data
Decreased blood pressure
Abdominal distention (K)
Soft, flabby muscles (K)
Muscle weakness (Na)
Poor skin turgor (Na)

Related Data
History of prolonged vomiting

Laboratory Findings:
Decreased blood potassium and sodium

Commonly Related Conditions:
Anorexia nervosa
Increased intracranial pressure

Commonly Related Diseases:
Gastritis
Peptic or duodenal ulcer
Volvulus
Subdural hematoma
Meniere's disease
Labrynthitis

POSSIBLE ETIOLOGY

Loss of gastric juices decreases the body's supply of chloride, potassium, and sodium found in the gastric mucus and magnesium found in the digestive enzymes.

NURSING DIAGNOSIS

Electrolyte imbalance related to vomiting: a decreased blood potassium and sodium level as a consequence of vomiting

PLANNING

Patient Needs	**Primary Nurse-Patient Goals**
Water-salt balance	To maintain fluid and electrolyte balance
Acid-base balance	To maintain regulating mechanisms and functions
Protection from physical harm	To prevent physical injury
Increased learning	To achieve awareness of needs

NURSING INTERVENTIONS

Nursing Treatments
Encourage increased potassium-food intake
Encourage increased sodium-food intake

Give high-potassium fluids orally
Give high-sodium fluids orally
Refrain from giving enemas (which further deplete potassium)

Nursing Observations
Monitor blood studies for abnormal electrolytes

Health Teaching
Explain the causes of the health problem
Explain the reason for and intended effect of the therapy

EVALUATION

See the evaluation criteria for each specific goal in Chapter 2.

Electrolyte Imbalance Related to Diarrhea (300,301,326)

ASSESSMENT

Subjective Data
Weakess (K)
Apathy (K)
Confusion (K)
Headache (Na)
Vertigo (Na)
Fatigue (Na)
Abdominal and muscle cramps (Na)

Objective Data
Decreased blood pressure
Abdominal distention (K)
Soft, flabby muscles (K)
Muscle weakness (Na)
Poor skin turgor (Na)

Related Data
History of prolonged physiologic diarrhea or prolonged bowel preparation
   for diagnostic studies
Laboratory Findings:
Decreased blood potassium and sodium
Commonly Related Diseases:
Gastritis
Ulcerative colitis
Diverticulitis
Ileitis

POSSIBLE ETIOLOGY

Potassium and sodium loss through excessive fluid and fecal elimination

NURSING DIAGNOSIS

Electrolyte imbalance related to diarrhea: a decreased blood potassium and
sodium level as a consequence of diarrhea

PLANNING

Patient Needs	**Primary Nurse-Patient Goals**
Water-salt balance	To maintain fluid and electrolyte balance
Acid-base balance	To maintain regulating mechanisms and functions
Protection from physical harm	To prevent physical injury
Increased learning	To achieve awareness of needs

NURSING INTERVENTIONS

Nursing Treatments
Encourage increased potassium-food intake
Encourage increased sodium-food intake
Give high-potassium fluids orally
Give high-sodium fluids orally
Refrain from giving enemas (which further deplete potassium)

Nursing Observations
Monitor blood studies for abnormal electrolytes

Health Teaching
Explain the causes of the health problem
Explain the reason for and intended effect of the therapy

EVALUATION

See the evaluation criteria for each specific goal in Chapter 2.

HYPONATREMIA-HYPOKALEMIA DISORDERS, POTENTIAL

Potential Electrolyte Imbalance Related to Adrenal-Steroid Therapy (70,326)

ASSESSMENT

Objective Data
Receiving adrenal-steroid therapy
Large steroid doses
Prolonged therapy

Related Data
Commonly Related Diseases:
Cushing's syndrome
Addison's disease
Rheumatoid arthritis

POSSIBLE ETIOLOGY

Corticosteroids increase the renal tubule reabsorption of sodium. The excessive availability of normal salts for reabsorption by the body prevents the electrolyte compounds from chemically combining positive and negative electrical charges with water molecules in normal concentration.

NURSING DIAGNOSIS

Potential electrolyte imbalance related to steroid therapy: the possibility that an unstable chemical body state will exist in which corticosteroids will change the electrolyte composition of body fluid so it is not in the normal proportion seen in a healthy state

PLANNING

Patient Needs	Primary Nurse-Patient Goals
Water-salt balance	To maintain fluid and electrolyte balance
Protection from physical harm	To prevent physical injury
Increased learning	To achieve awareness of needs

NURSING INTERVENTIONS

Nursing Treatments
Encourage decreased sodium-food intake
Encourage increased potassium-food intake
Give high-potassium fluids orally
Give low-sodium fluids orally
Refrain from giving enemas (which further deplete potassium)
Refrain from giving saline laxatives
Refrain from giving table salt
Substitute artificial salt

Nursing Observations
Measure the intake
Measure the output (for anuria or oliguria)
Inspect for edema (facial)
Inspect the (oral) mucous membranes for abnormalities (dryness)
Monitor blood studies for abnormal electrolytes (increased sodium, decreased potassium)
Observe for complaints of headache
Observe for complaints of thirst
Observe for complaints of weakness
Observe for confusion

Health Teaching
Explain the causes of the health problem
Explain the reason for and intended effect of the therapy

EVALUATION

See the evaluation criteria for each specific goal in Chapter 2.

Potential Electrolyte Imbalance Related to Colostomy Drainage (300,301,326)

ASSESSMENT

Objective Data
Excessive colostomy drainage
Prolonged liquid stools

Related Data
Commonly Related Diseases:
Intestinal carcinoma
Gunshot wound of the colon

POSSIBLE ETIOLOGY

The loss of 1000 cc of liquid stool results in an approximate sodium loss of 15 mEq and a potassium loss of 18 mEq.

NURSING DIAGNOSIS

Potential electrolyte imbalance related to colostomy drainage: the possibility that an unstable chemical body state will exist in which a decrease of salts, through external intestinal drainage, will change the electrolyte composition of body fluid so it is not in the normal proportion seen in a healthy state

PLANNING

Patient Needs	**Primary Nurse-Patient Goals**
Water-salt balance	To maintain fluid and electrolyte balance
Protection from physical harm	To prevent physical injury
Increased learning	To achieve awareness of needs

NURSING INTERVENTIONS

Nursing Treatments
Encourage increased potassium-food intake
Encourage increased sodium-food intake
Give high-potassium fluids orally
Give high-sodium fluids orally

Nursing Observations
Measure the intake
Measure the output
Monitor the blood pressure (for decrease)
Monitor blood studies for abnormal electrolytes (decreased sodium and potassium)
Observe for complaints of headache
Observe for complaints of weakness
Observe for complaints of pain (cramping)

Observe for fatigue
Observe for confusion

Health Teaching
Explain the causes of the health problem
Explain the reason for and intended effect of the therapy

EVALUATION

See the evaluation criteria for each specific goal in Chapter 2.

Potential Electrolyte Imbalance
Related to Diarrhea
(247,300,301,326)

ASSESSMENT

Objective Data
Frequent liquid stools
Prolonged physiologic diarrhea
Prolonged bowel preparation for extensive diagnostic studies

Related Data
Commonly Related Diseases:
Gastritis
Diverticulitis
Ileitis
Ulcerative colitis

POSSIBLE ETIOLOGY

In prolonged and frequent bowel elimination, sodium, magnesium, and potassium are lost in the feces. 1000 cc of liquid stool would result in a sodium loss of 15 mEq and a potassium loss of 18 mEq.

NURSING DIAGNOSIS

Potential electrolyte imbalance related to diarrhea: the possibility that an unstable chemical body state will exist in which frequent bowel elimination will change the electrolyte composition of body fluid so it is not in the normal proportion seen in a healthy state

PLANNING

Patient Needs	Primary Nurse-Patient Goals
Water-salt balance	To maintain fluid and electrolyte balance
Acid-base balance	To maintain regulating mechanisms and functions
Protection from physical harm	To prevent physical injury
Increased learning	To achieve awareness of needs

NURSING INTERVENTIONS

Nursing Treatments
Encourage increased potassium-food intake
Encourage increased sodium-food intake

Give high-magnesium fluids orally
Give high-potassium fluids orally
Give high-sodium fluids orally

Nursing Observations
Measure the intake
Measure the output
Inspect the hands for tremors
Monitor the blood pressure (increased or decreased)
Monitor blood studies for abnormal electrolytes (decreased sodium, potassium, magnesium)
Observe for complaints of headache
Observe for complaints of weakness
Observe for complaints of pain (cramping)
Observe for fatigue
Observe for confusion
Palpate the pulse for rate (tachycardia), rhythm, and volume

Health Teaching
Explain the causes of the health problem
Explain the reason for and intended effect of the therapy

EVALUATION

See the evaluation criteria for each specific goal in Chapter 2.

Potential Electrolyte Imbalance Related to T-Tube Drainage (300,301,326,391)

ASSESSMENT

Objective Data
Profuse bile flow through the T-tube
Prolonged insertion of the T-tube

Related Data

Commonly Related Conditions:
T-tube drainage following cholecystectomy
Commonly Related Diseases:
Cholelithiasis
Cholecystitis

POSSIBLE ETIOLOGY

Excessive loss of electrolyte (sodium and potassium) containing fluids through T-tube drainage

NURSING DIAGNOSIS

Potential electrolyte imbalance related to T-tube drainage: the possibility that an unstable chemical body state will exist in which a decrease of salts, through external bile drainage, will change the electrolyte composition of body fluids so it is not in the normal proportion seen in a healthy state

PLANNING

Patient Needs	Primary Nurse-Patient Goals
Water-salt balance	To maintain fluid and electrolyte balance
Protection from physical harm	To prevent physical injury
Increased learning	To achieve awareness of needs

NURSING INTERVENTIONS

Nursing Treatments
Encourage increased potassium-food intake
Encourage increased sodium-food intake
Give high-potassium fluids orally
Give high-sodium fluids orally

Nursing Observations
Measure the intake
Measure the output
Monitor the blood pressure (for decrease)
Monitor blood studies for abnormal electrolytes (decreased sodium and potassium)
Observe for complaints of headache
Observe for complaints of weakness
Observe for complaints of pain (cramping)
Observe for fatigue
Observe for confusion

Health Teaching
Explain the causes of the health problem
Explain the reason for and intended effect of the therapy

EVALUATION

See the evaluation criteria for each specific goal in Chapter 2.

Potential Electrolyte Imbalance Related to Vomiting (70,247)

ASSESSMENT

Objective Data
Severe vomiting
Prolonged vomiting

Related Data
Commonly Related Conditions:
Anorexia nervosa
Increased intracranial pressure

Commonly Related Diseases:
Gastritis
Volvulus

Subdural hematoma
Peptic or duodenal ulcer
Meniere's disease
Labrynthitis

POSSIBLE ETIOLOGY

Loss of gastric juices decreases the body's supply of chloride, potassium, and sodium found in the gastric mucus and magnesium found in the digestive enzymes. 1000 cc of lost gastric juices results in an approximate sodium loss of 55 mEq, potassium loss of 10 mEq, and chloride loss of 90 mEq.

NURSING DIAGNOSIS

Potential electrolyte imbalance related to vomiting: the possibility that an unstable chemical body state will exist in which loss of gastric juices will change the electrolyte composition of body fluid so it is not in the normal proportion seen in a healthy state

PLANNING

Patient Needs	Primary Nurse-Patient Goals
Water-salt balance	To maintain fluid and electrolyte balance
Protection from physical harm	To prevent physical injury
Increased learning	To achieve awareness of needs

NURSING INTERVENTIONS

Nursing Treatments
Encourage increased potassium-food intake
Encourage increased sodium-food intake
Give high-magnesium fluids orally
Give high-potassium fluids orally
Give high-sodium fluids orally
Refrain from giving enemas (which further deplete potassium)

Nursing Observations
Measure the intake
Measure the output
Inspect the hands for tremors
Monitor the blood pressure (increased or decreased)
Monitor blood studies for abnormal electrolytes (decreased sodium, potassium, and magnesium)
Observe for complaints of headache
Observe for complaints of pain (muscle spasm)
Observe for complaints of weakness
Observe for fatigue
Observe for confusion
Observe for muscle twitching
Palpate the pulse for rate (tachycardia), rhythm, and volume

Health Teaching
Explain the causes of the health problem
Explain the reason for and intended effect of the therapy

EVALUATION

See the evaluation criteria for each specific goal in Chapter 2.

HYPONATREMIA-HYPOKALEMIA-HYPOMAGNESEMIA DISORDERS, POTENTIAL

Potential Electrolyte Imbalance Related to Diaphoresis (300,301,247)

ASSESSMENT

Objective Data
Profuse perspiration
Prolonged perspiration

Related Data
Commonly Related Conditions:
Fever
Heat exhaustion
Extreme nervousness
Intense pain
Excessive exercise
High environmental temperature and humidity

Commonly Related Diseases:
Influenza
Rheumatic fever
Typhoid fever
Malaria

POSSIBLE ETIOLOGY

1000 cc of perspiration results in an approximate sodium loss of 82 mEq and a chloride loss of 12 mEq.

NURSING DIAGNOSIS

Potential electrolyte imbalance related to diaphoresis: the possibility that an unstable chemical body state will exist in which excessive perspiration will change the electrolyte composition of body fluid so it is not in the normal proportion seen in a healthy state

PLANNING

Patient Needs
Water-salt balance

Primary Nurse-Patient Goals
To maintain fluid and electrolyte balance

Protection from physical harm   To prevent physical injury
Increased learning   To achieve awareness of needs

NURSING INTERVENTIONS

Nursing Treatments
Encourage increased sodium-food intake
Give high-sodium fluids orally
Give low-magnesium fluids orally
Refrain from giving magnesium laxatives and antacids

Nursing Observations
Measure the intake
Measure the output
Monitor the blood pressure (for decrease)
Monitor blood studies for abnormal electrolytes (decreased sodium, increased magnesium)
Observe for complaints of headache
Observe for complaints of pain (abdominal cramps)
Observe for complaints of weakness
Observe for fatigue
Observe for confusion

Health Teaching
Explain the causes of the health problem
Explain the reason for and intended effect of the therapy

EVALUATION

See the evaluation criteria for each specific goal in Chapter 2.

Potential Electrolyte Imbalance Related to Ileal-Conduit Drainage (300,301,326)

ASSESSMENT

Objective Data
Excessive urine drainage from the conduit
Prolonged drainage

Related Data
Commonly Related Diseases:
Bladder carcinoma

POSSIBLE ETIOLOGY

Excessive loss of electrolyte-containing fluids through urine flow resulting from surgical implantation of the ureter into the ileum loop, rectum, or sigmoid. In the average 1500 cc daily urine output, 6 to 15 grams or 100 mEq of sodium are excreted, and 50 to 150 mEq of potassium are excreted. Under illness stress, the potassium output reaches 60 to 200 mEq.

NURSING DIAGNOSIS

Potential electrolyte imbalance related to ileal-conduit drainage: the possibility that an unstable chemical body state will exist in which a decrease of salts, through external urine flow from stomas or buds, will change the electrolyte composition of body fluid so it is not in the normal proportion seen in a healthy state

PLANNING

Patient Needs	**Primary Nurse-Patient Goals**
Water-salt balance	To maintain fluid and electrolyte balance
Protection from physical harm	To prevent physical injury
Increased learning	To achieve awareness of needs

NURSING INTERVENTIONS

Nursing Treatments
Encourage increased potassium-food intake
Encourage increased sodium-food intake
Give high-potassium fluids orally
Give high-sodium fluids orally
Refrain from giving magnesium laxatives and antacids

Nursing Observations
Measure the intake
Measure the output
Monitor the blood pressure (for decrease)
Monitor blood studies for abnormal electrolytes (decreased sodium and potassium)
Observe for complaints of headache
Observe for complaints of weakness
Observe for complaints of pain (cramping)
Observe for fatigue
Observe for confusion

Health Teaching
Explain the causes of the health problem
Explain the reason for and intended effect of the therapy

EVALUATION

See the evaluation criteria for each specific goal in Chapter 2.

Potential Electrolyte Imbalance Related to Ileostomy Drainage (300,301,326)

ASSESSMENT

Objective Data
Profuse ileostomy drainage
Prolonged drainage

Related Data

Commonly Related Diseases:
Carcinoma

POSSIBLE ETIOLOGY

Excessive loss of electrolyte-containing fluids through feces. 1000 cc of ileostomy drainage would result in an approximate sodium loss of 125 mEq and a potassium loss of 18 mEq.

NURSING DIAGNOSIS

Potential electrolyte imbalance related to ileostomy drainage: the possibility that an unstable chemical body state will exist in which a decrease of salts, through external intestinal drainage, will change the electrolyte composition of body fluid so it is not in the normal proportion seen in a healthy state

PLANNING

Patient Needs

Water-salt balance

Protection from physical harm

Increased learning

Primary Nurse-Patient Goals

To maintain fluid and electrolyte balance

To prevent physical injury

To achieve awareness of needs

NURSING INTERVENTIONS

Nursing Treatments
Encourage increased potassium-food intake
Encourage increased sodium-food intake
Give high-potassium fluids orally
Give high-sodium fluids orally
Refrain from giving magnesium laxatives and antacids

Nursing Observations
Measure the intake
Measure the output
Monitor the blood pressure (for decrease)
Monitor blood studies for abnormal electrolytes (decreased sodium and potassium)
Observe for complaints of headache
Observe for complaints of weakness
Observe for complaints of pain (cramping)
Observe for fatigue
Observe for confusion

Health Teaching
Explain the causes of the health problem
Explain the reason for and intended effect of the therapy

EVALUATION

See the evaluation criteria for each specific goal in Chapter 2.

HYPONATREMIA-HYPOKALEMIA-HYPOMAGNESEMIA DISORDERS, POTENTIAL

Potential Electrolyte Imbalance Related to Dextrose Infusion (247,300,326)

ASSESSMENT

Objective Data
Receiving dextrose intravenous therapy
Prolonged therapy

Related Data
Commonly Related Diseases:
Any disease or injury requiring intravenous fluid therapy

POSSIBLE ETIOLOGY

5% dextrose in water does not contain sodium, magnesium, potassium, or chloride. Large volumes of nonelectrolyte dextrose in water dilute the body's concentration of sodium, potassium, and magnesium.

NURSING DIAGNOSIS

Potential electrolyte imbalance related to dextrose infusion: the possibility that an unstable chemical body state will exist in which a large volume of infused dextrose in water will change the electrolyte composition of body fluid so it is not in the normal proportion seen in a healthy state

PLANNING

Patient Needs
Water-salt balance

Protection from physical harm
Increased learning

Primary Nurse-Patient Goals
To maintain fluid and electrolyte
  balance
To prevent physical injury
To achieve awareness of needs

NURSING INTERVENTIONS

Nursing Treatments
Give high-magnesium fluids orally
Give high-potassium fluids orally
Give high-sodium fluids orally

Nursing Observations
Inspect the hands for tremors
Monitor the blood pressure (increased or decreased)
Monitor blood studies for abnormal electrolytes (decreased sodium, potassium, magnesium)
Observe for complaints of headache
Observe for complaints of pain (muscle spasms)
Observe for complaints of weakness

Observe for confusion
Observe for fatigue
Observe for muscle twitching
Palpate the pulse for rate (tachycardia), rhythm, and volume

Health Teaching
Explain the causes of the health problem
Explain the reason for and intended effect of the therapy

EVALUATION
See the evaluation criteria for each specific goal in Chapter 2.

HYPERNATREMIA-HYPERMAGNESEMIA DISORDERS, POTENTIAL

Potential Electrolyte Imbalance Related to Inadequate Fluid Intake (70,247)

ASSESSMENT

Objective Data
Less than 1500 cc daily fluid intake
Prolonged inadequate intake

Related Data

Commonly Related Conditions:
Coma
Confusion

Commonly Related Diseases:
Cerebral vascular accident
Volvulus
Carcinoma

POSSIBLE ETIOLOGY

Dehydration increases the availability of normal salts for absorption by the body and prevents the electrolyte compounds from chemically combining positive and negative electrical charges with water molecules in normal concentration.

NURSING DIAGNOSIS

Potential electrolyte imbalance related to inadequate fluid intake: the possibility that an unstable chemical body state will exist in which a below-normal fluid intake will change the electrolyte composition of body fluid so it is not in the normal proportion seen in a healthy state

Patient Needs	**Primary Nurse-Patient Goals**
Water-salt balance	To maintain fluid and electrolyte balance
Protection from physical harm	To prevent physical injury
Increased learning	To achieve awareness of needs

NURSING INTERVENTIONS

Nursing Treatments
Encourage decreased sodium-food intake
Give low-magnesium fluids orally
Give low-sodium fluids orally
Refrain from giving magnesium laxatives and antacids
Refrain from giving saline laxatives
Refrain from giving table salt
Substitute artificial salt

Nursing Observations
Measure the intake
Measure the output (for anuria or oliguria)
Monitor blood studies for abnormal electrolytes (increased sodium and
    magnesium)
Observe for confusion
Observe for complaints of thirst
Observe for complaints of weakness
Inspect the (oral) mucous membranes for abnormalities (dryness)
Inspect the skin for discoloration (flushing)

Health Teaching
Explain the causes of the health problem
Explain the reason for and intended effect of the therapy

EVALUATION

See the evaluation criteria for each specific goal in Chapter 2.

HYPERNATREMIA-HYPOKALEMIA-HYPOMAGNESEMIA DISORDERS, POTENTIAL

Potential Electrolyte Imbalance Related to Normal Saline Infusion (70,247,300,326)

ASSESSMENT

Objective Data
Receiving normal saline intravenous therapy
Prolonged therapy

Related Data
Commonly Related Diseases:
Any disease or injury requiring intravenous fluid therapy

POSSIBLE ETIOLOGY

Large volumes of infused saline increase the body's sodium concentration.

NURSING DIAGNOSIS

Potential electrolyte imbalance related to normal saline infusion: the possibility that an unstable chemical body state will exist in which a large volume of infused saline will change the electrolyte composition of body fluid so it is not in the normal proportion seen in a healthy state

PLANNING

Patient Needs

Water-salt balance

Protection from physical harm

Increased learning

Primary Nurse-Patient Goals

To maintain fluid and electrolyte balance

To prevent physical injury

To achieve awareness of needs

NURSING INTERVENTIONS

Nursing Treatments

Give high-magnesium fluids orally
Give high-potassium fluids orally
Give low-sodium fluids orally
Refrain from giving saline laxatives

Nursing Observations

Inspect the skin for discoloration (flushing)
Inspect the hands for tremors
Inspect the mucous membranes for abnormalities (dryness)
Measure the intake
Measure the output (for anuria or oliguria)
Monitor the oral temperature (for elevation)
Monitor the blood pressure (increased)
Monitor blood studies for abnormal electrolytes (increased sodium, decreased potassium and magnesium)
Observe for complaints of thirst
Observe for complaints of weakness
Observe for muscle twitching
Observe for confusion

Health Teaching

Explain the causes of the health problem
Explain the reason for and intended effect of the therapy

EVALUATION

See the evaluation criteria for each specific goal in Chapter 2.

13.

NURSING DIAGNOSES RELATED TO
Environmental Conditions

ENVIRONMENT CONDUCIVE TO INJURY

Potential Accidental Automobile Injury (79,121,122)

ASSESSMENT

Subjective Data
Driving while emotionally upset
Reduced nighttime vision

Objective Data
Driving a mechanically unsafe vehicle
Driving after partaking of alcoholic beverages or drugs
Driving at excessive speed

Related Data
Commonly Related Diseases:
Skull fracture
Cervical spinal cord injury
Chest or abdominal trauma
Burn injury

POSSIBLE ETIOLOGY

Lack of education. Apathy.

NURSING DIAGNOSIS

Potential accidental automobile injury: the possibility that an automobile accident could occur, resulting in body injury

PLANNING

Patient Needs	**Primary Nurse-Patient Goals**
Protection from physical harm	To prevent accident, physical injury
Increased learning	To achieve awareness of needs

NURSING INTERVENTIONS

Nursing Treatments
Approach unhurriedly
Encourage patient questions

Nursing Observations
Observe for behavior modification

Health Teaching
Advise not to drive for three hours after two alcoholic drinks
Explain that corrective eye lenses require periodic adjustment
Emphasize that seat belts should be fastened
Recommend strict adherence to safety rules

EVALUATION

See the evaluation criteria for each specific goal in Chapter 2.

Potential Accidental Burn (79,121,122)

ASSESSMENT

Objective Data

Potential Scald Burn (Hot Fluid or Steam):
Facing pot handles toward the front of the stove
Pulling hot liquids off a table when accidentally pulling a tablecloth
Bathing in very hot water
Tripping and falling while carrying hot liquids
Being spattered by hot metals being poured

Potential Dry-Heat Flash Burn:
Igniting gas leaks
Experimenting with chemicals or gasoline

Potential Dry-Heat Flame Burn:
Unscreened fires and heaters igniting clothes
Wearing plastic aprons or long sleeves around an open flame
Playing with matches
Matches stored in paper or wood containers
Smoking in bed or around oxygen
Leaving unused electrical equipment plugged in
Allowing frying pans to catch fire from cooking fat
Allowing grease to collect on stoves
Using thin, worn pot holders or mits
Placing the hand on stove burners
Giving children toys made from flammable materials

Potential Dry-Heat Friction Burn:
Contact with rapid moving machinery, industrial pulleys or belts, restraints, coarse bed linens, irritating substances, falling and sliding on concrete or other hard surfaces when motorcycling or playing sports

Potential Electrical Burn:
Contact with faulty plugs and frayed wiring

Potential Chemical Burn:
Contact with acids or alkalis
Playing with fireworks or gunpowder

Potential Ice Burn:
Contact with intense cold

Potential Radiation Burn:
Overexposure to sun, heat, suntan lamps, radiotherapy, or nuclear war

POSSIBLE ETIOLOGY

Lack of safety precautions. Failure to recognize danger.

NURSING DIAGNOSIS

Potential accidental burn: the possibility that the person could be burned

PLANNING

Patient Needs

Protection from physical harm

Increased learning

Primary Nurse-Patient Goals

To prevent accident, physical injury

To achieve awareness of needs

NURSING INTERVENTIONS

Nursing Treatments
Minimize environmental dangers

Nursing Observations
Observe for behavior modification

Health Teaching
Advise against exposure to intense heat
Advise against prolonged skin exposure to the sun
Recommend the installation of a smoke alarm
Emphasize that fireplaces should be screened
Emphasize that matches should be stored in a metal container
Emphasize that open heaters should be screened
Explain that stoves should be kept free of grease
Emphasize the danger of smoking around oxygen
Emphasize the danger of smoking in bed
Inform that the skin should be protected from windburn
Recommend the use of well-padded pot holders
Recommend strict adherence to safety rules

EVALUATION

See the evaluation criteria for each specific goal in Chapter 2.

Potential Accidental Falling
(79,121,122)

ASSESSMENT

Objective Data
Highly waxed floors
Snow collected on stairs and walkways

Slippery throw rugs or tub mats
Use of unsteady ladders
Entering unlighted rooms
Nonsturdy stair rails
Unanchored extension cords
Litter or liquid spills on floors and stairways
Sleeping in high beds
Children playing, without stairgates, at the top of stairs

POSSIBLE ETIOLOGY

Nonadherence to safety in the environment

NURSING DIAGNOSIS

Potential accidental falling: the presence of environmental factors that increase the potential for body injury from falling

PLANNING

Patient Needs

Protection from physical harm

Increased learning

Primary Nurse-Patient Goals

To prevent accident, physical injury

To achieve awareness of needs

NURSING INTERVENTIONS

Nursing Treatments
Arrange orderly surroundings
Illuminate the room adequately
Place in an uncrowded area
Provide a low-height bed

Nursing Observations
Observe for behavior modification

Health Teaching
Recommend the use of suction tub mats
Emphasize that extension cords should be secured in place
Emphasize that floors and stairways should be litter-free
Emphasize that snow should be removed from stairs
Emphasize the need to maintain sturdy stair rails
Emphasize the danger of highly waxed floors
Recommend strict adherence to safety rules
Recommend the use of stairgates

EVALUATION

See the evaluation criteria for each specific goal in Chapter 2.

Potential Accidental Poisoning
(79,121,122)

ASSESSMENT
Objective Data
Large supplies of drugs have been prescribed

Medicines stored in unlocked cabinets are accessible to children and con-
    fused persons
Containers are poorly labeled
Products have been placed in containers that are marked and intended for
    other products
Dangerous products have been placed within the reach of children or con-
    fused persons
Medicinal products or drugs prescribed for another person are being used
    for self-medication
Incompatible drugs are being taken
Outdated drugs are being used

POSSIBLE ETIOLOGY

Apathy. Lack of instruction.

NURSING DIAGNOSIS

Potential accidental poisoning: the possibility that drugs or dangerous products could accidentally be taken in doses sufficient to cause poisoning

PLANNING

Patient Needs	Primary Nurse-Patient Goals
Protection from physical harm	To prevent physical injury
Increased learning	To achieve awareness of needs

NURSING INTERVENTIONS

Nursing Observations
Observe for behavior modification

Health Teaching
Emphasize that dangerous products should be stored out of reach
Emphasize that medicine cabinets should be locked
Explain that clear, correct product labeling is essential
Emphasize the danger of mixing drugs and alcohol
Emphasize the danger of sharing drugs between persons
Emphasize that outdated drugs should be discarded
Recommend that self-medication be avoided

EVALUATION

See the evaluation criteria for each specific goal in Chapter 2.

Potential Accidental Suffocation
(79,121,122)

ASSESSMENT

Objective Data
Placing pillows in an infant's crib
Placing infants in bed with adults
Warming automobiles in closed garages
Allowing children to play with plastic bags

Allowing children to play near discarded refrigerators and freezers
Leaving children unattended in bathtubs and pools
Household gas leaks
Smoking in bed
Using paint or lacquer in closed areas
Using heaters which are not vented to the outside
Placing clotheslines too low
Hanging a pacifier around an infant's neck

POSSIBLE ETIOLOGY

Inadequate education and poor judgment in matters of safety. Limited air space from which to draw oxygen.

NURSING DIAGNOSIS

Potential accidental suffocation: the likelihood that adequate air will not be available for inhalation

PLANNING

Patient Needs
Protection from physical harm
Increased learning

Primary Nurse-Patient Goals
To prevent physical injury
To achieve awareness of needs

NURSING INTERVENTIONS

Nursing Treatments
Minimize environmental dangers

Nursing Observations
Observe for behavior modification

Health Teaching
Emphasize that a car should never be started in a closed garage
Emphasize that clotheslines should be kept high to prevent strangulation
Emphasize that fume-producing substances should be used in the open air
Emphasize that heaters should be vented to the outside
Emphasize that plastic bags should be shredded and discarded
Emphasize that pools should be protected against entry
Emphasize that small children should always be attended
Emphasize that unused refrigerators should be locked or the doors removed
Emphasize the danger of sleeping with an infant
Emphasize the danger of smoking in bed
Inform that airway noise indicates obstruction
Explain that a pacifier should not be hung around an infant's neck
Instruct to place the infant in a pillow-free crib
Recommend strict adherence to safety rules

EVALUATION

See the evaluation criteria for each specific goal in Chapter 2.

Potential Accidental Wound
(79,121,122)

ASSESSMENT

Objective Data
Using cracked dishware or glasses
Placing uncovered knives in drawers
Placing guns and ammunition within easy reach
Leaving large icicles hanging from a roof
Allowing children to play in unfenced play areas
Exposure to dangerous machinery
Giving children toys that have sharp edges

POSSIBLE ETIOLOGY

Lack of instruction. Apathy.

NURSING DIAGNOSIS

Potential accidental wound: the possibility that a disruption of skin intactness could occur

PLANNING

Patient Needs
Protection from physical harm

Increased learning

Primary Nurse-Patient Goals
To prevent accident, physical injury
To achieve awareness of needs

NURSING INTERVENTIONS

Nursing Treatments
Minimize environmental dangers

Nursing Observations
Observe for behavior modification

Health Teaching
Emphasize that cracked dishware should be discarded
Emphasize that knife racks should be covered
Explain how to correctly store guns and ammunition
Emphasize that large icicles should be removed
Recommend wearing a hard hat for head protection
Emphasize that small children should always be attended
Recommend strict adherence to safety rules

EVALUATION

See the evaluation criteria for each specific goal in Chapter 2.

ENVIRONMENTAL INADEQUACY
Inadequate Physical Privacy

ASSESSMENT

Subjective Data
Embarrassment

Objective Data

Requests that curtains be pulled around the bed, the door be closed, or a
screen put up

Bathes under the bed sheet

Refuses to undress before others

Refuses to use the bedpan before others

Related Data

Commonly Related Diseases:

None

OR

Any disease or injury

POSSIBLE ETIOLOGY

Lack of facilities that support privacy. Threatened self-esteem due to the
inability to practice modesty and/or balance the social disadvantages of
being ill.

NURSING DIAGNOSIS

Inadequate physical privacy: lack of seclusion from others while taking care
of hygiene or health problems

PLANNING

Patient Needs

Comfort

Protection from psychologic threat

Primary Nurse-Patient Goals

To achieve comfort

To prevent emotional injury

NURSING INTERVENTIONS

Nursing Treatments

Keep the patient's door closed

Place in a private room

Place in an uncrowded area

Refrain from performing nonessential procedures

Screen the patient for privacy

EVALUATION

See the evaluation criteria for each specific goal in Chapter 2.

Unsafe Environment Related to
Suicide Ideation

ASSESSMENT

Objective Data

Unscreened windows

Unlocked drug cabinets

Large supplies of drugs, alcohol, or chemical products

Easily accessible glassware, knives, forks, etc.

Easily accessible rope, sheets, plastic bags, extension cords

Available guns, knives, clubs

Related Data

Commonly Related Diseases:
Schizophrenia
Manic-depressive psychosis

POSSIBLE ETIOLOGY

The presence of commonly used household objects perceived as methods for suicide

NURSING DIAGNOSIS

Unsafe environment related to suicide ideation: the presence of an environment that offers a person with suicidal tendencies an opportunity to perform the act

PLANNING

Patient Needs	**Primary Nurse-Patient Goals**
Protection from physical harm	To prevent physical injury
Increased learning	To achieve awareness of needs

NURSING INTERVENTIONS

Nursing Treatments
Remove harmful objects from the environment

Nursing Observations
Evaluate the safety of the environment
Evaluate the response to teaching

Health Teaching
Emphasize that dangerous products should be stored out of reach
Emphasize that medicine cabinets should be locked
Emphasize that plastic bags should be shredded and discarded
Explain how to correctly store guns and ammunition (out of reach)
Recommend strict adherence to safety rules

EVALUATION

See the evaluation criteria for each specific goal in Chapter 2.

ENVIRONMENTAL MAINTENANCE DEPENDENCE

Dependence on Maintenance of a Healthy Environment

ASSESSMENT

Subjective Data
Person relies on nurses for:
    environmental orderliness
    good ventilation

    odor control
    environmental cleanliness
    comfortable room temperature
    pleasant surroundings

Objective Data

Person is unable to maintain his immediate environment

Related Data

Commonly Related Conditions:
Aging

Commonly Related Diseases:
Any disease or injury that limits the person's capacity to maintain his own
    healthy environment

POSSIBLE ETIOLOGY

Inability to assume normal functions as a result of illness

NURSING DIAGNOSIS

Dependence on maintenance of a healthy environment: reliance on nurses
to maintain a healthy, immediate environment

PLANNING

Patient Needs	**Primary Nurse-Patient Goals**
Comfort	To achieve comfort
Cleanliness	To achieve good hygiene
Protection from physical harm	To prevent physical injury, infection
Dependence	To achieve comfort

NURSING INTERVENTIONS

Nursing Treatments
Arrange orderly surroundings
Arrange pleasant surroundings
Control offensive odors by removing the source
Maintain adequate room ventilation
Maintain a clean environment
Maintain a normal room temperature

Nursing Observations
Identify environmental discomforts

EVALUATION

See the evaluation criteria for each specific goal in Chapter 2.

Dependence on Convenient Toilet Facilities

ASSESSMENT

Subjective Data
Anxiety

Objective Data
Urinary frequency
Urinary urgency
Diarrhea
Incontinence
Inability to reach the bathroom facilities quickly

Related Data
Commonly Related Conditions:
Aging
Pregnancy
Commonly Related Diseases:
Uterine prolapse
Cerebral vascular accident
Spinal cord sarcoma
Rectal metastatic carcinoma
Cystitis
Benign prostatic hypertrophy
Prostatitis

POSSIBLE ETIOLOGY

Increased parasympathetic stimulation. Lack of or decreased sphincter control.

NURSING DIAGNOSIS

Dependence on convenient toilet facilities: reliance on nurses to provide readily available and close toilet facilities

PLANNING

Patient Needs
Comfort

Increased learning

Primary Nurse-Patient Goals
To achieve comfort

To achieve awareness of needs

NURSING INTERVENTIONS

Nursing Treatments
Arrange geographic placement (near a bathroom)
Dress in minimum clothing
Provide a bedpan (within the patient's reach)
   OR
Provide a bedside commode
Respond immediately to the patient's call
Toilet frequently

Nursing Observations
Identify environmental discomforts (related to the toilet facilities)

Health Teaching
Explain the reason for and intended effect of the therapy

EVALUATION

See the evaluation criteria for each specific goal in Chapter 2.

Dependence on Environmental Safety Related to Suicide Ideation

ASSESSMENT

Subjective Data
Person has thoughts of committing suicide
Is fearful of performing the act
Person relies on nurses for:
    prevention of the suicide act
    keeping the environment free of objects that could be used for suicide

Related Data
Commonly Related Diseases:
Schizophrenia
Manic-depressive psychosis

POSSIBLE ETIOLOGY

The inability to keep oneself or loved ones safe from suicidal impulses

NURSING DIAGNOSIS

Dependence on environmental safety related to suicide ideation: reliance on nurses to maintain an environment that offers safety for persons intent on performing the suicide act

PLANNING

Patient Needs
Protection from physical harm
Dependence
Increased learning

Primary Nurse-Patient Goals
To prevent physical injury
To achieve comfort
To achieve awareness of needs

NURSING INTERVENTIONS

Nursing Treatments
Arrange geographic placement (so the person can be seen by the nurses)
Remove harmful objects from the environment
Provide frequent patient contact

Nursing Observations
Evaluate the safety of the environment
Observe the person's activity pattern

Health Teaching
Explain the reason for and intended effect of the therapy

EVALUATION

See the evaluation criteria for each specific goal in Chapter 2.

ENVIRONMENTAL TEMPERATURE

Cold Intolerance

ASSESSMENT

Subjective Data
Usually feels chilly

Objective Data
Keeps windows closed
Frequently raises the room temperature
Tends to wear heavy clothing
If exposed to cold, may have a chill
Avoids cold showers and swimming in cold water

Related Data
Commonly Related Diseases:
Hypothryoidism
Myxedema
Creatinism
Simmonds' disease

POSSIBLE ETIOLOGY

Decreased metabolic rate provides inadequate body heat. Thin skin. Poor circulation.

NURSING DIAGNOSIS

Cold intolerance: inability to be comfortable in a cool environment

PLANNING

Patient Needs	**Primary Nurse-Patient Goals**
Normal temperature	To maintain regulating mechanisms and functions
Comfort	To achieve comfort
Protection from physical harm	To prevent physical injury
Increased learning	To achieve awareness of needs

NURSING INTERVENTIONS

Nursing Treatments
Cover with warm blankets
Decrease drafts
Drape for warmth
Dress in warm clothing
Give warm liquids
Keep the patient's windows closed
Maintain a warm room temperature
Place a blanket directly against the skin

Place only warm hands and objects on the patient
Refrain from giving iced liquids
Refrain from giving local cold applications
Discourage smoking

Nursing Observations
Identify environmental discomforts
Observe for chills

Health Teaching
Explain the causes of the health problem
Recommend the use of warm clothing
Explain the reason for and intended effect of the therapy

EVALUATION

See the evaluation criteria for each specific goal in Chapter 2.

Heat Intolerance

ASSESSMENT

Subjective Data
Complains of being hot
Headache
Nausea
Dizziness

Objective Data
Tachycardia
Abdominal cramps
Diarrhea
Profuse sweating
Neck and facial flushing
Tends to keep the windows open even in cold weather
Frequently lowers the room temperature

Related Data
Commonly Related Diseases:
Thyrotoxicosis
Cushing's syndrome

POSSIBLE ETIOLOGY

Increased metabolic rate due to excessive energy consumption by the body.
Hormone changes during menopause

NURSING DIAGNOSIS

Heat intolerance: inability to be comfortable in a warm environment or
with heat generated by physical exertion or stress

PLANNING

Patient Needs
Normal temperature

Primary Nurse-Patient Goals
To maintain regulating mechanisms
    and functions

Comfort
Protection from physical harm
Increased learning

To achieve comfort
To prevent physical injury
To achieve awareness of needs

NURSING INTERVENTIONS

Nursing Treatments
Cover with lightweight blankets
Dress in lightweight clothing
Give iced liquids
Increase drafts
Maintain adequate room ventilation
Maintain a cool room temperature
Place by a window
Place in an uncrowded area
Refrain from giving hot liquids
Refrain from giving oral stimulants
Refrain from giving local heat applications
Discourage oral stimulants
Discourage strenuous activities

Nursing Observations
Identify environmental discomforts

Health Teaching
Explain the causes of the health problem
Advise against exposure to intense heat
Explain the need to avoid overexertion
Recommend the use of lightweight clothing
Explain the reason for and intended effect of the therapy

EVALUATION

See the evaluation criteria for each specific goal in Chapter 2.

RESPONSES TO
THE ENVIRONMENT

Intolerance for Environmental
Disorder

ASSESSMENT

Subjective Data
Anxiety
Nervousness
Experiencing pain

Objective Data
Confusion
Irritability
Poor concentration ability

Related Data

Commonly Related Diseases:
Cerebral arteriosclerosis
Cerebral concussion
Simple senile psychosis
Alcoholism psychosis
Hypertension
Anxiety psychoneurosis
Schizophrenia
Epilepsy
Thyrotoxicosis

POSSIBLE ETIOLOGY

Intense stress. Mental disorganization.

NURSING DIAGNOSIS

Intolerance for environmental disorder: the inability to tolerate, without undesirable effects, haphazardly arranged environmental objects, excessive noise, and overcrowding

PLANNING

Patient Needs	Primary Nurse-Patient Goals
Comfort	To achieve comfort
Protection from physical harm	To prevent physical injury
Protection from psychologic threat	To prevent emotional injury
Predictable, orderly world	To achieve a therapeutic environment
Increased learning	To achieve awareness of needs

NURSING INTERVENTIONS

Nursing Treatments
Arrange orderly surroundings
Place in a private room
Place in an uncrowded area
Provide quiet
Refrain from performing nonessential procedures

Nursing Observations
Observe for an excessive stress level

Health Teaching
Explain the causes of the health problem
Explain the reason for and intended effect of the therapy

EVALUATION

See the evaluation criteria for each specific goal in Chapter 2.

Misperception of the Environment

ASSESSMENT

Subjective Data
Hears sounds in the environment that do not exist
Fearful

Objective Data
Misidentifies existing objects (lace perceived as a spider web)
Reacts to objects in the environment that do not actually exist

Related Data

Commonly Related Conditions:
Confusion
Uremia

Commonly Related Diseases:
Cerebral arteriosclerosis
Alcoholism
Cerebral tumor or concussion
Paranoid schizophrenia
Malaria

POSSIBLE ETIOLOGY

Drug side effects. In hallucinations, perceptions, sensations, and thoughts are projected into the environment as though they were independent of the individual. In illusions, the environment is misinterpreted as a result of a poorly integrated personality. Brain cell damage. High fever.

NURSING DIAGNOSIS

Misperception of the environment: a misinterpretation of that which exists in the environment

PLANNING

Patient Needs	Primary Nurse-Patient Goals
Comfort	To achieve comfort
Protection from psychologic threat	To prevent emotional injury
Increased learning	To achieve awareness of needs

NURSING INTERVENTIONS

Nursing Treatments
Arrange orderly surroundings
Illuminate the room adequately
Place in a private room
Place in an uncrowded area
Provide radio and television for diversion
Reassure verbally

Refrain from supporting the patient's illusions and hallucinations
Remove the stimuli which are supporting the misperception

Nursing Observations
Observe for an excessive stress level

Health Teaching
Explain the causes of the health problem
Advise against denouncing erroneous perceptions
Explain the reason for and intended effect of the therapy

EVALUATION

See the evaluation criteria for each specific goal in Chapter 2.

INADEQUATE INFORMATION RELATED TO THE ENVIRONMENT

Inadequate Information Related to Environmental Cleanliness

ASSESSMENT

Subjective Data
Person confirms a lack of information

Objective Data
Person's actions indicate a lack of information regarding the fact that:
   furniture, walls, windows, and floors require frequent dusting
   dishes and utensils should be washed and stored
   bed linens should be washed at least weekly
   bathrooms require scrupulous cleaning
   rodent and insect control is essential
   animals must be clean and controlled

Related Data
Commonly Related Diseases:
None
   OR
Any disease

POSSIBLE ETIOLOGY

Lack of education

NURSING DIAGNOSIS

Inadequate information related to environmental cleanliness: lack of information related to keeping the external surroundings free from soil or dust

PLANNING

Patient Needs	**Primary Nurse-Patient Goals**
Cleanliness	To achieve good hygiene
Protection from physical harm	To prevent physical injury
Increased learning	To achieve awareness of needs

NURSING INTERVENTIONS

Nursing Treatments
Approach unhurriedly
Encourage patient questions

Nursing Observations
Evaluate the response to teaching

Health Teaching
Explain how to maintain environmental cleanliness
Inform that cleanliness is basic to health

EVALUATION

See the evaluation criteria for each specific goal in Chapter 2.

Inadequate Information Related to Waste Sanitation (121,122)

ASSESSMENT

Subjective Data
Person confirms a lack of information

Objective Data
Person's actions indicate a lack of information regarding the fact that:
   exposed garbage allows flies and rats to carry infection
   human wastes should never be placed in areas where food and water can
      become contaminated by it
   human wastes should be buried out of reach of flies
   private sewage systems should never be closer than one acre apart
   cesspools should never be near limestone where the sewage can travel
      through the limestone crevices and contaminate underground wells
      and springs
   solids from septic tanks must be periodically removed and buried
   privies should be deep, have a floor above the ground, have an adequate
      seat cover, have screens over ventilation openings to prevent flies from
      entering, and have a tight door that prevents chickens, pigs, etc., from
      roaming inside

Related Data
Commonly Related Diseases:
Typhoid fever
Amebic dysentery
Bacillary dysentery
Cholera
Infectious hepatitis

POSSIBLE ETIOLOGY

Lack of instruction

NURSING DIAGNOSIS

Inadequate information related to waste sanitation: lack of information regarding satisfactory health measures for the disposal of human wastes

PLANNING

Patient Needs

Protection from physical harm

Increased learning

Primary Nurse-Patient Goals

To prevent physical injury, infection

To achieve awareness of needs and/or use of resources

NURSING INTERVENTIONS

Nursing Treatments

Approach unhurriedly

Encourage patient questions

Make a referral (to the city sanitation department)

Nursing Observations

Evaluate the response to teaching

Health Teaching

Emphasize that food wastes should be burned in animal-inhabited outdoor areas

Emphasize that garbage should be covered

Emphasize that, in outdoor living, human wastes should be buried

Emphasize the need to use only an approved sewage facility

Inform that cleanliness is basic to health

Recommend strict adherence to safety rules

EVALUATION

See the evaluation criteria for each specific goal in Chapter 2.

Inadequate Information Related to Water Sanitation (121,122)

ASSESSMENT

Subjective Data

Person confirms a lack of information

Objective Data

Person's actions indicate a lack of information regarding the fact that:
  river water should not be used for bathing
  unapproved water supplies should not be used
  unpurified water from lakes and streams is unsafe
  it is dangerous to use wells and springs located in limestone where pollution from nearby cesspools, privies, or flooded lakes and streams can occur
  safe wells and springs must be more than 50 feet from any source of contamination
  wells must have properly constructed casings, a drainage system away from the well, and not be connected to a sewer system
  ice cubes made from polluted water are as unsafe as the water itself

Related Data

Commonly Related Diseases:

Amebic dysentery

Cholera

Bacillary dysentery
Infectious hepatitis
Typhoid fever

POSSIBLE ETIOLOGY

Lack of instruction

NURSING DIAGNOSIS

Inadequate information related to water sanitation: inadequate information regarding satisfactory health measures involving the consumption of drinking water

PLANNING

Patient Needs

Protection from physical harm

Increased learning

Primary Nurse-Patient Goals

To prevent physical injury, infection

To achieve awareness of needs
  and/or use of resources

NURSING INTERVENTIONS

Nursing Treatments
Approach unhurriedly
Encourage patient questions
Make a referral (to the city sanitation department)

Nursing Observations
Evaluate the response to teaching

Health Teaching
Emphasize that potentially unsafe water should be boiled for ten minutes
Emphasize the need to use only an approved water supply
Inform that cleanliness is basic to health
Inform that Halazone tablets should be added to potentially unsafe water
Inform that the color and taste of outdoor water do not indicate its safety
Recommend strict adherence to safety rules

EVALUATION

See the evaluation criteria for each specific goal in Chapter 2.

INADEQUATE INFORMATION RELATED TO TRAVEL

Inadequate Information Related to Air-travel Fitness (497)

ASSESSMENT

Subjective Data
Person confirms a lack of information

Objective Data
Person's actions indicate a lack of information regarding the fact that:
  air travel is unsuitable for persons having severe anemia, leukemia,

sickle cell disease or trait, cardiac disease sufficiently severe to present discomfort after walking a city block or up a flight of stairs, respiratory disease, recent pneumothorax, recent (within 10 days) encephalography or ventriculography, a poorly regulated colostomy, a contagious disease, an extreme fear of flying, or who are highly emotionally disturbed

when a woman is 8 months' pregnant, she must have a physician's written permission to board a plane

infants less than 10 days old should not travel by plane

Related Data

Commonly Related Diseases:
Angina pectoris
Acute sinusitis
Cavitating tuberculosis, etc.

POSSIBLE ETIOLOGY

Lack of education regarding alterations in atmospheric pressure during ascent and descent. Decreased barometric pressure causing gas to be trapped in the hollow organs. Decreased barometric pressure reducing the alveolar oxygen pressure in the lungs which would require oxygen therapy for persons with respiratory disorders.

NURSING DIAGNOSIS

Inadequate information related to air-travel fitness: lack of information regarding the inadvisability of air travel in certain health conditions

PLANNING

Patient Needs
Protection from physical harm
Increased learning

Primary Nurse-Patient Goals
To prevent physical injury
To achieve awareness of needs

NURSING INTERVENTIONS

Nursing Treatments
Approach unhurriedly
Encourage modes of travel other than flying
Encourage patient questions

Nursing Observations
Evaluate the response to teaching

Health Teaching
Emphasize the need to fly in pressurized airplanes
Explain the causes of the health problem

EVALUATION

See the evaluation criteria for each specific goal in Chapter 2.

Inadequate Information Related to Foreign-Food Hazards (545)

ASSESSMENT

Subjective Data
Person confirms a lack of information

Objective Data
Person's actions indicate a lack of information regarding:
    the specific foods to avoid eating in foreign countries
    how to request that certain foods be cooked in foreign countries
    that the areas of highest food hazard are South or Central America, Asia,
        Africa, eastern Europe, the Orient, or Mexico

Related Data
Commonly Related Diseases:
Amebic dysentery
Bacillary dysentery

POSSIBLE ETIOLOGY

Lack of instruction

NURSING DIAGNOSIS

Inadequate information related to foreign-food hazards: lack of information
regarding the dangers of eating foreign foods

PLANNING

Patient Needs	**Primary Nurse-Patient Goals**
Protection from physical harm	To prevent physical injury
Increased learning	To achieve awareness of needs

NURSING INTERVENTIONS

Nursing Treatments
Approach unhurriedly
Encourage patient questions

Nursing Observations
Evaluate the response to teaching

Health Teaching
Advise against eating dairy products in foreign countries
Advise against eating in unlicensed restaurants
Advise against eating raw fruits and vegetables in foreign countries
Advise against using ice cubes made from potentially unsafe water
Emphasize that potentially unsafe water should be boiled for ten minutes
Explain the causes of the health problem
Inform that carbonated beverages are safe to drink in foreign countries
Inform that cleanliness is basic to health
Inform that Halazone tablets should be added to potentially unsafe water

Explain that teeth should not be brushed with potentially unsafe water

Recommend eating only well-cooked meat in foreign countries

EVALUATION

See the evaluation criteria for each specific goal in Chapter 2.

Inadequate Information Related to Jet Lag (489,542,545)

ASSESSMENT

Subjective Data

Person confirms a lack of information

Objective Data

Person's actions indicate a lack of information regarding the fact that:

jet lag does not occur when flying north or south because the time zones are unchanged

jet lag does occur when flying east or west because of multiple time zones

a 4- to 5-hour time difference requires minimal adjustment, while a gain or loss of more than 6 hours or a day requires considerable adjustment

adjustment is more difficult on flights away from home than on flights toward home

jet lag causes fatigue, sleeplessness, body temperature and blood pressure changes, irregular eating schedule, dehydration sometimes, and altered biophysiologic activity

physiologic changes are more persistent than psychologic changes

there are precautions to be taken with jet lag

POSSIBLE ETIOLOGY

Lack of instruction regarding the fact that rapid time changes temporarily disrupt the body's dependence of physiologic cycles on a well-ordered internal clock or daily rhythm

NURSING DIAGNOSIS

Inadequate information related to jet lag: lack of information regarding rapid adjustment to time changes in distant places while traveling by high speed airline

PLANNING

Patient Needs

Protection from physical harm

Increased learning

Primary Nurse-Patient Goals

To prevent physical injury

To achieve awareness of needs

NURSING INTERVENTIONS

Nursing Treatments

Approach unhurriedly

Discourage smoking (while in flight)

Encourage adequate rest (prior to and during the flight)
Encourage patient questions

Nursing Observations
Evaluate the response to teaching

Health Teaching
Explain the causes of the health problem
Advise that positions which impair circulation be avoided (while in flight)
Advise against wearing constrictive clothing
Instruct to increase fluid (water) intake (while in flight)
Recommend eating and drinking in moderation
Recommend limiting jet flying time to five consecutive hours when possible
Recommend that jet travelers reduce stress by arriving 24 hours before
    scheduled activity
Recommend the use of eye shields for sleeping (while in flight)

EVALUATION

See the evaluation criteria for each specific goal in Chapter 2.

14.

NURSING DIAGNOSES RELATED TO
The Gastrointestinal System

ORAL DISCOMFORTS

Oral Mucosa Irritation Related to Dentures

ASSESSMENT

Subjective Data
Some oral pain or discomfort

Objective Data
Slightly reddened gums
Gum tenderness and swelling
Denture pressure on gums or oral mucosa
Loose-fitting dentures slide around the mouth

POSSIBLE ETIOLOGY

Poorly fitting dentures

NURSING DIAGNOSIS

Oral mucosa irritation related to dentures: irritation of the oral mucosa by artificial teeth

PLANNING

Patient Needs
Comfort
Protection from physical harm
Increased learning

Primary Nurse-Patient Goals
To achieve comfort
To prevent physical injury
To achieve awareness of needs

NURSING INTERVENTIONS

Nursing Treatments
Remove the dentures
Make a referral (to a dentist)

Health Teaching
Explain the need for properly fitting dentures

EVALUATION

See the evaluation criteria for each specific goal in Chapter 2.

Poor Oral Secretion Control

ASSESSMENT

Objective Data
Drooling
Spitting
Lip or unilateral facial drooping

Related Data
Commonly Related Conditions:
Teething
Commonly Related Diseases:
Bulbar palsy
Mental retardation
Parkinson's disease
Cretinism
Stomatitis
Riley's syndrome
Iodide or mercury poisoning
Cerebral vascular accident

POSSIBLE ETIOLOGY

Facial nerve paralysis. Esophageal obstruction. Central nervous system disorder. Excessive salivation.

NURSING DIAGNOSIS

Poor oral secretion control: inability to control secretion flow from the mouth

PLANNING

Patient Needs	Primary Nurse-Patient Goals
Comfort	To achieve comfort
Cleanliness	To achieve good hygiene
Increased learning	To achieve awareness of needs

NURSING INTERVENTIONS

Nursing Treatments
Encourage decreased acid-food intake (for excessive salivation)
Place in the side-lying position (when in bed)
Protect with a plastic bib
Provide disposable tissue
Bathe locally

Provide standby emergency equipment (airway suction machine)
Suction the airway (as needed)

Nursing Observations
Observe for airway obstruction

Health Teaching
Explain the causes of the health problem
Explain the reason for and intended effect of the therapy

EVALUATION

See the evaluation criteria for each specific goal in Chapter 2.

POTENTIAL ORAL INJURY

Potential Teeth Discoloration

ASSESSMENT

Objective Data
Receives iron or iodine drugs in liquid form
Consumes excess coffee or tea
Smokes tobacco

POSSIBLE ETIOLOGY

Teeth staining from chemicals or foods

NURSING DIAGNOSIS

Potential teeth discoloration: the probability that the teeth will become discolored

PLANNING

Patient Needs	**Primary Nurse-Patient Goals**
Cleanliness	To achieve good hygiene
Protection from physical harm	To prevent physical injury
Increased learning	To achieve awareness of needs

NURSING INTERVENTIONS

Nursing Treatments
Discourage oral stimulants
Discourage smoking
Provide a drinking straw (when taking iron or iodine in liquid form)
Brush the teeth (after taking drugs)

Health Teaching
Explain the causes of the health problem
Explain the reason for and intended effect of the therapy

EVALUATION

See the evaluation criteria for each specific goal in Chapter 2.

Predisposition to Tooth Decay (40,96)

ASSESSMENT

Objective Data

Infrequent tooth brushing
Use of a nonfluoride toothpaste
Indulgence in high-starch and high-sugar foods
Crowded teeth
Profuse salivation
Infant sucks on a bottle of milk while going to sleep

Related Data

Most prevalent during childhood and adolescence

POSSIBLE ETIOLOGY

Inherited susceptibility. Poor dental hygiene. Character and amount of saliva. Poor nutrition. Contour of the mouth and position of the teeth.

NURSING DIAGNOSIS

Predisposition to tooth decay: a proneness toward decomposition of the teeth

PLANNING

Patient Needs	Primary Nurse-Patient Goals
Food balance	To maintain nutrition to all cells
Protection from physical harm	To prevent physical injury
Increased learning	To achieve awareness of needs

NURSING INTERVENTIONS

Nursing Treatments
Encourage decreased carbohydrate intake

Nursing Observations
Inspect the teeth for abnormalities

Health Teaching
Explain the causes of the health problem
Advise frequent and early dental attention
Advise against eating sweets
Advise early and consistent use of the toothbrush
Recommend the use of dental floss
Instruct that only water, not milk or juice, be given in the infant's bottle at
    bedtime
Recommend the use of a fluoride toothpaste
Explain the reason for and intended effect of the therapy

EVALUATION

See the evaluation criteria for each specific goal in Chapter 2.

GASTROINTESTINAL DISTRESS

Flatulence (247,414)

ASSESSMENT

Subjective Data
Feeling of fullness
Cramping pain, sometimes

Objective Data
Abdominal distention, usually mild
Gurgling bowel sounds
Abdominal tympany, if flatulence is severe

Related Data
Commonly Related Conditions:
Pregnancy
Commonly Related Diseases:
Spastic colon
Cholelithiasis
Sprue

POSSIBLE ETIOLOGY

Swallowed air. Production of air in the intestinal lumen due to bacterial fermentative action on proteins and carbohydrates. Compression of nonabsorbable sugars. Rapid eating.

NURSING DIAGNOSIS

Flatulence: excessive gas accumulation in the intestinal tract

PLANNING

Patient Needs	Primary Nurse-Patient Goals
Waste elimination	To maintain regulating mechanisms and functions
Exercise	To achieve exercise
Comfort	To achieve comfort
Protection from physical harm	To prevent physical injury
Increased learning	To achieve awareness of needs

NURSING INTERVENTIONS

Nursing Treatments
Change the patient's position frequently
Discourage smoking (especially at mealtime)
Encourage decreased gas-forming-food intake
Restrict fluids at mealtime
Give warm liquids after meals
Refrain from giving iced liquids
Refrain from giving carbonated beverages

Give nonprescription drugs (ExR) (Simethicone)
Insert a colon tube
Encourage moderate physical exercise

Nursing Observations
Inspect the abdomen for distention

Health Teaching
Explain the causes of the health problem
Advise against chewing gum
Instruct not to use a drinking straw
Recommend eating and drinking in moderation
Recommend thorough food chewing
Explain the reason for and intended effect of the therapy

EVALUATION

See the evaluation criteria for each specific goal in Chapter 2.

Gastric Irritation

ASSESSMENT

Subjective Data
Nausea
Cramping abdominal pain

Objective Data
Abdominal distention
Diarrhea
Anorexia

Related Data
Commonly Related Diseases:
None
    OR
Regional enteritis (milk)
Cholecystitis (fatty foods)
Stomach carcinoma (meat)

POSSIBLE ETIOLOGY

Intolerance for specific drugs or foods. Milk intolerance is due to an inability of the stomach or intestines to digest and absorb milk, or absence of the intestinal enzyme needed for milk digestion. Fatty food intolerance is due to insufficient bile being available to aid digestion by breaking fats into small globules so that intestinal enzymes can further digest it.

NURSING DIAGNOSIS

Gastric irritation: irritation of the digestive system by foods or drugs

PLANNING

Patient Needs	**Primary Nurse-Patient Goals**
Food balance	To maintain nutrition to all cells
Comfort	To achieve comfort

Protection from physical harm   To prevent physical injury

Increased learning   To achieve awareness of needs

NURSING INTERVENTIONS

Nursing Treatments

Specific to Foods:
Boil the milk
> OR

Dilute the milk
> OR

Give a whole milk substitute
Encourage decreased fatty-food intake
Give bland foods
Provide food selection

Specific to Drugs:
Dilute the medication
> OR

Give enteric-coated medications or enclose the medication in a gelatin capsule
> OR

Give milk with medications
> OR

Give medication by injection or in liquid form instead of pills

Nursing Observations
Observe for evidence of a favorable response to therapy

Health Teaching
Explain the causes of the health problem
Instruct to take medications immediately after meals
Explain the reason for and intended effect of the therapy

EVALUATION

See the evaluation criteria for each specific goal in Chapter 2.

Heartburn (414,453)

ASSESSMENT

Subjective Data
Burning, wavelike sensation slowly rising from the stomach to the throat, often extending into the jaw
Chest tightness

Objective Data
Onset following heavy, spicy meals and hurried eating
Mouth is opened for pain relief
Increased salivation

Related Data
Commonly Related Conditions:
Pregnancy

Commonly Related Diseases:
None
   OR
Peptic ulcer
Duodenal ulcer
Pyloric ulcer
Chronic gastritis
Esophageal hernia

POSSIBLE ETIOLOGY

Regurgitation of gastric contents into the esophagus. Esophageal distention by large amounts of food or drink. Habitual air swallowing.

NURSING DIAGNOSIS

Heartburn (pyrosis): a burning sensation in the mid-sternal area

PLANNING

Patient Needs	Primary Nurse-Patient Goals
Comfort	To achieve comfort
Increased learning	To achieve awareness of needs

NURSING INTERVENTIONS

Nursing Treatments
Discourage smoking (especially with meals)
Encourage decreased acid-food intake
Encourage decreased gas-forming-food intake
Give bland foods (if heartburn is chronic)
Give carbonated beverages
Give nonprescription drugs (ExR) (antacids, bicarbonates)

Nursing Observations
Observe for evidence of a favorable response to therapy

Health Teaching
Explain the causes of the health problem
Recommend eating and drinking in moderation
Recommend thorough food chewing
Explain the reason for and intended effect of the therapy

EVALUATION

See the evaluation criteria for each specific goal in Chapter 2.

Increased Intraabdominal Pressure Discomfort (70,71,391)

ASSESSMENT

Subjective Data
Severe pressure sensation
Abdominal tightness

Objective Data
Severe abdominal distention
Restlessness
Mild respiratory discomfort
Difficulty changing position

Related Data
Commonly Related Conditions:
Ascites
Pregnancy
Hepatomegaly
Splenomegaly
Commonly Related Diseases:
Laennec's cirrhosis
Abdominal carcinoma
Paralytic ileus
Pancreatic cyst
Ovarian cyst
Uterine tumor

POSSIBLE ETIOLOGY

Diminished peristalsis resulting from narcotic suppression or immobility.
Accumulated fluid or solid material within the abdominal cavity. Handling
of the intestines during surgery.

NURSING DIAGNOSIS

Increased intraabdominal pressure discomfort: the discomfort of increased
pressure within the abdominal cavity

PLANNING

Patient Needs
Comfort
Protection from physical harm
Increased learning

Primary Nurse-Patient Goals
To achieve comfort
To prevent physical injury
To achieve awareness of needs

NURSING INTERVENTIONS

Nursing Treatments
Change the patient's position frequently
Give small, frequent feedings (instead of full meals if bowel sounds are
    normal)
Handle gently
Place in the sitting position (for respiratory distress)
Remove constrictive clothing
Insert a colon tube

Nursing Observations
Auscultate the abdomen for abnormal bowel sounds

Health Teaching
Explain the causes of the health problem
Explain the reason for and intended effect of the therapy

EVALUATION

See the evaluation criteria for each specific goal in Chapter 2.

Indigestion (414,453)

ASSESSMENT

Subjective Data
Abdominal fullness
Dull, aching pain
Nausea

Objective Data
Belching
Flatulence
Mild abdominal distention, sometimes
Regurgitation
Onset during a meal or several hours later

Related Data
Commonly Related Diseases:
None
   OR
Gastritis
Peptic ulcer
Gastric carcinoma
Glomerulonephritis
Tuberculosis
Coronary sclerosis
Enteritis
Chronic pancreatitis
Sprue
Cholecystitis
Cholelithiasis

POSSIBLE ETIOLOGY

Faulty enzyme functioning. Gastric mucosa irritation or inflammation. Liver distention resulting from impaired cardiac or circulatory function. Difficulty in dissolving and breaking down food. Food allergy.

NURSING DIAGNOSIS

Indigestion (dyspepsia): a sense of fullness in the epigastrium

Nausea (28,113)

ASSESSMENT

Subjective Data
A queasy, unsettled gastric sensation

Objective Data
Difficulty eating
Prefers liquids and soft foods

Related Data

Commonly Related Conditions:
Drug toxicity
Carbon monoxide poisoning

Commonly Related Diseases:
Myocarditis
Myocardial infarction
Abdominal aneurysm
Addison's disease
Beriberi
Tularemia
Encephalitis
Endometritis
Acute and chronic gastritis
Pancreatitis
Glomerulonephritis
Hepatitis
Cerebral concussion
Cerebral contusion
Cerebral angioma
Meningioma
Laennec's cirrhosis
Cholecystitis
Cholelithiasis
Appendicitis
Pheochromocytoma
Meniere's disease
Stomach carcinoma
Gastric ulcer
Mesenteric vascular occlusion
Lupus erythematosus
Renal calculi
Smallpox
Poliomyelitis
Lymphocytic choriomeningitis
Cerebral vascular accident
Colorado tick fever
Strep throat
Salmonella gastroenteritis

POSSIBLE ETIOLOGY

Diminished gastric acid or enzyme activity. Reduced motility of the duodenum and large intestines. Displaced stomach from an intraabdominal mass or pregnant uterus. Equilibrium imbalance. Acidosis. Impaired cardiac circulation. Gastric irritation from foods and drugs. Viral or bacterial intestinal infection. Decreased blood pressure. Liver congestion. Adrenal insufficiency.

NURSING DIAGNOSIS

Nausea: a feeling that emesis is imminent

PLANNING

Patient Needs	**Primary Nurse-Patient Goals**
Comfort	To achieve comfort
Protection from physical harm	To prevent physical injury
Increased learning	To achieve awareness of needs

NURSING INTERVENTIONS

Nursing Treatments
Elevate the head
Encourage deep breathing
Feed slowly
Give bland foods
  OR
Give carbonated beverages
  OR
Give hot tea
Give small, frequent feedings
Withhold food until the patient requests it
Give nonprescription drugs (ExR) (Marezine, Dramamine, Emetrol)
Refrain from giving enemas

Nursing Observations
Auscultate the abdomen for abnormal bowel sounds

Health Teaching
Explain the causes of the health problem
Explain the reason for and intended effect of the therapy

Medical Treatments Performed by Nurses
Give the prescribed drugs

EVALUATION

See the evaluation criteria for each specific goal in Chapter 2.

POTENTIAL GASTROINTESTINAL DISTRESS

Potential Gastric Irritation

ASSESSMENT

Objective Data
Ingestion of drugs known to be gastric irritants
Eats highly spiced foods

Intake of substances that in the past have consistently caused gastric discomfort

Related Data

Commonly Related Diseases:
None
   OR
Gastritis
Enteritis
Peptic ulcer
Duodenal ulcer

POSSIBLE ETIOLOGY

Ingestion of irritating foods or chemicals

NURSING DIAGNOSIS

Potential gastric irritation: the probability that the gastric mucosa will become irritated

PLANNING

Patient Needs	**Primary Nurse-Patient Goals**
Protection from physical harm	To prevent physical injury
Increased learning	To achieve awareness of needs

NURSING INTERVENTIONS

Nursing Treatments
Dilute the medication
   OR
Give enteric-coated medications
   OR
Give medication by injection or in liquid form instead of pills
   OR
Give milk with medications
   OR
Give nonprescription drugs (ExR) (antacids with the irritating medication)
Provide food selection

Nursing Observations
Inspect the abdomen for distention
Observe for complaints of pain (cramping)
Observe for complaints of nausea
Observe for diarrhea

Health Teaching
Explain the reason for and intended effect of the therapy

EVALUATION

See the evaluation criteria for each specific goal in Chapter 2.

Predisposition to Stress Ulcer (387,487)

ASSESSMENT

Objective Data
Recent major infection
Recent multiple surgical procedures
Previous gastric ulcer
Extensive burns

Related Data
The potential increases in proportion to the percentage of the body area burned
Onset is most likely 3 to 10 days after thermal injury
In burns, the peak occurrence is 30 days after injury

Commonly Related Conditions:
Shock

Commonly Related Diseases:
Second- and third-degree burns
Cerebral vascular accident

POSSIBLE ETIOLOGY

The effect of acid hypersecretion, endotoxins, microemboli, and steroids. Rapid loss of protein. The stomach mucous cells undergo tissue breakdown and fail to duplicate themselves normally. This results in erosion of the stomach's superficial mucosa and causes ulceration.

NURSING DIAGNOSIS

Predisposition to stress ulcer: susceptibility to developing a gastric ulcer soon after receiving a serious injury

PLANNING

Patient Needs	**Primary Nurse-Patient Goals**
Protection from physical harm	To prevent physical injury
Protection from psychologic threat	To prevent emotional injury
Increased learning	To achieve awareness of needs

NURSING INTERVENTIONS

Nursing Treatments
Approach unhurriedly
Avoid causing intense emotional situations
Arrange pleasant surroundings
Encourage adequate rest
Encourage increased protein-food intake
Provide quiet
Reduce the demands placed upon the patient
Refrain from performing nonessential procedures
Give nonprescription drugs (ExR) (antacids)

Nursing Observations
Monitor blood studies for evidence of gastric ulceration

Health Teaching
Describe those symptoms which should be reported (pain, bleeding)
Explain the causes of the health problem
Explain the reason for and intended effect of the therapy

Medical Treatments Performed by Nurses.
Give the prescribed drugs (vitamin A parenterally)

EVALUATION

See the evaluation criteria for each specific goal in Chapter 2.

GASTROINTESTINAL ELIMINATION, EXCESSIVE

Chronic Regurgitation (325,391)

ASSESSMENT

Subjective Data
Sour taste

Objective Data
Food is swallowed
Returns to the mouth
Is unintentionally swallowed again
May occur only occasionally or after each meal

Related Data
Commonly Related Diseases:
Pyloric stenosis
Esophageal cancer

POSSIBLE ETIOLOGY

Stomach contents placing pressure against the cardiac sphincter

NURSING DIAGNOSIS

Chronic regurgitation: the return of food into the mouth from the stomach following eating

PLANNING

Patient Needs	**Primary Nurse-Patient Goals**
Comfort	To achieve comfort
Cleanliness	To achieve good hygiene
Protection from physical harm	To prevent physical injury
Increased learning	To achieve awareness of needs

NURSING INTERVENTIONS

Nursing Treatments
Feed slowly
Give small, frequent feedings
Place in the sitting position (while feeding)
Refresh with a mouthwash

Nursing Observations
Observe for airway obstruction (from aspiration)

Health Teaching
Explain the causes of the health problem
Explain the reason for and intended effect of the therapy

EVALUATION

See the evaluation criteria for each specific goal in Chapter 2.

Diarrhea (32,71,300,325)

ASSESSMENT

Subjective Data
Cramping pain
Weakness
Nausea

Objective Data
Frequent unformed stools
Gurgling bowel sounds

Related Data
Commonly Related Conditions:
Spastic colon
Arsenic poisoning

Commonly Related Diseases:
Amebic dysentery
Amyloidosis
Appendicitis
Cholera
Diabetes mellitus
Infectious hepatitis
Malaria
Pellegra
Peptic ulcer
Shigellosis
Sprue
Trichinosis
Typhoid fever
Gastritis
Escherichia coli

Diverticulitis
Ulcerative colitis
Intestinal metastatic carcinoma
Addison's disease
Tuberculosis
Lymphosarcoma
Celiac disease
Whipple's disease
Glomerulonephritis
Mesenteric vascular occlusion
Kwashiorkor
Trichuriasis
Histoplasmosis
Strongyloidiasis
Salmonella gastroenteritis
Epidemic neuromyasthenia
Bacillary dysentery
Thyrotoxicosis

POSSIBLE ETIOLOGY

Mechanical, chemical, or bacterial irritation of the intestinal mucosa causing rapid movement of feces through the intestinal tract. Emotional stress. Surgical procedures related to the gastrointestinal system. Contamination of food or drink with microorganisms such as *Escherichia coli*, *Salmonella*, *Shigella*, *Entamoeba histolytica*.

NURSING DIAGNOSIS

Diarrhea: the passage of unformed stools at frequent, successive intervals

PLANNING

Patient Needs	Primary Nurse-Patient Goals
Water-salt balance	To maintain fluid and electrolyte balance
Acid-base balance (if prolonged)	To maintain regulating mechanisms and functions
Rest	To achieve rest
Comfort	To achieve comfort
Protection from physical harm	To prevent physical injury
Increased learning	To achieve awareness of needs

NURSING INTERVENTIONS

Nursing Treatments
Balance fluid intake to equal output
Cover with warm blankets
Discourage oral stimulants
Encourage adequate rest
Encourage decreased residue-food intake

Give hot tea
  OR
Give carbonated beverages
  OR
Give clear liquid foods
  OR
Give full-liquid foods
  OR
Give dry crackers
Give nonprescription drugs (ExR) (antidiarrheal drugs)
Refrain from giving hot liquids
Refrain from giving iced liquids
Refrain from giving oral stimulants
Refrain from giving enemas
Refrain from giving laxatives
Refrain from inserting a rectal tube
Refrain from taking rectal temperatures

Nursing Observations
Auscultate the abdomen for abnormal bowel sounds
Measure the body weight (daily)
Measure the intake
Measure the output
Monitor blood studies for abnormal acid-base (if prolonged)
Monitor blood studies for abnormal electrolytes
Observe for complaints of pain
Obtain a bacterial culture (of stool, if bacteria suspected)

Health Teaching
Explain the causes of the health problem
Explain the reason for and intended effect of the therapy

Medical Treatments Performed by Nurses
Give the prescribed drugs (antidiarrheal drugs)

EVALUATION

See the evaluation criteria for each specific goal in Chapter 2.

Hyperemesis (325)

ASSESSMENT

Subjective Data
Headache
Dizziness
Weakness

Objective Data
Prolonged vomiting
Rapid weight loss
Dehydration
Rapid pulse

Related Data

Laboratory Findings:
Urine acetone
Decreased blood chloride

Commonly Related Conditions:
Pregnancy

Commonly Related Diseases:
Toxemia
Liver carcinoma
Alcoholic gastritis
Glomerulonephritis

POSSIBLE ETIOLOGY

Increased chorionic gonadotropin hormone blood level in pregnancy. Endocrine or metabolic imbalance.

NURSING DIAGNOSIS

Hyperemesis (morning sickness): excessive vomiting occurring primarily in the morning

PLANNING

Patient Needs	Primary Nurse-Patient Goals
Water-salt balance	To maintain fluid and electrolyte balance
Acid-base balance	To maintain regulating mechanisms and functions
Rest	To achieve rest
Comfort	To achieve comfort
Cleanliness	To achieve good hygiene
Protection from physical harm	To prevent physical injury
Increased learning	To achieve awareness of needs

NURSING INTERVENTIONS

Nursing Treatments
Restrict the intake to nothing by mouth (until the episode subsides)
Apply a cool, damp cloth to the face
Apply an ice collar
Bathe locally (around the mouth)
Balance fluid intake to equal output
Moisten the mouth with cracked ice
Refresh with a mouthwash
Encourage adequate rest
Give hot tea
   OR
Give carbonated beverages
   OR

Give clear liquid foods
   OR
Give full-liquid foods
   OR
Give dry crackers
Give small, frequent feedings
Give nonprescription drugs (ExR) (antiemetics)

Nursing Observations
Auscultate the abdomen for abnormal bowel sounds
Measure the body weight (daily)
Measure the intake
Measure the output
Monitor blood studies for abnormal acid-base
Monitor blood studies for abnormal electrolytes

Health Teaching
Explain the causes of the health problem
Explain the reason for and intended effect of the therapy

Medical Treatments Performed by Nurses
Give the prescribed drugs (antiemetics)

EVALUATION

See the evaluation criteria for each specific goal in Chapter 2.

Post-meal Diarrhea (70,247)

ASSESSMENT

Subjective Data
Weakness
Palpitations
Nausea

Objective Data
Stools occur 20–30 minutes after each meal
Sweating
Pallor

Related Data
Commonly Related Conditions:
Gastrectomy
Commonly Related Diseases:
Dumping syndrome

POSSIBLE ETIOLOGY

Rapid gastric emptying of stomach contents into the jejunum with jejunum distention resulting in increased peristalsis

NURSING DIAGNOSIS

Post-meal diarrhea: stools that occur shortly after ingestion of a meal

PLANNING

Patient Needs	Primary Nurse-Patient Goals
Water-salt balance	To maintain fluid and electrolyte balance
Food balance	To maintain nutrition to all cells
Rest	To achieve rest
Comfort	To achieve comfort .
Protection from physical harm	To prevent physical injury
Increased learning	To achieve awareness of needs

NURSING INTERVENTIONS

Nursing Treatments
Encourage decreased carbohydrate intake
Encourage increased fatty-food intake
Encourage increased protein-food intake
Feed slowly
Give small, frequent feedings
Place in the flat position (immediately after meals)
Refrain from giving hot liquids
Refrain from giving iced liquids
Restrict fluids at the mealtime

Nursing Observations
Measure the intake
Measure the output
Monitor the blood pressure
Monitor blood studies for abnormal electrolytes

Health Teaching
Explain the causes of the health problem
Explain the reason for and intended effect of the therapy

Medical Treatments Performed by Nurses
Give the prescribed drugs (tolbutamide)

EVALUATION

See the evaluation criteria for each specific goal in Chapter 2.

Vomiting (71,325,391)

ASSESSMENT

Subjective Data
Weakness
Sour taste

Objective Data
Loss of stomach contents
Consists of undigested food, clear fluid, bile, or pus
Of short duration

Related Data

Commonly Related Conditions:
Digitalis toxicity
Salicylate poisoning
Carbon monoxide poisoning
Radiation sickness

Commonly Related Diseases:
Gastric ulcer
Gastric carcinoma
Cholera
Acute or chronic gastritis
Thrombophlebitis
Myocardial infarction
Abdominal aneurysm
Beriberi
Diverticulitis
Diabetes mellitus
Encephalitis
Hepatitis
Pancreatitis
Meniere's disease
Cerebral angioma
Meningioma
Laennec's cirrhosis
Cholecystitis
Cholelithiasis
Appendicitis
Glomerulonephritis
Pheochromocytoma
Pneumococcal pneumonia
Myocarditis
Mesenteric vascular occlusion
Lupus erythematosus
Renal calculi
Cerebral vascular accident
Cerebral glioma
Kwashiorkor
Smallpox
Poliomyelitis
Lymphocytic choriomeningitis
Colorado tick fever
Epidemic neuromyasthenia
Salmonella gastroenteritis
Labyrinthitis
Hypertension
Pyloric stenosis
Ruptured esophageal abscess
Ruptured gastric abscess

POSSIBLE ETIOLOGY

Abdominal contractions due to stimulation of the afferent impulses in the medulla. Viral or bacterial intestinal infection. Liver congestion. Electrolyte imbalance. Gastric irritation from foods or drugs. Increased intracranial pressure. Equilibrium imbalance. Adrenal insufficiency. Internal organ irritation or inflammation. Acidosis. Impaired cardiac circulation. Increased pressure in the semicircular canal when the head is raised.

NURSING DIAGNOSIS

Vomiting: the ejection of stomach contents through the mouth

PLANNING

Patient Needs	Primary Nurse-Patient Goals
Water-salt balance	To maintain fluid and electrolyte balance
Rest	To achieve rest
Comfort	To achieve comfort
Cleanliness	To achieve good hygiene
Protection from physical harm	To prevent physical injury
Increased learning	To achieve awareness of needs

NURSING INTERVENTIONS

Nursing Treatments
Restrict the intake to nothing by mouth (until the episode subsides)
Apply a cool, damp cloth to the face
Apply an ice collar
Bathe locally (around the mouth)
Moisten the mouth with cracked ice
Refresh with a mouthwash
Balance fluid intake to equal output
Encourage adequate rest
Give hot tea
    OR
Give carbonated beverages
    OR
Give clear liquid foods
    OR
Give full-liquid foods
    OR
Give dry crackers
Give small, frequent feedings
Give nonprescription drugs (ExR) (antiemetics)
Refrain from giving enemas

Nursing Observations
Auscultate the abdomen for abnormal bowel sounds
Inspect the abdomen for distention
Palpate the abdomen for tenderness, rigidity, and masses

Percuss the abdomen for abnormal resonance
Measure the intake
Measure the output
Monitor the blood pressure
Monitor blood studies for abnormal electrolytes
Observe for complaints of pain

Health Teaching
Explain the causes of the health problem
Explain the reason for and intended effect of the therapy

Medical Treatments Performed by Nurses
Give the prescribed drugs

EVALUATION

See the evaluation criteria for each specific goal in Chapter 2.

GASTROINTESTINAL ELIMINATION, POTENTIAL EXCESSIVE

Potential Diarrhea

ASSESSMENT

Objective Data
Eating incompatible or spoiled foods
Receiving tube feedings
Recent, prolonged diarrhea

Related Data
Commonly Related Conditions:
Colostomy

POSSIBLE ETIOLOGY

Mechanical or chemical irritation of intestinal mucosa

NURSING DIAGNOSIS

Potential diarrhea: the probability that unformed stools in abnormal frequency will occur

PLANNING

Patient Needs
Protection from physical harm
Increased learning

Primary Nurse-Patient Goals
To prevent physical injury
To achieve awareness of needs

NURSING INTERVENTIONS

Nursing Treatments
Discourage oral stimulants
Encourage decreased residue-food intake

Give nonprescription drugs (ExR) (antidiarrheal)
Refrain from giving hot liquids
Refrain from giving iced liquids
Refrain from giving oral stimulants
Refrain from giving enemas
Refrain from giving laxatives
Refrain from inserting a rectal tube
Refrain from taking rectal temperatures
Withhold the drugs (which could cause intestinal irritation)

Nursing Observations
Observe for diarrhea

Health Teaching
Explain the causes of the health problem
Explain the reason for and intended effect of the therapy

EVALUATION

See the evaluation criteria for each specific goal in Chapter 2.

Potential Vomiting

ASSESSMENT

Subjective Data
Nausea
Severe headache
Gastric pain
Dizziness

Objective Data
Increased peristalsis

Related Data
Commonly Related Conditions:
Gastric hyperacidity
Motion sickness
Commonly Related Diseases:
Gastric ulcer
Gastric carcinoma
Gastritis
Pyloric obstruction
Hepatitis
Pancreatitis
Cholecystitis
Renal calculi

POSSIBLE ETIOLOGY

Gastric irritation or inflammation. Increased intracranial pressure. Drug toxicity. Metabolic imbalance. Recent surgery and anesthesia.

NURSING DIAGNOSIS

Potential vomiting: the probability that vomiting will occur

PLANNING

Patient Needs

Comfort

Protection from physical harm

Increased learning

Primary Nurse-Patient Goals

To achieve comfort

To prevent physical injury

To achieve awareness of needs

NURSING INTERVENTIONS

Nursing Treatments

Apply a cool, damp cloth to the face

Apply an ice collar

Elevate the head

Encourage deep breathing

Feed slowly

Give bland foods

   OR

Give clear liquid foods

   OR

Give full-liquid foods

   OR

Withhold food until the patient requests it

Give small, frequent feedings

Maintain a cool room temperature

Control offensive odors by removing the source

Give nonprescription drugs (ExR) (for pain or nausea)

Nursing Observations

Observe for vomiting

Health Teaching

Explain the causes of the health problem

Explain the reason for and intended effect of the therapy

Medical Treatments Performed by Nurses

Give the prescribed drugs (for pain or nausea)

EVALUATION

See the evaluation criteria for each specific goal in Chapter 2.

GASTROINTESTINAL ELIMINATION, INADEQUATE

Constipation (71,325,391)

ASSESSMENT

Subjective Data

Headache

Indigestion

Abdominal pain, fullness, or spasms
Abdominal tenderness in the right lower abdominal cecum area

Objective Data
Hard, small, round masses of stool
Alternating very large and very small stools
Dehydration
Flatulence

Related Data
Commonly Related Conditions:
Pregnancy
Rectocele

Commonly Related Diseases:
None
   OR
Hyperparathyroidism
Cerebral vascular accident
Diverticulitis
Cervical, thoracic, or lumbar spinal cord injury
Hypothyroidism

POSSIBLE ETIOLOGY

Excessive water absorption from the stool by the colon. Inattention to the defecation reflex. Sigmoid spasms. Emotional tension. Altered daily routine. Inadequate fluid intake. Barium fluoroscopy. Antacid therapy.

NURSING DIAGNOSIS

Constipation: decreased frequency of bowel elimination in relation to normal elimination

PLANNING

Patient Needs	**Primary Nurse-Patient Goals**
Water-salt balance	To maintain fluid and electrolyte balance
Waste elimination	To maintain regulating mechanisms and functions
Exercise	To achieve exercise
Comfort	To achieve comfort
Protection from physical harm	To prevent physical injury
Increased learning	To achieve awareness of needs

NURSING INTERVENTIONS

Nursing Treatments
Ambulate the patient (frequently)
Encourage moderate physical exercise
Encourage increased residue-food intake
Increase fluid intake to about 2000 cc daily
Give fresh fruits (daily)
   OR

Give prune juice (daily)
Give hot coffee
    OR
Give iced liquids
    OR
Give warm liquids (especially warm lemonade)
Place in the sitting position (for elimination)
Administer an enema
Give nonprescription drugs (ExR) (stool softeners, laxatives)

Nursing Observations
Measure the intake
Measure the output
Observe for evidence of a favorable response to therapy

Health Teaching
Advise not to take enemas and laxatives (chronically)
Explain that daily bowel elimination is not essential
Explain the need for scheduled bowel elimination
Instruct to immediately respond to the elimination reflex
Instruct to increase fluid intake
Explain the causes of the health problem
Explain the reason for and intended effect of the therapy

EVALUATION

See the evaluation criteria for each specific goal in Chapter 2.

Fecal Impaction (71,325)

ASSESSMENT

Subjective Data
Abdominal and rectal discomfort

Objective Data
Rectal distention
A hard, palpable, fecal mass
Oozing diarrhea around the rectum

Related Data
Commonly Related Conditions:
Aging
Prolonged bed rest
Commonly Related Diseases:
Paralytic ileus
Spastic colon
Cervical or thoracic spinal cord injury

POSSIBLE ETIOLOGY

Inadequate peristalsis or excessive reabsorption of water from the feces by
the colon

NURSING DIAGNOSIS

Fecal impaction: hardened feces collected in the rectum or sigmoid

PLANNING

Patient Needs	Primary Nurse-Patient Goals
Water-salt balance	To maintain fluid and electrolyte balance
Waste elimination	To maintain regulating mechanisms and functions
Exercise	To achieve exercise
Comfort	To achieve comfort
Protection from physical harm	To prevent physical injury
Increased learning	To achieve awareness of needs

NURSING INTERVENTIONS

Nursing Treatments
Remove the fecal impaction manually
Administer an enema (oil enema)
Encourage increased residue-food intake
Encourage moderate physical exercise
Increase fluid intake to about 2000 cc daily
Give nonprescription drugs (ExR) (stool softener)

Nursing Observations
Inspect for bleeding (rectal)
Measure the intake
Measure the output
Observe for complaints of pain (rectal)

Health Teaching
Explain the causes of the health problem
Explain the need for scheduled bowel elimination
Explain the reason for and intended effect of the therapy
Instruct to immediately respond to the elimination reflex
Instruct to increase fluid intake

EVALUATION

See the evaluation criteria for each specific goal in Chapter 2.

GASTROINTESTINAL ELIMINATION, POTENTIAL INADEQUATE

Potential Constipation (71)

ASSESSMENT

Objective Data
Prolonged immobility
Long-term bed rest

Sedentary life
Low-roughage diet
Poor fluid intake
On antacid therapy
Recent barium fluoroscopy

Related Data

Commonly Related Conditions:
Rectocele

Commonly Related Diseases:
Paralytic ileus
Megacolon
Metastatic carcinoma of descending colon
Myxedema
Hyperparathyroidism
Parkinson's disease
Cerebral vascular accident
Diverticulitis
Rectal stenosis
Cervical or thoracic spinal cord injury
Smallpox
Hypothyroidism

POSSIBLE ETIOLOGY

Excessive water absorption from the stool by the colon. Inattention to the defecation reflex. Sigmoid spasms. Emotional tension. Altered daily schedule.

NURSING DIAGNOSIS

Potential constipation: the probability that a decreased frequency of bowel elimination will occur

PLANNING

Patient Needs	**Primary Nurse-Patient Goals**
Water-salt balance	To maintain fluid and electrolyte balance
Waste elimination	To maintain regulating mechanisms and functions
Exercise	To achieve exercise
Comfort	To achieve comfort
Protection from physical harm	To prevent physical injury
Increased learning	To achieve awareness of needs

NURSING INTERVENTIONS

Nursing Treatments
Ambulate the patient (frequently)
Encourage moderate physical exercise
Encourage increased residue-food intake

Give fresh fruits (daily)
OR
Give prune juice (daily)
Give hot coffee
Increase fluid intake to about 2000 cc daily
Give nonprescription drugs (ExR) (stool softeners, laxatives)

Nursing Observations
Observe for complaints of constipation

Health Teaching
Describe those symptoms which should be reported (abdominal or rectal
    fullness, pain)
Explain the causes of the health problem
Explain the need for scheduled bowel elimination
Explain the reason for and intended effect of the therapy
Instruct to immediately respond to the elimination reflex
Instruct to increase fluid intake

EVALUATION

See the evaluation criteria for each specific goal in Chapter 2.

GASTROINTESTINAL-DRAINAGE THERAPY DEPENDENCE

Dependence on T-Tube Management (391)

ASSESSMENT

Subjective Data
Person relies on nurses for:
    observation of drainage
    dressing changes
    cleanliness

Objective Data
Person has a T-tube

Related Data
Commonly Related Diseases:
Cholelithiasis

POSSIBLE ETIOLOGY

The insertion of a T-tube as a precaution against bile flow obstruction. If the
bile duct goes into spasm, the tube will decompress the duct, allowing bile
to be secreted through the tube.

NURSING DIAGNOSIS

Dependence on T-tube management: reliance on nurses to care for a small
T-shaped tube placed in the common bile duct at the completion of a
cholecystectomy

PLANNING

Patient Needs	**Primary Nurse-Patient Goals**
Comfort	To achieve comfort
Cleanliness	To achieve good hygiene
Protection from physical harm	To prevent physical injury
Dependence	To achieve comfort
Increased learning	To achieve awareness of needs

NURSING INTERVENTIONS

Nursing Treatments
Change the dressing frequently
Attach the tube to straight drainage and a collection container
Keep the drainage container below T-tube level
Provide sufficiently long tubing to allow freedom of movement
Empty the collection container (as needed)
Position comfortably

Nursing Observations
Check the drainage system for leakage
Check the tube (T-tube) for patency
Measure the intake
Measure the output
Monitor blood studies for abnormal electrolytes

Health Teaching
Explain the reason for and intended effect of the therapy

EVALUATION

See the evaluation criteria for each specific goal in Chapter 2.

Dependence on Intestinal Tube Management (70,391)

ASSESSMENT

Subjective Data
Person relies on nurses for:
    observation of drainage
    periodic tube advancement
    tube irrigation
    relief of nasal irritation and throat soreness

Objective Data
Person has an intestinal tube

Related Data
Commonly Related Diseases:
Paralytic ileus

Volvulus
Metastatic carcinoma

POSSIBLE ETIOLOGY

Need for drainage of intestinal contents or release of intestinal obstruction.

NURSING DIAGNOSIS

Dependence on intestinal tube management: reliance on nurses for the care and functioning of a decompression tube inserted through the nose and stomach into the intestines, with aspiration by suction.

PLANNING

Patient Needs	Primary Nurse-Patient Goals
Comfort	To achieve comfort
Protection from physical harm	To prevent physical injury
Dependence	To achieve comfort
Increased learning	To achieve awareness of needs

NURSING INTERVENTIONS

Nursing Treatments
Anchor the tubing securely
Provide sufficiently long tubing to allow freedom of movement
Refrain from sealing the tube with a heavy clamp
Refrain from taping the intestinal tube until it is fully advanced
Irrigate the gastric tube with saline
Position comfortably
Lubricate the external nares
Apply a cold, moist compress (to the lips)
Lubricate the lips
Refresh with a mouthwash
Restrict the intake to nothing by mouth

Nursing Observations
Auscultate the abdomen for abnormal bowel sounds
Auscultate the abdomen for renewed bowel sounds (notify the physician
    when this occurs)
Check the tube (intestinal) for patency

Health Teaching
Explain the reason for and intended effect of the therapy

Medical Treatments Performed by Nurses
Advance the intestinal tube as ordered
Remove the therapeutic tube when the treatment is terminated

EVALUATION

See the evaluation criteria for each specific goal in Chapter 2.

Dependence on Nasogastric Tube Management (70,391)

ASSESSMENT

Subjective Data
Person relies on nurses for:
    drainage maintenance
    periodic tube irrigation
    prevention of drainage system leakage
    relief of nasal irritation and throat soreness

Objective Data
Person has a nasogastric tube

Related Data
Commonly Related Diseases:
Pancreatitis
Cholecystitis
Laennec's portal cirrhosis

POSSIBLE ETIOLOGY

Need for drainage of stomach contents

NURSING DIAGNOSIS

Dependence on nasogastric tube management: reliance on nurses for the care and functioning of a decompression tube inserted through the nose into the stomach, with or without aspiration by suction

PLANNING

Patient Needs	Primary Nurse-Patient Goals
Waste elimination	To maintain regulating mechanisms and functions
Comfort	To achieve comfort
Protection from physical harm	To prevent physical injury
Dependence	To achieve comfort
Increased learning	To achieve awareness of needs

NURSING INTERVENTIONS

Nursing Treatments
Anchor the tubing securely
Provide sufficiently long tubing to allow freedom of movement
Irrigate the gastric tube with saline
Introduce irrigating solutions slowly
Keep the drainage container below stomach level
Empty the collecion container (as needed)
Position comfortably
Lubricate the external nares
Apply a cold, moist compress (to the lips)
Lubricate the lips

Refresh with a mouthwash
Restrict the intake to nothing by mouth

Nursing Observations
Auscultate the abdomen for abnormal bowel sounds
Check the drainage system for leakage
Check the tube (gastric) for patency
Measure the intake
Measure the output
Monitor blood studies for abnormal electrolytes

Health Teaching
Explain the reason for and intended effect of the therapy

Medical Treatments Performed by Nurses
Attach the gastric tube to suction
Remove the therapeutic tube when the treatment is terminated

EVALUATION

See the evaluation criteria for each specific goal in Chapter 2.

GASTROINTESTINAL THERAPY DISCOMFORTS

NPO Discomfort

ASSESSMENT

Subjective Data
Preoccupation with thoughts of food and drink

Objective Data
Irritability
Restlessness
Begs for food and drink
Intermittently asks how long it will be before he can have food and drink

Related Data
Commonly Related Diseases:
Paralytic ileus
Acute gastritis
Acute pancreatitis
Hepatitis

POSSIBLE ETIOLOGY

Diagnostic studies. Presurgical and postsurgical fluid and food limitations. Intestinal disturbances. Gastric tube insertion. Presurgical drug administration of atropine, scopolamine, etc.

NURSING DIAGNOSIS

NPO discomfort: the discomfort resulting from a prescribed limitation of no food or drink to be taken by mouth for a particular length of time

PLANNING

Patient Needs

Comfort
Protection from physical harm
Increased learning

Primary Nurse-Patient Goals

To achieve comfort
To prevent physical injury
To achieve awareness of needs

NURSING INTERVENTIONS

Nursing Treatments

Apply a cold, moist compress (to the lips)
Provide cold water for mouth rinsing, but not swallowing
Refresh with a mouthwash
Lubricate the skin (lips) with petrolatum
Swab the mouth with diluted glycerine
Provide frequent patient contact
Provide radio and television for diversion (if possible)

Nursing Observations

Observe for an excessive stress level

Health Teaching

Explain the reason for and intended effect of the therapy

EVALUATION

See the evaluation criteria for each specific goal in Chapter 2.

GASTROINTESTINAL ELIMINATION THERAPY DEPENDENCE

Dependence on Colostomy (or Ileostomy) Management (70,391)

ASSESSMENT

Subjective Data

Person relies on nurses for:
    care and cleanliness
    control of ostomy odors
    appropriate diet to support ostomy control
    skin care

Objective Data

Person has a colostomy or ileostomy

Related Data

Commonly Related Diseases:
Metastatic carcinoma
Gunshot wound of the colon
Regional enteritis
Paralytic ileus
Volvulus

Ulcerative colitis
Intussusception

POSSIBLE ETIOLOGY

Surgical intervention of an intestinal obstruction. Lack of experience in caring for a colostomy or ileostomy.

NURSING DIAGNOSIS

Dependence on colostomy and/or ileostomy management: reliance on nurses to care for a colostomy (or ileostomy) until the patient can manage the ostomy independently

PLANNING

Patient Needs	Primary Nurse-Patient Goals
Water-salt balance	To maintain fluid and electrolyte balance
Waste elimination	To maintain regulating mechanisms and functions
Comfort	To achieve comfort
Cleanliness	To achieve good hygiene
Protection from physical harm	To prevent physical injury
Dependence	To achieve comfort
Mastery and competence in skills	To achieve optimum function
Increased learning	To achieve awareness of needs

NURSING INTERVENTIONS

Nursing Treatments
Apply an ostomy appliance
Empty the collection appliance (as needed)
Change the ostomy appliance as needed
Clean with surgical soap (around the ostomy)
Apply calamine lotion (around an ileostomy)
    OR
Apply milk of magnesia to the skin (around an ileostomy)
Apply aluminum paste to the skin (around a colostomy)
    OR
Apply zinc oxide to the skin (around a colostomy)
Introduce irrigating solutions slowly
Protect with absorbent padding
Encourage decreased residue-food intake
Refrain from giving laxatives
Provide needed supplies
Introduce to persons who have successfully undergone the same experience (if anxious)
Make a referral (to local ostomy association)

Nursing Observations
Inspect the skin for irritation

Health Teaching

Describe those symptoms which should be reported (excessive drainage, skin irritation, pain)

Explain the reason for and intended effect of the therapy

Teach how to apply the ostomy appliance

Teach how to irrigate a colostomy

Explain how to maintain cleanliness of the ostomy appliance

Instruct to maintain skin cleanliness

Explain how to obtain therapeutic supplies

Recommend that two ostomy appliances be alternately used

Recommend that extra therapeutic supplies be carried

Instruct to avoid foods having strong odors

Medical Treatments Performed by Nurses

Irrigate the ostomy

EVALUATION

See the evaluation criteria for each specific goal in Chapter 2.

EMERGENCY GASTROINTESTINAL CONDITIONS

Emergency Phase Abdominal Evisceration (391)

ASSESSMENT

Subjective Data

Bursting abdominal sensation

Objective Data

Incision separates

Surgical sutures break apart

Visible abdominal contents

Related Data

Commonly Related Conditions:

Abdominal surgery

POSSIBLE ETIOLOGY

Pressure from abdominal distention. Poor nutrition or aging which inhibits tissue healing. Abdominal trauma.

NURSING DIAGNOSIS

Emergency phase evisceration: the need for immediate health care as a result of the opening of an abdominal incision with protrusion of intestinal contents outside the abdominal cavity

PLANNING

Patient Needs	**Primary Nurse-Patient Goals**
Rest	To achieve rest
Comfort	To achieve comfort
Cleanliness	To achieve good hygiene
Protection from physical harm	To prevent physical injury, infection
Increased learning	To achieve awareness of needs

NURSING INTERVENTIONS

Nursing Treatments
Attend the patient constantly
Apply a sterile dressing (soaked with sterile saline)
Cover with warm blankets
Place in the flat position
Place on complete bed rest
Restrict the intake to nothing by mouth
Suture the wound (ExR) (if the physician is not available)
Consult with the physician (*immediately*)

Nursing Observations
Inspect the chest for respiratory rate and rhythm
Inspect for hemorrhage
Observe for shock
Monitor the blood pressure
Palpate the pulse for rate, rhythm, and volume

Health Teaching
Explain the causes of the health problem
Explain the reason for and intended effect of the therapy

EVALUATION

See the evaluation criteria for each specific goal in Chapter 2.

Emergency Phase Acute Gastric Dilatation (32,300,113)

ASSESSMENT

Subjective Data
Excessive thirst
Increased incisional pain
Chest pain
Heightened anxiety

Objective Data
Upper abdominal distention
Rapid, shallow respirations
Moist, cool skin
Ashen, gray skin

Decreased blood pressure
Decreased and thready pulse
Regurgitant vomiting every 15–20 minutes without distention relief
Hiccoughs
Percussion tympany
Abdominal rigidity
Diminished or absent bowel sounds
Visible peristalsis

Related Data

Commonly Related Conditions:
Abdominal surgery
Application of a hip spica cast
Prolonged respirator ventilation

Commonly Related Diseases:
None
  OR
Paralytic ileus

POSSIBLE ETIOLOGY

Gastric muscle paralysis. Immobility. Potassium depletion. Anesthesia and sedatives depressing peristaltic activity.

NURSING DIAGNOSIS

Emergency phase acute gastric dilatation: the need for immediate health care as a result of sudden, massive stomach distention with air and fluids that fail to pass through the gastrointestinal tract

PLANNING

Patient Needs	Primary Nurse-Patient Goals
Water-salt balance	To maintain fluid and electrolyte balance
Rest	To achieve rest
Comfort	To achieve comfort
Protection from physical harm	To prevent physical injury
Increased learning	To achieve awareness of needs

NURSING INTERVENTIONS

Nursing Treatments
Attend the patient constantly
Administer intravenous fluids (ET) (electrolyte solution)
Insert a gastric tube and attach to suction (ET)
Cover with lightweight blankets
Place in the slight sitting position
Place on complete bed rest
Restrict the intake to nothing by mouth
Withhold the drugs (sedatives)
Consult with the physician (*immediately*)

Nursing Observations
Monitor the blood pressure
Palpate the pulse for rate, rhythm, and volume

Health Teaching
Explain the causes of the health problem
Explain the reason for and intended effect of the therapy

EVALUATION

See the evaluation criteria for each specific goal in Chapter 2.

Emergency Phase Food Poisoning
(247,453)

ASSESSMENT

Subjective Data
Cramping abdominal pain
Nausea
Dizziness, blurred vision, and muscle weakness only occur with botulism

Objective Data
Chills
Fever
Diarrhea
Vomiting
No abdominal rigidity
Respiratory difficulty only occurs with botulism

Related Data
Onset in 2 to 4 hours indicates *Staphylococcus*; onset in 6 to 48 hours indicates *Salmonella*; onset in 15 hours indicates mushroom poisoning; onset
in 18 to 48 hours indicates botulism

Commonly Related Diseases:
None
    OR
Botulism

POSSIBLE ETIOLOGY

Lack of hygiene during food preparation, processing, or storage

NURSING DIAGNOSIS

Emergency phase food poisoning: the need for immediate health care as a
result of severe intestinal distress following the ingestion of bacteria-
contaminated foods

PLANNING

Patient Needs	**Primary Nurse-Patient Goals**
Water-salt balance	To maintain fluid and electrolyte balance
Rest	To achieve rest

Comfort

To achieve comfort

Cleanliness

To achieve good hygiene

Protection from physical harm

To prevent physical injury

Increased learning

To achieve awareness of needs

NURSING INTERVENTIONS

Nursing Treatments
Lavage the stomach (ET)
Place on complete bed rest
Restrict the intake to nothing by mouth (until nausea and vomiting subside)
Withhold the drugs (sedatives)
Save the poison (food) container for content analysis
Make a referral (to a physician)

Nursing Observations
Inspect for bleeding
Measure the intake
Measure the output
Monitor the blood pessure

Health Teaching
Explain the causes of the health problem
Explain the reason for and intended effect of the therapy

Medical Treatments Performed by Nurses
Give the prescribed drugs (botulism antitoxin)

EVALUATION

See the evaluation criteria for each specific goal in Chapter 2.

EMERGENCY INTRAABDOMINAL CONDITIONS, POTENTIAL

Potential Spleen Rupture (113,453)

ASSESSMENT

Subjective Data
Abdominal pressure sensation

Objective Data
Splenomegaly

Related Data
Commonly Related Diseases:
Chronic malaria
Typhoid fever
Infectious mononucleosis
Leukemia
Trauma injury

POSSIBLE ETIOLOGY

Blunt trauma to the left upper abdomen or left lower chest. Spleen infection.

NURSING DIAGNOSIS

Potential spleen rupture: the possibility that the spleen may break apart

PLANNING

Patient Needs

Sleep, rest

Comfort

Protection from physical harm

Increased learning

Primary Nurse-Patient Goals

To achieve sleep, rest

To achieve comfort

To prevent physical injury

To achieve awareness of needs

NURSING INTERVENTIONS

Nursing Treatments
Handle gently
Place on complete bed rest
Position comfortably
Give small, frequent feedings
Refrain from giving enemas
Remove constrictive clothing

Nursing Observations
Monitor the blood pressure (for hypotension)
Monitor the oral temperature (for decrease)
Observe for complaints of pain (severe abdominal or in the left scapular region)

Health Teaching
Inform that coughing should be avoided
Inform that elimination straining should be avoided
Explain the causes of the health problem
Explain the reason for and intended effect of the therapy

EVALUATION

See the evaluation criteria for each specific goal in Chapter 2.

INADEQUATE ARTIFICIAL BOWEL ELIMINATION MANAGEMENT

Inadequate Information Related to Colostomy (or Ileostomy) Care (70,391)

ASSESSMENT

Subjective Data
Person confirms a lack of information

Objective Data

Person's actions indicate a lack of information regarding:
    ostomy care and cleanliness
    control of ostomy odor
    appropriate diet
    skin care

Related Data

Commonly Related Diseases:
Metastatic carcinoma
Gunshot wound of the colon
Regional enteritis
Paralytic ileus
Volvulus
Ulcerative colitis
Intussusception

POSSIBLE ETIOLOGY

Lack of information. No previous experience with a colostomy or ileostomy.

NURSING DIAGNOSIS

Inadequate information related to colostomy (or ileostomy) care: lack of information regarding the care of a colostomy or ileostomy

PLANNING

Patient Needs	**Primary Nurse-Patient Goals**
Comfort	To achieve comfort
Protection from physical harm	To prevent physical injury
Mastery and competence in skills, independence	To achieve optimum function
Increased learning	To achieve awareness of needs

NURSING INTERVENTIONS

Nursing Treatments
Approach unhurriedly
Encourage patient questions

Nursing Observations
Evaluate the response to teaching

Health Teaching
Describe those symptoms which should be reported (excessive drainage, skin irritation, pain)
Teach how to apply the ostomy appliance
Teach how to irrigate a colostomy
Explain how to maintain cleanliness of the ostomy appliance
Instruct to maintain skin cleanliness
Explain how to obtain therapeutic supplies
Recommend that two ostomy appliances be alternately used

Recommend that extra therapeutic supplies be carried
Instruct to avoid foods having strong odors

EVALUATION

See the evaluation criteria for each specific goal in Chapter 2.

INADEQUATE NORMAL BOWEL ELIMINATION MANAGEMENT

Inadequate Information Related to Inappropriate Bowel Habits

ASSESSMENT

Subjective Data
Person confirms a lack of information

Objective Data
Person's actions indicate a lack of information regarding:
    the fact that daily bowel elimination is not essential
    the dangers of chronically taking laxatives and enemas
    the importance of responding immediately to the elimination reflex

POSSIBLE ETIOLOGY

Lack of instruction

NURSING DIAGNOSIS

Inadequate information related to inappropriate bowel habits: lack of information regarding daily bowel elimination

PLANNING

Patient Needs	**Primary Nurse-Patient Goals**
Comfort	To achieve comfort
Protection from physical harm	To prevent physical injury
Increased learning	To achieve awareness of needs

NURSING INTERVENTIONS

Nursing Treatments
Approach unhurriedly
Encourage patient questions

Nursing Observations
Evaluate the response to teaching

Health Teaching
Advise not to take enemas and laxatives
Explain that daily bowel elimination is not essential
Explain the need for scheduled bowel elimination
Inform that elimination straining should be avoided
Instruct to immediately respond to the elimination reflex

EVALUATION

See the evaluation criteria for each specific goal in Chapter 2.

Inadequate Information Related to Transmission of Intestinal Worms (453)

ASSESSMENT

Objective Data

Person's actions indicate a lack of information regarding:
    that intestinal worms are more prevalent in warm climates
    that the modes of transmission are the hands and bare feet
    the precautions that should be taken
    the signs and symptoms of intestinal worms

Related Data

Commonly Related Diseases:
Hookworm disease

POSSIBLE ETIOLOGY

Lack of instruction regarding contact with soil contaminated with worm larvae and eggs

NURSING DIAGNOSIS

Inadequate information related to transmission of intestinal worms: lack of information regarding the prevention of parasitic worm invasion into the intestinal tract

PLANNING

Patient Needs	**Primary Nurse-Patient Goals**
Cleanliness	To achieve good hygiene
Protection from physical harm	To prevent physical injury
Increased learning	To achieve awareness of needs

NURSING INTERVENTIONS

Nursing Treatments
Approach unhurriedly
Encourage patient questions

Nursing Observations
Evaluate the response to teaching

Health Teaching
Advise against walking barefoot
Advise handwashing after elimination
Advise handwashing before meals
Describe those symptoms which should be reported (anal itching)
Inform that cleanliness is basic to health
Explain the causes of the health problem

EVALUATION

See the evaluation criteria for each specific goal in Chapter 2.

15.
NURSING DIAGNOSES RELATED TO
The Genitourinary System

URINE ELIMINATION, EXCESSIVE

Excessive Urinary Output (70,391)

ASSESSMENT

Subjective Data
Fatigue

Objective Data
Excretes 3000 cc or more urine in 24 hours
Urinary frequency
Pale, dilute urine color

Related Data
Laboratory Findings:
Low urine specific gravity of 1.000 to 1.002
Commonly Related Diseases:
Diabetes mellitus
Diabetes insipidus
Pheochromocytoma
Hyperparathyroidism
Nephritis
Nephrosclerosis
Typhoid fever
Primary aldosteronism

POSSIBLE ETIOLOGY

Hypofunction of the posterior lobe of the pituitary gland. Infection.

NURSING DIAGNOSIS

Excessive urinary output (polyuria): the excretion of unusually large amounts of urine

PLANNING

Patient Needs	**Primary Nurse-Patient Goals**
Water-salt balance	To maintain fluid and electrolyte balance
Rest	To achieve rest
Protection from physical harm	To prevent physical injury
Increased learning	To achieve awareness of needs

NURSING INTERVENTIONS

Nursing Treatments
Balance fluid intake to equal output
Provide fresh drinking water (frequently)
Refrain from restricting fluids
Apply an external urinary catheter (if rest is constantly interrupted)

Nursing Observations
Inspect for dehydration
Measure the intake
Measure the output
Monitor blood studies for abnormal electrolytes
Monitor blood studies for abnormal pituitary function
Monitor blood studies for abnormal renal function

Health Teaching
Explain that fluid intake and output should be balanced
Explain the causes of the health problem
Explain the reason for and intended effect of the therapy

Medical Treatments Performed by Nurses
Give the prescribed drugs

EVALUATION

See the evaluation criteria for each specific goal in Chapter 2.

URINE ELIMINATION, INADEQUATE

Inadequate Urinary Output Related to Fluid Intake (70,325,391)

ASSESSMENT

Subjective Data
Thirst

Objective Data
Urine output of between 500 cc and 1000 cc in a 24-hour period
Fluid intake of less than 1200 cc to 1500 cc daily
Dehydration

Related Data

Commonly Related Conditions:
Fever
Profuse perspiration
Vomiting
Diarrhea

Commonly Related Diseases:
Gastritis
Cerebral vascular accident

POSSIBLE ETIOLOGY

Inadequate fluid intake. Increased fluid loss through systems other than the renal system

NURSING DIAGNOSIS

Inadequate urinary output related to fluid intake: an insufficient urine output related to an insufficient fluid intake

PLANNING

Patient Needs	**Primary Nurse-Patient Goals**
Water-salt balance	To maintain fluid and electrolyte balance
Waste elimination	To maintain regulating mechanisms and functions
Comfort	To achieve comfort
Protection from physical harm	To prevent physical injury
Increased learning	To achieve awareness of needs

NURSING INTERVENTIONS

Nursing Treatments
Increase fluid intake to about 2000 cc daily
Provide fresh drinking water
Provide small, frequent drinks
Distribute the fluid intake over 24 hours

Nursing Observations
Inspect for dehydration
Measure the body weight (daily)
Measure the intake
Measure the output

Health Teaching
Explain the causes of the health problem
Explain the reason for and intended effect of the therapy
Instruct to increase fluid intake

Medical Treatments Performed by Nurses
Administer intravenous fluids

EVALUATION

See the evaluation criteria for each specific goal in Chapter 2.

Inadequate Urinary Output Related to Urine Retention (70,325,391)

ASSESSMENT

Subjective Data

Lower abdominal pain or discomfort
Desire to urinate

Objective Data

Bladder distention
Restlessness

Related Data

Commonly Related Conditions:
Anesthesia
Prolonged bed rest

Commonly Related Diseases:
Cervical or thoracic spinal cord injury
Benign prostatic hypertrophy
Urethral stricture
Cystitis
Acute pyelonephritis

POSSIBLE ETIOLOGY

Decreased nerve stimulation to the bladder due to operative trauma or anesthesia. The reclining position fails to maintain normal bladder tone because of lack of the uniform hydrostatic pressure of urine on all bladder surfaces that usually exists when there is normal ambulation. Large amounts of rectal feces can cause sufficient pressure on the urethra to prevent urine flow. Obstruction between the bladder and the urethra. Loss of bladder muscle tone. Exposure to environmental cold. Urinary catheter obstruction or removal.

NURSING DIAGNOSIS

Inadequate urinary output related to urine retention: little or no urine output related to the bladder's inability to expel urine

PLANNING

Patient Needs	Primary Nurse-Patient Goals
Water-salt balance	To maintain fluid and electrolyte balance
Waste elimination	To maintain regulating mechanisms and functions
Comfort	To achieve comfort
Protection from physical harm	To prevent physical injury
Increased learning	To achieve awareness of needs

NURSING INTERVENTIONS

Nursing Treatments
Ambulate the patient (as much as possible)
Apply a heating pad
    OR   } (to the abdomen)
Apply a hot water bottle
Catheterize with an indwelling urinary catheter (only if other measures fail)
Do not withdraw by catheter more than 1000 cc of urine at one time
Increase fluid intake to about 2000 cc daily
Stand the patient for urination (if possible)

Nursing Observations
Inspect the abdomen for distention (periodically)
Palpate the bladder for distention
Measure the intake
Measure the output
Observe for complaints of pain

Health Teaching
Explain the causes of the health problem
Explain the reason for and intended effect of the therapy

EVALUATION

See the evaluation criteria for each specific goal in Chapter 2.

Inadequate Urinary Output Related to Urinary Catheter Obstruction (325,391)

ASSESSMENT

Subjective Data
Gradually increased bladder discomfort

Objective Data
Absence of urinary output
Bladder distention
Back pressure on the catheter with a sterile 50-cc syringe does not suction urine through and out of the catheter

POSSIBLE ETIOLOGY

Urine sediment plugs within the catheter

NURSING DIAGNOSIS

Inadequate urinary output related to urinary catheter obstruction: lack of urinary output related to a nonpatent urinary catheter

PLANNING

Patient Needs	**Primary Nurse-Patient Goals**
Waste elimination	To maintain regulating mechanisms and functions
Comfort	To achieve comfort

| Protection from physical harm | To prevent physical injury |
| Increased learning | To achieve awareness of needs |

NURSING INTERVENTIONS

Nursing Treatments
Irrigate the urinary catheter
  OR
Change the urinary catheter
Increase fluid intake to about 2000 cc daily

Nursing Observations
Check the tube (catheter) for patency (periodically)
Measure the intake
Measure the output

Health Teaching
Explain the causes of the health problem
Explain the reason for and intended effect of the therapy
Instruct to increase fluid intake

EVALUATION

See the evaluation criteria for each specific goal in Chapter 2.

URINE ELIMINATION, POTENTIAL INADEQUATE

Potential Inadequate Urinary Output (70,391)

ASSESSMENT

Subjective Data
Bladder fullness

Objective Data
Recent anesthesia
Prolonged bed rest
Poor fluid intake
Recent blood transfusion reaction
Hemorrhage
Shock
Streptococcus infection
Drug overdose

Related Data
Commonly Related Diseases:
Cervical or thoracic spinal cord injury
Benign prostatic hypertrophy
Renal calculi

POSSIBLE ETIOLOGY

Decreased nerve stimulation to the bladder due to trauma or anesthesia. The reclining position fails to maintain normal bladder tone because of lack of the uniform hydrostatic pressure of urine on all bladder surfaces that usually exists when there is normal ambulation. Large amounts of rectal feces can cause sufficient pressure on the urethra to prevent urine flow. Diminished fluid volume. Impaired renal circulation resulting from reduced blood pressure.

NURSING DIAGNOSIS

Potential inadequate urinary output: the possibility that an insufficient amount of urine will be voided

PLANNING

Patient Needs	Primary Nurse-Patient Goals
Water-salt balance	To maintain fluid and electrolyte balance
Protection from physical harm	To prevent physical injury
Increased learning	To achieve awareness of needs

NURSING INTERVENTIONS

Nursing Treatments
Ambulate the patient (as much as possible)
Change the patient's position frequently (if unable to ambulate)
Stand the patient for urination
Increase fluid intake to about 2000 cc daily

Nursing Observations
Measure the intake
Measure the output
Inspect the abdomen for distention
Palpate the bladder for distention
Observe for complaints of constipation

Health Teaching
Explain the causes of the health problem
Explain the reason for and intended effect of the therapy

EVALUATION

See the evaluation criteria for each specific goal in Chapter 2.

ELIMINATION CONTROL

Dependence on Retraining for Elimination Control (38,70,97,129)

ASSESSMENT

Subjective Data
Nonperception of defecation or urinary reflex
Person relies on nurses for retraining to reestablish bowel and bladder control

Objective Data
Involuntary bowel movement
Involuntary voiding

Related Data

Commonly Related Conditions:
Neurogenic bladder

Commonly Related Diseases:
Cerebral vascular accident
Cervical or thoracic spinal cord injury
Multiple sclerosis

POSSIBLE ETIOLOGY

Increased parasympathetic stimulation or lack of sphincter control. Loss of bladder muscle tone. Upper or lower motor neuron lesion.

NURSING DIAGNOSIS

Dependence on retraining for elimination control: reliance on nurses for guidance in reestablishing bowel and/or bladder control

PLANNING

Patient Needs	**Primary Nurse-Patient Goals**
Mastery and competence in skills, independence	To achieve optimum function
Increased learning	To achieve awareness of needs

NURSING INTERVENTIONS

Nursing Treatments

General Measures:
Place in the sitting position (for elimination)
Encourage the use of the bathroom
    OR
Provide a bedside commode
    OR
Provide a bedpan (placed on a chair)
Encourage moderate physical exercise

Bladder Training:
Give small, frequent drinks
Increase fluid intake to about 2000 cc daily
Clamp the indwelling urinary catheter intermittently (release clamp every 1–2 hours, progressing to 3–4 hours)
Schedule toileting (at regular intervals of every 2 hours, progressing to 3–4 hours; if a catheter has recently been removed, schedule every hour)
Stimulate the reflex bladder by applying cold to the abdomen, stroking the inner thigh, or running water
Restrict the intake (fluids) to nothing by mouth (after the evening meal)
Refrain from giving oral stimulants (until just prior to scheduled toileting)
Respond immediately to the patient's call (for assistance)
Dress in personal clothing

Bowel Training:
Schedule toileting (at the same time every day, preferably after a scheduled meal)

Balance nutritional intake

Increase fluid intake to about 3000 cc daily

Give nonprescription drugs (ExR) (glycerine suppository rectally 30 minutes prior to scheduled toileting)

Give prune juice (daily in the A.M.)

Stimulate the reflex bowel by abdominal stroking and anal stimulation

Refrain from giving enemas

Refrain from giving laxatives

Nursing Observations

Measure the intake

Measure the output

Measure the residual urine (if urine retention is suspected)

Health Teaching

Advise not to take enemas and laxatives

Advise not to stand for prolonged periods (when incontinent)

Explain the causes of the health problem

Explain the reason for and intended effect of the therapy

EVALUATION

See the evaluation criteria for each specific goal in Chapter 2.

GENITOURINARY CALCULI, POTENTIAL

Predisposition to Renal Calculi (71,391,453)

ASSESSMENT

Objective Data

Poor fluid intake

Prolonged bed rest

Eats a high-calcium diet

Highly alkaline urine, which supports calcium calculi

Highly acid urine, which supports cystine or uric acid calculi

Related Data

Laboratory Findings:

Previous small, yellow uric acid calculi

   OR

Previous waxy, translucent, stag-shaped cystine calculi

   OR

Previous small, dark calcium oxalate calculi

   OR

Previous soft, chalk white calcium phosphate calculi

Commonly Related Diseases:

Hyperparathyroidism

Milk alkali syndrome

Vitamin D intoxication

Cervical or thoracic spinal cord injury
Myeloid leukemia
Nephrocalcinosis
Gout

POSSIBLE ETIOLOGY

Increased excretion of calcium and phosphorus in the urine resulting from increased parathyroid activity. Increased milk and alkali intake. Prolonged immobility.

NURSING DIAGNOSIS

Predisposition to renal calculi: a susceptibility to the formation of kidney stones

PLANNING

Patient Needs	Primary Nurse-Patient Goals
Water-salt balance	To maintain fluid and electrolyte balance
Acid-base balance, waste elimination	To maintain regulating mechanisms and functions
Exercise	To achieve exercise
Comfort	To achieve comfort
Protection from physical harm	To prevent physical injury, infection
Increased learning	To achieve awareness of needs

NURSING INTERVENTIONS

Nursing Treatments
Ambulate the patient (as much as possible)
Change the patient's position frequently
Increase fluid intake to about 3000 cc daily
Encourage decreased calcium-food intake
  AND
Give urine-acidifying juices orally
  AND
Refrain from giving bicarbonates
  AND
Refrain from giving carbonated beverages
} (for potential calcium calculi)

Give carbonated beverages
  AND
Give urine-alkalinizing juices orally
} (for potential cystine or uric acid calculi)

Nursing Observations
Inspect for bleeding (hematuria)
Test the urine for pH (high urine alkalinity favors calcium calculi formation, while acidity favors cystine and uric acid calculi formation)

Health Teaching
Describe those symptoms which should be reported (dysuria, flank pain)
Explain the causes of the health problem

Explain the reason for and intended effect of the therapy

Recommend that alkalis be used conservatively (for potential calcium calculi)

EVALUATION

See the evaluation criteria for each specific goal in Chapter 2.

KIDNEY DYSFUNCTION, POTENTIAL

Predisposition to Progressive Renal Degeneration (32,70,247,271,325)

ASSESSMENT

Subjective Data
Easily fatigued

Objective Data
Some degree of renal nephron (glomerular filtration and/or renal tubule function) degeneration has been medically diagnosed

Related Data
May have a family history of renal insufficiency or failure

Laboratory Findings:
Creatinine clearance below 100 ml per minute
Proteinuria
Elevated blood urea nitrogen and serum creatinine levels

Commonly Related Diseases:
Glomerulonephritis
Nephrosclerosis
Nephrosis
Nephrotic syndrome
Chronic pyelonephritis
Malignant hypertension
Collagen disease

POSSIBLE ETIOLOGY

Hereditary predisposition. The damaging effects of infection (usually streptococcus) and inflammation of the glomeruli, renal tubules, and/or vascular system of the kidneys. An allergic response to an infection located elsewhere in the body (usually respiratory).

NURSING DIAGNOSIS

Predisposition to progressive renal degeneration: a susceptibility to developing impaired kidney function or increasing the degree of existing kidney dysfunction

PLANNING

Patient Needs	**Primary Nurse-Patient Goals**
Water-salt balance	To maintain fluid and electrolyte balance
Food balance	To maintain nutrition to all cells
Sleep and rest	To achieve rest
Exercise	To achieve exercise
Protection from physical harm	To prevent physical injury, infection
Increased learning	To achieve awareness of needs

NURSING INTERVENTIONS

Nursing Treatments

Balance nutritional intake

Encourage adequate rest (9 hours of sleep each night with 1–2 hours rest during the day; additional rest is essential during respiratory infection)

Encourage moderate physical exercise (never strenuous exercise)

Increase fluid intake to about 2000 cc daily (if the urine output is equal to the fluid intake and no fluid retention exists)

Give urine-acidifying juices orally (several times daily)

Assist the patient in restructuring his lifestyle (to one of moderation at all times)

Make a referral (to a physician if there is evidence of respiratory or genitourinary infection or changes in laboratory findings)

NURSING OBSERVATIONS

Inspect for bleeding (hematuria)

Inspect for edema

Measure the body weight (periodically for fluid retention)

Measure the intake
AND } (periodically to check for fluid retention)
Measure the output

Monitor blood studies for abnormal acid base

Monitor blood studies for abnormal electrolytes

Monitor blood studies for abnormal hematology (decreased hemoglobin and hematocrit)

Monitor blood studies for abnormal renal function (urea nitrogen and creatinine)   } (periodically every 3 to 6 months)

Monitor urine studies for abnormal renal function

Monitor urine studies for evidence of urinary tract infection (especially two weeks after any respiratory or streptococcus infection

Monitor the blood pressure (for hypertension or hypotension)
Monitor the oral temperature (for fever)
Observe for complaints of constipation
Observe for complaints of dysuria
Observe for complaints of malaise
Observe for complaints of nausea
Observe for dyspnea
Observe for urinary frequency (including nocturia or polyuria)
Observe the person's activity pattern (for decreased activity)
Observe the urine for abnormal color, content, and odor
Test the urine for protein

Health Teaching
Advise periodic examinations for known hereditary predispositions
Describe the specific dangerous effects of poor health practices (further renal degeneration)
Describe those symptoms which should be reported (hematuria, nausea, vomiting, respiratory infection, dysuria, urinary frequency, fever)
Explain how to measure intake and output (periodically)
Explain how to prevent cross infection
Explain how to prevent the common cold
Inform that cleanliness is basic to health
Explain the need to avoid overexertion
Instruct to increase fluid intake (to 2000 cc daily if there is no fluid retention)
Teach the principles of good nutrition
Recommend adherence to a moderate pace of living
Teach how to test the urine for protein
Explain the reason for and intended effect of the therapy

Medical Treatments Performed by Nurses
Give the prescribed diet (if any)
Give the prescribed drugs
Give the prescribed fluids (if there is fluid retention)

EVALUATION

See the evaluation criteria for each specific goal in Chapter 2.

URINARY-ELIMINATION THERAPY DEPENDENCE

Dependence on Decompression Urinary Drainage Management (129,391)

ASSESSMENT

Subjective Data
Person relies on nurses for:
    prevention of a sudden decrease in bladder pressure
    infection prevention

catheter patency
observation for leakage
discomfort relief

Objective Data
Person is receiving decompression urinary drainage therapy

Related Data
Commonly Related Diseases:
Bladder calculi
Benign prostatic hypertrophy
Prostate carcinoma

POSSIBLE ETIOLOGY

Need to prevent a sudden decrease in bladder pressure, so as to prevent bladder blood vessel rupture or hematuria. The antigravity setup causes urine to flow against the pull of gravity, so that bladder emptying does not occur rapidly.

NURSING DIAGNOSIS

Dependence on decompression urinary drainage management: reliance on nurses for the proper care and functioning of a urinary drainage system whereby rapid bladder emptying is prevented

PLANNING

Patient Needs	Primary Nurse-Patient Goals
Water-salt balance	To maintain fluid and electrolyte balance
Waste elimination	To maintain regulating mechanisms and functions
Comfort	To achieve comfort
Cleanliness	To achieve good hygiene
Protection from physical harm	To prevent physical injury, infection
Dependence	To achieve comfort
Increased learning	To achieve awareness of needs

NURSING INTERVENTIONS

Nursing Treatments
Anchor the tubing (catheter) securely
Provide sufficiently long tubing to allow freedom of movement
Keep the drainage container below bladder level
Empty the collection appliance (periodically)
Clean the urinary catheter externally at the meatus
Increase fluid intake to about 2000 cc daily
Attach the tube to straight drainage and a collection container (when the decompression therapy is terminated)

Nursing Observations
Check the drainage system for leakage
Check the tube for patency

Measure the intake
Measure the output
Observe for complaints of pain
Obtain a bacterial culture (of urine periodically)

Health Teaching
Explain the reason for and intended effect of the therapy
Instruct to increase fluid intake

Medical Treatments Performed by Nurses
Maintain the decompression drainage Y-tube at the ordered level

EVALUATION

See the evaluation criteria for each specific goal in Chapter 2.

Dependence on Indwelling Urinary Catheter Management (70,391)

ASSESSMENT

Subjective Data
Person relies on nurses for:
    insertion of the catheter
    maintenance of catheter patency
    infection prevention
    periodic catheter change
    maintenance of a sterile drainage system
    discomfort relief

Objective Data
Person needs or has an indwelling urinary catheter

Related Data
Commonly Related Diseases:
Cervical or thoracic spinal cord injury
Cerebral vascular accident
Urethral calculi
Bladder calculi

POSSIBLE ETIOLOGY

Need for waste elimination from the bladder. Urine incontinence.

NURSING DIAGNOSIS

Dependence on urinary catheter management: reliance on nurses for the proper care and functioning of an indwelling urinary catheter and bladder drainage system

PLANNING

Patient Needs
Water-salt balance

Primary Nurse-Patient Goals
To maintain fluid and electrolyte
    balance

Acid-base balance, waste
  elimination
Comfort
Cleanliness
Protection from physical harm
Dependence
Increased learning

To maintain regulating mechanisms
  and functions
To achieve comfort
To achieve good hygiene
To prevent physical injury, infection
To achieve comfort
To achieve awareness of needs

NURSING INTERVENTIONS

Nursing Treatments
Catheterize with an indwelling urinary catheter
Tape the urinary catheter onto the abdomen (if the catheter is inserted for a
    prolonged period)
Provide sufficiently long tubing to allow freedom of movement
Attach the tube to straight drainage and a collection container
    OR
Attach the tube to a leg urinal
Keep the drainage container below bladder level
Change the urinary catheter (as needed)
Change the urinary drainage apparatus (frequently)
Clean the urinary catheter externally at the meatus (daily)
Irrigate the urinary catheter (periodically)
Use sterile technique (when disconnecting the urinary drainage system)
Give urine-acidifying juices orally (four times daily)
Increase fluid intake to about 2000 cc daily

Nursing Observations
Check the drainage system for leakage
Check the tube (indwelling urinary catheter) for patency
Measure the intake
Measure the output
Monitor urine studies for evidence of urinary tract infection
Observe for complaints of pain
Observe the urine for abnormal color, content, and odor
Inspect for bleeding (hematuria)
Test the urine for pH

Health Teaching
Instruct that the drainage container should be held below the bladder level
Instruct to increase fluid intake
Teach how to apply a urinary-collection container
Teach how to do a catheterization
Teach how to irrigate a urinary catheter
Explain the reason for and intended effect of the therapy

EVALUATION
See the evaluation criteria for each specific goal in Chapter 2.

Dependence on Nephrostomy Drainage Management (71,391)

ASSESSMENT

Subjective Data
Person relies on nurses for:
  infection prevention
  periodic dressing changes
  prevention of leakage
  tube patency
  discomfort relief

Objective Data
Person has a nephrostomy tube

Related Data
Commonly Related Diseases:
Wilms' tumor
Fibrolipomyoma
Renal pelvis carcinoma
Renal calculi

POSSIBLE ETIOLOGY

The need for urinary drainage from the kidney following surgical intervention in renal disease

NURSING DIAGNOSIS

Dependence on nephrostomy drainage management: reliance on nurses to care for a urinary drainage tube, placed through a surgical incision into the renal pelvis, and to manage the drainage from the catheter

PLANNING

Patient Needs	Primary Nurse-Patient Goals
Waste elimination	To maintain regulating mechanisms and functions
Comfort	To achieve comfort
Cleanliness	To achieve good hygiene
Protection from physical harm	To prevent physical injury, infection
Dependence	To achieve comfort
Increased learning	To achieve awareness of needs

NURSING INTERVENTIONS

Nursing Treatments
Handle gently
Attach the tube to straight drainage and a collection container
Keep the drainage container below kidney level
Empty the collection container (periodically)

Use sterile technique (when disconnecting the urinary drainage system)
Provide sufficiently long tubing to allow freedom of movement
Change the urinary drainage apparatus (frequently)
Increase fluid intake to about 2000 cc daily
Change the dressing frequently
Clean with surgical soap (the skin around the nephrostomy tube when changing the dressing)
Position comfortably
Protect with absorbent padding
Refrain from jarring the bed

Nursing Observations
Check the drainage system for leakage
Check the tube (nephrostomy) for patency
Inspect for bleeding (around the nephrostomy incision)
Inspect for drainage
Inspect the skin for irritation (from the drainage)
Measure the urine output hourly (the first 48 hours)
Measure the intake
Measure the output
Monitor urine studies for evidence of urinary tract infection
Observe for complaints of pain
Observe the urine for abnormal color, content, and odor
Inspect for bleeding (hematuria)
Obtain a bacterial culture (of the urine periodically)

Health Teaching
Explain the reason for and intended effect of the therapy
Instruct that the drainage container should be held below the kidney level
Instruct to increase fluid intake

Medical Treatments Performed by Nurses
Irrigate the nephrostomy tube

EVALUATION

See the evaluation criteria for each specific goal in Chapter 2.

Dependence on Suprapubic Drainage Management (70,391)

ASSESSMENT

Subjective Data
Person relies on nurses for:
   infection prevention
   dressing changes
   skin care
   prevention of leakage
   maintenance of drainage apparatus
   discomfort relief

Objective Data
Person has a suprapubic catheter

Related Data

Commonly Related Diseases:
Prostatic hypertrophy
Bladder calculi

POSSIBLE ETIOLOGY

Drainage of the bladder in order to direct urine flow away from the urethra

NURSING DIAGNOSIS

Dependence on suprapubic drainage management (dependence on cystostomy drainage management): reliance on nurses to care for a catheter, placed through a surgical abdominal incision into the bladder, and to manage the drainage from the catheter

PLANNING

Patient Needs	**Primary Nurse-Patient Goals**
Waste elimination	To maintain regulating mechanisms and functions
Comfort	To achieve comfort
Cleanliness	To achieve good hygiene
Dependence	To achieve comfort
Increased learning	To achieve awareness of needs

NURSING INTERVENTIONS

Nursing Treatments
Handle gently
Tape the urinary catheter onto the abdomen
Attach the tube to straight drainage and a collection container
Keep the drainage container below bladder level
Empty the collection container (periodically, being sure the cystostomy tube contains urine before disconnecting the drainage system)
Use sterile technique (when disconnecting the urinary drainage system)
Change the urinary drainage apparatus (frequently)
Increase fluid intake to about 2000 cc daily
Apply a sterile dressing (after the catheter is removed)
Change the dressing frequently
Position comfortably
Protect with absorbent padding
Refrain from jarring the bed

Nursing Observations
Check the drainage system for leakage
Check the tube (suprapubic) for patency (periodically)
Measure the intake
Measure the output
Monitor urine studies for evidence of urinary tract infection
Observe for complaints of pain
Observe the urine for abnormal color, content, and odor
Inspect for bleeding (hematuria)

Health Teaching

Instruct that the drainage container should be held below the bladder level

Instruct to increase fluid intake

Explain the reason for and intended effect of the therapy

Medical Treatments Performed by Nurses

Clamp the suprapubic catheter (usually for 3–4 hours at a time) and have the patient attempt to void

EVALUATION

See the evaluation criteria for each specific goal in Chapter 2.

Dependence on Tidal Drainage Management (70,129)

ASSESSMENT

Subjective Data

Person relies on nurses for:

    alternate bladder irrigation and drainage

    regulation of drainage flow

    maintenance of catheter patency

    prevention of leakage

    maintenance of sterile technique

    discomfort relief

Objective Data

Person is receiving tidal drainage therapy

Related Data

Commonly Related Diseases:

Cervical or thoracic spinal cord injury

POSSIBLE ETIOLOGY

Need to stimulate normal bladder functioning by developing normal bladder capacity and tone

NURSING DIAGNOSIS

Dependence on tidal drainage management: reliance on nurses for the proper care and functioning of a drainage system that alternately fills and drains the bladder

PLANNING

Patient Needs	Primary Nurse-Patient Goals
Waste elimination	To maintain regulating mechanisms and functions
Comfort	To achieve comfort
Cleanliness	To achieve good hygiene
Protection from physical harm	To prevent physical injury, infection
Dependence	To achieve comfort
Increased learning	To achieve awareness of needs

NURSING INTERVENTIONS

Nursing Treatments
Catheterize with an indwelling urinary (double or triple lumen) catheter
Anchor the tubing securely
Provide sufficiently long tubing to allow freedom of movement
Introduce irrigating solutions slowly (40–60 drops a minute)
Keep the drainage container below bladder level
Protect with absorbent padding
Give urine-acidifying juices orally (four times daily)
Increase fluid intake to about 2000 cc daily

Nursing Observations
Check the drainage system for leakage
Check the tube(s) for patency
Measure the intake
Measure the output
Monitor urine studies for evidence of urinary tract infection
Observe for complaints of pain
Observe the urine for abnormal color, content, and odor
Obtain a bacterial culture (of the urine periodically)

Health Teaching
Instruct to increase fluid intake

Medical Treatments Performed by Nurses
Irrigate the bladder by tidal drainage

EVALUATION

See the evaluation criteria for each specific goal in Chapter 2.

Dependence on Ureteroileostomy Management (70,391)

ASSESSMENT

Subjective Data
Person relies on nurses for:
    cleanliness of body, clothing, and linens
    odor control
    catheter irrigation
    skin care
    infection prevention

Objective Data
Person has a ureteroileostomy

Related Data
Commonly Related Diseases:
Bladder carcinoma

POSSIBLE ETIOLOGY

Genitourinary tract obstruction below the ureters

NURSING DIAGNOSIS

Dependence on ureteroileostomy management (dependence on ileal conduit management) (dependence on Bricker procedure management): reliance on nurses to maintain proper care of an artificial abdominal opening in which the ureter has been surgically implanted into a loop of the ileum, with urine flowing externally from stomas or buds

PLANNING

Patient Needs	**Primary Nurse-Patient Goals**
Water-salt balance	To maintain fluid and electrolyte balance
Waste elimination	To maintain regulating mechanisms and functions
Comfort	To achieve comfort
Cleanliness	To achieve good hygiene
Protection from physical harm	To prevent physical injury
Dependence	To achieve comfort
Mastery and competence in skills	To achieve optimum function
Increased learning	To achieve awareness of needs

NURSING INTERVENTIONS

Nursing Treatments
Handle gently
Clean with surgical soap (around the ureteroileostomy)
Apply calamine lotion
   OR
Apply milk of magnesia to the skin } (around the ureteroileostomy)
   OR
Lubricate the skin with petrolatum
Apply an ostomy appliance (clear, plastic disposable type)
Attach the collection appliance to straight drainage and a collection container (if preferred, in order to protect the incision from urine contamination)
Empty the collection appliance (every 2–3 hours or when it contains 100 cc urine, if it is not attached to straight drainage)
Change the ostomy appliance as needed
Give urine-acidifying juices orally (four times a day)
Increase fluid intake to about 2000 cc daily
Introduce to persons who have successfully undergone the same experience (if the patient is anxious)
Make a referral (to the local ostomy association)

Nursing Observations
Check the drainage system for leakage
Inspect the skin for irritation
Measure the intake
Measure the output

Monitor urine studies for evidence of urinary tract infection
Observe for complaints of pain (in the lower abdomen)
Observe the urine for abnormal color, content, and odor
Inspect for bleeding (hematuria)
Obtain a bacterial culture (of urine periodically)

Health Teaching
Explain the reason for and intended effect of the therapy
Teach how to dilate the stoma with a sterile catheter
Explain how to obtain therapeutic supplies
Teach how to apply the ostomy appliance
Explain how to maintain cleanliness of the ostomy appliance
Recommend that two ostomy appliances be alternately used
Recommend that extra therapeutic supplies be carried
Instruct to avoid foods having strong odors
Instruct to increase fluid intake

Medical Treatments Performed by Nurses
Irrigate the ostomy

EVALUATION

See the evaluation criteria for each specific goal in Chapter 2.

Dependence on Ureterosigmoidostomy Management (70,391)

ASSESSMENT

Subjective Data
Person relies on nurses for:
    infection prevention
    cleanliness of body, clothing, and linens
    regulation of periodic toileting

Objective Data
Person has a ureterosigmoidostomy

Related Data
Commonly Related Diseases:
Benign prostatic hypertrophy
Prostate adenocarcinoma
Bladder neoplasm
Urethral calculi

POSSIBLE ETIOLOGY

Genitourinary obstruction below the ureters

NURSING DIAGNOSIS

Dependence on ureterosigmoidostomy management: reliance on nurses to maintain proper care of a surgical implantation of ureters in the anus, which resulted from anastomosis between the ureter and sigmoid colon

PLANNING

Patient Needs	Primary Nurse-Patient Goals
Waste elimination	To maintain regulating mechanisms and functions
Comfort	To achieve comfort
Cleanliness	To achieve good hygiene
Protection from physical harm	To prevent physical injury
Dependence	To achieve comfort
Mastery and competence in skills	To achieve optimum function
Increased learning	To achieve awareness of needs

NURSING INTERVENTIONS

Nursing Treatments
Handle gently
Encourage decreased residue-food intake (prior to and after surgery)
Toilet frequently (every 2–4 hours)
Remove the colon tube for bowel elimination and then reinsert about 4 inches
Anchor the tubing (colon) securely (to the buttocks)
Attach the tube to straight drainage and a collection container (during the night)
Increase fluid intake to about 3000 cc daily
Refrain from giving enemas
Refrain from giving laxatives
Lubricate the skin with petrolatum (around the rectal area if it becomes irritated)
Apply heat by a gooseneck lamp (for skin irritation)
Protect with plastic pants
Introduce to persons who have successfully undergone the same experience (if the patient is anxious)
Make a referral (to the local ostomy association)

Nursing Observations
Check the tube (ureterosigmoidostomy) for patency
Inspect the skin for irritation
Measure the urine output hourly (the first 24 hours postsurgery)
Measure the intake
Measure the output (after the first 24 hours)
Monitor blood studies for abnormal electrolytes
Monitor the oral temperature (for fever)
Monitor urine studies for evidence of urinary tract infection
Observe for complaints of nausea
Observe for complaints of pain
Observe for vomiting
Observe the urine for abnormal color, content, and odor
Inspect for bleeding (hematuria)
Obtain a bacterial culture (of urine periodically)

Health Teaching
Instruct to maintain skin cleanliness
Explain the reason for and intended effect of the therapy

EVALUATION

See the evaluation criteria for each specific goal in Chapter 2.

Dependence on Ureterostomy Management (70,391)

ASSESSMENT

Subjective Data
Person relies on nurses for:
    infection prevention
    periodic dressing changes
    skin care
    odor control

Objective Data
Person has a ureterostomy

Related Data
Commonly Related Diseases:
Retroperitoneal fibrosis
Ureteral carcinoma
Ureteral calculi
Rectocaval ureter
Nephrolithiasis

POSSIBLE ETIOLOGY

The surgical cutaneous implantation of the ureters in the abdomen as a result of ureteral obstruction

NURSING DIAGNOSIS

Dependence on ureterostomy management: reliance on nurses to maintain proper care of an artificial opening in the abdomen through which the ureter discharges urine

Patient Needs	Primary Nurse-Patient Goals
Water-salt balance	To maintain fluid and electrolyte balance
Waste elimination	To maintain regulating mechanisms and functions
Comfort	To achieve comfort
Cleanliness	To achieve good hygiene
Protection from physical harm	To prevent physical injury, infection
Dependence	To achieve comfort
Mastery and competence in skills	To achieve optimum function
Increased learning	To achieve awareness of needs

NURSING INTERVENTIONS

Nursing Treatments

First 5–10 Days When Catheter Is in the Ureter:
Apply a (sterile) saline compress (over the ureteral buds)
Apply a sterile dressing (over the saline compress)
Apply zinc oxide to the skin
   OR
Apply aluminum paste to the skin (around the ureterostomy)
   OR
Lubricate the skin with petrolatum

After Ureter Catheter Is Removed:
Apply an ostomy appliance
Empty the collection appliance (frequently during the day)
Attach the collection appliance to straight drainage and a collection container (during the night)
Change the ostomy appliance as needed (usually every 3–4 days)
Bathe locally (with soap and water when changing the appliance)
Apply tincture of benzoin (over the skin area covered by the appliance)
Give urine-acidifying juices orally (four times a day)
Increase fluid intake to about 2000 cc daily
Introduce to persons who have successfully undergone the same experience
   (if the patient is anxious)
Make a referral (to the local ostomy association)

Nursing Observations
Check the tube (ureterostomy) for patency
Inspect for edema (of the stoma)
Inspect the skin for irritation
Measure the intake
Measure the output
Observe for complaints of pain (backache which indicates that drainage is
   not flowing)
Observe the urine for abnormal color, content, and odor
Obtain a bacterial culture (of urine periodically)

Health Teaching
Explain the reason for and intended effect of the therapy
Teach how to dilate the stoma with a sterile catheter
Explain how to obtain therapeutic supplies
Teach how to apply the ostomy appliance
Explain how to maintain cleanliness of the ostomy appliance
Recommend that two ostomy appliances be alternately used
Recommend that extra therapeutic supplies be carried
Instruct to avoid foods having strong odors
Instruct to increase fluid intake

EVALUATION

See the evaluation criteria for each specific goal in Chapter 2.

DIALYSIS THERAPY DEPENDENCE

Dependence on Arteriovenous Shunt Management (391)

ASSESSMENT

Subjective Data
Person relies on nurses for:
- maintenance of sterile technique
- periodic dressing changes
- patency maintenance
- observation for and prevention of clotting

Objective Data
Person has an arteriovenous cannula

Related Data
Commonly Related Diseases:
Nephritis
Nephrosis
Glomerulonephritis

POSSIBLE ETIOLOGY

Need for hemodialysis

NURSING DIAGNOSIS

Dependence on arteriovenous shunt management: reliance on nurses to care for an arteriovenous cannula

PLANNING

Patient Needs	Primary Nurse-Patient Goals
Protection from physical harm	To prevent physical injury, infection
Dependence	To achieve comfort
Increased learning	To achieve awareness of needs

NURSING INTERVENTIONS

Nursing Treatments
Apply an antibiotic ointment
Apply a sterile dressing
Change the dressing frequently
Clean with surgical soap (around the cannula, using sterile technique)
Handle gently
Refrain from giving local cold applications
Refrain from tight bandaging

Nursing Observations
Auscultate and palpate the arteriovenous shunt for patency
Inspect for edema
Inspect for inflammation

Inspect for drainage
Monitor the oral temperature (for fever)
Obtain a bacterial culture (of any exudate)

Health Teaching
Explain the need to avoid sudden movements of an extremity having an
    arteriovenous shunt
Instruct to maintain skin dryness (on the extremity with the A-V shunt)
Instruct that it is essential to carry an arteriovenous shunt clamp
Teach how to care for an arteriovenous shunt
Explain the reason for and intended effect of the therapy

EVALUATION

See the evaluation criteria for each specific goal in Chapter 2.

Dependence on Hemodialysis Management (391)

ASSESSMENT

Subjective Data
Person relies on nurses for:
    maintenance of sterile technique
    maintenance of the kidney machine
    correct delivery of the hemodialysis treatment
    observation for and prevention of dangerous side effects

Objective Data
Person is receiving hemodialysis therapy

Related Data
Commonly Related Diseases:
Glomerulonephritis
Pyelonephritis
Polycystic kidney disease

POSSIBLE ETIOLOGY

Failure of the nonfunctioning kidney to filter body wastes

NURSING DIAGNOSIS

Dependence on hemodialysis management: reliance on nursing for the process of removing chemical wastes from the body by filtering blood through
a mechanical pump

PLANNING

Patient Needs	Primary Nurse-Patient Goals
Acid-base balance, waste elimination, normal temperature	To maintain regulating mechanisms and functions
Sleep, rest	To achieve sleep, rest
Comfort	To achieve comfort
Cleanliness	To achieve good hygiene

Protection from physical harm | To prevent physical injury, infection
Dependence | To achieve comfort
Increased learning | To achieve awareness of needs

NURSING INTERVENTIONS

Nursing Treatments
Attend the patient constantly
Position comfortably
Change the patient's position frequently
Place in the flat position (if the blood pressure drops)
Refrain from jarring the bed
Refrain from giving intravenous or intramuscular injections (postdialysis)

Nursing Observations
Auscultate the apical heartbeat for rate and rhythm
Check the dialysis circuit for leakage
Check the hemodialysis A-V shunt for cleanliness and patency
Check the hemodialysis equipment for mechanical breakdown
Inspect the chest for respiratory rate and rhythm
Inspect for bleeding (around dressings, in stools, gastric drainage, gums, nose)
Inspect the skin for perspiration abnormality (profuse perspiration)
Measure the body weight (before and after dialysis)
Monitor the blood pressure (before and at the start of dialysis, then every 15 minutes to 1 hour)
Observe for complaints of headache
Observe for complaints of itching
Observe for complaints of nausea
Observe for complaints of pain (muscle cramps or chest pain)
Observe for complaints of weakness
Observe for shock
Observe for vomiting
Monitor blood studies for abnormal clotting mechanism (decreased clotting time due to heparin)
Monitor blood studies for abnormal electrolytes (before and after dialysis)
Monitor blood studies for abnormal hematology (hematocrit)
Monitor blood studies for abnormal renal function (urea and creatinine before and after dialysis)
Monitor the oral temperature (for fever)

Health Teaching
Describe those symptoms which should be reported (pain, nausea, headache, weakness)
Explain the reason for and intended effect of the therapy

Medical Treatments Performed by Nurses
Administer the hemodialysis treatment
Give the prescribed drugs (heparin, protamine sulfate, dialysate fluid)

EVALUATION

See the evaluation criteria for each specific goal in Chapter 2.

Dependence on Peritoneal Dialysis Management (70,391)

ASSESSMENT

Subjective Data

Person relies on nurses for:
    maintenance of sterile technique
    supervision of the instillation and drainage of dialysate solution
    observation for and precaution against dangerous side effects
    relief from discomfort or pain

Objective Data

Person is receiving peritoneal dialysis therapy

Related Data

Commonly Related Diseases:
Hypertension
Glomerulonephritis
Nephrosis

POSSIBLE ETIOLOGY

Failure of the nonfunctioning kidney to filter body wastes. Need to remove excessive body fluid.

NURSING DIAGNOSIS

Dependence on peritoneal dialysis management: reliance on nurses for the procedure of removing chemical wastes from the blood by diffusing wastes (urea, phosphate, etc.) out of the blood, across the peritoneal membrane, and into the dialysate solution

PLANNING

Patient Needs	**Primary Nurse-Patient Goals**
Water-salt balance	To maintain fluid and electrolyte balance
Acid-base balance, waste elimination, normal temperature	To maintain regulating mechanisms and functions
Sleep, rest	To achieve sleep, rest
Comfort	To achieve comfort
Cleanliness	To achieve good hygiene
Protection from physical harm	To prevent physical injury, infection
Dependence	To achieve comfort
Increased learning	To achieve awareness of needs

NURSING INTERVENTIONS

Nursing Treatments

Attend the patient constantly
Place in the flat position

OR
Place in the slight sitting position
Warm the dialysis fluid before instillation (98.6 °F)
Do not allow air into the dialysis instillation tubing
Elevate the head
   OR   (if the dialysis fluid does not drain
Change the patient's position   adequately)
   frequently (from side to side)
Refrain from giving enemas (while the dialysis fluid is in the peritoneum)
Refrain from giving intravenous or intramuscular injections (postdialysis)
Refrain from jarring the bed
Change the dressing frequently (around the catheter)
Apply a sterile dressing (after the dialysis is completed)

Nursing Observations

Auscultate the apical heartbeat for rate and rhythm
Check the dialysis circuit for leakage
Check the peritoneal dialysis catheter for leakage or displacement
Check the peritoneal dialysis fluid for bloody or cloudy return
Check solution (dialysis) for flow rate (2000 cc per 10–15 minutes)
Check the peritoneal dialysis fluid for retention or drainage in excess of
   500 cc
Inspect the chest for respiratory rate and rhythm (drain the fluid from the
   peritoneum immediately if there is severe respiratory distress)
Inspect for bleeding (around the catheter)
Keep a dialysis flow sheet
Measure the body weight (before and after dialysis)
Measure the intake
Measure the output
Monitor the blood pressure (every 15 minutes for the first 2 hours, then
   every hour)
Monitor the oral temperature (every 4 hours)
Monitor blood studies for abnormal renal function (urea and albumin be-
   fore and during dialysis)
Observe for complaints of pain (severe abdominal pain, especially during
   fluid drainage)
Observe for complaints of pain radiation (to the left shoulder during instil-
   lation)
Observe for fatigue
Observe for shock
Obtain a bacterial culture (from the catheter tip and the last bottle of fluid
   drained)

Health Teaching

Describe those symptoms which should be reported (pain, fatigue)
Explain the reason for and intended effect of the therapy

Medical Treatments Performed by Nurses
Instill dialysate into the peritoneum (10–15 minutes), allow it to remain in
the abdomen (30–35 minutes), then drain dialysate (10–15 minutes)
Give the prescribed number of peritoneal dialysis exchanges
Give the prescribed drugs (heparin, potassium, antibiotics)

EVALUATION

See the evaluation criteria for each specific goal in Chapter 2.

DIALYSIS THERAPY DISCOMFORTS

Distress Related to Hemodialysis (318a)

ASSESSMENT

Subjective Data
Feels trapped and enslaved by the artificial kidney
Feels that the machine destroys his human identity, making him a
mechanized being
Resents the activity limitations imposed by the machine
Perceives the hours of treatment as uselessly wasted
Fears that if there is mechanical failure, a fatal blood loss will occur
Fears loss of strength or potency to the machine
May develop a phobia, or attribute magic powers or human motives to the
machine

Objective Data
Displays a frightened expression when looking at the machine
May avoid eye contact with the machine by staring at the ceiling, covering
his face, or sleeping during the treatment

Related Data
Commonly Related Conditions:
Uremia
Commonly Related Diseases:
Glomerulonephritis
Nephrotic syndrome
Chemically induced renal failure
Diabetes mellitus
Pyleonephritis

POSSIBLE ETIOLOGY

A need for the removal of body wastes as a result of kidney failure. An awareness that the maintenance of one's life is reliant upon a machine, with resulting intense anxiety.

NURSING DIAGNOSIS

Distress related to hemodialysis: intense misery regarding the use on oneself of an artificial kidney machine through which chemical substances are removed from the blood as a substitute for impaired kidney function

PLANNING

Patient Needs	Primary Nurse-Patient Goals
Comfort	To achieve comfort
Protection from psychologic threat	To prevent emotional injury
Dependence	To achieve comfort
Acceptance	To achieve productive interpersonal relationships
Warm, communicating relationships	To achieve effective verbal and nonverbal communications
Independence	To achieve optimum function
Increased learning	To achieve awareness of needs
Increased reality perception and problem solving	To achieve optimum function

NURSING INTERVENTIONS

Nursing Treatments

Approach unhurriedly
Demonstrate calmness
Reassure verbally (frequently)
Provide an atmosphere of acceptance
Attend the patient constantly
Anticipate needs
Arrange pleasant surroundings
Arrange situations which encourage patient autonomy
Ask the patient what makes him (her) comfortable
Encourage the expression of feelings
Listen attentively
Recognize the need for the use of appropriate defense mechanisms
Encourage the use of normal coping mechanisms
Explore with the patient his strengths and resources
Introduce to persons who have successfully undergone the same experience
Provide radio and television for di-
    version
        OR   } (during the treatment period if the
Provide reading material for diver-   patient desires such)
    sion
Encourage mutual problem solving

Nursing Observations

Determine the degree of insight

Evaluate the significance of emotional distress mannerisms

Identify abnormal perceptions (of the machine)

Identify disturbing conversation topics

Identify inappropriate use of defense mechanisms

Observe for an excessive stress level

Observe for impaired self-attitudes

Health Teaching

Explain that the person's emotional response is appropriate and commonly experienced

Explain how the equipment works (emphasizing its positive and safety features)

Recommend a habitual, positive mental attitude (that the artificial kidney, though often an object of fear and dependence, is primarily a source of improved health)

EVALUATION

See the evaluation criteria for each specific goal in Chapter 2.

INADEQUATE ARTIFICIAL BLADDER ELIMINATION MANAGEMENT

Inadequate Information Related to Urinary Catheter Care (71,391)

ASSESSMENT

Subjective Data

Person confirms a lack of information

Objective Data

Person's actions indicate a lack of information regarding:

how to insert a catheter

how to irrigate a catheter

how to maintain sterile technique

methods of odor control

the importance of adequate fluid intake

those symptoms that should be reported

Related Data

Commonly Related Diseases:

Thoracic or lumbar spinal cord injury

Spinal cord tumor

Bladder carcinoma

POSSIBLE ETIOLOGY

Lack of instruction

NURSING DIAGNOSIS

Inadequate information related to urinary catheter care: lack of information related to the care of a urinary catheter

PLANNING

Patient Needs	**Primary Nurse-Patient Goals**
Protection from physical harm	To prevent physical injury, infection
Mastery and competence in skills, independence	To achieve optimum function
Increased learning	To achieve awareness of needs

NURSING INTERVENTIONS

Nursing Treatments
Approach unhurriedly
Encourage patient questions

Nursing Observations
Evaluate the response to teaching

Health Teaching
Explain how to obtain therapeutic supplies
Explain that the urinary catheter should be taped to the abdomen
Inform that cleanliness is basic to health
Explain how to clean the external part of the indwelling urinary catheter
Instruct that the drainage container should be held below the bladder level
Instruct to anchor the urinary catheter
Teach how to apply a urinary collection container
Teach how to do a catheterization
Teach how to irrigate a urinary catheter
Teach how to test urine for pH
Explain the reason for and intended effect of the therapy

EVALUATION

See the evaluation criteria for each specific goal in Chapter 2.

INADEQUATE NORMAL BLADDER ELIMINATION MANAGEMENT

Inadequate Information Related to Juvenile Enuresis (400,453)

ASSESSMENT

Subjective Data
Person confirms a lack of information
Anxiety
Frustration

Objective Data

Person's (usually the mother's) actions indicate a lack of information regarding:

the measures to take to stop a child over age three from wetting the bed

the possible causes of the problem

POSSIBLE ETIOLOGY

Lack of instruction. First experience with the situation.

NURSING DIAGNOSIS

Inadequate information related to juvenile enuresis: lack of information regarding unintentional voiding at night by children who have no urologic disorder

PLANNING

Patient Needs	**Primary Nurse-Patient Goals**
Comfort	To achieve comfort
Increased learning	To achieve awareness of needs

NURSING INTERVENTIONS

Nursing Treatments

Approach unhurriedly

Encourage parent questions

Nursing Observations

Evaluate the response to teaching

Monitor urine studies for evidence of urinary tract infection

Health Teaching

Advise against participation in emotional situations before sleep

Describe those symptoms which should be reported (lack of urine control during the daytime or urine dribbling)

Explain that parental attitudes affect child development (teasing and punishment only make the child more tense)

Explain the causes of the health problem (excitement, tension, poor sphincter control)

Emphasize the need to develop self-reliance (in the child so that he can maintain control)

Instruct to toilet frequently (at night)

Recommend the use of warm clothing (when in bed)

EVALUATION

See the evaluation criteria for each specific goal in Chapter 2.

Inadequate Information Related to Toilet Training (400)

ASSESSMENT

Subjective Data

Person confirms a lack of information

Objective Data
Person's actions indicate a lack of information regarding:
    the correct age for toilet training a child
    the proper toilet training technique
    how to properly dress the child for training
    how much control the child is capable of maintaining

POSSIBLE ETIOLOGY

Socially and culturally imposed modes of conduct. Lack of instruction.

NURSING DIAGNOSIS

Inadequate information related to toilet training: lack of information as to
the proper method of teaching a child bladder and bowel control

Patient Needs	Primary Nurse-Patient Goals
Comfort	To achieve comfort
Mastery and competence in skills	To achieve optimum function
Increased learning	To achieve awareness of needs

NURSING INTERVENTIONS

Nursing Treatments

Approach unhurriedly
Encourage parent questions

Nursing Observations

Evaluate the response to teaching

Health Teaching

Advise that toilet training failures be ignored
Explain that a child should become accustomed to dry diapers during toilet
    training
Explain that commode sittings should be scheduled during toilet training
Explain that controlled elimination should be praised during toilet training
Inform as to the correct terminology for elimination
Inform that a child should be diapered only at night during toilet training
Inform that a child should be dressed in easily removable clothes for toilet-
    ing
Inform that a child should be fully awakened during nighttime toileting
Inform that children are receptive to stages of toilet training at different
    ages
Inform that toilet training should be delayed until the child can sit up
Inform that toilet training should be limited to short periods daily

EVALUATION

See the evaluation criteria for each specific goal in Chapter 2.

INADEQUATE DIALYSIS THERAPY MANAGEMENT

Inadequate Information Related to Arteriovenous Shunt Management (70,71,391)

ASSESSMENT

Subjective Data
Person confirms a lack of information
Anxiety

Objective Data
Person's actions indicate a lack of information regarding:
   how to clean the cannula
   how to change the dressing
   the precautions to be taken
   the signs and symptoms that should be reported

Related Data
Commonly Related Diseases:
Chronic glomerulonephritis
Nephrosis

POSSIBLE ETIOLOGY

Lack of instruction

NURSING DIAGNOSIS

Inadequate information related to arteriovenous shunt management: lack of knowledge as to the proper care and functioning of tubing surgically placed in an artery and vein for purposes of hemodialysis

PLANNING

Patient Needs	**Primary Nurse-Patient Goals**
Comfort	To achieve comfort
Protection from physical harm	To prevent physical injury, infection
Mastery and competence in skills	To achieve optimum function
Increased learning	To achieve awareness of needs

NURSING INTERVENTIONS

Nursing Treatments
Approach unhurriedly
Encourage patient questions

Nursing Observations
Evaluate the response to teaching

Health Teaching
Describe those symptoms which should be reported (pain, inflammation)
Explain the need to avoid sudden movements of an extremity having an
   arteriovenous shunt

Instruct to maintain skin dryness (on the extremity with the A-V shunt)
Instruct that it is essential to carry an arteriovenous shunt clamp
Teach how to care for an arteriovenous shunt
Explain the reason for and intended effect of the therapy

EVALUATION

See the evaluation criteria for each specific goal in Chapter 2.

Inadequate Information Related to Home Dialysis Management (70,391)

ASSESSMENT

Subjective Data
Person confirms a lack of information

Objective Data
Person's actions indicate a lack of information regarding:
> how to operate the artificial kidney
> how to fit hemodialysis into the daily living schedule
> which supplies are needed or the source of the supplies
> the dangerous signs to look for
> how to obtain health care assistance when it is needed

Related Data
Commonly Related Diseases:
Glomerulonephritis
Pyelonephritis
Polycystic kidney disease

POSSIBLE ETIOLOGY

Lack of instruction

NURSING DIAGNOSIS

Inadequate information related to home dialysis management: lack of information regarding home management of the hemodialysis treatment

PLANNING

Patient Needs	Primary Nurse-Patient Goals
Comfort	To achieve comfort
Protection from physical harm	To prevent physical injury, infection
Mastery and competence in skills, independence	To achieve optimum function
Increased learning	To achieve awareness of needs and/or use of resources

NURSING INTERVENTIONS

Nursing Treatments
Involve the family
Approach unhurriedly
Encourage patient questions
Introduce to persons who have successfully undergone the same experience

Nursing Observations
Evaluate the response to teaching

Health Teaching
Teach how to do home dialysis
Advise how to integrate the hemodialysis procedure into the home routine
Explain how to obtain therapeutic supplies
Teach how to care for an arteriovenous shunt
Teach how to take a blood pressure
Teach how to administer medications
Describe those symptoms which should be reported (weakness, pain, headache)
Explain the reason for and intended effect of the therapy

EVALUATION

See the evaluation criteria for each specific goal in Chapter 2.

INADEQUATE ORGAN TRANSPLANT INFORMATION

Inadequate Information Related to Organ Donation (391)

ASSESSMENT

Subjective Data
Person confirms a lack of information

Objective Data
Person's actions indicate a lack of information regarding:
    how or where organs are donated
    the procedure involved in organ donation
    how it is determined if the person is a suitable donor
    the state of health to expect following donation of an organ

Related Data
Commonly Related Diseases:
Glomerulonephritis
Polycystic kidney disease
Pyelonephritis

POSSIBLE ETIOLOGY

Lack of instruction

NURSING DIAGNOSIS

Inadequate information related to organ donation: lack of information regarding the giving of an organ for transplant to another person

PLANNING

Patient Needs	**Primary Nurse-Patient Goals**
Comfort	To achieve comfort
Protection from physical harm	To prevent physical injury
Increased learning	To achieve awareness of needs and/or use of resources

NURSING INTERVENTIONS

Nursing Treatments
Approach unhurriedly
Encourage patient questions
Discuss the anticipated procedure
Introduce to persons who have successfully undergone the same experience

Nursing Observations
Evaluate the response to teaching

Health Teaching
Explain the criteria for acceptance of an organ donor
Explain how and where organ donations are made
Explain how the loss of an organ will affect the donor's future health

EVALUATION

See the evaluation criteria for each specific goal in Chapter 2.

Inadequate Information Related to Organ (Kidney) Transplant Rejection (235,339,391)

ASSESSMENT

Subjective Data
Person confirms a lack of information

Objective Data
Person's actions indicate a lack of information regarding:
    why a transplant rejection could occur
    the signs and symptoms of transplant rejection
    how to test the urine
    when to seek medical help in relation to symptoms suggesting rejection

Related Data
Commonly Related Diseases:
Renal failure

POSSIBLE ETIOLOGY

Lack of instruction

NURSING DIAGNOSIS

Inadequate information related to kidney transplant rejection: lack of information regarding the rejection of a transplanted kidney

PLANNING

Patient Needs

Protection from physical harm

Increased learning

Primary Nurse-Patient Goals

To prevent physical injury, infection

To achieve awareness of needs
and/or use of resources

NURSING INTERVENTIONS

Nursing Treatments

Approach unhurriedly

Encourage patient questions

Nursing Observations

Evaluate the response to teaching

Health Teaching

Describe those symptoms which should be reported (fever, decreased urine
output, edema, pain, weight gain)

Explain the causes of the health problem

Explain the reason for and intended effect of the therapy

Explain how to measure intake and output

Instruct to immediately report serious symptoms

Teach how to test the urine for pH

Teach how to test the urine for protein

Teach how to test the urine for sugar-acetone

EVALUATION

See the evaluation criteria for each specific goal in Chapter 2.

16.

NURSING DIAGNOSES RELATED TO
Health Management

HEALTH MANAGEMENT DEPENDENCE

Dependence on Nursing Assessment of Health Status

ASSESSMENT

Subjective Data

Person relies on nurses for:
   physical examination
   laboratory studies
   evaluation of health status

Objective Data

Request for examination for normal health status

Related Data

Commonly Related Diseases:
None
   OR
Any disease

POSSIBLE ETIOLOGY

Concern for health status. Lack of available medical care.

NURSING DIAGNOSIS

Dependence on nursing assessment of health status: reliance on nurses to assess the person's health status and evaluate the findings as being within or out of normal limits

PLANNING

Patient Needs	**Primary Nurse-Patient Goals**
Comfort	To achieve comfort
Protection from physical harm	To prevent physical injury

Dependence   To achieve comfort
Increased learning   To achieve awareness of needs

NURSING INTERVENTIONS

Nursing Treatments
Position comfortably
Drape modestly
Maintain a warm room temperature
Listen attentively (to the information the patient presents)
Encourage patient questions
Make a referral (to a physician if there is any evidence of pathology)

Nursing Observations
Perform a physical examination and evaluate if the findings are normal (ExR)
Obtain standard laboratory studies and evaluate for normal levels

Health Teaching
Advise early correction of problems (if any are found)
Explain the meaning of the diagnostic reports

EVALUATION

See the evaluation criteria for each specific goal in Chapter 2.

Dependence on Predischarge Planning

ASSESSMENT

Subjective Data
Person relies on nurses for:
   planning continued care after discharge
   referral to available community resources
   coordination of both nursing and medical plans

Objective Data
Patient discharge is planned for the near future

Related Data
Commonly Related Conditions:
Any condition requiring hospitalization
Commonly Related Diseases:
Any disease or injury

POSSIBLE ETIOLOGY

Need for continued health care following hospital discharge.

NURSING DIAGNOSIS

Dependence on predischarge planning: reliance on nurses to plan for and coordinate health care following discharge

PLANNING

Patient Needs

Comfort
Protection from physical harm
Dependence
Independence
Increased learning

Primary Nurse-Patient Goals

To achieve comfort
To prevent physical injury
To achieve comfort
To achieve optimum function
To achieve awareness of needs
and/or use of resources

NURSING INTERVENTIONS

Nursing Treatments
Encourage patient questions
Encourage family-shared responsibilities (if they are to care for the patient)
Encourage mutual problem solving
Arrange a predischarge planning conference
Provide a home visit (to assess the home situation)
Suggest home adaptations appropriate to the health problem
Make a referral (to the appropriate community agencies)
Consult with the physician (regarding the medical plan for discharge)

Nursing Observations
Evaluate the response to teaching

Health Teaching
Inform of the resources available for health care
Advise that persons attending the sick economize their energies
Describe those symptoms which should be reported (specific to the condition)

EVALUATION

See the evaluation criteria for each specific goal in Chapter 2.

HEALTH MANAGEMENT DIFFICULTIES

Failure to Seek Health Care

ASSESSMENT

Subjective Data
Person perceives changes in his body that do not fit into the normal pattern
Ignores signs and symptoms as long as possible
May secretly be greatly concerned about his health

Objective Data
Family or friends openly recognize the need for health care for their loved one

Related Data

Commonly Related Diseases:
Any disease or injury

POSSIBLE ETIOLOGY

Fear of a dooming diagnosis, hospitalization, surgery, or painful treatment. A desire not to have one's lifestyle interrupted. The inability to recognize that early treatment usually leads to a cure. Denial that any abnormality could occur to him. Lack of financial resources to support health care. A sense of deep responsibility to family, job, etc., which the person feels must be fulfilled and cannot be set aside by illness. The perception of illness as shameful.

NURSING DIAGNOSIS

Failure to seek health care: the avoidance of seeking health care for oneself despite an awareness that such care is needed

PLANNING

Patient Needs	**Primary Nurse-Patient Goals**
Comfort	To achieve comfort
Protection from physical harm	To prevent physical injury
Acceptance	To achieve productive interpersonal relationships
Warm, communicating relationships	To achieve effective verbal and nonverbal communications
Increased learning	To achieve awareness of needs and/or use of resources

NURSING INTERVENTIONS

Nursing Treatments
Approach unhurriedly
Provide an atmosphere of acceptance
Reassure verbally
Express warmth and friendliness
Encourage the expression of feelings
Listen attentively
Explore with the patient the effects of his behavior on others
Support a realistic assessment of the situation
Provide emotionally safe experiences (such as assurance that the person will go home and will not be hospitalized immediately after seeing the doctor)
Introduce to persons who have successfully undergone the same experience
Discuss the anticipated procedure (associated with the person's problem)
Emphasize the person's value as an individual

Nursing Observations
Identify disturbing conversation topics
Determine the degree of insight (as to why health care is not sought)

Observe for an excessive stress level
Observe for behavior modification

Health Teaching
Advise early correction of problems

EVALUATION

See the evaluation criteria for each specific goal in Chapter 2.

Inability to Obtain Health Care

ASSESSMENT

Subjective Data
Concern
Anxiety

Objective Data
No available local health care facility
Fails to meet the criteria for admittance in a particular health care institution
Unable to leave daily responsibilities to obtain health care
Unable to transport self or obtain adequate transportation to health facilities

Related Data
Commonly Related Diseases:
None
    OR
Any disease or injury

POSSIBLE ETIOLOGY

Lack of instruction in how to obtain health care. Lack of facilities.

NURSING DIAGNOSIS

Inability to obtain health care: the presence of situations or circumstances that interfere with the ability to obtain health care

PLANNING

Patient Needs	**Primary Nurse-Patient Goals**
Protection from physical harm	To prevent physical injury
Increased learning	To achieve awareness of needs and/or use of resources
Increased problem-solving ability	To achieve optimum function

NURSING INTERVENTIONS

Nursing Treatments
Listen attentively
Encourage mutual problem solving
Provide a home visit
Make a referral (to social service, transportation pool, or any appropriate service)

Nursing Observations
Observe for an excessive stress level
Evaluate the response to teaching

Health Teaching
Inform of the resources available for health care

EVALUATION

See the evaluation criteria for each specific goal in Chapter 2.

Inadequate Motivation Related to Health Maintenance

ASSESSMENT

Subjective Data
Gives little or no thought to sound health practices
Has no health goals
Takes existing health for granted

Objective Data
Does not attempt the generally accepted sound health practices of exercise, good nutrition, adequate rest, etc.

Related Data
Commonly Related Conditions:
None
Commonly Related Diseases:
None

POSSIBLE ETIOLOGY

Lack of education. The existence of a reasonably sound health status. Lack of health-related interest on the part of significant others.

NURSING DIAGNOSIS

Inadequate motivation related to health maintenance: lack of striving toward goals that will maintain a sound health status

PLANNING

Patient Needs	Primary Nurse-Patient Goals
Protection from physical harm	To prevent physical injury
Sense of value, high evaluation of self	To achieve positive expressions, feelings, reactions
Goal achievement	To achieve optimum function
Increased learning	To achieve awareness of needs and/or use of resources

NURSING INTERVENTIONS

Nursing Treatments
Emphasize the person's value as an individual
Encourage a positive life approach

Encourage balanced long- and short-range goals (for health)

Encourage goals leading to self-enhancement (health makes one more attractive, etc.)

Encourage the substitution of undesirable habits with favorable habits

Explore with the patient his strengths and resources (for health maintenance)

Explore with the patient the effects of his behavior on others

Involve the family (in motivating the person)

Assist the patient in restructuring his lifestyle (so there is time for exercise, good nutrition, adequate rest, etc.)

Refrain from negatively criticizing

Nursing Observations

Determine the degree of insight

Determine the extent of lack of information (about health)

Evaluate the response to teaching

Observe for behavior modification

Health Teaching

Advise early correction of problems (related to health)

EVALUATION

See the evaluation criteria for each specific goal in Chapter 2.

Noncompliance to the Therapeutic Regime

ASSESSMENT

Subjective Data

Anger

Anxiety

Distrust of directions

Objective Data

Disregards the suggested health regime

Cooperates with part of the regime but disregards the rest

Gives multiple excuses for not complying

Related Data

Commonly Related Diseases:

Any disease or injury.

POSSIBLE ETIOLOGY

Lack of understanding. Hostility. Denial of illness. Desire to remain ill so as to maintain dependent status. Job demands. An irregular daily schedule. Home demands. Poverty.

NURSING DIAGNOSIS

Noncompliance to the therapeutic regime: not adhering to the health regime prescribed by health professionals

PLANNING

Patient Needs	**Primary Nurse-Patient Goals**
Protection from physical harm	To prevent physical injury
Protection from psychologic threat	To prevent emotional injury
Warm, communicating relationships	To achieve effective verbal and nonverbal communications
High evaluation of self	To achieve positive expressions, feelings, reactions
Increased learning	To achieve awareness of needs
Increased reality perception and problem-solving ability	To achieve optimum function
Less rigid conventionality	To achieve a therapeutic environment

NURSING INTERVENTIONS

Nursing Treatments

Approach unhurriedly
Ask questions which encourage answers that reflect reality perception
Avoid causing intense emotional situations
Emphasize the person's value as an individual
Encourage the expression of feelings
Encourage patient questions
Listen attentively
Explore with the patient the effects of his behavior on (significant) others
Provide an atmosphere of acceptance
Provide frequent patient contact
Provide reliable information
Refrain from forcing the treatment
Refrain from negatively criticizing

Nursing Observations

Determine the degree of insight
Observe for an excessive stress level

Health Teaching

Advise early correction of problems
Describe the specific dangerous effects of poor health practices
Explain the reason for and intended effect of the therapy

EVALUATION

See the evaluation criteria for each specific goal in Chapter 2.

Reluctance to Accept Health Treatment

ASSESSMENT

Subjective Data

Strong feelings of discomfort, tension, or threat when treatments are suggested or attempted

Objective Data
Person asks many questions about the treatment
Asks to have treatment postponed
Does not appear, or comes late for the scheduled treatment

Related Data
Commonly Related Diseases:
Any disease or injury

POSSIBLE ETIOLOGY

Inadequate explanations of what can be expected. Superstition. Physical discomfort that the situation produces. Inability to accept temporary dependence. Lack of trust in the persons involved. Threat of decreased self-esteem that the social disadvantage of illness presents.

NURSING DIAGNOSIS

Reluctance to accept health treatment: a cautious, incomplete willingness to accept treatments considered necessary for health

PLANNING

Patient Needs	**Primary Nurse-Patient Goals**
Comfort	To achieve comfort
Protection from physical harm	To prevent physical injury
Protection from psychologic threat	To prevent emotional injury
Warm, communicating relationships	To achieve effective verbal and nonverbal communications
High evaluation of self	To achieve positive expressions, feelings, reactions
Increased learning	To achieve awareness of needs

NURSING INTERVENTIONS

Nursing Treatments
Approach unhurriedly
Arrange pleasant surroundings
Arrange situations which encourage patient autonomy
Ask the patient what makes him/her comfortable
Avoid causing intense emotional situations
Demonstrate calmness
Discuss the anticipated procedure
Do not allow unpleasant surprise situations
Emphasize the person's value as an individual
Encourage acceptance of interdependence
Encourage mutual problem solving
Encourage patient questions
Encourage the expression of feelings
Listen attentively
Insure the patient's feeling of safety before introducing unpleasantness
Introduce to persons who have successfully undergone the same experience

Provide an atmosphere of acceptance
Provide reliable information
Refrain from forcing the treatment
Refrain from performing nonessential procedures
Refrain from negatively criticizing

Nursing Observations
Determine the degree of insight
Observe for an excessive stress level

Health Teaching
Explain the reason for and intended effect of the therapy

EVALUATION

See the evaluation criteria for each specific goal in Chapter 2.

INADEQUATE HEALTH THERAPY PROCEDURE INFORMATION

Inadequate Information Related to the Diagnostic Study

ASSESSMENT

Subjective Data
Person confirms a lack of information

Objective Data
Person's actions indicate a lack of information regarding:
    why the study is being done
    how to prepare for the study
    the procedure involved in the study
    what the results of the study mean

Related Data
Involves such studies as blood work, urinalysis, gastric analysis, pulmonary
    function studies, electrocardiogram, electroencephalogram, x-rays such
    as cholecystogram, upper GI series, barium enema, pyleogram, cystog-
    ram, arteriogram, pulmonary angiography, chest film, bone films, and
    liver, brain, thyroid, or renal scan
Commonly Related Diseases:
Any disease or suspected disease

POSSIBLE ETIOLOGY

Lack of instruction

NURSING DIAGNOSIS

Inadequate information related to the diagnostic study: lack of information
regarding tests performed for the purpose of diagnosis

PLANNING

Patient Needs	**Primary Nurse-Patient Goals**
Comfort	To achieve comfort
Increased learning	To achieve awareness of needs

NURSING INTERVENTIONS

Nursing Treatments
Approach unhurriedly
Discuss the anticipated procedure
Encourage patient questions

Nursing Observations
Evaluate the response to teaching

Health Teaching
Explain the reason for and intended effect of the study
Explain how to prepare for the diagnostic study
Explain the meaning of the diagnostic report

EVALUATION

See the evaluation criteria for each specific goal in Chapter 2.

Inadequate Information Related to the Physical Examination

ASSESSMENT

Subjective Data
Person confirms a lack of information

Objective Data
Person's actions indicate a lack of information regarding:
    the necessity for the physical examination
    how to prepare for the examination
    what the examination involves
    how often certain examinations are recommended

Related Data
Commonly Related Diseases:
None
   OR
Any disease or injury

POSSIBLE ETIOLOGY

Lack of instruction

NURSING DIAGNOSIS

Inadequate information related to the physical examination: lack of information regarding a general or specific physical examination of the body

PLANNING

Patient Needs

Comfort

Protection from physical harm

Increased learning

Primary Nurse-Patient Goals

To achieve comfort

To prevent physical injury

To achieve awareness of needs

NURSING INTERVENTIONS

Nursing Treatments
Approach unhurriedly
Discuss the anticipated procedure (or the examination)

Nursing Observations
Evaluate the response to teaching

Health Teaching
Advise early correction of problems
Advise an annual gynecologic examination
Instruct that douching be avoided (prior to pap smear for females)
Advise periodic examinations for known hereditary predispositions
Inform that elimination is advisable before abdominal examinations and
    procedures
Explain the reason for and intended effect of the examination

EVALUATION

See the evaluation criteria for each specific goal in Chapter 2.

Inadequate Information Related to
the Surgical Procedure

ASSESSMENT

Subjective Data
Person confirms a lack of information

Objective Data
Person's actions indicate a lack of information regarding:
    why the surgical procedure is to be done or was done
    what the surgical procedure actually involves
    how long recovery will take
    the extent of recovery

Related Data
Commonly Related Diseases:
Any disease requiring a surgical procedure

POSSIBLE ETIOLOGY

First experience with such a procedure. Lack of instruction.

NURSING DIAGNOSIS

Inadequate information related to the surgical procedure: lack of information regarding what may be involved in the performance of a surgical procedure and the effects of the procedure

PLANNING

Patient Needs

Comfort

Protection from physical harm

Increased learning

Primary Nurse-Patient Goals

To achieve comfort

To prevent physical injury

To achieve awareness of needs

NURSING INTERVENTIONS

Nursing Treatments

Approach unhurriedly
Discuss the anticipated procedure
Encourage patient questions
Introduce to persons who have successfully undergone the same experience

Nursing Observations
Evaluate the response to teaching
Observe for an excessive stress level

Health Teaching
Explain the reason for and intended effect of the therapy

EVALUATION

See the evaluation criteria for each specific goal in Chapter 2.

17.
NURSING DIAGNOSES RELATED TO
Hygiene and Dressing

INADEQUATE INDEPENDENT GENERAL HYGIENE PRACTICES

Inadequate General Hygiene

ASSESSMENT

Objective Data
Infrequent bathing
Uncombed, dirty hair
Dirty, uncut nails
Unclean mouth
Dirty ears
Unclean skin
Eyelid crusting
Offensive body odor

Related Data
Commonly Related Conditions:
Senility
Poverty
Commonly Related Diseases:
None
   OR
Any disease or injury

POSSIBLE ETIOLOGY

Lack of information. Poor motivation. Poor hygiene habits.

NURSING DIAGNOSIS

Inadequate general hygiene: failure to practice health habits of cleanliness of the entire body, despite the ability to do so

PLANNING

Patient Needs	**Primary Nurse-Patient Goals**
Comfort	To achieve comfort
Cleanliness	To achieve good hygiene
Protection from physical harm	To prevent physical injury, infection
Increased learning	To achieve awareness of needs

NURSING INTERVENTIONS

Nursing Treatments
Approach unhurriedly
Bathe daily
Apply an antiperspirant
Brush and comb the hair
Brush the teeth
Clean the nails
Clean the dentures
Clean the ears
Clean the eyes
Clear nasal secretions
Lubricate the skin with baby oil, bath oil, or body lotion
Provide clean clothing
Shampoo the hair

Nursing Observations
Observe for behavior modification

Health Teaching
Advise daily bathing
Recommend a daily change of clean clothing
Advise daily hair brushing
Instruct to maintain skin cleanliness
Explain the need for nail cleanliness
Explain the need for weekly hair shampoo
Inform that cleanliness is basic to health
Explain the reason for and intended effect of the therapy

EVALUATION

See the evaluation criteria for each specific goal in Chapter 2.

INADEQUATE INDEPENDENT SPECIFIC HYGIENE PRACTICES

Inadequate Disposal of Respiratory Excreta

ASSESSMENT

Objective Data
Excreta wiped on clothes, towels, sheets, pillowcases, etc.
Excreta spit onto floors, sidewalks, or out of car windows

Tissues containing excreta are left lying around
Lack of handwashing following contact with excreta

Related Data

Commonly Related Diseases:
Bronchiectasis
Bronchitis
Bronchopneumonia
Lobar pneumonia
Tuberculosis
Emphysema

POSSIBLE ETIOLOGY

Lack of instruction. Poor motivation. Poor hygiene habits.

NURSING DIAGNOSIS

Inadequate disposal of respiratory excreta: lack of cleanliness in the handling of respiratory excreta

PLANNING

Patient Needs	**Primary Nurse-Patient Goals**
Cleanliness	To achieve good hygiene
Protection from physical harm	To prevent physical injury, infection
Increased learning	To achieve awareness of needs

NURSING INTERVENTIONS

Nursing Treatments
Provide disposable tissue
Provide a paper bag for tissue disposal
Provide a sputum container
Refresh with a mouthwash (frequently if bringing up sputum)

Nursing Observations
Observe for behavior modification

Health Teaching
Inform that cleanliness is basic to health
Instruct to cover the mouth when coughing
Instruct to cover the nose when sneezing
Recommend the use of double-thickness tissue for infected sputum
Explain how to dispose of infectious expectoration
Explain the reason for and intended effect of the therapy

EVALUATION
See the evaluation criteria for each specific goal in Chapter 2.

Inadequate Feminine Hygiene

ASSESSMENT

Objective Data
Dirtiness
Genital odor

Genital skin irritation
Unclean clothing, especially undergarments

Related Data
Commonly Related Conditions:
Senility
Poverty

Commonly Related Diseases:
None

POSSIBLE ETIOLOGY

Lack of instruction. Poor motivation. Poor hygiene habits.

NURSING DIAGNOSIS

Inadequate feminine hygiene: lack of cleanliness of the external female genitalia

PLANNING

Patient Needs	**Primary Nurse-Patient Goals**
Comfort	To achieve comfort
Cleanliness	To achieve good hygiene
Protection from physical harm	To prevent physical injury, infection
Increased learning	To achieve awareness of needs

NURSING INTERVENTIONS

Nursing Treatments
Bathe daily
Bathe locally
Change the sanitary pads frequently
Provide clean clothing

Nursing Observations
Observe for behavior modification

Health Teaching
Inform that cleanliness is basic to health
Advise daily bathing
Recommend a daily change of clean clothing
Explain how to use toilet tissue correctly
Teach how to do perineal care
Teach how to give a douche
Explain the reason for and intended effect of the therapy

EVALUATION

See the evaluation criteria for each specific goal in Chapter 2.

Inadequate Hair Care

ASSESSMENT

Objective Data
Hair lacks luster
Is greasy
Is broken, split, or frizzy
Is dry, unmanageable
Is tangled

Related Data
Commonly Related Conditions:
Dandruff
Pediculosis
Commonly Related Diseases:
None

POSSIBLE ETIOLOGY

Lack of instruction. Poor motivation. Poor hygiene habits.

NURSING DIAGNOSIS

Inadequate hair care: lack of cleanliness and care of the hair

PLANNING

Patient Needs	**Primary Nurse-Patient Goals**
Comfort	To achieve comfort
Cleanliness	To achieve good hygiene
Protection from physical harm	To prevent physical injury
Increased learning	To achieve awareness of needs

NURSING INTERVENTIONS

Nursing Treatments
Brush and comb the hair
Encourage self-performance (of hair care)
Shampoo the hair
Soften the hair with a cream rinse

Nursing Observations
Observe for behavior modification

Health Teaching
Inform that cleanliness is basic to health
Advise daily hair brushing
Advise limited use of hair spray
Explain the need for weekly hair shampoo
Explain how to shampoo the hair
Recommend the use of dry shampoo (when unable to wash the hair)
Explain the reason for and intended effect of the therapy

EVALUATION

See the evaluation criteria for each specific goal in Chapter 2.

Inadequate Nail Care

ASSESSMENT

Objective Data
Dirty nails
Ragged, uneven nails
Nail overgrowth of more than 1/4 inch out from the finger
Dried skin surrounding the nails

Related Data
Commonly Related Conditions:
Ingrown nails
Commonly Related Diseases:
None

POSSIBLE ETIOLOGY

Lack of instruction. Poor motivation. Poor hygiene habits.

NURSING DIAGNOSIS

Inadequate nail care: lack of cleanliness and care of the nails

PLANNING

Patient Needs	**Primary Nurse-Patient Goals**
Comfort	To achieve comfort
Cleanliness	To achieve good hygiene
Protection from physical harm	To prevent physical injury, infection
Increased learning	To achieve awareness of needs

NURSING INTERVENTIONS

Nursing Treatments
Clean the nails
Soak the nails in warm oil
Encourage self-performance (of nail care)

Nursing Observations
Observe for behavior modification

Health Teaching
Advise that lanolin be applied to brittle nails
Explain how to file the nails correctly
Explain that nails should be soaked before trimming
Explain the need for nail cleanliness
Explain the reason for and intended effect of the therapy

EVALUATION

See the evaluation criteria for each specific goal in Chapter 2.

Inadequate Nasal Hygiene

ASSESSMENT

Objective Data
Dried exudate at the nasal opening or internal nares
Collected nasal secretions protruding from the nose on expiration
Difficulty breathing through the nose

Related Data
Commonly Related Diseases:
None

POSSIBLE ETIOLOGY

Lack of instruction. Poor motivation. Poor hygiene habits.

NURSING DIAGNOSIS

Inadequate nasal hygiene: lack of cleanliness of the internal and external
nose

PLANNING

Patient Needs	**Primary Nurse-Patient Goals**
Comfort	To achieve comfort
Cleanliness	To achieve good hygiene
Protection from physical harm	To prevent physical injury
Increased learning	To achieve awareness of needs

NURSING INTERVENTIONS

Nursing Treatments
Clear nasal secretions
Lubricate the external nares

Nursing Observations
Observe for behavior modification

Health Teaching
Inform that cleanliness is basic to health
Advise frequent nose blowing
Teach how to clean an infant's nose
Explain the reason for and intended effect of the therapy

EVALUATION

See the evaluation criteria for each specific goal in Chapter 2.

Inadequate Oral Hygiene

ASSESSMENT

Subjective Data
Unpleasant taste

Objective Data
Halitosis
Badly discolored teeth

Considerable tartar on the teeth
Thick oral secretions
Food particles lodged between the teeth
Infrequent teeth brushing
Infrequent mouthwash use

Related Data

Commonly Related Diseases:
None
  OR
Dental caries
Pyorrhea alveolaris
Peridontitis

POSSIBLE ETIOLOGY

Lack of instruction. Poor motivation. Poor hygiene habits.

NURSING DIAGNOSIS

Inadequate oral hygiene: lack of cleanliness of the mouth and teeth

PLANNING

Patient Needs	**Primary Nurse-Patient Goals**
Comfort	To achieve comfort
Cleanliness	To achieve good hygiene
Protection from physical harm	To prevent physical injury, infection
Increased learning	To achieve awareness of needs and/or use of resources

NURSING INTERVENTIONS

Nursing Treatments
Brush the teeth
Clean the dentures
Discourage smoking
Encourage self-performance (of mouth care)
Lubricate the lips
Make a referral (to a dentist for badly stained teeth)
Refresh with a mouth freshener
Refresh with a mouthwash
Swab the mouth with diluted glycerine

Nursing Observations
Observe for behavior modification

Health Teaching
Inform that cleanliness is basic to health
Advise early and consistent use of the toothbrush
Advise mouth rinsing when brushing is inconvenient
Recommend the use of dental floss
Recommend that the tongue be brushed (if necessary)
Teach how to brush the teeth correctly

Teach how to clean dentures
Explain the reason for and intended effect of the therapy

EVALUATION

See the evaluation criteria for each specific goal in Chapter 2.

Inadequate Skin Care

ASSESSMENT

Objective Data
Skin dryness or oiliness
Skin covered with bacteria, mud, grime, dust, blood, etc.
Discolored washcloth following skin cleansing

Related Data
Commonly Related Diseases:
None

POSSIBLE ETIOLOGY

Lack of instruction. Poor motivation. Poor hygiene habits.

NURSING DIAGNOSIS

Inadequate skin care: lack of cleanliness and care of the skin

PLANNING

Patient Needs	Primary Nurse-Patient Goals
Comfort	To achieve comfort
Cleanliness	To achieve good hygiene
Protection from physical harm	To prevent physical injury, infection
Increased learning	To achieve awareness of needs

NURSING INTERVENTIONS

Nursing Treatments
Bathe daily
Maintain dry skin
Lubricate the skin with baby oil, bath oil, or body lotion (for normal or dry
    skin)
Lubricate the skin with cocoa butter, glycerine, lanolin, mineral oil, or olive
    oil (for very dry skin)
Maintain dry, clean linen
Maintain wrinkle-free sheets

Nursing Observations
Observe for behavior modification

Health Teaching
Advise daily bathing
Instruct to maintain skin cleanliness
Instruct to inspect the skin
Instruct to lubricate the skin
Explain the reason for and intended effect of the therapy

EVALUATION

See the evaluation criteria for each specific goal in Chapter 2.

DEPENDENT GENERAL HYGIENE CARE

Dependence on General Hygiene

ASSESSMENT

Subjective Data

Person relies on nurses for:
    a bath
    hair care
    nail care
    mouth care
    skin care

Objective Data

Person is unable to maintain his own general hygiene

Related Data

Commonly Related Diseases:

Any disease or injury that results in inability to maintain self-care, such as
    the following:
    cerebral concussion
    cerebral vascular accident
    myasthenia gravis
    cervical spinal cord injury
    multiple sclerosis
    Parkinson's disease
    terminal carcinoma

POSSIBLE ETIOLOGY

Inability to maintain self-care as a result of weakness, loss of motor skills, infant dependence, or impaired cerebral function

NURSING DIAGNOSIS

Dependence on general hygiene: reliance on nurses for complete cleanliness and care of the body

PLANNING

Patient Needs	Primary Nurse-Patient Goals
Comfort	To achieve comfort
Cleanliness	To achieve good hygiene
Dependence	To achieve comfort
Increased learning	To achieve awareness of needs

NURSING INTERVENTIONS

Nursing Treatments
Acknowledge dependency
Anticipate needs
Screen the patient for privacy
Drape for warmth
Bathe daily
Brush and comb the hair
Brush the teeth
Clean the dentures
Clean the nails
Clean the eyes
Clear nasal secretions
Apply after-bath powder (if not lubricating the skin)
Apply an antiperspirant
Lubricate the skin with baby oil, bath oil, or body lotion
Provide clean clothing
Dress the patient

Nursing Observations
Observe for readiness to assume (some) activities of daily living

Health Teaching
Explain the reason for and intended effect of the therapy

EVALUATION

See the evaluation criteria for each specific goal in Chapter 2.

Dependence on General Hygiene Assistance

ASSESSMENT

Subjective Data
Person relies on nurses for:
    assistance with bathing
    assistance with hair care
    assistance with nail care
    assistance with mouth care
    assistance with skin care

Objective Data
Person is unable to fully maintain his own general hygiene

Related Data
Commonly Related Diseases:
Any disease or injury

POSSIBLE ETIOLOGY

The need for assistance in self-care as a result of weakness, loss of motor skills, or impaired cerebral function

NURSING DIAGNOSIS

Dependence on general hygiene assistance: reliance on nurses to assist the person in his attempt to provide complete cleanliness and care of his body

PLANNING

Patient Needs

Comfort

Cleanliness

Dependence

Independence

Increased learning

Primary Nurse-Patient Goals

To achieve comfort

To achieve good hygiene

To achieve comfort

To achieve optimum function

To achieve awareness of needs

NURSING INTERVENTIONS

Nursing Treatments

Acknowledge dependency

Anticipate needs

Screen the patient for privacy

Drape for warmth

Approach unhurriedly

Assist with hygiene

Assist with dressing

Encourage self-performance (partial self-hygiene)

Provide needed supplies

Nursing Observations

Observe for readiness to assume (more) activities of daily living

Health Teaching

Teach how to use assistive grooming devices

Explain the reason for and intended effect of the therapy

EVALUATION

See the evaluation criteria for each specific goal in Chapter 2.

DEPENDENT SPECIFIC HYGIENE CARE

Dependence on Artificial-Eye Care

ASSESSMENT

Subjective Data

Person relies on nurses for:

    insertion and removal of the artificial eye

    cleansing of the eye

    safe storage of the eye when unused

Objective Data

Person is unable to maintain care of his artificial eye

Related Data

Commonly Related Diseases:

Any disease or injury that results in inability to maintain self-care, such as the following:

cerebral concussion
cerebral vascular accident
myasthenia gravis
cervical spinal cord injury
multiple sclerosis
Parkinson's disease
terminal carcinoma

POSSIBLE ETIOLOGY

Inability to maintain self-care as a result of weakness, loss of motor skills, or impaired cerebral function

NURSING DIAGNOSIS

Dependence on artificial-eye care: reliance on nurses for daily cleanliness and care of an artificial eye

PLANNING

Patient Needs	**Primary Nurse-Patient Goals**
Comfort	To achieve comfort
Cleanliness	To achieve good hygiene
Protection from physical harm	To prevent physical injury, infection
Dependence	To achieve comfort
Increased learning	To achieve awareness of needs

NURSING INTERVENTIONS

Nursing Treatments

Acknowledge dependency
Clean the artificial eye
Insert and remove the artificial eye (as necessary)
Handle gently
Safeguard the patient's artificial eye

Nursing Observations

Observe for readiness to assume activities of daily living

Health Teaching

Teach how to care for an artificial eye
Explain the reason for and intended effect of the therapy

EVALUATION

See the evaluation criteria for each specific goal in Chapter 2.

Dependence on Body-Drainage Hygiene

ASSESSMENT

Subjective Data
Person relies on nurses for:
   removal of serous fluid, pus, or blood from eyes, ears, nose, mouth, vagina, or rectum
   removal of cerebral spinal fluid draining from ears or nose
   cleansing of body orifices following drainage removal

Objective Data
Person is unable to maintain cleanliness of drainage from body orifices

Related Data
Commonly Related Conditions:
Coma
Semicoma
Confusion
Hemiplegia
Quadriplegia

Commonly Related Diseases:
Any disease or injury that results in inability to maintain self-care, such as the following:
   cerebral concussion
   cerebral vascular accident
   myasthenia gravis
   cervical spinal cord injury
   multiple sclerosis
   Parkinson's disease
   terminal carcinoma

POSSIBLE ETIOLOGY

Inability to maintain self-care as a result of weakness, loss of motor skills, infant dependence, or impaired cerebral function

NURSING DIAGNOSIS

Dependence on body-drainage hygiene: reliance on nurses to maintain cleanliness of drainage that occurs from body orifices

PLANNING

Patient Needs	Primary Nurse-Patient Goals
Comfort	To achieve comfort
Cleanliness	To achieve good hygiene
Protection from physical harm	To prevent physical injury, infection
Dependence	To achieve comfort
Increased learning	To achieve awareness of needs

NURSING INTERVENTIONS

Nursing Treatments
Acknowledge dependency
Anticipate needs
Bathe locally
Change the dressing frequently
Maintain dry, clean linen
Maintain dry skin
Lubricate the skin with baby oil, bath oil, or body lotion (periodically)
Provide clean clothing
Position comfortably
Consult with the physician (for unusual or excess drainage)

Nursing Observations
Inspect the skin for irritation
Observe for readiness to assume activities of daily living

Health Teaching
Explain the reason for and intended effect of the therapy

EVALUATION

See the evaluation criteria for each specific goal in Chapter 2.

Dependence on Circumcision Care

ASSESSMENT

Subjective Data
Person relies on nurses for:
    periodic cleansing of the area
    periodic dressing changes

Objective Data
Person (usually an infant) is unable to maintain care and cleanliness of a
    circumcision

Related Data
Commonly Related Diseases:
None

POSSIBLE ETIOLOGY

Inability to maintain self-care as a result of weakness, loss of motor skills,
or infant dependence

NURSING DIAGNOSIS

Dependence on circumcision care: reliance on nurses for the cleanliness and
care of a circumcision wound

PLANNING

Patient Needs	**Primary Nurse-Patient Goals**
Comfort	To achieve comfort
Cleanliness	To achieve good hygiene

Protection from physical harm	To prevent physical injury, infection
Dependence	To achieve comfort
Increased learning	To achieve awareness of needs

NURSING INTERVENTIONS

Nursing Treatments
Acknowledge dependency
Anticipate needs
Apply an antibiotic ointment
Apply sterile petrolatum gauze (with each diaper change, or several times
     daily)
Bathe locally
Retract and clean the foreskin
Change the dressing frequently

Nursing Observations
Inspect for bleeding
Inspect for edema
Inspect for inflammation

Health Teaching
Explain the reason for and intended effect of the therapy

EVALUATION

See the evaluation criteria for each specific goal in Chapter 2.

Dependence on Contact-Lens Care

ASSESSMENT

Subjective Data
Person relies on nurses for:
     insertion and removal of the contact lens
     placement of the lens in solution
     safe storage of the lens when unused

Objective Data
Person is unable to maintain care of his contact lens

Related Data
Any disease or injury that results in inability to maintain self-care, such as
     the following:
     cerebral concussion
     cerebral vascular accident
     myasthenia gravis
     cervical spinal cord injury
     multiple sclerosis
     Parkinson's disease
     terminal carcinoma

POSSIBLE ETIOLOGY

Inability to maintain self-care as a result of weakness or loss of motor skills

NURSING DIAGNOSIS

Dependence on contact-lens care: reliance on nurses to care for one's contact lenses

PLANNING

Patient Needs	**Primary Nurse-Patient Goals**
Comfort	To achieve comfort
Cleanliness	To achieve good hygiene
Protection from physical harm	To prevent accident, physical injury, infection
Dependence	To achieve comfort
Increased learning	To achieve awareness of needs

NURSING INTERVENTIONS

Nursing Treatments
Acknowledge dependency
Anticipate needs
Clean the contact lenses
Insert and remove the contact lens (as needed)
Safeguard the patient's contact lenses

Nursing Observations
Observe for readiness to assume activities of daily living

Health Teaching
Teach how to clean contact lenses

EVALUATION

See the evaluation criteria for each specific goal in Chapter 2.

Dependence on Denture Care

ASSESSMENT

Subjective Data
Person relies on nurses for:
    insertion and removal of the dentures
    cleansing of the dentures
    safe storage of the dentures when unused

Objective Data
Person is unable to maintain care and cleanliness of his own dentures

Related Data
Commonly Related Diseases:
Any disease or injury that results in inability to maintain self-care, such as
  the following:
    cerebral concussion
    cerebral vascular accident
    myasthenia gravis
    cervical spinal cord injury

multiple sclerosis
Parkinson's disease
terminal carcinoma

POSSIBLE ETIOLOGY.

Inability to maintain self-care as a result of weakness, loss of motor skills, or impaired cerebral function

NURSING DIAGNOSIS

Dependence on denture care: reliance on nurses for the care and cleanliness of dentures

PLANNING

Patient Needs	Primary Nurse-Patient Goals
Comfort	To achieve comfort
Cleanliness	To achieve good hygiene
Protection from physical harm	To prevent physical injury
Dependence	To achieve comfort
Increased learning	To achieve awareness of needs

NURSING INTERVENTIONS

Nursing Treatments
Acknowledge dependency
Anticipate needs
Clean the dentures
Insert and remove the dentures (as needed)
Refresh with a mouthwash
Safeguard the patient's dentures

Nursing Observations
Observe for readiness to assume activities of daily living

Health Teaching
Teach how to clean dentures

EVALUATION

See the evaluation criteria for each specific goal in Chapter 2.

Dependence on Diaphoresis Hygiene

ASSESSMENT

Subjective Data
Wetness discomfort
Chilling
Person relies on nurses for:
    maintenance of dry skin
    frequent clothing change
    frequent linen change

Objective Data
Person is perspiring profusely

Related Data

Commonly Related Conditions:
Fever
Shock
Hypoglycemia

Commonly related Diseases:
Malaria
Pneumonia

POSSIBLE ETIOLOGY

Inability to maintain self-care

NURSING DIAGNOSIS

Dependence on diaphoresis hygiene: reliance on nurses to provide care and cleanliness during episodes of profuse perspiration

PLANNING

Patient Needs	**Primary Nurse-Patient Goals**
Comfort	To achieve comfort
Cleanliness	To achieve good hygiene
Protection from physical harm	To prevent physical injury
Dependence	To achieve comfort
Increased learning	To achieve awareness of needs

NURSING INTERVENTIONS

Nursing Treatments
Apply an antiperspirant
Bathe locally (or as needed)
Maintain dry, clean linen
Maintain dry skin
Protect with absorbent padding
Provide clean clothing

Nursing Observations
Inspect the skin for irritation

Health Teaching
Explain the reason for and intended effect of the therapy

EVALUATION

See the evaluation criteria for each specific goal in Chapter 2.

Dependence on Episiotomy Care

ASSESSMENT

Subjective Data
Woman relies on nurses for:
    periodic cleanliness
    observation for and prevention of infection

Objective Data

Woman is unable to maintain cleanliness and care of her episiotomy

Related Data

Commonly Related Diseases:
None

POSSIBLE ETIOLOGY

Lack of knowledge of a therapeutic procedure. Weakness.

NURSING DIAGNOSIS

Dependence on episiotomy care: reliance on nurses for the care and cleanliness of a surgical incision in perineal tissue

PLANNING

Patient Needs	**Primary Nurse-Patient Goals**
Comfort	To achieve comfort
Cleanliness	To achieve good hygiene
Protection from physical harm	To prevent physical injury, infection
Dependence	To achieve comfort
Increased learning	To achieve awareness of needs

NURSING INTERVENTIONS

Nursing Treatments
Acknowledge dependency
Anticipate needs
Change the sanitary pads frequently
Give perineal care
Maintain dry, clean linen
Position comfortably
Soak in a sitz bath

Nursing Observations
Inspect for bleeding
Inspect for edema
Inspect for inflammation
Obtain a bacterial culture (of any drainage)

Health Teaching
Teach how to do perineal care
Explain the reason for and intended effect of the therapy

EVALUATION

See the evaluation criteria for each specific goal in Chapter 2.

Dependence on Feminine Hygiene

ASSESSMENT

Subjective Data
Woman relies on nurses for:
    periodic external genitalia cleansing

intermittent sanitary pad change
appropriate douching

Objective Data

Woman is unable to maintain cleanliness of the genitalia and vagina

Related Data

Commonly Related Conditions:
Vaginal bleeding

Commonly Related Diseases:
Moniliasis

POSSIBLE ETIOLOGY

Inability to maintain self-care as a result of weakness, loss of motor skills, or impaired cerebral function

NURSING DIAGNOSIS

Dependence on feminine hygiene: reliance on nurses to maintain cleanliness of the female genitalia and vagina

PLANNING

Patient Needs	**Primary Nurse-Patient Goals**
Comfort	To achieve comfort
Cleanliness	To achieve good hygiene
Protection from physical harm	To prevent physical injury, infection
Increased learning	To achieve awareness of needs

NURSING INTERVENTIONS

Nursing Treatments
Acknowledge dependency
Anticipate needs
Administer a vaginal douche (if needed)
Bathe daily
Bathe locally
Change the sanitary pads frequently
Provide clean clothing

Nursing Observations
Observe for readiness to assume activities of daily living

Health Teaching
Explain the reason for and intended effect of the therapy

EVALUATION

See the evaluation criteria for each specific goal in Chapter 2.

Dependence on Hair Care

ASSESSMENT

Subjective Data
Person relies on nurses for:
    frequent hair washing

daily hair combing and brushing
application of appropriate hair conditioners

Objective Data

Person is unable to maintain cleanliness and care of his hair

Related Data

Commonly Related Diseases:

Any disease or injury that results in inability to maintain self-care, such as
the following:
cerebral concussion
cerebral vascular accident
myasthenia gravis
cervical spinal cord injury
multiple sclerosis
Parkinson's disease
terminal carcinoma

POSSIBLE ETIOLOGY

Inability to maintain self-care as a result of weakness, loss of motor skills,
infant dependence, or impaired cerebral function

NURSING DIAGNOSIS

Dependence on hair care: reliance on nurses for daily care and cleanliness
of the hair

PLANNING

Patient Needs	Primary Nurse-Patient Goals
Comfort	To achieve comfort
Cleanliness	To achieve good hygiene
Protection from physical harm	To prevent physical injury
Dependence	To achieve comfort
Increased learning	To achieve awareness of needs

NURSING INTERVENTIONS

Nursing Treatments
Acknowledge dependency
Anticipate needs
Brush and comb the hair
Shampoo the hair
Soften the hair with a cream rinse
Position comfortably
Handle gently

Nursing Observations
Observe for readiness to assume activities of daily living

Health Teaching
Explain the reason for and intended effect of the therapy
Explain how to shampoo the hair

EVALUATION

See the evaluation criteria for each specific goal in Chapter 2.

Dependence on Incontinence Hygiene

ASSESSMENT

Subjective Data

Discomfort

Chilling

Person relies on nurses for:

    cleansing of urine or feces from the skin

    removal of moist clothing from the body

    maintenance of dry linens

Objective Data

Person is incontinent

Related Data

Commonly Related Conditions:

Aging

Shock

Commonly Related Diseases:

Epilepsy

Hypothyroidism

Cervical or thoracic spinal cord lesions or injury

Spinal meningitis

Cystitis

Myasthenia gravis

Multiple sclerosis

Poliomyelitis

Bladder carcinoma

Prostate adenocarcinoma

Benign prostatic hypertrophy

Rectovaginal or ureterovaginal fistula

POSSIBLE ETIOLOGY

Bowel and urinary incontinence

NURSING DIAGNOSIS

Dependence on incontinence hygiene: reliance on nurses for the maintenance of cleanliness during conditions of incontinence

PLANNING

Patient Needs	Primary Nurse-Patient Goals
Comfort	To achieve comfort
Cleanliness	To achieve good hygiene
Protection from physical harm	To prevent physical injury
Dependence	To achieve comfort
Increased learning	To achieve awareness of needs

NURSING INTERVENTIONS

Nursing Treatments

Apply an external urinary catheter
OR
Place a urinal at the perineum
OR
Fold a towel between the legs during incontinence
Maintain dry, clean linen
Maintain dry skin
Bathe locally
Protect with absorbent padding
Protect with plastic pants
Provide clean clothing
Toilet frequently

Nursing Observations

Inspect the skin for breakdown

Health Teaching

Inform that cleanliness is basic to health
Instruct to maintain skin dryness

EVALUATION

See the evaluation criteria for each specific goal in Chapter 2.

Dependence on Local Drainage Tube Hygiene

ASSESSMENT

Subjective Data

Person relies on nurses for:
   periodic dressing changes
   skin care
   cleanliness of clothing and bedding
   odor control

Objective Data

Person has a local drainage tube

Related Data

Commonly Related Conditions:
Wound infections
Cholecystectomy

POSSIBLE ETIOLOGY

Therapeutic drainage of exudates

NURSING DIAGNOSIS

Dependence on local drainage tube hygiene: reliance on nurses for the care and cleanliness of a local drainage tube

PLANNING

Patient Needs	Primary Nurse-Patient Goals
Comfort	To achieve comfort
Cleanliness	To achieve good hygiene
Protection from physical harm	To prevent physical injury, infection
Dependence	To achieve comfort
Increased learning	To achieve awareness of needs

NURSING INTERVENTIONS

Nursing Treatments
Acknowledge dependency
Anticipate needs
Bathe locally
Bandage with a draining-wound dressing
Change the dressing frequently
Maintain dry, clean linen
Provide clean clothing (as needed)

Nursing Observations
Check the tube for patency
Inspect the skin for irritation

Health Teaching
Instruct to maintain skin cleanliness
Explain the reason for and intended effect of the therapy

EVALUATION

See the evaluation criteria for each specific goal in Chapter 2.

Dependence on Nail Care

ASSESSMENT

Subjective Data
Person relies on nurses for:
   nail cleanliness
   periodic nail shaping and trimming

Objective Data
Person is unable to maintain his own nail care

Related Data
Commonly Related Diseases:
Any disease or injury that results in inability to maintain self-care, such as
   the following:
   cerebral concussion
   cerebral vascular accident
   myasthenia gravis
   cervical spinal cord injury
   multiple sclerosis

Parkinson's disease
terminal carcinoma

POSSIBLE ETIOLOGY

Inability to maintain self-care as a result of weakness, loss of motor skills, infant dependence, or impaired cerebral function

NURSING DIAGNOSIS

Dependence on nail care: reliance on nurses for the cleanliness and care of the nails

PLANNING

Patient Needs	Primary Nurse-Patient Goals
Comfort	To achieve comfort
Cleanliness	To achieve good hygiene
Protection from physical harm	To prevent physical injury
Dependence	To achieve comfort
Increased learning	To achieve awareness of needs

NURSING INTERVENTIONS

Nursing Treatments
Acknowledge dependency
Anticipate needs
Clean the nails

Nursing Observations
Observe for readiness to assume activities of daily living

Health Teaching
Inform that cleanliness is basic to health

EVALUATION

See the evaluation criteria for each specific goal in Chapter 2.

Dependence on Oral Hygiene

ASSESSMENT

Subjective Data
Person relies on nurses for:
   cleansing of his teeth through brushing several times a day
   removal of thick oral secretions
   periodic use of mouthwash

Objective Data
Person is unable to maintain cleanliness of his own mouth

Related Data
Commonly Related Diseases:
Any disease or injury that results in inability to maintain self-care, such as the following:

cerebral concussion
cerebral vascular accident
myasthenia gravis
cervical spinal cord injury
multiple sclerosis
Parkinson's disease
terminal carcinoma

POSSIBLE ETIOLOGY

Inability to maintain self-care as a result of weakness, loss of motor skills, infant dependence, or impaired cerebral function

NURSING DIAGNOSIS

Dependence on oral hygiene: reliance on nurses for the daily cleanliness of the mouth

PLANNING

Patient Needs	Primary Nurse-Patient Goals
Comfort	To achieve comfort
Cleanliness	To achieve good hygiene
Protection from physical harm	To prevent physical injury
Dependence	To achieve comfort
Increased learning	To achieve awareness of needs

NURSING INTERVENTIONS

Nursing Treatments
Acknowledge dependency
Anticipate needs
Brush the teeth
Brush the tongue (if necessary)
Clean the dentures
Lubricate the lips
Refresh with a mouth freshener
    OR
Refresh with a mouthwash
    OR
Swab the mouth with diluted glycerine

Nursing Observations
Observe for readiness to assume activities of daily living

Health Teaching
Inform that cleanliness is basic to health
Explain the reason for and intended effect of the therapy

EVALUATION

See the evaluation criteria for each specific goal in Chapter 2.

Dependence on Skin Care

ASSESSMENT

Subjective Data

Person relies on nurses for:
skin cleansing
skin lubrication
skin massage

Objective Data

Person is unable to maintain the care and cleanliness of his own skin

Related Data

Commonly Related Diseases:

Any disease or injury that results in inability to maintain self-care, such as
the following:
cerebral concussion
cerebral vascular accident
myasthenia gravis
cervical spinal cord injury
multiple sclerosis
Parkinson's disease
terminal carcinoma

POSSIBLE ETIOLOGY

Inability to maintain self-care as a result of weakness, loss of motor skills,
infant dependence, or impaired cerebral function

NURSING DIAGNOSIS

Dependence on skin care: reliance on nurses for daily cleanliness and care
of the skin

PLANNING

Patient Needs	**Primary Nurse-Patient Goals**
Comfort	To achieve comfort
Cleanliness	To achieve good hygiene
Protection from physical harm	To prevent physical injury
Dependence	To achieve comfort
Increased learning	To achieve awareness of needs

NURSING INTERVENTIONS

Nursing Treatments

Acknowledge dependency
Anticipate needs
Drape for warmth
Bathe daily
Maintain dry skin
Maintain dry, clean linen
Maintain wrinkle-free sheets
Massage gently

OR

Massage vigorously

Nursing Observations
Inspect the skin for breakdown
Observe for readiness to assume activities of daily living

Health Teaching
Inform that cleanliness is basic to health
Explain the reason for and intended effect of the therapy

EVALUATION

See the evaluation criteria for each specific goal in Chapter 2.

Dependence on Umbilical Hygiene

ASSESSMENT

Subjective Data
Person relies on nurses for:
  umbilical cleanliness
  periodic dressing changes
  observation for and prevention of infection

Objective Data
Infant is unable to maintain cleanliness and care of his healing umbilicus
  following birth

Related Data
Commonly Related Diseases:
None

POSSIBLE ETIOLOGY

Infant dependence

NURSING DIAGNOSIS

Dependence on umbilical hygiene: reliance on nurses for the cleanliness
and care of the newborn's umbilicus

PLANNING

Patient Needs	**Primary Nurse-Patient Goals**
Comfort	To achieve comfort
Cleanliness	To achieve good hygiene
Protection from physical harm	To prevent physical injury, infection
Dependence	To achieve comfort
Increased learning (of the mother)	To achieve awareness of needs

NURSING INTERVENTIONS

Nursing Treatments
Acknowledge dependency
Anticipate needs

Bathe locally
Change the dressing frequently
Clean with alcohol
    OR
Clean with surgical soap
Maintain dry skin
Moisten the dressing before removal

Nursing Observations
Inspect for bleeding
Inspect for edema
Inspect for inflammation
Obtain a bacterial culture (if oozing occurs)

Health Teaching
Explain (to the mother) the reason for and intended effect of the therapy
Teach (the mother) how to do umbilical care

EVALUATION

See the evaluation criteria for each specific goal in Chapter 2.

Dependence on Wound Care

ASSESSMENT

Subjective Data
Person relies on nurses for:
    wound cleanliness
    periodic dressing change
    proper positioning of the wound
    observation for and prevention of infection

Objective Data
Person is unable to maintain cleanliness and care of his own wound

Related Data

Commonly Related Conditions:
Staphylococcus or *Streptococcus* wound infection

Commonly Related Diseases:
Any wound

POSSIBLE ETIOLOGY

Lack of information regarding a therapeutic procedure. Inability to maintain self-care as a result of weakness, loss of motor skills, or impaired cerebral function.

NURSING DIAGNOSIS

Dependence on wound care: reliance on nurses for the cleanliness and care of a wound

PLANNING

Patient Needs

Comfort

Cleanliness

Protection from physical harm

Dependence

Increased learning

Primary Nurse-Patient Goals

To achieve comfort

To achieve good hygiene

To prevent physical injury, infection

To achieve comfort

To achieve awareness of needs

NURSING INTERVENTIONS

Nursing Treatments

Acknowledge dependency

Anticipate needs

Bathe locally

Sponge the wound clean

    OR

Irrigate the wound

    OR

Clean with hydrogen peroxide

    OR

Clean with surgical soap

Apply an antibiotic ointment

Apply a sterile dressing

Change the dressing frequently

Moisten the dressing before removal

Remove adhesive tape and adhesive debris

Refrain from tight bandaging

Avoid placing tension on the wound

Pack the draining wound with gauze

    OR

Expose the draining wound to air

Maintain dry skin

Position comfortably

Nursing Observations

Inspect for bleeding

Inspect for edema

Inspect for foreign bodies

Inspect for inflammation

Inspect for drainage

Obtain a bacterial culture (of any drainage)

Health Teaching

Teach how to clean and dress a wound

Explain how to dispose of soiled dressings

Explain the need to avoid mechanical trauma

Instruct to carefully move the injured body part

Explain the reason for and intended effect of the therapy

Medical Treatments Performed by Nurses
Soak in a medicated solution

EVALUATION

See the evaluation criteria for each specific goal in Chapter 2.

DEPENDENT BODY CLOTHING

Dependence on Dressing

ASSESSMENT

Subjective Data
Person relies on nurses for:
    cleanliness of clothing
    clothing comfort
    the removal and putting on of clothing

Objective Data
Person is unable to clothe his body

Related Data

Commonly Related Conditions:
Impaired proprioception

Commonly Related Diseases:
Cerebral vascular accident
Cervical or thoracic spinal cord injury
Parkinson's disease
Cerebral palsy
Muscular dystrophy
Multiple sclerosis

POSSIBLE ETIOLOGY

Limited range of motion. Muscle spasticity or weakness. Impaired coordination. Impaired cerebral function.

NURSING DIAGNOSIS

Dependence on dressing: reliance on nurses to clothe the body as is appropriate

PLANNING

Patient Needs
Comfort
Dependence
Increased learning

Primary Nurse-Patient Goals
To achieve comfort
To achieve comfort
To achieve awareness of needs

NURSING INTERVENTIONS

Nursing Treatments
Acknowledge dependency
Anticipate needs

Handle gently
Dress the patient
Dress in personal clothing (whenever possible)

Nursing Observations
Observe for readiness to assume activities of daily living

Health Teaching
Explain how to adjust clothing to meet health problems

EVALUATION

See the evaluation criteria for each specific goal in Chapter 2.

Dependence on Dressing Assistance

ASSESSMENT

Subjective Data
Person relies on nurses for:
    assistance with keeping clothes clean
    assistance with choosing clothes
    assistance with the putting on and removal of clothes

Objective Data
Person is unable to completely dress himself

Related Data
Commonly Related Conditions:
Blindness
Commonly Related Diseases:
Cerebral vascular accident
Cervical or thoracic spinal cord injury
Parkinson's disease
Cerebral palsy
Muscular dystrophy
Multiple sclerosis

POSSIBLE ETIOLOGY

Limited range of motion. Muscle spasticity or weakness. Impaired coordination. Impaired cerebral function.

NURSING DIAGNOSIS

Dependence on dressing assistance: reliance on nurses to assist the person in his efforts to clothe himself

PLANNING

Patient Needs	Primary Nurse-Patient Goals
Comfort	To achieve comfort
Dependence	To achieve comfort
Independence	To achieve optimum function
Increased learning	To achieve awareness of needs and/or use of resources

NURSING INTERVENTIONS

Nursing Treatments
Acknowledge dependency
Anticipate needs
Assist with dressing
Encourage self-performance
Provide clean clothing

Nursing Observations
Observe for readiness to assume (more) activities of daily living

Health Teaching
Explain how to adjust clothing to meet health problems (extra large clothes facilitate ease in dressing)
Inform that when there is limited movement, the affected body side should be dressed first
Teach how to use assistive dressing devices
Explain that clothes should be laid out in the order of dressing for persons with impaired cerebral function
Recommend the use of knots to distinguish clothing color for the visually impaired

EVALUATION

See the evaluation criteria for each specific goal in Chapter 2.

INADEQUATE HYGIENE MANAGEMENT

Inadequate Information Related to Infant Bathing and Dressing

ASSESSMENT

Subjective Data
Person confirms a lack of information

Objective Data
Person's (usually the mother's) actions indicate a lack of information regarding:
    how to handle the infant during hygiene activities
    how to give the infant a bath
    how to dress the infant with the least discomfort to the infant

POSSIBLE ETIOLOGY

Lack of instruction. No previous experience with infants.

NURSING DIAGNOSIS

Inadequate information related to infant bathing and dressing: lack of information regarding how to bathe and dress a newborn or small infant

PLANNING

Patient Needs	Primary Nurse-Patient Goals
Comfort	To achieve comfort
Cleanliness	To achieve good hygiene
Protection from physical harm	To prevent physical injury
Increased learning	To achieve awareness of needs

NURSING INTERVENTIONS

Nursing Treatments
Approach unhurriedly
Encourage parent or family questions

Nursing Observations
Evaluate the response to teaching

Health Teaching
Teach how to bathe an infant
Teach how to clean an infant's ears
Teach how to clean an infant's nose
Teach how to dress an infant

EVALUATION

See the evaluation criteria for each specific goal in Chapter 2.

Inadequate Information Related to Hygienic Care of the Dependent Person

ASSESSMENT

Subjective Data
Person confirms a lack of information

Objective Data
Person's actions indicate a lack of information regarding:
    how to give a bed bath
    how to shampoo hair when the person is in bed or has limited mobility
    how to give skin care
    how to provide oral hygiene

Related Data
Commonly Related Diseases:
Cerebral vascular accident
Cervical or thoracic spinal cord injury
Myasthenia gravis
Multiple sclerosis
Terminal carcinoma
Parkinson's disease

POSSIBLE ETIOLOGY

Lack of instruction. No previous experience with the problem.

NURSING DIAGNOSIS

Inadequate information related to hygienic care of the dependent person: lack of knowledge as to how one maintains body cleanliness of a dependent person

PLANNING

Patient Needs

Comfort

Cleanliness

Increased learning

Primary Nurse-Patient Goals

To achieve comfort

To achieve good hygiene

To achieve awareness of needs

NURSING INTERVENTIONS

Nursing Treatments

Approach unhurriedly

Encourage patient or family questions

Nursing Observations

Evaluate the response to teaching

Health Teaching

Inform that cleanliness is basic to health

Advise daily bathing

Teach how to give a bed bath

Inform that clean linens are essential

Recommend a daily change of clean clothing

Teach how to brush the teeth correctly

Explain the need for nail cleanliness

Instruct to maintain skin cleanliness

Instruct to lubricate the skin

Instruct to inspect the skin

Advise daily hair brushing

Explain the need for weekly hair shampoo

Explain how to shampoo the hair

Teach how to make an occupied bed

EVALUATION

See the evaluation criteria for each specific goal in Chapter 2.

Inadequate Information Related to Premature-Infant Care

ASSESSMENT

Subjective Data

Person confirms a lack of information

Objective Data

Person's actions indicate a lack of information regarding:

    a premature infant's need for a stable temperature

    a premature infant's need for special foods

    the fact that premature infants are highly susceptible to infection

    the fact that premature infants cannot be left in day care centers

Related Data

Commonly Related Diseases.

None

POSSIBLE ETIOLOGY

Lack of instruction

NURSING DIAGNOSIS

Inadequate information related to premature-infant care: lack of information regarding special care needs of the premature infant in the home setting

PLANNING

Patient Needs	**Primary Nurse-Patient Goals**
Comfort	To achieve comfort
Protection from physical harm	To prevent physical injury
Increased learning	To achieve awareness of needs

NURSING INTERVENTIONS

Nursing Treatments

Approach unhurriedly

Encourage family or parent questions

Provide home visits

Suggest home adaptations appropriate to the health problem

Make a referral (to the visiting nurse)

Nursing Observations

Evaluate the response to teaching

Health Teaching

Explain that premature infants require at-home supervision

Explain the meaning of premature birth

Instruct that premature infants require moderate temperature

Instruct that premature infants require prescribed foods

Instruct that premature infants require protection against infection

EVALUATION

See the evaluation criteria for each specific goal in Chapter 2.

18.

NURSING DIAGNOSES RELATED TO
Infection, Inflammation, and Immune Responses

INFECTION:
POTENTIAL INFECTION

Infection Susceptibility (70,325,391)

ASSESSMENT

Subjective Data
Fatigue
Exhaustion

Objective Data
Recent infection
Receiving immunosuppressive drug therapy
Has contracted three or more colds a year for two or three consecutive years
Poor nutrition
Poor hygiene habits
Dehydration

Related Data
Laboratory Findings:
Decreased white blood cells
Increased white blood cells (in leukemia)
Commonly Related Conditions:
Splenectomy
Kidney transplant
Aging
Surgery
Respiratory embarrassment
Malnutrition
Commonly Related Diseases:
Chronic glomerulonephritis
Leukemia
Diabetes mellitus

Tonsilitis
Chronic bronchitis
Anemia
All inflammatory diseases

POSSIBLE ETIOLOGY

General state of poor health causing lowered body resistance. Drug therapy that causes immunologic suppression (Imuran, prednisone, actinomycin C). Recent infection. Lack of white blood cells to protect the body against infection. Increased white blood cells that are immature and unable to protect against infection, as in leukemia.

NURSING DIAGNOSIS

Infection susceptibility: loss of the normal strength of resistant factors needed to ward off infection

PLANNING

Patient Needs	**Primary Nurse-Patient Goals**
Food balance	To maintain nutrition to all cells
Sleep, rest	To achieve sleep, rest
Cleanliness	To achieve good hygiene
Protection from physical harm	To prevent infection
Increased learning	To achieve awareness of needs

NURSING INTERVENTIONS

Nursing Treatments
Encourage adequate rest
Encourage increased protein-food intake
Maintain a clean environment
Maintain reverse isolation
Immunize against infectious disease (ExR)

Nursing Observations
Monitor blood studies for evidence of infection

Health Teaching
Explain the causes of the health problem
Advise adherence to the immunization schedule
Advise against exposure to inclement weather
Advise against mingling in crowds
Inform that cleanliness is basic to health
Explain how to prevent cross infection
Teach the principles of good nutrition
Explain the reason for and intended effect of the therapy (especially the reverse isolation)

Medical Treatments Performed by Nurses
Give the prescribed drugs

EVALUATION

See the evaluation criteria for each specific goal in Chapter 2.

Delinquent Immunizations (620)

ASSESSMENT

Subjective Data

Apathy

Objective Data

Failure to follow the generally accepted immunization routine as recommended by the American Academy of Pediatrics and the National Foundation–March of Dimes (622):

Age	Immunization
2 months	First dose of diphtheria/tetanus/pertussis vaccine; first dose of polio vaccine
3 months	Second dose of diphtheria/tetanus/pertussis vaccine
4 months	Third dose of diphtheria/tetanus/pertussis vaccine; second dose of polio vaccine
6 months	Third dose of polio vaccine
12 months	Rubeola vaccine; tuberculin test
1–12 months	Rubella vaccine
15–18 months	Boosters for diphtheria/tetanus/pertussis and polio
4–6 years	Boosters for diphtheria/tetanus/pertussis and polio
12–14 years	Tetanus/diphtheria toxoid; mumps vaccine
Following years	Tetanus/diphtheria toxoid every 10 years

Related Data

Commonly Related Diseases:

None

   OR

Rubella

Smallpox

Diphtheria

Pertussis

Tetanus

POSSIBLE ETIOLOGY

Lack of instruction. Apathy. Misinformation. Lack of available facilities.

NURSING DIAGNOSIS

Delinquent immunizations: failure to adhere to the recommended immunization schedule

PLANNING

Patient Needs

Protection from physical harm

Increased learning

Primary Nurse-Patient Goals

To prevent physical injury, infection

To achieve awareness of needs and/or use of resources

NURSING INTERVENTIONS

Nursing Treatments
Immunize against infectious disease (ExR)
Make a referral (to the local health department)

Health Teaching
Advise adherence to the immunization schedule
Explain the reason for and intended effect of the therapy

Medical Treatments Performed by Nurses
Give the prescribed drugs

EVALUATION

See the evaluation criteria for each specific goal in Chapter 2.

Impending Systemic Infection (247,271,453)

ASSESSMENT

Subjective Data
Malaise
Mild aching
Fatigue

Objective Data
Anorexia
Irritability

Related Data
Recent exposure to an infected person
Commonly Related Diseases:
Influenza
Gastritis
Common cold

POSSIBLE ETIOLOGY

Exposure to infected persons or contaminated articles

NURSING DIAGNOSIS

Impending systemic infection: the presence of symptoms that indicate that a generalized infection is about to occur

PLANNING

Patient Needs	Primary Nurse-Patient Goals
Water-salt balance	To maintain fluid and electrolyte balance
Food balance	To maintain nutrition to all cells
Sleep, rest	To achieve sleep, rest
Comfort	To achieve comfort
Cleanliness	To achieve good hygiene
Protection from physical harm	To prevent physical injury
Increased learning	To achieve awareness of needs

NURSING INTERVENTIONS

Nursing Treatments
Encourage adequate rest
Encourage increased protein-food intake
Give nonprescription drugs (ExR) (aspirin)
Increase fluid intake to about 2000 cc daily

Nursing Observations
Monitor blood studies for evidence of infection
Monitor the oral temperature

Health Teaching
Inform that cleanliness is basic to health
Advise against exposure to inclement weather
Explain the reason for and intended effect of the therapy

EVALUATION

See the evaluation criteria for each specific goal in Chapter 2.

Potential Genitourinary Infection (71,451)

ASSESSMENT

Objective Data
Inadequate fluid intake
Prolonged bed rest or immobility
Chronic residual urine
Presence of an indwelling urinary catheter
Recent performance of diagnostic procedures related to the genitourinary tract

Related Data
Commonly Related Diseases:
Cervical or thoracic spinal cord injury
Syphilis
Gonorrhea

POSSIBLE ETIOLOGY

External introduction of microorganisms into the genitourinary tract. Urine stagnation in the genitourinary tract.

NURSING DIAGNOSIS

Potential genitourinary infection: the likelihood that pathogenic organisms will invade the kidney, ureter, bladder, or urethra

PLANNING

Patient Needs

Water-salt balance

Cleanliness

Protection from physical harm

Increased learning

Primary Nurse-Patient Goals

To maintain fluid and electrolyte balance

To achieve good hygiene

To prevent physical injury, infection

To achieve awareness of needs

NURSING INTERVENTIONS

Nursing Treatments

Ambulate the patient (as much as possible)
Change the patient's position frequently
Give urine-acidifying juices orally (four times daily)
Increase fluid intake to about 2000 cc daily
Sterilize the bedpan after each use
Change the urinary drainage apparatus (frequently)
Keep the drainage container below bladder level
Use sterile technique (when disconnecting urinary drainage system)

Nursing Observations

Monitor the oral temperature
Monitor urine studies for evidence of urinary tract infection
Test the urine for pH (urine acidity reduces the potential for infection)

Health Teaching

Explain the causes of the health problem
Describe those symptoms which should be reported (dysuria)
Explain the reason for and intended effect of the therapy
Explain how to use toilet tissue correctly

EVALUATION

See the evaluation criteria for each specific goal in Chapter 2.

Potential Infection Transmission
(71,247,271,325,358,391,453)

ASSESSMENT

Objective Data

Poor hygiene habits
Contact with infected persons
Contact with body discharges such as urine, feces, sputum, nose, throat, and mouth discharges, skin lesions, and blood

Contact with unpure water, spoiled foods, infection-carrying insects, contaminated articles, unclean bathroom facilities

Contact with infectious material such as waste, hair, or hide of animals with anthrax

Related Data

Commonly Related Diseases:
Nasopharyngitis
Pneumonia
Influenza
Tuberculosis
Cholera
Diphtheria
Dysentery
Hookworm
Measles
Mumps
Leprosy
Meningitis
Pertussis
Scarlet fever
Smallpox
Typhoid fever
Encephalitis
Hepatitis
Poliomyelitis
Gonorrhea
Syphilis

POSSIBLE ETIOLOGY

Lack of instruction. The facility of microorganisms to spread.

NURSING INTERVENTIONS

Potential infection transmission: the possibility that a person will be exposed to and will contract an infection

PLANNING

Patient Needs	**Primary Nurse-Patient Goals**
Sleep, rest	To achieve sleep, rest
Cleanliness	To achieve good hygiene
Protection from physical harm	To prevent physical injury, infection
Increased learning	To achieve awareness of needs and/or use of resources

NURSING INTERVENTIONS

Nursing Treatments
Maintain a clean environment
Disinfect contaminated articles
Encourage adequate rest
Isolate infected persons

Isolate persons exposed to communicable disease

Immunize against infectious disease (ExR)

Take nasal and oral secretion precautions (for diphtheria, influenza, meningitis, mumps, poliomyelitis, pneumonia, scarlet fever, smallpox, whooping cough)

Take needle-syringe precautions (for hepatitis, syphilis)

Take skin-contact precautions (for gonorrhea, leprosy, smallpox, syphilis, tuberculosis)

Take sputum precautions (for diphtheria, influenza, pneumonia, tuberculosis, whooping cough)

Take stool precautions (for cholera, dysentery, hepatitis, hookworm, poliomyelitis, tuberculosis, typhoid fever)

Take urine precautions (for typhoid fever)

Cover the bed with netting (when windows are unscreened against mosquitoes in malaria and encephalitis; for flies in meningitis, poliomyelitis, typhoid fever)

Detect communicable disease cases

Make a referral (to the local health department)

Nursing Observations

Inspect the mucous membranes for abnormalities (mouth, nose, and throat)

Inspect the skin for infectious lesions

Monitor blood studies for evidence of infection

Monitor the oral temperature

Observe for complaints of headache

Observe for complaints of itching

Observe for complaints of malaise

Observe for complaints of nausea

Observe for complaints of pain

Observe for complaints of weakness

Observe for coughing

Observe for diarrhea

Observe for irritability

Observe for lethargy

Observe for restlessness

Observe for vomiting

Obtain a bacterial culture (of blood and body discharges)

Health Teaching

Describe those symptoms which should be reported (fever, chills, malaise)

Explain the causes of the health problem

Explain the reason for and intended effect of the therapy

Advise handwashing after elimination

Explain the need to avoid contaminated soil (for hookworm and pinworm)

Explain how to dispose of infectious expectoration

Explain how to prevent cross infection

Explain how to prevent the common cold

Explain that the common cold is contagious for 48 hours after symptom onset

Instruct to cover the mouth when coughing
Instruct to cover the nose when sneezing
Explain how venereal disease is transmitted
Inform that immunity does not occur with venereal infection
Instruct to limit direct contact with infected persons
Recommend the use of disposable dishes for contagious diseases
Recommend the use of individual dishes, utensils, and drinking glasses
Recommend the use of individual towels and washcloths

EVALUATION

See the evaluation criteria for each specific goal in Chapter 2.

Potential Puerperal Infection (53)

ASSESSMENT

Subjective Data
Exhaustion from prolonged labor

Objective Data
Exposure of the uterine endometrium, pelvis, and peritoneum during child-
birth
Early membrane rupture
Retained placenta fragments

Related Data
Commonly Related Diseases:
Endometritis
Salpingitis
Pelvic thrombophlebitis
Salpingo-oophoritis
Parametritis
Gonorrhea

POSSIBLE ETIOLOGY

The exposure of the uterine endometrium, pelvis, and peritoneum during
childbirth increases the possibility of *Streptococcus* and *Staphlococcus* microorganism invasion. Infection of organs proximal to the uterus.

NURSING DIAGNOSIS

Potential puerperal infection: the possibility that a vaginal infection might
occur following childbirth

PLANNING

Patient Needs	Primary Nurse-Patient Goals
Rest	To achieve rest
Cleanliness	To achieve good hygiene
Protection from physical harm	To prevent physical injury, infection
Increased learning	To achieve awareness of needs

NURSING INTERVENTIONS

Nursing Treatments
Use sterile technique (during delivery)
Encourage adequate rest (of the mother)
Refrain from performing nonessential procedures

Nursing Observations
Inspect the placenta for abnormalities
Inspect the vagina for discharge
Monitor the oral tempertture
Monitor blood studies for evidence of infectoon

Health Teaching
Describe those symptoms which should be reported
Explain the reason for and intended effect of the therapy

EVALUATION

See the evaluation criteria for each specific goal in Chapter 2.

Potential Tetanus (71,247,453)

ASSESSMENT

Objective Data
A wound that has broken the skin
A rusty wound-causing object
Wound contamination with dirt from roads, streets, or earth or from animals or human feces
No basic tetanus immunizations or no tetanus booster within the past 5 years

Related Data
In the absence of an injury, if there has been no tetanus toxoid immunization in the past 10 years, the potential for tetanus from future minor injuries is heightened
Commonly Related Diseases:
Tetanus

POSSIBLE ETIOLOGY

The possibility of the introduction of *Clostridium tetani* into the body through a wound, burn, or fracture

NURSING DIAGNOSIS

Potential tetanus: the possibility that tetanus might occur

PLANNING

Patient Needs	**Primary Nurse-Patient Goals**
Cleanliness	To achieve good hygiene
Protection from physical harm	To prevent physical injury, infection
Increased learning	To achieve awareness of needs

NURSING INTERVENTIONS

Nursing Treatments

Clean with antiseptic solution
> OR

Clean with hydrogen peroxide
> OR

Clean with surgical soap

Give tetanus toxoid (ET) (0.5 ml I.M. within 24 hours after injury, if the patient has been previously immunized; if no previous immunizations have been given, give the initial dose and a second dose 4–6 weeks later)

Health Teaching

Advise adherence to the immunization schedule

Explain the reason for and intended effect of the therapy

Medical Treatments Performed by Nurses

Give the prescribed drugs

EVALUATION

See the evaluation criteria for each specific goal in Chapter 2.

Potential Wound Infection (71,325,391,468)

ASSESSMENT

Objective Data

Wound uncleanliness

Unclean dressings

Infrequent dressing changes

Dirty clothes contact with the wound

Frequent hand contact with the wound

Related Data

Commonly Related Conditions:

Skin graft procedures

Commonly Related Diseases:

First-, second-, or third-degree burns

POSSIBLE ETIOLOGY

Exposure of tissue to bacteria. Eschar formation.

NURSING DIAGNOSIS

Potential wound infection: the possibility that pathogenic organisms might enter a wound

PLANNING

Patient Needs	**Primary Nurse-Patient Goals**
Cleanliness	To achieve good hygiene
Protection from physical harm	To prevent physical injury, infection
Increased learning	To achieve awareness of needs

NURSING INTERVENTIONS

Nursing Treatments

Specific for Nonburn Wounds:
Apply an antibiotic ointment
Apply a sterile dressing
Change the dressing frequently
Clean with antiseptic solution
  OR
Clean with hydrogen peroxide
  OR
Clean with surgical soap
Irrigate the wound
Position to promote drainage of the infected area
Use sterile technique

Specific for Burn Wounds:
Apply an antibiotic ointment
Apply a sterile dressing
Change the dressing frequently
Clean with hydrogen peroxide
  OR
Clean with surgical soap
Maintain a clean environment
Maintain reverse isolation
Place on sterile linens
Use sterile technique

Nursing Observations
Inspect the skin for infectious lesions
Inspect for inflammation
Obtain a bacterial culture (of the wound)

Health Teaching
Describe those symptoms which should be reported (pus drainage)
Advise against pulling off scabs
Instruct to carefully move the injured body part
Teach how to clean and dress a wound
Teach how to irrigate a wound
Inform that cleanliness is basic to health
Explain the reason for and intended effect of the therapy

EVALUATION

See the evaluation criteria for each specific goal in Chapter 2.

INFECTION: SPECIFIC INFECTIONS

Localized Infection (32,414)

ASSESSMENT

Subjective Data
Pain

Objective Data
Redness
Heat
Swelling
Impaired function of the infected area
Fever, sometimes

POSSIBLE ETIOLOGY

Bacterial infection

NURSING DIAGNOSIS

Localized infection: the invasion of pathogenic organisms into tissue, localized to one area

PLANNING

Patient Needs	**Primary Nurse-Patient Goals**
Rest	To achieve rest
Comfort	To achieve comfort
Cleanliness	To achieve good hygiene
Protection from physical harm	To prevent physical injury, infection
Increased learning	To achieve awareness of needs

NURSING INTERVENTIONS

Nursing Treatments
Clean with antiseptic solution
   OR
Clean with hydrogen peroxide
   OR
Clean with surgical soap
Soak in saline solution
   OR
Apply a warm, moist compress
Apply an antibiotic ointment
Apply a sterile dressing
Refrain from tight bandaging
Change the dressing frequently
Give nonprescription drugs (ExR) (for pain)
Encourage adequate rest
Use sterile technique

Nursing Observations
Monitor the oral temperature

Health Teaching
Describe those symptoms which should be reported
Explain the causes of the health problem
Explain the reason for and intended effect of the therapy
Inform that cleanliness is basic to health
Teach how to apply heat therapy

Teach how to clean and dress a wound
Teach how to do therapeutic soaks

Medical Treatments Performed by Nurses
Give the prescribed drugs
Soak in a medicated solution

EVALUATION

See the evaluation criteria for each specific goal in Chapter 2.

INFECTION THERAPY DEPENDENCE

Dependence on Infection-Related Isolation Management (365)

ASSESSMENT

Subjective Data
Person relies on nurses for:
    restricted contact with other persons
    maintenance of sterile technique
    strict control of body excreta

Objective Data
Person is susceptible to infection or has a communicable infection

Related Data
Commonly Related Conditions:
Kidney transplant
Commonly Related Diseases:
Meningitis
Poliomyelitis
Measles
Influenza
Infectious mononucleosis
Tuberculosis
Hepatitis
Diphtheria
Leukemia
Aplastic anemia

POSSIBLE ETIOLOGY

Efforts to prevent the spread of infectious conditions. Efforts to protect susceptible persons from infection.

NURSING DIAGNOSIS

Dependence on infection-related isolation management: reliance on nurses to maintain standard isolation technique or reverse isolation

PLANNING

Patient Needs

Protection from physical harm
Dependence
Increased learning

Primary Nurse-Patient Goals

To prevent physical injury, infection
To achieve comfort
To achieve awareness of needs

NURSING INTERVENTIONS

Nursing Treatments
Isolate infected persons
Maintain isolation technique
Maintain reverse isolation

Health Teaching
Explain the causes of the health problem
Explain the limitations imposed by isolation
Explain the reason for and intended effect of the therapy

EVALUATION

See the evaluation criteria for each specific goal in Chapter 2.

INFLAMMATION

External Abscess (32,325,453)

ASSESSMENT

Subjective Data
Throbbing pain

Objective Data
Inflammation (redness)
Swelling
Purulent drainage
Well-defined borders
Fever, sometimes

Related Data

Commonly Related Conditions:
Boil (furuncle)
Carbuncle

Commonly Related Diseases:
Diabetes mellitus
Acne

POSSIBLE ETIOLOGY

Infectious microorganisms

NURSING DIAGNOSIS

External abscess: a local collection of pus anywhere on the body

PLANNING

Patient Needs	**Primary Nurse-Patient Goals**
Rest	To achieve rest
Comfort	To achieve comfort
Cleanliness	To achieve good hygiene
Protection from physical harm	To prevent physical injury, infection
Increased learning	To achieve awareness of needs

NURSING INTERVENTIONS

Nursing Treatments
Clean with antiseptic solution
    OR
Clean with hydrogen peroxide
    OR
Clean with surgical soap
Soak in saline solution
    OR
Apply a warm, moist compress
Soak in a sitz bath (for rectal or perineal abscess)
Apply an antibiotic ointment
Apply a sterile dressing
Refrain from tight bandaging
Change the dressing frequently
Give nonprescription drugs (ExR) (for pain)
Encourage adequate rest
Use sterile technique

Nursing Observations
Monitor the oral temperature
Obtain a bacterial culture (of drainage)

Health Teaching
Explain the causes of the health problem
Advise against piercing lesions
Inform that cleanliness is basic to health
Teach how to apply heat therapy
Teach how to clean and dress a wound
Teach how to do therapeutic soaks
Explain the reason for and intended effect of the therapy

Medical Treatments Performed by Nurses
Give the prescribed drugs
Soak in a medicated solution

EVALUATION

See the evaluation criteria for each specific goal in Chapter 2.

Limited Cellulitis (32,325,453)

ASSESSMENT

Subjective Data
Pain on palpation of skin
Headache
Lethargy
Chills

Objective Data
Area redness
Heat
Swelling
Poorly defined borders
Fever

Related Data
Commonly Related Conditions:
Drug reaction
Snakebite

POSSIBLE ETIOLOGY

Infectious microorganisms of a wide variety; streptococci and staphylococci are most common.

NURSING DIAGNOSIS

Limited cellulitis: a diffuse or spreading inflammation related to infection of cellular or connective tissue that is limited to a small area

PLANNING

Patient Needs	Primary Nurse-Patient Goals
Rest	To achieve rest
Comfort	To achieve comfort
Cleanliness	To achieve good hygiene
Protection from physical harm	To prevent physical injury, infection
Increased learning	To achieve awareness of needs

NURSING INTERVENTIONS

Nursing Treatments
Apply a warm, moist compress
   OR
Apply a hot water bottle
   OR
Soak in saline solution
Clean with antiseptic solution
   OR
Clean with hydrogen peroxide
   OR

Clean with surgical soap
Apply an antibiotic ointment
Apply a sterile dressing
Change the dressing frequently
Elevate the extremity
Encourage adequate rest
Refrain from tight bandaging
Use sterile technique

Nursing Observations
Monitor the oral temperature
Obtain a bacterial culture

Health Teaching
Explain the causes of the health problem
Explain the reason for and intended effect of the therapy
Inform that cleanliness is basic to health
Teach how to apply heat therapy
Teach how to clean and dress a wound
Teach how to do therapeutic soaks

Medical Treatments Performed by Nurses
Soak in a medicated solution

EVALUATION

See the evaluation criteria for each specific goal in Chapter 2.

IMMUNOLOGY THERAPY DEPENDENCE

Dependence on Nursing Supervision for Kidney-Transplant Rejection (70,71,391,451)

ASSESSMENT

Subjective Data
Person relies on nurses for:
    intense observation for several postoperative weeks
    periodic observation following hospital discharge
    recognition of the warning signs

Objective Data
Person has received a kidney transplant

Related Data
Commonly Related Diseases:
Renal failure

POSSIBLE ETIOLOGY

Immunologic rejection of a foreign body. The kidney becomes infiltrated with lymphocytes, which attempt to destroy the foreign kidney. As a result of the inflammation, the renal tubule epithelium develops necrosis, and small blood vessel thrombosis occurs in the kidney.

NURSING DIAGNOSIS

Dependence on nursing supervision for kidney-transplant rejection: reliance on nurses to observe for indications that rejection of the transplanted kidney is occurring

PLANNING

Patient Needs	Primary Nurse-Patient Goals
Waste elimination	To maintain regulating mechanisms and functions
Rest	To achieve rest
Comfort	To achieve comfort
Cleanliness	To achieve good hygiene
Protection from physical harm	To prevent physical injury, infection
Increased learning	To achieve awareness of needs

NURSING INTERVENTIONS

Nursing Treatments
Attend the patient constantly (during the early postoperative days)
Provide frequent patient contact (following hospital discharge)

Nursing Observations
Inspect for edema
Measure the body weight (daily)
Measure the intake
Measure the output (for decreased output)
Monitor the blood pressure (for increase)
Monitor the oral temperature (for fever)
Monitor blood studies for abnormal renal function
Observe for complaints of pain
Obtain a bacterial culture (of blood, stool, urine, respiratory secretions, and wounds if fever occurs in the first three postsurgical days)
Palpate for tenderness (and swelling over the kidney transplant area)
Test the urine for protein

Health Teaching
Explain the causes of the health problem
Explain the reason for and intended effect of the therapy

Medical Treatments Performed by Nurses
Give the prescribed drugs

EVALUATION

See the evaluation criteria for each specific goal in Chapter 2.

IMMUNOLOGY: EMERGENCY ANTIGEN-ANTIBODY RESPONSE

Emergency Phase Anaphylactic Shock, p. 452

Emergency Phase Blood Transfusion Reaction (70,391)

ASSESSMENT

Subjective Data
Sudden chest pain
Nausea
Headache

Objective Data
Chills
Fever
Hives
Cyanosis
Dyspnea
Vomiting
Facial flushing
Onset within 24 hours following blood transfusion

Related Data
Commonly Related Diseases:
Any disease or injury requiring blood replacement

POSSIBLE ETIOLOGY

Introduction of a foreign protein into the circulatory system

NURSING DIAGNOSIS

Emergency phase blood transfusion reaction: the need for immediate health care as a result of an antigen-antibody blood reaction

PLANNING

Patient Needs	Primary Nurse-Patient Goals
Rest	To achieve rest
Comfort	To achieve comfort
Protection from physical harm	To prevent physical injury
Increased learning	To achieve awareness of needs

NURSING INTERVENTIONS

Nursing Treatments
Discontinue the blood transfusion (*immediately*)
Attend the patient constantly
Cover with warm blankets
Provide standby emergency equipment (oxygen)

Return the blood to the blood bank after a reaction
Consult with the physician (*immediately*)

Nursing Observations
Measure the urine output hourly
Monitor the blood pressure
Monitor the oral temperature (for fever within the hour)

Health Teaching
Explain the causes of the health problem
Explain the reason for and intended effect of the therapy

Medical Treatments Performed by Nurses
Give the prescribed drugs

EVALUATION

See the evaluation criteria for each specific goal in Chapter 2.

INFECTION MANAGEMENT

Inadequate Information Related to Infection Prevention
(71,247,271,325,391,453)

ASSESSMENT

Subjective Data
Person confirms a lack of information

Objective Data
Person's actions indicate a lack of information regarding:
    that cleanliness is essential to infection prevention
    the means by which infection is transmitted
    the proper methods of disinfecting

Related Data
Commonly Related Diseases:
None

POSSIBLE ETIOLOGY

Lack of information

NURSING DIAGNOSIS

Inadequate information related to infection prevention: lack of information
as to the methods used for preventing infection and infection transmission

PLANNING

Patient Needs	**Primary Nurse-Patient Goals**
Protection from physical harm	To prevent infection
Increased learning	To achieve awareness of needs and/or use of resources

NURSING INTERVENTIONS

Nursing Treatments
Approach unhurriedly
Encourage patient questions

Nursing Observations
Evaluate the response to teaching

Health Teaching
Explain how to disinfect contaminated linen
Explain how to dispose of infectious expectoration
Explain how to dispose of soiled dressings
Explain how to prevent cross infection
Explain how venereal disease is transmitted
Inform that immunity does not occur with venereal infection
Instruct to cover the mouth when coughing
Instruct to cover the nose when sneezing
Instruct to limit direct contact with infected persons
Teach how to apply disinfecting solutions
Inform that cleanliness is basic to health

EVALUATION

See the evaluation criteria for each specific goal in Chapter 2.

IMMUNOLOGY MANAGEMENT

Inadequate Information Related to Drug Allergy (6)

ASSESSMENT

Subjective Data
Person confirms a lack of information

Objective Data
Person's actions indicate a lack of information regarding:
    the signs of drug allergy (respiratory difficulty, rash or hives, fever, swollen lymph glands)
    the symptoms of drug allergy (itching, generalized weakness, joint pain)
    the circumstances most likely to surround its occurrence (does not occur with the initial drug dose if on prolonged drug therapy; it will occur within 6 weeks of the initial dose; clears up within 2 days once the drug is stopped)
    the drugs with which it most frequently occurs (quinine, quinidine, antibiotics, tranquilizers, sulfonamides, antimalarial drugs, antihypertensive drugs, tetanus antitoxin)
    how to avoid allergic responses

Related Data
Commonly Related Diseases:
Aplastic anemia

POSSIBLE ETIOLOGY

Lack of instruction

NURSING DIAGNOSIS

Inadequate information related to drug allergy: lack of information regarding the cause, effects, and treatment of a hypersensitivity response to drugs

PLANNING

Patient Needs	Primary Nurse-Patient Goals
Comfort	To achieve comfort
Protection from physical harm	To prevent hypersensitivity response
Increased learning	To achieve awareness of needs

NURSING INTERVENTIONS

Nursing Treatments
Approach unhurriedly
Encourage patient questions

Nursing Observations
Evaluate the response to teaching

Health Teaching
Advise that the precipitating factor (the drug) be avoided
Describe those symptoms which should be reported
Explain the causes of the health problem

EVALUATION

See the evaluation criteria for each specific goal in Chapter 2.

Inadequate Information Related to Food Allergy (6,11,247,327,413)

ASSESSMENT

Subjective Data
Person confirms a lack of information

Objective Data
Person's actions indicate a lack of information regarding:
    the signs of food allergy (skin rash, hives, respiratory distress, nasal stuffiness, mouth and lip swelling, vomiting, diarrhea, slight fever)
    the symptoms of food allergy (nausea, severe abdominal pain, headache, malaise)
    the causes of food allergy
    how to avoid allergic responses

POSSIBLE ETIOLOGY

Lack of instruction

NURSING DIAGNOSIS

Inadequate information related to food allergy: lack of information regarding the cause, effects, and treatment of antibody-antigen reactions to ingested foods

PLANNING

Patient Needs	**Primary Nurse-Patient Goals**
Comfort	To achieve comfort
Protection from physical harm	To prevent hypersensitivity response
Increased learning	To achieve awareness of needs

NURSING INTERVENTIONS

Nursing Treatments
Approach unhurriedly
Encourage patient questions
Make a referral (to a physician for sensitivity testing and/or desensitizing)

Nursing Observations
Evaluate the response to teaching

Health Teaching
Explain the causes of the health problem
Describe those symptoms which should be reported
Inform of the therapies available for the specific condition
Inform that foods causing allergies fall into specific categories
Advise that the precipitating factor (specific food) be avoided

EVALUATION

See the evaluation criteria for each specific goal in Chapter 2.

Inadequate Information Related to Respiratory Allergy (6,11,247,327,413)

ASSESSMENT

Subjective Data
Person confirms a lack of information

Objective Data
Person's actions indicate a lack of information regarding:
> the signs of respiratory allergy (pale and swollen nasal mucous membranes, sneezing, excessive tearing, watery nasal secretion)
> the symptoms of respiratory allergy (malaise, headache, itching nose or eyes)
> the causes of respiratory allergy (in early spring, exposure to tree pollen precipitates response; in early summer, exposure to grass or weed pollen precipitates response; in early fall, exposure to ragweed pollen precipitates response; exposure to animal fur, dust particles, or feathers may precipitate response; usually worse on windy days)
> how to avoid allergic responses

Related Data
Commonly Related Diseases:
Hay fever
Rose fever
Allergic rhinitis

POSSIBLE ETIOLOGY

Lack of instruction

NURSING DIAGNOSIS

Inadequate information related to respiratory allergy: lack of information regarding the cause, effects, and treatment of antibody-antigen reaction to substances inhaled through the respiratory system

PLANNING

Patient Needs

Comfort

Protection from physical harm

Increased learning

Primary Nurse-Patient Goals

To achieve comfort

To prevent hypersensitivity response

To achieve awareness of needs

NURSING INTERVENTIONS

Nursing Treatments

Approach unhurriedly
Encourage patient questions
Discourage smoking
Make a referral (to a physician for sensitivity testing and/or desensitizing)

Nursing Observations

Evaluate the response to teaching

Health Teaching

Describe those symptoms which should be reported
Explain how to take allergy precautions
Explain the causes of the health problem
Inform of the therapies available for the specific condition
Explain the reason for and intended effect of the therapy

EVALUATION

See the evaluation criteria for each specific goal in Chapter 2.

Inadequate Information Related to Skin Allergy (6,11,247,327,413)

ASSESSMENT

Subjective Data

Person confirms a lack of information

Objective Data

Person's actions indicate a lack of information regarding:
    the signs of skin allergy (edema, hives, rash, redness, scaling or peeling skin surface)
    the symptoms of skin allergy (burning, stinging, itching skin)
    the causes of skin allergy (plants, metals, especially mercury, plastics, dyes, and soaps)
    how to avoid allergic responses

Related Data

Commonly Related Diseases:
Poison ivy

POSSIBLE ETIOLOGY

Lack of instruction

NURSING DIAGNOSIS

Inadequate information related to skin allergy: lack of information regarding the cause, effects, and treatment of antigen-antibody reaction following skin contact with irritating substances

PLANNING

Patient Needs	**Primary Nurse-Patient Goals**
Comfort	To achieve comfort
Protection from physical harm	To prevent hypersensitivity response
Increased learning	To achieve awareness of needs

NURSING INTERVENTIONS

Nursing Treatments
Approach unhurriedly
Encourage patient questions
Make a referral (to a physician for sensitivity testing)

Nursing Observations
Evaluate the response to teaching

Health Teaching
Explain how to take allergy precautions
Explain the causes of the health problem
Advise that the precipitating factor be avoided
Inform of the therapies available for the specific condition
Explain the reason for and intended effect of the therapy

EVALUATION

See the evaluation criteria for each specific goal in Chapter 2.

19.
NURSING DIAGNOSES RELATED TO
Integument:
Hair, Nails, and Skin

HAIR: SCALP DISORDERS

Cradle Cap (144,430)

ASSESSMENT

Objective Data
Yellowish substance on the scalp
Crusted area

Related Data
Commonly Related Diseases:
None

POSSIBLE ETIOLOGY

Excessive sebaceous gland secretion. Poor scalp hygiene.

NURSING DIAGNOSIS

Cradle cap: a crust formation on the infant's scalp

PLANNING

Patient Needs	**Primary Nurse-Patient Goals**
Comfort	To achieve comfort
Cleanliness	To achieve good hygiene
Increased learning (for the mother)	To achieve awareness of needs

NURSING INTERVENTIONS

Nursing Treatments
Shampoo the scalp (daily, with Fostex soap)
Brush the infant's hair with a soft hairbrush

Nursing Observations
Observe for evidence of a favorable response to therapy

Health Teaching
Explain the causes of the health problem
Inform that cleanliness is basic to health
Explain how to shampoo the scalp
Advise daily hair brushing
Explain the reason for and intended effect of the therapy

EVALUATION

See the evaluation criteria for each specific goal in Chapter 2.

Dandruff (145,161,430)

ASSESSMENT

Subjective Data
Severe itching
Irritating scalp

Objective Data
White, flaky, powdery scales scattered loosely in the hair (dry dandruff)
Slightly yellow, sticky scales clinging to the scalp in patches (oily dandruff)

Related Data
Commonly Related Diseases:
Seborrheic dermatitis
Hypothyroidism

POSSIBLE ETIOLOGY

The shedding of dead tissue from the epidermis. Endocrine disorders. Over-indulgence in fats or carbohydrates. Poor hygiene. Poor scalp circulation. Lack of nerve stimulation to the scalp.

NURSING DIAGNOSIS

Dandruff: scales in the hair or on the scalp

PLANNING

Patient Needs	Primary Nurse-Patient Goals
Water-salt balance	To maintain fluid and electrolyte balance
Food balance	To maintain nutrition to all cells
Comfort	To achieve comfort
Stimulation	To maintain stimulation
Cleanliness	To achieve good hygiene
Increased learning	To achieve awareness of needs

NURSING INTERVENTIONS

Nursing Treatments
Balance fluid intake to equal output
Massage vigorously (the scalp)
Shampoo the hair (with selenium or zinc pyrithione preparations)
Comb dandruff from the scalp

Nursing Observations
Inspect for dehydration

Health Teaching
Explain the causes of the health problem
Inform that cleanliness is basic to health
Advise against prolonged scalp exposure to the sun
Advise against prolonged scalp exposure to water
Explain the importance of individual use of a comb and brush
Instruct to comb dandruff up from the scalp
Teach the principles of good nutrition (fewer fats and carbohydrates)
Explain the reason for and intended effect of the therapy

EVALUATION

See the evaluation criteria for each specific goal in Chapter 2.

Parasite Infestation (144)

ASSESSMENT

Subjective Data
Itching

Objective Data
Presence of small, crawling organisms on the body
Found in the head, chest, axillary, and genital hair and in beard, eyebrows,
    and eyelashes

Related Data
Commonly Related Diseases:
Scabies
Pediculosis capitis
Pediculosis pubis

POSSIBLE ETIOLOGY

Contact with an infested person or environment. Poor hygiene.

NURSING DIAGNOSIS

Parasite infestation: the presence of lice, mites, or bedbugs on the body

PLANNING

Patient Needs	**Primary Nurse-Patient Goals**
Comfort	To achieve comfort
Cleanliness	To achieve good hygiene
Protection from physical harm	To prevent physical injury, infection
Increased learning	To achieve awareness of needs

NURSING INTERVENTIONS

Nursing Treatments
Apply a parasiticide
Shampoo the hair (frequently)
Brush and comb the hair (two or three times daily)

Maintain dry, clean linen (especially pillowcases)
Wash the brush and comb with a parasiticide

Nursing Observations
Observe for evidence of a favorable response to therapy

Health Teaching
Explain the causes of the health problem
Explain the importance of individual use of a comb and brush
Instruct to maintain scalp cleanliness
Instruct to inspect the scalp
Explain how to remove hair lice
Explain how to shampoo the hair (with a parasiticide)
Recommend the use of individual towels and washcloths
Inform that clean linens are essential
Explain the reason for and intended effect of the therapy

EVALUATION

See the evaluation criteria for each specific goal in Chapter 2.

HAIR: POTENTIAL SCALP DISORDERS

Potential Infestation Transmission

ASSESSMENT

Objective Data
Living with infested persons
Sharing infested clothing, beds, hair and brushes
Poor general hygiene

Related Data
Commonly Related Diseases:
Scabies
Pediculosis capitis
Pediculosis corporis
Pediculosis pubis
Bedbug infestation

POSSIBLE ETIOLOGY

The close proximity of persons infested with lice, mites, or bedbugs to a noninfested person

NURSING DIAGNOSIS

Potential infestation transmission: the possibility that lice, mites, or bedbugs may be transmitted from one person to another

PLANNING

Patient Needs
Cleanliness
Protection from physical harm
Increased learning

Primary Nurse-Patient Goals
To achieve good hygiene
To prevent physical injury
To achieve awareness of needs

NURSING INTERVENTIONS

Nursing Treatments
Shampoo the hair (frequently)
Brush and comb the hair (two or three times daily)
Maintain dry, clean linen

Nursing Observations
Inspect the hair for abnormalities (infestation)

Health Teaching
Explain the causes of the health problem
Instruct to limit direct contact with infected persons
Explain the importance of individual use of a comb and brush
Instruct to maintain scalp cleanliness
Instruct to inspect the hair (if in contact with persons who are infested)

Medical Treatments Performed by Nurses
Give the prescribed drugs

EVALUATION

See the evaluation criteria for each specific goal in Chapter 2.

NAILS

Ingrown Nail

ASSESSMENT

Subjective Data
Pain or tenderness around the nail bed

Objective Data
Nail margin penetrates the skin
Redness

Related Data
Commonly Related Diseases:
None

POSSIBLE ETIOLOGY

Increased cell growth. Injury. Prolonged pressure distorts the direction of nail growth.

NURSING DIAGNOSIS

Ingrown nail: nail tissue growing over its edges and pressing into soft skin tissue

PLANNING

Patient Needs

Comfort

Cleanliness

Protection from physical harm

Increased learning

Primary Nurse-Patient Goals

To achieve comfort

To achieve good hygiene

To prevent physical injury, infection

To achieve awareness of needs

NURSING INTERVENTIONS

Nursing Treatments

Clean with hydrogen peroxide
   OR
Clean with surgical soap
   OR
Soak in saline solution
Apply an antibiotic ointment
Pack sterile cotton between the ingrown nail and the skin

Nursing Observations

Inspect for inflammation

Health Teaching

Explain the causes of the health problem
Inform that cleanliness is basic to health
Instruct to cut the toenails straight across
Instruct to wear well-fitting shoes
Recommend the use of closed shoes for foot protection
Describe those symptoms which should be reported (inflammation, severe pain)

EVALUATION

See the evaluation criteria for each specific goal in Chapter 2.

SKIN: SKIN AND TISSUE DISORDERS

Erythema Skin Discomfort (144,145)

ASSESSMENT

Subjective Data

Itching
Burning sensation
Tenderness, sometimes

Objective Data
Color: dull red, which disappears with applied pressure
Shape: varied
Size: large or small
Content: no mass or fluid content
Elevation: none
Distribution: localized or diffuse
Other characteristics: dryness, if prolonged

Related Data
Commonly Related Conditions:
Any condition requiring drug therapy

Commonly Related Diseases:
Pellagra (early stage)
Scarlet fever
Lupus erythematosus
Erythema marginatum
Erythema circinatum
Erythema multiforme
Erythema nodosum

POSSIBLE ETIOLOGY

Capillary dilatation causing capillary congestion resulting from exposure to high environmental temperature, drug sensitivity, localized inflammation. Nervous responses.

NURSING DIAGNOSIS

Erythema skin discomfort: a condition in which reddened skin eruptions irritate the skin

PLANNING

Patient Needs

Comfort

Cleanliness

Protection from physical harm

Increased learning

Primary Nurse-Patient Goals

To achieve comfort

To achieve good hygiene

To prevent physical injury

To achieve awareness of needs

NURSING INTERVENTIONS

Nursing Treatments
Bathe in cool water
Clean with castile or lanolin soap
Apply calamine lotion
   OR
Apply cornstarch to the skin (where there are skin folds)
Do not allow skin surfaces to touch
Apply a bed cradle
Cover with lightweight blankets
Dress in minimum clothing

Give nonprescription drugs (ExR) (antihistamine for drug sensitivity)
Maintain a cool room temperature
Maintain dry skin
Avoid using rough-textured bed linens
Refrain from pulling the patient across the sheets
Place on a sheepskin
Withhold the drug (causing the erythema)

Nursing Observations
Observe for evidence of a favorable response to therapy

Health Teaching
Explain the causes of the health problem
Advise against scratching
Explain the reason for and intended effect of the therapy

EVALUATION

See the evaluation criteria for each specific goal in Chapter 2.

Jaundice Skin Discomfort (271,430)

ASSESSMENT

Subjective Data
Itching, often intense
Dryness

Objective Data
Color: yellow skin accompanied by yellow sclera (jaundice)
Shape: none
Size: none
Content: no mass or fluid content
Elevation: none
Distribution: complete skin coverage
Other characteristics: scaling

Related Data
Laboratory Findings:
Increased blood bilirubin
Increased urine urobilinogen
Commonly Related Conditions:
Prematurity
ABO and Rh blood incompatibility
Commonly Related Diseases:
Cholecystitis
Cholelithiasis
Infectious hepatitis

POSSIBLE ETIOLOGY

Abnormally high bilirubin pigments in the blood resulting from such conditions as liver dysfunction, excessive red blood cell distribution, or biliary obstruction and causing yellow staining of the skin

NURSING DIAGNOSIS

Jaundice skin discomfort: a condition in which bile pigment infiltrates and irritates the skin

PLANNING

Patient Needs

Water-salt balance

Rest

Comfort

Protection from physical harm

Increased learning

Primary Nurse-Patient Goals

To maintain fluid and electrolyte balance

To achieve rest

To achieve comfort

To prevent physical injury

To achieve awareness of needs

NURSING INTERVENTIONS

Nursing Treatments

Apply calamine lotion
  OR
Apply cornstarch to the skin
  OR
Apply soda bicarbonate to the skin
Bathe in cool water
Lubricate the skin with baby oil, bath oil, or body lotion
Dress in minimum clothing
Encourage adequate rest
Increase fluid intake to about 2000 cc daily
Maintain adequate atmospheric humidity
Maintain a cool room temperature
Expose the skin to sunlight

Nursing Observations

Observe for evidence of a favorable response to therapy

Health Teaching

Advise against scratching
Explain the causes of the health problem
Explain the reason for and intended effect of the therapy

Medical Treatments Performed by Nurses

Administer phototherapy treatment

EVALUATION

See the evaluation criteria for each specific goal in Chapter 2.

Macular Skin Discomfort (271,430)

ASSESSMENT

Subjective Data

No pain or tenderness
Itching, sometimes

Objective Data
Color: light red, purple, or bronze
Shape: round
Size: small
Content: no mass or fluid content
Elevation: level with the skin
Distribution: single or multiple
Other characteristics: none

Related Data
Commonly Related Diseases:
Varicella (chickenpox, early stage)
Rubella (German measles)
Leprosy (early stage)
Impetigo (early stage)
Variola (smallpox, first day)
Rubeola (measles)

POSSIBLE ETIOLOGY

Pigment deposits in the skin. Erythrocytes escaping from blood vessels into skin tissue. Dilatation of skin blood vessels.

NURSING DIAGNOSIS

Macular skin discomfort: a condition in which macules irritate the skin

PLANNING

Patient Needs	**Primary Nurse-Patient Goals**
Comfort	To achieve comfort
Cleanliness	To achieve good hygiene
Protection from physical harm	To prevent physical injury
Increased learning	To achieve awareness of needs

NURSING INTERVENTIONS

Nursing Treatments
Apply calamine lotion
Bathe in cool water
Cover with lightweight blankets
Dress in minimum clothing
Maintain a cool room temperature
Maintain dry skin

Nursing Observations
Observe for evidence of a favorable response to therapy

Health Teaching
Explain the causes of the health problem
Advise against exposure to intense heat
Advise against scratching
Instruct to maintain skin dryness
Explain the reason for and intended effect of the therapy

EVALUATION

See the evaluation criteria for each specific goal in Chapter 2.

Maculopapular Skin Discomfort
(60,144,271)

ASSESSMENT

Subjective Data
Itching
Burning pain

Objective Data
Color: brownish pink or red
Shape: irregular
Size: small
Content: solid, no fluid content
Elevation: none, or slightly raised above the skin
Distribution: single or multiple, often over the buttocks and genitalia
Other characteristics: none

Related Data
Commonly Related Conditions:
Diaper rash
Commonly Related Diseases:
Rubeola (measles)
Exanthema subitum (roseola)
Pityriasis rosea (mid-stage)

POSSIBLE ETIOLOGY

Viral infection. The use of harsh detergents to wash diapers. Infrequent
diaper change.

NURSING DIAGNOSIS

Maculopapular skin discomfort: a condition in which maculopapular lesions irritate the skin

PLANNING

Patient Needs

Comfort

Cleanliness

Protection from physical harm

Increased learning

Primary Nurse-Patient Goals

To achieve comfort

To achieve good hygiene

To prevent physical injury

To achieve awareness of needs

NURSING INTERVENTIONS

Nursing Treatments
Bathe in cool water
Bathe with water only
Cover with lightweight blankets
Dress in minimum clothing

Dust the skin with medicated powder (silicone preparation)
Maintain a cool room temperature
Maintain dry, clean linen
Maintain dry skin
Refrain from using an alkaline soap on the skin

Nursing Observations
Observe for evidence of a favorable response to therapy

Health Teaching
Advise against exposure to intense heat
Advise against piercing lesions
Advise against scratching
Advise against squeezing the skin
Advise limited use of powder on the infant's skin
Explain how to correctly wash diapers
Instruct to maintain skin dryness
Explain the causes of the health problem
Explain the reason for and intended effect of the therapy

EVALUATION

See the evaluation criteria for each specific goal in Chapter 2.

Nodular Skin Discomfort (145)

ASSESSMENT

Subjective Data
Tender, painful
Itching

Objective Data
Color: white, yellow, or red brown
Shape: round
Size: fairly large, greater than 5 mm in diameter
Content: solid, firm
Elevation: raised above the skin
Distribution: most frequent on the face and nose

Related Data
Commonly Related Conditions:
Infant milia
Cancer
Commonly Related Diseases:
Leprosy (mid-stage)

POSSIBLE ETIOLOGY

Tubercle bacilli. The formation of solid matter in the sebaceous glands.
Nutritional deficiency. Tissue proliferation or inflammation.

NURSING DIAGNOSIS

Nodular skin discomfort: a condition in which nodules irritate the skin

PLANNING

Patient Needs

Comfort

Cleanliness

Protection from physical harm

Increased learning

Primary Nurse-Patient Goals

To achieve comfort

To achieve good hygiene

To prevent physical injury, infection

To achieve awareness of needs

NURSING INTERVENTIONS

Nursing Treatments

Bathe in warm water
   OR
Apply a warm, moist compress
Clean the skin with a drying soap
   OR
Clean the skin with an astringent
   OR
Clean with surgical soap
Maintain dry skin
Use paper or transparent tape instead of adhesive on the skin
Refrain from using a cream-based soap

Nursing Observations

Observe for evidence of a favorable response to therapy

Health Teaching

Advise against piercing lesions
Advise against squeezing the skin
Instruct to maintain skin cleanliness
Recommend the use of individual towels and washcloths
Explain the causes of the health problem

EVALUATION

See the evaluation criteria for each specific goal in Chapter 2.

Papular Skin Discomfort (145,271)

ASSESSMENT

Subjective Data

Itching

Tenderness

Objective Data

Color: white with a black center, or violet color
Shape: round or angular
Size: small, less than 5 mm in diameter
Content: solid
Elevation: raised above the skin
Distribution: single lesions or in a rash
Other characteristics: pimple appearance; may have a flat or pointed top

Related Data

Commonly Related Diseases:
Varicella (chickenpox, mid-stage)
Variola (smallpox, second day)
Scabies
Cutaneous tuberculosis
Eczematous dermatitis (eczema)
Pityriasis rosea (mid-stage)
Acne vulgaris

POSSIBLE ETIOLOGY

Blockage of the sebaceous glands causing secretion solidification. Tissue proliferation or infiltration.

NURSING DIAGNOSIS

Papular skin discomfort: a condition in which papules irritate the skin

PLANNING

Patient Needs

Comfort

Cleanliness

Protection from physical harm

Increased learning

Primary Nurse-Patient Goals

To achieve comfort

To achieve good hygiene

To prevent physical injury, infection

To achieve awareness of needs

NURSING INTERVENTIONS

Nursing Treatments
Bathe in warm water
  OR
Apply a warm, moist compress
Clean the skin with a drying soap
  OR
Clean the skin with an astringent
  OR
Clean with hydrogen peroxide
  OR
Clean with surgical soap
Refrain from using a cream-based soap
Apply an antibiotic ointment
Apply a bed cradle (if the lesions are widespread)
Dress in minimum clothing
Maintain adequate atmospheric humidity (low humidity)
Maintain a cool room temperature
Maintain dry skin

Nursing Observations
Observe for evidence of a favorable response to therapy

Health Teaching
Advise against piercing lesions
Advise against scratching

Advise against squeezing the skin
Instruct to maintain skin cleanliness
Recommend the use of individual towels and washcloths
Explain the causes of the health problem
Explain the reason for and intended effect of the therapy

EVALUATION

See the evaluation criteria for each specific goal in Chapter 2.

Pruritus Discomfort (144,271,430)

ASSESSMENT

Subjective Data
Itching

Objective Data
Scratching
Restlessness
Irritability
Redness

Related Data

Commonly Related Conditions:
Pregnancy
Jaundice
Allergy
Insect bites
Drug reactions
Menopause
Hemorrhoids

Commonly Related Diseases:
Diabetes mellitus
Hyperthyroidism
Chickenpox
Poison ivy
Poison oak
Pediculosis
Ringworm
Mycosis fungoides
Scabies
Eczema
Psoriasis
Lichen planus
Pityriasis rosea
Chillblains
Leukemia
Chronic glomerulonephritis
Dermatitis venenata
Lichen simplex chronicus
Dermatitis medicamentosa

Exfoliative dermatitis
Seborrheic dermatitis
Urticaria
Angioneurotic edema
Stasis dermatitis
Impetigo
Folliculitis
Tinea corporis
Tinea cruris
Tinea versicolor
Tinea pedis
Dermatophytid
Cutaneous candidiasis
Allergic rhinitis
Pinworm disease
Moniliasis
Ear dermatitis
Chronic external otitis

POSSIBLE ETIOLOGY

An irritating stimuli affecting the epidermal nerve endings. Insect and parasite bites and infestation. Skin dryness. Inflammation and infection. Emotional stress. Allergic response. Impaired circulation. Drug reactions.

NURSING DIAGNOSIS

Pruritus discomfort: an irritating skin sensation that induces scratching

PLANNING

Patient Needs

Comfort

Cleanliness

Protection from physical harm

Increased learning

Primary Nurse-Patient Goals

To achieve comfort

To achieve good hygiene

To prevent physical injury

To achieve awareness of needs

NURSING INTERVENTIONS

Nursing Treatments

Bathe in cool water
    OR
Apply a cold, moist compress
Apply calamine lotion
    OR
Apply cornstarch to the skin
    OR
Apply soda bicarbonate to the skin
    OR
Dust the skin with medicated powder
Do not allow skin surfaces to touch
Apply a bed cradle

Cover with lightweight blankets
Dress in lightweight clothing
Dress in minimum clothing
Avoid using rough-textured bed linens
Decrease drafts
Lubricate the skin with baby oil, bath oil, or body lotion
   OR
Lubricate the skin with petrolatum
Maintain adequate atmospheric humidity
Maintain a cool room temperature
Refrain from jarring the bed
Refrain from local heat applications
Use paper or transparent tape instead of adhesive on the skin
Refrain from using an alkaline soap on the skin
Withhold the drugs (causing the pruritus)

Nursing Observations
Observe for evidence of a favorable response to therapy

Health Teaching
Advise against scratching
Explain the causes of the health problem
Explain the reason and intended effect of the therapy

EVALUATION

See the evaluation criteria for each specific goal in Chapter 2.

Pustular Skin Discomfort (144,271)

ASSESSMENT

Subjective Data
Tenderness
Painful, sometimes

Objective Data
Color: yellowish, milky, orange, or green
Shape: round, pimple
Size: varied
Content: pus or lymph
Elevation: raised above the skin
Distribution: single or multiple
Other characteristics: often develop around hair follicles or in sweat glands

Related Data
Commonly Related Diseases:
Variola (smallpox, fifth day)
Scabies
Acne vulgaris

POSSIBLE ETIOLOGY

Capillary congestion. Bacterial invasion.

NURSING DIAGNOSIS

Pustular skin discomfort: a condition in which pustules irritate the skin

PLANNING

Patient Needs

Comfort

Cleanliness

Protection from physical harm

Increased learning

Primary Nurse-Patient Goals

To achieve comfort

To achieve good hygiene

To prevent physical injury, infection

To achieve awareness of needs

NURSING INTERVENTIONS

Nursing Treatments

Bathe in warm water

OR

Apply a warm, moist compress

Clean with hydrogen peroxide

OR

Clean with surgical soap

Apply an antibiotic ointment

Apply a bed cradle (if the lesions are widespread)

Cover with lightweight blankets

Dress in lightweight clothing

Dress in minimum clothing

Place on sterile linens (if the lesions are widespread)

Use paper or transparent tape instead of adhesive on the skin

Refrain from using a cream-based soap

Nursing Observations

Observe for evidence of a favorable response to therapy

Health Teaching

Advise against piercing lesions

Advise against squeezing the skin

Instruct to maintain skin cleanliness

Recommend the use of individual towels and washcloths

Explain the causes of the health problem

Explain the reason for and intended effect of the therapy

EVALUATION

See the evaluation criteria for each specific goal in Chapter 2.

Scale Skin Discomfort (271,430)

ASSESSMENT

Subjective Data

Itching

Objective Data

Color: yellow, silvery

Shape: irregular

Size: irregular
Content: horny mass, no fluid content
Elevation: raised above the skin
Distribution: often on the knees, elbows, scalp, and trunk
Other characteristics: lighter or darker than normal skin; often develop on
    other lesions

Related Data

Commonly Related Diseases:
Contact dermatitis
Eczematous dermatitis (eczema)
Epidermophytosis (athlete's foot)
Seborrheic dermatitis
Psoriasis
Ichthyosis

POSSIBLE ETIOLOGY

Sebaceous gland inflammation. Androgen-estrogen imbalance.

NURSING DIAGNOSIS

Scale skin discomfort: a condition in which scales irritate the skin

PLANNING

Patient Needs	**Primary Nurse-Patient Goals**
Comfort	To achieve comfort
Cleanliness	To achieve good hygiene
Protection from physical harm	To prevent physical injury
Increased learning	To achieve awareness of needs

NURSING INTERVENTIONS

Nursing Treatments
Apply a warm, moist compress
    OR
Bathe in warm water
Clean with surgical soap
Apply an antibiotic ointment
Maintain a normal room temperature

Health Teaching
Advise against exposure to intense heat
Advise against exposure to inclement weather
Advise against prolonged skin exposure to the sun
Explain the causes of the health problem
Explain the reason for and intended effect of the therapy

Medical Treatments Performed by Nurses
Give the prescribed drugs

EVALUATION

See the evaluation criteria for each specific goal in Chapter 2.

Uremic-Frost Skin Discomfort (391)

ASSESSMENT

Subjective Data

Itching

Objective Data

Color: white, frosty
Shape: none
Size: none
Content: no mass or fluid content
Elevation: none
Distribution: mostly on the face and hands, but can cover entire body
Other characteristics: salt appearance

Related Data

Commonly Related Diseases:
Renal failure

POSSIBLE ETIOLOGY

Tissue retention of urea and sodium chloride

NURSING DIAGNOSIS

Uremic-frost skin discomfort: a condition in which body salts infiltrate and irritate the skin

PLANNING

Patient Needs	**Primary Nurse-Patient Goals**
Water-salt balance	To maintain fluid and electrolyte balance
Comfort	To achieve comfort
Cleanliness	To achieve good hygiene
Protection from physical harm	To prevent physical injury
Increased learning	To achieve awareness of needs

NURSING INTERVENTIONS

Nursing Treatments

Bathe in vinegar water
Cover with lightweight blankets
Dress in lightweight clothing
Dress in minimum clothing
Instruct to increase fluid intake (if allowed)
Maintain a cool room temperature
Maintain dry skin

Nursing Observations

Observe for evidence of a favorable response to therapy

Health Teaching

Advise against scratching
Explain the causes of the health problem
Explain the reason for and intended effect of the therapy

EVALUATION

See the evaluation criteria for each specific goal in Chapter 2.

Vesicular Skin Discomfort
(144,145,271,430)

ASSESSMENT

Subjective Data
Itching
Burning, stinging, or neuralgic pain, sometimes

Objective Data
Color: clear, translucent
Shape: round
Size: small, less than 5 mm in diameter (when larger than 5 mm, they are bullae)
Content: serum or water
Elevation: raised above the skin
Distribution: single or multiple, in groups or in chains
Other characteristics: hard, horny crusts during the healing phase

Related Data
Commonly Related Diseases:
Varicella (chickenpox, late stage)
Pellagra (mid-stage)
Impetigo (early stage)
Variola (smallpox, third day)
Herpes simplex (cold sore)
Herpes zoster (shingles)
Eczematous dermatitis (eczema)
Pemphigus
Poison ivy
Poison oak
Prickly heat

POSSIBLE ETIOLOGY

Local fluid collection under the skin due to tissue injury. Excessive heat exposure. Viral infection.

NURSING DIAGNOSIS

Vesicular skin discomfort: a condition in which vesicles irritate the skin

PLANNING

Patient Needs	Primary Nurse-Patient Goals
Comfort	To achieve comfort
Cleanliness	To achieve good hygiene
Protection from physical harm	To prevent physical injury, infection
Increased learning	To achieve awareness of needs

NURSING INTERVENTIONS

Nursing Treatments
Bathe in warm water
   OR
Apply a warm, moist compress
Clean with surgical soap
Apply a saline compress (several times daily)
Apply an analgesic ointment
Apply a bed cradle (if the lesions are widespread)
Cover with lightweight blankets
Dress in lightweight clothing
Dress in minimum clothing
Decrease drafts
Do not allow skin surfaces to touch
Maintain a cool room temperature
Maintain dry skin
Place on sterile linens (if the lesions are widespread)
Refrain from jarring the bed
Refrain from tight bandaging

Nursing Observations
Observe for evidence of a favorable response to therapy

Health Teaching
Advise against piercing lesions
Advise against squeezing the lesion
Recommend the use of individual towels and washcloths
Explain the causes of the health problem
Explain the reason for and intended effect of the therapy

EVALUATION

See the evaluation criteria for each specific goal in Chapter 2.

Vesiculopustular Skin Discomfort (144,430)

ASSESSMENT

Subjective Data
Itching
Burning

Objective Data
Color: cloudy
Shape: round
Size: small
Content: pus
Elevation: raised above the skin
Distribution: single or multiple
Other characteristics: hard, horny crusts during the healing phase

Related Data
Commonly Related Diseases:
Impetigo (late stage)

POSSIBLE ETIOLOGY

Bacterial infection

NURSING DIAGNOSIS

Vesiculopustular skin discomfort: a condition in which vesiculopustules irritate the skin

PLANNING

Patient Needs	Primary Nurse-Patient Goals
Comfort	To achieve comfort
Cleanliness	To achieve good hygiene
Protection from physical harm	To prevent physical injury
Increased learning	To achieve awareness of needs

NURSING INTERVENTIONS

Nursing Treatments
Bathe in warm water
   OR
Apply a warm, moist compress
Clean with surgical soap
Apply an antibiotic ointment (three or four times daily)
Apply a bed cradle (if the lesions are widespread)
Cover with lightweight blankets
Dress in lightweight clothing
Dress in minimum clothing
Decrease drafts
Do not allow skin surfaces to touch
Maintain a cool room temperature
Maintain dry skin
Refrain from tight bandaging

Nursing Observations
Observe for evidence of a favorable response to therapy

Health Teaching
Advise against piercing lesions
Advise against squeezing the lesions
Recommend the use of individual towels and washcloths
Explain the causes of the health problem
Explain the reason for and intended effect of the therapy

EVALUATION

See the evaluation criteria for each specific goal in Chapter 2.

Urticaria Skin Discomfort (144,430)

ASSESSMENT

Subjective Data
Itching

Objective Data
Color: white or pink edges
Shape: somewhat round
Size: varied
Content: soft; does not pit on pressure
Elevation: raised above the skin
Distribution: localized or generalized
Other characteristics: swelling appearance

Related Data
Commonly Related Conditions:
Food allergy
Blood transfusion reaction
Insect bites

POSSIBLE ETIOLOGY

Allergic response. Local fluid accumulation. Sudden climate changes.

NURSING DIAGNOSIS

Urticaria skin discomfort: a condition in which wheals (hives) irritate the skin

PLANNING

Patient Needs	**Primary Nurse-Patient Goals**
Comfort	To achieve comfort
Cleanliness	To achieve good hygiene
Protection from physical harm	To prevent physical injury
Increased learning	To achieve awareness of needs

NURSING INTERVENTIONS

Nursing Treatments
Apply a cold, moist compress
   OR
Bathe in cool water
Apply calamine lotion
Apply a bed cradle (if the lesions are widespread)
Cover with lightweight blankets
Dress in lightweight clothing
Give nonprescription drugs (ExR) (antihistamine)
Maintain a cool room temperature

Nursing Observations
Observe for evidence of a favorable response to therapy

Health Teaching
Advise against scratching
Explain the causes of the health problem
Explain the reason for and intended effect of the therapy

EVALUATION

See the evaluation criteria for each specific goal in Chapter 2.

SKIN: POTENTIAL SKIN DISORDERS

Potential Skin Irritation

ASSESSMENT

Subjective Data
Desire to scratch the skin

Objective Data
Excessive powdering of the skin
Skin exposure to coarse or wet sheets or diapers
Overexposure to water
Prolonged touching of two skin surfaces
Exposure to environmental heat
Use of new cosmetics

Related Data
Commonly Related Conditions:
Prolonged bed rest

POSSIBLE ETIOLOGY

Poor skin care or health practices

NURSING DIAGNOSIS

Potential skin irritation: the possibility that the skin could become irritated or further irritated by external factors

PLANNING

Patient Needs	**Primary Nurse-Patient Goals**
Comfort	To achieve comfort
Cleanliness	To achieve good hygiene
Protection from physical harm	To prevent physical injury
Increased learning	To achieve awareness of needs

NURSING INTERVENTIONS

Nursing Treatments
Avoid using rough-textured bed linens
Change the wet diaper immediately
Cover the hands with mittens

Cover with lightweight blankets
Do not allow skin surfaces to touch
Maintain a cool room temperature
Maintain dry, clean linen
Maintain dry skin
Place on a sheepskin
Refrain from pulling the patient across the sheets
Refrain from simultaneously powdering and lubricating the skin
Use paper or transparent tape instead of adhesive on the skin

Nursing Observations
Observe for evidence of a favorable response to therapy

Health Teaching
Advise against prolonged skin exposure to water
Advise against scratching
Advise limited use of powder on the infant's skin
Explain the importance of testing cosmetics for skin irritation
Instruct to maintain skin cleanliness
Explain how to correctly wash diapers
Explain the causes of the health problem
Explain the reason for and intended effect of the therapy

EVALUATION

See the evaluation criteria for each specific goal in Chapter 2.

SKIN: SPECIFIC SKIN NECROSIS

Decubitus Ulcer (71,271,391)

ASSESSMENT

Subjective Data
Pain

Objective Data
Color: deep redness
Size: small or large
Depth: surface or deep
Drainage: serous fluid, pus, or blood
Location: on buttocks, bony prominences, or other areas receiving pro-
    longed pressure
Other characteristics: raw appearance

Related Data
Commonly Related Conditions:
Prolonged bed rest
Immobility

Commonly Related Diseases:
Cerebral vascular accident
Cervical, thoracic, or lumbar spinal cord injury

Poliomyelitis
Parkinson's disease
Subarachnoid hemorrhage

POSSIBLE ETIOLOGY

Progressive destruction of cutaneous and underlying tissue. Prolonged local oxygen deficiency. Chemical injury. Prolonged pressure in one tissue area.

NURSING DIAGNOSIS

Decubitus ulcer (skin breakdown) (bedsore): an area of broken skin tissue

PLANNING

Patient Needs	Primary Nurse-Patient Goals
Circulation	To maintain oxygen to all cells
Comfort	To achieve comfort
Cleanliness	To achieve good hygiene
Protection from physical harm	To prevent physical injury, infection
Increased learning	To achieve awareness of needs

NURSING INTERVENTIONS

Nursing Treatments
Clean with hydrogen peroxide
   OR
Clean with surgical soap
Apply a saline compress
   OR
Soak in saline solution
   OR
Place in a whirlpool bath
Apply tincture of benzoin (to the tissue around the ulcer)
Massage vigorously (the tissue around the ulcer)
Apply a sterile dressing
   OR
Expose the decubitus wound to air
Apply heat by a gooseneck lamp
   OR
Apply a heat cradle
Change the patient's position frequently
Place on an alternating pressure mattress
   OR
Place on a CircOlectric bed
   OR
Place on a flotation mattress
   OR
Place on a Stryker frame
Place on a sheepskin
   OR
Place on a silicone pad

OR

Place on a split-foam mattress

OR

Place on a polyurethane foam pad

Place on sterile linens (if needed)

Refrain from giving local cold applications

Health Teaching

Instruct to maintain skin cleanliness

Teach decubitus ulcer care

Explain the causes of the health problem

Explain the reason for and intended effect of the therapy

EVALUATION

See the evaluation criteria for each specific goal in Chapter 2.

Stasis Ulcer

ASSESSMENT

Subjective Data

Painful, sometimes

Objective Data

Color: black; cyanotic

Size: small or large

Depth: fairly deep

Drainage: pus

Location: usually the foot or leg

Other characteristics: inflammation

Related Data

Commonly Related Diseases:

Diabetes mellitus

Third-degree burn

Sickle cell anemia

Thrombophlebitis

Varicose veins

Arteriosclerosis

Atherosclerosis

POSSIBLE ETIOLOGY

Severely impaired blood flow to tissue. Trauma. Arterial degeneration changes. Cell death.

NURSING DIAGNOSIS

Stasis ulcer: an open sore on a skin area of impaired circulation

PLANNING

Patient Needs	**Primary Nurse-Patient Goals**
Circulation	To maintain oxygen to all cells
Rest	To achieve rest

Comfort

Cleanliness

Protection from physical harm

Increased learning

To achieve comfort

To achieve good hygiene

To prevent physical injury

To achieve awareness of needs

NURSING INTERVENTIONS

Nursing Treatments

Clean with hydrogen peroxide

OR

Clean with surgical soap

Apply a saline compress

OR

Soak in saline solution

Apply an antibiotic ointment

Apply a sterile dressing

OR

Expose the draining wound to air

Apply heat by a gooseneck lamp

OR

Apply a heat cradle

Elevate the affected body part

Refrain from giving local cold applications

Nursing Observations

Observe for evidence of a favorable response to therapy

Health Teaching

Explain the causes of the health problem

Explain the reason for and intended effect of the therapy

EVALUATION

See the evaluation criteria for each specific goal in Chapter 2.

Threatening Decubitus Ulcer (271)

ASSESSMENT

Objective Data

Color: mild redness

Size: small or large

Depth: skin surface

Drainage: none

Location: on buttocks or bony prominences

Other characteristics: redness disappears on pressure application

Related Data

Commonly Related Conditions:

Prolonged bed rest

Immobility

Commonly Related Diseases:

Cerebral vascular accident

Cervical, thoracic, or lumbar spinal cord injury

Poliomyelitis
Parkinson's disease

POSSIBLE ETIOLOGY

Impaired local circulation. Prolonged pressure on tissue. Chemical injury.

NURSING DIAGNOSIS

Threatening decubitus ulcer (threatening skin breakdown) (threatening bedsore): a red, irritated skin area that could break down and form a decubitus ulcer

PLANNING

Patient Needs	Primary Nurse-Patient Goals
Circulation	To maintain oxygen to all cells
Comfort	To achieve comfort
Stimulation	To maintain stimulation
Cleanliness	To achieve good hygiene
Protection from physical harm	To prevent physical injury
Increased learning	To achieve awareness of needs

NURSING INTERVENTIONS

Nursing Treatments
Ambulate the patient (as much as possible)
Avoid using rough-textured bed linens
Change the patient's position frequently
Clean with castile or lanolin soap
     OR
Clean with surgical soap
Refrain from using an alkaline soap on the skin
Massage vigorously (the affected tissue)
Lubricate the skin with cocoa butter, glycerine, lanolin, mineral oil, or olive
     oil
Maintain dry, clean linen
Maintain wrinkle-free sheets
Pad the bony prominences
Place on an alternating pressure mattress
Place on a sheepskin
     OR
Place on a silicone pad
     OR
Place on a split-foam mattress
     OR
Place on a polyurethane foam pad
Refrain from simultaneously powdering and lubricating the skin

Nursing Observations
Observe for evidence of a favorable response to therapy

Health Teaching
Instruct to maintain skin cleanliness
Instruct to inspect the skin
Instruct to lubricate the skin
Instruct not to use rubber rings and doughnuts
Instruct to do wheelchair pushups
Instruct to maintain skin dryness
Recommend the use of a sheepskin
Explain the causes of the health problem
Explain the reason for and intended effect of the therapy

EVALUATION

See the evaluation criteria for each specific goal in Chapter 2.

Tissue Sloughing

ASSESSMENT

Objective Data
Color: normal skin tone
Size: small or large
Depth: surface
Drainage: some
Location: wound area
Other characteristics: skin cracks and separates from the wound edges,
    leaving skin patches in the middle

Related Data
Commonly Related Diseases:
First-, second-, or third-degree burns
Phlebothrombosis

POSSIBLE ETIOLOGY

Tissue cell death due to any severe injury. Ischemia. Drug infiltration into tissues. Infection, inflammation. As burned skin dries, a stiff skin slough forms from coagulated protein. Bacterial autolysis initiates the skin's separation from the wound.

NURSING DIAGNOSIS

Tissue sloughing: separation of necrotic tissue from living tissue

PLANNING

Patient Needs	Primary Nurse-Patient Goals
Comfort	To achieve comfort
Cleanliness	To achieve good hygiene
Protection from physical harm	To prevent physical injury, infection
Increased learning	To achieve awareness of needs

NURSING INTERVENTIONS

Nursing Treatments
Clean with hydrogen peroxide
   OR
Clean with surgical soap
Apply a saline compress
   OR
Soak in saline solution
   OR
Place in a whirlpool bath
Apply an antibiotic ointment
Apply a sterile dressing
   OR
Expose the draining wound to air
Do not allow skin surfaces to touch
Maintain adequate atmospheric humidity (40%–50% for burns)
Maintain a normal room temperature
Place on sterile linens
Refrain from giving local cold applications

Nursing Observations
Observe for evidence of a favorable response to therapy

Health Teaching
Advise against pulling off dead skin or scabs
Instruct to maintain skin cleanliness
Explain the causes of the health problem
Explain the reason for and intended effect of the therapy

EVALUATION

See the evaluation criteria for each specific goal in Chapter 2.

SKIN: NONSPECIFIC SKIN NECROSIS

Ulcerated Skin Tissue (271,391,430)

ASSESSMENT

Subjective Data
Tenderness
Pain

Objective Data
Color: deep redness
Size: small or large
Depth: surface or deep
Drainage: serous fluid, pus, or blood

Location: anywhere on the body
Other characteristics: raw appearance

Related Data
Commonly Related Conditions:
Chloral hydrate addiction
Bed rest
Immobility

POSSIBLE ETIOLOGY

Mechanical or chemical tissue trauma. Pathogenic organism invasion into tissues.

NURSING DIAGNOSIS

Ulcerated skin tissue: the presence of an open sore on skin tissue

PLANNING

Patient Needs	**Primary Nurse-Patient Goals**
Comfort	To achieve comfort
Cleanliness	To achieve good hygiene
Protection from physical harm	To prevent physical injury
Increased learning	To achieve awareness of needs

NURSING INTERVENTIONS

Nursing Treatments
Clean with hydrogen peroxide
    OR
Clean with surgical soap
Apply a warm, moist compress
    OR
Soak in saline solution
Apply an antibiotic ointment
Apply a sterile dressing
    OR
Expose the draining wound to air

Nursing Observations
Observe for evidence of a favorable response to therapy

Health Teaching
Advise against pulling off scabs (as healing occurs)
Explain the causes of the health problem
Explain the reason for and intended effect of the therapy

EVALUATION

See the evaluation criteria for each specific goal in Chapter 2.

SKIN: POTENTIAL SKIN NECROSIS

Potential Decubitus Ulcer (70)

ASSESSMENT

Objective Data
Stuporous
Emaciation
Incontinence
Debilitation
Therapeutic or paralytic immobility
Thin skin
Bone projections or protrusions

Related Data

Commonly Related Conditions:
Prolonged bed rest
Immobility

Commonly Related Diseases:
Cerebral vascular accident
Cervical, thoracic, or lumbar spinal cord injury
Parkinson's disease
Meningocele
Hydrocephalus
Astrocytoma
Meningioma
Medulloblastoma

POSSIBLE ETIOLOGY

Prolonged pressure on tissue. Impaired circulation. Chemical injury.

NURSING DIAGNOSIS

Potential decubitus ulcer (potential skin breakdown) (potential bedsore):
the probability that skin could undergo tissue destruction in a particular
area

PLANNING

Patient Needs	**Primary Nurse-Patient Goals**
Activity, exercise	To achieve activity and exercise
Stimulation	To maintain sensory function and stimulation
Cleanliness	To achieve good hygiene
Protection from physical harm	To prevent physical injury, infection
Increased learning	To achieve awareness of needs

NURSING INTERVENTIONS

Nursing Treatments
Ambulate the patient (as much as possible)

Change the patient's position frequently
Lubricate the skin with baby oil, bath oil, or body lotion
Maintain dry skin
Avoid using rough-textured bed linens
Maintain dry, clean linen
Maintain wrinkle-free sheets
Massage bony prominences
Pad the bony prominences
Pad the bedpan
Place on an alternating pressure mattress
    OR
Place on a CircOlectric bed
    OR
Place on a flotation mattress
    OR
Place on a Stryker frame
Place on a sheepskin
    OR
Place on a silicone pad
    OR
Place on a split-foam mattress
    OR
Place on a polyurethane foam pad
Refrain from pulling the patient across the sheets
Refrain from simultaneously powdering and lubricating the skin
Refrain from tight bandaging
Use paper or transparent tape instead of adhesive on the skin

Nursing Observations

Inspect the skin for breakdown

Health Teaching

Instruct to maintain skin cleanliness
Instruct to inspect the skin
Instruct to lubricate the skin
Explain how to pad bony prominences
Instruct not to use rubber rings and doughnuts
Instruct to do wheelchair pushups
Instruct to maintain skin dryness
Recommend the use of a sheepskin
Describe those symptoms which should be reported (skin redness, irritation)
Explain the causes of the health problem
Explain the reason for and intended effect of the therapy

EVALUATION

See the evaluation criteria for each specific goal in Chapter 2.

SKIN: IRREGULAR SKIN TEXTURE
Dermal Coarseness
ASSESSMENT
Objective Data
Thick skin
Heavily lined
Lacks normal elasticity
Leathery appearance

Related Data
Commonly Related Diseases:
None
  OR
Ichthyosis
Leprosy
Myxedema
Scleroderma
Third-degree burns
Elephantiasis

POSSIBLE ETIOLOGY

Changes in small arterioles. Collagen fibrosis. Epidermal atrophy. In granulation tissue, there is development of new capillaries from already existing capillaries, with the eventual combing of capillary loops and cells to form a thick scar tissue and replace lost skin.

NURSING DIAGNOSIS

Dermal coarseness: rough-textured skin

PLANNING

Patient Needs	Primary Nurse-Patient Goals
Water-salt balance	To maintain fluid and electrolyte balance
Comfort	To achieve comfort
Cleanliness	To achieve good hygiene
Protection from physical harm	To prevent physical injury
Increased learning	To achieve awareness of needs

NURSING INTERVENTIONS

Nursing Treatments
Clean with castile or lanolin soap
Refrain from using an alkaline soap on the skin
Refrain from cleansing with alcohol
Lubricate the skin with cocoa butter, glycerine, lanolin, mineral oil, or olive oil
Increase fluid intake to about 2000 cc daily

Nursing Observations
Observe for evidence of a favorable response to therapy

Health Teaching
Advise against prolonged skin exposure to the sun
Advise against prolonged skin exposure to water
Instruct to maintain skin cleanliness
Instruct to lubricate the skin
Explain the causes of the health problem
Explain the reason for and intended effect of the therapy

EVALUATION

See the evaluation criteria for each specific goal in Chapter 2.

Dermal Fragility

ASSESSMENT

Objective Data
Thin skin
Visible veins and arteries
Light color
Tense, taut skin

Related Data
Commonly Related Conditions:
Edema
Ascites
Commonly Related Diseases:
None
   OR
Cushing's disease
Laennec's cirrhosis
Diffuse scleroderma

POSSIBLE ETIOLOGY

A congenital decrease in the number of tissue cells

NURSING DIAGNOSIS

Dermal fragility: skin that is easily injured or irritated

PLANNING

Patient Needs	**Primary Nurse-Patient Goals**
Comfort	To achieve comfort
Cleanliness	To achieve good hygiene
Protection from physical harm	To prevent physical injury
Increased learning	To achieve awareness of needs

NURSING INTERVENTIONS

Nursing Treatments
Clean with castile or lanolin soap
Refrain from using an alkaline soap on the skin
Refrain from cleansing with alcohol
Lubricate the skin with baby oil, bath oil, or body lotion
Avoid using rough-textured bed linens
Maintain dry, clean linen
Maintain wrinkle-free sheets
Massage gently
Use paper or transparent tape instead of adhesive on the skin

Nursing Observations
Observe for evidence of a favorable response to therapy

Health Teaching
Advise against prolonged skin exposure to the sun
Advise against prolonged skin exposure to water
Instruct to maintain skin cleanliness
Instruct to lubricate the skin
Inform that the skin should be protected from windburn
Explain the causes of the health problem
Explain the reason for and intended effect of the therapy

EVALUATION

See the evaluation criteria for each specific goal in Chapter 2.

SKIN: POTENTIAL ALTERED SKIN TONE

Potential Skin Striae

ASSESSMENT

Objective Data
Rapid weight gain
Poor skin lubrication

Related Data
Commonly Related Conditions:
Ascites
Pregnancy
Commonly Related Diseases:
Cushing's disease

POSSIBLE ETIOLOGY

Prolonged skin stretching

NURSING DIAGNOSIS

Potential skin striae: the probability that the skin will develop depressed
grooves in the breasts, thighs, or abdomen

PLANNING

Patient Needs

Protection from physical harm

Increased learning

Primary Nurse-Patient Goals

To prevent physical injury

To achieve awareness of needs

NURSING INTERVENTIONS

Nursing Treatments

Lubricate the skin with cocoa butter, glycerine, lanolin, mineral oil, or olive
   oil

Nursing Observations

Observe for evidence of a favorable response to therapy

Health Teaching

Explain the causes of the health problem

Instruct to lubricate the skin

Explain the reason for and intended effect of the therapy

EVALUATION

See the evaluation criteria for each specific goal in Chapter 2.

SKIN: POTENTIAL SKIN INJURY FROM ALTERED PIGMENTATION

Potential Skin Injury Related to Decreased Pigmentation (145,271)

ASSESSMENT

Objective Data

Very fair skin

White skin patches evident against normal skin color

Related Data

Skin is frequently exposed to sunlight

Commonly Related Conditions:

Vitiligo

Albinism

Commonly Related Diseases:

Addison's disease

Hyperthyroidism

Hypoparathyroidism

Pernicious anemia

POSSIBLE ETIOLOGY

The presence of genetic skin defects in melanocyte structure resulting in
inability to form normal amounts of melanin pigmentation

NURSING DIAGNOSIS

Potential skin injury related to decreased pigmentation: the possibility of
damage to skin that is more susceptible to injury from sunlight because of
lack of skin color

PLANNING

Patient Needs	**Primary Nurse-Patient Goals**
Comfort	To achieve comfort
Protection from physical harm	To prevent physical injury
Increased learning	To achieve awareness of needs

NURSING INTERVENTIONS

Nursing Observations
Observe for evidence of a favorable response to therapy

Health Teaching
Explain the causes of the health problem
Advise against prolonged skin exposure to the sun
Explain how to adjust clothing to meet health problems (wear long sleeves, hats, and pants to cover the skin)
Instruct to lubricate the skin

EVALUATION

See the evaluation criteria for each specific goal in Chapter 2.

Potential Skin Injury Related to Increased Pigmentation (145,271)

ASSESSMENT

Objective Data
Yellowish brown pregnancy mask
Brownish butterfly marking on the nose and cheeks
Tan freckle spots
Reddish brown or copper skin
Strawberry, ruby, or port-wine skin discoloration

Related Data
Skin is frequently exposed to sunlight
Commonly Related Conditions:
Pregnancy
Commonly Related Diseases:
Lupus erythematosus
Addison's disease
Wilson's disease

POSSIBLE ETIOLOGY

Erythrocytes escaping from blood vessels into skin tissue. Dilatation of skin blood vessels. Endocrine imbalance. Drug side effects (progesterone). Abnormal epidermal copper deposits resulting from abnormal copper metabolism. Congenital vascular malformation and/or incomplete development of embryonic tissue (in angiomas).

NURSING DIAGNOSIS

Potential skin injury related to increased pigmentation: the possibility of damage to skin that is more susceptible to injury from sunlight because of increased skin color

PLANNING

Patient Needs	**Primary Nurse-Patient Goals**
Comfort	To achieve comfort
Protection from physical harm	To prevent physical injury
Increased learning	To achieve awareness of needs

NURSING INTERVENTIONS

Nursing Observations
Observe for evidence of a favorable response to therapy

Health Teaching
Explain the causes of the health problem
Advise against prolonged skin exposure to the sun
Explain how to adjust clothing to meet health problems (wear long sleeves, hats, and pants to cover the skin)

EVALUATION

See the evaluation criteria for each specific goal in Chapter 2.

SKIN: DISRUPTION OF SKIN INTACTNESS

Inadequate Wound Closure

ASSESSMENT

Objective Data
Unsutured tracheostomy wound following removal of the tracheostomy
    tube
Unsutured chest wound following removal of chest tubes

Related Data
Commonly Related Conditions:
Airway obstruction

Commonly Related Diseases:
Poliomyelitis
Cervical spinal cord injury
Cerebral vascular accident
Myasthenia gravis
Pneumothorax

POSSIBLE ETIOLOGY

An effort at natural wound healing without the support of sutures

NURSING DIAGNOSIS

Inadequate wound closure: the presence of a surgical wound that has not been sutured and is in the healing process

PLANNING

Patient Needs	**Primary Nurse-Patient Goals**
Comfort	To achieve comfort
Cleanliness	To achieve good hygiene
Protection from physical harm	To prevent infection
Increased learning	To achieve awareness of needs

NURSING INTERVENTIONS

Nursing Treatments

Clean with hydrogen peroxide
   OR
Clean with surgical soap
Compress the wound edges together
   AND
Use sterile adhesive strips for wound closure
Apply an antibiotic ointment
Apply a sterile dressing
Change the dressing frequently
Apply a warm, moist compress (if the area becomes crusted)
Avoid placing tension on the wound
Handle gently

Nursing Observations

Inspect for edema
Inspect for inflammation
Inspect the wound dressing frequently
Inspect for drainage
Observe for delayed healing

Health Teaching

Describe those symptoms which should be reported (pain, drainage)
Inform that cleanliness is basic to health
Teach how to clean and dress a wound
Explain the reason for and intended effect of the therapy

EVALUATION

See the evaluation criteria for each specific goal in Chapter 2.

SKIN: POTENTIAL DISRUPTION OF SKIN INTACTNESS

Potential Incisional Tension

ASSESSMENT
Objective Data
Abdominal distention

Persistent coughing
Elimination straining
Heavy lifting
Jarring body movements

Related Data
Commonly Related Conditions:
Any surgical procedure

Commonly Related Diseases:
Trauma-related wounds

POSSIBLE ETIOLOGY

Indulgence in activities that place tension on wounds

NURSING DIAGNOSIS

Potential incisional tension: the possibility that severe tension could be placed on a wound and disrupt its closure

PLANNING

Patient Needs
Protection from physical harm
Increased learning

Primary Nurse-Patient Goals
To prevent physical injury
To achieve awareness of needs

NURSING INTERVENTIONS

Nursing Treatments
Handle gently
Approach unhurriedly
Avoid placing tension on the wound
Change the patient's position gradually
Refrain from jarring the bed
Elevate the head
      AND   } (for abdominal incisions)
Do not place in the flat position
Ambulate the patient (as much as possible to reduce abdominal distention)
Refrain from giving enemas (when abdominal wounds exist)

Nursing Observations
Observe for dehiscence
Observe for complaints of pain

Health Teaching
Instruct to change position gradually
Inform that coughing should be avoided
Inform that elimination straining should be avoided
Inform that heavy lifting should be avoided

EVALUATION

See the evaluation criteria for each specific goal in Chapter 2.

SKIN: HEALING

Immobility Requirement
Related to Tissue Healing

ASSESSMENT

Subjective Data
Discomfort

Objective Data
Unhealed wound or bone at a joint or vertebral area
Skin graft in the healing stage

Related Data
Commonly Related Conditions:
Puncture, incisional, or laceration wounds
Skin graft
Commonly Related Diseases:
Bone fracture
Second- or third-degree burns

POSSIBLE ETIOLOGY

A wound that cannot heal correctly unless stabilized in a fixed position

NURSING DIAGNOSIS

Immobility requirement related to tissue healing: the need to maintain a fixed body position so that healing tissue can knit together

PLANNING

Patient Needs
Protection from physical harm
Increased learning

Primary Nurse-Patient Goals
To prevent physical injury
To achieve awareness of needs

NURSING INTERVENTIONS

Nursing Treatments
Apply an arm sling
    OR
Apply an elastic bandage
    OR
Apply a supportive splint
    OR
Position with pillows
    OR
Position with sandbags
Position comfortably
Refrain from jarring the bed
Provide radio and television for diversion
Provide frequent patient contact

Nursing Observations
Observe for fatigue
Observe for restlessness

Health Teaching
Explain the reason for and intended effect of the therapy

EVALUATION

See the evaluation criteria for each specific goal in Chapter 2.

SKIN: SKIN BITES

Animal Bite (271)

ASSESSMENT

Subjective Data
Pain

Objective Data
Break in the skin
Bleeding
Deep or superficial
Teeth marks are frequently evident

Related Data
Inflicted by cat, dog, squirrel, mouse, rat, etc.
Commonly Related Diseases:
Rabies (hydrophobia)

POSSIBLE ETIOLOGY

Animal contact. Animal self-defense.

NURSING DIAGNOSIS

Animal bite: a wound inflicted by a small animal

PLANNING

Patient Needs	**Primary Nurse-Patient Goals**
Rest	To achieve rest
Comfort	To achieve comfort
Cleanliness	To achieve good hygiene
Protection from physical harm	To prevent physical injury, infection
Freedom from pain	To achieve comfort
Increased learning	To achieve awareness of needs and/or use of resources

NURSING INTERVENTIONS

Nursing Treatments
Clean with antiseptic solution
  OR

Clean with hydrogen peroxide
OR
Clean with surgical soap
Soak in Betadine solution
Apply an antibiotic ointment
Apply a sterile dressing
Encourage adequate rest
Give nonprescription drugs (ExR) (analgesics)
Confine suspected infected animals
Make a referral (to the public health department)

Nursing Observations
Inspect the mouth for abnormal (excessive) salivation
Observe for complaints of malaise
Observe for complaints of pain (laryngeal spasms)
Observe for emotional instability (especially mental depression)
Observe for restlessness
Monitor the oral temperature (for fever)

Health Teaching
Teach how to clean and dress a wound
Instruct not to kill animals suspected of being infected
Explain the reason for and intended effect of the therapy

Medical Treatments Performed by Nurses
Give the prescribed drugs (rabies immunization)

EVALUATION

See the evaluation criteria for each specific goal in Chapter 2.

Human Bite

ASSESSMENT

Subjective Data
Painful

Objective Data
Break in the skin
Bleeding
Deep or superficial
Teeth marks are frequently evident

Related Data
Inflicted by a highly agitated person
Commonly Related Diseases:
None

POSSIBLE ETIOLOGY

Contact with a person who is emotionally disturbed

NURSING DIAGNOSIS

Human bite: a wound inflicted by human teeth

PLANNING

Patient Needs
Comfort
Cleanliness
Protection from physical harm
Freedom from pain
Increased learning

Primary Nurse-Patient Goals
To achieve comfort
To achieve good hygiene
To prevent physical injury, infection
To achieve comfort
To achieve awareness of needs

NURSING INTERVENTIONS

Nursing Treatments
Clean with antiseptic solution
   OR
Clean with hydrogen peroxide
   OR
Clean with surgical soap
Soak in Betadine solution
Apply an antibiotic ointment
Apply a sterile dressing
Give nonprescription drugs (ExR) (analgesics)

Nursing Observations
Inspect for bleeding
Inspect for edema
Monitor the oral temperature (for fever)
Obtain a bacterial culture (of the wound)

Health Teaching
Teach how to clean and dress a wound
Explain the reason for and intended effect of the therapy

EVALUATION

See the evaluation criteria for each specific goal in Chapter 2.

Insect Bite (271)

ASSESSMENT

Subjective Data
Stinging, burning pain
Itching

Objective Data
Swelling
Redness

Related Data
Inflicted by bee, wasp, yellow jacket, mosquito, or fly
Commonly Related Diseases:
Malaria
Poliomyelitis

POSSIBLE ETIOLOGY

Contact with an insect

NURSING DIAGNOSIS

Insect bite: a wound inflicted by a small invertebrate animal

PLANNING

Patient Needs	**Primary Nurse-Patient Goals**
Comfort	To achieve comfort
Cleanliness	To achieve good hygiene
Protection from physical harm	To prevent physical injury, infection
Freedom from pain	To achieve comfort
Increased learning	To achieve awareness of needs

NURSING INTERVENTIONS

Nursing Treatments

Apply a cold, moist compress
   OR
Apply an ice bag
   OR
Apply soda bicarbonate to the skin
Clean with alcohol
   OR
Clean with antiseptic solution
   OR
Clean with surgical soap
Elevate the extremity
Give nonprescription drugs (ExR) (analgesics)
Remove the insect stinger

Nursing Observations

Inspect for bleeding
Inspect for edema
Inspect for inflammation
Observe for complaints of itching

Health Teaching

Explain the reason for and intended effect of the therapy

EVALUATION

See the evaluation criteria for each specific goal in Chapter 2.

Nonpoisonous Snakebite (192,271)

ASSESSMENT

Subjective Data
Little pain

Objective Data
No fang marks on the skin
Minimal swelling within 30 minutes

POSSIBLE ETIOLOGY
Self-defense on the part of the snake

NURSING DIAGNOSIS
Nonpoisonous snakebite: a skin wound inflicted by a nonpoisonous snake

PLANNING

Patient Needs	**Primary Nurse-Patient Goals**
Comfort	To achieve comfort
Cleanliness	To achieve good hygiene
Protection from physical harm	To prevent physical injury, infection
Freedom from pain	To achive comfort
Increased learning	To achieve awareness of needs

NURSING INTERVENTIONS

Nursing Treatments
Attend the patient constantly
Immobilize the affected body part
Apply a tourniquet between the extremity wound and the body
Position the affected limb lower than the rest of the body
Clean with alcohol
    OR
Clean with antiseptic solution
    OR
Clean with surgical soap
Apply an antibiotic ointment
Apply a sterile dressing
Apply a cold, moist compress   ⎫
    OR   ⎬ (to the wound)
Apply an ice bag   ⎭
Cover with lightweight blankets
Place on complete bed rest
Place in the flat position
Suction the snake venom

Nursing Observations
Inspect for inflammation
Observe for complaints of pain
Observe the level of consciousness
Observe for shock

Health Teaching
Explain the reason for and intended effect of the therapy

Medical Treatments Performed by Nurses
Give the prescribed drugs (antibiotics, tetanus antitoxin)

EVALUATION
See the evaluation criteria for each specific goal in Chapter 2.

Nonpoisonous Spider Bite (192,271)

ASSESSMENT

Subjective Data
Stinging pain

Objective Data
Local swelling

Related Data
Spider may or may not be present
Commonly Related Diseases:
None

POSSIBLE ETIOLOGY

Contact with a spider

NURSING DIAGNOSIS

Nonpoisonous spider bite: a skin wound inflicted by a nonpoisonous arachnid

PLANNING

Patient Needs	Primary Nurse-Patient Goals
Comfort	To achieve comfort
Cleanliness	To achieve good hygiene
Protection from physical harm	To prevent physical injury, infection
Freedom from pain	To achieve comfort
Increased learning	To achieve awareness of needs

NURSING INTERVENTIONS

Nursing Treatments
Apply a cold, moist compress
   OR
Apply an ice bag
Clean with antiseptic solution
   OR
Clean with hydrogen peroxide
   OR
Clean with surgical soap
Apply soda bicarbonate to the skin
   OR
Apply calamine lotion

Nursing Observations
Inspect for bleeding
Inspect for edema
Inspect for inflammation
Observe for shock
Observe for complaints of pain

Health Teaching
Explain the reason for and intended effect of the therapy

EVALUATION

See the evaluation criteria for each specific goal in Chapter 2.

Tick Bite (271)

ASSESSMENT

Objective Data
Examination reveals tick burrowed into the skin
Paralysis if bite is in the neck

Related Data
Commonly Related Diseases:
Rocky Mountain spotted fever
Tularemia

POSSIBLE ETIOLOGY

Contact with ticks

NURSING DIAGNOSIS

Tick bite: a wound inflicted by a tick

PLANNING

Patient Needs	**Primary Nurse-Patient Goals**
Comfort	To achieve comfort
Cleanliness	To achieve good hygiene
Protection from physical harm	To prevent physical injury
Freedom from pain	To achieve comfort
Increased learning	To achieve awareness of needs and/or use of resources

NURSING INTERVENTIONS

Nursing Treatments
Apply a greasy substance over the tick
    OR
Place a smoldering match on the imbedded tick
Remove the tick with tweezers
Apply a cold, moist compress
Clean with antiseptic solution
    OR
Clean with surgical soap
Elevate the extremity

Nursing Observations
Observe for chills
Inspect for bleeding
Inspect for edema

Inspect for inflammation
Observe for complaints of headache
Observe for complaints of malaise
Monitor the oral temperature (for fever)

Health Teaching
Describe those symptoms which should be reported (chills, headache, malaise)
Explain the reason for and intended effect of the therapy

EVALUATION

See the evaluation criteria for each specific goal in Chapter 2.

SKIN: EMERGENCY SKIN BITE

Emergency Phase Poisonous Snakebite (192,271)

ASSESSMENT

Subjective Data
Immediate, intense pain
Nausea
Dyspnea

Objective Data
Two small fang marks on the skin
Rows of scratches on the skin
Swelling
Tachycardia
Vomiting
Shock

Related Data
The snake has bands of red, black, and yellow across its body
Commonly Related Conditions:
Snake poisoning

POSSIBLE ETIOLOGY

Self-defense on the part of the snake

NURSING DIAGNOSIS

Emergency phase poisonous snakebite: the need for immediate health care following a bite by a poisonous snake

PLANNING

Patient Needs	Primary Nurse-Patient Goals
Rest	To achieve rest
Comfort	To achieve comfort
Cleanliness	To achieve good hygiene

Protection from physical harm   To prevent physical injury, infection

Freedom from pain   To achieve comfort

Increased learning   To achieve awareness of needs

NURSING INTERVENTIONS

Nursing Treatments

Attend the patient constantly

Immobilize the affected body part

Apply a tourniquet between the extremity wound and the body

Position the affected limb lower than the rest of the body

Clean with alcohol

OR

Clean with antiseptic solution

OR

Clean with surgical soap

Apply an antibiotic ointment

Apply a sterile dressing

Apply a cold, moist compress

Apply an ice bag (to the wound)

Cover with lightweight blankets

Place on complete bed rest

Place in the flat position

Refrain from giving oral stimulants

Suction the snake venom

Give tetanus toxoid (ET)

Nursing Observations

Inspect for inflammation

Observe for complaints of pain (severe)

Observe the level of consciousness

Observe for shock

Health Teaching

Explain the reason for and intended effect of the therapy

Medical Treatments Performed by Nurses

Give the prescribed drugs (antivenom serum)

EVALUATION

See the evaluation criteria for each specific goal in Chapter 2.

Emergency Phase Poisonous
Spider Bite (192,271)

ASSESSMENT

Subjective Data

Pain begins 15–60 minutes after the bite

Pain moves to the extremities, then to the abdomen

Headache

Numbness of the hands and feet

Objective Data
Rigid abdomen
Labored respirations
Vomiting
Sweating
Excessive salivation
Hyperactive reflexes
Twitching
Tremors
Local tissue necrosis
Two small puncture marks on the skin (black widow spider)
A black spot on the skin (brown recluse spider)

Related Data (Spider or Scorpion)
Coal black with red hourglass design on underside (black widow spider)
Black with red legs (red-legged widow spider)
Brown and hairy, legspread about 4.5 inches (tarantula)
Brown, with legs about 1.5 inches long (brown recluse spider)
Crablike feet and a tail (scorpion)

POSSIBLE ETIOLOGY

Contact with the spider

NURSING DIAGNOSIS

Emergency phase poisonous spider bite: a skin wound inflicted by a poisonous arachnid

PLANNING

Patient Needs	**Primary Nurse-Patient Goals**
Comfort	To achieve comfort
Cleanliness	To achieve good hygiene
Protection from physical harm	To prevent physical injury, infection
Freedom from pain	To achieve comfort
Increased learning	To achieve awareness of needs and/or use of resources

NURSING INTERVENTIONS

Nursing Treatments
Apply a cold, moist compress
   OR
Apply an ice bag
Give hot coffee
Apply a tourniquet between the extremity wound and the body
Position the affected limb lower than the rest of the body
Suction the spider venom
Clean with antiseptic solution
   OR
Clean with hydrogen peroxide
   OR
Clean with surgical soap

Apply soda bicarbonate to the skin
  OR
Apply calamine lotion
Make a referral (to a physician or an emergency room)

Nursing Observations
Inspect for bleeding
Inspect for edema
Inspect for inflammation
Observe for shock
Observe for complaints of pain

Health Teaching
Explain the reason for and intended effect of the therapy

Medical Treatments Performed by Nurses
Give the prescribed drugs (antivenom serum)

EVALUATION

See the evaluation criteria for each specific goal in Chapter 2.

INTEGUMENT THERMAL INJURY: RESUSCITATION PERIOD FOLLOWING THERMAL INJURY

Note: Many of the nursing diagnoses associated with burn injuries are also significant to other systems. To avoid duplication, these nursing diagnoses are listed by title only with a referral to their page location.

Dependence on Airway Patency Maintenance, p. 1119

Predisposition to Shock, p. 462

Emergency Phase Hemorrhagic Shock, p. 459

Dependence on Intravenous Infusion Management, p. 374

Potential Edema Related to Localized Tissue Injury, p. 367

Emergency Phase Burn Injury (47,71,192,271,391,618)

ASSESSMENT

Subjective Data
Second-Degree Burn (Partial-Thickness Burn):
Very painful wound

Third-Degree Burn (Full-Thickness Burn):
Insensitive to pinprick

Objective Data

Person Has a Second- or Third-Degree Burn or Combined Degrees of Burn on the Body Surface:

Minor (may be treated as an outpatient): covers an area of less than 10% in children and 15% in adults of the total body surface; a full-thickness wound covers an area of less than 2%, excepting burns of the face, legs, feet, hands, genitalia, inhalation injury, fractures or soft tissue injury

Moderate (treated in a general hospital): covers an area of from 10% in children and 15% to 25% in adults

Critical (treated in a burn unit): any patient with involvement of the face, eyes, feet, hands, genitalia, or evidence of inhalation injury, soft tissue injury, fractures, etc.

First-Degree Burn in Which the Injury Extends Only to the Outer Layer (Epidermis) of the Skin:

Dry skin surface
Skin redness or flush
Heals in a few days

Second-Degree Burn (Partial-Thickness Burn) in Which the Injury Extends Into the Second Layer (Dermis) of the Body:

Weeping, moist wound with blister formation
Mottled redness
Skin feels soft on palpation
Edema
Scarring with deep second-degree wounds

Third-Degree Burn (Full-Thickness Burn) in Which the Injury Extends Through All Three Skin Layers:

Dry skin surface
Pearly white or charred appearance
Leathery, without moisture, or may have bullae from steam trapped in the dermis
Thrombosed blood vessels
Function may be lost if the injured area is over a joint
Tissue sloughing
Scarring

POSSIBLE ETIOLOGY

Burn trauma resulting from skin contact with flames, hot objects, scalds, flash, chemicals, and electrical injuries (electrical injuries not covered under this heading)

NURSING DIAGNOSIS

Emergency phase burn injury: the need for immediate health care as a result of a second- or third-degree burn.

PLANNING

Patient Needs	**Primary Nurse-Patient Goals**
Oxygen	To maintain oxygen to all cells
Water-salt balance	To maintain fluid and electrolyte balance
Comfort	To achieve comfort
Cleanliness (of the wound)	To achieve good hygiene
Protection from physical harm	To prevent physical injury, infection

NURSING INTERVENTIONS

Nursing Treatments (Minor Burns)
(May be treated on an outpatient basis)
Apply a cold, moist compress ⎱
   OR   ⎬ (for about 30 minutes)
Bathe in cool water ⎰
Apply a sterile dressing
Make a referral (to a physician or the emergency room as needed both for immediate care or follow-up)

Nursing Treatments (Moderate or Critical Burns)
Airway:
Hold the jaw forward to maintain an airway ⎱
   OR   ⎬ (as needed)
Place in the side-lying position ⎰
Provide standby emergency equipment (endotracheal tube)
Insert a nasal airway ⎱
   OR   ⎬ (as needed)
Insert an oral airway ⎰
Administer humidified oxygen (ET) (as needed)
Place in the slight sitting (semi-Fowler's) position (if cyanosis and dyspnea are present)
Fluid Resuscitation:
Administer intravenous fluids (ET) (according to one of several formulas: crystalloid, Evans, Moore's, hypertonic, or Brooke, if the burn size is greater than 20% of the total body surface. Crystalloid formula is calculated by the following equation: 4 cc Ringers Lactate × weight in kilograms × percent of burn = fluid for a 24-hour period postinjury. One half of the calculated amount is given in the first eight hours, 1/4 in the second eight hours, and 1/4 in the third eight hours)
Catheterize with an indwelling urinary catheter (to measure output)
Restrict the intake to nothing by mouth
Insert a gastric tube and attach to suction (ET)
Pain Relief:
Decrease drafts (in the room)
Maintain a warm room temperature (above 80°F or a degree comfortable to the patient)

Infection Prevention and Wound Care:
Maintain a clean environment
Use sterile technique
Maintain dry, clean linen
    OR
Place on sterile linens
Irrigate the wound (gently with water or saline)
    AND
Wash with a germicidal agent
Shave the hair surrounding the burned area
Remove the loose burned skin with a gauze pad and slight pressure
Remove foreign objects from the skin
Remove blisters from the burned area (expect those on the palms and soles)
Maintenance of Function:
Elevate the (burned) extremities (above the level of the heart)
Elevate the head (if the head or neck are burned)
Exercise (the extremities) in range of motion (gently every 2 hours)
Do not allow skin surfaces to touch (especially in areas of the groin, axilla, and neck, to prevent maceration of the wound)

Nursing Observations
Observe for airway obstruction
Observe the level of consciousness
Measure the intake (intravenous fluids)
Measure the urine output hourly (should be 50–70 cc per hour)
Monitor the central venous pressure (and/or pulmonary artery pressures)
Palpate the pulse for rate, rhythm, and volume
Observe for shock
Inspect the chest for respiratory rate and rhythm
Observe for cyanosis
Inspect the nose, mouth, and throat for evidence of burns (singed nasal hairs, reddened dry buccal mucosa, soot in the sputum)
Auscultate the chest for lung aeration
Monitor the blood pressure
Inspect for the percentage of burned area (upon arrival at the hospital and again following wound cleansing)
Observe for restlessness (assess for hypoxia or pain)
Inspect the extremities for adequate circulation (especially full-thickness burned tissue, every 30 minutes)
Observe for evidence of pressure on the skin
Observe for complaints of pain (deep aching)
Inspect the skin for impaired feeling perception
Observe the extremities for motor function
Test the urine for sugar and acetone (every four hours)
Monitor blood studies for abnormal acid base
Monitor blood studies for abnormal hematology
Monitor blood studies for abnormal electrolytes
Monitor blood studies for abnormal glucose

Monitor blood studies for abnormal gas exchange
Monitor blood studies for abnormal renal function (urea nitrogen)

Medical Treatments Performed by Nurses

Pain Relief:
Apply the prescribed topical agent (silver sulfadiazine)
Give the prescribed drugs (small doses of narcotics intravenously)

Fluid Resuscitation:
Administer intravenous fluids
Administer a blood transfusion

Infection Prevention and Wound Care:
Apply the prescribed topical agent
Apply a biologic dressing (heterograft or hemograft for partial thickness injuries)
Give the prescribed drugs (antibiotics, tetanus toxoid, antacids)

EVALUATION

See the evaluation criteria for each specific goal in Chapter 2.

INTEGUMENT THERMAL INJURY: ACUTE CARE PERIOD FOLLOWING THERMAL INJURY

Increased Nutritional Requirement Related to Tissue Healing, p. 924

Increased Nutritional Requirement Related to Metabolism, p. 922

Predisposition to Bleeding, p. 408

Potential Wound Infection, p. 747

Potential Limited Range of Motion, p. 861

Potential Joint Contracture, p. 878

Painful Dressing Change, p. 1061

Dependence on General Hygiene, p. 708

Predisposition to Stress Ulcer, p. 610

Dependence on Feeding, p. 943

Difficult Adaptation to Illness Dependency, p. 151

Potential Depression, p. 180

Dependence on Burn Wound Management (47,71,192,271,391,618)

ASSESSMENT

Subjective Data

Person relies on nurses for:
    precautions against burn wound complications
    bathing and debridement of the burn wound
    comfort measures
    dressing changes

Objective Data

Person has a first-, second-, or third-degree burn or combined degrees of burn on the body surface

First-Degree Burn in Which the Injury Extends Only to the Outer Layer (Epidermis) of the Skin:

Dry skin surface

Skin redness or flush

Heals in a few days

Second-Degree Burn (Partial-Thickness Burn) in Which the Injury Extends Into the Second Layer (Dermis) of the Body:

Weeping, moist wound with blister formation

Mottled redness

Skin feels soft on palpation

Edema

Scarring with deep second-degree wounds

Third-Degree Burn (Full-Thickness Burn) in Which the Injury Extends Through All Three Skin Layers:

Dry skin surface

Pearly white or charred appearance

Leathery without moisture or may have bullae from steam trapped in the dermis

Thrombosed blood vessels

Function may be lost if the injured area is over a joint

Tissue sloughing

Scarring

POSSIBLE ETIOLOGY

Burn trauma resulting from skin contact with flames, hot objects, scalds, flash, chemicals, and electrical injuries

NURSING DIAGNOSIS

Dependence on burn wound management: reliance on nurses for the care of a wound resulting from a burn injury

PLANNING

Patient Needs	Primary Nurse-Patient Goals
Comfort	To achieve comfort
Cleanliness	To achieve good hygiene
Protection from physical harm	To prevent physical injury, (control of) infection
Dependence	To achieve comfort
Increased learning	To achieve awareness of needs

NURSING INTERVENTIONS

Nursing Treatments
Wash with a germicidal solution (Betadine)
Bathe in bed
   OR
Bathe in a shower   (to remove the prescribed topical
   OR   agent before reapplication of the
Bathe in a tub (submerge the patient   agent)
   in water for closed wounds)
Expose the burn wound to air (open method)
Apply a sterile dressing (fine mesh gauze, Kling, or Surgiflex applying
   lightly)
   OR
Apply an occlusive dressing (closed method)
Moisten the dressing before removal (if the dressing is not intended for de-
   bridement)
Apply a bed cradle (if the trunk and legs are burned)
Cover with lightweight blankets (unless a heat lamp is used)
Do not allow skin surfaces to touch (if at all possible)
Handle gently
Maintain body alignment
Maintain a warm room temperature (about 80°F or a degree comfortable
   to the patient)
   OR
Apply a heat cradle
   OR
Apply heat by a gooseneck lamp
Maintain adequate atmospheric humidity (40% to 50% or a percentage
   comfortable to the patient)
Maintain a clean environment
Maintain reverse isolation (if the burn covers a large area)

Maintain dry, clean linen
OR
Place on sterile linens (if the burn covers a large area)

Nursing Observations
Monitor the oral temperature
Palpate the pulse for rate, rhythm, and volume
Inspect the chest for respiratory rate and rhythm
Auscultate the chest for abnormal breath sounds
Inspect the wound dressing (if a dressing is applied)
Inspect for signs of infection (wound infection and systemic sepsis)
Observe for evidence of pressure on the skin
Observe for signs of healing
Observe for delayed healing
Obtain a bacterial culture (of the burned surface)

Health Teaching
Explain the reason for and intended effect of the therapy
Teach how to clean and dress a wound (if necessary)

Medical Treatments Performed by Nurses
Apply the prescribed topical agent (silver nitrate, Sulfamylon, Sulfidiazine, Betadine, cerium nitrate)
Apply a medicated dressing (wet-wet dressing: a thick dressing that has been saturated with a prescribed solution; wet the dressing with the solution every four hours and change the dressing every eight hours; this dressing is not intended for debridement) (wet-dry dressing: apply the dressing as above; remove the dry dressing every four hours and reapply for debridement purposes)

EVALUATION

See the evaluation criteria for each specific goal in Chapter 2.

INTEGUMENT THERMAL INJURY: REHABILITATION PERIOD FOLLOWING THERMAL INJURY

Immobility Requirement Related to Healing, p. 806

Difficulty Ambulating, p. 851

Inadequate Emotional Support Related to the Endurance of Health Treatments, p. 261

Difficult Adaptation to Altered Body Image, p. 279

Embarrassment Related to Social Exposure, p. 184

Inadequate Emotional Support Related to Grieving, p. 207

Frustration Related to Slow Cure Progression, p. 192

Guilt Related to the Burden of Illness on Others, p. 236

EMERGENCY EYE THERMAL INJURY

Emergency Phase Chemical Eye Burn (71,192)

ASSESSMENT

Subjective Data
Severe pain
Impaired vision

Objective Data
Eye contact with a chemical
Inflammation
Drainage

Related Data
Commonly Related Diseases:
Burn injury

POSSIBLE ETIOLOGY

Accidental or intentional injury

NURSING DIAGNOSIS

Emergency phase chemical eye burn: the need for immediate health care when harsh chemical substances come in contact with the eye

PLANNING

Patient Needs	Primary Nurse-Patient Goals
Rest	To achieve rest
Comfort	To achieve good hygiene
Protection from physical harm	To prevent physical injury
Increased learning	To achieve awareness of needs

NURSING INTERVENTIONS

Nursing Treatments
Do not neutralize the chemical injuring the eye
Irrigate the eye (with saline or plain water)
Apply a sterile dressing
Make a referral (to a physician *immediately*)

Nursing Observations
Observe for complaints of pain

Health Teaching
Explain the reason for and intended effect of the therapy
Instruct to avoid rubbing the eyes

EVALUATION

See the evaluation criteria for each specific goal in Chapter 2.

Emergency Phase Heat Eye Burn (192)

ASSESSMENT

Subjective Data
Severe pain

Objective Data
Unable to voluntarily open the eyes
Eye redness
Swelling
Drainage
Burned eyelids, sclera, or cornea

Related Data
Commonly Related Diseases:
First-, second-, or third-degree burns

POSSIBLE ETIOLOGY

Exposure to steam or welding arc heat. Flash burns.

NURSING DIAGNOSIS

Emergency phase heat eye burn: the need for immediate health care when the eye is injured from intense heat

PLANNING

Patient Needs	Primary Nurse-Patient Goals
Rest	To achieve rest
Comfort	To achieve comfort
Protection from physical harm	To prevent physical injury
Increased learning	To achieve awareness of needs

NURSING INTERVENTIONS

Nursing Treatments
Apply a cold, moist compress (intermittently until the pain subsides)
Lubricate the eyes (both eyes with mineral oil)

Apply a sterile dressing (over the eye)
Make a referral (to a physician *immediately*)

Nursing Observations
Observe for complaints of pain

Health Teaching
Explain the reason for and intended effect of the therapy

EVALUATION

See the evaluation criteria for each specific goal in Chapter 2.

EMERGENCY COLD-RELATED SKIN INJURY

Emergency Phase Frostbite (192)

ASSESSMENT

Subjective Data
Decreased feeling sensation
Tenderness

Objective Data
Pallor (early sign)
Bluish red skin discoloration (later sign)
Edema

Related Data
Location:
Primarily affects the hands and feet
Commonly Related Conditions:
Chillblain

POSSIBLE ETIOLOGY

Destruction of superficial tissues exposed to extreme cold. Crystallization of fluids in tissue cells. Impaired circulation.

NURSING DIAGNOSIS

Emergency phase frostbite: the need for immediate health care as a result of skin exposure to intense cold

PLANNING

Patient Needs	Primary Nurse-Patient Goals
Normal temperature	To maintain regulating mechanisms and functions
Comfort	To achieve comfort
Protection from physical harm	To prevent physical injury
Increased learning	To achieve awareness of needs

NURSING INTERVENTIONS

Nursing Treatments
Soak in saline solution (at 103–107.5°F [39.4°C–41.9°C])
Give hot coffee
   OR
Give hot tea
Discourage smoking
Cover with warm blankets
Do not massage
Exercise in range of motion (once the limb is rewarmed)

Nursing Observations
Inspect for bleeding
Inspect for edema
Inspect the extremities for adequate circulation
Monitor the blood pressure
Monitor the oral temperature

Health Teaching
Advise against exposure to inclement weather
Recommend the use of warm clothing
Explain the reason for and intended effect of the therapy

EVALUATION

See the evaluation criteria for each specific goal in Chapter 2.

SKIN MANAGEMENT

Inadequate Information Related to Carotene Skin Discoloration

ASSESSMENT

Subjective Data
Person confirms a lack of information

Objective Data
Person's actions indicate a lack of information regarding:
   the relationship of food intake to the yellow or orange skin discoloration
   how to reduce the discoloration

Related Data
Commonly Related Diseases:
Myxedema
Diabetes mellitus
Panhypopituitarism

POSSIBLE ETIOLOGY

Lack of information regarding balanced nutrition

NURSING DIAGNOSIS

Inadequate information related to carotene skin discoloration: lack of information regarding skin discoloration from excessive carotene intake

PLANNING

Patient Needs

Comfort

Protection from physical harm

Increased learning

Primary Nurse-Patient Goals

To achieve comfort

To prevent physical injury

To achieve awareness of needs

NURSING INTERVENTIONS

Nursing Treatments
Approach unhurriedly
Encourage patient questions
Encourage decreased yellow fruit and vegetable intake

Nursing Observations
Observe for evidence of a favorable response to therapy

Health Teaching
Explain the causes of the health problem
Explain the reason for and intended effect of the therapy

EVALUATION

See the evaluation criteria for each specific goal in Chapter 2.

Inadequate Information Related to Diabetic Skin Care

ASSESSMENT

Subjective Data
Person confirms a lack of information

Objective Data
Person's actions indicate a lack of information regarding:
    how to properly clean skin
    proper skin lubrication
    the dangers of pressure on the skin
    that constant observation for diabetic skin problems is essential

Related Data
Commonly Related Diseases:
Diabetes mellitus

POSSIBLE ETIOLOGY

Lack of instruction

NURSING DIAGNOSIS

Inadequate information related to diabetic skin care: lack of information regarding the special care of a diabetic's skin

PLANNING

Patient Needs

Protection from physical harm

Increased learning

Primary Nurse-Patient Goals

To prevent physical injury, infection

To achieve awareness of needs

NURSING INTERVENTIONS

Nursing Treatments

Approach unhurriedly

Encourage patient questions

Nursing Observations

Inspect the skin for breakdown

Evaluate the response to teaching

Health Teaching

Explain that the diabetic's feet should be washed gently

Instruct that a soft towel should be used to dry the diabetic's feet

Instruct to thoroughly dry the skin between the diabetic's toes

Instruct to lanolize the diabetic's feet, but not the toes

Instruct to lightly rub the diabetic's feet with alcohol (if there is extreme perspiration)

Explain that powder should be applied between the diabetic's toes after bathing

Advise against walking barefoot

Emphasize the danger of cutting calloused skin

Instruct to maintain skin dryness

Recommend the use of closed shoes for foot protection

Instruct to wear well-fitting shoes

Instruct to maintain skin cleanliness

Instruct to inspect the skin

Instruct to lubricate the skin

EVALUATION

See the evaluation criteria for each specific goal in Chapter 2.

Inadequate Information Related to Skin Care

ASSESSMENT

Subjective Data

Person confirms a lack of information

Objective Data

Person's actions indicate a lack of information regarding:
    skin cleansing
    skin lubrication
    prevention of skin trauma

POSSIBLE ETIOLOGY

Lack of instruction

NURSING DIAGNOSIS

Inadequate information related to skin care: lack of information regarding the proper care of the skin

PLANNING

Patient Needs	**Primary Nurse-Patient Goals**
Comfort	To achieve comfort
Cleanliness	To achieve good hygiene
Protection from physical harm	To prevent physical injury
Increased learning	To achieve awareness of needs

NURSING INTERVENTIONS

Nursing Treatments
Approach unhurriedly
Encourage patient questions

Nursing Observations
Observe for evidence of pressure on the skin

Health Teaching
Instruct to maintain skin cleanliness
Instruct to maintain skin dryness
Instruct to lubricate the skin
Instruct to inspect the skin (periodically)
Emphasize the danger of cutting calloused skin
Explain the need to avoid mechanical trauma
Advise against squeezing the skin
Advise against prolonged skin exposure to the sun
Advise against prolonged skin exposure to water
Inform that the skin should be protected from windburn

EVALUATION

See the evaluation criteria for each specific goal in Chapter 2.

Inadequate Information Related to Nail Care

ASSESSMENT

Subjective Data
Person confirms a lack of information

Objective Data
Person's actions indicate a lack of information regarding:
    how to clean the nails
    how to shape the nails
    proper nail lubrication

POSSIBLE ETIOLOGY

Lack of information

NURSING DIAGNOSIS

Inadequate information related to nail care: lack of information regarding general nail care

PLANNING

Patient Needs

Comfort

Cleanliness

Protection from physical harm

Increased learning

Primary Nurse-Patient Goals

To achieve comfort

To achieve good hygiene

To prevent physical injury

To achieve awareness of needs

NURSING INTERVENTIONS

Nursing Treatments
Approach unhurriedly
Encourage patient questions

Nursing Observations
Inspect the nails for abnormalities
Evaluate the response to teaching

Health Teaching
Advise that lanolin be applied to brittle nails
Explain how to file the nails correctly
Explain that nails should be soaked before trimming
Explain the need for nail cleanliness
Instruct to cut the toenails straight across
Instruct to lubricate the nails

EVALUATION

See the evaluation criteria for each specific goal in Chapter 2.

Inadequate Information Related to Diabetic Nail Care

ASSESSMENT

Subjective Data
Person confirms a lack of information

Objective Data
Person's actions indicate a lack of information regarding:
    how to shape the diabetic's nails
    how to clean the diabetic's nails
    proper nail lubrication
    special precautions for diabetics

Related Data
Commonly Related Diseases:
Diabetes mellitus

POSSIBLE ETIOLOGY

Lack of instruction

NURSING DIAGNOSIS

Inadequate information related to diabetic nail care: lack of information regarding the special care of a diabetic's nails

PLANNING

Patient Needs	**Primary Nurse-Patient Goals**
Comfort	To achieve comfort
Cleanliness	To achieve good hygiene
Protection from physical harm	To prevent physical injury
Increased learning	To achieve awareness of needs

NURSING INTERVENTIONS

Nursing Treatments
Approach unhurriedly
Encourage patient questions

Nursing Observations
Evaluate the response to teaching

Health Teaching
Advise that lanolin be applied to brittle nails
Explain how to file the nails correctly
Explain that nails should be soaked before trimming
Instruct to clean the nails with a cotton-tipped stick (after soaking)
Instruct to cut the toenails straight across
Instruct to lubricate the nails
Explain the need for nail cleanliness
Explain the reason for and intended effect of the therapy

EVALUATION

See the evaluation criteria for each specific goal in Chapter 2.

20.
NURSING DIAGNOSES RELATED TO
Metabolism

Note: Many of the nursing diagnoses associated with the metabolic system are also significant to other systems. To avoid duplication, these nursing diagnoses are listed in this chapter by title only, with referral to their page location.

ADRENAL HYPERFUNCTION

Predisposition to Cardiovascular Pathology, p. 434

Predisposition to Hypertension, p. 426

Predisposition to Stress Ulcer, p. 610

ADRENAL HYPOFUNCTION

Adrenal-Steroid Intolerance, p. 489

Difficult Adaptation to Altered Body Image, p. 279

Inability to Control Body Temperature, p. 386

Increased Nutritional Requirement Related to Metabolism, p. 922

Additional Rest Requirement, p. 1221

Infection Susceptibility, p. 737

Insulin Intolerance, p. 500

Intolerance to Stress, p. 330

Postural Hypotension, p. 422

Potential Skin Injury Related to Increased Skin Pigmentation, p. 802

**Predisposition to Accidental Injury,
p. 899**

Predisposition to Diabetes, p. 840

ADRENAL HYPOFUNCTION, POTENTIAL EMERGENCY

Emergency Phase Impending Adrenal Shock (70,391)

ASSESSMENT

Subjective Data
Generalized weakness
Headache
Nausea

Objective Data
Restlessness
Weak, rapid pulse
Sudden increased temperature
Sudden hypotension
Cold, cyanotic extremities
Vomiting
Increased respirations
Diarrhea

Related Data
Commonly Related Conditions:
Systemic shock
Commonly Related Diseases:
Addison's disease

POSSIBLE ETIOLOGY

Inability of the adrenal glands to secrete adequate amounts of cortical hormones. Adrenal atrophy. Insufficient adrenal hormones for normal body adaptation to stress, severe trauma, infection, or intense environmental heat.

NURSING DIAGNOSIS

Emergency phase impending adrenal shock (emergency phase impending adrenal crisis): the need for immediate health care indicated by signs and symptoms that warn that a severe, decreased production of epinephrine and cortical hormones is threatening to occur

PLANNING

Patient Needs	Primary Nurse-Patient Goals
Oxygen	To maintain oxygen to all cells
Water-salt balance	To maintain fluid and electrolyte balance
Acid-base balance, normal temperature	To maintain regulating mechanisms and functions
Sleep, rest	To achieve sleep, rest
Comfort	To achieve comfort
Protection from physical harm	To prevent physical injury, infection
Increased learning	To achieve awareness of needs

NURSING INTERVENTIONS

Nursing Treatments
Administer intravenous fluids (ET) (sodium chloride)
Administer humidified oxygen (ET) (as needed)
Give hot coffee
   OR
Give hot tea
Withhold the drugs (morphine or barbiturates until cortisone is given)
Place on complete bed rest
Cover with lightweight blankets
Maintain normal room temperature
Provide quiet
Attend the patient constantly
Anticipate needs
Refrain from performing nonessential procedures
Avoid causing intense emotional situations
Consult with the physician (*immediately*)

Nursing Observations
Auscultate the chest for abnormal heart sounds
Auscultate the chest for abnormal breath sounds
Measure the intake
Measure the output (save for a 24-hour urine)
Monitor the blood pressure
Monitor blood studies for abnormal adrenal function
Monitor the oral temperature (for decrease)
Observe for shock

Health Teaching
Explain the causes of the health problem
Explain the reason for and intended effect of the therapy

Medical Treatments Performed by Nurses
Give the prescribed drugs (hydrocortisone)

EVALUATION

See the evaluation criteria for each specific goal in Chapter 2.

PANCREATIC HYPOFUNCTION

Dependence on Nursing Supervision
of Controlled Diabetes
(70,300,301,325)

ASSESSMENT

Subjective Data
Person relies on nurses for:
    frequent blood sugar and urine tests
    weight checkups
    assurance that the prescribed diet and drugs are being taken correctly
    prevention of skin infection
    assurance that a balanced health state exists
    guidance in an exercise and activity regime

Related Data
Commonly Related Diseases:
Diabetes mellitus

POSSIBLE ETIOLOGY

Confirmed diagnosis of diabetes. Patient is on diabetic therapy regime.

NURSING DIAGNOSIS

Dependence on nursing supervision of controlled diabetes: reliance on nurses to periodically evaluate the health status of the patient whose diabetes is relatively stabilized

PLANNING

Patient Needs	Primary Nurse-Patient Goals
Comfort	To achieve comfort
Protection from physical harm	To prevent physical injury
Increased learning	To achieve awareness of needs

NURSING INTERVENTIONS

Nursing Treatments
Approach unhurriedly
Encourage moderate activity

Nursing Observations
Inspect for edema
Inspect the skin for infectious lesions
Inspect the skin for breakdown
Measure the body weight (for excessive gain or loss)
Monitor the blood pressure
Monitor blood studies for abnormal carbohydrate metabolism
Observe for complaints of dizziness
Observe for complaints of headache
Observe for complaints of malaise
Observe for complaints of nausea

Observe for complaints of pain (abdominal)
Observe for complaints of thirst
Observe for weakness
Observe for delayed healing
Observe for fatigue
Observe personal hygiene habits
Review the dietary intake with the patient to determine adherence to the
    prescribed diet
Observe the person's activity pattern
Test the urine for sugar and acetone
Test the urine for pH
Observe for evidence of a favorable response to therapy

Health Teaching
Describe the characteristics of controlled diabetes
Describe those symptoms which should be reported (nausea, headache,
    thirst, weakness)
Instruct to immediately report serious symptoms
Explain the need to avoid overexertion
Explain the reason for and intended effect of the therapy

EVALUATION

See the evaluation criteria for each specific goal in Chapter 2.

Predisposition to Diabetes
(71,123,398)

ASSESSMENT

Objective Data
Patient is overweight or obese
Has high carbohydrate intake
Woman has had multiple pregnancies
Woman has delivered children weighing 10 pounds or more
Woman has had a myocardial infarction prior to menopause
Man has had a myocardial infarction before age 40

Related Data
More prevelant in adults than children, in women than in men
Age 45 to 70
Family history of diabetes
With each succeeding generation, in a family where diabetes exists, onset
    occurs at an earlier age
Medical treatment with cortisone preparations for other diseases
Commonly Related Diseases:
None
    OR
Cushing's disease
Gigantism

Acromegaly
Pancreatitis

POSSIBLE ETIOLOGY

Chronic, excessive carbohydrate consumption overstimulates insulin secretion, which predisposes the pancreatic beta cells to be unable to supply adequate insulin to metabolize carbohydrates. In obesity, the fat cells are distended, which decreases their ability to utilize glucose. Stress of pregnancy. Menopause hormone imbalance.

NURSING DIAGNOSIS

Predisposition to diabetes: a susceptibility for developing diabetes

PLANNING

Patient Needs

Protection from physical harm

Increased learning

Primary Nurse-Patient Goals

To prevent physical injury

To achieve awareness of needs

NURSING INTERVENTIONS

Nursing Treatments
Encourage decreased calorie intake
Encourage decreased carbohydrate intake

Nursing Observations
Measure the body weight (for excessive gain or loss)
Monitor the blood pressure
Monitor blood studies for abnormal carbohydrate metabolism
Observe the breath for abnormal odors
Observe for complaints of dizziness
Observe for complaints of headache
Observe for complaints of malaise
Observe for complaints of nausea
Observe for complaints of pain (abdominal)
Observe for complaints of thirst
Observe for complaints of weakness
Test the urine for sugar and acetone

Health Teaching
Inform that a predisposition to the illness exists
Advise periodic examinations for known hereditary predispositions
Describe those symptoms which should be reported (slow healing wounds, increased appetite with weight loss, increased urine output)
Emphasize the danger of excessive body weight
Teach how to test the urine for sugar-acetone

EVALUATION

See the evaluation criteria for each specific goal in Chapter 2.

PANCREATIC HYPOFUNCTION, EMERGENCY

Emergency Phase Insulin Shock (32,70,71,300,325)

ASSESSMENT

Subjective Data
Generalized weakness
Headache
Nervousness
Hunger
Dizziness

Objective Data
Pallor
Tremors
Restlessness
Irritability
Sweating
Drowsiness or confusion

Related Data
Laboratory Findings:
Decreased blood glucose
Commonly Related Diseases:
Diabetes mellitus

POSSIBLE ETIOLOGY

Incompatibility of or failure to adhere to the prescribed diabetic diet and insulin dosage. Decreased activity level with unadjusted insulin dosage.

NURSING DIAGNOSIS

Emergency phase insulin shock: the need for immediate health care as a result of a critical decrease in the blood glucose of a diabetic receiving insulin therapy

PLANNING

Patient Needs	Primary Nurse-Patient Goals
Food balance	To maintain nutrition to all cells
Rest	To achieve rest
Comfort	To achieve comfort
Protection from physical harm	To prevent physical injury
Increased learning	To achieve awareness of needs

NURSING INTERVENTIONS

Nursing Treatments
Give hard candy (*immediately*)
   OR

Give high-glucose fluids orally (*immediately*)
  OR
Administer intravenous fluids (ET) (glucose)
Follow quick-acting glucose with long-acting carbohydrates
Place on complete bed rest
Cover with warm blankets
Maintain a warm room temperature
Refrain from giving insulin
Attend the patient constantly
Consult with the physician (*immediately*)

Nursing Observations
Monitor the blood pressure
Monitor blood studies for abnormal glucose
Test the urine for sugar and acetone

Health Teaching
Explain the causes of the health problem
Explain the reason for and intended effect of the therapy

EVALUATION

See the evaluation criteria for each specific goal in Chapter 2.

Emergency Phase Diabetic Acidosis, p. 110

PARATHYROID HYPERFUNCTION

Predisposition to Bone Fracture, p.900

Potential Constipation, p. 625

Predisposition to Hypertension, p. 426

Predisposition to Renal Calculi, p. 651

Predisposition to Stress Ulcer (Peptic), p. 610

PARATHYROID HYPOFUNCTION

Cramping Pain, p. 966

Light Intolerance Discomfort, p. 1206

Potential Airway Obstruction, p. 1123

Potential Muscle Spasms, p. 1056

Predisposition to Alkalosis, p. 107

Predisposition to Shock (Cardiogenic), p. 462

PITUITARY HYPERFUNCTION

Difficult Adaptation to Altered Body Image, p. 279

Increased Nutritional Requirement Related to Metabolism, p. 922

Potential Drug Intolerance, p. 503

Predisposition to Diabetes, p. 840

Predisposition to Shock (Cardiogenic), p. 462

PITUITARY HYPOFUNCTION

Cold Intolerance, p. 583

Difficult Adaptation to Altered Body Image, p. 279

Excessive Urinary Output, p. 643

Reduced Female Sexual Response, p. 302

Infection Susceptibility, p. 737

Intolerance to Stress, p. 330

Physical Irritability, p. 339

Postural Hypotension, p. 422

Potential Drug Intolerance, p. 503

THYROID HYPERFUNCTION

Caffeine Intolerance, p. 496

Dependence on Cardiac Workload Reduction, p. 428

Epinephrine Intolerance, p. 497

Heat Intolerance, p. 584

Increased Nutritional Requirement Related to Metabolism, p. 922

Additional Rest Requirement, p. 1221

Intolerance to Stress, p. 330

Physical Irritability, p. 339

Physical Nervousness, p. 342

Potential Diarrhea, p. 620

Potential Drug Intolerance, p. 503

Potential Simple Goiter (32,70,325)

ASSESSMENT

Subjective Data
Feeling of throat fullness

Objective Data
Use of noniodized salt
Unbalanced diet
Palpable, minimal thyroid enlargement

Related Data
Person lives in a region of the Pacific Northwest or Great Lakes
Commonly Related Conditions:
Adolescence
Pregnancy
Commonly Related Diseases:
Nontoxic goiter

POSSIBLE ETIOLOGY

Insufficient iodine in the diet

NURSING DIAGNOSIS

Potential simple goiter: the probability that severe thyroid enlargement will occur from iodine deficiency

PLANNING

Patient Needs

Protection from physical harm

Increased learning

Primary Nurse-Patient Goals

To prevent physical injury

To achieve awareness of needs

NURSING INTERVENTIONS

Nursing Observations

Monitor blood studies for abnormal thyroid function
Palpate the thyroid gland for enlargement (periodically)
Inspect the chest for respiratory rate and rhythm (wheezing)
Inspect the throat for an impaired swallowing reflex

Health Teaching

Teach the principles of good nutrition
Recommend the use of iodized salt
Describe those symptoms which should be reported (wheezing, difficulty swallowing)
Explain the reason for and intended effect of the therapy

EVALUATION

See the evaluation criteria for each specific goal in Chapter 2.

THYROID HYPOFUNCTION

Analgesic Intolerance, p. 491

Anorexia, p. 925

Cold Intolerance, p. 583

Difficult Adaptation to Altered Body Image, p. 279

Excessive Lactation, p. 1095

Physical Nervousness, p. 342

Potential Constipation, p. 625

Potential Drug Intolerance, p. 503

Sedative Intolerance, p. 502

CRISIS OF THYROID FUNCTION

Emergency Phase Impending Thyroid Crisis (32,71,271)

Subjective Data
Weakness
Fatigue

Objective Data
Tachycardia (140–200 beats each minute)
Increased respirations
Restlessness
Irritability
Gradually rising temperature

Related Data
If related to a thyroidectomy, it occurs within 12 hours following surgery
Commonly Related Conditions:
Emotional stress
Infectious conditions
Commonly Related Diseases:
Thyrotoxicosis

POSSIBLE ETIOLOGY

The body's attempt to adapt to stress without adequate thyroid hormone to meet the stress. Surgical removal of the thyroid gland reducing the body's thyroxine level.

NURSING DIAGNOSIS

Emergency phase impending thyroid crisis: the need for immediate health care indicated by signs and symptoms that warn that a thyroid crisis is threatening to occur

PLANNING

Patient Needs	Primary Nurse-Patient Goals
Water-salt balance	To maintain fluid and electrolyte balance
Normal temperature	To maintain regulating mechanisms and functions
Rest	To achieve rest
Comfort	To achieve comfort
Protection from physical harm	To prevent physical injury
Increased learning	To achieve awareness of needs

NURSING INTERVENTIONS

Nursing Treatments
Administer humidified oxygen (ET) (cool, not heated)

Administer intravenous fluids (ET) (10% dextrose in distilled water)
Place on complete bed rest
Cover with lightweight blankets
Maintain a cool room temperature
Bathe in cool water
Provide quiet
Attend the patient constantly
Anticipate needs
Refrain from giving oral stimulants
Refrain from giving hot liquids
Refrain from performing nonessential procedures
Avoid causing intense emotional situations
Consult with the physician (*immediately*)

Nursing Observations
Monitor the blood pressure (for decrease)
Monitor the oral temperature (for fever)
Observe for airway obstruction
Observe for shock
Palpate the pulse for rate (tachycardia), rhythm, and volume

Health Teaching
Explain the causes of the health problem
Explain the reason for and intended effect of the therapy

Medical Treatments Performed by Nurses
Give the prescribed drugs (sodium iodide, corticosteroids, propylthiouracil)
Place on a hypothermia blanket

EVALUATION

See the evaluation criteria for each specific goal in Chapter 2.

INADEQUATE INFORMATION RELATED TO METABOLISM

Inadequate Information Related to Diabetes Management (71)

ASSESSMENT

Subjective Data
Person confirms a lack of information

Objective Data
Person's actions indicate a lack of information regarding:
    what diabetes is
    what causes the disease
    that there is a hereditary predisposition
    how to follow the prescribed diabetic regime
    the possible complications associated with diabetes

Related Data

Commonly Related Diseases:
Diabetes mellitus

POSSIBLE ETIOLOGY

No previous experience with the condition. Lack of instruction.

NURSING DIAGNOSIS

Inadequate information related to diabetes management: lack of information regarding the causes, effects, and therapeutic plan associated with diabetes

PLANNING

Patient Needs	**Primary Nurse-Patient Goals**
Comfort	To achieve comfort
Protection from physical harm	To prevent physical injury
Increased learning	To achieve awareness of needs

NURSING INTERVENTIONS

Nursing Treatments
Approach unhurriedly
Encourage patient questions
Encourage adequate rest
Encourage moderate physical exercise

Nursing Observations
Evaluate the response to teaching

Health Teaching
Describe the characteristics of controlled diabetes
Describe the manifestations of impending diabetic coma
Describe the manifestations of impending insulin shock
Explain how impending insulin shock can be interrupted
Recommend that a high-glucose source be carried at all times
Describe those symptoms which should be reported (dizziness, headache, nausea, thirst, weakness, malaise)
Explain the causes of the health problem
Inform that a predisposition to the illness exists
Teach how to give insulin
Teach how to test the urine for sugar-acetone
Teach how to test the blood for glucose using the finger-stick method

EVALUATION

See the evaluation criteria for each specific goal in Chapter 2.

21.
NURSING DIAGNOSES RELATED TO
Mobility

IMPAIRED MOBILITY

Difficulty Ambulating (416)

ASSESSMENT

Subjective Data
Fatigue after limited ambulation
Generalized weakness
Pain

Objective Data
Person walks slowly
Leans toward one side while walking
Holds onto chairs, railings, etc.
Takes short, wide-based steps and sways from side to side (waddling gait)
Raises the thigh excessively high, slapping the heel down before the foot
 (steppage gait)
Walks with choppy, stiff movements, dragging the toes, holding the legs
 together, while flexing the hips, knees, and joints (spastic gait)
Walks by crossing the legs (scissor gait)
Propels the body forward with short shuffling steps that become faster and
 faster (Parkinsonian gait)
Walks by drooping one side of the body (limping gait)
Takes one or two normal steps, then one or two long hopping steps (chorea
 gait)
Lifts the feet too high and places them down with excessive force in a stag-
 gering, wavering, lurching walk (atactic gait)
Collides with furniture, etc.

Related Data
Commonly Related Conditions:
Hemiplegia

Monoplegia
Ataxia
Motion sickness
Impaired proprioception
Commonly Related Diseases:
Thoracic spinal cord injury
Poliomyelitis
Multiple sclerosis
Cerebral palsy
Dissecting aortic aneurysm
Ruptured cervical disk
Cervical spondylosis
Tibia fracture
Meniere's disease
Cerebral vascular accident
Parkinson's disease
Alcoholism
Posterolateral sclerosis
Acute labyrinthitis
Huntington's chorea
Tabes dorsalis
Sydenham's chorea
Bone tuberculosis
Central nervous system syphilis
Peripheral neuritis
Landouzy-Dejerine dystrophy

POSSIBLE ETIOLOGY

Cerebral cortex injury. Central nervous system disease. Muscle weakness.
Nerve impairment. Aging. Impaired muscle coordination. Painful walking.
Unequal leg length. Joint limitations. Left cerebral hemisphere lesion.
Paralysis. Frontal lobe atrophy. Hip dislocation. Pain.

NURSING DIAGNOSIS

Difficulty ambulating: inability to walk sure-footed and without unusual
effort

PLANNING

Patient Needs	Primary Nurse-Patient Goals
Activity, exercise	To achieve activity and exercise
Protection from physical harm	To prevent physical injury, deformities
Dependence	To achieve comfort
Mastery and competence in skills, independence	To achieve optimum function
Increased learning	To achieve awareness of needs

NURSING INTERVENTIONS

Nursing Treatments
Approach unhurriedly
Assist with mobility
Attend the patient constantly (while ambulating)
Mobilize by walker
　OR
Mobilize by wheelchair
　OR
Mobilize with a cane
Place in an uncrowded area
Minimize environmental barriers
Limit the patient's mobility distance
Encourage normal use of the involved limb
Apply a safety helmet to the head
Use a waist safety strap during mobility

Nursing Observations
Observe for mobility capabilities
Observe for complaints of weakness
Observe for abnormal gait
Test for impaired coordination

Health Teaching
Explain the causes of the health problem
Instruct to use a wide supportive stance for good body balance
Instruct to wear well-fitting shoes
Recommend the use of low-heeled shoes
Teach good body mechanics
Teach that weight-bearing should be done on the unaffected side

EVALUATION

See the evaluation criteria for each specific goal in Chapter 2.

Difficulty Sitting Up (416)

ASSESSMENT

Subjective Data
Unsteadiness

Objective Data
Person falls forward or to one side when sitting in a chair
Cannot pull the body up to a sitting position
Cannot sit up without some back support
Cannot tolerate prolonged sitting

Related Data
Commonly Related Conditions:
Hemiplegia

Paraplegia
Quadriplegia
Aging
Commonly Related Diseases:
Cerebral vascular accident
Cerebral palsy
Muscular dystrophy
Parkinson's disease
Poliomyelitis

POSSIBLE ETIOLOGY

Muscle weakness or atrophy. Nerve degeneration.

NURSING DIAGNOSIS

Difficulty sitting up: inability to sit without unusual effort

PLANNING

Patient Needs
Protection from physical harm
Dependence
Mastery and competence in skills
Increased learning

Primary Nurse-Patient Goals
To prevent physical injury
To achieve comfort
To achieve optimum function
To achieve awareness of needs

NURSING INTERVENTIONS

Nursing Treatments
Maintain body alignment
Approach unhurriedly
Mobilize by invalid chair
    OR
Mobilize by stretcher
Position with pillows
    OR
Prop with a back rest
Sit the patient in an armchair

Nursing Observations
Observe for fatigue

Health Teaching
Explain the causes of the health problem
Explain how to use a bed rope
Teach how to use the forearm to push up from a lying position when hemi-
    plegic

EVALUATION

See the evaluation criteria for each specific goal in Chapter 2.

Difficulty Standing Up (416)

ASSESSMENT

Subjective Data
Leg weakness
Unsteadiness

Objective Data
Person struggles to a standing position
Sways body
Uses bent posture
Leans on supportive objects while standing

Related Data
Commonly Related Conditions:
Aging
Commonly Related Diseases:
Muscular dystrophy
Multiple sclerosis
Poliomyelitis

POSSIBLE ETIOLOGY

Muscle weakness or atrophy. Nerve degeneration.

NURSING DIAGNOSIS

Difficulty standing up (dysstasia): inability to stand up without unusual effort

PLANNING

Patient Needs	Primary Nurse-Patient Goals
Protection from physical harm	To prevent physical injury
Dependence	To achieve comfort
Mastery and competence in skills	To achieve optimum function
Increased learning	To achieve awareness of needs

NURSING INTERVENTIONS

Nursing Treatments
Approach unhurriedly
Attend the patient constantly
Change the patient's position gradually
Provide a low-height bed

Nursing Observations
Inspect for abnormal body movements
Observe for fatigue
Observe for complaints of weakness

Health Teaching
Instruct that the nonhemiplegic leg be placed down first when getting out of
    bed

Instruct to wear well-fitting shoes

Recommend the use of a shower chair (when unable to stand up in the shower)

Recommend the use of low-heeled shoes

Teach good body mechanics

Teach that weight-bearing should be done on the unaffected side

Teach how to move from a sitting to a standing position when hemiplegic

Teach how to remove a brace

Teach how to use the forearm to push up from a lying position when hemiplegic

EVALUATION

See the evaluation criteria for each specific goal in Chapter 2.

Difficulty Transferring (416)

ASSESSMENT

Objective Data

Difficulty raising the body off a bed or chair

Cannot comfortably move the body from a bed to a chair, chair to a car, etc.

Has to be transferred by other persons

Related Data

Commonly Related Diseases:

Cerebral vascular accident

Thoracic spinal cord injury

Cervical spinal cord injury

Arteriosclerotic disease amputation

POSSIBLE ETIOLOGY

Nervous system disorder. Poor motor coordination. Muscle weakness. Lack of instruction in transferring skills. Lack of appropriate assistance devices.

NURSING DIAGNOSIS

Difficulty transferring: difficulty moving oneself from the bed to the wheelchair, car, regular chair, bathtub, etc., or back to the bed

PLANNING

Patient Needs	**Primary Nurse-Patient Goals**
Protection from physical harm	To prevent physical injury
Dependence	To achieve comfort
Mastery and competence in skills, independence	To achieve optimum function
Increased learning	To achieve awareness of needs

NURSING INTERVENTIONS

Nursing Treatments

Anticipate needs

Approach unhurriedly

Assist with mobility
Minimize environmental barriers
Place on an orthopedic bed
> AND

Provide a trapeze bar
> OR

Provide a low-height bed
Provide a transfer board
Lift with a hydraulic hoist
Refrain from pulling the patient across the sheets
Suggest home adaptations appropriate to the health problem

Nursing Observations
Observe for fatigue
Observe for complaints of weakness

Health Teaching
Explain the causes of the health problem
Instruct to lock the wheelchair before transferring
Teach good body mechanics
Teach that weight-bearing should be done on the unaffected side
Instruct that the nonhemiplegic leg be placed down first when getting out of
> bed

Teach how to move from a bed to a chair when hemiplegic
Teach how to get into a bathtub when hemiplegic
Teach how to transfer from a bathtub to a wheelchair
Teach how to transfer from a bed to a wheelchair
Teach how to transfer from a chair to a wheelchair
Teach how to transfer from a wheelchair to an automobile
Teach how to transfer from a wheelchair to a bed
Teach how to transfer from a wheelchair to a chair
Teach how to transfer from an automobile to a wheelchair
Teach how to use the forearm to push up from a lying position when hemi-
> plegic

Teach how to use the unaffected leg to move the hemiplegic leg
Teach how to use a hydraulic hoist

EVALUATION

See the evaluation criteria for each specific goal in Chapter 2.

Difficulty Turning Self (416)

ASSESSMENT

Objective Data
Person remains in one position unless turned by others
Attempts to turn self without success
May be able to turn self but soon falls back into the former position

Related Data
Commonly Related Conditions:
Hemiplegia

Quadriplegia
Unconsciousness

Commonly Related Diseases:
Cervical spinal cord injury
Cerebral vascular accident
Cerebral palsy
Muscular dystrophy

POSSIBLE ETIOLOGY

Muscle weakness or atrophy. Paralysis. Therapeutic procedures such as casting, traction, etc. Limited range of motion. Lack of appropriate assistance devices.

NURSING DIAGNOSIS

Difficulty turning self: difficulty moving one's body from side to side when in bed

PLANNING

Patient Needs

Protection from physical harm

Dependence

Mastery and competence in skills, independence

Increased learning

Primary Nurse-Patient Goals

To prevent physical injury

To achieve comfort

To achieve optimum function

To achieve awareness of needs

NURSING INTERVENTIONS

Nursing Treatments
Anticipate needs
Approach unhurriedly
Place on a CircOlectric bed
    OR
Place on a Stryker frame
Change the patient's position frequently

Nursing Observations
Observe for complaints of weakness

Health Teaching
Explain the causes of the health problem
Instruct to change position frequently
Teach good body mechanics
Teach how to turn over when hemiplegic

EVALUATION

See the evaluation criteria for each specific goal in Chapter 2.

Limited Hand Dexterity

ASSESSMENT
Subjective Data
Frustration
Pain, sometimes

Objective Data
Involuntary hand quivering or shaking
Bandaged hands
Absence of one or more fingers
Person frequently drops objects placed in the hand

Related Data
Commonly Related Conditions:
Aging
Tetany
Commonly Related Diseases:
Parkinson's disease
Thyrotoxicosis
Alcoholism
Cerebral vascular accident
Trauma
Amputation

POSSIBLE ETIOLOGY

Trauma. Nerve deterioration.

NURSING DIAGNOSIS

Limited hand dexterity: decreased ability to perform hand activities

PLANNING

Patient Needs	**Primary Nurse-Patient Goals**
Dependence	To achieve comfort
Mastery and competence in skills, independence	To achieve optimum function
Increased learning	To achieve awareness of needs

NURSING INTERVENTIONS

Nursing Treatments
Anticipate needs
Approach unhurriedly
Assist with skilled hand activities
Encourage normal use of the involved limb
Place objects within reach
Place the work at a comfortable level
Provide firm eating utensils
Provide lightweight utensils
Provide unbreakable objects
Tape implements to the bandaged hands

Nursing Observations
Observe for readiness to assume activities of daily living

Health Teaching
Explain the causes of the health problem
Teach how to use assistive eating devices

Teach how to use assistive grooming devices
Teach how to use assistive holding-reaching devices

EVALUATION

See the evaluation criteria for each specific goal in Chapter 2.

Limited Range of Motion (416)

ASSESSMENT
Subjective Data
Pain
Frustration

Objective Data

Impaired circular motion: the head, neck, arms, hands, fingers, legs, feet, or toes cannot be moved in a circular motion

Impaired straight joint motion: the lower arm or leg or the fingers cannot be stretched straight outward; the neck cannot be completely straightened upward from the chest

Impaired rotation joint motion: the head cannot be turned from side to side; the shoulders cannot be turned without moving the hips; the entire arm cannot be moved from above the head down to the leg and up again

Impaired inward joint motion: the head, trunk, leg, or arm cannot be bent toward the center of the body; the fingers or toes cannot be moved toward the center of the hand or foot

Impaired forward motion: the lower arm cannot be bent upward toward the upper arm; the lower leg cannot be bent upward toward the back of the thigh; the neck cannot be bent downward toward the chest; the fingers cannot be bent inward toward the palm of the hand

Related Data

Commonly Related Diseases:
Closed fracture
Compound fracture
Compound dislocation
Rheumatoid arthritis
Osteogenic sarcoma
Cervical or thoracic spinal cord injury
Bone tuberculosis or syphilis
Second- or third-degree burns
Cerebral vascular accident
Rheumatoid spondylitis
Whiplash
Poliomyelitis
Arteriosclerotic disease

POSSIBLE ETIOLOGY

Congenital defect. Joint fibrous tissue becoming bony and immobile. Nerve damage. Joint inflammation. Therapeutic need to immobilize a joint, as with a cast, traction, or cervical collar.

NURSING DIAGNOSIS

Limited range of motion: difficulty moving a joint or joints within the normal capacity to move

PLANNING

Patient Needs	**Primary Nurse-Patient Goals**
Exercise	To achieve exercise
Protection from physical harm	To prevent physical injury
Dependence	To achieve comfort
Mastery and competence in skills, independence	To achieve optimum function
Increased learning	To achieve awareness of needs

NURSING INTERVENTIONS

Nursing Treatments
Anticipate needs
Approach unhurriedly
Handle gently
Change the patient's position gradually
Encourage normal use of the involved limb
Exercise in range of motion
Place in a whirlpool bath

Nursing Observations
Observe for readiness to assume activities of daily living

Health Teaching
Explain the causes of the health problem
Instruct to carefully move the injured body part
Teach how to do range-of-motion exercises
Explain the reason for and intended effect of the therapy

EVALUATION

See the evaluation criteria for each specific goal in Chapter 2.

POTENTIAL IMPAIRED MOBILITY

Potential Limited Range of Motion

ASSESSMENT

Subjective Data
Pain on movement

Objective Data
Muscle weakness
Muscle spasms
Increasing disuse of joints
Confinement to cast or traction

Related Data

Commonly Related Conditions:
Joint stiffness
Joint inflammation
Paralysis

Commonly Related Diseases:
Fibromyositis
Rheumatoid arthritis
Wryneck disease
Tuberculosis of the joint

POSSIBLE ETIOLOGY

Long-term immobility

NURSING DIAGNOSIS

Potential limited range of motion: the possibility that the motion capabilities of a joint will become less than normal

PLANNING

Patient Needs	**Primary Nurse-Patient Goals**
Exercise	To achieve exercise
Protection from physical harm	To prevent physical injury
Increased learning	To achieve awareness of needs

NURSING INTERVENTIONS

Nursing Treatments
Maintain body alignment
Encourage normal use of the involved limb
Exercise the fingers with a ball
Exercise in range of motion

Nursing Observations
Inspect the joints for abnormalities
Inspect the muscles for impaired tone
Observe for readiness to assume activities of daily living
Observe the extremities for motor function
Observe for mobility capabilities

Health Teaching
Explain the causes of the health problem
Advise early correction of problems
Teach how to do isometric exercises
Teach how to do range-of-motion exercises
Explain the reason for and intended effect of the therapy

EVALUATION

See the evaluation criteria for each specific goal in Chapter 2.

IMPAIRED MOBILITY RELATED TO THE ENVIRONMENT

Immobility Related to Architectural Barriers

ASSESSMENT

Subjective Data
Frustration

Objective Data
Inability to push open heavy doors
Inability to move a wheelchair through narrow doors and halls, through revolving doors, around small rooms, up curbs without ramps, over thick carpets
Inability to walk up steep stairs
Inability to reach cabinets, sinks, stoves, refrigerators, etc.
Inability to see reflection in mirrors placed too high

Related Data
Commonly Related Diseases:
Thoracic or cervical spinal cord injury
Cerebral palsy
Multiple sclerosis
Fractured tibia

POSSIBLE ETIOLOGY

Lack of recognition of the needs of the disabled. Dwellings and buildings built prior to recognition of such barriers.

NURSING DIAGNOSIS

Immobility related to architectural barriers: the existence of obstructions, within the structural design of a dwelling or building, that inhibit independent, normal activity of disabled persons

PLANNING

Patient Needs	Primary Nurse-Patient Goals
Comfort	To achieve comfort
Independence	To achieve optimum function
Increased learning	To achieve awareness of needs and/or use of resources
Increased problem-solving ability	To achieve optimum function

NURSING INTERVENTIONS

Nursing Treatments
Arrange orderly surroundings
Minimize environmental barriers
Place in an uncrowded area

Place objects within reach
Place the work at a comfortable level

Nursing Observations
Observe for mobility capabilities
Evaluate the response to teaching

Health Teaching
Recommend living in a single-level, ground-floor dwelling
Inform that deep carpeting should be avoided by persons in a wheelchair
Recommend housing with few doors and hallways for persons in a wheelchair
Recommend low window sills for persons in a wheelchair
Recommend that doorknobs and switches be placed 36 inches above the floor
Recommend that electrical outlets be placed 18 inches above the floor
Recommend polyethylene door sills for persons in a wheelchair
Recommend the use of front-loading washers and dryers for persons in a wheelchair
Recommend the use of front stove controls for persons in a wheelchair
Recommend the use of high storage cabinets for persons unable to stoop
Recommend the use of low clothes racks for persons in a wheelchair
Recommend the use of low storage cabinets for persons in a wheelchair
Recommend the use of revolving cabinet shelves
Recommend the use of top-loading washers and dryers for persons unable to stoop
Recommend the use of top stove controls for persons unable to stoop

EVALUATION

See the evaluation criteria for each specific goal in Chapter 2.

INADEQUATE MOBILITY-DEVICE MANAGEMENT

Inadequate Information Related to Brace Maintenance (317,416)

ASSESSMENT

Subjective Data
Person confirms a lack of information

Objective Data
Person's actions indicate a lack of information regarding the fact that:
    braces must be kept in alignment when not in use
    brace joints need oiling
    lint must be removed from brace joints
    brace shoe heels should not be allowed to run down

Related Data
Commonly Related Diseases:
Cerebral vascular accident

Poliomyelitis
Cerebral palsy
Muscular dystrophy
Cervical, thoracic, and lumbar spinal cord injury

POSSIBLE ETIOLOGY

Inadequate instruction in brace care

NURSING DIAGNOSIS

Inadequate information related to brace maintenance: lack of information regarding the proper care of a brace by the person wearing it

PLANNING

Patient Needs	**Primary Nurse-Patient Goals**
Protection from physical harm	To prevent physical injury
Mastery and competence in skills, independence	To achieve optimum function
Increased learning	To achieve awareness of needs

NURSING INTERVENTIONS

Nursing Treatments
Approach unhurriedly
Encourage patient questions

Nursing Observations
Evaluate the response to teaching

Health Teaching
Explain how to recognize the outgrowth of a brace
Inform that an unused leg brace should be stored in an aligned position
Inform that brace locks and joints need to be oiled
Inform that brace straps require cleanliness and repair
Inform that lint should be removed from brace locks and joints
Explain the need to maintain balanced brace shoe heels

EVALUATION

See the evaluation criteria for each specific goal in Chapter 2.

Inadequate Information Related to Brace Manipulation (317,416)

ASSESSMENT

Subjective Data
Person confirms a lack of information

Objective Data
Person's actions indicate a lack of information regarding:
    how to apply and remove a brace
    the proper clothing to be worn with a brace
    the safety precautions related to wearing a brace
    how to attain maximum mobility with a brace

Related Data

Commonly Related Diseases:
Cerebral vascular accident
Poliomyelitis
Cerebral palsy
Muscular dystrophy
Cervical, thoracic, and lumbar spinal cord injury

POSSIBLE ETIOLOGY

Lack of instruction

NURSING DIAGNOSIS

Inadequate information related to brace manipulation: lack of information regarding proper mobility with a therapeutic brace

PLANNING

Patient Needs	**Primary Nurse-Patient Goals**
Comfort	To achieve comfort
Protection from physical harm	To prevent physical injury
Mastery and competence in skills, independence	To achieve optimum function
Increased learning	To achieve awareness of needs

NURSING INTERVENTIONS

Nursing Treatments
Approach unhurriedly
Encourage patient questions

Nursing Observations
Evaluate the response to teaching
Observe for mobility capabilities

Health Teaching
Explain how to adjust clothing to meet health problems
Instruct to use a wide supportive stance for good body balance
Teach how to apply and remove a leg brace
Teach how to elevate from a sitting to a standing position with leg braces
Teach mobility down stairs and curbs with leg braces
Teach mobility from a standing to a sitting position with leg braces
Teach mobility up a curb with leg braces
Teach mobility up stairs with leg braces

Medical Treatments Performed by Nurses
Mobilize with the prescribed brace

EVALUATION

See the evaluation criteria for each specific goal in Chapter 2.

Inadequate Information Related to Cane Use (317,116)

ASSESSMENT

Subjective Data
Person confirms a lack of information

Objective Data
Person's actions indicate a lack of information regarding:
    when to use a cane
    how to properly use a cane
    the safety precautions related to using a cane
    how to recognize an incorrect cane length

Related Data
Commonly Related Diseases:
Cerebral vascular accident
Rheumatoid arthritis
Lumbar spinal cord injury
Closed fracture
Compound fracture

POSSIBLE ETIOLOGY

Therapeutic prescription of a cane to provide body support in balancing and weight-bearing

NURSING DIAGNOSIS

Inadequate information related to cane use: lack of information regarding the proper use of a therapeutic cane

PLANNING

Patient Needs	**Primary Nurse-Patient Goals**
Comfort	To achieve comfort
Protection from physical harm	To prevent physical injury
Mastery and competence in skills, independence	To achieve optimum function
Increased learning	To achieve awareness of needs

NURSING INTERVENTIONS

Nursing Treatments
Approach unhurriedly
Encourage patient questions

Nursing Observations
Check the cane for correct length
Evaluate the response to teaching

Health Teaching
Explain how to determine proper cane length
Teach how to use a cane for balancing
Teach how to use a cane for weight-bearing

EVALUATION

See the evaluation criteria for each specific goal in Chapter 2.

Inadequate Information Related to Crutch Manipulation (317,416)

ASSESSMENT

Subjective Data

Person confirms a lack of information

Objective Data

Person's actions indicate a lack of information regarding:
the type of crutches to use
how to prepare for crutch walking
when crutches are too long or too short
how to attain maximum mobility with crutches

Related Data

Commonly Related Diseases:
Cerebral vascular accident
Thoracic or lumbar spinal cord injury
Closed fracture
Compound fracture

POSSIBLE ETIOLOGY

Lack of instruction

NURSING DIAGNOSIS

Inadequate information related to crutch manipulation: lack of information regarding the use of crutches for mobility

PLANNING

Patient Needs	**Primary Nurse-Patient Goals**
Comfort	To achieve comfort
Protection from physical harm	To prevent physical injury
Mastery and competence in skills	To achieve optimum function
Increased learning	To achieve awareness of needs and/or use of resources

NURSING INTERVENTIONS

Nursing Treatments
Approach unhurriedly
Encourage patient questions
Make a referral (to crutch fitter, if the size is incorrect)

Nursing Observations
Check the crutches for correct length
Check the crutches for intact rubber tips
Check the crutch handbar for position
Evaluate the response to teaching
Observe for mobility capabilities

Health Teaching

Explain how to determine proper crutch length
Inform that the use of unadjustable crutches for heavyweight persons is
   preferable
Instruct to use a wide supportive stance for good body balance
Recommend the use of low-heeled shoes
Teach the proper gait to use with crutches
Teach correct weight-bearing on the crutch handbar
Teach good crutch-walking posture
Teach how to elevate from a sitting to a standing position with crutches
Teach mobility down a curb with crutches
Teach mobility down stairs with crutches
Teach mobility from a standing to a sitting position with crutches
Teach mobility up a curb with crutches
Teach mobility up stairs with crutches
Teach how to do pre-crutch-walking exercises

Medical Treatments Performed by Nurses

Mobilize with the prescribed crutches

EVALUATION

See the evaluation criteria for each specific goal in Chapter 2.

Inadequate Information Related to Limb Prosthesis (317,416)

ASSESSMENT

Subjective Data

Person confirms a lack of information

Objective Data

Person's actions indicate a lack of information regarding:
   how to prepare for use of a prosthesis
   the precautions to be taken when wearing a prosthesis
   how to properly use the prosthesis

Related Data

Commonly Related Diseases:
Frostbite
Crushing injury
Arteriosclerosis
Metastatic carcinoma
Buerger's disease
Raynaud's disease

POSSIBLE ETIOLOGY

Lack of instruction

NURSING DIAGNOSIS

Inadequate information related to limb prosthesis: lack of information regarding an artificial limb

PLANNING

Patient Needs

Comfort

Protection from physical harm

Mastery and competence in skills,
    independence

Increased learning

Primary Nurse-Patient Goals

To achieve comfort

To prevent physical injury

To achieve optimum function

To achieve awareness of needs

NURSING INTERVENTIONS

Nursing Treatments
Approach unhurriedly
Encourage patient questions

Nursing Observations
Evaluate the response to teaching
Determine if the prosthesis is effective

Health Teaching
Advise not to stand for prolonged periods (initially)
Instruct to gradually increase the wearing time of the prosthesis
Instruct to avoid artificial leg abduction
Instruct to avoid hiking the shoulder when walking with a leg prosthesis
Instruct to use a wide supportive stance for good body balance
Recommend the use of low-heeled shoes
Teach how to apply a stump sock
Instruct that several stump socks should not be worn simultaneously
Instruct to frequently wash the stump sock
Teach how to percuss the amputation stump
Teach how to use a temporary prosthesis
Explain the reason for delaying the prosthesis application

Medical Treatments Performed by Nurses
Apply the prescribed prosthesis

EVALUATION

See the evaluation criteria for each specific goal in Chapter 2.

Inadequate Information Related to
Walker Manipulation (317,416)

ASSESSMENT

Subjective Data
Person confirms a lack of information

Objective Data
Person's actions indicate a lack of information regarding:
    the kind of walker to use
    how to determine if the walker height is correct
    how to manipulate the walker

Related Data

Commonly Related Diseases:
Cerebral vascular accident
Closed fracture
Compound fracture

POSSIBLE ETIOLOGY

Lack of instruction

NURSING DIAGNOSIS

Inadequate information related to walker manipulation: lack of information regarding mobility with a therapeutic walker

PLANNING

Patient Needs	Primary Nurse-Patient Goals
Comfort	To achieve comfort
Protection from physical harm	To prevent physical injury
Mastery and competence in skills	To achieve optimum function
Increased learning	To achieve awareness of needs

NURSING INTERVENTIONS

Nursing Treatments
Approach unhurriedly
Encourage patient questions

Nursing Observations
Check the walker for proper height
Evaluate the response to teaching
Observe for mobility capabilities

Health Teaching
Advise not to stand for prolonged periods
Explain how to determine proper walker height
Inform that the use of a walker without wheels is preferable
Instruct to wear well-fitting shoes
Recommend the use of low-heeled shoes
Teach good body mechanics
Teach the proper gait to use with a walker

EVALUATION

See the evaluation criteria for each specific goal in Chapter 2.

Inadequate Information Related to Wheelchair Manipulation (317,416)

ASSESSMENT

Subjective Data
Person confirms a lack of information

Objective Data

Person's actions indicate a lack of information regarding:
the kind of a wheelchair to use
how to avoid the dangers associated with using a wheelchair
how to most effectively propel the wheelchair

Related Data

Commonly Related Diseases:
Cerebral vascular accident
Cervical, thoracic, or lumbar spinal cord injury
Closed or compound fracture

POSSIBLE ETIOLOGY

Lack of instruction

NURSING DIAGNOSIS

Inadequate information related to wheelchair manipulation: lack of information regarding the use of a wheelchair

PLANNING

Patient Needs

Comfort

Protection from physical harm

Mastery and competence in skills,
   independence

Increased learning

Primary Nurse-Patient Goals

To achieve comfort

To prevent accident, physical injury

To achieve optimum function

To achieve awareness of needs

NURSING INTERVENTIONS

Nursing Treatments
Approach unhurriedly
Encourage patient questions

Nursing Observations
Evaluate the response to teaching
Observe for mobility capabilities

Health Teaching
Inform that powered wheelchairs are available
Inform that the use of a lightweight wheelchair is preferable
Inform that the use of a wheelchair with good brakes is preferable
Instruct in the use of projections on wheelchair wheel rims
Instruct to lock the wheelchair before transferring
Recommend the use of long, even strokes to propel the wheelchair

EVALUATION

See the evaluation criteria for each specific goal in Chapter 2.

22.

NURSING DIAGNOSES RELATED TO
The Musculoskeletal and Neurologic Systems

BODY ALIGNMENT, INCORRECT

Joint Contracture (71,391)

ASSESSMENT

Subjective Data

Pain on movement

Objective Data

Twisted position of hand, finger, elbow, shoulder, foot, knee, or toe
Flexed (bent) position
Limited movement or inability to move
Abnormal alignment

Related Data

Commonly Related Conditions:
Hip flexion after amputation
Knee flexion after orthotomy
Knee flexion after prolonged use of a cast or corrective splint

Commonly Related Diseases:
Cerebral vascular accident
Cervical spinal cord injury
Thoracic spinal cord injury
Second- and third-degree burns
Multiple sclerosis
Muscular dystrophy

POSSIBLE ETIOLOGY

Resistance of muscle tissue around joints caused by immobility or inflammation and infection

NURSING DIAGNOSIS

Joint contracture: muscle and/or tendon shortening with impaired muscle and/or tendon use

PLANNING

Patient Needs	**Primary Nurse-Patient Goals**
Activity, exercise	To achieve activity and exercise
Comfort	To achieve comfort
Protection from physical harm	To prevent physical injury, deformities
Increased learning	To achieve awareness of needs

NURSING INTERVENTIONS

Nursing Treatments
Maintain body alignment
Ambulate the patient (as much as possible)
Change the patient's position frequently
Exercise in range of motion
Place in a whirlpool bath (during exercise, if possible)
 OR
Bathe in warm water
Massage gently
Place a footboard at the feet
Place a hand roll under the fingers
Place a trochanter roll for positioning
 OR
Position with sandbags
Encourage normal use of the involved limb

Nursing Observations
Inspect the bones for alignment
Inspect the muscles for impaired tone
Observe for evidence of a favorable response to therapy

Health Teaching
Explain the causes of the health problem
Explain how to maintain body alignment
Teach how to apply preventive splints

Medical Treatments Performed by Nurses
Apply the prescribed preventive splint

EVALUATION

See the evaluation criteria for each specific goal in Chapter 2.

Footdrop (32,71,391)

ASSESSMENT

Objective Data
Sole of the foot falls downward
Person cannot hold the foot in a normal position or in the dorsiflexion position
Foot inversion may or may not occur

Person drags foot
Heel fails to touch the ground if walking is attempted
Person walks on his toes

Related Data
Commonly Related Conditions:
Impaired mobility
Commonly Related Diseases:
Cervical, thoracic, or lumbar spinal cord injury
Subdural hematoma
Polyneuritis
Cerebral vascular accident

POSSIBLE ETIOLOGY

Prolonged bed rest without proper alignment, pressure from heavy bed clothes on the foot, and paralysis of the ankle's flexion muscle produce shortened Achilles tendon

NURSING DIAGNOSIS

Footdrop (plantar flexion): bending of the ankle in the direction of the sole of the foot

PLANNING

Patient Needs

Protection from physical harm

Increased learning

Primary Nurse-Patient Goals

To prevent physical injury, deformities

To achieve awareness of needs

NURSING INTERVENTIONS

Nursing Treatments
Maintain body alignment
Apply a bed cradle
Cover with lightweight blankets
Provide loose bedding with toe pleats
Exercise in range of motion
Place in a whirlpool bath (during exercise, if possible)
Place the feet in hard-soled ankle-top shoes
   OR
Place a footboard at the feet
Position with sandbags

Nursing Observations
Observe for evidence of a favorable response to therapy

Health Teaching
Explain how to maintain body alignment
Teach how to do range-of-motion exercises
Explain the causes of the health problem
Explain the reason for and intended effect of the therapy

Medical Treatments Performed by Nurses
Apply the prescribed preventive splint

EVALUATION

See the evaluation criteria for each specific goal in Chapter 2.

Irregular Joint Rotation (71)

ASSESSMENT

Subjective Data
Pain on movement, sometimes

Objective Data
Legs or arms point toward the body (internal rotation)
Legs or arms point away from the body (external rotation)
Person has difficulty in walking
Person has impaired range of movement

Related Data
Commonly Related Diseases:
Cerebral vascular accident
Cervical or thoracic spinal cord injury
Femur fracture
Second- or third-degree burns

POSSIBLE ETIOLOGY

Nerve impairment. Muscle shortening. Congenital defect. Prolonged bed rest without proper alignment.

NURSING DIAGNOSIS

Irregular joint rotation: the inward or outward curvature of a limb from the body

PLANNING

Patient Needs

Exercise

Comfort

Protection from physical harm

Increased learning

Primary Nurse-Patient Goals

To achieve exercise

To achieve comfort

To prevent physical injury, deformities

To achieve awareness of needs

NURSING INTERVENTIONS

Nursing Treatments
Maintain body alignment
Exercise in range of motion
Place a pillow between the knees
Place a trochanter roll for positioning
   OR
Position with pillows
   OR

Position with sandbags
Encourage normal use of the involved limb

Nursing Observations
Inspect the bones for alignment
Observe for evidence of a favorable response to therapy

Health Teaching
Explain how to maintain body alignment
Teach how to do range-of-motion exercises
Explain the causes of the health problem
Explain the reason for and intended effect of the therapy

EVALUATION

See the evaluation criteria for each specific goal in Chapter 2.

Wristdrop (70,391)

ASSESSMENT

Objective Data
Palm of the hand falls downward
Hand cannot be extended at the wrist
Person has limited movement or inability to move

Related Data
Commonly Related Conditions:
Alcohol, arsenic, or lead poisoning
Commonly Related Diseases:
Poliomyelitis
Cerebral vascular accident
Cervical spinal cord injury

POSSIBLE ETIOLOGY

Radial or cervical nerve injury. Paralysis of wrist and hand extensor muscles.

NURSING DIAGNOSIS

Wristdrop (palmar flexion): bending of the wrist in a downward direction

PLANNING

Patient Needs	**Primary Nurse-Patient Goals**
Exercise	To achieve exercise
Protection from physical harm	To prevent physical injury, deformities
Increased learning	To achieve awareness of needs

NURSING INTERVENTIONS

Nursing Treatments
Maintain body alignment
Apply a supportive splint

Exercise in range of motion
Place in a whirlpool bath (during exercise, if possible)
   OR
Bathe in warm water
Place a hand roll under the fingers
Encourage normal use of the involved limb

Nursing Observations
Observe for evidence of a favorable response to therapy

Health Teaching
Explain how to maintain body alignment
Teach how to do range-of-motion exercises
Explain the causes of the health problem
Explain the reason for and intended effect of the therapy

Medical Treatments Performed by Nurses
Apply the prescribed preventive splint

EVALUATION

See the evaluation criteria for each specific goal in Chapter 2.

BODY ALIGNMENT, POTENTIAL INCORRECT

Potential Joint Contracture (32,97,391)

ASSESSMENT

Objective Data
Poor position alignment
Infrequent position change
Insufficient range-of-motion exercises
Muscle weakness
Paralysis

Related Data

Commonly Related Diseases:
Cerebral vascular accident
Cervical or thoracic spinal cord injury
Second- or third-degree burns
Multiple sclerosis
Muscular dystrophy

POSSIBLE ETIOLOGY

Muscle spasm. Poor body alignment.

NURSING DIAGNOSIS

Potential joint contracture: the probability that the muscle will become so inflexible that it will resist stretching in normal functional movement

PLANNING

Patient Needs	**Primary Nurse-Patient Goals**
Exercise	To achieve exercise
Protection from physical harm	To prevent physical injury, deformities
Increased learning	To achieve awareness of needs

NURSING INTERVENTIONS

Nursing Treatments
Maintain body alignment
Change the patient's position frequently
Exercise the fingers with a ball
Exercise in range of motion
Massage gently
Place a footboard at the feet
Place a hand roll under the fingers
Elevate the affected body part (elevate the forearm on the chest if the elbow or shoulder is affected)
Encourage normal use of the involved limb

Nursing Observations
Inspect the joints for impending contractures

Health Teaching
Explain the causes of the health problem
Explain how to maintain body alignment
Teach how to apply preventive splints
Teach how to do range-of-motion exercises
Explain the reason for and intended effect of the therapy

Medical Treatments Performed by Nurses
Apply the prescribed preventive splint

EVALUATION

See the evaluation criteria for each specific goal in Chapter 2.

Potential Footdrop (32,71,391)

ASSESSMENT

Objective Data
Prolonged bed rest
No footboard
Heavy bed clothing weighting the feet
Poor foot alignment
Muscle weakness
Paralysis

Related Data
Commonly Related Diseases:
Spinal cord injury

Subdural hematoma
Polyneuritis
Cerebral vascular accident

POSSIBLE ETIOLOGY

Poor therapeutic measures to prevent ankle flexion and Achilles tendon shortening, resulting in gastrocnemius and soleus muscle contracture

NURSING DIAGNOSIS

Potential footdrop (potential plantar flexion): the likelihood that the ankle will become bent in the direction of the sole of the foot

PLANNING

Patient Needs

Exercise

Protection from physical harm

Increased learning

Primary Nurse-Patient Goals

To achieve exercise

To prevent physical injury, deformities

To achieve awareness of needs

NURSING INTERVENTIONS

Nursing Treatments
Maintain body alignment
Apply a bed cradle
Cover with lightweight blankets
Provide loose bedding with toe pleats
Exercise in range of motion
Place in the functional position
Place the feet in hard-soled ankle-top shoes
    OR
Place a footboard at the feet
Position with pillows
    OR
Position with sandbags

Nursing Observations
Observe for evidence of a favorable response to therapy

Health Teaching
Explain how to maintain body alignment
Teach how to do range-of-motion exercises
Explain the causes of the health problem
Explain the reason for and intended effect of the therapy

Medical Treatments Performed by Nurses
Apply the prescribed preventive splint

EVALUATION

See the evaluation criteria for each specific goal in Chapter 2.

Potential Wristdrop (70,391)

ASSESSMENT

Objective Data
Poor hand alignment
Prolonged hand immobility
Lack of wrist support
Muscle weakness
Paralysis

Related Data
Commonly Related Conditions:
Alcohol, arsenic, or lead poisoning

Commonly Related Diseases:
Poliomyelitis
Cerebral vascular accident
Cervical spinal cord injury
Polyneuritis

POSSIBLE ETIOLOGY

Cervical and radial nerve injury. Paralysis of wrist and hand extensor muscles.

NURSING DIAGNOSIS

Potential wristdrop (potential palmar flexion): the probability that the wrist will become bent and deformed in a downward position

PLANNING

Patient Needs	Primary Nurse-Patient Goals
Exercise	To achieve exercise
Protection from physical harm	To prevent physical injury, deformities
Increased learning	To achieve awareness of needs

NURSING INTERVENTIONS

Nursing Treatments
Maintain body alignment
Exercise in range of motion
Place a hand roll under the fingers
Place in the functional position
Encourage normal use of the involved limb

Nursing Observations
Observe for evidence of a favorable response to therapy

Health Teaching
Explain how to maintain body alignment
Teach how to do range-of-motion exercises
Explain the causes of the health problem
Explain the reason for and intended effect of the therapy

Medical Treatments Performed by Nurses
Apply the prescribed preventive splint

EVALUATION

See the evaluation criteria for each specific goal in Chapter 2.

BONE DEGENERATION, POTENTIAL

Potential Bone Demineralization (32,453)

ASSESSMENT

Objective Data
Prolonged bed rest
Prolonged immobility
Poor protein, vitamin D, and calcium intake

Related Data
Commonly Related Diseases:
Hyperparathyroidism
Scurvy
Cushing's syndrome
Hyperthyroidism
Hypothyroidism
Acromegaly

POSSIBLE ETIOLOGY

Bone atrophy from lack of exercise and weight-bearing. Failure of bone matrix to form. Decreased bone formation with increased bone reabsorption.

NURSING DIAGNOSIS

Potential bone demineralization: the probability that lime salts will be withdrawn from the bone and cause decreased bone density

PLANNING

Patient Needs
Food balance

Activity, exercise

Protection from physical harm

Increased learning

Primary Nurse-Patient Goals
To maintain nutrition to all cells

To achieve activity and exercise

To prevent physical injury

To achieve awareness of needs

NURSING INTERVENTIONS

Nursing Treatments
Change the patient's position frequently
Exercise in range of motion

Encourage moderate physical exercise
Encourage increased calcium food intake
Encourage increased protein-food intake
Encourage increased high-vitamin-food intake (vitamin D)
Make a referral (to a physician for periodic bone x-ray)

Nursing Observations
Measure the body weight (periodically for weight loss)
Measure the girth of the bone (for atrophy)
Observe for complaints of pain

Health Teaching
Explain the causes of the health problem
Instruct to change position frequently
Teach how to do range-of-motion exercises
Teach the principles of good nutrition
Explain the reason for and intended effect of the therapy

EVALUATION

See the evaluation criteria for each specific goal in Chapter 2.

CONVULSIVE DISORDERS

Dependence on Nursing Supervision of Controlled Seizures (71,271,453)

ASSESSMENT

Subjective Data
Person relies on nurses for:
    observation for drug side effects
    evaluation of the significance of signs and symptoms
    guidance toward living a normal life
    safety related to daily occupation
    direction toward good health habits and positive attitudes

Objective Data
Person has been on a medical regimen for treatment of seizures

Related Data
Commonly Related Diseases:
Epilepsy

POSSIBLE ETIOLOGY

Confirmed diagnosis of epilepsy. On epilepsy treatment regimen.

NURSING DIAGNOSIS

Dependence on nursing supervision of controlled seizures: reliance on nurses to periodically evaluate the health status of the person whose seizures are relatively stabilized

PLANNING

Patient Needs	Primary Nurse-Patient Goals
Comfort	To achieve comfort
Protection from physical harm	To prevent physical injury
Dependence	To achieve comfort
Increased learning	To achieve awareness of needs

NURSING INTERVENTIONS

Nursing Treatments
Encourage adequate rest
Encourage moderate physical exercise
Encourage acceptance of self-limitations
Discourage oral stimulants (especially alcohol)

Nursing Observations
Observe for (antiepileptic) drug reactions (gum hypertrophy, nervousness, rash, drowsiness)

Health Teaching
Describe the manifestations of impending seizure
Describe those symptoms which should be reported (seizures, dizziness, visual disturbances)
Explain how to manage seizure episodes
Inform of those conditions which precipitate seizures
Recommend adherence to a moderate pace of living
Teach the principles of good nutrition
Explain the reason for and intended effect of the therapy

EVALUATION

See the evaluation criteria for each specific goal in Chapter 2.

CONVULSIVE DISORDER, POTENTIAL

Impending Seizure (247,271,453)

ASSESSMENT

Subjective Data
Headache
Visualization of flashing lights
Tingling of any body area
Disagreeable tastes or odors

Objective Data
Previous seizures
Several hours prior to seizure onset, the patient appears:
    apathetic
    depressed

irritable
> OR

unusually alert
ecstatic
Extremity muscle twitching

Related Data

Commonly Related Conditions:
Hypoglycemia

Commonly Related Diseases:
Epilepsy
Eclampsia
Tetanus
Malaria
Toxemia
Cerebral astrocytoma
Meningioma
Medulloblastoma
Neurofibroma
Glomerulonephritis
Lupus erythematosus
Cerebral vascular accident
Phenylketonuria
Von Gierke's disease
Roseola infantum
Encephalitis
Meningococcal meningitis
Tuberculous meningitis

POSSIBLE ETIOLOGY

Cerebral cortex central nervous system disease. Response to toxicity.

NURSING DIAGNOSIS

Impending seizure: the presence of signs and symptoms indicating that a seizure is about to occur

PLANNING

Patient Needs

Comfort
Protection from physical harm
Increased learning

Primary Nurse-Patient Goals

To achieve comfort
To prevent accident, physical injury
To achieve awareness of needs

NURSING INTERVENTIONS

Nursing Treatments
Place on complete bed rest
Provide quiet
Subdue the room lighting
Remove constrictive clothing

Minimize environmental dangers
Restrict the intake to nothing by mouth (temporarily)
Provide standby emergency equipment (padded tongue blade)
Refrain from performing nonessential procedures
Attend the patient constantly (until the episode subsides)

Nursing Observations
Inspect for abnormal body movements (twitching)
Observe for confusion
Observe the level of consciousness
Observe the seizure characteristics (if they occur)

Health Teaching
Explain the causes of the health problem
Explain the reason for and intended effect of the therapy
Instruct to remove dentures

Medical Treatments Performed by Nurses
Give the prescribed drugs

EVALUATION

See the evaluation criteria for each specific goal in Chapter 2.

CRANIAL PRESSURE, ALTERED

Minimal Intracranial Pressure Requirement (32,70)

ASSESSMENT

Subjective Data
Severe headache
Pain from light glare

Objective Data
Hypertensive blood pressure
Gradually increasing infant's head circumference
Enlarging cerebral tumor
Recent head trauma
Cerebral hemorrhage

Related Data
Commonly Related Diseases:
Cerebral concussion
Cerebral contusion
Subdural hematoma
Subarachnoid hemorrhage
Ruptured cerebral aneurysm
Encephalitis
Hypertensive encephalopathy

Hydrocephalus
Cerebral tumor
Hypertension

POSSIBLE ETIOLOGY

Increased intracranial bulk from bleeding, edema, tumor, or abscess. Increased spinal fluid within the brain ventricles.

NURSING DIAGNOSIS

Minimal intracranial pressure requirement: a need to keep the intracranial pressure as low as possible

PLANNING

Patient Needs	Primary Nurse-Patient Goals
Sleep, rest	To achieve sleep, rest
Comfort	To achieve comfort
Protection from physical harm	To prevent physical injury
Freedom from pain	To achieve comfort
Increased learning	To achieve awareness of needs

NURSING INTERVENTIONS

Nursing Treatments
Place on complete bed rest
Provide quiet
Subdue the room lighting
Elevate the head
Do not place in the flat position
Change the patient's position gradually
Discourage oral stimulants
Handle (the head) gently
Slow the intravenous infusion flow rate
Limit infant crying by feeding on schedule and immediately changing soiled diapers
Refrain from jarring the bed
Refrain from performing nonessential procedures

Nursing Observations
Inspect the chest for respiratory rate and rhythm (alternating rapid breathing and breathing cessation)
Inspect the eyes for papilledema
Inspect the eyes for pupil equality and response changes
Monitor the blood pressure (for increase)
Observe for confusion
Observe for lethargy
Observe for restlessness
Observe for vomiting
Observe for complaints of headache
Observe for complaints of nausea
Palpate the pulse for rate (tachycardia), rhythm, and volume (bounding)

Health Teaching
Describe those symptoms which should be reported (severe pain)
Explain the causes of the health problem
Explain the reason for and intended effect of the therapy
Instruct to change position gradually
Advise gentle nose blowing
Inform that coughing should be avoided
Inform that elimination straining should be avoided

Medical Treatments Performed by Nurses
Give the prescribed drugs

EVALUATION

See the evaluation criteria for each specific goal in Chapter 2.

MUSCLE DEGENERATION, POTENTIAL

Potential Muscle Weakness (71,113)

ASSESSMENT

Objective Data
Prolonged bed rest
Sedentary life
Prolonged therapeutic immobility, such as when in a cast
Lack of exercise

Related Data
Commonly Related Conditions:
Aging

POSSIBLE ETIOLOGY

Immobility. Disease processes causing muscle degeneration.

NURSING DIAGNOSIS

Potential muscle weakness: the possibility that the muscle could lose strength and functioning capacity

PLANNING

Patient Needs	**Primary Nurse-Patient Goals**
Activity, exercise	To achieve activity and exercise
Protection from physical harm	To prevent physical injury
Increased learning	To achieve awareness of needs

NURSING INTERVENTIONS

Nursing Treatments
Ambulate the patient (as much as possible)
Encourage moderate physical exercise

Exercise in range of motion
Massage (the muscles) vigorously

Nursing Observations
Test for the degree of muscle strength

Health Teaching
Explain the causes of the health problem
Teach how to do range-of-motion exercises
Explain the reason for and intended effect of the therapy

EVALUATION

See the evaluation criteria for each specific goal in Chapter 2.

MUSCULOSKELETAL AND NEUROLOGIC DISCOMFORTS

Involuntary Muscle Twitching (247,453)

ASSESSMENT

Subjective Data
Pain, sometimes

Objective Data
Spontaneous and intermittent muscle jerking
Twitching may be accentuated with voluntary movement
Twitching may involve any body area, but usually the arm, leg, or head

Related Data
Commonly Related Conditions:
Muscular atrophy
Hypocalcemia
Respiratory alkalosis from hyperventilation

Commonly Related Diseases:
Amyotrophic lateral sclerosis
Bulbar palsy
Peripheral neuropathy
Poliomyelitis
Sydenham's chorea
Huntington's chorea
Uremia

POSSIBLE ETIOLOGY

Muscle depolarization before repolarization is complete. Disease of the basal ganglion. Decreased blood calcium level.

NURSING DIAGNOSIS

Involuntary muscle twitching: uncontrollable muscle contractions

PLANNING

Patient Needs	**Primary Nurse-Patient Goals**
Relaxation	To achieve relaxation
Comfort	To achieve comfort
Protection from physical harm	To prevent physical injury
Increased learning	To achieve awareness of needs

NURSING INTERVENTIONS

Nursing Treatments

Apply a heating pad
  OR   } (to the area)
Apply a hot water bottle
  OR
Bathe in warm water
Cover with warm blankets
Maintain a warm room temperature
Decrease drafts
Handle gently
Massage gently
Refrain from jarring the bed
Encourage increased calcium-food intake
  AND   } (if the blood calcium is low)
Give high-calcium fluids orally

Nursing Observations

Monitor blood studies for abnormal electrolytes (decreased calcium)
Inspect for abnormal body movements (twitching)
Observe for evidence of a favorable response to therapy

Health Teaching

Teach how to apply heat therapy
Explain the causes of the health problem
Explain the reason for and intended effect of the therapy

EVALUATION

See the evaluation criteria for each specific goal in Chapter 2.

Motion Sickness (247,453)

ASSESSMENT

Subjective Data

Nausea

Objective Data

Dizziness
Vomiting
Sweating
Onset is associated with motion

Related Data

Commonly Related Diseases:
None

POSSIBLE ETIOLOGY

The labyrinth of the inner ear is stimulated by motion, which affects the vomiting center in the medulla of the brain

NURSING DIAGNOSIS

Motion sickness: a sensation of sickness occurring when in motion in a car, airplane, boat, or train

PLANNING

Patient Needs	**Primary Nurse-Patient Goals**
Rest	To achieve rest
Comfort	To achieve comfort
Protection from physical harm	To prevent physical injury
Increased learning	To achieve awareness of needs

NURSING INTERVENTIONS

Nursing Treatments
Apply a cool, damp cloth to the face
Place in the slight sitting position
Change the patient's position gradually
Encourage adequate rest
Give nonprescription drugs (ExR) (Dramamine, Marezine)

Nursing Observations
Observe for evidence of a favorable response to therapy

Health Teaching
Advise against reading or looking out the window while in a moving vehicle
Explain the causes of the health problem
Explain the reason for and intended effect of the therapy

EVALUATION

See the evaluation criteria for each specific goal in Chapter 2.

Phantom-Limb Discomfort (32,391)

ASSESSMENT

Subjective Data
Person feels sensation as if it was in the amputated body part
Focuses attention on the amputated area
May fear going insane because of awareness that, although the limb is not whole, feeling is still perceived

Objective Data
Often attempts to walk on the missing leg, but falls

Related Data

Commonly Related Diseases:
Frostbite
Crushing injury
Arteriosclerosis
Metastatic carcinoma
Buerger's disease
Raynaud's disease

POSSIBLE ETIOLOGY

Autonomic nervous system responses

NURSING DIAGNOSIS

Phantom-limb discomfort: a feeling that a body part still exists even though the body part has been amputated

PLANNING

Patient Needs	**Primary Nurse-Patient Goals**
Activity, exercise	To achieve activity and exercise
Comfort	To achieve comfort
Protection from psychologic threat	To prevent emotional injury
Increased learning	To achieve awareness of needs

NURSING INTERVENTIONS

Nursing Treatments
Reassure verbally
Apply a bed cradle
Cover with lightweight blankets
Decrease drafts
Handle gently
Encourage moderate physical exercise
Exercise in range of motion
Percuss the amputation stump to increase firmness
Wrap the amputation stump
Position comfortably

Nursing Observations
Observe for evidence of a favorable response to therapy

Health Teaching
Explain the causes of the health problem
Teach how to percuss the amputation stump
Teach how to wrap an amputation stump
Explain the reason for and intended effect of the therapy

EVALUATION

See the evaluation criteria for each specific goal in Chapter 2.

Restless Leg Discomfort

ASSESSMENT

Subjective Data
Prickly, creeping leg sensation
Aches or pains, sometimes

Objective Data
Onset 15–30 minutes after sitting or lying down
Constant leg activity
Leg spasmodically and involuntarily kicks and jerks about
Leg jerks only one or two times, or may last for hours
Person is awakened from sleep by the jerking limb
Discomfort is intermittent, in that it occurs, then disappears for several months, then returns again

Related Data
Frequently associated with riding on trains or airplanes
Commonly Related Conditions:
Pregnancy
Commonly Related Diseases:
Iron-deficiency anemia

POSSIBLE ETIOLOGY

Unknown, but believed to be a disorder of either the spinal cord or affected limb. Nervous system excitement.

NURSING DIAGNOSIS

Restless leg discomfort: a creeping, crawling, jerking leg sensation, occurring only when the limb is at rest

PLANNING

Patient Needs	Primary Nurse-Patient Goals
Sleep, rest, relaxation	To achieve sleep, rest, relaxation
Comfort	To achieve comfort
Protection from physical harm	To prevent physical injury
Increased learning	To achieve awareness of needs

NURSING INTERVENTIONS

Nursing Treatments
Ambulate the patient
Apply a heating pad (to the limb)
    OR
Bathe in warm water
    OR
Cover with warm blankets
Maintain a warm room temperature
Give nonprescription drugs (ExR) (aspirin)
Massage gently (the jerking limb)

Nursing Observations
Monitor blood studies for abnormal hematology
Observe for evidence of a favorable response to therapy

Health Teaching
Explain the causes of the health problem
Teach how to apply heat therapy
Explain the reason for and intended effect of the therapy

EVALUATION

See the evaluation criteria for each specific goal in Chapter 2.

Vertigo (271,453)

ASSESSMENT

Subjective Data
When the eyes are open, a sensation that the environment is whirling
    around
When the eyes are closed, a sensation that the body is whirling around
Nausea

Objective Data
Unsteady gait
Vomiting

Related Data
Commonly Related Conditions:
Hypoglycemia
Commonly Related Diseases:
Otitis media
Labyrinthitis
Meniere's disease
Cerebral concussion or contusion
Encephalitis
Cerebral tumor

POSSIBLE ETIOLOGY

Middle ear imbalance. Decreased cardiac output.

NURSING DIAGNOSIS

Vertigo: the sensation that the environment is whirling around the person
or that the person is whirling around

PLANNING

Patient Needs	Primary Nurse-Patient Goals
Sleep, rest	To achieve sleep, rest
Comfort	To achieve comfort
Protection from physical harm	To prevent physical injury
Increased learning	To achieve awareness of needs

NURSING INTERVENTIONS

Nursing Treatments
Sit the patient in an armchair
OR
Place in the slight sitting position (in bed)
OR
Place in the flat position (if due to labyrinthitis)
Change the patient's position gradually
Encourage adequate rest
Give nonprescription drugs (ExR) (Dramamine)
Attend the patient constantly (until the episode subsides)
Refrain from jarring the bed
Withhold the drugs (streptomycin, salicylates, alcohol)

Nursing Observations
Observe for evidence of a favorable response to therapy

Health Teaching
Explain the causes of the health problem
Instruct to change position gradually
Explain the reason for and intended effect of the therapy

EVALUATION

See the evaluation criteria for each specific goal in Chapter 2.

MINOR MUSCULOSKELETAL AND NEUROLOGIC INJURY

Sprain (71,192,453)

ASSESSMENT

Subjective Data
Tenderness
Painful joint movement
Muscle spasm

Objective Data
Sudden joint swelling
Joint heat
Discoloration
Impaired function

Related Data
Commonly Related Diseases:
Lumbosacral sprain
Achilles tendon sprain

POSSIBLE ETIOLOGY

Trauma

NURSING DIAGNOSIS

Sprain: tearing or traumatizing of the fibrous connective tissue surrounding a joint

PLANNING

Patient Needs	**Primary Nurse-Patient Goals**
Comfort	To achieve comfort
Protection from physical harm	To prevent physical injury
Increased learning	To achieve awareness of needs

NURSING INTERVENTIONS

Nursing Treatments
Elevate the affected body part
Apply an ice bag (at the time of injury and intermittently for the first 36 hours)
Apply a hot water bottle (after 36 hours)
Apply an arm sling (for an upper extremity sprain)
Apply an elastic bandage
Give nonprescription drugs (ExR) (analgesics)

Nursing Observations
Inspect for edema
Observe for complaints of pain

Health Teaching
Describe those symptoms which should be reported (severe pain)
Explain the causes of the health problem
Instruct to elevate the body part
Teach that weight-bearing should be done on the unaffected side (when able to ambulate)
Explain the reason for and intended effect of the therapy

EVALUATION

See the evaluation criteria for each specific goal in Chapter 2.

MUSCULOSKELETAL AND NEUROLOGIC INJURY, POTENTIAL

Potential Bone Deformity

ASSESSMENT

Objective Data
Prolonged bed rest
Prolonged immobility
Poor bone alignment
Cast indentation or deformity
Abnormal, early walking trends of children

Related Data

Commonly Related Diseases:
Rickets
Hypothyroidism
Hypogonadism
Hyperparathyroidism
Osteogenesis imperfecta
Hypopituitarism
Closed fracture
Compound fracture

POSSIBLE ETIOLOGY

Poor body alignment. Hereditary factors. When a wet cast becomes indented or deformed and then hardens, its irregular formation will cause the bone to heal in a nonaligned position.

NURSING DIAGNOSIS

Potential bone deformity: the probability that bone alignment will be distorted

PLANNING

Patient Needs

Activity, exercise

Protection from physical harm

Increased learning

Primary Nurse-Patient Goals

To achieve activity and exercise

To prevent physical injury

To achieve awareness of needs

NURSING INTERVENTIONS

Nursing Treatments
Maintain body alignment
Place a bedboard under the mattress
Position with sandbags
Ambulate the patient (as much as possible)
AND
Exercise in range of motion
} (if on prolonged bed rest)
Consult with the physician (regarding a new cast if the current one is indented)

Health Teaching
Explain the causes of the health problem
Teach how to do range-of-motion exercises
Explain the reason for and intended effect of the therapy

Medical Treatments Performed by Nurses
Apply the prescribed preventive splint
Apply the prescribed traction

EVALUATION

See the evaluation criteria for each specific goal in Chapter 2.

Potential Paralysis Related to Spinal Cord Injury (84,192,391)

ASSESSMENT

Subjective Data

Weakness and numbness below the point of injury

Objective Data

Inability to move either the arms or legs
Respiratory distress
Loss of bowel or bladder control

Related Data

Person has sustained an injury in which the head has been bent backward or forward, such as falling down stairs, diving into a shallow pool, or a car accident

Commonly Related Diseases:

Cervical, thoracic, or lumbar spinal cord injury
Whiplash injury

POSSIBLE ETIOLOGY

Fractured vertebrae that could squeeze or shear the spinal cord nerves

NURSING DIAGNOSIS

Potential paralysis related to spinal cord injury: the possibility that paralysis could occur as a result of a spinal cord injury

PLANNING

Patient Needs

Protection from physical harm

Increased learning

Primary Nurse-Patient Goals

To prevent physical injury

To achieve awareness of needs

NURSING INTERVENTIONS

Nursing Treatments

Maintain body alignment
Immobilize the affected body part (spine)
   AND
Position with sandbags (to assure immobility)
Place in the flat position
Place in the face-upward (supine) position (in cervical vertebrae injury)
Place on complete bed rest
Move the entire body as a single unit (using a board to support the body)

Nursing Observations

Inspect the chest for respiratory rate and rhythm (dyspnea, diaphragmatic breathing, respiratory failure)
Observe the extremities for motor function
Observe for complaints of numbness and tingling

Health Teaching
Describe those symptoms which should be reported (sensation loss)
Explain the reason for and intended effect of the therapy

EVALUATION

See the evaluation criteria for each specific goal in Chapter 2.

Predisposition to Accidental Injury

ASSESSMENT

Subjective Data
Dizziness
Vertigo
Generalized weakness
High-level anxiety
Preoccupation

Objective Data
Poor coordination
Muscle weakness
Unsteady gait
Hyperactivity
Impaired vision
Impaired hearing
Confusion
Disorientation
Poor control of body movements from excessive body weight

Related Data
Most prevelant in children and the aged
Commonly Related Conditions:
Late stages of pregnancy
Mental retardation
Proprioception
Commonly Related Diseases:
None
OR
Multiple sclerosis
Cerebral palsy
Muscular dystrophy
Cushing's disease
Addison's disease
Bone fracture

POSSIBLE ETIOLOGY

Limited perception of environmental dangers. Diminished ability to control
one's movement through and about the environment.

NURSING DIAGNOSIS

Predisposition to accidental injury: a proneness to an unusually high rate of unfortunate, physically harmful occurrences

PLANNING

Patient Needs

Protection from physical harm

Increased learning

Primary Nurse-Patient Goals

To prevent accident, physical injury

To achieve awareness of needs

NURSING INTERVENTIONS

Nursing Treatments
Arrange orderly surroundings
Minimize environmental barriers
Minimize environmental dangers
Assist with mobility
Provide safe play equipment for children
Restrain the patient (for safety purposes)
Safeguard with a crib dome
Safeguard with siderail padding
Safeguard with siderails
Apply a safety helmet to the head
Cover the bed with netting
Encourage participation in safe, thrilling experiences

Health Teaching
Recommend strict adherence to safety rules
Explain the reason for and intended effect of the therapy

EVALUATION

See the evaluation criteria for each specific goal in Chapter 2.

Predisposition to Bone Fracture
(71,247,271)

ASSESSMENT

Subjective Data
Bone pain

Objective Data
Malnutrition
Blue sclera
Prolonged immobility

Related Data
Often associated with adrenal-steroid therapy and the pursuit of contact
  sports

Laboratory Findings:
Increased or decreased blood calcium
Commonly Related Conditions:
Aging
Commonly Related Diseases:
Osteoporosis
Osteomalacia
Multiple myeloma
Osteogenic sarcoma
Endothelial myeloma
Reticulum cell sarcoma
Osteogenesis imperfecta
Anemia

POSSIBLE ETIOLOGY

Disease invasion at the specific bone site. Generalized bone disease.

NURSING DIAGNOSIS

Predisposition to bone fracture: the likelihood that a bone will break under circumstances that normally would not cause bone breakage

PLANNING

Patient Needs
Food balance

Protection from physical harm

Increased learning

Primary Nurse-Patient Goals
To maintain nutrition to all cells

To prevent accident, physical injury

To achieve awareness of needs

NURSING INTERVENTIONS

Nursing Treatments
Handle gently
Change the patient's position gradually
Refrain from jarring the bed
Encourage increased calcium-food intake (if the blood calcium is low)

Health Teaching
Explain the causes of the health problem
Instruct to change position gradually
Inform that heavy lifting should be avoided
Emphasize the danger of excessive body weight (pressure on the bones)
Teach good body mechanics
Teach the principles of good nutrition
Explain the reason for and intended effect of the therapy

EVALUATION

See the evaluation criteria for each specific goal in Chapter 2.

MUSCULOSKELETAL AND NEUROLOGIC INJURY DEPENDENCE

Dependence on Amputation Stump Care (71,391)

ASSESSMENT

Subjective Data

Person relies on nurses for:
   frequent dressing change
   correct positioning
   proper exercises
   preparation for prosthesis

Objective Data

Person has an amputation stump of recent origin

Related Data

Commonly Related Diseases:
Frostbite
Crushing injury
Arteriosclerosis
Metastatic carcinoma
Buerger's disease
Raynaud's disease
Gas gangrene
Diabetes mellitus

POSSIBLE ETIOLOGY

Lack of instruction in amputation care

NURSING DIAGNOSIS

Dependence on amputation stump care: reliance on nurses for the care and cleanliness of an amputation stump and preparation of the stump for a prosthesis

PLANNING

Patient Needs	Primary Nurse-Patient Goals
Exercise	To achieve exercise
Comfort	To achieve comfort
Cleanliness	To achieve good hygiene
Protection from physical harm	To prevent accident, physical injury, deformities, infection
Dependence	To achieve comfort
Increased learning	To achieve awareness of needs

NURSING INTERVENTIONS

Nursing Treatments
Clean with surgical soap

Change the dressing frequently
Wrap the amputation stump
Apply a stump sock
Percuss the amputation stump to increase firmness
Place the amputation stump in the extension position
Do not place the amputation stump in the flexion position
Exercise in range of motion
Place a bedboard under the mattress

Nursing Observations
Inspect for bleeding
Inspect the skin for irritation
Observe the amputation stump for odor
Determine if the prosthesis is effective

Health Teaching
Explain the need for maintaining a firm surface under the hip of an amputated leg
Instruct that the flexion stump position be avoided
Instruct to lie in the prone position
Instruct that pillows not be placed under the knee
Instruct that the amputation stump should not be rested on the crutch handrail
Teach how to apply a stump sock
Instruct to frequently wash the stump sock
Instruct that several stump socks should not be worn stimultaneously
Instruct to gradually increase the wearing time of the prosthesis
Teach good prosthesis-walking posture
Instruct to avoid hiking the shoulder when walking with a leg prosthesis
Teach how to use a temporary prosthesis
Teach how to do above-knee stump exercises
Teach how to do below-knee stump exercises
Teach how to percuss the amputation stump
Teach how to wrap an amputation stump
Teach how to do range-of-motion exercises
Explain the reason for and intended effect of the therapy

EVALUATION

See the evaluation criteria for each specific goal in Chapter 2.

MUSCULOSKELETAL AND NEUROLOGIC THERAPY DEPENDENCE

Dependence on Traction Management (70,391)

ASSESSMENT

Subjective Data
Person relies on nurses for:
    traction alignment

maintenance of correct traction weights
protection from infection at the traction pin or tong sites
freedom from rope, halter, or tape irritation

Objective Data

Person is receiving traction therapy

Related Data

Commonly Related Diseases:
Closed fracture
Compound fracture
Cervical vertebra fracture

POSSIBLE ETIOLOGY

Need to bring bones into correct position for healing or correct body alignment

NURSING DIAGNOSIS

Dependence on traction management: reliance on nurses for the care and proper functioning of an applied, weighted, pulling device on bones and muscles

PLANNING

Patient Needs	**Primary Nurse-Patient Goals**
Rest	To achieve rest
Exercise	To achieve exercise
Comfort	To achieve comfort
Protection from physical harm	To prevent physical injury, deformities, infection
Dependence	To promote comfort
Increased learning	To achieve awareness of needs

NURSING INTERVENTIONS

Nursing Treatments

Maintain body alignment
Change the patient's position gradually
Clean with surgical soap (around the tong or pin insertion sites)
Maintain countertraction force
Place a bedboard under the mattress
Provide a firm mattress
Position comfortably
Refrain from jarring the bed
Encourage adequate rest

Nursing Observations

Check that the traction weights are hanging free
Check the traction ropes and pulleys for alignment
Inspect the skin for breakdown
Inspect the orthopedic pin for position and for cleanliness
Observe for cyanosis (of the area in traction)

Health Teaching
Instruct to change position gradually
Explain the causes of the health problem
Explain the reason for and intended effect of the therapy

Medical Treatments Performed by Nurses
Apply the prescribed traction

EVALUATION

See the evaluation criteria for each specific goal in Chapter 2.

MUSCULOSKELETAL AND NEUROLOGIC THERAPY DISCOMFORT

Cast Discomfort (70,391)

ASSESSMENT

Subjective Data
Itching under the cast
Muscle cramps

Objective Data
Skin irritation from the cast
Limited mobility
Cast heaviness and cumbersomeness
Disagreeable odors from a soiled cast

Related Data
Commonly Related Diseases:
Closed or compound fracture
Spondylosyndesis
Osteogenesis imperfecta

POSSIBLE ETIOLOGY

Need for bone immobility to support healing

NURSING DIAGNOSIS

Cast discomfort: annoyances or mild pain resulting from wearing a cast

PLANNING

Patient Needs	**Primary Nurse-Patient Goals**
Comfort	To achieve comfort
Protection from physical harm	To prevent physical injury
Increased learning	To achieve awareness of needs

NURSING INTERVENTIONS

Nursing Treatments
Elevate the affected body part (in the cast)
Massage gently (the area around the cast)

Pad the rough cast edges
Position comfortably
Position with pillows
Provide a scratching device
Consult with the physician (about a new cast if the current one is odoriferous)
Waterproof the cast surface (to prevent soiling)
Bivalve and spread the cast to relieve pressure (ET) (if necessary)

Nursing Observations
Inspect the skin for irritation
Observe for cyanosis (of the casted area)

Health Teaching
Explain how to pad rough cast edges
Teach good body mechanics (for easier mobility)
Explain the reason for and intended effect of the therapy

EVALUATION

See the evaluation criteria for each specific goal in Chapter 2.

Cervical Collar Discomfort

ASSESSMENT

Subjective Data
Muscle soreness
Muscle spasms
Neck stiffness

Objective Data
Skin irritation from the collar
Impaired mobility

Related Data
Commonly Related Diseases:
Cervical vertebra injury
Whiplash injury

POSSIBLE ETIOLOGY

Need for neck immobility for healing

NURSING DIAGNOSIS

Cervical collar discomfort: annoyances or mild pain resulting from wearing a cervical collar

PLANNING

Patient Needs	**Primary Nurse-Patient Goals**
Comfort	To achieve comfort
Protection from physical harm	To prevent physical injury
Increased learning	To achieve awareness of needs

NURSING INTERVENTIONS

Nursing Treatments

Apply a heating pad
   OR
Apply a hot water bottle ⎫ (to the area for stiffness, soreness, or spasm)

Pad the bony prominences (around the jaw)
Position comfortably

Nursing Observations
Observe for evidence of a favorable response to therapy

Health Teaching
Teach good body mechanics (while wearing the cervical collar)
Explain the reason for and intended effect of the therapy

EVALUATION

See the evaluation criteria for each specific goal in Chapter 2.

NONFUNCTIONING MUSCULOSKELETAL AND NEUROLOGIC THERAPEUTIC DEVICE

Disrupted Traction (70,391)

ASSESSMENT

Subjective Data
Loss of pulling, traction sensation

Objective Data
Traction weights have been placed on a chair
Weights have stretched to the floor
Loose or untied ropes
Nonaligned traction
Tongs have been displaced from the scalp

Related Data
Commonly Related Diseases:
Compound fracture

POSSIBLE ETIOLOGY

Accident. Poor fitting of the traction parts.

NURSING DIAGNOSIS

Disrupted traction: traction that because of breaks or disarrangement no longer functions properly

PLANNING

Patient Needs	**Primary Nurse-Patient Goals**
Comfort	To achieve comfort
Protection from physical harm	To prevent accident, physical injury, deformities
Increased learning	To achieve awareness of needs

NURSING INTERVENTIONS

Nursing Treatments
Handle gently
Immobilize the affected body part (until the traction is reapplied properly)

Nursing Observations
Check that the traction weights are hanging free
Check the traction ropes and pulleys for alignment
Observe the extremities for motor function
Observe for complaints of numbness and tingling

Health Teaching
Explain the causes of the health problem
Explain the reason for and intended effect of the therapy

EVALUATION

See the evaluation criteria for each specific goal in Chapter 2.

EMERGENCY MUSCULOSKELETAL AND NEUROLOGIC CONDITIONS, POTENTIAL

Potential Postfracture Fat Embolus (70,391,453)

ASSESSMENT

Objective Data
Recent fracture of a long bone
Dehydration

Related Data
Person was in a highly traumatic event such as an automobile accident, falling from a great distance, etc.
Commonly Related Conditions:
Heavy consumption of alcohol
Commonly Related Diseases:
Any bone fracture
Diabetes mellitus
Severe second- or third-degree burns

POSSIBLE ETIOLOGY

Following injury to the bone, fat is released from the bone marrow, enters the circulation, and affects vital organs

NURSING DIAGNOSIS

Potential postfracture fat embolus: the possibility that a patient with a recent bone fracture will develop fat embolus

PLANNING

Patient Needs	**Primary Nurse-Patient Goals**
Water-salt balance	To maintain fluid and electrolyte balance
Protection from physical harm	To prevent physical injury
Increased learning	To achieve awareness of needs

NURSING INTERVENTIONS

Nursing Treatments
Handle gently (the injured area)
Increase fluid intake to about 2000 cc daily
Provide frequent patient contact

Nursing Observations
Auscultate the chest for rales (bubbling, crackling) and rhonchi
Inspect the chest for respiratory rate and rhythm
Inspect for bleeding (hemoptysis)
Inspect the skin for petechiae (over the chest and shoulders)
Monitor the blood pressure
Monitor the oral temperature (for fever)
Observe for complaints of visual disturbance
Observe for confusion
Observe for convulsions
Observe for cyanosis
Observe for dyspnea
Observe for irritability
Observe for restlessness
Observe for shock

Health Teaching
Explain the reason for and intended effect of the therapy

EVALUATION

See the evaluation criteria for each specific goal in Chapter 2.

Potential Tissue Injury Related to Fracture (71,192)

ASSESSMENT

Subjective Data
Acute pain at the injury site

Objective Data
Bone projection from normal alignment
Bone crepitation
Loss of voluntary movement
Swelling
Hemorrhage
Bone has not been put in a cast
Requires movement for therapeutic treatment

Related Data

Commonly Related Diseases:
Closed fracture
Compound fracture
Extracapsular fracture
Intracapsular fracture
Commuted fracture
Longitudinal fracture
Greenstick fracture
Depressed fracture
Impacted fracture
Pathologic fracture
Spiral fracture
Oblique fracture
Transverse fracture
Skull fracture
Cervical spine fracture
Mandible fracture
Clavicle fracture
Rib fracture
Humerus fracture
Pelvis fracture
Femur fracture
Tibia fracture
Fibula fracture
Patella fracture
Phalanx fracture
Metatarsal fracture

POSSIBLE ETIOLOGY

Trauma

NURSING DIAGNOSIS

Potential tissue injury related to fracture: the possibility that a fractured bone will tear into and injure the soft tissue surrounding the bone

PLANNING

Patient Needs	**Primary Nurse-Patient Goals**
Comfort	To achieve comfort
Protection from physical harm	To prevent physical injury
Increased learning	To achieve awareness of needs

NURSING INTERVENTIONS

Nursing Treatments
Maintain body alignment
Apply a supportive splint
Handle gently
Immobilize the affected body part
Mobilize by stretcher (until the bone is placed in a cast)
Remove constrictive clothing

Nursing Observations
Observe the extremities for motor function
Observe for complaints of numbness and tingling
Observe for complaints of pain
Palpate for arterial pulsations (in the injured area)

Health Teaching
Explain the causes of the health problem
Explain the reason for and intended effect of the therapy

EVALUATION

See the evaluation criteria for each specific goal in Chapter 2.

INADEQUATE INFORMATION RELATED TO CONVULSIVE DISORDERS

Inadequate Information Related to Seizures (71,271,453)

ASSESSMENT

Subjective Data
Person confirms a lack of information
May believe in the traditional superstitions related to seizures

Objective Data
Person's actions indicate a lack of information regarding:
    why seizures occur
    dangers associated with seizures
    reasons for or anticipated effects of treatments
    how to handle impending seizures

Related Data
Commonly Related Diseases:
Epilepsy

POSSIBLE ETIOLOGY

Lack of instruction

NURSING DIAGNOSIS

Inadequate information related to seizures: lack of information regarding the cause, effects, and treatment of seizures

PLANNING

Patient Needs

Protection from physical harm

Increased learning

Primary Nurse-Patient Goals

To prevent physical injury

To achieve awareness of needs

NURSING INTERVENTIONS

Nursing Treatments

Approach unhurriedly

Encourage patient questions

Nursing Observations

Evaluate the response to teaching

Health Teaching

Describe the manifestations of impending seizure

Explain how to manage seizure episodes

Inform of those conditions which precipitate seizures

Inform that seizures are not contagious

Explain the causes of the health problem

Explain the reason for and intended effect of the therapy

EVALUATION

See the evaluation criteria for each specific goal in Chapter 2.

23.
NURSING DIAGNOSIS RELATED TO
Nutrition

NUTRITIONAL INTAKE DISORDERS

Malnutrition (70,365,391,453)

ASSESSMENT

Subjective Data
Weakness
Muscle tenderness
Hunger
Nausea
Peripheral neuritis
Fatigue

Objective Data
Underweight
Chronic weight loss
Restlessness
Pallor
Tachycardia
Sunken abdomen
Pica, sometimes

Related Data
Commonly Related Conditions:
Cachexia
Commonly Related Diseases:
Sprue
Rickets
Beriberi
Iron-deficiency anemia
Pellagra
Laennec's cirrhosis
Scurvy

Osteomalacia
Cystic fibrosis
Ulcerative colitis

POSSIBLE ETIOLOGY

Poor eating habits. Unavailability of proper foods. Malabsorption in which inflammation or fibrosis of the intestinal mucosa disturbs the mechanisms of transport, diffusion, and liquid absorption by phagocyte cells.

NURSING DIAGNOSIS

Malnutrition (balanced nutritional requirement): improper intake or absorption of balanced food substances with a resulting tissue deficiency of carbohydrates, fats, proteins, and vitamins

PLANNING

Patient Needs	Primary Nurse-Patient Goals
Food balance	To maintain nutrition to all cells
Sleep, rest	To achieve sleep, rest
Protection from physical harm	To prevent physical injury
Increased learning	To achieve awareness of needs

NURSING INTERVENTIONS

Nursing Treatments
Balance nutritional intake
Supplement protein intake
Estimate the required daily calories
Give small, frequent feedings
Give snacks
Give buttermilk or yogurt (to improve absorption)
Grant special requests (for food)
Encourage the substitution of undesirable (eating) habits with favorable habits
Encourage adequate rest
Discourage smoking

Nursing Observations
Measure the body weight (daily)
Observe and record the food intake
Observe the eating pattern for abnormality

Health Teaching
Explain the causes of the health problem
Advise against using mineral oil laxatives (which further deplete vitamins)
Explain how to budget
Inform that underweight persons require additional sleep
Teach the principles of good nutrition
Explain the reason for and intended effect of the therapy

Medical Treatments Performed by Nurses
Give the prescribed diet

EVALUATION

See the evaluation criteria for each specific goal in Chapter 2.

Obesity (70,365,391,453)

ASSESSMENT

Subjective Data
Chronic fatigue

Objective Data
A 20% or more excess of body weight
Single skin fold thickness of more than 1 inch
Dyspnea on exertion

Related Data
Commonly Related Diseases:
Hypothyroidism
Hypopituitarism
Hypothalamus lesion
Diabetes mellitus
Rheumatoid arthritis
Essential or malignant hypertension
Myocardial infarction

POSSIBLE ETIOLOGY

Endocrine imbalance. Calorie intake that exceeds caloric requirement. Body storage of excessive carbohydrates as fat. Cultural and family habits of overeating. Damage to the satiation center in the hypothalamus, which regulates eating. A desire to enjoy the sedative, relaxing effect and satisfaction gained from food. Substitution of food for love perceived as not being given to the person.

NURSING DIAGNOSIS

Obesity: an excessive amount of body weight with an accumulation of fatty or adipose tissue

PLANNING

Patient Needs
Food balance
Activity, exercise
Protection from physical harm
Increased learning

Primary Nurse-Patient Goals
To maintain nutrition to all cells
To achieve activity and exercise
To prevent physical injury
To achieve awareness of needs

NURSING INTERVENTIONS

Nursing Treatments
Encourage decreased calorie intake
Encourage decreased carbohydrate intake
Encourage moderate physical exercise
Estimate the required daily calories

Provide a nontempting environment
Refrain from giving between-meal feedings
Encourage the substitution of undesirable (eating) habits with favorable habits

Nursing Observations
Measure the body weight (weekly)
Observe and record the food intake
Observe the eating pattern for abnormality

Health Teaching
Explain the causes of the health problem
Emphasize the danger of excessive body weight
Advise against eating sweets
Advise that between-meal snacks be avoided
Recommend eating and drinking in moderation
Teach the principles of good nutrition
Explain the reason for and intended effect of the therapy

Medical Treatments Performed by Nurses
Give the prescribed diet

EVALUATION

See the evaluation criteria for each specific goal in Chapter 2.

NUTRITIONAL INTAKE DISORDERS, POTENTIAL

Potential Malnutrition (70,365,391,453)

ASSESSMENT

Subjective Data
Prolonged nausea

Objective Data
Anorexia
Prolonged vomiting
Chronically poor eating habits
Difficulty in swallowing or sucking

Related Data
Common among teenagers and the aged
Commonly Related Conditions:
Wired jaw
Severe trauma or major surgery
Commonly Related Diseases:
Sprue
Addison's disease
Peptic ulcer
Metastatic carcinoma
Ulcerative colitis

Gastritis
Alcoholism
Celiac disease

POSSIBLE ETIOLOGY

Unavailability of adequate food. Improper intake or absorption of normally required food substances.

NURSING DIAGNOSIS

Potential malnutrition: the probability that a state of malnutrition can or will exist

PLANNING

Patient Needs

Food balance

Protection from physical harm

Increased learning

Primary Nurse-Patient Goals

To maintain nutrition to all cells

To prevent physical injury

To achieve awareness of needs

NURSING INTERVENTIONS

Nursing Treatments
Balance nutritional intake
Supplement protein intake
Estimate the required daily calories
Give small, frequent feedings
Give snacks
Grant special requests
Provide food selection

Nursing Observations
Measure the body weight (periodically)
Observe and record the food intake
Observe the eating pattern for abnormality
Observe for diet intolerance
Observe for increased nutritional requirements

Health Teaching
Explain the causes of the health problem
Recommend a regular mealtime schedule
Teach the principles of good nutrition
Explain the reason for and intended effect of the therapy

EVALUATION

See the evaluation criteria for each specific goal in Chapter 2.

Potential Obesity (70,365,391,453)

ASSESSMENT

Subjective Data
Person gains emotional satisfaction from food

Objective Data
Excessive food intake

Excessive carbohydrate intake
Considerable between-meal snacking
Sedentary living habits

POSSIBLE ETIOLOGY

Calorie intake in excess of caloric requirements

NURSING DIAGNOSIS

Potential obesity: the possibility that a condition of 20%–30% or more excess body weight will occur

PLANNING

Patient Needs	Primary Nurse-Patient Goals
Food balance	To maintain nutrition to all cells
Activity, exercise	To achieve activity and exercise
Protection from physical harm	To prevent physical injury
Increased learning	To achieve awareness of needs

NURSING INTERVENTIONS

Nursing Treatments
Balance nutritional intake
Estimate the required daily calories
Encourage decreased calorie intake
Encourage decreased carbohydrate intake
Refrain from giving between-meal feedings
Encourage moderate physical exercise

Nursing Observations
Measure the body weight
Observe and record the food intake
Observe the eating pattern for abnormality

Health Teaching
Explain the causes of the health problem
Emphasize the danger of excessive body weight
Advise against eating sweets
Advise that between-meal snacks be avoided
Recommend eating and drinking in moderation
Teach the principles of good nutrition
Explain the reason for and intended effect of the therapy

EVALUATION

See the evaluation criteria for each specific goal in Chapter 2.

NUTRITIONAL EXCESSES

Excessive Caffeine Intake (309)

ASSESSMENT

Subjective Data
Person relies on coffee to offset fatigue

Objective Data
Person consumes five or more cups of coffee a day
Prefers coffee black
Needs coffee to get started in the morning
Is irritable without coffee

Related Data
Commonly Related Diseases:
Peptic ulcer
Duodenal ulcer
Gastric ulcer
Arteriosclerosis
Hypertension
Glaucoma
Myocardial infarction

POSSIBLE ETIOLOGY

A daily living habit. Need for stimulation.

NURSING DIAGNOSIS

Excessive caffeine intake: the daily intake of large amounts of coffee

PLANNING

Patient Needs	**Primary Nurse-Patient Goals**
Protection from physical harm	To prevent physical injury
Increased learning	To achieve awareness of needs

NURSING INTERVENTIONS

Nursing Treatments
Encourage increased protein-food intake (to offset fatigue)
Substitute caffeine-free coffee

Health Teaching
Emphasize the danger of excessive coffee consumption

EVALUATION

See the evaluation criteria for each specific goal in Chapter 2.

NUTRITIONAL REQUIREMENTS, ABOVE NORMAL

Increased Nutritional Requirement Related to Blood Loss (247,271)

ASSESSMENT

Subjective Data
Dyspnea
Malaise

Fatigue
Palpitations
Dizziness
Thirst

Objective Data
Pallor
Sweating
Tachycardia
Blood loss of less than 500 cc a week
No gastrointestinal bleeding

Related Data
Laboratory Findings:
Low blood hemoglobin, red blood cell count, and iron
Elevated total iron binding capacity

Commonly Related Conditions:
Prolonged excessive menstrual flow
Prolonged hemorrhoid bleeding
Chronic epistaxis
Excessive blood donations

Commonly Related Diseases:
Iron-deficiency anemia

POSSIBLE ETIOLOGY

The loss of blood decreases the blood volume, causing fluid from the tissues to enter the circulatory system. This dilutes the existing blood and decreases its capacity to carry oxygen.

NURSING DIAGNOSIS

Increased nutritional requirement related to chronic blood loss: an above-normal need for one or more nutrients as a result of prolonged loss of blood

PLANNING

Patient Needs	**Primary Nurse-Patient Goals**
Food balance	To maintain nutrition to all cells
Protection from physical harm	To prevent physical injury
Increased learning	To achieve awareness of needs

NURSING INTERVENTIONS

Nursing Treatments
Encourage increased iron-food intake
Encourage increased protein-food intake
Give nonprescription drugs (ExR) (iron compound)
Make a referral (to a physician if the hemoglobin remains low after 3 weeks of iron therapy)

Nursing Observations
Monitor blood studies for abnormal hematology
Observe for a favorable response to therapy

Health Teaching
Explain the causes of the health problem
Explain the reason for and intended effect of the therapy

EVALUATION

See the evaluation criteria for each specific goal in Chapter 2.

Increased Nutritional Requirement Related to Lactation (460)

ASSESSMENT

Objective Data
Mother is producing breast milk
Infant is nursing at the breast

Related Data
Commonly Related Conditions:
Postpartum period
Commonly Related Diseases:
None

POSSIBLE ETIOLOGY

The need of the mother to maintain her own nutrition and in addition provide nutrition for her infant

NURSING DIAGNOSIS

Increased nutritional requirement related to lactation: an above-normal need for one or more nutrients as a result of producing breast milk for infant nursing

NURSING INTERVENTIONS

Nursing Treatments
Balance nutritional intake
Encourage increased caloric intake (2800–3000 calories daily)
Encourage increased calcium-food intake
Give small, frequent feedings
Give snacks

Nursing Observations
Observe and record food intake
Observe for a favorable response to therapy

Health Teaching
Explain the causes of the health problem
Teach the principles of good nutrition
Explain the reason for and intended effect of the therapy

EVALUATION

See the evaluation criteria for each specific goal in Chapter 2.

Increased Nutritional Requirement
Related to Metabolism (70,71,365,391)

ASSESSMENT

Subjective Data
Craving for excess food quantity
Craving for specific foods
Fatigue

Objective Data
Fever
Hyperactivity

Related Data
Commonly Related Diseases:
Thyrotoxicosis
Addison's disease

POSSIBLE ETIOLOGY

An accelerated body metabolism requires excessive amounts of nutritional fuel to meet the body's rapid energy consumption. Insufficient adrenal function reduces the body's available energy, some of which can be supplemented nutritionally.

NURSING DIAGNOSIS

Increased nutritional requirement related to metabolism: an above-normal need for one or more nutrients as a result of accelerated metabolic requirements

PLANNING

Patient Needs	Primary Nurse-Patient Goals
Food balance	To maintain nutrition to all cells
Energy	To maintain regulating mechanisms and functions
Protection from physical harm	To prevent physical injury
Increased learning	To achieve awareness of needs

NURSING INTERVENTIONS

Nursing Treatments
Balance nutritional intake
Encourage increased carbohydrate intake
Encourage increased protein-food intake
Supplement protein intake
Give small, frequent feedings
Give snacks
Provide extra food helpings at mealtimes
Grant special requests

Nursing Observations
Measure the body weight (daily for weight stabilization)

Observe and record the food intake
Observe for a favorable response to therapy

Health Teaching
Explain the causes of the health problem
Explain the reason for and intended effect of the therapy

Medical Treatments Performed by Nurses
Give the prescribed diet

EVALUATION

See the evaluation criteria for each specific goal in Chapter 2.

Increased Nutritional Requirement Related to Smoking Habituation (271,333,453)

ASSESSMENT

Subjective Data
Fatigue

Objective Data
Person smokes three or more cigarettes daily or smokes cigars or a pipe

Related Data
Laboratory Findings:
Low blood ascorbic acid
Decreased blood levels of B vitamins

Commonly Related Diseases:
Amblyopia

POSSIBLE ETIOLOGY

The toxic substances that enter the body with cigarette smoking deplete the body of vitamin C. Cigar and pipe smoking lead to B vitamin deficiencies. The acetaldehyde in cigarette smoke combines rapidly with protein and causes disturbed protein function.

NURSING DIAGNOSIS

Increased nutritional requirement related to smoking habituation: an above-normal need for one or more nutrients or amounts of nutrients as a result of heavy smoking

PLANNING

Patient Needs	**Primary Nurse-Patient Goals**
Food balance	To maintain nutrition to all cells
Protection from physical harm	To prevent physical injury
Increased learning	To achieve awareness of needs

NURSING INTERVENTIONS

Nursing Treatments
Encourage increased high-vitamin-food intake (vitamins B and C)

Encourage increased protein-food intake

Nursing Observations
Observe for a favorable response to therapy

Health Teaching
Advise against using mineral oil laxatives (which further deplete vitamins)
Explain the causes of the health problem
Explain the reason for and intended effect of the therapy

EVALUATION

See the evaluation criteria for each specific goal in Chapter 2.

Increased Nutritional Requirement
Related to Tissue Healing (70,365,391)

ASSESSMENT

Objective Data
Healing surgical incision
Healing burn wound
Healing trauma wound
Healing of an infected site

Related Data
Commonly Related Diseases:
First-, second-, or third-degree burns
Tuberculosis
Peptic ulcer

POSSIBLE ETIOLOGY

Tissue healing requires an additional consumption of body energy available through food intake

NURSING DIAGNOSIS

Increased nutritional requirement related to tissue healing: an above-normal need for one or more nutrients as a result of the ongoing healing process

PLANNING

Patient Needs	**Primary Nurse-Patient Goals**
Food balance	To maintain nutrition to all cells
Energy	To maintain regulating mechanisms and functions
Protection from physical harm	To prevent physical injury
Increased learning	To achieve awareness of needs

NURSING INTERVENTIONS

Nursing Treatments
Balance nutritional intake
Encourage increased protein-food intake
Supplement protein intake

Give small, frequent feedings
Give snacks
Provide extra food helpings at mealtimes

Nursing Observations
Measure the body weight (daily)
Observe and record the food intake
Observe for a favorable response to therapy

Health Teaching
Explain the causes of the health problem
Explain the reason for and intended effect of the therapy

Medical Treatments Performed by Nurses
Give the prescribed diet

EVALUATION

See the evaluation criteria for each specific goal in Chapter 2.

EATING DISORDERS

Anorexia (70,391)

ASSESSMENT

Subjective Data
No enthusiasm for food
Unconcerned about poor appetite

Objective Data
Prefers not to eat
Requires coaxing
May eat a little
Prefers certain foods

Related Data
Commonly Related Conditions:
Drug toxicity, such as digitalis intoxication
Hypokalemia
Vitamin deficiency
Aging
Commonly Related Diseases:
Rheumatic fever
Bacterial endocarditis
Glomerulonephritis
Gastritis
Hepatitis
Leukemia
Pellagra
Sprue
Pernicious anemia
Second- and third-degree burns

Laennec's cirrhosis
Hypothyroidism
Pheochromocytoma
Kwashiorkor
Colorado tick fever
Infectious mononucleosis
Brucellosis
Fasciolopsiasis
Coccidioidomycosis
Malignancies

POSSIBLE ETIOLOGY

Displeasurable feelings of illness inhibit the normally pleasurable desire to enjoy food. Emotional stress.

NURSING DIAGNOSIS

Anorexia: lack of a desire for food

PLANNING

Patient Needs
Food balance
Comfort
Protection from physical harm
Increased learning

Primary Nurse-Patient Goals
To maintain nutrition to all cells
To achieve comfort
To prevent physical injury
To achieve awareness of needs

NURSING INTERVENTIONS

Nursing Treatments
Approach unhurriedly
Arrange pleasant surroundings (during meals)
Provide an attractive meal tray
Postpone feeding when the patient is fatigued
    OR
Withhold food until the patient requests it
Balance nutritional intake
Give small, frequent feedings
Provide food selection
Provide foods at their most appetizing temperature
Encourage the bringing in of outside food
Season the food for individual taste
Give high-potassium fluids orally (if the blood potassium is low)
Discourage smoking

Nursing Observations
Measure the body weight (daily)
Monitor blood studies for abnormal electrolytes (decreased potassium)
Observe and record the food intake
Observe for increased nutritional requirements

Health Teaching
Explain the causes of the health problem

Explain the need for pleasant mealtimes
Recommend that food servings be in proportion to the appetite
Teach the principles of good nutrition

EVALUATION

See the evaluation criteria for each specific goal in Chapter 2.

Blunted Appetite

ASSESSMENT

Subjective Data
Person desires food, but only in small quantities
Is concerned about decreased appetite

Objective Data
Person eats small amounts of food
Eats at frequent intervals

Related Data
Commonly Related Conditions:
Drug toxicity
Electrolyte imbalance

Commonly Related Diseases:
Rheumatic fever
Bacterial endocarditis
Glomerulonephritis
Gastritis
Hepatitis
Leukemia
Pellagra
Sprue
Pernicious anemia
Second- and third-degree burns
Mitral stenosis

POSSIBLE ETIOLOGY

Displeasurable feelings of illness inhibit the normally pleasurable desire to enjoy food. Emotional stress.

NURSING DIAGNOSIS

Blunted appetite: a dull desire for food

PLANNING

Patient Needs	Primary Nurse-Patient Goals
Water-salt balance	To maintain fluid and electrolyte balance
Food balance	To maintain nutrition to all cells
Comfort	To achieve comfort
Protection from physical harm	To prevent physical injury
Increased learning	To achieve awareness of needs

NURSING INTERVENTIONS

Nursing Treatments
Approach unhurriedly
Arrange pleasant surroundings (during meals)
Provide an attractive meal tray
Postpone feeding when the patient is fatigued
Balance nutritional intake
Give small, frequent feedings
Give snacks
Give wine before meals
Provide food selection
Season the food for individual taste
Encourage the bringing in of outside food
Discourage smoking

Nursing Observations
Measure the body weight (daily)
Observe and record the food intake
Observe for increased nutritional requirements

Health Teaching
Explain the causes of the health problem
Explain the need for pleasant mealtimes
Recommend that food servings be in proportion to the appetite
Teach the principles of food nutrition

EVALUATION

See the evaluation criteria for each specific goal in Chapter 2.

Impaired Ability to Taste Food (113)

ASSESSMENT

Subjective Data
Food tastes dull or flat
Most foods taste the same

Objective Data
Increased seasoning of food
Inability to distinguish tastes such as bitter, sweet, sour, salty, etc.
Decreased appetite

Related Data
Commonly Related Conditions:
Laryngectomy
Commonly Related Diseases:
Chronic rhinitis
Olfactory and glossopharyngeal nerve paralysis
Bell's palsy
Basal skull fracture

POSSIBLE ETIOLOGY

VII (facial), IX (glossopharyngeal), and X (vagus) cranial nerve impairment.

Temporal lobe lesion. Nasal infection. Frequent use of tobacco deadens the taste bud receptors. Injury or disease to olfactory end organs or nerves leading to the cerebral cortex.

NURSING DIAGNOSIS

Impaired ability to taste food: decreased ability to perceive the normal flavor of food

PLANNING

Patient Needs	**Primary Nurse-Patient Goals**
Food balance	To maintain nutrition to all cells
Comfort	To achieve comfort
Protection from physical harm	To prevent physical injury
Increased learning	To achieve awareness of needs

NURSING INTERVENTIONS

Nursing Treatments
Approach unhurriedly
Arrange pleasant surroundings (during meals)
Give flavor-intensified food
Give strongly seasoned foods
Provide food selection
Provide foods at their most appetizing temperature
Provide an attractive meal tray
Withhold food until the patient requests it
Discourage smoking

Nursing Observations
Observe for evidence of a favorable response to therapy

Health Teaching
Explain the causes of the health problem
Explain the reason for and intended effect of the therapy

EVALUATION

See the evaluation criteria for each specific goal in Chapter 2.

Poor Feeder (460)

ASSESSMENT

Subjective Data
Generalized weakness

Objective Data
Infant takes only small amounts of food
Spits up some of the food taken
Eats only certain foods

Related Data
Commonly Related Diseases:
Cystic fibrosis

Down's syndrome

POSSIBLE ETIOLOGY

Formula incompatibility. Small stomach capacity.

NURSING DIAGNOSIS

Poor feeder: an infant who takes only small amounts of food

PLANNING

Patient Needs
Food balance
Comfort
Protection from physical harm
Increased learning

Primary Nurse-Patient Goals
To maintain nutrition to all cells ·
To achieve comfort
To prevent physical injury
To achieve awareness of needs

NURSING INTERVENTIONS

Nursing Treatments
Arrange pleasant surroundings (while eating)
Feed slowly
Give small, frequent feedings
Gradually increase the amount of feedings
Hold the infant while feeding
Postpone feeding when the patient is fatigued
Stimulate the infant with back stroking or foot thumping
Use a large-holed nipple for feeding

Nursing Observations
Measure the body weight (daily)
Observe and record the food intake
Observe for fatigue
Observe for increased nutritional requirements

Health Teaching
Explain the causes of the health problem
Explain how to stimulate an infant during feeding
Teach how to bottle-feed an infant
Teach how to spoon-feed an infant

EVALUATION

See the evaluation criteria for each specific goal in Chapter 2.

EATING DIFFICULTIES

Chewing Difficulty

ASSESSMENT

Subjective Data
Painful chewing, sometimes

Objective Data
Inability to clench the teeth
Impaired jaw movement
Poor control of food when chewing

Related Data
Commonly Related Conditions:
Paralysis
Commonly Related Diseases:
Fractured mandible
Trench mouth
Myasthenia gravis
Trigeminal (V) nerve paralysis
Encephalitis
Tetanus
Tic douloureux
Pyorrhea
Chorea
Cerebral vascular accident

POSSIBLE ETIOLOGY

Loss of natural teeth through disease or injury. Decreased contraction strength of the masseter muscle. Injury or disease of the hypoglossal nerve fibers. Injured or inflamed oral mucous membrane. Involuntary tongue movements, or sensation loss from paralysis, limits food manipulation when chewing. Ill-fitting dentures.

NURSING DIAGNOSIS

Chewing difficulty: the inability to effectively reduce food to small particles in the mouth

PLANNING

Patient Needs
Food balance
Comfort
Protection from physical harm
Increased learning

Primary Nurse-Patient Goals
To maintain nutrition to all cells
To achieve comfort
To prevent physical injury
To achieve awareness of needs

NURSING INTERVENTIONS

Nursing Treatments
Assist with eating
Give full-liquid foods
   OR
Give mechanically soft foods
   OR
Give pureed foods
Cut the food into small bites

Feed slowly
Give small, frequent feedings
Postpone feeding when the patient is fatigued
Provide food selection

Nursing Observations
Observe and record the food intake
Observe for increased nutritional requirements

Health Teaching
Explain the causes of the health problem
Explain the reason for and intended effect of the therapy

EVALUATION

See the evaluation criteria for each specific goal in Chapter 2.

Chronic Rumination

ASSESSMENT

Objective Data
Infant sucks his fingers
Brings food up into the mouth and throat with suction pressure, then re-
chews the food and swallows

Related Data
Seen primarily in children, but also occurs in some senile adults
Commonly Related Diseases:
Pyloric stenosis
Diphtheria
Soft palate paralysis

POSSIBLE ETIOLOGY

The presence of the stomach contents against the cardiac sphincter along
with the inability of the person to cope hygienically with the occurrence

NURSING DIAGNOSIS

Chronic rumination: the return of food into the mouth from the stomach
with rechewing and reswallowing

PLANNING

Patient Needs
Comfort
Cleanliness
Protection from physical harm
Increased learning

Primary Nurse-Patient Goals
To achieve comfort
To achieve good hygiene
To prevent physical injury
To achieve awareness of needs

NURSING INTERVENTIONS

Nursing Treatments
Attend the patient constantly (while eating)

Hold the infant while feeding
Place in the sitting position
Feed slowly
Give soft foods
Remove food from the mouth (immediately, before rechewing can occur)
Restrain the patient (only his hands)

Nursing Observations
Observe for a favorable response to therapy

Health Teaching
Explain the causes of the health problem
Explain (to the mother) the reason for and intended effect of the therapy

EVALUATION

See the evaluation criteria for each specific goal in Chapter 2.

Diminished Sucking (53,220,460)

ASSESSMENT

Subjective Data
General apathy

Objective Data
When stimulated, the infant sucks only one to six times Stroking the lips or cheeks of the infant does not stimulate the normal food-seeking response

Related Data
Commonly Related Conditions:
Cerebral anoxia

POSSIBLE ETIOLOGY

Depressed nervous function. Gastrointestinal disturbance. Weakness.

NURSING DIAGNOSIS

Diminished sucking: a decreased infant sucking reflex in response to normal lip stimulation

PLANNING

Patient Needs	**Primary Nurse-Patient Goals**
Stimulation	To maintain stimulation
Protection from physical harm	To prevent physical injury
Increased learning	To achieve awareness of needs

NURSING INTERVENTIONS

Nursing Treatments
Stimulate the sucking reflex through jaw or lip pressure
Feed slowly
Give small, frequent feedings

Use a large-holed nipple for feeding

Nursing Observations
Observe and record the food intake
Observe for increased nutritional requirements
Test the infant for the rooting reflex

Health Teaching
Explain the causes of the health problem
Teach how to bottle-feed an infant

EVALUATION

See the evaluation criteria for each specific goal in Chapter 2.

Impaired Swallowing

ASSESSMENT

Subjective Data
Lump-in-the-throat sensation
Throat tightness
Painful swallowing

Objective Data
Person swallows slowly
Puts only small amounts of food in the mouth at a time
Accumulates saliva in the mouth, rather than swallowing it
Drools

Related Data
Commonly Related Conditions:
Laryngeal edema
Presence of a tracheostomy or laryngectomy tube
Commonly Related Diseases:
Esophageal hernia
Botulism
Streptococcus throat infection
Metastatic throat carcinoma
Cerebral vascular accident
Cerebral palsy
Streptococcal pharyngitis
Infectious mononucleosis
Vincent's angina
Diphtheria
Measles
Tonsilitis
Scarlet fever
Parkinson's disease

POSSIBLE ETIOLOGY

Obstruction, inflammation, irritation, or edema of the throat. Emotional stress. Throat surgery.

NURSING DIAGNOSIS

Impaired swallowing: inability to swallow or discomfort when swallowing

PLANNING

Patient Needs	**Primary Nurse-Patient Goals**
Comfort	To achieve comfort
Protection from physical harm	To prevent physical injury
Increased learning	To achieve awareness of needs·

NURSING INTERVENTIONS

Nursing Treatments
Attend the patient constantly (while eating)
Give clear liquid foods
    OR
Give full-liquid foods
    OR
Give pureed foods
    OR
Give soft foods
Cut the food into small bites
Feed slowly
Give small, frequent feedings
Refrain from giving hot liquids
Refrain from giving iced liquids
Place in the sitting position
    OR
Hold the infant while feeding
Discourage talking while eating
Refrain from distracting the patient while he swallows

Nursing Observations
Observe for airway obstruction (when eating)
Observe and record the food intake
Observe for diet intolerance
Observe for increased nutritional requirements

Health Teaching
Advise not to partake of very hot or cold foods and drinks
Explain that fluids should not be given to persons unable to swallow
Recommend thorough food chewing
Explain the causes of the health problem
Explain the reason for and intended effect of the therapy

EVALUATION

See the evaluation criteria for each specific goal in Chapter 2.

Sucking Difficulty (53,220,460)

ASSESSMENT

Objective Data
Normal sucking reflex
Difficulty in controlling liquids sucked into the mouth
Swallowing of large amounts of air
Spread of sucked liquids into the nose
Aspiration, sometimes

Related Data
Commonly Related Diseases:
Cleft palate
Harelip

POSSIBLE ETIOLOGY

Congenital mouth deformity. Neurologic disorders.

NURSING DIAGNOSIS

Sucking difficulty: difficulty in sucking and controlling liquids in the mouth

PLANNING

Patient Needs	**Primary Nurse-Patient Goals**
Food balance	To maintain nutrition to all cells
Comfort	To achieve comfort
Protection from physical harm	To prevent physical injury
Increased learning	To achieve awareness of needs

NURSING INTERVENTIONS

Nursing Treatments
Attend the patient constantly (while eating)
Hold the infant while feeding
Place in the sitting position
Feed by cup
　　OR
Feed by medicine dropper
　　OR
Feed by syringe
Feed slowly
Use a large-holed nipple for feeding (if able to control liquids)
　　OR
Use a small-holed nipple for feeding (if unable to control liquids)
Suction the airway (as needed)

Nursing Observations
Observe and record the food intake
Observe for evidence of a favorable response to therapy

Health Teaching
Explain the causes of the health problem
Inform that airway noise indicates obstruction
Teach how to bottle-feed an infant
Explain the reason for and intended effect of the therapy

EVALUATION

See the evaluation criteria for each specific goal in Chapter 2.

Eating Difficulty Related to Hyperactivity

ASSESSMENT

Subjective Data
Intense internal restlessness

Objective Data
Person sits down to eat
May take one or two bites of food
Immediately gets up and moves about, leaving the food behind

Related Data
Commonly Related Conditions:
Hyperactivity
Commonly Related Diseases:
Manic psychosis

POSSIBLE ETIOLOGY

Neurologic disorders. Emotional distress.

NURSING DIAGNOSIS

Eating difficulty related to hyperactivity: the inability to sit at the table for a meal as a result of uncontrollable continuous physical movement

PLANNING

Patient Needs	**Primary Nurse-Patient Goals**
Food balance	To maintain nutrition to all cells
Protection from physical harm	To prevent physical injury
Increased learning	To achieve awareness of needs

NURSING INTERVENTIONS

Nursing Treatments
Provide finger food
Feed by bottle ⎫
    OR   ⎬ (which can be carried about)
Feed by cup ⎭

Provide food selection
Give small, frequent feedings
Give small, frequent drinks

Nursing Observations
Observe and record the food intake
Observe for evidence of a favorable response to therapy

Health Teaching
Explain the causes of the health problem
Explain the reason for and intended effect of the therapy

EVALUATION

See the evaluation criteria for each specific goal in Chapter 2.

DIETARY DISSATISFACTION

Food Selection Dissatisfaction

ASSESSMENT

Subjective Data
Anger
Frustration

Objective Data
No therapeutic dietary limitations
Frequent complaints about the food or its preparation
Refusal to eat the available food
Irritability

Related Data
Commonly Related Diseases:
None

POSSIBLE ETIOLOGY

An attempt to gain attention. A desire to maintain control in a dependent situation. Perception of food as having emotional significance. Cultural eating habits. Use of food as the scapegoat for internal dissatisfaction or discontent.

NURSING DIAGNOSIS

Food selection dissatisfaction: dissatisfaction with the available selection of food, how it is prepared, or how it is served

PLANNING

Patient Needs	**Primary Nurse-Patient Goals**
Food balance	To maintain nutrition to all cells
Comfort	To achieve comfort
Increased learning	To achieve awareness of needs

NURSING INTERVENTIONS

Nursing Treatments
Anticipate needs
Approach unhurriedly
Arrange pleasant surroundings (while eating)
Provide an attractive meal tray
Provide food selection
Grant special requests
Provide foods at their most appetizing temperature
Season the food for individual taste
Encourage the bringing in of outside food
Provide frequent patient contact (to assure satisfaction)

Nursing Observations
Observe and record the food intake
Observe the eating pattern for abnormality
Observe for increased nutritional requirements
Observe for evidence of a favorable response to therapy

Health Teaching
Teach the principles of good nutrition

EVALUATION

See the evaluation criteria for each specific goal in Chapter 2.

Therapeutic Diet Dissatisfaction

ASSESSMENT

Subjective Data
Anger
May deny the disease that necessitates the therapeutic diet
Objective Data
Receiving a prescribed, therapeutic diet
Complains about food preparation, inconvenience, and expense
May refuse to eat the diet
Related Data
Common with diabetes and low-salt and low-calorie diets
Commonly Related Diseases:
Diabetes mellitus
Hypertension
Myocardial infarction
Cirrhosis of the liver

POSSIBLE ETIOLOGY

Therapeutic food restrictions altering normal food habits and pleasures obtained from food

NURSING DIAGNOSIS

Therapeutic diet dissatisfaction: unhappiness and discontent with a prescribed diet

PLANNING

Patient Needs	**Primary Nurse-Patient Goals**
Food balance	To maintain nutrition to all cells
Comfort	To achieve comfort
Protection from physical harm	To prevent physical injury
Increased learning	To achieve awareness of needs

NURSING INTERVENTIONS

Nursing Treatments
Anticipate needs
Approach unhurriedly
Arrange pleasant surroundings (while eating)
Provide an attractive meal tray
Provide food selection ⎫
    AND   ⎬ (whenever possible)
Grant special requests ⎭
Provide foods at their most appetizing temperature
Season the food for individual taste
Provide frequent patient contact (to assure satisfaction)

Nursing Observations
Observe and record the food intake
Observe the eating pattern for abnormality
Observe for diet intolerance
Observe for evidence of a favorable response to therapy

Health Teaching
Explain the reason for and intended effect of the therapy
Teach the principles of good nutrition

Medical Treatments Performed by Nurses
Give the prescribed diet

EVALUATION

See the evaluation criteria for each specific goal in Chapter 2.

Unsatisfied Sucking (2,9,29)

ASSESSMENT

Subjective Data
Frustration

Objective Data
Infant sucks well during bottle feeding
Sucks continuously 15 to 30 times before resting
Sucks fingers after feeding despite adequate milk intake

Related Data
Commonly Related Diseases:
None

POSSIBLE ETIOLOGY

Insufficient sucking during bottle feeding. An attempt to offset the discomfort of hunger, boredom, fatigue, frustration, illness, or teething.

NURSING DIAGNOSIS

Unsatisfied sucking: an increased need for prolonged sucking

PLANNING

Patient Needs

Comfort

Protection from physical harm

Increased learning

Primary Nurse-Patient Goals

To achieve comfort

To prevent physical injury

To achieve awareness of needs

NURSING INTERVENTIONS

Nursing Treatments
Decrease the time interval between infant feedings
Feed slowly
Give a pacifier to the infant
Hold the infant while feeding (for comfort)
Provide finger food (to suck on)
Use a small-holed nipple for feeding

Nursing Observations
Observe for increased nutritional requirements
Observe for evidence of a favorable response to therapy

Health Teaching
Explain the causes of the health problem
Explain the reason for and intended effect of the therapy
Teach how to bottle-feed an infant

EVALUATION

See the evaluation criteria for each specific goal in Chapter 2.

DEPENDENT FEEDING

Dependence on Eating Assistance

ASSESSMENT

Subjective Data
Person relies on nurses for:
    cutting food
    opening packaged foods
    providing eating assistance devices
    proper positioning

Objective Data
Person frequently spills food
Is unable to cut food

Struggles with packaged foods (cereal boxes, milk cartons, etc.)
Has difficulty in manipulating standard eating utensils
Is unable to see the food
Immobilized position makes it difficult to reach for food and bring it to the
mouth

Related Data

Commonly Related Conditions:
Impaired proprioception
Blindness

Commonly Related Diseases:
Cerebral palsy
Muscular dystrophy
Cervical or thoracic spinal cord injury
Cerebral vascular accident
Bone fracture
First-, second-, or third-degree burn

POSSIBLE ETIOLOGY

Limited range of motion. Weakness. Paralysis. Impaired coordination. Muscle spasticity. Immobility from a cast or traction.

NURSING DIAGNOSIS

Dependence on eating assistance: reliance on nurses to assist with preparatory activities so that the person may feed himself

PLANNING

Patient Needs	**Primary Nurse-Patient Goals**
Food balance	To maintain nutrition to all cells
Comfort	To achieve comfort
Cleanliness	To achieve good hygiene
Protection from physical harm	To prevent physical injury
Independence	To achieve optimum function
Increased learning	To achieve awareness of needs

NURSING INTERVENTIONS

Nursing Treatments
Acknowledge dependency
Anticipate needs
Approach unhurriedly
Provide a convenient meal tray
Cut the food into small bites
Open packaged foods
Protect with a plastic bib
Provide firm eating utensils
Provide lightweight utensils
Provide unbreakable objects (dishes)
Assist with eating (as needed)

Provide frequent patient contact (during the meal in case needs arise)
Encourage self-performance

Nursing Observations
Observe for fatigue

Health Teaching
Teach how to use assistive eating devices
Recommend methods for eating suggested for the visually impaired

EVALUATION

See the evaluation criteria for each specffic goal in Chapter 2.

Dependence on Feeding

ASSESSMENT

Subjective Data
Person relies on nurses for:
 handwashing prior to meals
 food preparation
 comfortable position for eating
 being fed

Objective Data
Person is unable to feed himself

Related Data
Commonly Related Diseases:
Cervical spinal cord injury
Cerebral vascular accident
Bilateral arm fractures
Bilateral arm and hand second- and third-degree burns

POSSIBLE ETIOLOGY

Inability to maintain self-care as a result of weakness, loss of motor skills, or infant dependence

NURSING DIAGNOSIS

Dependence on feeding: reliance on nurses to feed the person

PLANNING

Patient Needs	Primary Nurse-Patient Goals
Food balance	To maintain nutrition to all cells
Comfort	To achieve comfort
Protection from physical harm	To prevent physical injury
Dependence	To achieve comfort
Increased learning	To achieve awareness of needs

NURSING INTERVENTIONS

Nursing Treatments
Acknowledge dependency

Anticipate needs
Approach unhurriedly
Arrange pleasant surroundings (at meals)
Provide an attractive meal tray
Provide food selection
Grant special requests
Provide foods at their most appetizing temperature
Position comfortably
Wash the patient's hands (before feeding)
Feed the patient

Nursing Observations
Observe for readiness to assume activities of daily living

EVALUATION

See the evaluation criteria for each specific goal in Chapter 2.

ARTIFICIAL-FEEDING THERAPY DEPENDENCE

Dependence on Hyperalimentation Management (455,503)

ASSESSMENT

Subjective Data
Person relies on nurses for:
   administration of prescribed dextrose, protein, amino acids, electrolytes,
      and vitamins
   maintenance of sterile technique
   cleanliness maintenance
   protection against dangerous side effects
   discomfort relief

Objective Data
Person is receiving hyperalimentation therapy

Related Data
Commonly Related Conditions:
Cachexia
Coma
Intestinal malabsorption
Commonly Related Diseases:
Metastatic carcinoma
Intestinal ileus
Third-degree burns
Cerebral vascular accident

POSSIBLE ETIOLOGY

Inability to maintain adequate nutrition through the oral route. Rapid blood flow of the subclavian vein quickly dilutes the hyperalimentation solution, making it readily absorbable. Effort to provide concentrated calories (2000–4000 daily), protein, dextrose, electrolytes, vitamins, and trace elements. Effort to maintain positive nitrogen balance, wound healing, and weight gain.

NURSING DIAGNOSIS

Dependence on hyperalimentation management: reliance on nurses for routine feedings through a venous Intracath with a concentrated nutrient solution

PLANNING

Patient Needs	Primary Nurse-Patient Goals
Water-salt balance	To maintain fluid and electrolyte balance
Food balance	To maintain nutrition to all cells
Comfort	To achieve comfort
Cleanliness	To achieve good hygiene
Protection from physical harm	To prevent physical injury, infection
Dependence	To achieve comfort
Increased learning	To achieve awareness of needs

NURSING INTERVENTIONS

Nursing Treatments
Position comfortably
Change the patient's position gradually
Clean with surgical soap (the skin around the catheter insertion site)
Apply an antibiotic ointment (to the catheter insertion site)
Apply a sterile dressing
Wear sterile gloves (during a dressing change)
Change the dressing frequently (three or four times a week)
Change the hyperalimentation tubing with each dressing change
Use separate hyperalimentation infusion sets for incompatible solutions
Keep the hyperalimentation tube patent with 5% dextrose in water
Refrain from drawing blood studies via the subclavian Intracath
Do not give a blood transfusion via a subclavian Intracath
Do not give medications via a subclavian Intracath
Refrain from rapid replacement of lagging hyperalimentation solution
Remove the therapeutic tube when the treatment is terminated
Provide frequent patient contact

Nursing Observations
Check the tube (hyperalimentation Intracath) for patency
Check the hyperalimentation solution for cloudiness and precipitation
Check the solution (hyperalimentation) for flow rate
Check the solution (hyperalimentation) for infiltration
Inspect the arms and hands for venous distention
Inspect the chest for respiratory rate and rhythm
Inspect the neck veins for distention

Measure the body weight (daily)
Measure the intake
Measure the output (for excessive urine output if rapid infusion occurs)
Monitor the blood pressure
Monitor blood studies for abnormal (decreased) glucose (if slow infusion occurs)
Monitor the oral temperature (for fever)
Observe for complaints of headache ⎫
Observe for confusion   ⎪
Observe for lethargy   ⎬ (if rapid infusion occurs)
Observe the level of consciousness   ⎪
Observe for complaints of nausea   ⎭
Obtain a bacterial culture (of the catheter tip and bottle if fever occurs)
Test the urine for sugar and acetone

Health Teaching
Explain how to prevent cross infection
Explain the reason for and intended effect of the therapy

Medical Treatments Performed by Nurses
Give the prescribed hyperalimentation feeding

EVALUATION

See the evaluation criteria for each specific goal in Chapter 2.

Dependence on Gastrostomy-Feeding Management (70,391)

ASSESSMENT

Subjective Data
Person relies on nurses for:
    tube feeding administration
    cleanliness maintenance
    proper positioning
    adequate fluid intake
    prevention of complications
    dressing changes
    discomfort relief

Objective Data
Person has a gastrostomy

Related Data
Commonly Related Conditions:
Prolonged coma
Commonly Related Diseases:
Esophageal metastatic carcinoma
Esophageal stricture
Cerebral vascular accident
Severe cerebral trauma

POSSIBLE ETIOLOGY

Inability to obtain adequate nutrition through normal routes. Lack of skill in administering one's own gastrostomy feeding.

NURSING DIAGNOSIS

Dependence on gastrostomy-feeding management: reliance on nurses for routine feedings through a surgical opening through the abdominal wall into the stomach

PLANNING

Patient Needs	Primary Nurse-Patient Goals
Water-salt balance	To maintain fluid and electrolyte balance
Food balance	To maintain nutrition to all cells
Comfort	To achieve comfort
Cleanliness	To achieve good hygiene
Protection from physical harm	To prevent physical injury, infection
Dependence	To achieve comfort
Increased learning	To achieve awareness of needs

NURSING INTERVENTIONS

Nursing Treatments
Approach unhurriedly
Attend the patient constantly (during the feeding)
Balance fluid intake to equal output
   AND
Balance nutritional intake
Estimate the required daily calories
Feed slowly
Place in the sitting position (during feeding)
Position comfortably (during feeding)
Refrain from giving iced liquids
Refrain from sealing the tube with a heavy clamp (to avoid dislodging the tube)
Apply a sterile dressing (after the feeding)

Nursing Observations
Measure the intake
Measure the output
Inspect the abdomen for distention
Observe for complaints of nausea
Observe for diarrhea
Observe for diet intolerance
Observe for increased nutritional requirements

Medical Treatments Performed by Nurses
Give the prescribed tube feeding

EVALUATION

See the evaluation criteria for each specific goal in Chapter 2.

Dependence on Jejunostomy-Feeding Management (70,391)

ASSESSMENT

Subjective Data

Person relies on nurses for:
   tube feeding administration
   cleanliness maintenance
   proper positioning
   adequate fluid intake
   prevention of complications
   dressing changes
   discomfort relief

Objective Data

Person has a jejunostomy

Related Data

Esophageal, gastric, or duodenal metastatic carcinoma

POSSIBLE ETIOLOGY

Inability to obtain nutrition through normal routes. Lack of skill in administering one's own jejunostomy feeding.

NURSING DIAGNOSIS

Dependence on jejunostomy-feeding management: reliance on nurses for routine feedings through an opening into the jejunum of the small intestine

PLANNING

Patient Needs	Primary Nurse-Patient Goals
Water-salt balance	To maintain fluid and electrolyte balance
Food balance	To maintain nutrition to all cells
Comfort	To achieve comfort
Cleanliness	To achieve good hygiene
Protection from physical harm	To prevent physical injury, infection
Dependence	To achieve comfort
Increased learning	To achieve awareness of needs

NURSING INTERVENTIONS

Nursing Treatments

Approach unhurriedly
Attend the patient constantly (during feeding)
Balance fluid intake to equal output
Balance nutritional intake
Estimate the required daily calories
Feed slowly
Place in the sitting position (during the feeding)
Position comfortably
Refrain from giving iced liquids

Refrain from sealing the tube with a heavy clamp (to avoid dislodging the tube)

Apply a sterile dressing (when the feeding is completed)

Nursing Observations
Inspect the abdomen for distention
Measure the intake
Measure the output
Observe for complaints of nausea
Observe for diarrhea
Observe for diet intolerance
Observe for increased nutritional requirements

Health Teaching
Recommend a regular meal schedule
Describe those symptoms which should be reported (nausea, diarrhea)
Teach how to administer tube feeding
Teach how to prepare a formula (for tube feeding)
Explain the reason for and intended effect of the therapy

Medical Treatments Performed by Nurses
Give the prescribed tube feeding

EVALUATION

See the evaluation criteria for each specific goal in Chapter 2.

Dependence on Nasogastric-Tube-Feeding Management (70,391)

ASSESSMENT

Subjective Data
Person relies on nurses for:
    tube feeding administration
    cleanliness maintenance
    proper positioning
    adequate fluid intake
    prevention of complications
    dressing changes
    discomfort relief

Objective Data
Person has a nasogastric feeding tube

Related Data
Commonly Related Conditions:
Coma
Commonly Related Diseases:
Laryngeal metastatic carcinoma
Cerebral vascular accident

POSSIBLE ETIOLOGY

Inability to obtain adequate nutrition through the normal route

NURSING DIAGNOSIS

Dependence on nasogastric-tube-feeding management: reliance on nurses for routine feeding through a tube inserted through the nose into the stomach

PLANNING

Patient Needs	Primary Nurse-Patient Goals
Water-salt balance	To maintain fluid and electrolyte balance
Food balance	To maintain nutrition to all cells
Comfort	To achieve comfort
Cleanliness	To achieve good hygiene
Protection from physical harm	To prevent physical injury
Dependence	To achieve comfort
Increased learning	To achieve awareness of needs

NURSING INTERVENTIONS

Nursing Treatments

Approach unhurriedly
Attend the patient constantly (during the feeding)
Balance fluid intake to equal output
Balance nutritional intake
Estimate the required daily calories
Feed slowly
Place in the sitting position (during feeding)
Position comfortably
Refrain from giving iced liquids
Refrain from sealing the tube with a heavy clamp (to avoid dislodging the tube)

Nursing Observations

Check the tube's placement before giving tube feeding
Inspect the abdomen for distention
Measure the intake
Measure the output
Observe for complaints of nausea
Observe for diarrhea
Observe for diet intolerance
Observe for increased nutritional requirements

Health Teaching

Recommend a regular meal schedule
Describe those symptoms which should be reported (nausea, diarrhea)
Teach how to administer tube feeding
Teach how to prepare a formula (for tube feeding)
Explain the reason for and intended effect of the therapy

Medical Treatments Performed by Nurses

Give the prescribed tube feeding

EVALUATION

See the evaluation criteria for each specific goal in Chapter 2.

INADEQUATE FEEDING MANAGEMENT

Inadequate Information Related to Infant Bottle Feeding (53,220,460)

ASSESSMENT

Subjective Data
Person confirms a lack of information

Objective Data
Person's actions indicate a lack of information regarding:
    the type of bottles and nipples to use
    how to mix formula preparations
    how to prepare bottles for formula
    the correct amounts to feed the infant
    how to hold the infant during feeding
    the age at which to terminate bottle feeding

Related Data
Commonly Related Diseases:
None

POSSIBLE ETIOLOGY

Lack of instruction

NURSING DIAGNOSIS

Inadequate information related to infant bottle feeding: lack of information regarding the nourishing of an infant with milk from a bottle

PLANNING

Patient Needs	Primary Nurse-Patient Goals
Food balance	To maintain nutrition to all cells
Comfort	To achieve comfort
Protection from physical harm	To prevent physical injury
Mastery and competence in skills, independence	To achieve optimum function
Increased learning	To achieve awareness of needs

NURSING INTERVENTIONS

Nursing Treatments
Approach unhurriedly
Encourage patient questions

Nursing Observations
Evaluate the response to teaching

Health Teaching
Explain the need for pleasant mealtimes
Recommend that infants be fed on a self-demand schedule
Teach how to bottle-feed an infant
Teach how to prepare a formula
Explain how to stimulate an infant during feeding
Describe the signs of infant readiness to be weaned

EVALUATION

See the evaluation criteria for each specific goal in Chapter 2.

Inadequate Information Related to Infant Breast Feeding (53,220,460)

ASSESSMENT

Subjective Data
Person confirms a lack of information

Objective Data
Person's actions indicate a lack of information regarding:
    when to start breast feeding
    how often to breast-feed
    the preferable length of nursing periods
    the proper positioning of mother and infant
    good breast hygiene
    the types of clothing appropriate for breast feeding
    the dangers of taking drugs during breast feeding
    the need for balanced nutrition

Related Data
Commonly Related Diseases:
None

POSSIBLE ETIOLOGY

Lack of instruction

NURSING DIAGNOSIS

Inadequate information related to infant breast feeding: lack of knowledge regarding the nourishing of an infant with milk from the mother's breast

PLANNING

Patient Needs	**Primary Nurse-Patient Goals**
Food balance	To maintain nutrition to all cells
Comfort	To achieve comfort
Cleanliness	To achieve good hygiene

Protection from physical harm

To prevent physical injury, infection

Mastery and competence in skills, independence

To achieve optimum function

Increased learning

To achieve awareness of needs

NURSING INTERVENTIONS

Nursing Treatments
Approach unhurriedly
Encourage patient questions

Nursing Observations
Evaluate the response to teaching

Health Teaching
Explain the advantages and disadvantages of breast feeding
Correct misinformation regarding breast feeding
Teach prenursing nipple hygiene
Teach how to breast-feed an infant
Inform of the recommended length of infant nursing periods
Recommend that infants be fed on a self-demand schedule
Explain that mothers have a choice of single or double breast feeding
Explain that nursing the infant on alternate breasts reduces tenderness
Inform that extended breast sucking indicates hunger
Explain how to stimulate an infant during feeding
Describe the signs of infant readiness to be weaned
Recommend the use of a nipple shield
Recommend the use of nipple padding
Explain how to adjust clothing to meet health problems
Explain the need for pleasant mealtimes (during breast feeding)

EVALUATION

See the evaluation criteria for each specific goal in Chapter 2.

Inadequate Information Related to Infant Solid-Food Feeding

ASSESSMENT

Subjective Data
Person confirms a lack of information

Objective Data
Person's actions indicate a lack of information regarding:
    the specific solid foods a child can eat at different ages
    how to prepare foods for the child
    the food preferences of children
    the correct sequence for introducing new foods
    the necessity of positive attitudes toward new food

Related Data

Commonly Related Diseases:
None

POSSIBLE ETIOLOGY

Lack of instruction. Lack of previous experience with child feeding.

NURSING DIAGNOSIS

Inadequate information related to infant solid-food feeding: lack of information regarding methods of introducing solid foods to infants

PLANNING

Patient Needs	**Primary Nurse-Patient Goals**
Food balance	To maintain nutrition to all cells
Comfort	To achieve comfort
Increased learning	To achieve awareness of needs

NURSING INTERVENTIONS

Nursing Treatments
Approach unhurriedly
Encourage patient questions

Nursing Observations
Evaluate the response to teaching

Health Teaching
Recommend a regular meal schedule
Advise that infants be started on solid foods no later than 6 months
Explain that parental attitudes affect child development
Explain the need for pleasant mealtimes
Inform that new foods should be introduced to children at the beginning of
    the meal
Inform that vegetables should be introduced to children before fruits at the
    meal
Recommend that children be introduced to a wide variety of food
Recommend that food servings be in proportion to the appetite
Recommend the preferable age for introducing specific foods to children
Teach how to spoon-feed an infant
Teach the principles of good nutrition

EVALUATION

See the evaluation criteria for each specific goal in Chapter 2.

Inadequate Information Related to Tube Feeding (70,391)

ASSESSMENT

Subjective Data
Person confirms a lack of information

Objective Data

Person's actions indicate a lack of information regarding:
how to prepare tube feeding formula
the correct method of administering tube feeding
how to care for the tube feeding aparatus
the common side effects of tube feedings

Related Data

Commonly Related Diseases:
Carcinoma
Esophageal stricture

POSSIBLE ETIOLOGY

Lack of instruction

NURSING DIAGNOSIS

Inadequate information related to tube feeding: lack of information regarding the correct method of administering tube feeding

PLANNING

Patient Needs	Primary Nurse-Patient Goals
Water-salt balance	To maintain fluid and electrolyte balance
Food balance	To maintain nutrition to all cells
Protection from physical harm	To prevent physical injury
Mastery and competence in skills, independence	To achieve optimun function
Increased learning	To achieve awareness of needs

NURSING INTERVENTIONS

Nursing Treatments

Approach unhurriedly
Encourage patient questions

Nursing Observations
Evaluate the response to teaching

Health Teaching
Describe those symptoms which should be reported (nausea, diarrhea)
Explain how to obtain therapeutic supplies
Teach how to administer tube feeding
Teach how to prepare a formula (for tube feeding)
Teach the principles of good nutrition
Explain the reason for and intended effect of the therapy

EVALUATION

See the evaluation criteria for each specific goal in Chapter 2.

INADEQUATE NUTRITION MANAGEMENT

Inadequate Information Related to Balanced Nutrition (244,309)

ASSESSMENT

Subjective Data
Person confirms a lack of information

Objective Data
Person's actions indicate a lack of information regarding:
the essential daily nutritional requirements
which foods contain specific nutrients
how to prepare food so as to preserve maximum nutrients
how to plan well-balanced meals from day to day
how to balance nutrition when there are minimum financial resources

Related Data
Commonly Related Conditions:
Malnutrition
Obesity
Commonly Related Diseases:
Pellagra
Scurvy

POSSIBLE ETIOLOGY

Lack of instruction. Adherence to cultural food habits.

NURSING DIAGNOSIS

Inadequate information related to balanced nutrition: lack of information regarding the planning and preparation of a well-balanced food intake

PLANNING

Patient Needs	**Primary Nurse-Patient Goals**
Food balance	To maintain nutrition to all cells
Comfort	To achieve comfort
Protection from physical harm	To prevent physical injury
Mastery and competence in skills, independence	To achieve optimum function
Increased learning	To achieve awareness of needs

NURSING INTERVENTIONS

Nursing Treatments
Approach unhurriedly
Encourage patient questions

Nursing Observations
Evaluate the response to teaching

Health Teaching
Recommend a regular meal schedule
Describe the specific dangerous effects of poor health practices
Explain how to budget (for food value)
Explain how to maintain maximum nutrients in food
Teach how to prepare balanced meals
Teach the principles of good nutrition

EVALUATION

See the evaluation criteria for each specific goal in Chapter 2.

Inadequate Information Related to Fad Dieting (309)

ASSESSMENT

Subjective Data
Person confirms a lack of information

Objective Data
Person's actions indicate a lack of information regarding:
    the unhealthiness of alternating from one diet to another
    the fact that weight loss by diet should be professionally supervised
    the fact that excessive vitamin and mineral intake can have serious side
        effects
    the fact that consistent, balanced nutrition is essential to health

Related Data
Commonly Related Diseases:
None

POSSIBLE ETIOLOGY

Lack of instruction. Willingness to accept any idea that appears to promote health restoration.

NURSING DIAGNOSIS

Inadequate information related to fad dieting: lack of information regarding the use of diets that are passing fancies

PLANNING

Patient Needs	**Primary Nurse-Patient Goals**
Food balance	To maintain nutrition to all cells
Comfort	To achieve comfort
Protection from physical harm	To prevent physical injury
Increased learning	To achieve awareness of needs

NURSING INTERVENTIONS

Nursing Treatments
Approach unhurriedly
Encourage patient questions

Nursing Observations
Evaluate the response to teaching

Health Teaching
Recommend a regular meal schedule
Emphasize the danger of crash-dieting
Teach how to prepare balanced meals
Teach the principles of good nutrition

EVALUATION

See the evaluation criteria for each specific goal in Chapter 2.

Inadequate Information Related to the Prescribed Diet (244,309)

ASSESSMENT

Subjective Data
Person confirms a lack of information

Objective Data
Person's actions indicate a lack of information regarding:
    why a special diet was prescribed and its physiologic effects
    how to calculate the diet
    how to plan meals around the diet
    how to maintain the diet when there are minimum financial resources

Related Data
Commonly Related Diseases:
Hypertension
Diabetes mellitus
Diverticulosis
Gout
Peptic ulcer

POSSIBLE ETIOLOGY

Lack of instruction

NURSING DIAGNOSIS

Inadequate information related to the prescribed diet: lack of information regarding the planning and preparation of a prescribed diet

PLANNING

Patient Needs	**Primary Nurse-Patient Goals**
Food balance	To maintain nutrition to all cells
Comfort	To achieve comfort

Protection from physical harm   To prevent physical injury

Mastery and competence in skills, independence   To achieve optimum function

Increased learning   To achieve awareness of needs

NURSING INTERVENTIONS

Nursing Treatments
Approach unhurriedly
Encourage patient questions

Nursing Observations
Evaluate the response to teaching

Health Teaching
General Teaching:
Explain how to budget (for food value)
Teach how to calculate a diet
Teach how to prepare balanced meals
Instruct to eat only prescribed foods and amounts of foods
Instruct to measure foods after cooking
Explain the reason for and intended effect of the therapy
Specific to Diabetic Diet:
Instruct to eat only at the mealtime
Instruct that diabetics should not fry foods
Instruct to measure foods after cooking
Explain how to maintain a diabetic diet when away from home
Specific to Low Sodium Diet:
Explain the difference between salt and sodium diet restriction

EVALUATION

See the evaluation criteria for each specific goal in Chapter 2.

INADEQUATE FOOD HANDLING

Inadequate Information Related to Safe Food Handling (309)

ASSESSMENT

Subjective Data
Person confirms a lack of information

Objective Data
Person's actions indicate a lack of information regarding:
    the necessity for handwashing prior to food handling
    how to properly clean raw fruits and vegetables
    how to adequately refrigerate food
    the importance of using clean cooking utensils
    how to perform safe canning methods

Related Data

Commonly Related Diseases:
Typhoid fever
Amebic dysentery
Bacillary dysentery
Botulism

POSSIBLE ETIOLOGY

Lack of education. Apathy

NURSING DIAGNOSIS

Inadequate information related to safe food handling: lack of information regarding satisfactory measures in the preparation and storage of food

PLANNING

Patient Needs	**Primary Nurse-Patient Goals**
Protection from physical harm	To prevent physical injury
Increased learning	To achieve awareness of needs

NURSING INTERVENTIONS

Nursing Treatments
Approach unhurriedly
Encourage patient questions

Nursing Observations
Evaluate the response to teaching

Health Teaching
Recommend adequate food refrigeration
Advise handwashing before meals (and meal preparation)
Advise that fresh foods should be thoroughly washed
Emphasize that bulging food cans should be discarded
Emphasize that outdated foods should be discarded
Inform that cleanliness is basic to health

EVALUATION

See the evaluation criteria for each specific goal in Chapter 2.

24.

NURSING DIAGNOSES RELATED TO
Pain

NONSPECIFIC PAIN

Aching Pain (70,247,271,326,391,453)

ASSESSMENT

Subjective Data
Pain distribution: generalized or localized
Duration: continuous or intermittent
Onset: gradual
Intensity: mild or moderate; increased by body movements
Level: superficial or deep
Quality: sore sensation

Objective Data
Irritability
Restlessness

Related Data
Commonly Related Conditions:
Dysmenorrhea
Commonly Related Diseases:
Buerger's disease
Influenza
Dengue
Plague
Rocky Mountain spotted fever
Gastritis
Thrombophlebitis
Rickets
Varicose veins

POSSIBLE ETIOLOGY

Cell and tissue receptors carry pain stimuli by way of the nerves and spinal cord to the thalamus. Sensation is conducted along nerve fibers and pain perception occurs in the cerebral cortex. Infection. Inflammation.

NURSING DIAGNOSIS

Aching pain: a warning sign of potential or existing tissue cell damage manifested in a dull, distressful hurting

PLANNING

Patient Needs	Primary Nurse-Patient Goals
Rest, relaxation	To achieve rest, relaxation
Comfort	To achieve comfort
Protection from physical harm	To prevent physical injury
Freedom from pain	To achieve comfort
Increased learning	To achieve awareness of needs

NURSING INTERVENTIONS

Nursing Treatments
Approach unhurriedly
Reassure that the pain will subside
Communicate nurse sensitivity to the person's pain
Handle gently
Position comfortably
Apply a heating pad
    OR
Apply a hot water bottle
    OR
Apply a warm, moist compress
    OR
Bathe in warm water
Apply mentholated ointment
Massage gently
Ask the patient what makes him (or her) comfortable
Discuss possible pain-reducing measures
Provide a pain-relief measure of the patient's choice
Give nonprescription drugs (ExR) (analgesics)
Offer assurance of other measures if the pain-relief method fails
Encourage adequate rest

Nursing Observations
Observe for complaints of pain duration
Observe for complaints of pain radiation
Evaluate the effectiveness of the pain-relief measures
Monitor the oral temperature (for fever)

Health Teaching
Explain the causes of pain
Teach how to apply heat therapy
Explain the reason for and intended effect of the therapy

Medical Treatments Performed by Nurses
Give the prescribed drugs (analgesics)

EVALUATION

See the evaluation criteria for each specific goal in Chapter 2.

Burning Pain (70,247,271,326,391,453)

ASSESSMENT

Subjective Data
Pain distribution: localized and referred
Duration: continuous or intermittent
Onset: acute
Intensity: severe; increased intensity when there are temperature changes
    or movement
Level: deep or superficial
Quality: fiery sensation

Objective Data
Irritability
Restlessness

Related Data

Commonly Related Conditions:
Indigestion

Commonly Related Diseases:
Dissecting aortic aneurysm
Uremia
Duodenal ulcer
Gastric ulcer
Hiatus hernia
Urinary tract tuberculosis
Athlete's foot
First degree burn
Contact dermatitis
Erythema multiforme
Hemorrhoids
Herpes simplex
Malaria
Beriberi
Herpes zoster
Polyneuritis
Varicose veins

POSSIBLE ETIOLOGY

Inadequate circulation to peripheral nerves. Injury to the peripheral nerve trunk. Impaired digestion. Impaired kidney function elevates the serum phosphate which decreases the calcium level causing neuritis pain.

NURSING DIAGNOSIS

Burning pain: a warning sign of potential or existing tissue cell damage manifested by a hot, distressful hurting

PLANNING

Patient Needs

Rest, relaxation

Comfort

Protection from physical harm

Freedom from pain

Increased learning

Primary Nurse-Patient Goals

To achieve rest, relaxation

To achieve comfort

To prevent physical injury

To achieve comfort

To achieve awareness of needs

NURSING INTERVENTIONS

Nursing Treatments

Approach unhurriedly

Reassure that the pain will subside

Communicate nurse sensitivity to the person's pain

Handle gently

Position comfortably

Apply a cold, moist compress

OR

Apply an ice bag

OR

Bathe in cool water

OR

Soak in cold water

Apply an analgesic ointment (to burns or lesions)

Remove constrictive clothing

Remove tight bandaging

Apply a bed cradle (for skin lesions)

Cover with lightweight blankets (for skin lesions)

Decrease drafts

Ask the patient what makes him (or her) comfortable

Discuss possible pain-reducing measures

Provide a pain-relief measure of the patient's choice

Give nonprescription drugs (ExR) (analgesics, antacids)

Encourage adequate rest

Encourage increased calcium-food intake (if the serum phosphate is elevated)

Nursing Observations

Observe for complaints of pain duration

Evaluate the effectiveness of the pain-relief measures

Health Teaching

Explain the causes of pain

Teach how to apply cold therapy

Explain the reason for and intended effect of the therapy

Medical Treatments Performed by Nurses

Give the prescribed drugs

EVALUATION

See the evaluation criteria for each specific goal in Chapter 2.

Constrictive Pain
(70,247,271,326,391,453)

ASSESSMENT

Subjective Data
Pain distribution: localized
Duration: continuous or intermittent
Onset: acute
Intensity: moderate or severe
Level: deep
Quality: squeezing sensation

Objective Data
Irritability
Restlessness

Related Data
Commonly Related Conditions:
Angina
Commonly Related Diseases:
Syphilis
Esophageal stricture
Myocardial infarction
Arteriosclerotic heart disease

POSSIBLE ETIOLOGY

Sensory nerve fiber irritation

NURSING DIAGNOSIS

Constrictive pain: a warning sign of potential or existing tissue cell damage manifested in a binding, distressful hurting

PLANNING

Patient Needs	**Primary Nurse-Patient Goals**
Rest, relaxation	To achieve rest, relaxation
Comfort	To achieve comfort
Protection from physical harm	To prevent physical injury
Freedom from pain	To achieve comfort
Increased learning	To achieve awareness of needs

NURSING INTERVENTIONS

Nursing Treatments
Approach unhurriedly
Reassure that the pain will subside
Communicate nurse sensitivity to the person's pain

Handle gently
Position comfortably
Apply a heating pad
    OR
Apply a hot water bottle
    OR
Apply a warm, moist compress
Give warm liquids (for internal pain)
Refrain from giving iced liquids
Remove constrictive clothing
Ask the patient what makes him (or her) comfortable
Discuss possible pain-reducing measures
Provide a pain-relief measure of the patient's choice
Give nonprescription drugs (ExR) (analgesics)
Encourage adequate rest

Nursing Observations
Observe for complaints of pain duration
Observe for complaints of pain radiation
Evaluate the effectiveness of the pain-relief measures

Health Teaching
Explain the causes of pain
Teach how to apply heat therapy
Explain the reason for and intended effect of the therapy

Medical Treatments Performed by Nurses
Give the prescribed drugs (analgesics)

EVALUATION

See the evaluation criteria for each specific goal in Chapter 2.

Cramping Pain (70,247,326,391,453)

ASSESSMENT

Subjective Data
Pain duration: localized and/or shifting
Duration: intermittent
Onset: acute
Intensity: severe, sometimes excruciating
Level: deep or superficial
Quality: gripping sensation

Objective Data
Irritability
Restlessness
Spasm feels hard
Shrill cry (especially in infants)

Related Data
Commonly Related Conditions:
Food poisoning

Menstruation
Muscle spasm
Flatulence
Afterbirth pains
Commonly Related Diseases:
Dysentery
Cholecystitis
Renal calculi
Strongyloidosis
Intussusception
Choledocholithiasis
Diverticulitis
Duodenal ulcer
Intestinal tuberculosis
Sprue
Regional enteritis
Ulcerative colitis
Ectopic pregnancy
Primary dysmenorrhea
Salpingitis
Ureteral stone
Varicose veins

POSSIBLE ETIOLOGY

Reduced blood supply to tissues. Alternate contraction and relaxation of muscle tissue.

NURSING DIAGNOSIS

Cramping pain (colicky pain): a warning sign of potential or existing tissue cell damage manifested in a spasm type, distressful hurting

PLANNING

Patient Needs	**Primary Nurse-Patient Goals**
Rest, relaxation	To achieve rest, relaxation
Comfort	To achieve comfort
Protection from physical harm	To prevent physical injury
Freedom from pain	To achieve comfort
Increased learning	To achieve awareness of needs

NURSING INTERVENTIONS

Nursing Treatments
Approach unhurriedly
Reassure that the pain will subside
Communicate nurse sensitivity to the person's pain
Handle gently
Position comfortably
Apply a heating pad
   OR

Apply a hot water bottle
   OR
Apply a saline compress
   OR
Bathe in warm water
Massage gently
Remove constrictive clothing
Give warm liquids (for internal cramping)
Refrain from giving iced liquids
Introduce irrigating solutions slowly (if cramping pain is due to enema administration or the like)
Ask the patient what makes him (or her) comfortable
Discuss possible pain-reducing measures
Provide a pain-relief measure of the patient's choice
Give nonprescription drugs (ExR) (analgesics)
Encourage adequate rest

Nursing Observations
Observe for complaints of pain duration
Observe for complaints of pain radiation
Evaluate the effectiveness of the pain-relief measures

Health Teaching
Explain the causes of pain
Teach how to apply heat therapy
Explain the reason for and intended effect of the therapy

Medical Treatments
Give the prescribed drugs (analgesics)

EVALUATION

See the evaluation criteria for each specific goal in Chapter 2.

Gnawing Pain (70,247,271,326,391,453)

ASSESSMENT

Subjective Data
Pain distribution: localized
Duration: continuous or intermittent
Onset: acute or gradual
Intensity: mild or moderate
Level: deep
Quality: growling, empty sensation

Objective Data
Irritability
Restlessness

Related Data
Commonly Related Conditions:
Hunger

Commonly Related Diseases:
Peptic ulcer
Gastric ulcer
Duodenal ulcer

POSSIBLE ETIOLOGY

Cell and tissue receptors carry irritation stimuli by way of the nerves and spinal cord to the thalamus. Sensation is conducted to the cerebral cortex where pain perception occurs.

NURSING DIAGNOSIS

Gnawing pain: a warning sign of potential or existing tissue cell damage manifested in a gnarling, distressful hurting

PLANNING

Patient Needs	Primary Nurse-Patient Goals
Acid-base balance	To maintain regulating mechanisms and functions
Rest, relaxation	To achieve rest, relaxation
Comfort	To achieve comfort
Protection from physical harm	To prevent physical injury
Freedom from pain	To achieve comfort
Increased learning	To achieve awareness of needs

NURSING INTERVENTIONS

Nursing Treatments
Approach unhurriedly
Reassure that the pain will subside
Communicate nurse sensitivity to the person's pain
Give milk
Give warm liquids
Refrain from giving iced liquids
Encourage decreased acid-food intake
Ask the patient what makes him (or her) comfortable
Provide a pain-relief measure of the patient's choice
Give nonprescription drugs (ExR) (antacids)

Nursing Observations
Observe for complaints of pain duration
Evaluate the effectiveness of the pain-relief measures

Health Teaching
Explain the causes of pain
Explain the reason for and intended effect of the therapy

Medical Treatments Performed by Nurses
Give the prescribed drugs

EVALUATION

See the evaluation criteria for each specific goal in Chapter 2.

Neuralgic Pain
(70,247,271,326,391,453)

ASSESSMENT

Subjective Data

Pain distribution: localized and/or referred
Duration: intermittent
Onset: acute
Intensity: severe
Level: superficial
Quality: lancinating pain

Objective Data

Irritability
Restlessness

Related Data

Commonly Related Diseases:
Herpes zoster
Polyarteritis nodosa
Rheumatoid arthritis
Tic douloureux
Trigeminal neuralgia
Rheumatic heart disease

POSSIBLE ETIOLOGY

Inflammation of, trauma to, pressure on, or degeneration of nerves or nerve cells

NURSING DIAGNOSIS

Neuralgic pain: a warning sign of potential or existing tissue cell damage manifested in a sharp, cutting, distressful hurting

PLANNING

Patient Needs	**Primary Nurse-Patient Goals**
Rest, relaxation	To achieve rest, relaxation
Comfort	To achieve comfort
Protection from physical harm	To prevent physical injury
Freedom from pain	To achieve comfort
Increased learning	To achieve awareness of needs

NURSING INTERVENTIONS

Nursing Treatments
Approach unhurriedly
Reassure that the pain will subside
Communicate nurse sensitivity to the person's pain
Handle gently
Position comfortably
Apply heat by a gooseneck lamp
  OR

Apply a heat cradle
OR
Apply a heating pad
OR
Apply a hot water bottle
OR
Apply a warm, moist compress
OR
Apply a cold, moist compress
OR
Apply an ice bag
Massage gently
Refrain from tight bandaging
Remove constrictive clothing
Apply a bed cradle
Cover with lightweight blankets
Decrease drafts
Refrain from jarring the bed
Ask the patient what makes him (or her) comfortable
Discuss possible pain-reducing measures
Provide a pain-relief measure of the patient's choice
Give nonprescription drugs (ExR) (analgesics)
Encourage adequate rest

Nursing Observations
Observe for complaints of pain duration
Observe for complaints of pain radiation
Evaluate the effectiveness of the pain-relief measures

Health Teaching
Explain the causes of pain
Teach how to apply cold therapy
Teach how to apply heat therapy

Medical Treatments Performed by Nurses
Give the prescribed drugs (analgesics, steroids, antibiotics)

EVALUATION

See the evaluation criteria for each specific goal in Chapter 2.

Stabbing Pain (70,247,271,326,391,453)

ASSESSMENT

Subjective Data
Pain distribution: localized and/or shifting
Duration: intermittent
Onset: acute
Intensity: severe
Level: deep or superficial
Quality: knifelike

Objective Data
Irritability
Restlessness
Jerky respirations

Related Data

Commonly Related Conditions:
Pleural effusion
Angina pectoris
Spontaneous pneumathorax

Commonly Related Diseases:
Acute pericarditis
Bronchitis
Pneumococcal pneumonia
Tuberculosis
Renal calculi
Ruptured bladder
Trigeminal neuralgia
Pulmonary embolism

POSSIBLE ETIOLOGY

Short intervals of stimuli to sensory pain fibers

NURSING DIAGNOSIS

Stabbing pain (sharp pain): a warning sign of potential or existing tissue cell damage manifested in a piercing, distressful hurting

PLANNING

Patient Needs	**Primary Nurse-Patient Goals**
Rest, relaxation	To achieve rest, relaxation
Comfort	To achieve comfort
Protection from physical harm	To prevent physical injury
Freedom from pain	To achieve comfort
Increased learning	To achieve awareness of needs

NURSING INTERVENTIONS

Nursing Treatments
Approach unhurriedly
Reassure that the pain will subside
Communicate nurse sensitivity to the person's pain
Handle gently
Position comfortably
Place a pillow on the affected side
Remove constrictive clothing
Ask the patient what makes him (or her) comfortable
Provide a pain-relief measure of the patient's choice
Give nonprescription drugs (ExR) (analgesics)
Encourage adequate rest

Nursing Observations
Observe for complaints of pain duration
Observe for complaints of pain radiation
Evaluate pain for intensity and quality
Evaluate the effectiveness of the pain-relief measures

Health Teaching
Explain the causes of pain
Explain the reason for and intended effect of the therapy

Medical Treatments Performed by Nurses
Give the prescribed drugs

EVALUATION

See the evaluation criteria for each specific goal in Chapter 2.

Stinging Pain (70,247,271,326,391,453)

ASSESSMENT

Subjective Data
Pain distribution: localized
Duration: continuous
Onset: acute
Intensity: mild or moderate
Level: superficial
Quality: smarting sensation

Objective Data
Irritability
Restlessness

Related Data
Commonly Related Conditions:
Insect, spider, and pest bites
Commonly Related Diseases:
Contact dermatitis
Herpes simplex
First degree burns

POSSIBLE ETIOLOGY

Cell and tissue receptors carry irritation stimuli by way of the nerves and spinal cord to the thalamus. Sensation is conducted to the cerebral cortex where pain perception occurs.

NURSING DIAGNOSIS

Stinging pain: a warning sign of potential or existing tissue cell damage manifested in a pricking, piercing, distressful hurting

PLANNING

Patient Needs	**Primary Nurse-Patient Goals**
Rest, relaxation	To achieve rest, relaxation

Comfort

Protection from physical harm

Freedom from pain

Increased learning

To achieve comfort

To prevent physical injury

To achieve comfort

To achieve awareness of needs

NURSING INTERVENTIONS

Nursing Treatments

Approach unhurriedly

Reassure that the pain will subside

Communicate nurse sensitivity to the person's pain

Handle gently

Position comfortably

Apply a cold, moist compress

OR

Apply an ice bag

OR

Soak in cold water

Apply sodium bicarbonate to the skin

OR

Apply cornstarch to the skin

Apply an analgesic ointment

Ask the patient what makes him (or her) comfortable

Provide a pain-relief measure of the patient's choice

Give nonprescription drugs (ExR) (analgesics)

Encourage adequate rest

Nursing Observations

Observe for complaints of pain duration

Evaluate the effectiveness of the pain-relief measures

Health Teaching

Explain the causes of pain

Explain the reason for and intended effect of the therapy

Medical Treatments Performed by Nurses

Give the prescribed drugs

EVALUATION

See the evaluation criteria for each specific goal in Chapter 2.

Tenderness (113)

ASSESSMENT

Subjective Data

Pain distribution: localized

Duration: continuous

Onset: acute

Intensity: mild, moderate, or severe

Level: deep or superficial

Quality: sore sensation only when pressure is applied

Objective Data
Redness, sometimes

Related Data
Commonly Related Conditions:
Acute peritonitis
Commonly Related Diseases:
(LLQ) Diverticulosis
Diverticulitis
(RLQ) Regional enteritis
Appendicitis
Acute mesenteric lymphadinitis
(RUQ) Infectious hepatitis
Serum hepatitis
Laennec's cirrhosis
Biliary cirrhosis
Acute cholecystitis
Chronic cholecystitis
Choledocholithiasis
(LUQ) Splenic rupture
Splenic infarction
Renal calculi
(Diffuse) Acute pancreatitis
Intestinal obstruction
Mesenteric vascular occlusion
(Lower Abdomen) Ulcerative colitis
(Epigastric) Duodenal or gastric ulcer
Chronic gastritis

NURSING DIAGNOSIS

Tenderness: the perception of mild pain upon gentle pressure against the skin

POSSIBLE ETIOLOGY

Pressure against cell and tissue receptors carries irritation stimuli by way of the nerves and spinal cord to the thalamus. Sensation is conducted to the cerebral cortex where pain perception occurs. Infection. Inflammation. Muscle strain.

PLANNING

Patient Needs	**Primary Nurse-Patient Goals**
Rest, relaxation	To achieve rest, relaxation
Comfort	To achieve comfort
Protection from physical harm	To prevent physical injury
Freedom from pain	To achieve comfort
Increased learning	To achieve awareness of needs

NURSING INTERVENTIONS

Nursing Treatments
Approach unhurriedly
Reassure that the pain will subside
Communicate nurse sensitivity to the person's pain
Handle gently
Position comfortably (off the tender area)
Remove constrictive clothing
Refrain from tight bandaging
Refrain from jarring the bed
Ask the patient what makes him (or her) comfortable
Discuss possible pain-reducing measures
Provide a pain-relief measure of the patient's choice
Give nonprescription drugs (ExR) (analgesics)

Nursing Observations
Observe for complaints of pain duration
Evaluate the effectiveness of the pain-relief measures

Health Teaching
Explain the causes of pain
Explain the reason for and intended effect of the therapy

Medical Treatments Performed by Nurses
Give the prescribed drugs

EVALUATION

See the evaluation criteria for each specific goal in Chapter 2.

Throbbing Pain
(70,247,271,326,391,453)

ASSESSMENT

Subjective Data
Pain distribution: localized
Duration: intermittent, occurs with each pulse beat; subsides between pulse
    beats
Onset: acute
Intensity: moderate or severe
Level: deep or superficial
Quality: pounding sensation

Objective Data
Irritability
Restlessness

Related Data
Commonly Related Conditions:
Dental caries
Commonly Related Diseases:
Thrombophlebitis

Phlebothrombosis
Arteriovenous fistula
Lymphangitis
Lymphadenitis
Temporal arteritis

POSSIBLE ETIOLOGY

Irritation stimuli to sensory pain fibers. Vasodilatation or vasoconstriction.

NURSING DIAGNOSIS

Throbbing pain: a warning sign of potential or existing tissue cell damage manifested in a pulsating, distressful hurting

PLANNING

Patient Needs	Primary Nurse-Patient Goals
Rest, relaxation	To achieve rest, relaxation
Comfort	To achieve comfort
Protection from physical harm	To prevent physical injury
Freedom from pain	To achieve comfort
Increased learning	To achieve awareness of needs

NURSING INTERVENTIONS

Nursing Treatments
Approach unhurriedly
Reassure that the pain will subside
Communicate nurse sensitivity to the person's pain
Handle gently
Position comfortably
Change the patient's position gradually
Support the affected body part
Apply a cold, moist compress
      OR
Apply an ice bag
Refrain from tight bandaging
Remove constrictive clothing
Ask the patient what makes him (or her) comfortable
Elevate the affected body part
Encourage adequate rest
Provide a pain-relief measure of the patient's choice
Give nonprescription drugs (ExR) (analgesics)

Nursing Observations
Observe for complaints of pain duration
Evaluate the effectiveness of the pain-relief measures

Health Teaching
Explain the causes of pain
Explain the reason for and intended effect of the therapy

Medical Treatments Performed by Nurses
Give the prescribed drugs

EVALUATION

See the evaluation criteria for each specific goal in Chapter 2.

Tingling Pain (70,247,271,326,391,453)

ASSESSMENT

Subjective Data
Pain distribution: generalized or localized
Duration: intermittent
Onset: acute
Intensity: mild or moderate
Level: superficial
Quality: sensation of tiny, sharp pinpoints dancing on the skin

Related Data
Commonly Related Conditions:
B vitamin deficiency
Hyperventilation
Hypoglycemia
Commonly Related Diseases:
Polyneuritis
Rabies
Hypothyroidism
Tetanus
Posterolateral sclerosis

POSSIBLE ETIOLOGY

Drug toxicity. Nerve injury. Excessive loss of carbon dioxide through expiratory breathing. Impaired peripheral circulation. Vascular insufficiency due to unrelieved swelling. Tight cast.

NURSING DIAGNOSIS

Tingling pain: a warning sign of potential or existing tissue cell damage manifested in a pin-pricking, distressful hurting

PLANNING

Patient Needs	Primary Nurse-Patient Goals
Rest, relaxation	To achieve rest, relaxation
Comfort	To achieve comfort
Protection from physical harm	To prevent physical injury
Freedom from pain	To achieve comfort
Increased learning	To achieve awareness of needs

NURSING INTERVENTIONS

Nursing Treatments
Approach unhurriedly

Reassure that the pain will subside
Communicate nurse sensitivity to the person's pain
Handle gently
Position comfortably
Change the patient's position frequently
Apply heat by a gooseneck lamp
    OR
Apply a heating pad
Refrain from tight bandaging
Apply a bed cradle
Cover with lightweight blankets
Ask the patient what makes him (or her) comfortable
Provide a pain-relief measure of the patient's choice
Give nonprescription drugs (ExR) (analgesics)
Bivalve and spread the cast to relieve pressure (ET) (if the cast is the cause
    of the tingling)

Nursing Observations
Observe for complaints of pain duration
Evaluate the effectiveness of the pain-relief measures

Health Teaching
Advise that positions which impair circulation be avoided
Explain the causes of pain
Explain the reason for and intended effect of the therapy

Medical Treatments Performed by Nurses
Give the prescribed drugs

EVALUATION

See the evaluation criteria for each specific goal in Chapter 2.

SPECIFIC CARDIAC PAIN

Angina (247,453)

ASSESSMENT

Subjective Data
Dyspnea
Pain distribution: localized and/or referred; pain starts near the heart or
    behind the sternum; radiates down the left shoulder and arm to the
    fourth and little fingers; sometimes radiates up the neck to the back or
    right side
Duration: intermittent
Onset: acute
Intensity: severe
Level: deep
Quality: a pressing, squeezing, or choking sensation

Objective Data
Increased or decreased blood pressure

Increased respirations
Profuse sweating
Pallor
Lies motionless
Cyanosis

Related Data

Commonly Related Conditions:
Cardiac arrhythmias
Angina pectoris

Commonly Related Diseases:
Coronary occlusion
Atherosclerosis
Myocardial infarction

POSSIBLE ETIOLOGY

Impaired circulation to the heart muscle

NURSING DIAGNOSIS

Angina: a pressing, squeezing, choking chest pain

PLANNING

Patient Needs	**Primary Nurse-Patient Goals**
Oxygen, circulation	To maintain oxygen to all cells
Sleep, rest, relaxation	To achieve sleep, rest, relaxation
Comfort	To achieve comfort
Protection from physical harm	To prevent physical injury
Freedom from pain	To achieve comfort
Increased learning	To achieve awareness of needs

NURSING INTERVENTIONS

Nursing Treatments
Approach unhurriedly
Reassure that the pain will subside
Communicate nurse sensitivity to the person's pain
Demonstrate calmness
Administer humidified oxygen (ET)
Position comfortably
Place in the sitting position
Place on complete bed rest
Remove constrictive clothing
Refrain from giving hot liquids
Refrain from giving iced liquids
Refrain from performing nonessential procedures
Avoid causing intense emotional situations
Ask the patient what makes him (or her) comfortable
Discuss possible pain-reducing measures
Provide a pain-relief measure of the patient's choice

Nursing Observations
Auscultate the apical heartbeat for rate and rhythm
Evaluate the effectiveness of the pain-relief measures
Estimate the degree of pain experienced
Monitor the blood pressure
Monitor blood studies for abnormal cardiac enzymes
Monitor the cardiogram
Monitor the pulse pressure
Observe for complaints of pain radiation (recurring)
Observe for nonverbal communication of pain
Palpate the pulse for rate, rhythm, and volume

Health Teaching
Teach how to administer medications (nitroglycerine)
Describe those symptoms which should be reported (recurring pain)
Explain the causes of pain
Explain the reason for and intended effect of the therapy

Medical Treatments Performed by Nurses
Give the prescribed drugs (nitroglycerine)

EVALUATION

See the evaluation criteria for each specific goal in Chapter 2.

SPECIFIC EAR PAIN

Earache (70)

ASSESSMENT

Subjective Data
Pain distribution: localized to the ear
Duration: intermittent or chronic
Onset: acute
Intensity: mild to severe
Level: deep
Quality: aching, sharp, throbbing sensation

Objective Data
Restlessness
Irritability
Holds the ear with the hand

Related Data

Commonly Related Diseases:
Herpes zoster
Carcinoma
Meatitis
Trigeminal neuralgia
Otitis media
Mastoiditis

Temperomandibular arthritis
Tonsillitis
Thyroiditis

POSSIBLE ETIOLOGY

Trauma. Extreme environmental temperature. Impacted earwax. Foreign body pressure. Infection. Tooth decay.

NURSING DIAGNOSIS

Earache: a painful ear

PLANNING

Patient Needs	Primary Nurse-Patient Goals
Sleep, rest, relaxation	To achieve sleep, rest, relaxation
Comfort	To achieve comfort
Cleanliness	To achieve good hygiene
Protection from physical harm	To prevent physical injury
Freedom from pain	To achieve comfort
Increased learning	To achieve awareness of needs

NURSING INTERVENTIONS

Nursing Treatments
Approach unhurriedly
Reassure that the pain will subside
Communicate nurse sensitivity to the person's pain
Handle gently
Position comfortably
Apply a heating pad
    OR
Apply a hot water bottle
    OR
Apply a warm, moist compress (to the ear)
Instill warm oil into the ear
Maintain a warm room temperature
Ask the patient what makes him (or her) comfortable
Discuss possible pain-reducing measures
Provide a pain-relief measure of the patient's choice
Give nonprescription drugs (ExR) (analgesics)
Encourage adequate rest

Nursing Observations
Observe for complaints of pain duration
Observe for complaints of pain radiation
Evaluate the effectiveness of the pain-relief measures
Inspect the ears with an otoscope
Monitor the oral temperature (for fever)
Obtain a bacterial culture (if drainage exists)

Health Teaching
Explain the causes of pain
Teach how to apply heat therapy
Teach how to instill ear drops
Explain the reason for and intended effect of the therapy

Medical Treatments Performed by Nurses
Give the prescribed drugs

EVALUATION

See the evaluation criteria for each specific goal in Chapter 2.

SPECIFIC ELIMINATION PAIN

Bladder Spasms (70,326,391)

ASSESSMENT

Subjective Data
Pain distribution: localized, abdominal
Duration: intermittent, for several seconds
Onset: acute
Intensity: mild, moderate, or severe
Level: deep
Quality: cramping pain

Objective Data
Urinary incontinence
Abdominal muscular contractions

Related Data
Commonly Related Conditions:
Suprapubic prostatectomy
Commonly Related Diseases:
Prostatic hypertrophy
Bladder calculi
Prostate carcinoma

POSSIBLE ETIOLOGY

Severe bladder contractions

NURSING DIAGNOSIS

Bladder spasms: colicky pain in the bladder area accompanied by muscular contraction

PLANNING

Patient Needs	**Primary Nurse-Patient Goals**
Relaxation	To achieve relaxation
Comfort	To achieve comfort
Protection from physical harm	To prevent physical injury

Freedom from pain

Increased learning

To achieve comfort

To achieve awareness of needs

NURSING INTERVENTIONS

Nursing Treatments

Approach unhurriedly

Reassure that the pain will subside

Communicate nurse sensitivity to the person's pain

Handle gently

Position comfortably

Apply a heating pad

  OR

Apply a hot water bottle (to the abdomen)

Give warm liquids

Refrain from giving iced liquids

Massage gently (the lumbar area)

Cover with warm blankets

Place only warm hands and objects on the patient

Refrain from jarring the bed

Discourage oral stimulants

Discourage smoking

Ask the patient what makes him (or her) comfortable

Discuss possible pain-reducing measures

Provide a pain-relief measure of the patient's choice

Give nonprescription drugs (ExR) (analgesics)

Nursing Observations

Observe for complaints of pain duration

Evaluate pain for intensity and quality

Evaluate the effectiveness of the pain-relief measures

Health Teaching

Explain the causes of pain

Teach how to apply heat therapy

Explain the reason for and intended effect of the therapy

Medical Treatments Performed by Nurses

Give the prescribed drugs (antispasmodics)

EVALUATION

See the evaluation criteria for each specific goal in Chapter 2.

Painful Defecation (70,326,391)

ASSESSMENT

Subjective Data

Pain distribution: localized, rectal or abdominal

Duration: intermittent, during and/or after elimination

Onset: acute

Intensity: mild, moderate, or severe

Level: deep

Quality: burning pain

Objective Data
Delayed bowel elimination in anticipation of pain

Related Data
Commonly Related Conditions:
Anal or rectal fissure, abscess, ulcer, stricture, or polyps
Hemorrhoids
Commonly Related Diseases:
Carcinoma
Acute salpingitis
Endometriosis
Rectal stenosis
Metastic carcinoma

POSSIBLE ETIOLOGY

Pressure from fecal bulk irritates sensory nerve endings in an area of already existing sensitivity. Lower bowel or rectal spasm. Obstructive growth.

NURSING DIAGNOSIS

Painful defecation: a distressful hurting that occurs during or after bowel elimination

PLANNING

Patient Needs	**Primary Nurse-Patient Goals**
Waste elimination	To maintain regulating mechanisms and functions
Comfort	To achieve comfort
Protection from physical harm	To prevent physical injury
Freedom from pain	To achieve comfort
Increased learning	To achieve awareness of needs

NURSING INTERVENTIONS

Nursing Treatments
Approach unhurriedly
Reassure that the pain will subside
Communicate nurse sensitivity to the person's pain
Position comfortably
Apply a warm, moist compress (to the anal area)
    OR
Soak in a sitz bath
Increase fluid intake to about 2000 cc daily
Encourage decreased residue-food intake
Ask the patient what makes him (or her) comfortable
Discuss possible pain-reducing measures
Provide a pain-relief measure of the patient's choice
Give nonprescription drugs (ExR) (analgesics, stool softener)

Nursing Observations
Observe for complaints of pain duration
Evaluate pain for intensity and quality
Evaluate the effectiveness of the pain-relief measures

Health Teaching
Describe those symptoms which should be reported (bleeding)
Explain the causes of pain
Instruct to increase fluid intake
Teach how to take a sitz bath
Explain the reason for and intended effect of the therapy

Medical Treatments Performed by Nurses
Give the prescribed drugs

EVALUATION

See the evaluation criteria for each specific goal in Chapter 2.

Painful Urination (70,326,391)

ASSESSMENT

Subjective Data
Pain distribution: localized, in the area of the urinary meatus
Duration: intermittent, during or following voiding
Onset: acute
Intensity: mild, moderate, or severe
Level: deep
Quality: burning, stinging sensation

Objective Data
Urinary frequency
Urinary urgency
Urinary hesitancy

Related Data

Commonly Related Diseases:
Urethritis
Cystitis
Bladder calculi
Prostatitis
Urethral stricture
Uterine prolapse
Cervical cancer
Meatal stenosis
Ureteral calculi
Prostate adenocarcinoma
Benign prostatic hypertrophy

POSSIBLE ETIOLOGY

Pressure or irritation of the nerve fiber endings. High urine acidity.
Inflammation. Genitourinary infection.

NURSING DIAGNOSIS

Painful urination (dysuria): discomfort in the area of the urinary meatus during or after urination

PLANNING

Patient Needs	Primary Nurse-Patient Goals
Water-salt balance	To maintain fluid and electrolyte balance
Acid-base balance	To maintain regulating mechanisms and functions
Comfort	To achieve comfort
Cleanliness	To achieve good hygiene
Protection from physical harm	To prevent physical injury, infection
Freedom from pain	To achieve comfort
Increased learning	To achieve awareness of needs

NURSING INTERVENTIONS

Nursing Treatments
Approach unhurriedly
Reassure that the pain will subside
Communicate nurse sensitivity to the person's pain
Soak in a sitz bath
Increase fluid intake to about 3000 cc daily
Discuss possible pain-reducing measures
Give urine-acidifying juices orally (if infection is suspected)

Nursing Observations
Observe for complaints of pain duration
Evaluate pain for intensity and quality
Evaluate the effectiveness of the pain-relief measures
Measure the intake
Measure the output
Monitor the oral temperature (for fever)
Monitor urine studies for evidence of urinary tract infection
Observe for urinary frequency
Observe the urine for abnormal color, content, and odor
Inspect for bleeding (hematuria)
Obtain a bacterial culture (of the urine)
Test the urine for pH

Health Teaching
Describe those symptoms which should be reported
Explain the causes of pain
Instruct to increase fluid intake

Medical Treatments Performed by Nurses
Give the prescribed drugs

EVALUATION

See the evaluation criteria for each specific goal in Chapter 2.

Renal Colic Pain (247,271,453)

ASSESSMENT

Subjective Data

Pain distribution: localized and referred; pain begins on the side and in the back; radiates to the lower abdomen, genitals, and inner thighs; tenderness over the lower back and sides

Duration: a few minutes or several hours

Onset: acute

Intensity: severe

Level: deep

Quality: extreme, cramping pain

Objective data

Restlessness

Fever

Hematuria sometimes occurs

Vomiting

Irritability

Doubled up with pain

Related Data

Commonly Related Diseases:

Calcium renal calculi

Cystine renal calculi

Uric acid renal calculi

POSSIBLE ETIOLOGY

Kidney or ureter obstruction from stones, blood clots, or pus. Renal or ureteral spasms attempting to force the obstructing object through the urinary system.

NURSING DIAGNOSIS

Renal colic pain: agonizing, spasmodic pain in the area of the kidney and abdomen

PLANNING

Patient Needs	**Primary Nurse-Patient Goals**
Water-salt balance	To maintain fluid and electrolyte balance
Sleep, rest	To achieve sleep, rest
Activity, exercise	To achieve activity and exercise
Comfort	To achieve comfort
Protection from physical harm	To prevent physical injury
Freedom from pain	To achieve comfort
Increased learning	To achieve awareness of needs

NURSING INTERVENTIONS

Nursing Treatments

Approach unhurriedly

Reassure that the pain will subside
Communicate nurse sensitivity to the person's pain
Handle gently
Attend the patient constantly
Ambulate the patient (during the initial pain, if possible)
Position comfortably (once the severe pain subsides)
Apply a heating pad   ⎫
     OR   ⎬ (to the abdomen)
Apply a hot water bottle ⎭
     OR
Soak in a sitz bath
Increase fluid intake to about 3000 cc daily
Remove constrictive clothing
Refrain from jarring the bed
Ask the patient what makes him (or her) comfortable
Discuss possible pain-reducing measures
Provide a pain-relief measure of the patient's choice
Give nonprescription drugs (ExR) (analgesics)
Encourage adequate rest

Nursing Observations
Observe for complaints of pain duration
Observe for complaints of pain radiation
Observe for the sudden absence of severe pain
Estimate the degree of pain experienced
Evaluate the effectiveness of the pain-relief measures
Observe for shock
Strain the urine (until the stone is passed)

Health Teaching
Describe those symptoms which should be reported (sudden pain cessation)
Explain the causes of pain
Instruct to increase fluid intake
Explain the reason for and intended effect of the therapy

Medical Treatments Performed by Nurses
Give the prescribed drugs (analgesics, antispasmotics)

EVALUATION

See the evaluation criteria for each specific goal in Chapter 2.

SPECIFIC HEAD PAIN

Cluster Headache (247,453)

ASSESSMENT

Subjective Data
Pain distribution: localized, unilateral; located near the eye orbit, temple, or side of the face; sometimes radiates to the jaw and neck
Duration: constant, lasting about one hour; may occur each night for several nights, weeks, or months, but then disappears for a time

Onset: acute, usually occurs several hours after falling asleep
Intensity: severe
Level: deep
Quality: throbbing, boring pain

Objective Data
Reddened eyes
Nasal congestion or stuffiness followed by watery discharge
Ptosis
Cheek edema
Miosis

Related Data

Commonly Related Diseases:
Carotid aneurysm
Intracranial tumor
Sinusitis
Hemangioma

POSSIBLE ETIOLOGY

Dilatation of the branches of the internal carotid artery. Histamine reaction.

NURSING DIAGNOSIS

Cluster headache (histamine headache): headaches that occur consistently each night for a limited period and then disappear for a while

PLANNING

Patient Needs	**Primary Nurse-Patient Goals**
Rest, relaxation	To achieve rest, relaxation
Comfort	To achieve comfort
Protection from physical harm	To prevent physical injury
Freedom from pain	To achieve comfort
Increased learning	To achieve awareness of needs

NURSING INTERVENTIONS

Nursing Treatments
Approach unhurriedly
Reassure that the pain will subside
Communicate nurse sensitivity to the person's pain
Position comfortably
Change the patient's position gradually
Elevate the head
Apply a cold, moist compress (to the forehead)
     OR
Apply an ice bag (to the head)
Massage gently (the neck and shoulders)
Subdue the room lighting
Provide quiet

Encourage adequate rest
Ask the patient what makes him (or her) comfortable
Discuss possible pain-reducing measures
Provide the pain-relief measure of the patient's choice
Give nonprescription drugs (ExR) (analgesics, antihistamines)

Nursing Observations
Evaluate pain for intensity and quality
Observe for complaints of pain duration
Evaluate the effectiveness of the pain-relief measures
Inspect the eyes for pupil equality and response changes
Monitor the blood pressure

Health Teaching
Explain the causes of pain
Advise not to take hot baths
Inform that coughing should be avoided
Inform that elimination straining should be avoided
Explain the reason for and intended effect of the therapy

Medical Treatments Performed by Nurses
Give the prescribed drugs (analgesics)

EVALUATION

See the evaluation criteria for each specific goal in Chapter 2.

Eyestrain Headache (271,453)

ASSESSMENT

Subjective Data
Pain distribution: forehead, eye orbit, or above the eye
Duration: intermittent
Onset: gradual, during prolonged close eye work
Intensity: moderate or severe
Level: deep
Quality: aching pain

Related Data
Commonly Related Diseases:
Hypermetropia
Astigmatism

POSSIBLE ETIOLOGY

Prolonged contraction of the temporal, occipital, frontal, and/or extraocular muscles

NURSING DIAGNOSIS

Eyestrain headache: head pain associated with intense use of the eyes

PLANNING

Patient Needs	**Primary Nurse-Patient Goals**
Rest, relaxation	To achieve rest, relaxation

Comfort	To achieve comfort
Protection from physical harm	To prevent physical injury
Freedom from pain	To achieve comfort
Increased learning	To achieve awareness of needs

NURSING INTERVENTIONS

Nursing Treatments
Approach unhurriedly
Reassure that the pain will subside
Communicate nurse sensitivity to the person's pain
Position comfortably
Massage gently (the neck and shoulders)
Provide quiet
Ask the patient what make him (or her) comfortable
Discuss possible pain-reducing measures
Provide a pain-relief measure of the patient's choice
Give nonprescription drugs (ExR) (analgesics)
Encourage adequate rest
Make a referral (to an opthalmologist)

Nursing Observations
Observe for complaints of pain duration
Evaluate pain for intensity and quality
Evaluate the effectiveness of the pain-relief measures

Health Teaching
Explain the causes of pain
Explain the reason for and intended effect of the therapy

Medical Treatments Performed by Nurses
Give the prescribed drugs (analgesics)

EVALUATION

See the evaluation criteria for each specific goal in Chapter 2.

Febrile Headache (453)

ASSESSMENT

Subjective Data
Pain distribution: forehead, back of the head, or generalized
Duration: constant
Onset: gradual, as fever rises
Intensity: mild, moderate or severe
Level: deep
Quality: throbbing or stabbing sensation

Objective Data
Fever

Related Data
Commonly Related Diseases:
Tonsillitis

Typhoid fever
Malaria
Yellow fever
Rocky Mountain spotted fever
Q-fever
Influenza
Encephalitis
Pneumonia
Scarlet fever

POSSIBLE ETIOLOGY

Cerebral vasodilatation

NURSING DIAGNOSIS

Febrile headache: generalized head pain associated with fever

PLANNING

Patient Needs	Primary Nurse-Patient Goals
Rest	To achieve rest
Comfort	To achieve comfort
Protection from physical harm	To prevent physical injury
Freedom from pain	To achieve comfort
Increased learning	To achieve awareness of needs

NURSING INTERVENTIONS

Nursing Treatments
Approach unhurriedly
Reassure that the pain will subside
Communicate nurse sensitivity to the person's pain
Position comfortably
Change the patient's position gradually
Elevate the head
Apply a cold, moist compress (to the forehead)
    OR
Apply an ice bag (to the head)
Provide quiet
Encourage adequate rest
Ask the patient what makes him (or her) comfortable
Discuss possible pain-reducing measures
Provide a pain-relief measure of the patient's choice
Give nonprescription drugs (ExR) (analgesics, antipyretics)

Nursing Observations
Observe for complaints of pain duration
Evaluate pain for intensity and quality
Evaluate the effectiveness of the pain-relief measures

Health Teaching
Explain the causes of pain
Explain the reason for and intended effect of the therapy

Medical Treatments Performed by Nurses
Give the prescribed drugs (analgesics)

EVALUATION

See the evaluation criteria for each specific goal in Chapter 2.

Hypertensive Headache (271,453)

ASSESSMENT

Subjective Data
Pain distribution: localized, covering the skull cap area, or generalized
Duration: intermittent
Onset: gradual or acute
Intensity: moderate or severe
Level: deep
Quality: throbbing
Other characteristics: often most prevalent in the morning

Objective Data
Diastolic blood pressure above 110 mm Hg
Papilledema

Related Data
Commonly Related Diseases:
Hypertension

POSSIBLE ETIOLOGY

Increased intracranial pressure or cerebral vasodilatation. Increased pressure within the brain when the flat position elevates the blood pressure.

NURSING DIAGNOSIS

Hypertensive headache: throbbing head pain associated with an elevated blood pressure

PLANNING

Patient Needs	**Primary Nurse-Patient Goals**
Rest, relaxation	To achieve rest, relaxation
Comfort	To achieve comfort
Protection from physical harm	To prevent physical injury
Freedom from pain	To achieve comfort
Increased learning	To achieve awareness of needs

NURSING INTERVENTIONS

Nursing Treatments
Approach unhurriedly
Reassure that the pain will subside
Communicate nurse sensitivity to the person's pain
Position comfortably
Change the patient's position gradually

Elevate the head
Apply a cold, moist compress (to the forehead)
  OR
Apply an ice bag (to the head)
Give hot coffee (black)
Massage gently (the neck and shoulders)
Subdue the room lighting
Provide quiet
Encourage adequate rest
Ask the patient what makes him (or her) comfortable
Discuss possible pain-reducing measures
Provide a pain-relief measure of the patient's choice
Give nonprescription drugs (ExR) (acetylsalicylic acid simultaneous with coffee)

Nursing Observations
Observe for complaints of pain duration
Evaluate pain for intensity and quality
Evaluate the effectiveness of the pain-relief measures
Monitor the blood pressure

Health Teaching
Explain the causes of pain
Advise not to take hot baths
Advise that highly emotional situations be avoided
Inform that coughing should be avoided
Inform that elimination straining should be avoided
Explain the reason for and intended effect of the therapy

Medical Treatments Performed by Nurses
Give the prescribed drugs (analgesics)

EVALUATION

See the evaluation criteria for each specific goal in Chapter 2.

Meningeal Headache (271,453)

ASSESSMENT

Subjective Data
Pain distribution: generalized; covers entire head
Duration: constant
Onset: acute
Intensity: severe, especially at the base of the skull
Level: deep
Quality: throbbing

Objective Data
Neck stiffness
Vomiting, sometimes
Irritability
Restlessness

Related Data

Commonly Related Diseases:
Acute meningitis

POSSIBLE ETIOLOGY

Chemical irritation of nerve fiber endings in the meninges

NURSING DIAGNOSIS

Meningeal headache: throbbing head pain associated with inflammation of the meninges

PLANNING

Patient Needs	Primary Nurse-Patient Goals
Rest, relaxation	To achieve rest, relaxation
Comfort	To achieve comfort
Protection from physical harm	To prevent physical injury
Freedom from pain	To achieve comfort
Increased learning	To achieve awareness of needs

NURSING INTERVENTIONS

Nursing Treatments
Approach unhurriedly
Reassure that the pain will subside
Communicate nurse sensitivity to the person's pain
Position comfortably
Change the patient's position gradually
Apply a cold, moist compress
    OR
Apply an ice bag (to the head)
Massage gently (the neck and shoulders)
Subdue the room lighting
Provide quiet
Encourage adequate rest
Refrain from jarring the bed
Reduce the demands placed upon the patient
Refrain from performing nonessential procedures
Ask the patient what makes him (or her) comfortable
Discuss possible pain-reducing measures
Provide a pain-relief measure of the patient's choice
Give nonprescription drugs (ExR) (analgesics)

Nursing Observations
Observe for complaints of pain duration
Evaluate pain for intensity and quality
Evaluate the effectiveness of the pain-relief measures

Health Teaching
Explain the causes of pain
Advise not to take hot baths

Inform that coughing should be avoided
Inform that elimination straining should be avoided
Explain the reason for and intended effect of the therapy

Medical Treatments Performed by Nurses
Give the prescribed drugs (analgesics)

EVALUATION

See the evaluation criteria for each specific goal in Chapter 2.

Menstrual-Migraine Headache (453)

ASSESSMENT

Subjective Data
Pain distribution: localized; usually confined to one side of the head; temporal or occipital
Duration: intermittent or continuous
Onset: acute; begins several days prior to menstrual onset, reaching greatest intensity at the onset of flow
Intensity: severe
Level: deep
Quality: boring, sharp pain

Objective Data
Irritability
Body edema

Related Data
Commonly Related Diseases:
None

POSSIBLE ETIOLOGY

Excessive secretion of the follicle-stimulating hormone by the pituitary increases the estrogen secretion and inhibits the gonadotropic function of the pituitary, causing abnormal estrogen and gonadotropin excretion. Allergy to one's own hormones. Fluid retention causing intermittent cranial edema.

NURSING DIAGNOSIS

Menstrual-migraine headache: a boring headache just prior to menstruation onset

PLANNING

Patient Needs	Primary Nurse-Patient Goals
Water-salt balance	To maintain fluid and electrolyte balance
Rest, relaxation	To achieve rest, relaxation
Comfort	To achieve comfort
Protection from physical harm	To prevent physical injury
Freedom from pain	To achieve comfort
Increased learning	To achieve awareness of needs

NURSING INTERVENTIONS

Nursing Treatments

Approach unhurriedly

Reassure that the pain will subside

Communicate nurse sensitivity to the person's pain

Position comfortably

Apply a cold, moist compress

    OR

Apply an ice bag

Provide quiet

Encourage adequate rest

Ask the patient what makes her comfortable

Discuss possible pain-reducing measures

Provide a pain-relief measure of the patient's choice

Give nonprescription drugs (ExR) (analgesics)

Encourage decreased sodium-food intake (one week prior to menstruation onset)

Restrict the fluid intake according to the weight gain (one week prior to menstruation onset)

Nursing Observations

Observe for complaints of pain duration

Evaluate pain for intensity and quality

Evaluate the effectiveness of the pain-relief measures

Health Teaching

Describe those symptoms which should be reported

Explain the causes of pain

Explain the reason for and intended effect of the therapy

Medical Treatments Performed by Nurses

Give the prescribed drugs (analgesics)

EVALUATION

See the evaluation criteria for each specific goal in Chapter 2.

Migraine Headache (247,271,453)

ASSESSMENT

Subjective Data

Pain distribution: unilateral or generalized

Duration: continuous

Onset: acute; prior to onset there is visualization of stars or zig-zag flashes of light of white, blue, yellow, or green color; patient can then see only half of all objects; vision clears in 15–30 minutes, and the headache follows

Intensity: severe

Level: deep

Quality: throbbing, boring pain

Objective Data
Nausea
Vomiting, sometimes
Light sensitivity
Sound sensitivity

Related Data
Family history of migraine headaches
Commonly Related Diseases:
Allergic response (chocolate, etc.)

POSSIBLE ETIOLOGY

Cause is uncertain at this time. Believed to be due to impaired cranial circulation that causes vasoconstriction followed by vasodilatation that causes the pain.

NURSING DIAGNOSIS

Migraine headache: extremely severe, constant head pain, following an aura

PLANNING

Patient Needs	**Primary Nurse-Patient Goals**
Sleep, rest, relaxation	To achieve sleep, rest, relaxation
Comfort	To achieve comfort
Protection from physical harm	To prevent physical injury
Freedom from pain	To achieve comfort
Increased learning	To achieve awareness of needs

NURSING INTERVENTIONS

Nursing Treatments
Approach unhurriedly
Reassure that the pain will subside
Communicate nurse sensitivity to the person's pain
Elevate the head
Position comfortably
Change the patient's position gradually
Apply a cold, moist compress (to the forehead)
   OR
Apply an ice bag (to the head)
Massage gently (the neck and shoulders)
Subdue the room lighting
Provide quiet
Encourage adequate rest
Refrain from performing nonessential procedures
Ask the patient what makes him (or her) comfortable
Discuss possible pain-reducing measures
Provide a pain-relief measure of the patient's choice
Give hot coffee (before the headache becomes severe)
Give nonprescription drugs (ExR) (acetylsalicylic acid with the coffee)
Provide frequent patient contact

Nursing Observations
Observe for complaints of pain duration
Observe for complaints of pain radiation
Estimate the degree of pain experienced
Evaluate the effectiveness of the pain-relief measures

Health Teaching
Advise not to take hot baths
Describe those symptoms which should be reported
Explain the causes of pain
Inform that coughing should be avoided
Inform that elimination straining should be avoided

Medical Treatments Performed by Nurses
Give the prescribed drugs (Ergotamine)

EVALUATION

See the evaluation criteria for each specific goal in Chapter 2.

Sinus Headache (8,10,18,247,271,453)

ASSESSMENT

Subjective Data
Pain distribution: forehead; between, behind, or over the eyes; patient's face
    may hurt; sometimes the teeth hurt; pain may spread to the base of the
    neck
Duration: continuous
Onset: gradual; pain is worse in the morning, decreasing when the head is
    elevated; it may again appear in late morning and disappear in the eve-
    ning
Intensity: mild, moderate, or severe
Level: deep
Quality: throbbing pain; a stooping posture increases the pain

Objective Data
Sinus tenderness
Nasal congestion
Purulent nasal discharge, sometimes
Postnasal drainage sometimes causes a cough or sore throat

Related Data
Most common in cold, damp weather
Commonly Related Diseases:
Sinusitis

POSSIBLE ETIOLOGY

Infection or irritation of the sinus cavities

NURSING DIAGNOSIS

Sinus headache: throbbing head pain related to the sinuses

PLANNING

Patient Needs	**Primary Nurse-Patient Goals**
Rest, relaxation	To achieve rest, relaxation
Comfort	To achieve comfort
Protection from physical harm	To prevent physical injury
Freedom from pain	To achieve comfort
Increased learning	To achieve awareness of needs

NURSING INTERVENTIONS

Nursing Treatments
Approach unhurriedly
Reassure that the pain will subside
Communicate nurse sensitivity to the person's pain
Elevate the head
Position comfortably
Administer vaporized air
Apply a heating pad
   OR
Apply a warm, moist compress
Provide quiet
Subdue the room lighting
Encourage adequate rest
Ask the patient what makes him (or her) comfortable
Provide a pain-relief measure of the patient's choice
Give nonprescription drugs (ExR) (analgesics)

Nursing Observations
Observe for complaints of pain duration
Observe for complaints of pain radiation
Evaluate pain for intensity and quality
Evaluate the effectiveness of the pain-relief measures

Health Teaching
Explain the causes of pain
Explain the reason for and intended effect of the therapy

Medical Treatments Performed by Nurses

Give the prescribed drugs (analgesics)

EVALUATION

See the evaluation criteria for each specific goal in Chapter 2.

Spinal Puncture Headache (453)

ASSESSMENT

Subjective Data
Pain distribution: generalized, occipital pain
Duration: continuous

Onset: acute, shortly after a spinal puncture

Intensity: severe; increases when in the upright position; decreases when horizontal

Level: deep

Quality: throbbing

Related Data

Commonly Related Diseases:
None

POSSIBLE ETIOLOGY

Following a spinal puncture, spinal fluid leaks through the puncture site and escapes from the spinal canal into surrounding tissues. This reduces the normal supply of spinal fluid to the brain, causing traction on the dural attachments to the venous sinuses, resulting in a headache.

NURSING DIAGNOSIS

Spinal-puncture headache: a severe headache occurring after a spinal puncture

PLANNING

Patient Needs	**Primary Nurse-Patient Goals**
Rest, relaxation	To achieve rest, relaxation
Comfort	To achieve comfort
Protection from physical harm	To prevent physical injury
Freedom from pain	To achieve comfort
Increased learning	To achieve awareness of needs

NURSING INTERVENTIONS

Nursing Treatments

Approach unhurriedly

Reassure that the pain will subside

Communicate nurse sensitivity to the person's pain

Place in the flat position (12–24 hours after spinal puncture)

Position comfortably

Apply a cold, moist compress
    OR
Apply an ice bag

Provide quiet

Subdue the room lighting

Encourage adequate rest

Refrain from performing nonessential procedures

Ask the patient what makes him (or her) comfortable

Discuss possible pain-reducing measures

Provide a pain-relief measure of the patient's choice

Give nonprescription drugs (ExR) (analgesics)

Provide frequent patient contact

Nursing Observations
Observe for complaints of pain duration
Estimate the degree of pain experienced
Evaluate the effectiveness of the pain-relief measures

Health Teaching
Explain the causes of pain
Explain the reason for and intended effect of the therapy

Medical Treatments Performed by Nurses
Give the prescribed drugs (analgesics)

EVALUATION

See the evaluation criteria for each specific goal in Chapter 2.

Tension Headache (247,271,453)

ASSESSMENT

Subjective Data
Pain distribution: back of the head, above both eyes, top of the head
Duration: continuous, often during both the day and night for several days
Onset: gradual, often associated with stress
Intensity: severe
Level: deep
Quality: head fullness; sensation of a band or vicelike squeezing pain; nonthrobbing, dull, sometimes burning sensation; possibly a creeping sensation over the head

Objective Data
Patient may appear apathetic or tense and anxious

Related Data
Analgesics do not give complete pain relief. Common during the menopause.
Commonly Related Diseases:
None

POSSIBLE ETIOLOGY

Cerebral vasodilatation. Stress. Fatigue. Prolonged contraction of head and neck muscles.

NURSING DIAGNOSIS

Tension headache: a tight, viselike head pain

PLANNING

Patient Needs	Primary Nurse-Patient Goals
Rest, relaxation	To achieve rest, relaxation
Comfort	To achieve comfort
Protection from physical harm	To prevent physical injury
Freedom from pain	To achieve comfort
Increased learning	To achieve awareness of needs

NURSING INTERVENTIONS

Nursing Treatments
Approach unhurriedly
Reassure that the pain will subside
Communicate nurse sensitivity to the person's pain
Elevate the head
Position comfortably
Change the patient's position gradually
Apply a heating pad
   OR
Apply a hot water bottle
Bathe in warm water (for relaxation)
Massage gently (the neck and shoulders)
Subdue the room lighting
Provide quiet
Encourage adequate rest
Ask the patient what makes him (or her) comfortable
Discuss possible pain-reducing measures
Provide a pain relief measure of the patient's choice
Give nonprescription drugs (ExR) (analgesics)
Encourage the expression of feelings (about current stress)
Reduce the demands placed upon the patient

Nursing Observations
Observe for complaints of pain duration
Observe for complaints of pain radiation
Evaluate pain for intensity and quality
Evaluate the effectiveness of the pain-relief measures
Monitor the blood pressure

Health Teaching
Explain the causes of pain
Explain that fatigue should be recognized as a stress factor
Explain how to reduce muscular tension
Recommend adherence to a moderate pace of living
Explain the reason for and intended effect of the therapy

Medical Treatments Performed by Nurses
Give the prescribed drugs (analgesics)

EVALUATION

See the evaluation criteria for each specific goal in Chapter 2.

Toxic Headache (271)

ASSESSMENT

Subjective Data
Pain distribution: generalized
Duration: constant
Onset: acute, upon exposure to toxins

Intensity: severe
Level: deep
Quality: throbbing

Objective Data
Unstable gait

Related Data
Recent exposure to lead or carbon monoxide. Recent ingestion of alcohol, arsenic, or certain drugs.

Commonly Related Diseases:
None

POSSIBLE ETIOLOGY

The poisonous effects of certain agents cause nerve irritation resulting in headache.

NURSING DIAGNOSIS

Toxic headache: head pain resulting from recent exposure to toxic substances

PLANNING

Patient Needs	**Primary Nurse-Patient Goals**
Waste elimination	To maintain regulating mechanisms and functions
Rest, relaxation	To achieve rest, relaxation
Comfort	To achieve comfort
Protection from physical harm	To prevent physical injury
Freedom from pain	To achieve comfort
Increased learning	To achieve awareness of needs

NURSING INTERVENTIONS

Nursing Treatments
Approach unhurriedly
Reassure that the pain will subside
Communicate nurse sensitivity to the person's pain
Position comfortably
Encourage deep breathing
Apply a cold, moist compress
　OR
Apply an ice bag
Increase fluid intake to about 3000 cc daily (for ingested toxins)
Subdue the room lighting
Provide quiet
Encourage adequate rest
Ask the patient what makes him (or her) comfortable
Discuss possible pain-reducing measures
Provide a pain-relief measure of the patient's choice
Give nonprescription drugs (ExR) (analgesics)

Nursing Observations
Observe for complaints of pain duration
Evaluate pain for intensity and quality
Evaluate the effectiveness of the pain-relief measures

Health Teaching
Explain the causes of pain
Explain the reason for and intended effect of the therapy

Medical Treatments Performed by Nurses
Give the prescribed drugs (analgesics)

EVALUATION

See the evaluation criteria for each specific goal in Chapter 2.

Trauma Headache (453)

ASSESSMENT

Subjective Data
Pain distribution: generalized or localized
Duration: continuous or intermittent; lasts anywhere from several days to
    one or 2 weeks
Onset: acute, with the injury
Intensity: severe
Level: deep
Quality: throbbing

Objective Data
Tenderness at the injury site

Related Data
Commonly Related Diseases:
Cerebral contusion
Cerebral concussion

POSSIBLE ETIOLOGY

Pressure from trauma on the cranium

NURSING DIAGNOSIS

Trauma headache: a headache resulting from injury to the cranium

PLANNING

Patient Needs	Primary Nurse-Patient Goals
Rest	To achieve rest
Comfort	To achieve comfort
Protection from physical harm	To prevent physical injury
Freedom from pain	To achieve comfort
Increased learning	To achieve awareness of needs

NURSING INTERVENTIONS

Nursing Treatments
Approach unhurriedly
Reassure that the pain will subside
Communicate nurse sensitivity to the person's pain
Elevate the head
Change the patient's position gradually
Apply a cold, moist compress
> OR

Apply an ice bag
Place on complete bed rest
Refrain from jarring the bed
Ask the patient what makes him (or her) comfortable
Discuss possible pain-reducing measures
Provide a pain-relief measure of the patient's choice
Give nonprescription drugs (ExR) (analgesics)
Provide frequent patient contact

Nursing Observations
Observe for complaints of pain duration
Observe for complaints of pain radiation
Evaluate the effectiveness of the pain-relief measures
Inspect the eyes for pupil equality and response changes
Inspect the hands for impaired grasp
Observe the level of consciousness

Health Teaching
Explain the causes of pain
Explain the reason for and intended effect of the therapy

Medical Treatments Performed by Nurses
Give the prescribed drugs (analgesics)

EVALUATION

See the evaluation criteria for each specific goal in Chapter 2.

SPECIFIC NEUROMUSCULAR PAIN

Backache (90,243)

ASSESSMENT

Subjective Data
Pain distribution: localized and/or referred; pain in the lumbar or sacral
   area, which may radiate down the leg
Duration: intermittent or continuous
Onset: gradual or acute
Intensity: mild, moderate, or severe
Level: deep

Quality: muscle tenderness, spasm, or rigidity; patient has difficulty standing straight

Objective Data
Irritability
Backholding
Frequent position change
Frequently seen sitting on desks and tables or leaning against supporting objects

Related Data
Commonly Related Conditions:
Sprained ligaments
Pregnancy
Commonly Related Diseases:
Herniated disk
Lumbar fracture
Ankylosing spondylitis
Bone fracture
Rheumatoid arthritis
Osteoporosis

POSSIBLE ETIOLOGY

Lack of exercise. Poor posture. Pressure on the spine from uterine or prostate abnormalities. Poorly developed muscle tone. Injury to vertebrae or ligaments in the spine. Infection. Inflammation. Excessive muscle tension due to stress.

NURSING DIAGNOSIS

Backache: a distressful hurting in the lower lumbar, lumbosacral, or sacroiliac region

PLANNING

Patient Needs	Primary Nurse-Patient Goals
Rest, relaxation	To achieve rest, relaxation
Comfort	To achieve comfort
Protection from physical harm	To prevent physical injury, deformities
Freedom from pain	To achieve comfort
Increased learning	To achieve awareness of needs

NURSING INTERVENTIONS

Nursing Treatments
Approach unhurriedly
Reassure that the pain will subside
Communicate nurse sensitivity to the person's pain
Position comfortably
Change the patient's position gradually
Maintain body alignment

Apply a heating pad
   OR
Apply a hot water bottle
   OR
Apply a warm, moist compress
   OR
Bathe in warm water
Massage gently
Place a bedboard under the mattress
Provide a firm mattress
Encourage adequate rest
Ask the patient what makes him (or her) comfortable
Discuss possible pain-reducing measures
Provide a pain-relief measure of the patient's choice
Give nonprescription drugs (ExR) (analgesics)

Nursing Observations
Observe for complaints of pain duration
Observe for complaints of pain radiation
Estimate the degree of pain experienced
Evaluate the effectiveness of the pain-relief measures

Health Teaching
Explain the causes of pain
Explain how to maintain body alignment
Explain that fatigue should be recognized as a stress factor
Explain how to reduce muscular tension
Inform that heavy lifting should be avoided
Recommend the use of a back-support garment
Recommend the use of a car back rest
Recommend the use of low-heeled shoes
Teach good body mechanics
Explain the reason for and intended effect of the therapy

Medical Treatments Performed by Nurses
Give the prescribed drugs (analgesics)

EVALUATION

See the evaluation criteria for each specific goal in Chapter 2.

Bone Pain (453)

ASSESSMENT

Subjective Data
Pain distribution: localized in the bone area
Duration: intermittent or continuous
Onset: gradual or acute
Intensity: severe, increased by weight-bearing or movement
Level: deep
Quality: aching pain; muscles over the bone do not hurt ·

Objective Data
Irritability
Localized edema, sometimes

Related Data
Commonly Related Diseases:
Hyperparathyroidism
Multiple myeloma
Paget's bone disease
Leukemia
Staphylococcus osteomyelitis
Streptococcus osteomyelitis
Tuberculosis
Syphilis
Closed fracture
Compound fracture
Aplastic anemia

POSSIBLE ETIOLOGY

Bone trauma. Bone disease. Excessive white blood cell production results in expansion (hyperplasia) of the bone marrow. Increased destruction or decreased production of red blood cells results in compensatory blood marrow expansion as the body attempts to offset the deficiency of RBCs and WBCs in the bone marrow.

NURSING DIAGNOSIS

Bone pain: a distressful hurting felt within the bone itself

PLANNING

Patient Needs	Primary Nurse-Patient Goals
Rest	To achieve rest
Protection from physical harm	To prevent physical injury
Freedom from pain	To achieve comfort
Increased learning	To achieve awareness of needs

NURSING INTERVENTIONS

Nursing Treatments
Approach unhurriedly
Reassure that the pain will subside
Communicate nurse sensitivity to the person's pain
Handle gently
Position comfortably
Change the patient's position gradually
Support the affected body part
Apply a warm, moist compress (to a localized area)
   OR
Place in a whirlpool bath
Encourage adequate rest

Ask the patient what makes him (or her) comfortable
Discuss possible pain-reducing measures
Provide a pain-relief measure of the patient's choice
Give nonprescription drugs (ExR) (analgesics)

Nursing Observations
Observe for complaints of pain duration
Observe for complaints of pain radiation
Estimate the degree of pain experienced
Evaluate the effectiveness of the pain-relief measures

Health Teaching
Explain the causes of pain
Explain the reason for and intended effect of the therapy

Medical Treatments Performed by Nurses
Give the prescribed drugs (analgesics)

EVALUATION

See the evaluation criteria for each specific goal in Chapter 2.

Muscle Spasm (70,326,453)

ASSESSMENT

Subjective Data
Pain distribution: localized
Duration: intermittent
Onset: acute
Intensity: severe
Level: deep
Quality: cramping pain

Objective Data
Irritability
Muscle tightness
Grasping or rubbing the area of spasm

Related Data

Laboratory Findings:
Decreased blood calcium, magnesium
Increased blood phosphorous

Commonly Related Conditions:
Respiratory or metabolic alkalosis
Hypocalcemia
Hypomagnesemia

Commonly Related Diseases:
Cervical or thoracic spinal cord injury
Uremia
Tetanus
Hypoparathyroidism

POSSIBLE ETIOLOGY

Increased nervous and muscular excitability due to changes in blood calcium level and blood pH. Repetitive activation of efferent nerve fibers carrying motor impulses to muscle fibers before relaxation can occur.

NURSING DIAGNOSIS

Muscle spasm: a continuous state of muscle contraction with intense pain

PLANNING

Patient Needs	Primary Nurse-Patient Goals
Water-salt balance	To maintain fluid and electrolyte balance
Relaxation	To achieve relaxation
Comfort	To achieve comfort
Protection from physical harm	To prevent accident, physical injury
Freedom from pain	To achieve comfort
Increased learning	To achieve awareness of needs

NURSING INTERVENTIONS

Nursing Treatments
Approach unhurriedly
Reassure that the pain will subside
Communicate nurse sensitivity to the person's pain
Handle gently
Position comfortably
Change the patient's position gradually
Remove constrictive clothing
Apply a heating pad
   OR
Apply a hot water bottle
   OR
Apply a warm, moist compress
   OR
Place in a whirlpool bath
Refrain from local cold applications
Massage gently (the area of spasm)
Cover with warm blankets
Maintain a warm room temperature
Decrease drafts
Place only warm hands and objects on the patient
Place a footboard at the feet (to press against during the spasm)
Place a pillow between the knees
Control excessive spasticity with firm hand pressure
Refrain from jarring the bed
Refrain from performing nonessential procedures
Ask the patient what makes him (or her) comfortable
Discuss possible pain-reducing measures

Provide a pain-relief measure of the patient's choice
Give nonprescription drugs (ExR) (analgesics)
Encourage increased calcium-food intake ⎫
   AND   ⎬ (if the blood calcium is low)
Give high calcium fluids orally ⎭
Give high-magnesium fluids orally (if the blood magnesium is low)

Nursing Observations
Observe for complaints of pain duration
Evaluate pain for intensity and quality
Evaluate the effectiveness of the pain-relief measures
Monitor blood studies for abnormal acid-base
Monitor blood studies for abnormal electrolytes
Monitor blood studies for abnormal (decreased) parathyroid function
Test for Chvostek's sign
Test for a positive Trousseau's sign

Health Teaching
Explain the causes of pain
Teach how to apply heat therapy
Explain the reason for and intended effect of the therapy

Medical Treatments Performed by Nurses
Give the prescribed drugs (analgesics, antispasmodics)

EVALUATION

See the evaluation criteria for each specific goal in Chapter 2.

Painful Joint Motion (247,326,453)

ASSESSMENT

Subjective Data
Pain distribution: localized
Duration: intermittent
Onset: acute, with attempted joint movement
Intensity: mild, moderate, or severe
Level: deep
Quality: aching pain; usually worse in the morning

Objective Data
Joint rigidity
Little or no joint function

Related Data
Commonly Related Diseases:
Meningitis
Whiplash injury
Fibromyositis
Rheumatoid arthritis
Wryneck disease
Tuberculosis of the joint
Spondylitis

POSSIBLE ETIOLOGY

Prolonged immobility. Joint cartilage degeneration. Muscle rigidity or spasm. Trauma. Nervous system infection. Inflammation.

NURSING DIAGNOSIS

Painful joint motion: inability to freely move a joint without pain

PLANNING

Patient Needs	Primary Nurse-Patient Goals
Exercise	To achieve exercise
Comfort	To achieve comfort
Protection from physical harm	To prevent physical injury, deformities
Freedom from pain	To achieve comfort
Increased learning	To achieve awareness of needs

NURSING INTERVENTIONS

Nursing Treatments
Approach unhurriedly
Reassure that the pain will subside
Communicate nurse sensitivity to the person's pain
Handle gently
Position comfortably
Change the patient's position gradually
Maintain body alignment
Apply a heating pad
    OR
Apply a hot water bottle
    OR
Apply a warm, moist compress
    OR
Apply mentholated ointment
    OR
Place in a whirlpool bath
Massage gently
Exercise in range of motion (gently)
Ask the patient what makes him (or her) comfortable
Discuss possible pain-reducing measures
Provide a pain-relief measure of the patient's choice
Give nonprescription drugs (ExR) (analgesics)

Nursing Observations
Observe for complaints of pain duration
Observe for complaints of pain radiation
Evaluate pain for intensity and quality
Evaluate the effectiveness of the pain-relief measures

Health Teaching
Explain the causes of pain

Teach how to apply heat therapy
Explain how to maintain body alignment
Explain that immobility related to pain causes further pain
Teach how to do range-of-motion exercises
Explain the reason for and intended effect of the therapy

Medical Treatments Performed by Nurses
Give the prescribed drugs (analgesics, steroids)

EVALUATION

See the evaluation criteria for each specific goal in Chapter 2.

Phantom Pain (391,453)

ASSESSMENT

Subjective Data
Pain distribution: localized; in a body area where tissue no longer exists
Duration: continuous
Onset: acute (with amputation)
Intensity: severe
Level: deep
Quality: burning pain
Fear of being labeled "crazy" for experiencing pain where there is no tissue
Anxiety
Nervousness

Objective Data
Irritability

Related Data
Commonly Related Conditions:
Limb amputation
Commonly Related Diseases:
Gas gangrene
Crushing injury

POSSIBLE ETIOLOGY

Stimuli that continue to arise from severed sensory nerves

NURSING DIAGNOSIS

Phantom pain: a distressful hurting felt in the amputated area of a limb

PLANNING

Patient Needs	Primary Nurse-Patient Goals
Comfort	To achieve comfort
Protection from physical harm	To prevent physical injury
Freedom from pain	To achieve comfort
Increased learning	To achieve awareness of needs

NURSING INTERVENTIONS

Nursing Treatments
Approach unhurriedly
Reassure that the pain will subside
Communicate nurse sensitivity to the person's pain
Provide an atmosphere of acceptance
Handle gently
Position comfortably
Avoid placing tension on the wound
Support the affected body part
Refrain from tight bandaging
Ask the patient what makes him (or her) comfortable
Provide a pain-relief measure of the patient's choice
Give nonprescription drugs (ExR) (analgesics)

Nursing Observations
Observe for complaints of pain duration
Evaluate pain for intensity and quality
Evaluate the effectiveness of the pain-relief measures

Health Teaching
Explain that it is acceptable to admit the existence of pain
Explain the causes of pain
Explain the reason for and intended effect of the therapy

Medical Treatments Performed by Nurses
Give the prescribed drugs (analgesics)

EVALUATION

See the evaluation criteria for each specific goal in Chapter 2.

SPECIFIC ORAL
AND GASTRIC PAIN

Biliary Colic Pain (247,271,453)

ASSESSMENT

Subjective Data
Pain distribution: localized and/or referred; right upper quadrant and/or
    abdominal pain; pain may radiate to the right shoulder and back
Duration: continuous
Onset: acute
Intensity: severe
Level: deep
Quality: cramping pain; abdominal tenderness

Objective Data
Severe belching
Vomiting of yellow-green emesis

Gurgling bowel sounds
Abdominal hyperesthesia or rigidity sometimes
Gallbladder enlargement sometimes

Related Data

Commonly Related Diseases:
Choledocholithiasis
Cholecystitis
Cholelithiasis

POSSIBLE ETIOLOGY

Bile duct obstruction causing infection and impaired bile flow

NURSING DIAGNOSIS

Biliary colic pain: intensely painful spasms of the gallbladder bile ducts

PLANNING

Patient Needs	**Primary Nurse-Patient Goals**
Rest, relaxation	To achieve rest, relaxation
Comfort	To achieve comfort
Protection from physical harm	To prevent physical injury
Freedom from pain	To achieve comfort
Increased learning	To achieve awareness of needs

NURSING INTERVENTIONS

Nursing Treatments
Approach unhurriedly
Reassure that the pain will subside
Communicate nurse sensitivity to the person's pain
Position comfortably
Give warm liquids
Refrain from giving iced liquids
Apply a heating pad
   OR   } (slightly warm only)
Apply a hot water bottle
Give bland foods
Encourage decreased fatty-food intake
Encourage adequate rest
Refrain from performing nonessential procedures
Ask the patient what makes him (or her) comfortable
Discuss possible pain-reducing measures
Provide a pain-relief measure of the patient's choice
Give nonprescription drugs (ExR) (analgesics)

Nursing Observations
Observe for complaints of pain duration
Observe for complaints of pain radiation
Estimate the degree of pain experienced
Evaluate the effectiveness of the pain-relief measures
Inspect the abdomen for distention

Inspect the stool for abnormalities (clay-colored)
Monitor blood studies for biliary obstruction
Monitor urine studies for biliary obstruction

Health Teaching
Explain the causes of pain
Explain the reason for and intended effect of the therapy

Medical Treatments Performed by Nurses
Give the prescribed drugs (analgesics)

EVALUATION

See the evaluation criteria for each specific goal in Chapter 2.

Gastrointestinal-Cardiac Pain (359,453)

ASSESSMENT

Subjective Data
Pain distribution: localized and/or referred
  Gallbladder: radiation to substernal area
  Pancreatic: right epigastric, mid-epigastric, left lower epigastric pain, or across the epigastrium radiating to the back; radiation to the sternum, or either scapula
  Stomach ulceration: lower anterior chest, dorsal or right anterior chest, intrascapular area, lateral chest wall, abdomen, or right shoulder.
Duration: continuous (gallbladder) or intermittent
Onset: gradual or acute
Intensity: severe
Level: deep
Quality:
  Gallbladder: cramping pain
  Pancreatic: boring, bandlike pain
  Stomach ulceration: aching, burning, gnawing pain

Objective Data
Vomiting
Anorexia
Abdominal distention and/or rigidity
Fever, sometimes
Normal cardiogram

Related Data
Laboratory Findings:
Normal cardiac enzymes
Blood studies indicate pancreatic or biliary dysfunction or gastric ulcer
Commonly Related Diseases:
Cholecystitis
Common bile duct spasm

Pancreatitis
Pancreatic cyst
Pancreatic carcinoma
Gastric ulcer
Duodenal ulcer

POSSIBLE ETIOLOGY

Gallbladder pain impulses and cardiac pain impulses may be transmitted to the same or overlapping spinal cord areas. Pancreatic enzymes directly act on cardiac muscles and pancreatic nerve reflexes cause coronary artery spasm. In peptic ulcer, the vagal nerve impulses pick up local inflammatory reactions, and the afferent impulse of visceral pain is transmitted through the intercostal nerves in the chest to the spinal cord and brain.

NURSING DIAGNOSIS

Gastrointestinal cardiac pain: pain that has its source in the abdomen but is felt as cardiac pain

PLANNING

Patient Needs	**Primary Nurse-Patient Goals**
Rest, relaxation	To achieve rest, relaxation
Comfort	To achieve comfort
Protection from physical harm	To prevent physical injury
Freedom from pain	To achieve comfort
Increased learning	To achieve awareness of needs

NURSING INTERVENTIONS

Nursing Treatments
Approach unhurriedly
Reassure that the pain will subside
Communicate nurse sensitivity to the person's pain
Position comfortably
Give warm liquids
Provide quiet
Encourage adequate rest
Ask the patient what makes him (or her) comfortable
Discuss possible pain-reducing measures
Provide a pain-relief measure of the patient's choice
Give nonprescription drugs (ExR) (analgesics, antacids)

Nursing Observations
Observe for complaints of pain duration
Observe for complaints of pain radiation
Evaluate pain for intensity and quality
Evaluate the effectiveness of the pain-relief measures
Auscultate the apical heartbeat for rate and rhythm
Monitor the blood pressure
Palpate the pulse for rate, rhythm, and volume

Health Teaching
Explain the causes of pain
Explain the reason for and intended effect of the therapy

Medical Treatments Performed by Nurses
Give the prescribed drugs (analgesics)

EVALUATION

See the evaluation criteria for each specific goal in Chapter 2.

Gastrointestinal Spasms (247,271,453)

ASSESSMENT

Subjective Data
Pain distribution: localized, abdominal
Duration: intermittent
Onset: acute
Intensity: severe
Level: deep
Quality: cramping pain

Objective Data
Hyperperistalsis
Alternate diarrhea and constipation

Related Data
Commonly Related Diseases:
Peptic ulcer
Spastic colon

POSSIBLE ETIOLOGY

Vagus nerve overstimulation. Overwork. Severe stress or excitement.

NURSING DIAGNOSIS

Gastrointestinal spasms: painful, involuntary contraction of the smooth muscles of the gastrointestinal mucosa

PLANNING

Patient Needs	Primary Nurse-Patient Goals
Water-salt balance	To maintain fluid and electrolyte balance
Waste elimination	To maintain regulating mechanisms and functions
Rest, relaxation	To achieve rest, relaxation
Comfort	To achieve comfort
Protection from physical harm	To prevent physical injury
Freedom from pain	To achieve comfort
Increased learning	To achieve awareness of needs

NURSING INTERVENTIONS

Nursing Treatments
Approach unhurriedly
Reassure that the pain will subside
Communicate nurse sensitivity to the person's pain
Apply a heating pad
   OR   } (to the abdomen)
Apply a hot water bottle
   OR
Give warm liquids
Refrain from giving hot liquids
Refrain from giving iced liquids
Massage gently (for the relaxation effect)
Give bland foods
Encourage decreased gas-forming-food intake
Encourage decreased residue-food intake
Balance fluid intake to equal output
Refrain from giving enemas
Discourage oral stimulants
Discourage smoking
Encourage adequate rest
Ask the patient what makes him (or her) comfortable
Discuss possible pain-reducing measures
Provide a pain-relief measure of the patient's choice
Give nonprescription drugs (ExR) (antacids, stool softners)

Nursing Observations
Observe for complaints of pain duration
Observe for complaints of pain radiation
Evaluate pain for intensity and quality
Evaluate the effectiveness of the pain-relief measures

Health Teaching
Explain the causes of pain
Advise not to take enemas and laxatives
Inform that elimination straining should be avoided
Instruct to immediately respond to the elimination reflex
Instruct to increase fluid intake
Recommend thorough food chewing
Advise that highly emotional situations be avoided
Explain the reason for and intended effect of the therapy

Medical Treatments Performed by Nurses
Give the prescribed drugs (antispasmodics)

EVALUATION

See the evaluation criteria for each specific goal in Chapter 2.

Hemorrhoidal Pain (247,271,453)

ASSESSMENT

Subjective Data

Pain distribution: localized; rectal
Duration: intermittent or continuous
Onset: acute
Intensity: mild, moderate, or severe
Level: superficial
Quality: burning pain with itching

Objective Data

Inflamed hemorrhoids
Irritability

Related Data

Commonly Related Conditions:
Pregnancy
Ascites
Diarrhea
Constipation

Commonly Related Diseases:
Portal hypertension

POSSIBLE ETIOLOGY

Increased intravascular pressure on and weakening of the rectal veins. Increased intraabdominal pressure.

NURSING DIAGNOSIS

Hemorrhoidal pain: painful dilated and thrombosed rectal veins

PLANNING

Patient Needs	**Primary Nurse-Patient Goals**
Water-salt balance	To maintain fluid and electrolyte balance
Comfort	To achieve comfort
Protection from physical harm	To prevent physical injury
Freedom from pain	To achieve comfort
Increased learning	To achieve awareness of needs

NURSING INTERVENTIONS

Nursing Treatments

Approach unhurriedly
Reassure that the pain will subside
Communicate nurse sensitivity to the person's pain
Apply a heating pad
   OR   } (to the anal area)
Apply a hot water bottle
   OR

Apply a warm, moist compress
   OR
Soak in a sitz bath
} (to the anal area)

Arrange pillows comfortably (under the buttocks)
Place in the flat position (when hemorrhoids are severely dilated)
Refrain from giving enemas
Refrain from inserting a rectal tube
Refrain from taking rectal temperatures
Refrain from doing a rectal examination
Increase fluid intake to about 2000 cc daily
Encourage decreased residue-food intake
Ask the patient what makes him (or her) comfortable
Discuss possible pain-reducing measures
Provide a pain-relief measure of the patient's choice
Give nonprescription drugs (ExR) (analgesics, stool softner)

Nursing Observations
Observe for complaints of pain duration
Evaluate pain for intensity and quality
Evaluate the effectiveness of the pain-relief measures
Inspect for bleeding

Health Teaching
Explain the causes of pain
Describe those symptoms which should be reported (bleeding)
Advise not to stand for prolonged periods
Inform that coughing should be avoided
Inform that elimination straining should be avoided
Teach how to take a sitz bath
Explain the reason for and intended effect of the therapy

Medical Treatments Performed by Nurses
Give the prescribed drugs (analgesics)

EVALUATION

See the evaluation criteria for each specific goal in Chapter 2.

Oral Tenderness

ASSESSMENT

Subjective Data
Pain distribution: localized; mouth
Duration: intermittent or continuous
Onset: acute or gradual
Intensity: mild, moderate, or severe
Level: superficial
Quality: soreness or burning

Objective Data
Swollen oral mucosa, tongue, or gums
Redness

Oral ulceration, sometimes
Oral sutures, sometimes

Related Data

Commonly Related Conditions:
Tongue biting
Dilantin and antibiotic sensitivity

Commonly Related Diseases:
Carcinoma
Syphilis
Leukoplakia
First, second or third degree burn
Glossitis
Pellegra
Anemia
Scurvy
Leukemia
Collagen disease
Chronic glomerulonephritis
Scarlet fever
Lichen planus
Herpes simplex

POSSIBLE ETIOLOGY

Chronic tissue irritation. Malignant cells. Surgical procedures performed on the mouth. Chemical, thermal, or mechanical trauma. Radiation cell degeneration from radium treatments. Injury to local nerves. Drug effects.

NURSING DIAGNOSIS

Oral tenderness: soreness and pain of the oral cavity

PLANNING

Patient Needs	**Primary Nurse-Patient Goals**
Comfort	To achieve comfort
Protection from physical harm	To prevent physical injury
Freedom from pain	To achieve comfort
Increased learning	To achieve awareness of needs

NURSING INTERVENTIONS

Nursing Treatments
Approach unhurriedly
Reassure that the pain will subside
Communicate nurse sensitivity to the person's pain
Give bland foods
    OR
Give full-liquid foods
    OR
Give mechanically soft foods
    OR

Give pureed foods
OR
Give soft foods
Encourage decreased acid-food intake
Give small, frequent feedings
Refrain from giving hot liquids
Refrain from giving iced liquids
Brush the teeth with a soft toothbrush
Ask the patient what makes him (or her) comfortable
Discuss possible pain-reducing measures
Provide a pain-relief measure of the patient's choice
Give nonprescription drugs (ExR) (analgesics)

Nursing Observations
Observe for complaints of pain duration
Evaluate pain for intensity and quality
Evaluate the effectiveness of the pain-relief measures

Health Teaching
Explain the causes of pain
Advise not to partake of very hot or cold foods and drinks
Explain the reason for and intended effect of the therapy

Medical Treatments Performed by Nurses
Give the prescribed drugs (analgesics)

EVALUATION

See the evaluation criteria for each specific goal in Chapter 2.

Parotid-Gland Pain (247,453)

ASSESSMENT

Subjective Data
Pain distribution: localized; under both ears or under the chin when chew-
ing
Duration: continuous
Onset: acute
Intensity: severe
Level: deep
Quality: tenderness; aching pain

Objective Data
Swelling around the jaw

Related Data
Increased when eating acid foods
Commonly Related Diseases:
Mumps

POSSIBLE ETIOLOGY

An irritation reaction of the parotid gland tissue to a filterable virus

NURSING DIAGNOSIS

Parotid-gland pain: painful swelling of the parotid gland

PLANNING

Patient Needs

Comfort

Protection from physical harm

Freedom from pain

Increased learning

Primary Nurse-Patient Goals

To achieve comfort

To prevent physical injury

To achieve comfort

To achieve awareness of needs

NURSING INTERVENTIONS

Nursing Treatments

Approach unhurriedly

Reassure that the pain will subside

Communicate nurse sensitivity to the person's pain

Apply an ice bag

    OR   } (to the side of the face)

Apply an ice collar

Give bland foods

Encourage decreased acid-food intake

Ask the patient what makes him (or her) comfortable

Provide a pain-relief measure of the patient's choice

Give nonprescription drugs (ExR) (analgesics)

Nursing Observations

Observe for complaints of pain duration

Observe for complaints of pain radiation

Evaluate pain for intensity and quality

Evaluate the effectiveness of the pain-relief measures

Health Teaching

Explain the causes of pain

Explain the reason for and intended effect of the therapy

Medical Treatments Performed by Nurses

Give the prescribed drugs (analgesics)

EVALUATION

See the evaluation criteria for each specific goal in Chapter 2.

Peritoneal Irritation Pain (247,271,453)

ASSESSMENT

Subjective Data

Pain distribution: localized; abdominal

Duration: continuous

Onset: gradual or acute

Intensity: severe

Level: deep

Quality: fiery pain; accentuated by pressure, movement, coughing, or sneezing

Objective Data
Tendency to lie still

Related Data

Commonly Related Conditions:
Peritonitis

Commonly Related Diseases:
Appendicitis
Diverticulitis
Perforated duodenal ulcer
Regional enteritis
Pancreatitis
Ruptured bladder

POSSIBLE ETIOLOGY

Inflammation of organs within the peritoneal cavity. Irritation of the lining of the abdomen.

NURSING DIAGNOSIS

Peritoneal irritation pain: severe, burning abdominal pain

PLANNING

Patient Needs	**Primary Nurse-Patient Goals**
Rest, relaxation	To achieve rest, relaxation
Comfort	To achieve comfort
Protection from physical harm	To prevent physical injury
Freedom from pain	To achieve comfort
Increased learning	To achieve awareness of needs

NURSING INTERVENTIONS

Nursing Treatments
Approach unhurriedly
Reassure that the pain will subside
Communicate nurse sensitivity to the person's pain
Handle gently (avoiding all pressure on the painful area)
Position comfortably (off the painful area)
Change the patient's position gradually
Massage gently (the lumbar area)
Place on complete bed rest
Remove constrictive clothing
Refrain from jarring the bed
Provide quiet
Ask the patient what makes him (or her) comfortable
Discuss possible pain-reducing measures
Provide a pain-relief measure of the patient's choice

Nursing Observations
Observe for complaints of pain duration
Observe for complaints of pain radiation
Evaluate pain for intensity and quality

Evaluate the effectiveness of the pain-relief measures
Monitor the oral temperature
Palpate the pulse for rate, rhythm, and volume
Observe for the sudden absence of severe pain

Health Teaching
Explain the causes of pain
Inform that coughing should be avoided
Explain the reason for and intended effect of the therapy

Medical Treatments Performed by Nurses
Give the prescribed drugs (analgesics)

EVALUATION

See the evaluation criteria for each specific goal in Chapter 2.

Sensitive Teeth (96)

ASSESSMENT

Subjective Data
Pain distribution: generalized; in all the teeth, not in a single tooth
Duration: intermittent
Onset: acute; stimulated by hot or cold foods and the pressure of hard foods
Intensity: moderate or severe
Level: deep
Quality: burning, sharp pain

Objective Data
Patient avoids eating hot, cold, or hard foods

Related Data
Commonly Related Diseases:
None

POSSIBLE ETIOLOGY

Loss of enamel on the crown of the tooth, which can be caused by faulty brushing or abrasion. When gums recede below the neck of the tooth, the gums no longer protect the tooth. When nerves in the pulp of the tooth become exposed because of loss of the protective covering, pain is easily stimulated.

NURSING DIAGNOSIS

Sensitive teeth: teeth which hurt when exposed to cold, heat, sour, sweetness, or pressure

PLANNING

Patient Needs	Primary Nurse-Patient Goals
Comfort	To achieve comfort
Protection from physical harm	To prevent physical injury
Freedom from pain	To achieve comfort
Increased learning	To achieve awareness of needs

NURSING INTERVENTIONS

Nursing Treatments
Approach unhurriedly
Reassure that the pain will subside
Communicate nurse sensitivity to the person's pain
Give bland foods
Give soft foods
Refrain from giving carbonated beverages
Refrain from giving hot liquids
Refrain from giving iced liquids
Brush the teeth with a soft toothbrush
Discuss possible pain-reducing measures
Give nonprescription drugs (ExR) (analgesics, strontium chloride tooth-
    paste)
Make a referral (to a dentist if the pain persists)

Nursing Observations
Observe for complaints of pain duration
Observe for complaints of pain radiation
Evaluate pain for intensity and quality
Evaluate the effectiveness of the pain-relief measures

Health Teaching
Explain the causes of pain
Advise against eating sweets
Advise not to partake of very hot or cold foods and drinks
Instruct to use a soft, new toothbrush and to apply only mild toothbrush
    pressure
Explain the reason for and intended effect of the therapy

EVALUATION

See the evaluation criteria for each specific goal in Chapter 2.

Stomachache

ASSESSMENT

Subjective Data
Pain distribution: localized; abdominal
Duration: continuous, but of short duration
Onset: acute
Intensity: mild or moderate
Level: deep
Quality: aching pain

Objective Data
No vomiting
No fever
Slight abdominal distention

Related Data

Commonly Related Diseases:
None
OR
Gastritis

POSSIBLE ETIOLOGY

Overeating. Eating incompatible food combinations. Rapid eating.

NURSING DIAGNOSIS

Stomachache: distressful hurting in the stomach

PLANNING

Patient Needs	**Primary Nurse-Patient Goals**
Comfort	To achieve comfort
Protection from physical harm	To prevent physical injury
Freedom from pain	To achieve comfort
Increased learning	To achieve awareness of needs

NURSING INTERVENTIONS

Nursing Treatments
Approach unhurriedly
Reassure that the pain will subside
Communicate nurse sensitivity to the person's pain
Give bland foods
OR
Give full-liquid foods
Give warm liquids
Refrain from giving iced liquids
Give carbonated beverages
Ask the patient what makes him (or her) comfortable
Discuss possible pain-reducing measures
Provide a pain-relief measure of the patient's choice
Give nonprescription drugs (ExR) (bismuth preparations)

Nursing Observations
Observe for complaints of pain duration
Evaluate pain for intensity and quality
Evaluate the effectiveness of the pain-relief measures
Inspect the abdomen for distention (severe)
Monitor the oral temperature (for fever)
Observe for complaints of pain (increased)
Observe for complaints of nausea
Observe for vomiting
Observe for diarrhea

Health Teaching
Explain the causes of pain
Describe those symptoms which should be reported (increased pain, vomiting, diarrhea)

Recommend eating and drinking in moderation
Recommend thorough food chewing
Explain the reason for and intended effect of the therapy

Medical Treatments Performed by Nurses
Give the prescribed drugs

EVALUATION

See the evaluation criteria for each specific goal in Chapter 2.

Teething Pain (96)

ASSESSMENT

Subjective Data
Pain distribution: localized; in areas of specific erupting tooth
Duration: continuous
Onset: gradual
Intensity: mild, moderate, or severe
Level: deep
Quality: tenderness

Objective Data
Drooling
Irritability
Crying
Anorexia
Appearance of teeth between age 6–9 months

Related Data
Commonly Related Diseases:
None

POSSIBLE ETIOLOGY

Normal teeth development

NURSING DIAGNOSIS

Teething pain: pain occurring in the area in which teeth break through the gums

PLANNING

Patient Needs	**Primary Nurse-Patient Goals**
Sleep, rest	To achieve sleep, rest
Comfort	To achieve comfort
Protection from physical harm	To prevent physical injury
Freedom from pain	To achieve comfort
Increased learning	To achieve awareness of needs

NURSING INTERVENTIONS

Nursing Treatments
Approach unhurriedly
Reassure (the mother) that pain will subside (when the teeth are through)

Communicate nurse sensitivity to the person's pain
Massage the infant's gums
Give soft foods
Encourage adequate rest (to reduce irritability)
Give nonprescription drugs (ExR) (mild analgesics)

Nursing Observations
Observe for complaints of pain duration
Evaluate pain for intensity and quality
Evaluate the effectiveness of the pain-relief measures
Inspect the gums for abnormalities
Inspect the teeth for abnormalities

Health Teaching
Explain the causes of pain
Explain the reason for and intended effect of the therapy

EVALUATION

See the evaluation criteria for each specific goal in Chapter 2.

Throat Soreness

ASSESSMENT

Subjective Data
Pain distribution: localized; throat
Duration: continuous
Onset: acute
Intensity: mild, moderate, or severe; increased with swallowing
Level: deep
Quality: burning, stinging pain

Objective Data
Throat redness
Swelling
Fever, sometimes
Lymph node enlargement, sometimes
Throat exudate, sometimes

Related Data

Commonly Related Conditions:
Common cold

Commonly Related Diseases:
Streptococcal pharyngitis
Infectious mononucleosis
Typhoid fever
Vincent's angina
Diptheria
Measles
Tonsillitis
Scarlet fever
Rocky Mountain spotted fever

Hookworm disease
Poliomyelitis
Encephalitis
Dengue
Thyrotoxicosis

POSSIBLE ETIOLOGY

Infectious microorganisms

NURSING DIAGNOSIS

Throat soreness: a distressful hurting of the throat

PLANNING

Patient Needs	Primary Nurse-Patient Goals
Rest	To achieve rest
Comfort	To achieve comfort
Protection from physical harm	To prevent physical injury
Freedom from pain	To achieve comfort
Increased learning	To achieve awareness of needs

NURSING INTERVENTIONS

Nursing Treatments
Approach unhurriedly
Reassure that the pain will subside
Communicate nurse sensitivity to the person's pain
Apply an ice bag (to the throat)
    OR
Moisten the mouth with cracked ice
Give full-liquid foods
    OR
Give soft foods
    OR
Give bland foods
Feed slowly
Give small, frequent feedings
Refrain from giving hot liquids
Encourage adequate rest
Ask the patient what makes him (or her) comfortable
Provide a pain-relief measure of the patient's choice
Give coughdrops
Give nonprescription drugs (ExR) (analgesics)

Nursing Observations
Observe for complaints of pain duration
Evaluate pain for intensity and quality
Evaluate the effectiveness of the pain-relief measures
Inspect (the throat) for inflammation
Monitor the oral temperature
Obtain a bacterial culture (of the throat)

Health Teaching
Recommend throat gargling (with warm saline solution)
Describe those symptoms which should be reported (severe difficulty swallowing)
Explain the causes of pain
Explain the reason for and intended effect of the therapy

Medical Treatments Performed by Nurses
Give the prescribed drugs

EVALUATION

See the evaluation criteria for each specific goal in Chapter 2.

Toothache (96)

ASSESSMENT

Subjective Data
Pain distribution: localized; in areas surrounding the tooth
Duration: continuous
Onset: acute
Intensity: severe
Level: deep
Quality: throbbing pain

Objective Data
Restlessness
Inability to sleep
Jaw holding
Jaw swelling, sometimes

Related Data
Commonly Related Diseases:
None

POSSIBLE ETIOLOGY

Bacterial invasion and decay. Dental pulp and surrounding tissue inflammation.

NURSING DIAGNOSIS

Toothache: pain in the tooth and surrounding area

PLANNING

Patient Needs	Primary Nurse-Patient Goals
Rest	To achieve rest
Comfort	To achieve comfort
Protection from physical harm	To prevent physical injury
Freedom from pain	To achieve comfort
Increased learning	To achieve awareness of needs

NURSING INTERVENTIONS

Nursing Treatments
Approach unhurriedly
Reassure that the pain will subside
Communicate nurse sensitivity to the person's pain
Apply an ice bag (to the cheek)
Give full-liquid foods
    OR
Give soft foods
Refrain from giving hot liquids
Refrain from giving iced liquids
Encourage adequate rest
Ask the patient what makes him (or her) comfortable
Discuss possible pain-reducing measures
Provide a pain-relief measure of the patient's choice
Give nonprescription drugs (ExR) (analgesics)
Make a referral (to a dentist)

Nursing Observations
Observe for complaints of pain duration
Estimate the degree of pain experienced
Evaluate the effectiveness of the pain-relief measures

Health Teaching
Explain the causes of pain
Advise frequent and early dental attention
Advise not to partake of very hot or cold foods and drinks
Instruct to use a soft, new toothbrush and to apply only mild toothbrush
    pressure
Encourage the use of a warm, saline gargle
Explain the reason for and intended effect of the therapy

Medical Treatments Performed by Nurses
Give the prescribed drugs (analgesics)

EVALUATION

See the evaluation criteria for each specific goal in Chapter 2.

SPECIFIC REPRODUCTIVE-ORGAN PAIN

After-Birth Pain (53,112,271)

ASSESSMENT

Subjective Data
Pain distribution: localized; abdominal
Duration: intermittent; sometimes occurs only during breast feeding
Onset: acute

Intensity: severe
Level: deep
Quality: cramping pain

Objective Data
Restlessness

Related Data
Women who have had twin or multiple births are most prone to after-birth
   pain

Commonly Related Diseases:
None

POSSIBLE ETIOLOGY

Uterine retraction and contraction resulting from lochia discharge and
gradual return of the uterus to normal size. Breast feeding stimulation.

NURSING DIAGNOSIS

After-birth pain: uterine pain following delivery

PLANNING

Patient Needs	**Primary Nurse-Patient Goals**
Rest, relaxation	To achieve rest, relaxation
Comfort	To achieve comfort
Protection from physical harm	To prevent physical injury
Freedom from pain	To achieve comfort
Increased learning	To achieve awareness of needs

NURSING INTERVENTIONS

Nursing Treatments
Approach unhurriedly
Reassure that the pain will subside
Communicate nurse sensitivity to the person's pain
Handle gently
Position comfortably
Change the patient's position gradually
Apply a heating pad
   OR   } (to the abdomen)
Apply a hot water bottle
   OR
Soak in a sitz bath (warm)
Give warm liquids
Refrain from giving iced liquids
Massage gently (the lumbar area)
Refrain from giving enemas
Refrain from jarring the bed
Provide quiet

Encourage adequate rest
Refrain from performing nonessential procedures
Ask the patient what makes her comfortable
Discuss possible pain-reducing measures
Provide a pain-relief measure of the patient's choice
Give nonprescription drugs (ExR) (analgesics)

Nursing Observations
Observe for complaints of pain duration
Observe for complaints of pain radiation
Evaluate pain for intensity and quality
Evaluate the effectiveness of the pain-relief measures

Health Teaching
Explain the causes of pain
Inform that after-birth pains following delivery are normal
Teach how to apply heat therapy
Explain the reason for and intended effect of the therapy

Medical Treatments Performed by Nurses
Give the prescribed drugs (analgesics, antispasmodics)

EVALUATION
See the evaluation criteria for each specific goal in Chapter 2.

Breast Engorgement (53,112,253)

ASSESSMENT
Subjective Data
Pain distribution: localized, breast
Duration: continuous
Onset: gradual
Intensity: moderate or severe
Level: deep
Quality: severe tenderness, breast heaviness

Objective Data
Breast distention
Breast hardness
Fever
Irritability

Related Data
Commonly Related Diseases:
None

POSSIBLE ETIOLOGY
Obstruction of mammary gland ducts. Lymphatic and venous congestion.

NURSING DIAGNOSIS
Breast engorgement: painful fluid congestion in the breast

PLANNING

Patient Needs	Primary Nurse-Patient Goals
Rest	To achieve rest
Comfort	To achieve comfort
Protection from physical harm	To prevent physical injury
Freedom from pain	To achieve comfort
Increased learning	To achieve awareness of needs

NURSING INTERVENTIONS

Nursing Treatments
Approach unhurriedly
Reassure that the pain will subside
Communicate nurse sensitivity to the person's pain
Handle gently
Position comfortably
Elevate the head
Apply a brassiere
    OR
Apply a breast binder
Apply an ice bag
Apply hot packs to the breast before breast feeding
Express breast milk manually
Express breast milk mechanically
Provide quiet
Encourage adequate rest
Ask the patient what makes her comfortable
Discuss possible pain-reducing measures
Provide a pain-relief measure of the patient's choice
Give nonprescription drugs (ExR) (analgesics)

Nursing Observations
Observe for complaints of pain duration
Evaluate pain for intensity and quality
Evaluate the effectiveness of the pain-relief measures

Health Teaching
Explain the causes of pain
Teach how to apply a breast binder
    OR
Recommend the use of a brassiere for breast support
Instruct not to massage the breast
Teach how to apply cold therapy
Teach how to apply heat therapy
Explain the reason for and intended effect of the therapy

Medical Treatments Performed by Nurses
Give the prescribed drugs (diethylstilbestrol, atropine)

EVALUATION

See the evaluation criteria for each specific goal in Chapter 2.

Breast Tenderness (54,112,253)

ASSESSMENT

Subjective Data
Pain distribution: localized in the breast
Duration: continuous
Onset: gradual
Intensity: mild or moderate
Level: deep
Quality: soreness

Related Data
When it occurs prior to menstruation, it is most frequent in women who
  have borne children

Commonly Related Conditions:
Menstruation
Pregnancy

Commonly Related Diseases:
Chronic cystic mastitis
Fibrocystic disease

POSSIBLE ETIOLOGY

Increased hormone activity 7–10 days prior to menstruation, causes fluid
accumulation in breast tissue. Abnormal tissue fluid causing pressure
against breast nerve fibers.

NURSING DIAGNOSIS

Breast tenderness: cutaneous sensitivity of the breast

PLANNING

Patient Needs	**Primary Nurse-Patient Goals**
Comfort	To achieve comfort
Protection from physical harm	To prevent physical injury
Freedom from pain	To achieve comfort
Increased learning	To achieve awareness of needs

NURSING INTERVENTIONS

Nursing Treatments
Approach unhurriedly
Reassure that the pain will subside
Communicate nurse sensitivity to the person's pain
Handle gently
Position comfortably (off the tender area)
Apply a brassiere
  OR   } (to the breast)
Apply an ice bag
Remove constrictive clothing
Encourage decreased sodium-food intake (7–10 days prior to menstruation
  onset)

Restrict the fluid intake according to weight gain
Ask the patient what makes her comfortable
Discuss possible pain-reducing measures
Provide a pain-relief measure of the patient's choice
Give nonprescription drugs (ExR) (analgesics)

Nursing Observations
Observe for complaints of pain duration
Evaluate pain for intensity and quality
Evaluate the effectiveness of the pain-relief measures

Health Teaching
Explain the causes of pain
Teach how to apply cold therapy
Explain the reason for and intended effect of the therapy

Medical Treatments Performed by Nurses
Give the prescribed drugs (testosterone, 7–10 days prior to menstruation onset)

EVALUATION

See the evaluation criteria for each specific goal in Chapter 2.

Cracked-Nipple Pain (54,112,253)

ASSESSMENT

Subjective Data
Pain disribution: localized, breast nipple
Duration: continuous
Onset: gradual or acute
Intensity: mild, moderate, or severe
Level: superficial
Quality: soreness

Objective Data
Nipple cracking

Related Data
Commonly Related Diseases:
Mastitis

POSSIBLE ETIOLOGY

Infant sucking pressure. Irritation.

NURSING DIAGNOSIS

Cracked-nipple pain: a painful cracking or splitting of the breast nipple

PLANNING

Patient Needs	**Primary Nurse-Patient Goals**
Comfort	To achieve comfort
Protection from physical harm	To prevent physical injury, infection

Freedom from pain

Increased learning

To achieve comfort

To achieve awareness of needs

NURSING INTERVENTIONS

Nursing Treatments

Approach unhurriedly

Reassure that the pain will subside

Communicate nurse sensitivity to the person's pain

Handle gently

Position comfortably

Apply a warm, moist compress

Remove constrictive clothing

Lubricate the skin with cocoa butter, glycerine, lanolin, mineral oil, or olive
  oil

Apply an antibiotic ointment

Place a shield over the breast nipple

Caution about breast feeding

Ask the patient what makes her comfortable

Discuss possible pain-reducing measures

Provide a pain-relief measure of the patient's choice

Give nonprescription drugs (ExR) (analgesics)

Nursing Observations

Observe for complaints of pain duration

Evaluate pain for intensity and quality

Evaluate the effectiveness of the pain-relief measures

Inspect for bleeding

Health Teaching

Explain the causes of pain

Describe those symptoms which should be reported (bleeding)

Explain the reason for and intended effect of the therapy

Medical Treatments Performed by Nurses

Give the prescribed drugs (analgesics)

EVALUATION

See the evaluation criteria for each specific goal in Chapter 2.

False Labor Pain (54,112,253)

ASSESSMENT

Subjective Data

Pain distribution: localized; abdominal; does not radiate from the back to
  the front

Duration: intermittent and short; the frequency of pains does not increase;
  walking may cause cessation of pain

Onset: acute

Intensity: mild; fails to become progressively stronger

Level: deep

Quality: cramping pain

Objective Data
Restlessness

Related Data
Commonly Related Diseases:
None

POSSIBLE ETIOLOGY

Fetal activity. Intestinal flatulence.

NURSING DIAGNOSIS

False labor pain: pains that at first appear to be labor pains but are not

PLANNING

Patient Needs	**Primary Nurse-Patient Goals**
Comfort	To achieve comfort
Protection from physical harm	To prevent physical injury
Freedom from pain	To achieve comfort
Increased learning	To achieve awareness of needs

NURSING INTERVENTIONS

Nursing Treatments
Approach unhurriedly
Reassure that the pain will subside
Communicate nurse sensitivity to the person's pain
Ambulate the patient
Give warm liquids
Refrain from giving iced liquids
Massage gently (the lumbar area)
Remove constrictive clothing
Ask the patient what makes her comfortable
Discuss possible pain-reducing measures
Provide a pain-relief measure of the patient's choice
Give nonprescription drugs (ExR) (analgesics)

Nursing Observations
Observe for complaints of pain duration
Observe for complaints of pain radiation
Evaluate pain for intensity and quality
Evaluate the effectiveness of the pain-relief measures

Health Teaching
Explain the causes of pain
Describe those symptoms which should be reported (true labor pains)
Explain the difference between true and false labor pains
Explain the reason for and intended effect of the therapy

EVALUATION

See the evaluation criteria for each specific goal in Chapter 2.

Labor Pain (53,112,253)

ASSESSMENT

Subjective Data

Pain distribution: localized, primarily in the center of the back during the first stage of labor; generalized, in the anterior abdomen during the second stage of labor

Duration: intermittent, every 10–15 minutes apart during the first stage of labor; continuous, every 2–3 minutes, lasting 50–100 seconds during the second stage of labor, finally becoming constant

Onset: acute

Intensity: mild during the first stage of labor, gradually becoming more severe; during the second stage of labor and full cervical dilatation, the pains are very severe and frequently excruciating

Level: deep

Quality: cramping pains during the first stage of labor; constrictive, girdlelike pain in the second stage

Objective Data

Restlessness

Related Data

Commonly Related Conditions:
Termination of pregnancy

Commonly Related Diseases:
None

POSSIBLE ETIOLOGY

Uterine contractions and cervical dilatation that occurs in an effort to expel the infant from the uterus

NURSING DIAGNOSIS

Labor pain: maternal, distressful hurting that occurs during the process of delivery of a child

PLANNING

Patient Needs	Primary Nurse-Patient Goals
Rest, relaxation	To achieve rest, relaxation
Comfort	To achieve comfort
Protection from physical harm	To prevent physical injury
Freedom from pain	To achieve comfort
Increased learning	To achieve awareness of needs

NURSING INTERVENTIONS

Nursing Treatments

Approach unhurriedly
Reassure that the pain will subside
Communicate nurse sensitivity to the person's pain

Attend the patient constantly
Demonstrate calmness
Provide an atmosphere of acceptance
Handle gently
Position comfortably
Change the patient's position gradually
Ambulate the patient
Apply a heating pad
   OR   } (to the abdomen)
Apply a hot water bottle
Encourage deep breathing
Remove constrictive clothing
Give warm liquids
Refrain from giving iced liquids
Refrain from jarring the bed
Provide quiet
Encourage adequate rest
Ask the patient what makes her comfortable
Discuss possible pain-reducing measures
Provide a pain-relief measure of the patient's choice
Give nonprescription drugs (ExR) (analgesics)
Massage gently (lumbar area)

Nursing Observations
Observe for complaints of pain duration
Observe for complaints of pain radiation
Estimate the degree of pain experienced
Evaluate the effectiveness of the pain-relief measures

Health Teaching
Describe those symptoms which should be reported
Explain that it is acceptable to admit the existence of pain
Explain the causes of pain

Medical Treatments Performed by Nurses
Give the prescribed drugs (analgesics)

EVALUATION
See the evaluation criteria for each specific goal in Chapter 2.

Menstrual Pain (247,271)
ASSESSMENT
Subjective Data
Pain distribution: localized and/or referred; abdominal, suprapubic, back pain; sometimes radiates into the thighs
Duration: intermittent or continuous; lasts from one to several days
Onset: acute; usually occurs before or at the onset of menstruation
Intensity: mild, moderate, or severe
Level: deep
Quality: cramping, associated primarily with flow; dull, heavy backache

Objective Data
Irritability
Vomiting, sometimes

Related Data
Commonly Related Diseases:
Endometriosis
Uterine retroversion
Uterine fibroid
Tuberculosis
Syphilis
Anemia

POSSIBLE ETIOLOGY

Imbalanced estrogen-progesterone levels. Incomplete disintegration of abnormally thick endometrium resulting from corpus luteum overactivity. Exceptionally long cervix. Uterine underdevelopment. Uterine malposition. Poor posture. Nerve ending sensitivity in the uterine isthmus resulting in uncoordinate, highly irritable uterine contractions. Vasoconstriction causing myometrium ischemia. Vagus nerve hyperexcitability because of hypersensitive autonomic nerves supplying the uterus. Blood leaving the uterus in spasmodic spurts as the uterus contracts irregularly every 1–15 minutes. Failure of the liver to destroy excessive hormone production by an overactive ovarian follicle. Decreased blood calcium level that supports muscle spasm.

NURSING DIAGNOSIS

Menstrual pain: sharp, colicky pain associated with menstruation

PLANNING

Patient Needs	Primary Nurse-Patient Goals
Rest, relaxation	To achieve rest, relaxation
Exercise	To achieve exercise
Comfort	To achieve comfort
Protection from physical harm	To prevent physical injury
Freedom from pain	To achieve comfort
Increased learning	To achieve awareness of needs

NURSING INTERVENTIONS

Nursing Treatmens
Approach unhurriedly
Reassure that the pain will subside
Communicate nurse sensitivity to the person's pain
Position comfortably
Place in the knee-chest position
Apply a heating pad ⎫
   OR   ⎬ (to the abdomen)
Apply a hot water bottle ⎭

Administer a hot foot bath
Give warm liquids
Refrain from giving iced liquids
Massage gently (the lumbar area)
Encourage increased calcium-food intake (one week prior to menstruation
    onset)
Encourage increased protein-food intake (daily)
Encourage adequate rest
Encourage moderate physical exercise
Ask the patient what makes her comfortable
Discuss possible pain-reducing measures
Provide a pain-relief measure of the patient's choice
Give nonprescription drugs (ExR) (analgesics)

Nursing Observations
Observe for complaints of pain duration
Observe for complaints of pain radiation
Evaluate pain for intensity and quality
Evaluate the effectiveness of the pain-relief measures

Health Teaching
Explain the causes of pain
Advise not to stand for prolonged periods
Teach how to apply heat therapy
Explain the reason for and intended effect of the therapy

Medical Treatments Performed by Nurses
Give the prescribed drugs (analgesics, hormones, antispasmodics)

EVALUATION

See the evaluation criteria for each specific goal in Chapter 2.

Ovulation Pain (247)

ASSESSMENT

Subjective Data
Pain distribution: localized; lower abdomen, on either or both sides; some-
    times appears on alternate sides each month
Duration: intermittent; lasts about 24 hours
Onset: gradual; about 14 days prior to menstruation onset
Intensity: mild or moderate
Level: deep
Quality: cramping pain; residual lower abdominal soreness for 24–48 hours

Objective Data
Vomiting
May have a palpable enlarged, tender ovary
Clear vaginal discharge

Related Data
Commonly Related Diseases:
None

POSSIBLE ETIOLOGY

Graafian follicle rupture and blood oozing from the ovulation site into the peritoneal cavity. When the egg escapes from the ovary during ovulation, the fluid in the sack surrounding the egg is discharged and temporarily irritates the sensitive inside lining of the pelvic cavity, causing a mild peritonitis.

NURSING DIAGNOSIS

Ovulation pain: pain associated with the rupture of the graafian follicle and the discharge of the ovum from the ovary

PLANNING

Patient Needs	Primary Nurse-Patient Goals
Rest	To achieve rest
Comfort	To achieve comfort
Protection from physical harm	To prevent physical injury
Freedom from pain	To achieve comfort
Increased learning	To achieve awareness of needs

NURSING INTERVENTIONS

Nursing Treatments
Approach unhurriedly
Reassure that the pain will subside
Communicate nurse sensitivity to the person's pain
Position comfortably
Apply a hot water bottle
   OR
Soak in a sitz bath (warm)
Give warm liquids
Refrain from giving iced liquids (if cramping)
Encourage adequate rest
Ask the patient what makes her comfortable
Discuss possible pain-reducing measures
Provide a pain-relief measure of the patient's choice
Give nonprescription drugs (ExR) (analgesics)

Nursing Observations
Observe for complaints of pain duration
Evaluate pain for intensity and quality
Evaluate the effectiveness of the pain-relief measures

Health Teaching
Explain the causes of pain
Teach how to apply heat therapy
Teach how to take a sitz bath
Explain the reason for and intended effect of the therapy

EVALUATION

See the evaluation criteria for each specific goal in Chapter 2.

Pelvic Heaviness

ASSESSMENT

Subjective Data

Pain distribution: localized; lower abdomen
Duration: intermittent or continuous
Onset: gradual; often follows prolonged standing
Intensity: mild or moderate
Level: deep
Quality: weighted sensation; feeling that one's insides are about to fall out

Objective Data

Urinary incontinence with sneezing or coughing, sometimes

Related Data

Most fequent in women who have had large babies, numerous pregnancies, or difficult labor

Commonly Related Conditions:
Aging
Menstruation

Commonly Related Diseases:
Bladder prolapse (cystocele)
Uterine prolapse
Ovarian cyst

POSSIBLE ETIOLOGY

Weakened musculature of the bladder and/or uterus as a result of traumatic childbirth. Pelvic fluid congestion prior to menstruation onset.

NURSING DIAGNOSIS

Pelvic heaviness: a feeling of congestion or weighted discomfort in the lower abdomen

PLANNING

Patient Needs	**Primary Nurse-Patient Goals**
Comfort	To achieve comfort
Protection from physical harm	To prevent physical injury
Freedom from pain	To achieve comfort
Increased learning	To achieve awareness of needs

NURSING INTERVENTIONS

Nursing Treatments

Approach unhurriedly
Reassure that the pain will subside
Communicate nurse sensitivity to the person's pain
Apply an abdominal support garment
Place in the foot-elevated head-lowered (Trendelenburg) position
Place in the knee-chest position

Apply a heating pad ⎱
    OR   ⎰ (to the abdomen)
Apply a hot water bottle ⎰
    OR
Soak in a sitz bath (warm)
Give warm liquids
Remove constrictive clothing
Ask the patient what makes her comfortable
Discuss possible pain-reducing measures
Provide a pain-relief measure of the patient's choice
Give nonprescription drugs (ExR) (analgesics)

Nursing Observations
Observe for complaints of pain duration
Evaluate the effectiveness of the pain-relief measures

Health Teaching
Explain the causes of pain
Advise not to stand for prolonged periods
Recommend the use of an abdominal-support garment
Recommend the use of low-heeled shoes
Teach how to apply heat therapy
Teach how to take a sitz bath
Explain the reason for and intended effect of the therapy

Medical Treatments Performed by Nurses
Give the prescribed drugs (analgesics)

EVALUATION

See the evaluation criteria for each specific goal in Chapter 2.

Pendulous Breast Discomfort

ASSESSMENT

Subjective Data
Pain distribution: localized; breast
Duration: continuous
Onset: gradual
Intensity: mild or moderate
Level: deep
Quality: heavily weighted sensation; pulling at the shoulders

Objective Data
Breast enlargement
Coarse, thick breast skin, sometimes
Brassiere straps cut into the shoulders

Related Data
Commonly Related Conditions:
Pregnancy

Commonly Related Diseases:
Females:
Hypothalamus lesion
Primary hyperaldosteronism
Single follicle ovarian cysts
Polycystic ovaries
Granulosa-theca cell ovarian tumor
Males:
Laennec's cirrhosis
Testicle teratomas
Testicle choriocarcinomas

POSSIBLE ETIOLOGY

Increased size and number of breast tissue cells

NURSING DIAGNOSIS

Pendulous breast discomfort: a discomforting heaviness associated with excessive enlargement of one or both breasts

PLANNING

Patient Needs	Primary Nurse-Patient Goals
Comfort	To achieve comfort
Protection from physical harm	To prevent physical injury
Freedom from pain	To achieve comfort
Increased learning	To achieve awareness of needs

NURSING INTERVENTIONS

Nursing Treatments
Approach unhurriedly
Reassure that the pain will subside
Communicate nurse sensitivity to the person's pain
Apply a brassiere (for females)
Apply an elastic bandage (for males)
Position comfortably

Nursing Observations
Evaluate the effectiveness of the pain-relief measures

Health Teaching
Recommend the use of a brassiere for breast support
Explain how to apply an elastic bandage
Explain the reason for and intended effect of the therapy

EVALUATION

See the evaluation criteria for each specific goal in Chapter 2.

Postpartal Perineal Pain (54,112,253)

ASSESSMENT

Subjective Data
Pain distribution: localized; perineum

Duration: continuous
Onset: acute, following delivery
Intensity: mild or moderate; increased when sitting
Level: superficial
Quality: burning, itching pain

Objective Data
Perineal sutures
Perineal suture marks

Related Data
Commonly Related Conditions:
Termination of pregnancy
Commonly Related Diseases:
None

POSSIBLE ETIOLOGY

Stretching of the birth canal and perineal structures. Swelling from an episiotomy.

NURSING DIAGNOSIS

Postpartal perineal pain: a painful, discomforting sensation in the perineal area following childbirth

PLANNING

Patient Needs	**Primary Nurse-Patient Goals**
Comfort	To achieve comfort
Protection from physical harm	To prevent physical injury
Freedom from pain	To achieve comfort
Increased learning	To achieve awareness of needs

NURSING INTERVENTIONS

Nursing Treatments
Approach unhurriedly
Reassure that the pain will subside
Communicate nurse sensitivity to the person's pain
Handle gently
Position comfortably
Apply heat by a gooseneck lamp
    OR
Apply a heating pad
    OR   (to the perineum)
Apply a hot water bottle
    OR
Apply a warm, moist compress
    OR
Soak in a sitz bath (warm)
Apply an analgesic ointment
Arrange pillows comfortably (under the buttocks)

Avoid placing tension on the wound
Refrain from jarring the bed
Ask the patient what makes her comfortable
Discuss possible pain-reducing measures
Provide a pain-relief measure of the patient's choice
Give nonprescription drugs (ExR) (analgesics)

Nursing Observations
Observe for complaints of pain duration
Evaluate pain for intensity and quality
Evaluate the effectiveness of the pain-relief measures
Inspect for inflammation

Health Teaching
Explain the causes of pain
Teach how to apply heat therapy
Teach how to take a sitz bath
Explain the reason for and intended effect of the therapy

Medical Treatments Performed by Nurses
Give the prescribed drugs (analgesics)

EVALUATION

See the evaluation criteria for each specific goal in Chapter 2.

SPECIFIC RESPIRATORY PAIN

Painful Respirations (70,391)

ASSESSMENT

Subjective Data
Dyspnea, sometimes
Pain distribution: localized or referred
Duration: intermittent, with each breath
Onset: acute
Intensity: mild, moderate, or severe; increased pain during coughing or laughing
Level: deep
Quality: sharp, stabbing pain

Objective Data
Shallow respirations
Restricted chest movements
Friction rub

Related Data
Commonly Related Conditions:
Chest surgery
Pulmonary embolism
Pleural effusion

Commonly Related Diseases:
Pleurisy
Rib fracture
Tuberculosis
Pulmonary carcinoma
Pneumonia
Empyema
Acute pericarditis

POSSIBLE ETIOLOGY

Rubbing pleural spaces. Tension on an incisional area. Pleura inflammation.

NURSING DIAGNOSIS

Painful respirations (ponopnea): distressful hurting accompanying breathing

PLANNING

Patient Needs	Primary Nurse-Patient Goals
Rest	To achieve rest
Comfort	To achieve comfort
Protection from physical harm	To prevent physical injury
Freedom from pain	To achieve comfort
Increased learning	To achieve awareness of needs

NURSING INTERVENTIONS

Nursing Treatments
Approach unhurriedly
Reassure that the pain will subside
Communicate nurse sensitivity to the person's pain
Handle gently
Position comfortably
Change the patient's position gradually
Apply an elastic bandage (to the chest)
   OR
Place on the affected side
Splint the incisional area
Apply a heating pad
   OR   } (for pleuritic pain)
Apply a hot water bottle
Massage gently (the posterior thorax area)
Maintain a warm room temperature
Refrain from performing nonessential procedures
Ask the patient what makes him (or her) comfortable
Discuss possible pain-reducing measures
Encourage adequate rest
Provide a pain-relief measure of the patient's choice
Give nonprescription drugs (ExR) (analgesics)

Nursing Observations
Observe for complaints of pain duration
Observe for complaints of pain radiation
Evaluate pain for intensity and quality
Auscultate the chest for lung aeration
Evaluate the effectiveness of the pain-relief measures

Health Teaching
Explain the causes of pain
Describe those symptoms which should be reported (increased pain or air hunger)
Explain how to splint an incision
Teach how to apply heat therapy
Explain the reason for and intended effect of the therapy

Medical Treatments Performed by Nurses
Give the prescribed drugs (analgesics)

EVALUATION

See the evaluation criteria for each specific goal in Chapter 2.

PAINFUL CONDITIONS, POTENTIAL

Potential Painful Defecation (70,391)

ASSESSMENT

Subjective Data
Recent painful defecation
Chronic constipation

Objective Data
Hemorrhoid inflammation
Anal stricture
Fecal impaction

Related Data
Commonly Related Diseases:
Rectal carcinoma

POSSIBLE ETIOLOGY

Sensitive areas around the anus where pressure from fecal bulk will cause irritation. Rectal obstruction.

NURSING DIAGNOSIS

Potential painful defecation: the probability that a distressful hurting will occur with bowel elimination

PLANNING

Patient Needs
Comfort

Primary Nurse-Patient Goals
To achieve comfort

Protection from physical harm	To prevent physical injury
Freedom from pain	To achieve comfort
Increased learning	To achieve awareness of needs

NURSING INTERVENTIONS

Nursing Treatments
Encourage decreased residue-food intake
Give bland foods
Increase fluid intake to about 3000 cc daily
Give nonprescription drugs (ExR) (stool softeners)
Administer an (oil) enema (if needed)
Remove the fecal impaction manually (if one exists)

Nursing Observations
Observe for complaints of pain

Health Teaching
Explain the causes of pain
Inform that elimination straining should be avoided
Instruct to increase fluid intake
Explain the reason for and intended effect of the therapy

EVALUATION

See the evaluation criteria for each specific goal in Chapter 2.

Potential Headache (70,391)

ASSESSMENT

Subjective Data
Mild, discomforting head sensations that previously signaled oncoming
· headache

Objective Data
Recent spinal tap or puncture
Increasing blood pressure
Recent blow to the head

Related Data

Commonly Related Conditions:
Drug therapy
Spinal tap
Anesthesia
Severe emotional stress

Commonly Related Diseases:
Gastritis
Hypertension
Cerebral concussion

POSSIBLE ETIOLOGY

Any nonhealth situation where there is increased intracranial pressure,
inflammation, brain tissue irritation, or physiochemical disturbance

NURSING DIAGNOSIS

Potential headache: the likelihood that a headache will occur

PLANNING

Patient Needs	Primary Nurse-Patient Goals
Sleep, rest, relaxation	To achieve sleep, rest, relaxation
Comfort	To achieve comfort
Protection from physical harm	To prevent physical injury
Increased learning	To achieve awareness of needs

NURSING INTERVENTIONS

Nursing Treatments

Encourage adequate rest
Elevate the head
    OR
Place in the flat position (12–24 hours following spinal puncture)
Position comfortably
Change the patient's position gradually
Massage gently (the neck and shoulders)
Provide quiet
Subdue the room lighting
Refrain from jarring the bed
Discourage oral stimulants
Discourage smoking
Give nonprescription drugs (ExR) (analgesics, if the headache is threatening)

Nursing Observations

Observe for complaints of pain

Health Teaching

Explain the causes of pain
Advise not to take hot baths
Advise that highly emotional situations be avoided
Inform that coughing should be avoided
Inform that elimination straining should be avoided
Recommend adherence to a moderate pace of living
Explain the reason for and intended effect of the therapy

EVALUATION

See the evaluation criteria for each specific goal in Chapter 2.

Potential Muscle Spasm (70,391)

ASSESSMENT

Subjective Data

Fears recurring spasms

Objective Data

Tense muscles
Recent muscle spasms

Related Data

Laboratory Findings.
Decreased blood calcium

Commonly Related Diseases:
Thomsen's disease
Spinal cord injury
Hypoparathyroidism
Tetanus
Hypothyroidism
Addison's disease
Cerebral palsy

POSSIBLE ETIOLOGY

Repetitive activation of efferent nerve fibers carrying motor impulses to muscle fibers before relaxation can occur

NURSING DIAGNOSIS

Potential muscle spasm: the probability that muscle spasms will occur

PLANNING

Patient Needs	**Primary Nurse-Patient Goals**
Relaxation	To achieve relaxation
Comfort	To achieve comfort
Protection from physical harm	To prevent accident, physical injury
Freedom from pain	To achieve comfort
Increased learning	To achieve awareness of needs

NURSING INTERVENTIONS

Nursing Treatments
Handle gently
Change the patient's position gradually
Remove constrictive clothing
Apply a bed cradle (to prevent the bed clothes from stimulating spasms)
Drape for warmth
Place only warm hands and objects on the patient
Decrease drafts
Maintain a warm room temperature
Refrain from giving local cold applications
Refrain from jarring the bed
Refrain from performing nonessential procedures
Give high-calcium fluids orally
    AND   } (if the blood calcium is low)
Encourage increased calcium-food intake

Nursing Observations
Observe for complaints of pain

Health Teaching
Explain the causes of pain
Explain the reason for and intended effect of the therapy

EVALUATION

See the evaluation criteria for each specific goal in Chapter 2.

PAIN OF PSYCHIC ORIGIN

Psychogenic Pain (463,548)

ASSESSMENT

Subjective Data
Pain distribution: generalized; involves numerous body regions
Duration: continuous during the day; pain does not disturb sleep at night
Onset: gradual or acute
Intensity: severe; pain is actually experienced
Level: deep or superficial
Quality: described in terms of grief, anguish, emotional conflict, or distress

Objective Data
Crying
Attention seeking
Hysteria, sometimes

Related Data
Commonly Related Diseases:
None
   OR
Anxiety psychoneurosis
Hysteria psychoneurosis
Manic-depressive psychoneurosis

POSSIBLE ETIOLOGY

Mentally experiencing pain as a means of symbolically attempting to solve emotional conflict. Need to focus on some physical distress as a temporary escape from emotional distress. Unconscious association of pain with punishment.

NURSING DIAGNOSIS

Psychogenic pain: a distressful hurting that occurs in the absence of any physical disorder

PLANNING

Patient Needs	Primary Nurse-Patient Goals
Relaxation	To achieve relaxation
Comfort	To achieve comfort
Protection from physical harm	To prevent physical injury
Protection from psychologic threat	To prevent emotional injury
Freedom from pain	To achieve comfort
Personal growth and maturity	To achieve optimum function
Increased learning	To achieve awareness of needs

Increased reality perception and   To achieve optimum function
   problem solving

NURSING INTERVENTIONS

Nursing Treatments
Approach unhurriedly
Reassure that the pain will subside
Communicate nurse sensitivity to the person's pain
Demonstrate calmness
Accept and attempt to relieve unexplainable body complaints
Avoid causing painful emotional situations
Listen attentively
Encourage the expression of feelings
Reveal the patient's ambivalent feelings
Encourage mutual problem solving
Encourage self-explanation of the causes of pain
Support a realistic assessment of the situation
Massage gently (for its relaxation effect)
Touch the patient judiciously
Provide an atmosphere of acceptance
Provide frequent patient contact
Ask the patient what makes him (or her) comfortable
Provide a pain-relief measure of the patient's choice
Reduce the demands placed upon the patient
Refrain from performing nonessential procedures
Use positive suggestion in pain relief
Make a referral (to a psychiatric nurse specialist)

Nursing Observations
Determine the precipitating factors
Determine the relieving factors
Observe for complaints of pain duration
Evaluate pain for intensity and quality
Evaluate the effectiveness of the pain-relief measures
Observe for an excessive stress level
Determine the degree of insight

Health Teaching
Explain how to obtain release from emotional stress
Emphasize the importance of recognizing tension within oneself
Explain the relationship between conflict and psychogenic pain
Recommend more effective methods of coping

EVALUATION

See the evaluation criteria for each specific goal in Chapter 2.

Psychosomatic Pain (463,548)

ASSESSMENT

Subjective Data
Pain distribution: generalized or localized

Duration: continuous or intermittent

Onset: gradual or acute; frequently follows emotional trauma; seldom related to activity but tends to occur during periods of rest

Intensity: mild, moderate, or severe

Level: deep or superficial

Quality: varied, depending on the organic disorder

Objective Data

Irritability

Heavy coffee drinking

Heavy tobacco use

Nervous behavior

Related Data

Commonly Related Conditions:

Nonbacterial diarrhea

Headache

Neck soreness

Muscle spasms

Commonly Related Diseases:

Peptic or duodenal ulcer

POSSIBLE ETIOLOGY

Organic pain results from muscle tension and nerve stimulation due to stress situations. Psychologic stress has been translated into physical stress. Constitutional physical weakness is accentuated by intense stress and causes physical disorders. The pain itself results from nerve excitation and is considered an autonomic nervous system disorder.

NURSING DIAGNOSIS

Psychosomatic pain: a distressful hurting that occurs in the presence of a physical disorder, that has been brought on by intense stress

PLANNING

Patient Needs	Primary Nurse-Patient Goals
Sleep, rest, relaxation	To achieve sleep, rest, relaxation
Comfort	To achieve comfort
Protection from physical harm	To prevent physical injury
Protection from psychologic threat	To prevent emotional injury
Freedom from pain	To achieve comfort
Personal growth and maturity	To achieve optimum function
Increased learning	To achieve awareness of needs
Increased reality perception and problem solving	To achieve optimum function

NURSING INTERVENTIONS

Nursing Treatments

Approach unhurriedly

Reassure that the pain will subside
Communicate nurse sensitivity to the person's pain
Demonstrate calmness
Listen attentively
Provide an atmosphere of acceptance
Provide frequent patient contact
Massage gently (for the relaxation effect)
Encourage adequate rest
Avoid causing painful emotional situations
Reduce the demands placed upon the patient
Refrain from performing nonessential procedures
Encourage the expression of feelings
Encourage self-explanation of the causes of pain
Support a realistic assessment of the situation
Ask the patient what makes him (or her) comfortable
Discuss possible pain-reducing measures
Provide a pain-relief measure of the patient's choice
Give nonprescription drugs (ExR) (analgesics)

Nursing Observations
Observe for complaints of pain duration
Evaluate pain for intensity and quality
Determine the degree of insight
Evaluate the effectiveness of the pain-relief measures
Observe for an excessive stress level

Health Teaching
Explain the psychologic causes of organic pain
Explain how to obtain release from emotional stress
Emphasize the importance of recognizing tension within oneself
Explain how to reduce muscular tension

EVALUATION

See the evaluation criteria for each specific goal in Chapter 2.

PAINFUL THERAPY

Painful Dressing Change

ASSESSMENT

Subjective Data
Pain distribution: localized
Duration: intermittent
Onset: acute
Intensity: mild, moderate, or severe
Level: superficial
Quality: burning pain

Objective Data
Dressings adhere to the wound
Wound bleeds when dressing is removed

Related Data
Commonly Related Conditions:
Any surgical incision
Commonly Related Diseases:
Second- or third-degree burns

POSSIBLE ETIOLOGY

Pulling pressure applied to open nerve endings. Debridement of burns.

NURSING DIAGNOSIS

Painful dressing change: the recurring procedure of changing dressings
which results in repetitive, distressful hurting

PLANNING .

Patient Needs	Primary Nurse-Patient Goals
Comfort	To achieve comfort
Protection from physical harm	To prevent physical injury
Freedom from pain	To achieve comfort
Increased learning	To achieve awareness of needs

NURSING INTERVENTIONS

Nursing Treatments
Approach unhurriedly
Reassure that the pain will subside
Communicate nurse sensitivity to the person's pain
Handle gently
Attend the patient constantly
Decrease drafts
Give nonprescription drugs (ExR) (analgesics)
Maintain a warm room temperature
Moisten the dressing before removal
Prepare the patient for a painful experience

Nursing Observations
Evaluate pain for intensity and quality
Evaluate the effectiveness of the pain-relief measures

Health Teaching
Explain the causes of pain
Explain the reason for and intended effect of the therapy

Medical Treatments Performed by Nurses
Give the prescribed drugs

EVALUATION

See the evaluation criteria for each specific goal in Chapter 2.

REACTIONS TO PAIN

High Pain Threshold (477,495,548)

ASSESSMENT

Subjective Data
Patient experiences high levels of pain
Mentally tries to minimize the pain

Objective Data
Patient seldom, if ever, complains
Continues activities despite intense pain
Will not give in until pain is excruciating
Hesitates to ask for pain relief
Withdraws and prefers to cry alone
Even after communicating the existence of pain, patient outwardly expresses pain minimally

Related Data
Commonly Related Diseases:
Any painful disease or injury

POSSIBLE ETIOLOGY

Cultural influence

NURSING DIAGNOSIS

High pain threshold: a high tolerance for pain with minimum external communication of the pain

PLANNING

Patient Needs	Primary Nurse-Patient Goals
Comfort	To achieve comfort
Protection from physical harm	To prevent physical injury
Freedom from pain	To achieve comfort
Increased learning	To achieve awareness of needs

NURSING INTERVENTIONS

Nursing Treatments
Approach unhurriedly
Provide an atmosphere of acceptance
Anticipate needs
Provide frequent patient contact
Refrain from equating sleep with the absence of pain
Encourage the expression of feelings
Ask the patient what makes him (or her) comfortable
Discuss possible pain-reducing measures
Provide a pain-relief measure of the patient's choice
Give nonprescription drugs (ExR) (analgesics)

Nursing Observations
Observe for nonverbal communication of pain
Determine the influence of culture on the pain reaction

Health Teaching
Explain how to describe pain
Explain that it is acceptable to admit the existence of pain

Medical Treatments Performed by Nurses
Give the prescribed drugs (analgesics)

EVALUATION

See the evaluation criteria for each specific goal in Chapter 2.

Low Pain Threshold (477,495,548)

ASSESSMENT

Subjective Data
Anxiety

Objective Data
Patient frequently complains
Demands early, adequate pain relief
Often exaggerates the pain experienced
Accepts drug therapy willingly
Gives into pain easily
Is content when pain is relieved

Related Data
Commonly Related Diseases:
Any painful disease or injury

POSSIBLE ETIOLOGY

The threshold for emotional reaction to pain varies according to culture. Repeated stimulation of pain perception does not increase the tolerance for pain but instead results in a hypersensitivity to pain. Inflammatory disease lowers pain tolerance. Fatigue, malnutrition, or debilitation make pain less tolerable.

NURSING DIAGNOSIS

Low pain threshold: a decreased tolerance for inhibiting the expression of pain, with uninhibited external communication of pain

PLANNING

Patient Needs	Primary Nurse-Patient Goals
Sleep, rest, relaxation	To achieve sleep, rest, relaxation
Comfort	To achieve comfort
Protection from physical harm	To prevent physical injury
Freedom from pain	To achieve comfort
Increased learning	To achieve awareness of needs

NURSING INTERVENTIONS

Nursing Treatments
Approach unhurriedly
Reassure that the pain will subside
Communicate nurse sensitivity to the person's pain
Demonstrate calmness
Listen attentively
Provide an atmosphere of acceptance
Anticipate needs
Respond immediately to the patient's call
Provide frequent patient contact
Encourage the expression of feelings
Refrain from performing nonessential procedures
Ask the patient what makes him (or her) comfortable
Discuss possible pain-reducing measures
Provide a pain-relief measure of the patient's choice
Give nonprescription drugs (ExR) (analgesics)
Use positive suggestion in pain relief

Nursing Observations
Determine the urgency of pain relief
Evaluate pain for intensity and quality
Evaluate the effectiveness of the pain-relief measures
Determine the influence of culture on the pain reaction

Health Teaching
Explain the causes of pain
Explain the reason for the delay in giving a pain-relief drug (if a delay is
  necessary)

Medical Treatments Performed by Nurses
Give the prescribed drugs (analgesics)

EVALUATION

See the evaluation criteria for each specific goal in Chapter 2.

Heightened Nighttime Pain (477,495)

ASSESSMENT

Subjective Data
Pain intensity increases at night
Patient experiences heightened anxiety

Objective Data
Patient is unable to sleep
Seeks the company of others
Complains more frequently at night than during the day

Related Data
Commonly Related Diseases:
Any disease or injury

POSSIBLE ETIOLOGY

Increased perception of pain due to fewer distractions during nighttime quiet

NURSING DIAGNOSIS

Heightened nighttime pain: an increase in pain perception during the normal hours of sleep

PLANNING

Patient Needs

Sleep, rest, relaxation

Comfort

Protection from physical harm

Freedom from pain

Increased learning

Primary Nurse-Patient Goals

To achieve sleep, rest, relaxation

To achieve comfort

To prevent physical injury

To achieve comfort

To achieve awareness of needs

NURSING INTERVENTIONS

Nursing Treatments

Approach unhurriedly

Reassure that the pain will subside

Communicate nurse sensitivity to the person's pain

Handle gently

Anticipate needs

Provide frequent patient contact

  OR

Sit with the patient

Touch the patient judiciously

Arrange geographic placement (so the patient can see the nurses)

Position comfortably

Massage gently ⎫

  OR ⎬ (for the relaxation effect)

Bathe in warm water ⎭

Provide a nightlight

Ask the patient what makes him (or her) comfortable

Discuss possible pain-reducing measures

Provide a pain-relief measure of the patient's choice

Give nonprescription drugs (ExR) (analgesics)

Nursing Observations

Observe for complaints of pain duration

Evaluate the pain for intensity and quality

Evaluate the effectiveness of the pain-relief measures

Health Teaching

Explain the causes of pain (lack of distraction at night)

EVALUATION

See the evaluation criteria for each specific goal in Chapter 2.

Pain Anticipation

ASSESSMENT

Subjective Data
Intense fear of pain
Feeling of pain before it occurs
Fatigue

Objective Data
Nervous behavior
Weeping
Seeking of drug relief before the painful experience

Related Data
Commonly Related Diseases:
None
  OR
Any disease or injury

POSSIBLE ETIOLOGY

Expressions of anxiety and fear in anticipation of an expected painful event.
Previous past experience with a similar painful situation.

NURSING DIAGNOSIS

Pain anticipation: a dread of pain that has not yet occurred, but threatens
to occur

PLANNING

Patient Needs	**Primary Nurse-Patient Goals**
Relaxation	To achieve relaxation
Comfort	To achieve comfort
Protection from physical harm	To prevent physical injury
Protection from psychologic threat	To prevent emotional injury
Increased learning	To achieve awareness of needs
Increased reality perception and problem solving	To achieve optimum function

NURSING INTERVENTIONS

Nursing Treatments
Approach unhurriedly
Reassure verbally (that the nurse will stay with the patient during the pro-
    cedure)
Attend the patient constantly (during the procedure)
Demonstrate calmness
Listen attentively
Discuss the anticipated procedure
Prepare the patient for a painful experience
Encourage the expression of feelings

Provide objects which symbolize safeness
Introduce to persons who have successfully undergone the same experience
Involve the family
Provide an atmosphere of acceptance
Refrain from forcing the treatment
Refrain from performing nonessential procedures

Nursing Observations
Determine the degree of insight
Observe for an excessive stress level

Health Teaching
Explain the causes of fear of pain

EVALUATION

See the evaluation criteria for each specific goal in Chapter 2.

Pain Avoidance (477,495,548)

ASSESSMENT

Subjective Data
Intense anxiety, when forced into the painful situation

Objective Data
Irritability
Refusal to participate in an experience perceived as painful
Unavailability at the scheduled time of the experience
If certain persons are associated with the pain, they will be rejected and
    persons perceived more favorably will be sought

Related Data
Commonly Related Diseases:
Any painful disease or injury

POSSIBLE ETIOLOGY

A desire to protect oneself against unpleasant events, sights, or persons

NURSING DIAGNOSIS

Pain avoidance: withdrawal from painful experiences or objects

PLANNING

Patient Needs	**Primary Nurse-Patient Goals**
Comfort	To achieve comfort
Protection from physical harm	To prevent physical injury
Freedom from pain	To achieve comfort
Adequacy	To achieve positive expressions, feelings, reactions
Increased learning	To achieve awareness of needs

NURSING INTERVENTIONS

Nursing Treatments
Approach unhurriedly

Reassure verbally
Demonstrate calmness
Attend the patient constantly
Arrange situations that encourage patient autonomy
Discuss the anticipated procedure
Prepare the patient for a painful experience
Encourage acceptance of unpleasantness
Encourage the expression of feelings
Explore with the patient previous displays of courage
Support a realistic assessment of the situation
Introduce to persons who have successfully undergone the same experience
Provide objects which symbolize safeness
Refrain from forcing the treatment

Nursing Observations
Determine the degree of insight
Determine the precipitating factors
Determine the relieving factors
Observe for an excessive stress level

Health Teaching
Explain the causes of fear of pain

EVALUATION

See the evaluation criteria for each specific goal in Chapter 2.

INADEQUATE PAIN MANAGEMENT

Inadequate Information Related to Pain-Relief Methods

ASSESSMENT

Subjective Data
Person is deeply concerned about relieving his own or the pain of another
Confirms a lack of information

Objective Data
Person's actions indicate a lack of information regarding:
    which drugs are appropriate for pain relief
    the fact that there are nondrug methods of pain relief
    which pain relief methods are most suitable to specific types of pain

Related Data
Commonly Related Diseases:
Any painful disease or injury

POSSIBLE ETIOLOGY

Lack of instruction

NURSING DIAGNOSIS

Inadequate information related to pain-relief methods: lack of information regarding the many ways in which pain can be relieved

PLANNING

Patient Needs

Comfort

Protection from physical harm

Freedom from pain

Increased learning

Primary Nurse-Patient Goals

To achieve comfort

To prevent physical injury

To achieve comfort

To achieve awareness of needs

NURSING INTERVENTIONS

Nursing Treatments

Approach unhurriedly

Encourage patient questions

Nursing Observations

Evaluate the response to teaching

Health Teaching

Explain that there are nondrug methods available for pain relief

Teach how to administer medications

EVALUATION

See the evaluation criteria for each specific goal in Chapter 2.

25.
NURSING DIAGNOSES RELATED TO
Physical Activity

ACTIVITY TOLERANCE

Minimum Activity Tolerance
(70,274,391)

ASSESSMENT

Subjective Data
Dyspnea on exertion
Fatigue
Nervousness
Inability to deal with simple problems

Objective Data
Person stays in bed most of the time
Has little interest in performing activity

Related Data
Commonly Related Conditions:
Cardiac failure
Muscular atrophy

Commonly Related Diseases:
Myocardial infarction
Guillian-Barre syndrome
Poliomyelitis
Myasthenia gravis
Cerebrovascular accident

POSSIBLE ETIOLOGY

Endocrine disturbances. Tissue toxicity. Inadequate tissue oxygenation. Recovery from surgical procedures. Poor nutrition. Depression.

NURSING DIAGNOSIS

Minimum activity tolerance: the inability to tolerate any physical activity without the presence of discomforts

PLANNING

Patient Needs

Sleep, rest, relaxation

Energy

Comfort

Dependence

Increased learning

Primary Nurse-Patient Goals

To achieve sleep, rest, relaxation

To maintain regulating mechanisms and functions

To achieve comfort

To achieve comfort

To achieve awareness of needs

NURSING INTERVENTIONS

Nursing Treatments

Acknowledge dependency

Anticipate needs

Approach unhurriedly

Encourage adequate rest

Encourage alternate rest and activity

Place the call light within reach

Place objects within reach

Reduce the demands placed upon the patient

Refrain from performing nonessential procedures

Nursing Observations

Observe for readiness to assume activities of daily living

Observe for dyspnea

Palpate the pulse for rate, rhythm, and volume

Health Teaching

Advise a gradual return to activity

Describe those symptoms which should be reported (increased dyspnea or fatigue)

EVALUATION

See the evaluation criteria for each specific goal in Chapter 2.

Mild Activity Tolerance (70,274,391)

ASSESSMENT

Subjective Data

Dyspnea on moderate exertion

Nervousness

Ability to deal only with simple problems

Objective Data

Person is out of bed for multiple short periods

Comfortably performs some activity but requires intermittent rest

Cannot maintain the daily routine of a healthy person
Has rapid pulse on moderate exertion
Is irritable

Related Data

Commonly Related Conditions:
Hypokalemia

Commonly Related Diseases:
Bacterial endocarditis
Pericarditis
Myocarditis
Addison's disease
Myasthenia gravis
Glomerulonephritis

POSSIBLE ETIOLOGY

Endocrine disturbances. Tissue toxicity. Inadequate tissue oxygenation.
Poor nutrition. Recovery from a surgical procedure.

NURSING DIAGNOSIS

Mild activity tolerance: the ability to tolerate only a very limited amount of
physical activity without the presence of discomforts

PLANNING

Patient Needs	Primary Nurse-Patient Goals
Sleep, rest, relaxation	To achieve sleep, rest, relaxation
Energy	To maintain regulating mechanisms and functions
Comfort	To achieve comfort
Dependence	To achieve comfort
Increased learning	To achieve awareness of needs

NURSING INTERVENTIONS

Nursing Treatments
Acknowledge dependency
Anticipate needs
Approach unhurriedly
Provide frequent patient contact
Encourage acceptance of self-limitations
Encourage adequate rest
Encourage alternate rest and activity
Encourage self-performance
Place the call light within reach
Place objects within reach
Place the work at a comfortable level
Provide a low-height bed
Reduce the demands placed upon the patient

Refrain from performing nonessential procedures
Sit the patient in an armchair

Nursing Observations
Observe for readiness to assume activities of daily living
Observe for dyspnea
Palpate the pulse for rate, rhythm, and volume (during activity)

Health Teaching
Advise a gradual return to activity
Describe the characteristics of fatigue
Recommend living in a single-level, ground-floor dwelling
Explain the causes of the health problem
Explain the need to avoid overexertion
Instruct to immediately report serious symptoms
Recommend adherence to a moderate pace of living
Recommend distributing heavy tasks throughout the week
Recommend that time be divided between energy- and nonenergy-consuming activities
Recommend the duplication of equipment in work areas
Recommend the elimination of unnecessary work

EVALUATION

See the evaluation criteria for each specific goal in Chapter 2.

Moderate Activity Tolerance (70,274,391)

ASSESSMENT

Subjective Data
Dyspnea on prolonged exertion
Nervousness
Ability to deal fairly well with complex problems

Objective Data
Person comfortably performs activity
Maintains the daily routine of a healthy person but requires occasional rest
Has rapid pulse on prolonged exertion
Is irritable, sometimes

Related Data
Commonly Related Conditions:
Aging
Mitral or pulmonary stenosis
Commonly Related Diseases:
Myocardial infarction
Myasthenia gravis
Guillian-Barre syndrome
Hypertension
Rheumatic fever

Bacterial endocarditis
Pericarditis
Myocarditis
Addison's disease
Glomerulonephritis

POSSIBLE ETIOLOGY

Endocrine disturbances. Tissue toxicity. Inadequate tissue oxygenation.
Poor nutrition. Recovery from a surgical procedure.

NURSING DIAGNOSIS

Moderate activity tolerance: the ability to tolerate a moderate, but not a
full day of, physical activity without the presence of discomfort

PLANNING

Patient Needs	Primary Nurse-Patient Goals
Sleep, rest	To achieve sleep, rest
Activity, exercise	To achieve activity and exercise
Energy	To maintain regulating mechanisms and functions
Comfort	To achieve comfort
Increased learning	To achieve awareness of needs

NURSING INTERVENTIONS

Nursing Treatments
Anticipate needs
Approach unhurriedly
Discourage strenuous activities
Encourage acceptance of self-limitations
Encourage adequate rest
Encourage alternate rest and activity
Encourage moderate physical exercise
Encourage self-performance
Place the work at a comfortable level
Reduce the demands placed upon the patient
Refrain from performing nonessential procedures

Nursing Observations
Observe for readiness to assume activities of daily living
Observe for dyspnea
Observe for fatigue
Palpate the pulse for rate, rhythm, and volume

Health Teaching
Explain the causes of the health problem
Recommend a regular sleeping schedule
Advise a gradual return to activity
Describe the characteristics of fatigue
Explain the need to avoid overexertion

Inform that heavy lifting should be avoided
Instruct to avoid pushing and pulling activities
Instruct to immediately report serious symptoms
Recommend consideration of occupation change (if it is energy depleting)
Recommend distributing heavy tasks throughout the week
Recommend napping whenever possible
Recommend that time be divided between energy- and nonenergy-
    consuming activities
Recommend the duplication of equipment in work areas
Recommend the elimination of unnecessary work

EVALUATION

See the evaluation criteria for each specific goal in Chapter 2.

SPECIFIC STRENGTH DEPLETION ACTIVITIES

Eating Fatigue

ASSESSMENT

Subjective Data
Dyspnea after minimal food intake
Extreme fatigue

Objective Data
Person chews food slowly
Refuses to eat more than one or two bites of food

Related Data
Commonly Related Conditions:
Cachexia
Commonly Related Diseases:
Glomerulonephritis
Guillian-Barre syndrome
Myasthenia gravis
Myocardial infarction
Cerebral vascular accident

POSSIBLE ETIOLOGY

Endocrine disturbance. Tissue toxicity. Extremely poor nutritional status. Energy depletion from prolonged illness.

NURSING DIAGNOSIS

Eating fatigue: extreme fatigue resulting from eating

PLANNING

Patient Needs
Water-salt balance

Primary Nurse-Patient Goals
To maintain fluid and electrolyte
    balance

Food balance

To maintain nutrition to all cells

Comfort

To achieve comfort

Dependence

To achieve comfort

Increased learning

To achieve awareness of needs

NURSING INTERVENTIONS

Nursing Treatments
Acknowledge dependency
Approach unhurriedly
Discourage talking while eating
Encourage rest periods while eating
Feed the patient
Feed slowly
Give mechanically soft foods
    OR
Give pureed foods
Give small, frequent feedings
Postpone feeding when the patient is fatigued
Provide a short drinking straw
Provide small frequent drinks
Refrain from performing nonessential procedures (around mealtime)

Nursing Observations
Determine the precipitating factors
Determine the relieving factors

Health Teaching
Explain the causes of the health problem
Explain the reason for and intended effect of the therapy

EVALUATION

See the evaluation criteria for each specific goal in Chapter 2.

Emotional Fatigue (89,118)

ASSESSMENT

Subjective Data
Fatigue upon rising in the morning, which decreases as the day progresses
Nervousness
Anxiety
Depression
Weakness
Palpitations
Headache
Difficulty concentrating
Difficulty sleeping

Objective Data
Anorexia
Irritability

Related Data

Commonly Related Conditions:
None

Commonly Related Diseases:
None
  OR
Psychoneurosis

POSSIBLE ETIOLOGY

The use of physical energy to meet emotional conflict. Exposure to prolonged and intensely stressful emotional situations. Reluctance to face problems and difficulties.

NURSING DIAGNOSIS

Emotional fatigue: bodily weariness or loss of strength following emotional stress

PLANNING

Patient Needs	Primary Nurse-Patient Goals
Sleep, rest, relaxation	To achieve sleep, rest and relaxation
Comfort	To achieve comfort
Protection from physical harm	To prevent physical injury
Protection from psychologic threat	To prevent emotional injury
Warm, communicating relationships	To achieve effective verbal and nonverbal communications
Increased learning	To achieve awareness of needs
Increased reality perception and problem solving	To achieve optimum function

NURSING INTERVENTIONS

Nursing Treatments
Approach unhurriedly
Reassure verbally
Listen attentively
Arrange a structured environment
Ask questions which encourage answers that reflect reality perception
Avoid causing intense emotional situations
Encourage adequate rest
Encourage alternate rest and activity
Encourage active diversional activities
Encourage mutual problem solving
Encourage planned one-day-at-a-time living
Encourage a positive life approach
Reduce the demands placed upon the patient
Refrain from performing nonessential procedures

Nursing Observations
Determine the degree of insight
Determine the precipitating factors

Determine the relieving factors
Estimate the degree of stress experienced
Identify disturbing conversation topics
Identify the current dominant emotion
Observe for an excessive stress level

Health Teaching
Explain the causes of the health problem
Advise early correction of problems
Advise that highly emotional situations be avoided
Explain how to obtain release from emotional stress
Emphasize the importance of recognizing tension within oneself
Explain the need to recognize highly stressful situations
Explain the importance of offering emotional support to one another
Explain the reason for and intended effect of the therapy

EVALUATION

See the evaluation criteria for each specific goal in Chapter 2.

Wheelchair Fatigue

ASSESSMENT

Subjective Data
Fatigue

Objective Data
Person takes long rests after propelling the wheelchair a short distance
Coaxes others to push his wheelchair
Is irritable when forced to remain in the wheelchair for prolonged periods

Related Data
Commonly Related Diseases:
Lumbar or thoracic spinal cord injury
Myocardial infarction
Cerebral vascular accident
    OR
Any disease or injury resulting in wheelchair confinement

POSSIBLE ETIOLOGY

Depletion of body cell energy. Poor muscle tone. Impaired nerve function.

NURSING DIAGNOSIS

Wheelchair fatigue: tiredness and weariness resulting from pushing one's
own wheelchair

PLANNING

Patient Needs	**Primary Nurse-Patient Goals**
Rest	To achieve rest
Energy	To maintain regulating mechanisms and functions
Comfort	To achieve comfort

Protection from physical harm   To prevent accident, physical injury

Increased learning   To achieve awareness of needs

NURSING INTERVENTIONS

Nursing Treatments
Acknowledge dependency
Encourage alternate rest and activity
Mobilize by wheelchair (for short periods only)
Provide frequent patient contact (while up in wheelchair)

Nursing Observations
Observe for fatigue (increased)

Health Teaching
Inform that powered wheelchairs are available
Inform that the use of a lightweight wheelchair is preferable
Instruct in the use of projections on wheelchair wheel rims
Recommend the use of long, even strokes to propel the wheelchair

EVALUATION

See the evaluation criteria for each specific goal in Chapter 2.

STRENGTH DEPLETION, POTENTIAL

Potential Generalized Weakness (326,350,391)

ASSESSMENT

Subjective Data
Intense emotional stress

Objective Data
Poor nutrition
Prolonged bed rest
Lack of exercise
Inadequate sleep and rest

Related Data
Commonly Related Conditions:
Long-term bedrest or immobility
Commonly Related Diseases:
Cerebral vascular accident
Bone fracture

POSSIBLE ETIOLOGY

Disease of body musculature. Impaired circulation from inactivity. Stress-related energy depletion. Severe metabolic changes.

NURSING DIAGNOSIS

Potential generalized weakness: the possibility that there will be a loss of normal strength

PLANNING

Patient Needs	**Primary Nurse-Patient Goals**
Circulation	To maintain oxygen to all cells
Food balance	To maintain nutrition to all cells
Sleep, rest	To achieve sleep, rest
Activity, exercise	To achieve activity and exercise
Energy	To maintain regulating mechanisms and functions
Protection from physical harm	To prevent physical injury
Increased learning	To achieve awareness of needs

NURSING INTERVENTIONS

Nursing Treatments
Ambulate the patient (as much as possible)
   OR
Sit the patient in an armchair
Encourage moderate physical exercise
Encourage adequate rest
Encourage alternate rest and activity
Encourage self-performance
Exercise in range of motion
Balance nutritional intake
Supplement protein intake

Nursing Observations
Observe for increased nutritional requirements
Observe for complaints of weakness

Health Teaching
Explain the causes of the health problem
Advise a gradual return to activity
Describe those symptoms which should be reported (weakness)
Explain the reason for and intended effect of the therapy

EVALUATION

See the evaluation criteria for each specific goal in Chapter 2.

INADEQUATE PHYSICAL ENERGY MANAGEMENT

Inadequate Information Related to Conserving Physical Energy (317,593)

ASSESSMENT

Subjective Data
Fatigue
Frustration
Person confirms a lack of information

Objective Data

Person's actions indicate a lack of information regarding:
    how to employ methods that ease the workload
    available resources for conserving physical energy

Related Data

Commonly Related Diseases:
Any disease that causes energy depletion

POSSIBLE ETIOLOGY

Lack of instruction

NURSING DIAGNOSIS

Inadequate information related to conserving physical energy: a lack of information regarding those activity methods that can be used to conserve human energy as it relates to the person's state of health

PLANNING

Patient Needs	**Primary Nurse-Patient Goals**
Comfort	To achieve comfort
Protection from physical harm	To prevent physical injury
Independence	To achieve optimum function
Increased learning	To achieve awareness of needs

NURSING INTERVENTIONS

Nursing Treatments
Approach unhurriedly
Encourage adequate rest
Encourage alternate rest and activity
Encourage patient questions

Nursing Observations
Evaluate the response to teaching

Health Teaching
Advise that persons attending the sick economize energies
Explain that socialization depletes the ill patient's energy
Recommend living in a single-level, ground-floor dwelling
Explain the need to avoid overexertion
Inform that heavy lifting should be avoided
Instruct to avoid pushing and pulling activities
Recommend adherence to a moderate pace of living
Recommend distributing heavy tasks throughout the week
Recommend limiting one's involvement in monotonous tasks
Recommend that work activities be combined
Recommend that time be divided between energy- and nonenergy-
    consuming activities
Recommend the duplication of equipment in work areas
Recommend the elimination of unnecessary work
Recommend the pursuit of only one activity at a time

Recommend the use of a cannister vacuum for energy conservation
Recommend the use of an electric garage door for energy conservation
Recommend the use of lightweight utensils
Recommend the use of push-bar windows for energy conservation
Recommend the use of rolling tables to ease work

EVALUATION

See the evaluation criteria for each specific goal in Chapter 2.

26.

NURSING DIAGNOSES RELATED TO
The Reproductive System

Note: Many of the nursing diagnoses associated with the reproductive system are also significant to other systems. To avoid duplication, these nursing diagnoses are listed in this chapter by title only with a referral to their page location.

PREGNANCY DISCOMFORTS

Postural Hypotension, p. 422

Potential Varicose Veins, p. 404

ANTEPARTAL CARE DEPENDENCE

Dependence on Nursing Supervision of Normal Pregnancy (258,357,429,460)

ASSESSMENT

Subjective Data

Woman relies on nurses for guidance regarding:
    weight control
    adequate hygiene
    breast care
    proper rest and exercise
    nutritional balance
    skin care
    comfortable clothing
    observation for and prevention of pregnancy complications

Objective Data

Woman is pregnant

Related Data

Commonly Related Diseases:
None

POSSIBLE ETIOLOGY

The existence of a pregnancy

NURSING DIAGNOSIS

Dependence on nursing supervision of normal pregnancy: reliance on nurses for guidance in the maintenance of health during the period from conception to the onset of labor

PLANNING

Patient Needs	**Primary Nurse-Patient Goals**
Comfort	To achieve comfort
Protection from physical harm	To prevent physical injury
Dependence	To achieve comfort
Increased learning	To achieve awareness of needs

NURSING INTERVENTIONS

Nursing Treatments
Encourage adequate rest
Encourage moderate physical exercise

Encourage increased calcium-food intake
Encourage increased protein-food intake
Encourage increased residue-food intake
Encourage increased high-vitamin-food intake
Discourage oral stimulants
Discourage smoking

Nursing Observations

Specific to the Initial Visit:
Measure the pelvic size
Monitor blood studies for blood type
Monitor blood studies for Rh factor
Monitor blood studies for positive VDRL
Monitor the Pap smear study for positive findings
Monitor culture for positive evidence of gonorrhea

Initial and Follow-up Visits:
Monitor the fetal heart sounds
Palpate the uterus for normal enlargement during pregnancy
Inspect the breasts for abnormalities
Inspect for edema
Inspect for bleeding
Inspect the vagina for discharge (especially bleeding)
Measure the body weight
Monitor the blood pressure
Monitor blood studies for abnormal hematology
Observe for complaints of constipation
Observe for complaints of backache
Observe for complaints of itching (vaginal)
Test the urine for protein
Test the urine for sugar and acetone

Health Teaching
Inform that cleanliness is basic to health
Explain when showering should be substituted for tub bathing during pregnancy
Teach good breast hygiene during pregnancy
Describe the breast changes expected during pregnancy
Recommend the use of a brassiere for breast support
Explain the advantages and disadvantages of breast feeding
Explain how to adjust clothing to meet health problems
Recommend the use of an abdominal-support garment (if back problem is of major concern)
Advise against wearing constrictive clothing
Recommend the use of low-heeled shoes
Explain how to apply elastic stockings or an elastic bandage
Instruct to increase fluid intake (especially water)
Instruct that douching be avoided
Advise not to take enemas and laxatives (habitually)
Advise against using mineral oil laxatives

Explain that sexual activity should be temporarily limited (if there is a history of abortion, membrane rupture, or mucous plug passage)
Recommend that self-medication be avoided
Teach the principles of good nutrition
Explain how to control weight gain during pregnancy
Inform that heavy lifting should be avoided
Emphasize the danger of x-ray exposure during early pregnancy
Describe the danger signs of pregnancy
Describe the normal behavior pattern common during pregnancy
Explain how to calculate the delivery date
Explain how the infant grows in utero
Explain how to prepare the breasts during pregnancy for postdelivery breast feedings
Instruct to immediately report serious symptoms
Explain the reason for and intended effect of the therapy

EVALUATION

See the evaluation criteria for each specific goal in Chapter 2.

Dependence on Preparation for Approaching Childbirth (258,357,429,460)

ASSESSMENT

Subjective Data
Woman relies on nurses for guidance regarding:
    how to recognize the onset of labor
    the physical changes to expect as labor progresses
    the procedures that will be carried out during labor and delivery
    methods the mother can use to ease childbirth
    common behavior associated with childbirth

Objective Data
Woman is pregnant

Related Data
Commonly Related Diseases:
None

POSSIBLE ETIOLOGY

Anticipated termination of pregnancy

NURSING DIAGNOSIS

Dependence on preparation for childbirth: reliance on nurses to prepare the potential mother for labor and delivery

PLANNING

Patient Needs	Primary Nurse-Patient Goals
Comfort	To achieve comfort
Protection from physical harm	To prevent physical injury

Protection from psychologic threat   To prevent emotional injury

Dependence   To achieve comfort

Increased learning   To achieve awareness of needs

NURSING INTERVENTIONS

Nursing Treatments

Approach unhurriedly

Encourage patient questions

Discuss the anticipated procedure (such as perineal shave, cleansing enema, rectal and vaginal examinations, monitoring fetal heart sounds, I.V. therapy)

Nursing Observations

Evaluate the response to teaching

Observe for an excessive stress level

Health Teaching

Describe the manifestations of labor onset

Explain the difference between true and false labor pains

Explain the significance of premature membrane rupture and that it does not indicate difficult labor

Describe the process of labor and delivery

Explain that childbirth is a normal process

Describe the normal behavior pattern common during labor

Teach how to control breathing to aid the labor process

Recommend methods for achieving total relaxation

EVALUATION

See the evaluation criteria for each specific goal in Chapter 2.

INTRAPARTAL CARE
DEPENDENCE

Dependence on Nursing Supervision of Normal Labor and Delivery (192,258,357,429,460)

ASSESSMENT

Subjective Data

First Stage Labor:

Woman relies on nurses for:

    evaluation of uterine contractions

    monitoring of fetal heart sounds

    evaluation of cervical dilatation

    monitoring of vital signs

    maintenance of good hygiene and sterile technique

    protection from complications

    protection against exhaustion

Second Stage Labor:
Woman relies on nurses for:
    monitoring of fetal heart sounds
    maintenance of sterile technique
    guidance toward appropriate bearing down
    observation for presentation of the infant
Third Stage Labor:
Woman relies on nurses for:
    supervision of placenta expulsion
    observation for and prevention of hemorrhage
    evaluation of fundus contractability
    monitoring of the blood pressure and pulse
Pain
Anxiety

Objective Data
Woman is in the first, second, or third stage of labor

Related Data
Commonly Related Diseases:
None

POSSIBLE ETIOLOGY

The termination of pregnancy

NURSING DIAGNOSIS

Dependence on nursing supervision of normal labor and delivery: reliance on nurses to supervise and assist the mother during labor and delivery

PLANNING

Patient Needs	**Primary Nurse-Patient Goals**
Rest, relaxation	To achieve rest, relaxation
Comfort	To achieve comfort
Cleanliness	To achieve good hygiene
Protection from physical harm	To prevent physical injury, infection
Protection from psychologic threat	To prevent emotional injury
Freedom from pain	To achieve comfort
Dependence	To achieve comfort
Increased learning	To achieve awareness of needs

NURSING INTERVENTIONS

Nursing Treatments
First Stage Labor:
Attend the patient constantly
Reassure verbally
Provide a clean, comfortable bed
Provide quiet
Do perineal prep

Administer an enema (cleansing enema given slowly and as comfortably as
   possible)
Ambulate the patient (as much as possible during early first stage)
Give small, frequent drinks (during early first stage)
Restrict the intake to nothing by mouth (food restriction during entire first
   stage; fluid restriction during advanced first stage)
Position comfortably (as first stage advances)
Massage gently (the lumbar-sacral area and effeurage the abdomen)
Toilet frequently
Touch the patient judiciously
Refrain from performing nonessential procedures
Provide radio and television for diversion (if the patient desires)
Encourage visiting by significant others

Second Stage Labor:
Place in the lithotomy (dorsosacral) position (on the delivery table)
Place on sterile linens
Drape modestly
Position comfortably (as much as possible)
Restrain the patient (for safety)
Do perineal prep (cleansing only)
Facilitate delivery by gently guiding the infant through the vulva (ExR)

Third Stage Labor:
Tie off and cut the umbilical cord (ExR)
Await placenta delivery (ExR)
Refrain from pulling the umbilical cord during placenta expulsion
Refrain from removing the placenta except during uterine contraction
Massage the uterine fundus (if it fails to contract)

Nursing Observations

First Stage Labor:
Monitor the fetal heart sounds
Palpate the cervix for dilatation
Palpate the uterus for contraction quality
Time the uterine contractions
Monitor the blood pressure (every hour)
Monitor the oral temperature
Palpate the pulse for rate, rhythm, and volume
Inspect the chest for respiratory rate and rhythm
Observe for uterine membrane rupture
Inspect the amniotic fluid for meconium
Inspect the vagina for a prolapsed umbilical cord
Observe for complaints of pain
Observe for an excessive stress level
Observe for fatigue
Test the urine for protein
Test the urine for sugar and acetone

Second Stage Labor:
Monitor the fetal heart sounds (until birth occurs)

Third Stage Labor:
Inspect for bleeding
Inspect the placenta for abnormalities
Inspect the umbilical cord for abnormalities
Palpate the uterus for firmness
Monitor the blood pressure
Palpate the pulse for rate, rhythm, and volume

Health Teaching

First Stage Labor:
Explain the reason for and intended effect of the therapy
Describe those symptoms which should be reported
Teach how to control breathing to aid the labor process
Recommend methods for achieving total relaxation

Second Stage Labor:
Inform that bearing down aids the process of second stage labor

EVALUATION

See the evaluation criteria for each specific goal in Chapter 2.

INTRAPARTAL PROBLEMS

False Labor Pain, p. 1041

Inadequate Emotional Support Related to the Endurance of Pain, p. 253

Labor Pain, p. 1043

Potential Puerperal Infection, p. 745

POSTPARTAL CARE DEPENDENCE

Dependence on Episiotomy Care, p. 717

Dependence on Feminine Hygiene, p. 718

Dependence on Nursing Supervision of Immediate Postpartal Period (258,357,429)

ASSESSMENT

Subjective Data
Woman relies on nurses for protection against postdelivery complications

Maternal exhaustion
Hunger
Thirst
Dependency

Objective Data
Woman has completed delivery

Related Data
Commonly Related Diseases:
None

POSSIBLE ETIOLOGY

Termination of pregnancy

NURSING DIAGNOSIS

Dependence on nursing supervision of immediate postpartal period: reliance on nurses for care during the period immediately following childbirth

PLANNING

Patient Needs	**Primary Nurse-Patient Goals**
Water-salt balance	To maintain fluid and electrolyte balance
Sleep, rest, relaxation	To achieve sleep, rest, and relaxation
Comfort	To achieve comfort
Protection from physical harm	To prevent physical injury
Dependence	To achieve comfort
Increased learning	To achieve awareness of needs

NURSING INTERVENTIONS

Nursing Treatments
Encourage adequate rest
Cover with warm blankets
Give warm liquids
Provide quiet
Massage the uterine fundus (if it becomes relaxed)

Nursing Observations
Inspect for bleeding (every 15 minutes)
Inspect the skin for perspiration abnormality (profuse perspiration)
Measure the intake
Measure the output (if there have been pregnancy complications)
Monitor the blood pressure (every 15 minutes until stable, then every hour)
Monitor the oral temperature
Inspect for edema
Inspect for inflammation } (of the incision site if an episiotomy
Inspect for bleeding   } is done)
Observe for complaints of thirst
Palpate the uterus for firmness (every 15 minutes)

Palpate the bladder for distention
Palpate the pulse for rate, rhythm, and volume

Health Teaching
Describe those symptoms which should be reported (bleeding, pain, etc.)
Explain the reason for and intended effect of the therapy
Teach how to massage the uterine fundus

Medical Treatments Performed by Nurses
Give the prescribed drugs

EVALUATION

See the evaluation criteria for each specific goal in Chapter 2.

Dependence on Nursing Supervision of Normal Puerperium (258,357,429)

ASSESSMENT

Subjective Data
Woman relies on nurses for guidance regarding:
    maintenance of good hygiene
    breast care
    breast feeding
    reestablishment of prepregnancy body shape
    infant care
    observation for and prevention of complications

Objective Data
Woman is recovering from childbirth

Related Data
Commonly Related Diseases:
None

POSSIBLE ETIOLOGY

The body's adjustment to normalcy following delivery

NURSING DIAGNOSIS

Dependence on nursing supervision of normal puerperium: reliance on nurses for guidance and care during the postpregnancy stage

PLANNING

Patient Needs	Primary Nurse-Patient Goals
Food balance	To maintain nutrition to all cells
Rest	To achieve rest
Activity, exercise	To achieve activity and exercise
Cleanliness	To achieve good hygiene
Protection from physical harm	To prevent physical injury
Dependence	To achieve comfort
Increased learning	To achieve awareness of needs

NURSING INTERVENTIONS

Nursing Treatments
Balance nutritional intake
Encourage adequate rest
Encourage moderate physical exercise
Provide frequent patient contact

Nursing Observations
Inspect the breasts for abnormalities
Inspect for edema (of the perineum)
Inspect for (vaginal) bleeding
Inspect the vagina for discharge
Palpate the uterus for fundus height
Measure the body weight (loss is normal)
Monitor the blood pressure
Monitor the oral temperature
Monitor blood studies for abnormal hematology
Monitor urine studies for evidence of urinary tract infection
Observe for complaints of constipation
Palpate the pulse for rate, rhythm, and volume

Health Teaching
Describe the characteristics of normal lochia
Explain when the postpartum flow normally resumes
Describe those symptoms which should be reported (abnormal bleeding)
Inform that cleanliness is basic to health
Inform that heavy lifting should be avoided
Teach how to do postpartum exercises
Teach the principles of good nutrition
Explain the reason for and intended effect of the therapy

EVALUATION

See the evaluation criteria for each specific goal in Chapter 2.

POSTPARTAL PROBLEMS

After-Birth Pain, p. 1035

Breast Engorgement, p. 1037

Constipation, p. 622

Cracked-Nipple Pain, p. 1040

Excessive Lactation (258,460)

ASSESSMENT

Objective Data
Spontaneous flow of breast milk

Fissured nipples
Fever
Insomnia
Breast inflammation

Related Data

Commonly Related Diseases:
Pituitary tumor
Acromegaly
Hypothyroidism

POSSIBLE ETIOLOGY

Mammary gland oversecretion due to excessive estrogen and progesterone production. Repeated breast stimulation.

NURSING DIAGNOSIS

Excessive lactation: overabundant flow of breast milk

PLANNING

Patient Needs	**Primary Nurse-Patient Goals**
Food balance	To maintain nutrition to all cells
Rest	To achieve rest
Comfort	To achieve comfort
Cleanliness	To achieve good hygiene
Protection from physical harm	To prevent physical injury, infection
Mastery and competence in skills	To achieve optimum function
Increased learning	To achieve awareness of needs

NURSING INTERVENTIONS

Nursing Treatments
Apply a breast binder
Apply an ice bag (to the breasts)
Do not pump the breasts

Nursing Observations
Observe for complaints of pain

Health Teaching
Explain the causes of the health problem
Instruct not to massage the breast
Recommend the use of a nipple shield
Recommend the use of nipple padding
Teach how to apply a breast binder
Explain the reason for and intended effect of the therapy

Medical Treatments Performed by Nurses
Give the prescribed drugs

EVALUATION

See the evaluation criteria for each specific goal in Chapter 2.

Lactation Deficiency (258,460)

ASSESSMENT

Subjective Data
Breast pain radiating to the back

Objective Data
Breast fullness with milk
Failure of milk to flow

Related Data
Commonly Related Diseases:
Simmonds' disease

POSSIBLE ETIOLOGY

Mammary gland undersecretion due to decreased estrogen and progesterone secretion. Inadequate sucking stimulus. Poor maternal nutrition.

NURSING DIAGNOSIS

Lactation deficiency: inadequate secretion of breast milk

PLANNING

Patient Needs	Primary Nurse-Patient Goals
Water-salt balance	To maintain fluid and electrolyte balance
Food balance	To maintain nutrition to all cells
Activity, exercise	To achieve activity and exercise
Comfort	To achieve comfort
Cleanliness	To achieve good hygiene
Protection from physical harm	To prevent physical injury
Increased learning	To achieve awareness of needs

NURSING INTERVENTIONS

Nursing Treatments
Apply hot packs to the breast before breast feeding
Massage gently (the breasts)
Encourage increased carbohydrate intake
Increase fluid intake to about 3000 cc daily

Nursing Observations
Inspect the breasts for abnormalities

Health Teaching
Explain the causes of the health problem
Explain the reason for and intended effect of the therapy

Medical Treatments Performed by Nurses
Give the prescribed drugs

EVALUATION

See the evaluation criteria for each specific goal in Chapter 2.

Lactation Suppression (258)

ASSESSMENT

Subjective Data
Pain, sometimes

Objective Data
Breasts are initially full with milk
Drugs are given to suppress lactation
Breast milk dries up in a few days

Related Data
Commonly Related Diseases:
None

POSSIBLE ETIOLOGY

Maternal decision not to breast feed

NURSING DIAGNOSIS

Lactation suppression: the prevention of breast milk formation by therapeutic means

PLANNING

Patient Needs	Primary Nurse-Patient Goals
Comfort	To achieve comfort
Cleanliness	To achieve good hygiene
Protection from physical harm	To prevent physical injury, infection
Increased learning	To achieve awareness of needs

NURSING INTERVENTIONS

Nursing Treatments
Apply a brassiere
Apply an ice bag (to the breasts)
Do not massage
Do not pump the breasts

Nursing Observations
Observe for evidence of a favorable response to teaching

Health Teaching
Instruct not to massage the breast
Explain the reason for and intended effect of the therapy

Medical Treatments Performed by Nurses
Give the prescribed drugs

EVALUATION

See the evaluation criteria for each specific goal in Chapter 2.

Postpartal Diminished Abdominal Muscle Tone (258,460)

ASSESSMENT

Subjective Data
Abdominal sagging sensation
Weakened back muscles

Objective Data
Muscles appear loose with poor tone
Diminished muscle tone is most prominent the first few days following delivery

Related Data
Commonly Related Diseases:
None

POSSIBLE ETIOLOGY

Muscle stretching during pregnancy from the enlarged and heavy uterus

NURSING DIAGNOSIS

Postpartal diminished abdominal muscle tone: loss of abdominal muscle tone following delivery

PLANNING

Patient Needs	Primary Nurse-Patient Goals
Activity, exercise	To achieve activity and exercise
Comfort	To achieve comfort
Protection from physical harm	To prevent physical injury
Increased learning	To achieve awareness of needs

NURSING INTERVENTIONS

Nursing Treatments
Encourage moderate physical exercise

Nursing Observations
Observe for evidence of a favorable response to therapy

Health Teaching
Explain the causes of the health problem
Instruct to lie in the prone position (following delivery)
Teach how to do postpartum exercises
Recommend use of an abdominal-support garment
Explain the reason for and intended effect of the therapy

EVALUATION

See the evaluation criteria for each specific goal in Chapter 2.

Postpartal Perineal Pain, p. 1050

Uterine Fundus Nondescent (357,460)

ASSESSMENT

Objective Data

Uterus fails to descend, from just below the umbilicus, by one or two fingerbreadths a day

Fundus remains palpable

Lochia flow is excessive

Related Data

Commonly Related Diseases:

None

POSSIBLE ETIOLOGY

Retained blood clots, lochia, fetal membrane, placental tissue. Distended bladder. Full rectum.

NURSING DIAGNOSIS

Uterine fundus nondescent (subinvolution): the postpartum uterine fundus does not descend the normal 1 cm a day for 10 days following birth

PLANNING

Patient Needs	Primary Nurse-Patient Goals
Protection from physical harm	To prevent physical injury
Increased learning	To achieve awareness of needs

NURSING INTERVENTIONS

Nursing Treatments

Apply a hot water bottle (to the abdomen)

Massage the uterine fundus

Place in the sitting position

Soak in a sitz bath (warm)

Nursing Observations

Palpate the uterus for fundus height

Health Teaching

Explain the causes of the health problem

Teach how to massage the uterine fundus

Explain the reason for and intended effect of the therapy

Medical Treatments Performed by Nurses

Give the prescribed drugs (Methergene, ergotrate)

EVALUATION

See the evaluation criteria for each specific goal in Chapter 2.

MENSTRUATION

RADIATION THERAPY DEPENDENCE

Dependence on Radiation Related Isolation Management (70,391)

ASSESSMENT

Subjective Data
Person relies on nurses for:
>the removal of irradiated clothes, urine, etc.
>the protection of visitors from unnecessary radiation
>guidance regarding the proper procedure to follow

Objective Data
Person is receiving radiation therapy

Related Data
Commonly Related Diseases:
Uterine cancer
Oral cancer

POSSIBLE ETIOLOGY

The danger that persons receiving radiation therapy will emit radiation rays harmful to others

NURSING DIAGNOSIS

Dependence on radiation related isolation management: reliance on nurses to maintain adequate isolation of the person receiving radium therapy

PLANNING

Patient Needs	Primary Nurse-Patient Goals
Comfort	To achieve comfort
Protection from physical harm	To prevent physical injury
Increased learning	To achieve awareness of needs

NURSING INTERVENTIONS

Nursing Treatments

Anticipate needs

Place in a private room

Collect radiation-contaminated linen in a special laundry bag

Collect radiation-contaminated urine in a lead-lined container

Limit the amount of time visitors are exposed to radiation

Limit the distance from which visitors approach the irradiated patient

Shield visitors from exposure to radiation

Nursing Observations

Observe for an excessive stress level

Observe for evidence of a favorable response to (nursing) therapy

Health Teaching

Explain the causes of the health problem

Explain the reason for and intended effect of the therapy

EVALUATION

See the evaluation criteria for each specific goal in Chapter 2.

INADEQUATE INFORMATION RELATED TO REPRODUCTIVE SYSTEM CANCER

Inadequate Information Related to Breast Cancer (143)

ASSESSMENT

Subjective Data

Person confirms a lack of information

Objective Data

Person's actions indicate a lack of information regarding:

the signs and symptoms of breast cancer

the factors associated with the occurrence of breast cancer

the type of therapy suggested (usually a mastectomy or radiation therapy) and its effect

Related Data

Commonly Related Diseases:

Fibroadenoma

Lymphosarcoma

Fibrosarcoma

POSSIBLE ETIOLOGY

Lack of instruction

NURSING DIAGNOSIS

Inadequate information related to breast cancer: lack of information regarding the signs, symptoms, causes, and treatment of breast cancer

PLANNING

Patient Needs

Comfort

Protection from physical harm

Increased learning

Primary Nurse-Patient Goals

To achieve comfort

To prevent physical injury

To achieve awareness of needs

NURSING INTERVENTIONS

Nursing Treatments
Approach unhurriedly
Encourage patient questions
Discuss the anticipated procedure (x-rays, surgery, etc.)

Nursing Observations
Evaluate the response to teaching

Health Teaching
Advise early correction of problems
Describe those symptoms which should be reported (breast lumps, nipple discharge, breast asymmetry)
Explain the importance of periodic breast inspection
Describe the factors associated with the occurrence of the problem (occurs most frequently between the ages of 20 and menopause and after age 65, in childless women with late menopause, in obese women, in the use of hormone therapy beyond menopause; occurs least frequently in women with multiple pregnancies and prolonged nursing)
Explain the causes of the health problem
Explain the reason for and intended effect of the therapy
Evaluate the response to teaching

EVALUATION

See the evaluation criteria for each specific goal in Chapter 2.

Inadequate Information Related to Prostate Cancer (143)

ASSESSMENT

Subjective Data
Person confirms a lack of information

Objective Data
Person's actions indicate a lack of information regarding:
    the signs and symptoms of prostate cancer
    the factors associated with the occurrence of prostate cancer

the value of a prostatectomy

Related Data

Commonly Related Diseases:
Metatastic or primary carcinoma

POSSIBLE ETIOLOGY

Lack of information

NURSING DIAGNOSIS

Inadequate information related to prostate cancer: lack of information regarding the signs, symptoms, causes, and treatment of prostate cancer

PLANNING

Patient Needs	**Primary Nurse-Patient Goals**
Comfort	To achieve comfort
Protection from physical harm	To prevent physical injury
Increased learning	To achieve awareness of needs

NURSING INTERVENTIONS

Nursing Treatments
Approach unhurriedly
Encourage patient questions
Discuss the anticipated procedure (diagnostic studies or surgery)

Nursing Observations
Evaluate the response to teaching

Health Teaching
Advise early correction of problems
Describe those symptoms which should be reported (urinary frequency, severe backache, pain down the back of the leg)
Describe the factors associated with the occurrence of the problem (most frequent in men between the ages of 60–90)
Explain the causes of the health problem
Explain the reason for and intended effect of the therapy

EVALUATION

See the evaluation criteria for each specific goal in Chapter 2.

Inadequate Information Related to Uterine Cancer (143)

ASSESSMENT

Subjective Data
Person confirms a lack of information

Objective Data
Person's actions indicate a lack of information regarding:

the signs and symptoms of uterine cancer
the factors associated with the occurrence of uterine cancer
the meaning of different classes of Pap smear results
the value of having the uterus removed when cancer is suspected

Related Data

Commonly Related Diseases:
Cervical cancer
Uterine carcinoma
Endometriosis

POSSIBLE ETIOLOGY

Lack of instruction

NURSING DIAGNOSIS

Inadequate information related to uterine cancer: lack of information regarding the signs, symptoms, causes, and treatment of uterine cancer

PLANNING

Patient Needs	**Primary Nurse-Patient Goals**
Comfort	To achieve comfort
Protection from physical harm	To prevent physical injury
Increased learning	To achieve awareness of needs

NURSING INTERVENTIONS

Nursing Treatments
Approach unhurriedly
Encourage patient questions
Discuss the anticipated procedure (Pap smear, surgery)

Nursing Observations
Evaluate the response to teaching

Health Teaching
Advise an annual gynecologic examination
Advise early correction of problems
Describe those symptoms which should be reported (abnormal vaginal
    bleeding, brown vaginal discharge, foul vaginal odor)
Describe the factors associated with the occurrence of the problem (occurs
    most frequently between the ages of 30 and 50 in women who have had
    multiple pregnancies and who have a family history of uterine cancer)
Explain the meaning of the diagnostic report (Pap smear)
Explain the causes of the health problem
Explain the reason for and intended effect of the therapy

EVALUATION

See the evaluation criteria for each specific goal in Chapter 2.

INADEQUATE INFORMATION RELATED TO NORMAL BODY CHANGES ASSOCIATED WITH MENSTRUATION

Inadequate Information Related to Menstruation (143,175,367)

ASSESSMENT

Subjective Data

Person confirms a lack of information

Objective Data

Person's actions indicate a lack of information regarding:
   when menstruation onset normally occurs
   the physiology of menstruation
   abnormalities associated with menstruation
   normal emotional changes associated with the menstrual cycle
   the principles of good menstrual hygiene
   general health practices recommended during menstruation

Related Data

Commonly Related Diseases:
None

POSSIBLE ETIOLOGY

Lack of instruction

NURSING DIAGNOSIS

Inadequate information related to menstruation: lack of information regarding menstruation

PLANNING

Patient Needs	**Primary Nurse-Patient Goals**
Comfort	To achieve comfort
Protection from physical harm	To prevent physical injury
Increased learning	To achieve awareness of needs

NURSING INTERVENTIONS

Nursing Treatments
Approach unhurriedly
Encourage patient questions
Encourage adequate rest
Encourage moderate physical exercise

Nursing Observations
Evaluate the response to teaching

Health Teaching

Describe the emotional changes which normally occur during the menstrual cycle

Explain those menstrual variations which indicate abnormality

Describe the factors associated with the occurrence of the problem (onset usually occurs when the young woman reaches 105 pounds of body weight, between the ages of 9 to 15)

Teach menstrual cycle physiology

Teach menstrual hygiene

Advise against using tampons (during a vaginal infection)

Teach the principles of good nutrition

EVALUATION

See the evaluation criteria for each specific goal in Chapter 2.

Inadequate Information Related to Premenstrual Tension (175)

ASSESSMENT

Subjective Data

Person confirms a lack of information

Objective Data

Person's actions indicate a lack of information regarding:

the signs and symptoms of premenstrual tension

the factors related to its occurrence

general health practices recommended to minimize the discomfort

Related Data

Commonly Related Diseases:

Secondary aldosteronism

Hyperpituitarism

POSSIBLE ETIOLOGY

Lack of instruction regarding the increase in the estrogen, but especially the progesterone level, which causes water retention throughout the body, especially in the brain and nerve tissue

NURSING DIAGNOSIS

Inadequate information related to premenstrual tension: lack of information regarding discomforting signs and symptoms prior to menstruation

PLANNING

Patient Needs	Primary Nurse-Patient Goals
Comfort	To achieve comfort
Protection from physical harm	To prevent physical injury
Protection from psychologic threat	To prevent emotional injury
Increased learning	To achieve awareness of needs

NURSING INTERVENTIONS

Nursing Treatments
Approach unhurriedly
Encourage patient questions
Encourage adequate rest
Encourage moderate physical activity
Encourage intake of diuretic fluids
Encourage decreased sodium-food intake
Restrict the fluid intake according to the weight gain
Discourage oral stimulants

Nursing Observations
Evaluate the response to teaching

Health Teaching
Advise that highly emotional situations be avoided (during this period)
Describe the manifestations of premenstrual tension
Describe the factors associated with the occurrence of the problem (onset
   usually occurs 4–10 days prior to menstrual onset and primarily between
   the ages of 24 and 40)
Explain the causes of the health problem
Teach the princples of good nutrition (especially during this period)
Explain the reason for and intended effect of the therapy

EVALUATION

See the evaluation criteria for each specific goal in Chapter 2.

INADEQUATE INFORMATION RELATED TO NORMAL BODY CHANGES ASSOCIATED WITH MENOPAUSE

Inadequate Information Related to Premenopause (143,175,367)

ASSESSMENT

Subjective Data
Person confirms a lack of information

Objective Data
Person's actions indicate a lack of information regarding:
   the signs and symptoms of premenopause
   the many alterations in the menstrual cycle that can occur
   the factors related to its occurrence
   general health practices recommended to minimize the discomfort

Related Data

Commonly Related Diseases:
None

POSSIBLE ETIOLOGY

Lack of instruction regarding the temporary progesterone-pituitary gonadotropic hormone imbalance that occurs as the body adapts to the new hormone balance of menopause

NURSING DIAGNOSIS

Inadequate information related to premenopause: lack of information regarding the life stage prior to and leading up to menstruation cessation

PLANNING

Patient Needs	**Primary Nurse-Patient Goals**
Comfort	To achieve comfort
Protection from physical harm	To prevent physical injury
Protection from psychologic threat	To prevent emotional injury
Increased learning	To achieve awareness of needs

NURSING INTERVENTIONS

Nursing Treatments
Approach unhurriedly
Encourage patient questions
Encourage adequate rest
Encourage moderate physical exercise

Health Teaching
Advise that highly emotional situations be avoided
Describe the normal changes associated with premenopause
Describe the normal menstrual cycle changes during premenopause
Describe the factors associated with the occurrence of the problem (onset usually occurs after age 40 but normally occurs earlier in women who have not been pregnant; it usually indicates that menopause is 2–4 years in the future)
Explain the causes of the health problem
Teach the principles of good nutrition

EVALUATION

See the evaluation criteria for each specific goal in Chapter 2.

Inadequate Information Related to Menopause (143,175,367)

ASSESSMENT

Subjective Data
Person confirms a lack of information

Objective Data

Person's actions indicate a lack of information regarding:
the signs and symptoms of menopause
the normal behavior patterns associated with menopause
the effect of menopause on sexual desire or response
the factors related to its occurrence
general health practices recommended to minimize the discomfort

Related Data

Commonly Related Diseases:
None

POSSIBLE ETIOLOGY

Lack of instruction regarding decreased ovarian activity and increased pituitary activity, resulting in estrogen deficiency or menopause

NURSING DIAGNOSIS

Inadequate information related to menopause: lack of information regarding the life stage in which cessation of menstruation has occurred for one year

PLANNING

Patient Needs	**Primary Nurse-Patient Goals**
Comfort	To achieve comfort
Protection from physical harm	To prevent physical injury
Protection from psychologic threat	To prevent emotional injury
Increased learning	To achieve awareness of needs

NURSING INTERVENTIONS

Nursing Treatments
Approach unhurriedly
Encourage patient questions
Encourage adequate rest

Nursing Observations
Evaluate the response to teaching

Health Teaching
Advise that highly emotional situations be avoided
Describe the normal changes associated with menopause
Describe the normal psychic changes common during menopause
Inform that menopause does not interfere with sex life
Describe the factors associated with the occurrence of the problem (usually occurs between ages 44 and 55 but normally occurs earlier in women who have not been pregnant)
Teach the principles of good nutrition
Explain the causes of the health problem
Explain the reason for and intended effect of the therapy

EVALUATION

See the evaluation criteria for each specific goal in Chapter 2.

INADEQUATE INFORMATION RELATED TO SURGICAL BODY CHANGES ASSOCIATED WITH THE FEMALE REPRODUCTIVE SYSTEM

Inadequate Information Related to Postmastectomy Management (71,391)

ASSESSMENT

Subjective Data
Person confirms a lack of information

Objective Data
Person's actions indicate a lack of information regarding:
how or where to obtain breast prosthesis
the need to support the unamputated breast
the need for careful, periodic examination of the remaining breast
the importance of postmastectomy range-of-motion exercises

Related Data
Commonly Related Diseases:
Fibrosarcoma
Lymphosarcoma
Hemangiosarcoma

POSSIBLE ETIOLOGY

Lack of instruction

NURSING DIAGNOSIS

Inadequate information related to postmastectomy management: lack of information regarding how to care for oneself following a mastectomy

PLANNING

Patient Needs	**Primary Nurse-Patient Goals**
Exercise	To achieve exercise
Comfort	To achieve comfort
Protection from physical harm	To prevent physical injury
Mastery and competence in skills	To achieve optimum function
Increased learning	To achieve awareness of needs

NURSING INTERVENTIONS

Nursing Treatments
Approach unhurriedly
Encourage patient questions

Health Teaching
Recommend an appropriate breast prosthesis
Recommend the use of a brassiere for breast support (of the unamputated breast)

Explain the importance of periodic breast inspection (of the unamputated breast)

Teach how to do postmastectomy exercises

Explain the reason for and intended effect of the therapy

EVALUATION

See the evaluation criteria for each specific goal in Chapter 2.

INADEQUATE INFORMATION RELATED TO NORMAL BODY CHANGES ASSOCIATED WITH THE MALE REPRODUCTIVE SYSTEM

Inadequate Information Related to Male Puberty (367)

ASSESSMENT

Subjective Data

Person confirms a lack of information

Objective Data

Person's actions indicate a lack of information regarding:

when male puberty onset normally occurs

the signs and symptoms of male puberty onset

the physiology of male puberty

normal emotional changes associated with male puberty

good health practices recommended during male puberty

Related Data

Commonly Related Diseases:

None

POSSIBLE ETIOLOGY

Lack of instruction regarding the onset of androgen excretion from the adrenal cortex of male youths

NURSING DIAGNOSIS

Inadequate information related to male puberty: lack of information regarding that life stage when male reproductive organs become functionally mature

PLANNING

Patient Needs	**Primary Nurse-Patient Goals**
Comfort	To achieve comfort
Protection from physical harm	To prevent physical injury
Increased learning	To achieve awareness of needs

NURSING INTERVENTIONS

Nursing Treatments
Approach unhurriedly
Encourage patient questions
Encourage adequate rest
Encourage moderate physical exercise

Nursing Observations
Evaluate the response to teaching

Health Teaching
Describe the normal changes associated with male puberty
Describe the normal behavior pattern common during male puberty
Describe the factors associated with the occurrence of the problem (onset of
   male puberty occurs about age 14–15)
Teach the principles of good nutrition

EVALUATION

See the evaluation criteria for each specific goal in Chapter 2.

Inadequate Information Related to Male Climacteric (367)

ASSESSMENT

Subjective Data
Person confirms a lack of information

Objective Data
Person's actions indicate a lack of information regarding:
   when male climacteric onset normally occurs
   the signs and symptoms of male climacteric
   the cause of male climacteric
   good health practices recommended during male climacteric

Related Data
Commonly Related Diseases:
None

POSSIBLE ETIOLOGY

Lack of instruction regarding the onset of decreased androgen excretion
from the adrenal cortex

NURSING DIAGNOSIS

Inadequate information related to male climacteric: lack of information regarding that life stage when there is gradual reduction of male sexual potency

PLANNING

Patient Needs   **Primary Nurse-Patient Goals**
Comfort   To achieve comfort

Protection from physical harm   To prevent physical injury
Protection from psychologic threat   To prevent emotional injury
Increased learning   To achieve awareness of needs

NURSING INTERVENTIONS

Nursing Treatments
Approach unhurriedly
Encourage patient questions
Encourage adequate rest
Encourage moderate physical exercise

Nursing Observations
Evaluate the response to teaching

Health Teaching
Describe the normal changes associated with male climacteric
Describe the factors associated with the occurrence of the problem (onset
    occurs around age 50 with almost complete quieting by age 60)
Explain the causes of the health problem
Teach the principles of good nutrition

EVALUATION

See the evaluation criteria for each specific goal in Chapter 2.

INADEQUATE INFORMATION RELATED TO REPRODUCTIVE SYSTEM BLEEDING

Inadequate Information Related to Abnormal Vaginal Bleeding (224,391)

ASSESSMENT

Objective Data
Person's actions indicate a lack of information regarding:
    when menstrual bleeding is abnormal
    that vaginal bleeding during pregnancy requires immediate medical at-
        tention
    that any abnormal vaginal bleeding should be brought to the physician's
        attention
    the causes of abnormal vaginal bleeding

Related Data
Commonly Related Conditions:
Cervical, endocervical, or endometrial polyps
Commonly Related Diseases:
Uterine carcinoma
Endometriosis
Ectopic pregnancy

Ovarian granulosa cell tumor
Cervical carcinoma
Fundus carcinoma

POSSIBLE ETIOLOGY

Lack of instruction

NURSING DIAGNOSIS

Inadequate information related to abnormal vaginal bleeding: lack of information regarding vaginal bleeding occurring in unusual amounts or at unusual intervals

PLANNING

Patient Needs	**Primary Nurse-Patient Goals**
Comfort	To achieve comfort
Protection from physical harm	To prevent physical injury
Increased learning	To achieve awareness of needs

NURSING INTERVENTIONS

Nursing Treatments
Approach unhurriedly
Encourage patient questions

Nursing Observations
Evaluate the response to teaching

Health Teaching
Describe the characteristics of abnormal vaginal bleeding
Instruct to immediately report serious symptoms
Explain the causes of the health problem

EVALUATION

See the evaluation criteria for each specific goal in Chapter 2.

Inadequate Information Related to Extragenital Menstrual Bleeding

ASSESSMENT

Subjective Data
Person confirms a lack of information

Objective Data
Person's actions indicate a lack of information regarding:
    bleeding from the nose, mouth, bladder, eyes, ears, breast, skin, or gums
        occurring during or just prior to menstruation
    the cause of the bleeding

POSSIBLE ETIOLOGY

Lack of instruction regarding a decreased platelet count that occurs 14 days prior to menstruation possibly resulting in extragenital bleeding

NURSING DIAGNOSIS

Inadequate information related to extragenital menstrual bleeding: lack of information regarding bleeding that occurs in other body areas, simultaneous with, or just prior to menstruation

PLANNING

Patient Needs

Protection from physical harm

Increased learning

Primary Nurse-Patient Goals

To prevent physical injury

To achieve awareness of needs

NURSING INTERVENTIONS

Nursing Treatments

Approach unhurriedly

Encourage patient questions

Reassure verbally (that it is a normal occurrence)

Nursing Observations

Evaluate the response to teaching

Health Teaching

Explain the causes of the health problem

EVALUATION

See the evaluation criteria for each specific goal in Chapter 2.

Inadequate Information Related to Postsurgical Vaginal Bleeding (224)

ASSESSMENT

Subjective Data

Person confirms a lack of information

Objective Data

Person's actions indicate a lack of information regarding:

the fact that following a dilatation and currettement procedure, a red-brown bloody discharge can be expected for several days

the fact that following a hysterectomy, bright blood, a red-brown discharge, or spotting can occur for as long as 6 weeks

the causes of the bleeding

recommended methods for minimizing the bleeding

Related Data

Commonly Related Diseases:

Uterine carcinoma

Endometriosis

POSSIBLE ETIOLOGY

Lack of instruction regarding the fact that post-D&C bleeding is caused by surgical scraping of the uterine lining; that posthysterectomy bleeding is caused by slow healing of the surgical incision made at the top of the vagina in order to free the cervix from the vagina

NURSING DIAGNOSIS

Inadequate information related to postsurgical vaginal bleeding: lack of information regarding bleeding that normally occurs following vaginal surgery

PLANNING

Patient Needs	Primary Nurse-Patient Goals
Comfort	To achieve comfort
Protection from physical harm	To prevent physical injury
Increased learning	To achieve awareness of needs

NURSING INTERVENTIONS

Nursing Treatments
Approach unhurriedly
Encourage patient questions
Reassure verbally (that it is a normal occurrence)
Encourage adequate rest

Nursing Observations
Evaluate the response to teaching

Health Teaching
Explain the causes of the health problem
Describe those symptoms which should be reported (profuse bleeding)
Advise not to stand for prolonged periods
Inform that heavy lifting should be avoided
Instruct to avoid pushing and pulling activities
Advise against using tampons
Advise not to take enemas and laxatives
Inform that elimination straining should be avoided
Instruct that douching be avoided
Advise daily bathing (in the shower, not the tub)

EVALUATION

See the evaluation criteria for each specific goal in Chapter 2.

27.
NURSING DIAGNOSES RELATED TO
The Respiratory
System

AIRWAY PATENCY DEPENDENCE

Dependence on Airway Patency Maintenance (32,300)

ASSESSMENT

Subjective Data

Person relies on nurses for:
  intermittent suctioning or removal of secretions
  liquification of thick, tenacious secretions
  positioning for maximum oxygenation

Objective Data

Person has a tracheostomy, endotracheal tube, airway tube, or is unable to
  clear the throat, blow his nose, or cough

Related Data

Commonly Related Conditions:
Quadraplegia
Monoplegia

Commonly Related Diseases:
Myasthenia gravis
Multiple sclerosis
Cerebral concussion
Cerebral vascular accident
Cancer of throat
Chest trauma
Pneumothorax

POSSIBLE ETIOLOGY

The need for an artificial airway. Muscle weakness or paralysis that prevents clearing of one's own airway.

NURSING DIAGNOSIS

Dependence on airway patency maintenance: reliance on nurses to maintain an open, clear airway for adequate breathing

PLANNING

Patient Needs	**Primary Nurse-Patient Goals**
Oxygen	To maintain oxygen to all cells
Comfort	To achieve comfort
Protection from physical harm	To prevent physical injury
Dependence	To achieve comfort
Increased learning	To achieve awareness of needs

NURSING INTERVENTIONS

Nursing Treatments
Suction the airway (as needed)
Encourage coughing
Encourage deep breathing
Clear nasal secretions
Place in the sitting position (when possible)
Place in the side-lying (Sim's) position (during sleep or unconsciousness)
Administer vaporized air (for thick secretions)
Provide standby emergency equipment (suction machine, airway tube, tracheostomy tray, etc.)
Attend the patient constantly

Nursing Observations
Inspect the chest for respiratory rate and rhythm
Inspect the chest for symmetrical expansion
Auscultate the chest for abnormal breath sounds
Auscultate the chest for abnormal voice sounds
Auscultate the chest for lung aeration
Auscultate the chest for rales and rhonchi
Percuss the chest for abnormal resonance
Percuss the posterior chest for decreased diaphragmatic descent
Monitor blood studies for abnormal gas exchange
Observe for dyspnea
Observe for mouth breathing
Observe for nasal congestion
Observe for nasal flare
Palpate the chest for abnormal vocal fremitus

Health Teaching
Describe those symptoms which should be reported (dyspnea)
Explain the reason for and intended effect of the therapy

Medical Treatments Performed by Nurses
Administer heated humidified oxygen
   OR
Administer humidified oxygen

EVALUATION

See the evaluation criteria for each specific goal in Chapter 2.

AIRWAY PATENCY, INCOMPLETE

Airway Obstruction (32,300)

ASSESSMENT

Subjective Data
Dyspnea
Intense anxiety
Air hunger

Objective Data
Drowsiness
Wheezing, snoring, or grunting respirations
Cyanosis
Rib retraction
Absent or decreased breath sounds
Mouth breathing
Nasal flare
Respiratory stridor
Choking
Sweating
Twitching
Coarse tremor

Related Data
Commonly Related Conditions:
Analgesic or sedative overdose
Commonly Related Diseases:
None
    OR
Cerebral vascular accident
Cervical spinal cord injury
Guillian-Barre syndrome
Epilepsy

POSSIBLE ETIOLOGY

Inhalation of a foreign body into the respiratory passage. Infection.
Laryngeal spasm. Poor control over respiratory and swallowing reflexes.

NURSING DIAGNOSIS

Airway obstruction: the inability of air to pass through the respiratory passage

PLANNING

Patient Needs	**Primary Nurse-Patient Goals**
Oxygen	To maintain oxygen to all cells

Waste elimination

To maintain regulating mechanisms and functions

Comfort

To achieve comfort

Protection from physical harm

To prevent physical injury

Increased learning

To achieve awareness of needs

NURSING INTERVENTIONS

Nursing Treatments

Remove foreign objects
Suction the airway
   OR
Hold the jaw forward to maintain an airway
   OR
Insert an oral airway
   OR
Apply the Heimlich maneuver
Resuscitate breathing (ET)
   OR
Perform a tracheostomy (ET) (as a last resort)
Place in the sitting position
Encourage deep breathing (once the airway is cleared)
Administer humidified oxygen (ET) (for a short period once the airway is cleared)
Remove constrictive clothing
Attend the patient constantly (until the episode subsides)
Provide standby emergency equipment (oxygen, suction machine)

Nursing Observations

Inspect the chest for respiratory rate and rhythm
Inspect the chest for symmetrical expansion
Auscultate the chest for abnormal breath sounds
Auscultate the chest for abnormal voice sounds
Auscultate the chest for lung aeration
Auscultate the chest for rales and rhonchi
Palpate the chest for abnormal vocal fremitus
Percuss the chest for abnormal resonance
Percuss the posterior chest for decreased diaphragmatic descent
Monitor blood studies for abnormal gas exchange

Health Teaching

Explain the causes of the health problem
Describe those symptoms which should be reported (dyspnea, pain)
Inform that airway noise indicates obstruction
Recommend that bones be removed from foods before eating
Recommend that food be cut into small bite sizes
Explain the reason for and intended effect of the therapy

EVALUATION

See the evaluation criteria for each specific goal in Chapter 2.

AIRWAY PATENCY, POTENTIAL INCOMPLETE

Potential Airway Obstruction (32,300,325)

ASSESSMENT

Subjective Data
Dyspnea

Objective Data
Coma
Paralysis
Seizure
Cyanosis
Drowsiness
Large or swollen tongue
Wired jaw
Nasal edema
Adenoid enlargement
Nasal polyps
Thick airway secretions
Constricting objects about the neck
Foreign objects in the mouth
Postanesthesia vomiting
Rapid eating or drinking
Laughing, deep breathing, or severe coughing while eating
Eating while lying down

Related Data
Commonly Related Diseases:
Esophageal stricture
Cerebral vascular accident
Epilepsy
Alcoholism
Cerebral palsy

POSSIBLE ETIOLOGY

Structural abnormality of a respiratory organ. Poor control over respiratory and swallowing reflexes. Poor preventive health practices.

NURSING DIAGNOSIS

Potential airway obstruction: the possibility that air will be unable to pass through the respiratory tract

PLANNING

Patient Needs
Protection from physical harm
Increased learning

Primary Nurse-Patient Goals
To prevent physical injury
To achieve awareness of needs

NURSING INTERVENTIONS

Nursing Treatments

Administer vaporized air (for thick secretions)
Insert an oral airway (as needed)
Suction the airway (as needed)
Elevate the head (especially while eating)
Feed slowly
Inflate the airway tube cuff (before feeding)
Discourage talking while eating
Refrain from distracting the patient while he swallows
Restrict the intake to nothing by mouth (when there is cerebral impairment)
Place in the side-lying (Sim's) position (postanesthesia, during coma, or seizure)
Encourage coughing
  AND
Encourage deep breathing
Refrain from using a cotton-filled gauze tracheostomy dressing
Drain condensation from the nebulizer tubing periodically
Provide standby emergency equipment (suction machine, airway tube, tracheostomy tray, wire cutters)

Nursing Observations

Inspect the chest for respiratory rate and rhythm
Inspect the chest for symmetrical expansion
Auscultate the chest for abnormal breath sounds
Auscultate the chest for abnormal voice sounds
Auscultate the chest for lung aeration
Auscultate the chest for rales and rhonchi
Palpate the chest for abnormal vocal fremitus
Percuss the chest for abnormal resonance
Percuss the posterior chest for decreased diaphragmatic descent
Inspect for foreign bodies
Observe for cyanosis
Observe for dyspnea
Observe for mouth breathing
Observe for nasal congestion
Observe for nasal flare

Health Teaching

Explain that fluids should not be given to persons unable to swallow
Inform that airway noise indicates obstruction
Recommend that bones be removed from foods before eating
Recommend thorough food chewing
Explain the reason for and intended effect of the therapy

EVALUATION

See the evaluation criteria for each specific goal in Chapter 2.

PULMONARY AERATION, ALTERED

Inadequate Pulmonary Ventilation (30,300)

ASSESSMENT

Subjective Data
Anxiety
Dyspnea

Objective Data
Cyanosis
Drowsiness
Coma
Decreased movement of the chest
Absent, decreased, or wheezing breath sounds
Absent voice sounds
Thoracic dullness
Rate less than eight times a minute
Sweating
Coarse tremor
Twitching

Related Data
Commonly Related Diseases:
Bronchial asthma
Emphysema
Pneumonia
Lung abscess
Croup
Tuberculosis
Myasthenia gravis
Congestive heart failure
Pleurisy

POSSIBLE ETIOLOGY

Decreased respiratory muscle strength. Pain inhibited normal respiratory depth. Severe abdominal pressure causing pressure on the diaphragm. Drug-depressed respirations. Thoracic tumor. Excessively enlarged heart. A fluid-distended pericardium compressing the lung.

NURSING DIAGNOSIS

Inadequate pulmonary ventilation (respiratory depression): a diminished incomplete or partial inflation of one or both lungs with air

PLANNING

Patient Needs	Primary Nurse-Patient Goals
Oxygen	To maintain oxygen to all cells

Protection from physical harm	To prevent physical injury
Increased learning	To achieve awareness of needs

NURSING INTERVENTIONS

Nursing Treatments
Change the patient's position frequently
Encourage coughing
    AND   } (periodically and frequently)
Encourage deep breathing
Place in the sitting position
Ambulate the patient (as soon and as often as possible)
Withhold the drugs (sedatives)

Nursing Observations
Inspect the chest for respiratory rate and rhythm
Inspect the chest for symmetrical expansion
Auscultate the chest for abnormal breath sounds
Auscultate the chest for abnormal voice sounds
Auscultate the chest for lung aeration
Auscultate the chest for rales and rhonchi
Palpate the chest for abnormal vocal fremitus
Percuss the chest for abnormal resonance
Percuss the posterior chest for decreased diaphragmatic descent
Monitor blood studies for abnormal gas exchange
Observe for cyanosis

Health Teaching
Explain the causes of the health problem
Explain the reason for and intended effect of the therapy

Medical Treatments Performed by Nurses
Administer heated humidified oxygen
Administer intermittent positive pressure breathing

EVALUATION

See the evaluation criteria for each specific goal in Chapter 2.

Excessive Carbon Dioxide Retention (325)

ASSESSMENT

Subjective Data
Dyspnea

Objective Data
Cyanosis
Coma
Drowsiness
Twitching
Sweating
Coarse tremor

Absent or decreased breath sounds
Prolonged expiratory breath sounds
Decreased voice sounds
Thick secretions

Related Data

Laboratory Findings:
Increased blood CO_2 content

Commonly Related Diseases:
Emphysema
Asthma

POSSIBLE ETIOLOGY

Loss of elastic tissue in alveoli. Bronchiol or bronchiolar obstruction or narrowing. Increased lung volume from trapped air. Allergic reaction.

NURSING DIAGNOSIS

Excessive carbon dioxide retention: the inability to adequately eliminate carbon dioxide from the lungs

PLANNING

Patient Needs	**Primary Nurse-Patient Goals**
Waste elimination	To maintain regulating mechanisms and functions
Comfort	To achieve comfort
Protection from physical harm	To prevent physical injury
Increased learning	To achieve awareness of needs

NURSING INTERVENTIONS

Nursing Treatments
Place in the sitting position
Do not place in the flat position
Remove constrictive clothing
Withhold the oxygen therapy (if the blood CO_2 content is 70–75vol/100ml)

Nursing Observations
Inspect the chest for respiratory rate and rhythm
Inspect the chest for symmetrical expansion
Auscultate the chest for abnormal breath sounds
Auscultate the chest for lung aeration
Auscultate the chest for rales and rhonchi
Percuss the chest for abnormal resonance
Monitor blood studies for abnormal gas exchange

Health Teaching
Explain the causes of the health problem
Describe those symptoms which should be reported (severe respiratory distress)
Teach how to do abdominal breathing

Teach how to do resistive breathing exercises
Explain the reason for and intended effect of the therapy

Medical Treatments Performed by Nurses
Administer heated humidified oxygen (at no more than 1–2 liters per minute)
Administer intermittent positive pressure breathing
Give the prescribed drugs (sedatives, bronchodilators)

EVALUATION

See the evaluation criteria for each specific goal in Chapter 2.

PULMONARY AERATION, POTENTIAL ALTERED

Potential Inadequate Pulmonary Ventilation (30,32)

ASSESSMENT

Subjective Data
Generalized weakness
Respiratory muscle weakness
Pain at the site of surgery

Objective Data
Recent administration of anesthesia
Heavy sedation
Prolonged bed rest
Prolonged immobility

Related Data
Commonly Related Diseases:
Any disease requiring surgical intervention
Cerebral vascular accident
Cervical spinal cord injury
Thoracic spinal cord injury

POSSIBLE ETIOLOGY

Respiratory depression. Inability to control breathing.

NURSING DIAGNOSIS

Potential inadequate pulmonary ventilation: the possibility that there will be diminished, incomplete, or partial inflation of one or both lungs with air

PLANNING

Patient Needs	**Primary Nurse-Patient Goals**
Oxygen	To maintain oxygen to all cells
Waste elimination	To maintain regulating mechanisms and functions

Activity	To achieve activity
Protection from physical harm	To prevent physical injury
Increased learning	To achieve awareness of needs

NURSING INTERVENTIONS

Nursing Treatments
Ambulate the patient (as much and as soon as possible)
Change the patient's position frequently
Suction the airway (periodically)
Encourage coughing
   AND
Encourage deep breathing
Encourage alternate rest and activity
Withhold the drugs (sedatives)

Nursing Observations
Inspect the chest for respiratory rate and rhythm
Inspect the chest for symmetrical expansion
Auscultate the chest for abnormal breath sounds
Auscultate the chest for abnormal voice sounds
Auscultate the chest for lung aeration
Auscultate the chest for rales and rhonchi
Palpate the chest for abnormal vocal fremitus
Percuss the chest for abnormal resonance
Percuss the posterior chest for decreased diaphragmatic descent
Monitor blood studies for abnormal gas exchange
Observe for complaints of pain (chest)
Observe for cyanosis
Observe for dyspnea
Observe for fatigue
Palpate the pulse for rate (tachycardia), rhythm, and volume

Health Teaching
Explain the causes of the health problem
Explain the reason for and intended effect of the therapy

EVALUATION

See the evaluation criteria for each specific goal in Chapter 2.

RESPIRATORY EFFORT, IRREGULAR

Distressed Respiratory Effort (32,300,325)

ASSESSMENT

Subjective Data
Air hunger

Anxiety
Weakness
Fatigue
Painful breathing

Objective Data
Restlessness
Irregular or difficult chest movements
Abnormal respiratory rate, rhythm, or depth

Related Data
Commonly Related Conditions:
Orthopnea
Flail chest
Chest lag
Pleural effusion
Pulmonary atelectasis
Increased intracranial pressure

Commonly Related Diseases:
Pneumonia
Congestive heart failure
Pleurisy
Pericarditis
Rib fracture
Bronchiectasis
Tuberculosis
Poliomyelitis
Myasthenia gravis
Guillian-Barre syndrome

POSSIBLE ETIOLOGY

Cardiac insufficiency. Inadequate airway. Diaphragmatic paralysis. Cyclic respiratory understimulation or overstimulation. Impaired respiratory musculature. Drug oversedation.

NURSING DIAGNOSIS

Distressed respiratory effort: an uncomfortable, increased effort during respiratory inspiration and expiration

PLANNING

Patient Needs	**Primary Nurse-Patient Goals**
Oxygen	To maintain oxygen to all cells
Waste elimination	To maintain regulating mechanisms and functions
Rest	To achieve rest
Comfort	To achieve comfort

Protection from physical harm
Increased learning

To prevent physical injury
To achieve awareness of needs

NURSING INTERVENTIONS

Nursing Treatments
Position comfortably
Elevate the head
   OR
Place in the sitting position
Encourage deep breathing
Suction the airway (as needed)
Administer vaporized air
Encourage adequate rest
Remove constrictive clothing
Maintain a cool room temperature
Maintain adequate atmospheric humidity
Maintain adequate room ventilation
Refrain from performing nonessential procedures
Discourage smoking

Nursing Observations
Inspect the chest for respiratory rate and rhythm
Inspect the chest for symmetrical expansion
Auscultate the chest for abnormal breath sounds
Auscultate the chest for abnormal voice sounds
Auscultate the chest for lung aeration
Auscultate the chest for rales and rhonchi
Palpate the chest for abnormal vocal fremitus
Percuss the chest for abnormal resonance
Percuss the chest for cracked-pot sounds
Percuss the posterior chest for decreased diaphragmatic descent
Monitor blood studies for abnormal gas exchange
Observe for complaints of pain
Observe for cyanosis
Observe for dyspnea
Observe for fatigue

Health Teaching
Explain the causes of the health problem
Explain the reason for and intended effect of the therapy

Medical Treatments Performed by Nurses
Administer heated humidified oxygen
Administer intermittent positive pressure breathing
Give the prescribed drugs

EVALUATION

See the evaluation criteria for each specific goal in Chapter 2.

RESPIRATORY DISCOMFORTS

Cough Discomfort (325,391)

ASSESSMENT

Subjective Data
Fatigue
Pain, sometimes
Dyspnea

Objective Data
Prolonged, persistent coughing
Productive or unproductive

Related Data
Commonly Related Diseases:
Aortic aneurysm
Laryngeal diptheria
Bronchogenic carcinoma
Acute laryngitis (inflammatory croup)
Tuberculosis
Pleurisy
Asthma
Emphysema
Mitral stenosis
Pneumonia

POSSIBLE ETIOLOGY

Pulmonary irritation from lesions. Bronchial irritation from tobacco smoking. Respiratory obstruction. Laryngeal spasms or irritation.

NURSING DIAGNOSIS

Cough discomfort: the discomfort of persistent coughing

PLANNING

Patient Needs	Primary Nurse-Patient Goals
Waste elimination	To maintain regulating mechanisms and functions
Rest	To achieve rest
Comfort	To achieve comfort
Protection from physical harm	To prevent physical injury
Increased learning	To achieve awareness of needs

NURSING INTERVENTIONS

Nursing Treatments
Elevate the head
    OR
Place in the sitting position
Increase fluid intake to about 2000 cc daily
Administer vaporized air

Give warm liquids
Refrain from giving iced liquids
Refrain from giving milk or milk products (if they stimulate coughing)
Give coughdrops
Give nonprescription drugs (ExR) (antitussives)
Encourage adequate rest
Discourage smoking
Remove constrictive clothing (around the neck and chest)
Maintain adequate atmospheric humidity
Maintain a warm room temperature

Nursing Observations
Inspect the chest for respiratory rate and rhythm
Inspect the chest for symmetrical expansion
Auscultate the chest for abnormal breath sounds
Auscultate the chest for abnormal voice sounds
Auscultate the chest for lung aeration
Auscultate the chest for rales and rhonchi
Percuss the chest for abnormal resonance
Percuss the posterior chest for decreased diaphragmatic descent
Monitor the laboratory findings of sputum analysis
Observe the characteristics of the cough
Observe for complaints of pain
Observe for fatigue

Health Teaching
Advise against exposure to airborne irritants
Explain how to prevent coughing
Emphasize the danger of breathing cold air
Instruct to increase fluid intake
Instruct to change position frequently
Explain the causes of the health problem
Explain the reason for and intended effect of the therapy

Medical Treatments Performed by Nurses
Give the prescribed drugs
Place on the prescribed bed rest

EVALUATION

See the evaluation criteria for each specific goal in Chapter 2.

Hiccough Discomfort (32,113,247)

ASSESSMENT

Subjective Data
Fatigue or exhaustion
Nausea

Objective Data
Persistent hiccough spasm
Coarse "hic" sound
Vomiting, sometimes

Related Data

Commonly Related Conditions:
Indigestion
Tobacco smoking

Commonly Related Diseases:
None
  OR
Alcoholism
Conversion hysteria psychoneurosis
Meningitis
Encephalitis
Subdural hematoma
Myocardial infarction
Esophageal obstruction
Pneumonia pleurisy
Diaphragmatic hernia
Splenic infarction
Pancreatitis
Cholera
Glomerulonephritis
Peritonitis

POSSIBLE ETIOLOGY

Contractions of the diaphragm caused by irritation of the phrenic nerve which controls the muscles separating the chest from the abdomen

NURSING DIAGNOSIS

Hiccough discomfort: the discomfort of prolonged, spasmodic contractions of the diaphragm

PLANNING

Patient Needs	Primary Nurse-Patient Goals
Acid-base balance	To maintain regulating mechanisms and functions
Rest	To achieve rest
Comfort	To achieve comfort
Increased learning	To achieve awareness of needs

NURSING INTERVENTIONS

Nursing Treatments
Position comfortably
Encourage adequate rest
Encourage deep breathing
Give nonprescrition drugs (ExR) (antacids)
  OR
Give sugar (one teaspoon, dry)
  OR

Give warm liquids
 OR
Provide a paper bag for breathing (3–5 minutes)
Maintain adequate atmospheric humidity
Maintain adequate room ventilation
Provide standby emergency equipment (oxygen)
Reduce the demands placed upon the patient

Nursing Observations
Inspect the chest for respiratory rate and rhythm
Inspect the abdomen for distention
Observe for fatigue

Health Teaching
Explain the causes of the health problem
Teach how to do breath-holding
Explain the reason for and intended effect of the therapy

Medical Treatments Performed by Nurses
Give the prescribed drugs (sedatives if other measures fail)

EVALUATION

See the evaluation criteria for each specific goal in Chapter 2.

Mouth-Breathing Discomfort (32)

ASSESSMENT

Subjective Data
Mouth and throat dryness

Objective Data
Chronically open mouth
Dry, cracked lips
Anorexia

Related Data

Commonly Related Conditions:
Common cold

Commonly Related Diseases:
Nasal carcinoma
Nasopharyngitis

POSSIBLE ETIOLOGY

Inability to obtain sufficient air through an obstructed nasal passage. Respiratory disorder.

NURSING DIAGNOSIS

Mouth-breathing discomfort: the discomfort of having to keep the mouth open to breathe

PLANNING

Patient Needs

Oxygen

Comfort

Protection from physical harm

Increased learning

Primary Nurse-Patient Goals

To maintain oxygen to all cells

To achieve comfort

To prevent physical injury

To achieve awareness of needs

NURSING INTERVENTIONS

Nursing Treatments

Clear nasal secretions

Lubricate the lips

Moisten the mouth with cracked ice

Refresh with a mouthwash

Administer vaporized air

Increase fluid intake to about 2000 cc daily

Place in the sitting position

Position comfortably

Discourage smoking

Nursing Observations

Inspect the chest for respiratory rate and rhythm

Inspect the chest for symmetrical expansion

Auscultate the chest for lung aeration

Inspect the nose for asymmetry

Inspect the nose for polyps

Observe for dyspnea

Observe for fatigue

Observe for mouth breathing

Observe for nasal flare

Health Teaching

Advise against exposure to airborne irritants

Advise gentle nose blowing

Explain the causes of the health problem

Explain the reason for and intended effect of the therapy

EVALUATION

See the evaluation criteria for each specific goal in Chapter 2.

Nasal Congestion (113,325)

ASSESSMENT

Subjective Data

Crusty, dry nasal sensation

Difficult nasal breathing

Objective Data

Nasal cartilage redness

Nasal tissue edema

Nasal drainage
Mouth breathing, sometimes

Related Data

Commonly Related Diseases:
Acute sinusitis
Rhinitis

POSSIBLE ETIOLOGY

Increased blood and fluid volume within the vessels in the tissue surrounding the nasal bones resulting in mucosa swelling

NURSING DIAGNOSIS

Nasal congestion: inability to breathe through one or both sides of the nose

PLANNING

Patient Needs	**Primary Nurse-Patient Goals**
Oxygen	To maintain oxygen to all cells
Rest	To achieve rest
Comfort	To achieve comfort
Cleanliness	To achieve good hygiene
Protection from physical harm	To prevent physical injury
Increased learning	To achieve awareness of needs

NURSING INTERVENTIONS

Nursing Treatments
Administer vaporized air
Increase fluid intake to about 2000 cc daily
Give warm liquids
Refrain from giving milk or milk products
Give nonprescription drugs (ExR) (decongestants)
Maintain adequate atmospheric humidity
Maintain a warm room temperature
Discourage smoking

Nursing Observations
Inspect the chest for respiratory rate and rhythm
Auscultate the chest for lung aeration
Observe for cyanosis
Observe for dyspnea
Observe for fatigue

Health Teaching
Emphasize the danger of excessive use of nosedrops
Advise gentle nose blowing
Explain the causes of the health problem
Explain the reason for and intended effect of the therapy

EVALUATION

See the evaluation criteria for each specific goal in Chapter 2.

Postnasal Drainage (137)

ASSESSMENT

Subjective Data
Throat tickling sensation

Objective Data
Hacking
Coughing
Nasal mucous membrane edema

Related Data
Commonly Related Diseases:
Chronic rhinitis
Allergic rhinitis
Acute sinusitis
Bronchitis

POSSIBLE ETIOLOGY

Thick, fluid-filled mucous membranes causing drainage. Allergic response.
Nasal irritation from smoke. Emotional stress. A long, soft palate.

NURSING DIAGNOSIS

Postnasal drainage: the drainage of nasal secretions to the back of the nasal
cavity and down into the throat

PLANNING

Patient Needs	**Primary Nurse-Patient Goals**
Comfort	To achieve comfort
Cleanliness	To achieve good hygiene
Protection from physical harm	To prevent physical injury, infection
Increased learning	To achieve awareness of needs

NURSING INTERVENTIONS

Nursing Treatments
Elevate the head
   OR
Place in the sitting position
Administer vaporized air
Give nonprescription drugs (ExR) (antihistamines)
Maintain adequate atmospheric humidity
Discourage smoking

Nursing Observations
Inspect the chest for respiratory rate and rhythm
Inspect the nasal turbinates for abnormalities
Inspect the nose for symmetry
Observe for nasal congestion

Health Teaching
Advise against exposure to airborne irritants

Advise against drawing secretions to the back of the throat
Advise frequent nose blowing
Advise gentle nose blowing
Explain the causes of the health problem
Explain the reason for and intended effect of the therapy

EVALUATION

See the evaluation criteria for each specific goal in Chapter 2.

Sinus Congestion (137,452)

ASSESSMENT

Subjective Data
Malaise
Morning headache
Sensitivity to light
Dizziness
Pain in the forehead or above the eye (frontal sinus)
Pain in the upper teeth, cheek, or side of the nasal bridge (maxillary sinus)
Pain behind the eye or in the neck (sphenoid or ethmoid sinus)

Objective Data
Sinus tenderness
Periorbital or forehead edema
Swollen nasal turbinates
Nasal drainage

Related Data
Discomfort is increased by smoking, drinking alcohol, eating spicy foods, and damp, chilling weather
Commonly Related Diseases:
Acute or chronic sinusitis
Aerosinusitis

POSSIBLE ETIOLOGY

Thickened sinus mucosa resulting in inadequate drainage of the cavity. Allergic response. Viral or bacterial (usually streptococcal, pneumococcal, or staphylococcal) infection. Emotional stress.

NURSING DIAGNOSIS

Sinus congestion: increased fluid or swollen mucosa of the sinus cavity

PLANNING

Patient Needs	**Primary Nurse-Patient Goals**
Water-salt balance	To maintain fluid and electrolyte balance
Waste elimination	To maintain regulating mechanisms and functions
Rest	To achieve rest

Comfort	To achieve comfort
Cleanliness	To achieve good hygiene
Protection from physical harm	To prevent physical injury, infection
Increased learning	To achieve awareness of needs

NURSING INTERVENTIONS

Nursing Treatments
Apply a warm, moist compress (to the sinus area)
Administer vaporized air
Give warm liquids
Increase fluid intake to about 2000 cc daily
Elevate the head (especially during sleep)
Position comfortably (on the unaffected side)
Give nonprescription drugs (ExR) (decongestants and vasoconstricting nasal spray)
Discourage oral stimulants
Discourage smoking
Maintain adequate atmospheric humidity

Nursing Observations
Inspect the chest for respiratory rate and rhythm
Inspect the nasal turbinates for abnormalities
Observe for complaints of headache
Observe for fatigue
Observe for mouth breathing
Observe for nasal congestion

Health Teaching
Advise against exposure to airborne irritants
Advise against exposure to inclement weather
Advise gentle nose blowing
Explain the causes of the health problem
Explain the reason for and intended effect of the therapy

EVALUATION

See the evaluation criteria for each specific goal in Chapter 2.

Sneezing Discomfort (11,413)

ASSESSMENT

Subjective Data
Fatigue
Burning nasal irritation

Objective Data
Prolonged persistent sneezing
Nasal secretions

Related Data
Commonly Related Conditions:
Sinusitis

Allergic rhinitis
Rhinitis

POSSIBLE ETIOLOGY

Spasmodic contraction of expiratory muscles. An attempt to clear the nasal passage. Irritation from bright sunlight.

NURSING DIAGNOSIS

Sneezing discomfort: the discomfort of persistent sneezing

PLANNING

Patient Needs	Primary Nurse-Patient Goals
Rest	To achieve rest
Comfort	To achieve comfort
Cleanliness	To achieve good hygiene
Protection from physical harm	To prevent physical injury, infection
Increased learning	To achieve awareness of needs

NURSING INTERVENTIONS

Nursing Treatments
Clear nasal secretions
Lubricate the external nares
Damp-dust the room of allergy-prone persons daily
Discourage smoking
Encourage adequate rest
Give nonprescription drugs (ExR) (antihistamines)
Maintain a cool room temperature
Maintain adequate atmospheric humidity

Nursing Observations
Inspect the chest for respiratory rate and rhythm
Inspect for foreign bodies
Inspect the nasal turbinates for abnormalities
Inspect the nose for asymmetry
Inspect the nose for polyps
Observe for fatigue

Health Teaching
Advise against exposure to airborne irritants
Advise gentle nose blowing
Explain how to prevent sneezing
Inform that cleanliness is basic to health
Explain the causes of the health problem
Explain the reason for and intended effect of the therapy

EVALUATION

See the evaluation criteria for each specific goal in Chapter 2.

RESPIRATORY SECRETIONS, ABNORMAL

Copious Airway Secretions (300,301)

ASSESSMENT

Subjective Data
Dyspnea, if secretions are not removed

Objective Data
Irregular chest movement
Grunting respirations
Profuse drainage from an airway passage
Thin secretions
Gurgling sound
Coughing

Related Data
Commonly Related Diseases:
Pneumonia
Nasopharangitis

POSSIBLE ETIOLOGY

Infection or irritation of the respiratory mucosa. Foreign body.

NURSING DIAGNOSIS

Copious airway secretions: the production of large amounts of drainage from the respiratory airway

PLANNING

Patient Needs	Primary Nurse-Patient Goals
Water-salt balance	To maintain fluid and electrolyte balance
Waste elimination	To maintain regulating mechanisms and functions
Comfort	To achieve comfort
Cleanliness	To achieve good hygiene
Protection from physical harm	To prevent physical injury, infection
Increased learning	To achieve awareness of needs

NURSING INTERVENTIONS

Nursing Treatments
Suction the airway
Increase fluid intake to about 2000 cc daily
Administer vaporized air
Place in the sitting position (as much as possible)
Bathe locally (if secretions come in contact with the skin)
Provide disposable tissue
Maintain adequate atmospheric humidity

Nursing Observations
Inspect the chest for respiratory rate and rhythm
Inspect the chest for symmetrical expansion
Auscultate the chest for lung aeration
Inspect the sputum for characteristics
Monitor the oral temperature
Observe the characteristics of the cough
Observe for complaints of pain
Observe for complaints of respiratory muscle weakness
Observe for dyspnea
Observe for fatigue
Observe for complaints of weakness

Health Teaching
Advise against exposure to airborne irritants
Advise against exposure to inclement weather
Instruct to lean forward for improved ventilation
Teach postural drainage
Inform that cleanliness is basic to health
Explain the causes of the health problem
Explain the reason for and intended effect of the therapy

Medical Treatments Performed by Nurses
Give the prescribed drugs

EVALUATION

See the evaluation criteria for each specific goal in Chapter 2.

Pulmonary Secretion Congestion (113,453)

ASSESSMENT

Subjective Data
Fatigue
Malaise

Objective Data
Loose, productive cough
Purulent sputum
Bubbling, crackling, musical rales
Fever, sometimes

Related Data
Commonly Related Conditions:
Pulmonary edema
Commonly Related Diseases:
Myocardial infarction
Bronchiectasis
Bronchitis
Lung abscess
Pneumonia

Pulmonary embolus
Tuberculosis
Emphysema
Asthma
Congestive heart failure

POSSIBLE ETIOLOGY

Failure of the respiratory and cough reflexes to clear secretions from the respiratory system

NURSING DIAGNOSIS

Pulmonary secretion congestion: the presence of fluid or thick exudate in the lungs

PLANNING

Patient Needs	**Primary Nurse-Patient Goals**
Oxygen	To maintain oxygen to all cells
Waste elimination	To maintain regulating mechanisms and functions
Sleep, rest	To achieve sleep, rest
Comfort	To achieve comfort
Cleanliness	To achieve good hygiene
Protection from physical harm	To prevent physical injury, infection
Increased learning	To achieve awareness of needs

NURSING INTERVENTIONS

Nursing Treatments
Apply a hot water bottle
   OR
Apply a warm, moist compress (to the chest)
Administer vaporized air
Give warm liquids
Place in postural drainage
Change the patient's position frequently
Encourage coughing
   AND
Encourage deep breathing
Give nonprescription drugs (ExR) (decongestants)
Encourage adequate rest
Discourage smoking
Maintain adequate atmospheric humidity

Nursing Observations
Inspect the chest for respiratory rate and rhythm
Inspect the chest for symmetrical expansion
Auscultate the chest for abnormal breath sounds
Auscultate the chest for abnormal voice sounds

Auscultate the chest for lung aeration
Auscultate the chest for rales and rhonchi
Palpate the chest for abnormal vocal fremitus
Percuss the chest for abnormal resonance
Percuss the chest for cracked-pot sounds
Percuss the posterior chest for decreased diaphragmatic descent
Inspect the sputum for characteristics
Monitor the oral temperature
Observe for complaints of pain
Observe for dyspnea
Observe for fatigue
Observe for complaints of weakness

Health Teaching
Advise against exposure to airborne irritants
Advise against exposure to inclement weather
Teach how to give vaporized air inhalation
Inform that cleanliness is basic to health
Describe those symptoms which should be reported (dyspnea, pain)
Explain the causes of the health problem
Explain the reason for and intended effect of the therapy

Medical Treatments Performed by Nurses
Administer heated humidified oxygen
Administer intermittent positive pressure breathing

EVALUATION

See the evaluation criteria for each specific goal in Chapter 2.

Tenacious Airway Secretions (70,300,301)

ASSESSMENT

Subjective Data
Feeling of fullness in the airway

Objective Data
Secretions are thick and jellylike
Difficult to cough up or suction
Form plugs in the airway

Related Data

Commonly Related Diseases:
Bronchial asthma
Bronchitis
Bronchiectasis
Pneumonia
Rabies

POSSIBLE ETIOLOGY

Inadequate airway humidification

NURSING DIAGNOSIS

Tenacious airway secretions: thick, adhering material excreted from an airway

PLANNING

Patient Needs	Primary Nurse-Patient Goals
Water-salt balance	To maintain fluid and electrolyte balance
Waste elimination	To maintain regulating mechanisms and functions
Cleanliness	To achieve good hygiene
Protection from physical harm	To prevent physical injury, infection
Increased learning	To achieve awareness of needs

NURSING INTERVENTIONS

Nursing Treatments
Suction the airway
Increase fluid intake to about 2000 cc daily
Administer vaporized air
Maintain adequate atmospheric humidity
Encourage coughing
    AND
Encourage deep breathing
Place in the sitting position (as much as possible)
Bathe locally (if secretions come in contact with the skin)
Discourage smoking

Nursing Observations
Inspect the chest for respiratory rate and rhythm
Inspect the chest for symmetrical expansion
Auscultate the chest for abnormal breath sounds
Auscultate the chest for abnormal voice sounds
Auscultate the chest for lung aeration
Auscultate the chest for rales and rhonchi
Palpate the chest for abnormal vocal fremitus
Percuss the chest for abnormal resonance
Percuss the posterior chest for decreased diaphragmatic descent
Observe for cyanosis
Observe for dyspnea

Health Teaching
Teach how to give vaporized air inhalation
Explain the causes of the health problem
Explain the reason for and intended effect of the therapy

Medical Treatments Performed by Nurses
Administer aerosol mist by nebulizer
Administer heated humidified oxygen

EVALUATION

See the evaluation criteria for each specific goal in Chapter 2.

RESPIRATORY SECRETIONS, POTENTIAL ABNORMAL

Potential Pulmonary Secretion Congestion (113,453)

ASSESSMENT

Subjective Data
Weakness
Fatigue

Objective Data
Recent anesthesia
Prolonged bed rest
Immobility
Debilitation
Muscle weakness
Shallow chest movements

Related Data
Commonly Related Conditions:
Common cold
Commonly Related Diseases:
Influenza

POSSIBLE ETIOLOGY

Failure to ventilate the lungs adequately. Insufficient use of the cough reflex to clear secretions in the respiratory system.

NURSING DIAGNOSIS

Potential pulmonary secretion congestion: the possibility that increased exudate will develop in the lungs

PLANNING

Patient Needs
Protection from physical harm
Increased learning

Primary Nurse-Patient Goals
To prevent physical injury
To achieve awareness of needs

NURSING INTERVENTIONS

Nursing Treatments
Ambulate the patient (as much and as soon as possible)
Change the patient's position frequently (every 2 hours)
Encourage coughing
    AND
Encourage deep breathing
Suction the airway (as needed)

Nursing Observations
Inspect the chest for respiratory rate and rhythm
Inspect the chest for symmetrical expansion
Auscultate the chest for abnormal breath sounds

Auscultate the chest for abnormal voice sounds
Auscultate the chest for lung aeration
Auscultate the chest for rales and rhonchi
Palpate the chest for abnormal vocal fremitus
Percuss the chest for abnormal resonance
Percuss the posterior chest for decreased diaphragmatic descent
Monitor the oral temperature (for fever)
Observe for coughing
Observe for fatigue
Observe for complaints of malaise

Health Teaching
Instruct to change position frequently
Describe those symptoms which should be reported (fever, cough, fatigue)
Explain the causes of the health problem
Explain the reason for and intended effect of the therapy

EVALUATION

See the evaluation criteria for each specific goal in Chapter 2.

RESPIRATORY THERAPY DEPENDENCE

Dependence on Endotracheal Tube Management (71,391)

ASSESSMENT

Subjective Data
Person relies on nurses for:
    removal of secretions by suctioning
    proper tube placement for adequate ventilation
    provision of adequate humidification or oxygenation
    mouth care

Objective Data
Person has an endotracheal tube

Related Data
Commonly Related Diseases:
Cerebral vascular accident
Cerebral neoplasm
Subdural hematoma
Second or third degree burns
Guillian-Barre syndrome

POSSIBLE ETIOLOGY

Surgical anesthesia. Respiratory distress. Need to maintain a clean airway.

NURSING DIAGNOSIS

Dependence on endotracheal tube management: reliance on nurses for the care and cleanliness of an airway tube placed through the nose or mouth into the trachea

PLANNING

Patient Needs	Primary Nurse-Patient Goals
Oxygen	To maintain oxygen to all cells
Comfort	To achieve comfort
Cleanliness	To achieve good hygiene
Protection from physical harm	To prevent physical injury, infection
Dependence	To achieve comfort
Increased learning	To achieve awareness of needs

NURSING INTERVENTIONS

Nursing Treatments
Suction the airway (as needed)
Change the catheter each time the airway is suctioned
Place in the side-lying position
Administer vaporized air (with an endotracheal adaptor)
Inflate the airway tube cuff
Swab the mouth with diluted glycerine (periodically)

Nursing Observations
Inspect the chest for respiratory rate and rhythm
Inspect the chest for symmetrical expansion
Auscultate the chest for abnormal breath sounds (absent breath sounds may
    indicate tube obstruction)
Check the tube (endotracheal) for patency
Monitor blood studies for abnormal gas exchange
Monitor blood studies for abnormal hematology
Monitor blood studies for evidence of infection
Monitor the laboratory findings of sputum analysis
Observe for cyanosis
Observe for dyspnea
Observe for fatigue

Health Teaching
Explain the reason for and intended effect of the therapy

Medical Treatments Performed by Nurses
Administer heated humidified oxygen
Give the prescribed drugs

EVALUATION

See the evaluation criteria for each specific goal in Chapter 2.

Dependence on Laryngectomy Management (70,391,523,554,573,574,575)

ASSESSMENT
Subjective Data
Person relies on nurses for:
    laryngectomy tube cleanliness

adequate humidification
safety precautions against respiratory distress
mouth care

Objective Data
Person has a laryngectomy

Related Data
Commonly Related Diseases:
Laryngeal carcinoma

POSSIBLE ETIOLOGY

Inability to care for oneself. No previous experience caring for a laryngectomy. Removal of the larynx (voice box) as a result of cancer.

NURSING DIAGNOSIS

Dependence on laryngectomy management: reliance on nurses for the care of an opening surgically placed in the anterior neck and joined to the trachea following removal of the larynx

PLANNING

Patient Needs	**Primary Nurse-Patient Goals**
Oxygen	To maintain oxygen to all cells
Comfort	To achieve comfort
Cleanliness	To achieve good hygiene
Protection from physical harm	To prevent physical injury, infection
Dependence	To achieve comfort
Increased learning	To achieve awareness of needs

NURSING INTERVENTIONS

Nursing Treatments
Defer speech communication for 72 hours after partial laryngectomy
Clean the laryngectomy tube inner cannula
Suction the airway (as needed)
Administer vaporized air
Shield the laryngectomy stoma from water
Rinse the mouth with diluted hydrogen peroxide
    OR
Swab the mouth with diluted glycerine
    OR
Refresh with a mouthwash

Nursing Observations
Check the laryngectomy tube for patency and cleanliness
Inspect the chest for respiratory rate and rhythm
Inspect the chest for symmetrical expansion
Auscultate the chest for lung aeration
Observe for coughing
Inspect for bleeding
Monitor the blood pressure

Health Teaching
Advise against exposure to airborne irritants
Explain how to adjust clothing to meet health problems
Inform that heavy lifting should be avoided
Inform that handwashing is essential before touching the laryngectomy stoma
Teach how to clean a laryngectomy tube
Inform that the laryngectomy stoma should be protected against sunburning
Instruct that soap should not be used on the laryngectomy stoma
Instruct to apply a warm, moist compress to the laryngectomy stoma for
   dyspnea
Instruct to maintain a moist laryngectomy bib
Instruct to protect the laryngectomy from water
Instruct to use a water-base lubricant around the laryngectomy stoma
Recommend the use of a laryngectomy bib
Recommend that the tongue be brushed
Teach how to give vaporized air inhalation
Explain the importance of wearing a Medic Alert tag
Describe those symptoms which should be reported (respiratory distress)

Medical Treatments Performed by Nurses
Give the prescribed tube feeding

EVALUATION

See the evaluation criteria for each specific goal in Chapter 2.

Dependence on Closed-Chest
Drainage Management (71,391)

ASSESSMENT

Subjective Data
Person relies on nurses for:
   maintenance of chest tube patency
   measurement and observation of drainage
   maintenance of sterile technique
   prevention of air leaks or disruption of the drainage system

Related Data
Commonly Related Conditions:
Pneumothorax
Commonly Related Diseases:
Penetrating chest wound

POSSIBLE ETIOLOGY

Need for continued removal of blood and secretions from the chest cavity

NURSING DIAGNOSIS

Dependence on closed-chest drainage management: reliance on nurses for
the care and functioning of a tube placed into the pleural chest cavity to allow
for lung reexpansion

PLANNING

Patient Needs	Primary Nurse-Patient Goals
Rest	To achieve rest
Comfort	To achieve comfort
Cleanliness	To achieve good hygiene
Protection from physical harm	To prevent physical injury, infection
Dependence	To achieve comfort
Increased learning	To achieve awareness of needs

NURSING INTERVENTIONS

Nursing Treatments
Attach the chest tube to a water-seal drainage
Strip the chest tubing (periodically)
Keep the drainage container below chest level
Protect the water-seal drainage apparatus from damage
Clamp the chest tube but for only a short time (if there is any interruption of
the drainage system)
Encourage coughing
AND
Encourage deep breathing
Place in the sitting position (as much as possible)
Place on the affected side
Change the patient's position frequently
Provide standby emergency equipment (rubber-tipped hemostats)

Nursing Observations
Check the chest-bottle drainage for quality and quantity
Check the drainage system for leakage
Check for fluctuation of the fluid level in the water-seal container
Inspect for bleeding (around the chest tube insertion site)
Measure the output (by means of a marking tape on the outside of the water-
seal container)
OR
Measure the chest drainage after clamping the chest tube and attaching a new
drainage system
Inspect the chest for respiratory rate and rhythm (rapid, shallow respirations)
Auscultate the chest for lung aeration (when lack of fluid fluctuation indicates
lung reexpansion)
Monitor the blood pressure (for decrease)
Monitor the oral temperature
Observe for cyanosis
Observe for dyspnea

Health Teaching
Describe those symptoms which should be reported (dyspnea)
Explain the reason for and intended effect of the therapy

Medical Treatments Performed by Nurses
Give the prescribed drugs

EVALUATION

See the evaluation criteria for each specific goal in Chapter 2.

Dependence on Tracheostomy Management (71,391)

ASSESSMENT

Subjective Data

Person relies on nurses for:
  removal of accumulated secretions
  periodic tube cleansing
  periodic dressing changes
  cleansing of the skin surrounding the tracheostomy
  protection against infection
  provision of adequate humidification or oxygenation

Objective Data

Person has a tracheostomy

Related Data

Commonly Related Diseases:
Diptheria
Laryngeal carcinoma
Cervical spinal cord injury
Cerebral vascular accident
Guillian-Barre syndrome

POSSIBLE ETIOLOGY

Need for a surgical airway where an airway obstruction exists

NURSING DIAGNOSIS

Dependence on tracheostomy management: reliance on nurses for the care and cleanliness of a tracheostomy airway

PLANNING

Patient Needs	**Primary Nurse-Patient Goals**
Oxygen	To maintain oxygen to all cells
Comfort	To achieve comfort
Cleanliness	To achieve good hygiene
Protection from physical harm	To prevent physical injury, infection
Dependence	To achieve comfort
Increased learning	To achieve awareness of needs

NURSING INTERVENTIONS

Nursing Treatments

Administer vaporized air (by tracheostomy collar)
Maintain adequate atmospheric humidity
Maintain a warm room temperature (80°F)
Suction the airway (as needed)

Change the catheter each time the airway is suctioned
Wear a mask when suctioning
Wear sterile gloves (when suctioning)
Change the dressing frequently
Change the tracheostomy tube (if plugged)
Clean the tracheostomy tube inner cannula (every 4 hours)
Clean with surgical soap (the skin around the tracheostomy site)
Shield the tracheostomy from water
Encourage coughing
Encourage deep breathing
Inflate the airway-tube cuff
Deflate the airway-tube cuff periodically
Place in the sitting position (unless contraindicated)
Rinse the mouth with dilute hydrogen peroxide
   OR
Swab the mouth with diluted glycerine
   OR
Refresh with a mouthwash

Nursing Observations
Check the tracheostomy tube for patency and cleanliness
Inspect for bleeding (around the tracheostomy site)
Inspect the chest for respiratory rate and rhythm
Inspect the chest for symmetrical expansion
Auscultate the chest for lung aeration
Monitor blood studies for abnormal gas exchange
Observe for cyanosis
Observe for dyspnea

Health Teaching
Describe those symptoms which should be reported (dyspnea)
Explain the reason for and intended effect of the therapy

Medical Treatments Performed by Nurses
Administer humidified oxygen

EVALUATION

See the evaluation criteria for each specific goal in Chapter 2.

NONFUNCTIONING RESPIRATORY THERAPY DEVICES

Interrupted Closed-Chest Drainage (71,391)

ASSESSMENT

Subjective Data
Pain

Objective Data
Grunting respirations
Chest tube that has slipped from the chest
Tube leakage
Kinked tubing
Blood clots in the tubing
Chest bottle breakage or drainage bag puncture
Chest bottle or bag elevation above the chest level
Insufficient sterile water in the drainage container
Constant water level in the drainage container, despite lack of lung reexpansion

Related Data
Commonly Related Diseases:
Penetrating chest wound
Pneumothorax

POSSIBLE ETIOLOGY

Drainage system breakdown

NURSING DIAGNOSIS

Interrupted closed-chest drainage: a break in the closed-chest drainage system

PLANNING

Patient Needs	**Primary Nurse-Patient Goals**
Comfort	To achieve comfort
Cleanliness	To achieve good hygiene
Protection from physical harm	To prevent physical injury
Increased learning	To achieve awareness of needs

NURSING INTERVENTIONS

Nursing Treatments
Cover the sucking wound immediately (if the tube slips from the chest)
Clamp the chest tube but only for a short time (*immediately* if water-seal pressure is lost or the container is elevated above the chest level)
Attach the chest tube to a water-seal drainage (if a new tube is inserted)
Strip the chest tubing (if drainage ceases)

Nursing Observations
Check the drainage system for leakage (and replace if leakage exists)
Check the tube for patency
Inspect the chest for respiratory rate and rhythm
Inspect the chest for symmetrical expansion

Health Teaching
Explain the reason for and intended effect of the therapy

EVALUATION

See the evaluation criteria for each specific goal in Chapter 2.

RESPIRATORY THERAPY DISCOMFORTS

Artificial-Ventilation Discomfort (70,391)

ASSESSMENT

Subjective Data

Smothering sensation when a mask or nose clip is applied
Choking sensation with high ventilator pressure
Fear that oxygen will explode or the pressure will rupture the lungs
Fear of infection transfer from other patients using the machine

Objective Data

Patient has difficulty synchronizing breathing with the respirator
Is disturbed by high aerosol mist
May refuse to use a ventilator or a nose clip

Related Data

Commonly Related Diseases:
Pneumonia
Asthma
Emphysema
Bronchitis
Bronchiectasis
Lung neoplasm
Tuberculosis
Myocardial infarction

POSSIBLE ETIOLOGY

Lack of instruction in how to use the ventilation. Lack of gradual introduction to the use of the ventilator.

NURSING DIAGNOSIS

Artificial-ventilation discomfort: discomfort related to the use of a mechanical device to assist with lung hygiene or respiratory maintenance

PLANNING

Patient Needs	Primary Nurse-Patient Goals
Oxygen	To maintain oxygen to all cells
Waste elimination	To maintain regulating mechanisms and functions
Comfort	To achieve comfort
Cleanliness	To achieve good hygiene
Protection from physical harm	To prevent physical injury
Increased learning	To achieve awareness of needs

NURSING INTERVENTIONS

Nursing Treatments

Attend the patient constantly (during the treatment)

Reassure verbally
Demonstrate calmness
Limit IPPB treatments to short periods
Gradually increase the amount of ventilator pressure
Place in the sitting position
Do not place in the flat position
Refrain from strapping the ven-
    tilator mask in place   (until the patient feels more
    AND   comfortable)
Refrain from using a ventilator nose clip

Nursing Observations
Inspect the chest for respiratory rate and rhythm (during treatment)
Inspect the chest for symmetrical expansion (during treatment)
Monitor the blood pressure
Monitor blood studies for abnormal acid-base
Observe for complaints of pain
Observe for an excessive stress level

Health Teaching
Teach how to give positive pressure breathing
Explain the reason for and intended effect of the therapy

EVALUATION

See the evaluation criteria for each specific goal in Chapter 2.

Nasal-Pack Discomfort

ASSESSMENT

Subjective Data
Nasal dryness
Air hunger
Anxiety

Objective Data
Nasal distention
Difficulty swallowing

Related Data
Commonly Related Diseases:
Nasal fracture
Hypertension
Leukemia
Sickle cell anemia
Hemophilia
Laennec's cirrhosis

POSSIBLE ETIOLOGY

Therapy to stop nasal bleeding

NURSING DIAGNOSIS

Nasal-pack discomfort: annoyances or mild discomfort related to the presence of gauze strips therapeutically inserted into the nose

PLANNING

Patient Needs

Comfort

Protection from physical harm

Increased learning

Primary Nurse-Patient Goals

To achieve comfort

To prevent physical injury

To achieve awareness of needs

NURSING INTERVENTIONS

Nursing Treatments
Administer vaporized air (if mouth breathing)
Feed slowly
Elevate the head
   OR
Place in the sitting position
Reassure verbally
Provide frequent patient contact
Discourage smoking

Nursing Observations
Observe for dyspnea
Observe for an excessive stress level

Health Teaching
Explain the reason for and intended effect of the therapy

EVALUATION

See the evaluation criteria for each specific goal in Chapter 2.

EMERGENCY PULMONARY GAS EXCHANGE IMBALANCES

Emergency Phase Carbon Dioxide Insufficiency (271,391)

ASSESSMENT

Subjective Data
Numbness and tingling of the nose, ears, fingertips, or toes
Lightheadedness

Objective Data
Depressed respirations or hyperventilation
Muscle twitching

Related Data
Laboratory Findings:
Decreased levels of blood CO_2 and $PaCO_2$

Commonly Related Conditions:
Salicylate poisoning
Fever
Commonly Related Diseases:
Pulmonary embolism
Anxiety neurosis
Lesions in the regions of the pons
Hyperthyroidism

POSSIBLE ETIOLOGY

Reduced respiratory center stimulation due to reduced carbon dioxide level. Failure of the respiratory center impulses to discharge. Drug depression. Respirator, emotional, or high-altitude hyperventilation.

NURSING DIAGNOSIS

Emergency phase carbon dioxide insufficiency (emergency phase hypocapnia) (emergency phase hypocarbia) (emergency phase hypocarbemia): the need for immediate health care as a result of insufficient carbon dioxide within the blood

PLANNING

Patient Needs	**Primary Nurse-Patient Goals**
Acid-base balance	To maintain regulating mechanisms and functions
Stimulation	To maintain stimulation
Protection from physical harm	To prevent physical injury
Increased learning	To achieve awareness of needs

NURSING INTERVENTIONS

Nursing Treatments
Attend the patient constantly (until the episode subsides)
Provide a paper bag for breathing (if patient is hyperventilating)

Nursing Observations
Inspect the chest for respiratory rate and rhythm
Auscultate the chest for lung aeration
Monitor the blood pressure
Monitor blood studies for abnormal acid base
Monitor blood studies for abnormal gas exchange (decreased CO_2)
Observe for complaints of dizziness
Observe for complaints of pain
Observe for complaints of respiratory muscle weakness

Health Teaching
Explain the causes of the health problem
Explain how to use a paper bag to reduce hyperventilation
Teach how to do breath-holding
Explain the reason for and intended effect of the therapy

Medical Treatments Performed by Nurses
Administer carbon dioxide whiffs

EVALUATION

See the evaluation criteria for each specific goal in Chapter 2.

Emergency Phase Carbon Dioxide Toxicity (300,391)

ASSESSMENT

Subjective Data
Headache
Visual disturbances

Objective Data
Drowsiness
Listlessness
Coma
Recurrent yawning
Rapid, deep breathing followed by respiratory depression
Muscle twitching
Rapid pulse
Erythema
Sweating

Related Data

Laboratory Findings:
Increased blood CO_2 and $PaCO_2$

Commonly Related Diseases:
Pulmonary emphysema
Myasthenia gravis
Guillian-Barre syndrome
Poliomyelitis
Congestive heart failure

POSSIBLE ETIOLOGY

Decreased ability of the lung alveoli to ventilate. The administration of high oxygen concentrations causing further carbon dioxide retention.

NURSING DIAGNOSIS

Emergency phase carbon dioxide toxicity (emergency phase hypercapnia) (emergency phase hypercarbia) (emergency phase hypercarbemia) (emergency phase carbon dioxide narcosis): the need for immediate health care as a result of excess carbon dioxide in the blood

PLANNING

Patient Needs	Primary Nurse-Patient Goals
Waste elimination	To maintain regulating mechanisms and functions
Rest	To achieve rest
Stimulation	To maintain stimulation
Protection from physical harm	To prevent physical injury

Increased learning   To achieve awareness of needs

NURSING INTERVENTIONS

Nursing Treatments
Administer intermittent positive pressure breathing (ET) (with O_2 no higher
   than 1 or 2 liters per minute)
Encourage deep breathing
Withhold the drugs (sedatives)
Withhold the oxygen therapy (of high concentrations)
Attend the patient constantly (until the episode subsides)

Nursing Observations
Inspect the chest for respiratory rate and rhythm
Inspect the chest for symmetrical expansion
Auscultate the chest for abnormal breath sounds
Auscultate the chest for abnormal voice sounds
Auscultate the chest for lung aeration
Palpate the chest for abnormal vocal fremitus
Percuss the chest for abnormal resonance
Percuss the posterior chest for decreased diaphragmatic descent
Monitor blood studies for abnormal acid base
Monitor blood studies for abnormal gas exchange (increased CO_2)
Monitor the oral temperature
Observe the characteristics of the cough
Observe for confusion
Palpate the pulse for rate (tachycardia), rhythm, and volume

Health Teaching
Teach how to do resistive breathing exercises
Explain the causes of the health problem
Explain the reason for and intended effect of the therapy

Medical Treatments Performed by Nurses
Administer oxygen by Venturi mask
Give the prescribed drugs

EVALUATION

See the evaluation criteria for each specific goal in Chapter 2.

Emergency Phase Oxygen Toxicity (271,391)

ASSESSMENT

Objective Data
Rosy, pink skin
Depressed respirations
Confusion
Restlessness

Related Data
Laboratory Findings:
Increased level of blood PO_2

Commonly Related Conditions:
Pulmonary atelectasis

Commonly Related Diseases:
Any disease requiring prolonged oxygen therapy such as:
Myocardial infarction
Pneumonia
Pulmonary carcinoma
Cerebral vascular accident

POSSIBLE ETIOLOGY

Prolonged, high levels of oxygen inhalation

NURSING DIAGNOSIS

Emergency phase oxygen toxicity (emergency phase hyperoxia): the need for immediate health care as a result of an above normal increase in oxygen content, tension, or concentration

PLANNING

Patient Needs	**Primary Nurse-Patient Goals**
Waste elimination	To maintain regulating mechanisms and functions
Stimulation	To maintain sensory function and stimulation
Protection from physical harm	To prevent physical injury
Increased learning	To achieve awareness of needs

NURSING INTERVENTIONS

Nursing Treatments
Withhold the oxygen therapy
Attend the patient constantly (until the episode subsides)
Withhold the drugs (causing respiratory depression)
Provide standby emergency equipment (oxygen at very low flow rate of 1–2 liters per minute)

Nursing Observations
Inspect the chest for respiratory rate and rhythm
Inspect the chest for symmetrical expansion
Auscultate the chest for abnormal breath sounds
Auscultate the chest for abnormal voice sounds
Auscultate the chest for lung aeration
Percuss the chest for abnormal resonance
Percuss the posterior chest for decreased diaphragmatic descent
Monitor the blood pressure
Monitor blood studies for abnormal gas exchange (increased O_2 saturation)
Observe for complaints of dizziness
Observe for complaints of headache
Observe for confusion

Health Teaching
Explain the causes of the health problem

Explain the reason for and intended effect of the therapy

Medical Treatments Performed by Nurses
Administer carbon dioxide whiffs

EVALUATION

See the evaluation criteria for each specific goal in Chapter 2.

Emergency Phase Oxygen Insufficiency (271,300)

ASSESSMENT

Subjective Data
Nausea
Headache
Anxiety
Dyspnea

Objective Data
Cyanosis
Lethargy
Confusion
Vomiting
Restlessness
Rapid pulse in early stage
Slow pulse in late stage
Speaks in short, broken sentences
Decreased blood pressure

Related Data
Laboratory Findings:
Decreased blood O_2 saturation

Commonly Related Conditions:
Pneumothorax

Commonly Related Diseases:
Myocardial infarction
Pneumonia
Pulmonary carcinoma
Cerebral vascular accident
Iron deficiency anemia
Arteriosclerosis
Aortic or mitral stenosis
Aortic regurgitation
Congestive heart failure
Pulmonary embolus

POSSIBLE ETIOLOGY

Impaired circulation. Reduced hemoglobin to transport the oxygen. Reduced oxygen content or tension within the body. Living in high altitudes.

NURSING DIAGNOSIS

Emergency phase oxygen insufficiency (emergency phase hypoxia) (emergency phase hopoxemia) (emergency phase anoxia): the need for immediate health care as a result of inadequate oxygen available to body cells

PLANNING

Patient Needs	**Primary Nurse-Patient Goals**
Oxygen	To maintain oxygen to all cells
Rest	To achieve rest
Comfort	To achieve comfort
Protection from physical harm	To prevent physical injury
Increased learning	To achieve awareness of needs

NURSING INTERVENTIONS

Nursing Treatments
Administer heated humidified oxygen (ET)
   OR
Administer intermittent positive pressure breathing (ET)
Elevate the head
   OR
Place in the sitting position
Place on complete bed rest
Encourage coughing
   AND
Encourage deep breathing
Withhold the drugs (causing respiratory depression)
Attend the patient constantly (until the episode subsides)

Nursing Observations
Inspect the chest for respiratory rate and rhythm
Inspect the chest for symmetrical expansion
Auscultate the chest for abnormal breath sounds
Auscultate the chest for abnormal voice sounds
Auscultate the chest for lung aeration
Auscultate the chest for rales and rhonchi
Palpate the chest for a thrill
Palpate the chest for abnormal vocal fremitus
Percuss the chest for abnormal resonance
Percuss the chest for decreased diaphragmatic descent
Monitor the blood pressure
Monitor blood studies for abnormal gas exchange (decreased O_2 saturation)
Observe for confusion
Observe for cyanosis
Observe for dyspnea
Palpate the pulse for rate, rhythm, and volume

Health Teaching
Explain the causes of the health problem
Explain the reason for and intended effect of the therapy

Medical Treatments Performed by Nurses
Administer controlled positive pressure breathing

EVALUATION

See the evaluation criteria for each specific goal in Chapter 2.

EMERGENCY PULMONARY GAS EXCHANGE IMBALANCES, POTENTIAL

Potential Carbon Dioxide Insufficiency (271,391)

ASSESSMENT

Subjective Data
Anxiety

Objective Data
Rapid breathing supported by a ventilator
Rapid breathing precipitated by high altitude
Emotional hyperventilation

Related Data
Laboratory Findings:
Decreased blood erythrocytes
Commonly Related Conditions:
Fever
Commonly Related Diseases:
Pulmonary embolism
Anxiety neurosis
Lesions in the regions of the pons
Hyperthyroidism

POSSIBLE ETIOLOGY

Excessive loss of carbon dioxide through rapid expiration. Areas of uneven distribution of inspired air resulting from altered elasticity of the lungs.

NURSING DIAGNOSIS

Potential carbon dioxide insufficiency: the probability that there will be inadequate carbon dioxide in the lungs

PLANNING

Patient Needs
Protection from physical harm
Increased learning

Primary Nurse-Patient Goals
To prevent physical injury
To achieve awareness of needs

NURSING INTERVENTIONS

Nursing Treatments
Attend the patient constantly (if breathing rapidly)
Elevate the head
    OR   } (to ease breathing)
Place in the sitting position }

Encourage deep breathing (at a slow rate)

Refrain from giving continuous positive pressure breathing (at a rapid rate)

Maintain adequate atmospheric humidity

Maintain adequate room ventilation

Nursing Observations

Inspect the chest for respiratory rate and rhythm

Auscultate the chest for lung aeration

Monitor the blood pressure

Monitor blood studies for abnormal gas exchange (decreased CO_2)

Observe for complaints of dizziness

Observe for complaints of numbness and tingling

Observe for complaints of pain

Observe for dyspnea

Observe for muscle twitching

Health Teaching

Explain the causes of the health problem

Describe those symptoms which should be reported (numbness and tingling, muscle twitching, lightheadedness)

Advise that highly emotional situations be avoided (if the person is prone to hyperventilation)

Teach how to do breath-holding

Explain how to use a paper bag to reduce hyperventilation

Recommend that high altitudes be avoided after cardiac damage

Explain the reason for and intended effect of the therapy

EVALUATION

See the evaluation criteria for each specific goal in Chapter 2.

Potential Carbon Dioxide Toxicity (300,391)

ASSESSMENT

Objective Data

Respiratory depression

Chest hyperinflation with prolonged inspiratory position

Participating in intense exercise

Receiving high doses of therapeutic oxygen when there is an increased CO_2 blood level

Related Data

Laboratory Findings:

Increasing level of blood CO_2

Commonly Related Diseases:

Emphysema

Poliomyelitis

Guillian-Barre syndrome

Myasthenia gravis

POSSIBLE ETIOLOGY

The administration of CO_2 therapy. Increased cell metabolism during mus cle exercise. Inability of the lung to expire sufficient CO_2.

NURSING DIAGNOSIS

Potential carbon dioxide toxicity: the possibility that an abnormally high level of carbon dioxide could accumulate in the blood

PLANNING

Patient Needs	Primary Nurse-Patient Goals
Waste elimination	To maintain regulating mechanisms and functions
Protection from physical harm	To prevent physical injury
Increased learning	To achieve awareness of needs

NURSING INTERVENTIONS

Nursing Treatments
Encourage deep breathing (frequently)
Encourage moderate physical exercise (not strenuous exercise)
Refrain from giving carbonated beverages
Withhold the oxygen therapy (if the blood O_2 level is elevated)

Nursing Observations
Inspect the chest for respiratory rate and rhythm (depression)
Auscultate the chest for lung aeration
Monitor blood studies for abnormal gas exchange (increased CO_2 and O_2)
Observe for complaints of headache
Observe for complaints of visual disturbance
Observe for muscle twitching
Palpate the pulse for rate (tachycardia), rhythm, and volume

Health Teaching
Teach how to do abdominal breathing
Teach how to do resistive breathing exercises
Describe those symptoms which should be reported (headache, visual disturbances, muscle twitching, tachycardia)
Explain the causes of the health problem
Explain the reason for and intended effect of the therapy

EVALUATION

See the evaluation criteria for each specific goal in Chapter 2.

Potential Oxygen Insufficiency (271,300)

ASSESSMENT

Objective Data
Decreased blood pressure
Rapid or slow pulse

Dysrhythmic heart rate or rhythm
Recent myocardial damage

Related Data

Laboratory Findings:
Decreased level of blood hemoglobin, erythrocytes

Commonly Related Conditions:
Shock

Commonly Related Diseases:
Aplastic anemia
Myocardial infarction
Iron deficiency anemia
Arteriosclerosis
Leukemia

POSSIBLE ETIOLOGY

Inability of the red blood cells to transport oxygen to body organs. Inability of the heart to pump adequate blood for the oxygenation of body cells. Impaired circulation in one or more body areas.

NURSING DIAGNOSIS

Potential oxygen insufficiency: the possibility that there will be inadequate oxygen available to body cells

PLANNING

Patient Needs	**Primary Nurse-Patient Goals**
Protection from physical harm	To prevent physical injury
Increased learning	To achieve awareness of needs

NURSING INTERVENTIONS

Nursing Treatments
Encourage adequate rest
Encourage alternate rest and activity
Provide standby emergency equipment (oxygen)

Nursing Observations
Inspect the chest for respiratory rate and rhythm
Inspect the chest for symmetrical expansion
Auscultate the chest for abnormal breath sounds
Auscultate the chest for abnormal voice sounds
Auscultate the chest for lung aeration
Auscultate the chest for rales and rhonchi
Palpate the chest for abnormal vocal fremitus
Percuss the chest for abnormal resonance
Percuss the posterior chest for decreased diaphragmatic descent
Monitor the blood pressure (for decrease)
Monitor blood studies for abnormal gas exchange (decreased O_2 saturation)
Observe for complaints of headache
Observe for complaints of nausea

Observe for confusion
Observe for cyanosis
Observe for dyspnea
Observe for lethargy
Observe for restlessness
Observe for vomiting
Palpate the pulse for rate (bradycardia or tachycardia), rhythm, and volume

Health Teaching
Describe those symptoms which should be reported (headache, nausea, con-
  fusion, cyanosis, dyspnea, lethargy, restlessness, vomiting)
Explain the need to avoid overexertion
Recommend that high altitudes be avoided after cardiac damage
Emphasize the need to fly in pressurized airplanes
Teach how to give oxygen therapy
Explain the causes of the health problem
Explain the reason for and intended effect of the therapy

EVALUATION

See the evaluation criteria for each specific goal in Chapter 2.

Potential Oxygen Toxicity (271,391)

ASSESSMENT

Objective Data
Prolonged, high-level oxygen therapy
Decreasing respiratory rate

Related Data
Laboratory Findings:
Increasing blood O_2 saturation
Commonly Related Diseases:
Any disease requiring oxygen therapy
  OR
Poliomyelitis
Guillian-Barre syndrome
Myasthenia gravis

POSSIBLE ETIOLOGY

Respiratory depression. Tendency of the body to accumulate O_2.

NURSING DIAGNOSIS

Potential oxygen toxicity: the possibility that an above normal increase in
oxygen content, tension, or concentration could occur

PLANNING

Patient Needs	**To Primary Nurse-Patient Goals**
Protection from physical harm	To prevent physical injury
Increased learning	To achieve awareness of needs

NURSING INTERVENTIONS

Nursing Treatments
Limit therapeutic oxygen concentrations to below 40%

Nursing Observations
Inspect the chest for respiratory rate and rhythm (depression)
Inspect the chest for symmetrical expansion
Auscultate the chest for lung aeration
Inspect the skin for discoloration (rosy, pink)
Monitor blood studies for abnormal gas exchange (increased O_2 saturation)
Observe for confusion
Observe for restlessness

Health Teaching
Explain the causes of the health problem
Explain the reason for and intended effect of the therapy

EVALUATION

See the evaluation criteria for each specific goal in Chapter 2.

EMERGENCY RESPIRATORY CONDITIONS

Emergency Phase Carbon Monoxide Poisoning (247,453)

ASSESSMENT

Subjective Data
Headache
Nausea
Visual disturbances
Tinnitis

Objective Data
Shallow respirations
Cherry-red skin color, nail-beds, and mucous membranes
Increasing drowsiness
Giddiness
Fainting
Eventual respiratory cessation

Related Data
Commonly Related Diseases:
None
　OR
Manic depressive psychosis
Involutional psychosis

POSSIBLE ETIOLOGY

Enclosed exposure to the gas

NURSING DIAGNOSIS

Emergency phase carbon monoxide poisoning: the need for immediate health care as a result of inhalation of high amounts of carbon monoxide

PLANNING

Patient Needs

Oxygen

Stimulation

Protection from physical harm

Increased learning

Primary Nurse-Patient Goals

To maintain oxygen to all cells

To maintain sensory function and stimulation

To prevent physical injury

To achieve awareness of needs

NURSING INTERVENTIONS

Nursing Treatments

Remove immediately to a safe area

Resuscitate breathing (ET) (as needed)

Administer heated humidified oxygen (ET)

    OR

Administer intermittent positive pressure breathing (ET)

Cover with warm blankets

Encourage coughing

    AND

Encourage deep breathing

Give hot coffee ⎫

    OR   ⎬ (if conscious)

Give hot tea ⎭

Stimulate by movement, touch, sternal pressure, or speech

Remove constrictive clothing

Make a referral (to a physician)

Nursing Observations

Inspect the chest for respiratory rate and rhythm

Inspect the chest for symmetrical expansion

Auscultate the chest for abnormal breath sounds

Auscultate the chest for lung aeration

Auscultate the chest for rales and rhonchi

Percuss the chest for abnormal resonance

Percuss the posterior chest for decreased diaphragmatic descent

Monitor the blood pressure

Monitor blood studies for abnormal gas exchange

Monitor the oral temperature (for fever)

Observe the level of consciousness

Palpate the pulse for rate, rhythm, and volume

Health Teaching

Explain the reason for and intended effect of the therapy

EVALUATION

See the evaluation criteria for each specific goal in Chapter 2.

Emergency Phase Drowning (247,453)

ASSESSMENT

Objective Data

Salt Water Drowning:
Unconsciousness
Cyanosis
Cold skin
Barely perceptible or absent pulse
Decreased blood pressure
Pulmonary edema

Fresh Water Drowning:
Unconsciousness
Cyanosis
Cold skin
Barely perceptible or absent pulse
Increased blood pressure
Ventricular fibrillation

Related Data

Laboratory Findings (Salt Water Drowning):
Increased blood erythrocytes and sodium
Decreased blood protein

Laboratory Findings (Fresh Water Drowning):
Decreased blood erythrocytes and sodium

Commonly Related Diseases:
None
    OR
Cerebral concussion

POSSIBLE ETIOLOGY

Salt water drowning: accidental or intentional submersion in ocean water for a prolonged period. Hypertonic salt water rapidly diffuses salt into the bloodstream resulting in pulmonary edema and hemoconcentration. Fresh water drowning: accidental or intentional submersion in lakes, pools, streams, or any inland water for a prolonged period. Hypotonic fresh water is rapidly absorbed into the blood and causes a sudden increase in blood volume.

NURSING DIAGNOSIS

Emergency phase drowning: the need for immediate health care as a result of decreased oxygen and increased carbon dioxide within the blood resulting from water in the lungs

PLANNING

Patient Needs

Oxygen, circulation
Stimulation

Primary Nurse-Patient Goals

To maintain oxygen to all cells
To maintain sensory function and
    stimulation

Protection from physical harm

Increased learning

To prevent physical injury

To achieve awareness of needs

NURSING INTERVENTIONS

Nursing Treatments

Remove foreign objects (from the airway)

Resuscitate breathing (ET)

Suction the airway

Insert an oral airway

Administer humidified oxygen (ET)

Administer intermittent positive pressure breathing (ET) (in fresh water drowning)

Place in the foot-elevated head-lowered (Trendelenberg) position

Cover with warm blankets

Remove constrictive clothing

Stimulate by movement, touch, sternal pressure, or speech

Make a referral (to a physician)

Nursing Observations

Inspect the chest for respiratory rate and rhythm

Inspect the chest for symmetrical expansion

Auscultate the chest for abnormal breath sounds (wheezing)

Auscultate the chest for lung aeration

Auscultate the chest for rales (bubbling) and rhonchi

Percuss the chest for abnormal resonance

Percuss the posterior chest for decreased diaphragmatic descent

Inspect the sputum for characteristics (frothy pink)

Monitor the blood pressure

Monitor blood studies for abnormal gas exchange

Observe for cyanosis

Observe for dyspnea

Observe the level of consciousness

Palpate the pulse for rate (tachycardia), rhythm, and volume

Health Teaching

Explain the reason for and intended effect of the therapy

Medical Treatments Performed by Nurses

Administer intermittent positive pressure by expiratory positive pressure mask (in pulmonary edema from salt water drowning)

EVALUATION

See the evaluation criteria for each specific goal in Chapter 2.

Emergency Phase Pulmonary Irritant Inhalation (192)

ASSESSMENT

Subjective Data

Dyspnea

Nausea

Objective Data
Severe coughing
Choking
Hoarseness
Nasal membrane swelling or redness
Singed nasal hairs

POSSIBLE ETIOLOGY

Breathing in smoke from fire. Inhalation of smog (smoke and fog). Breathing dust blown about by the wind. Inhalation of leaking gas or chemicals. Exposure to dust in mines.

NURSING DIAGNOSIS

Emergency phase pulmonary irritant inhalation: the need for immediate health care as a result of the breathing in of large amounts of smoke, smog, gases, or dust which interfere with or irritate the respiratory system

PLANNING

Patient Needs	Primary Nurse-Patient Goals
Oxygen	To maintain oxygen to all cells
Waste elimination	To maintain regulating mechanisms and functions
Comfort	To achieve comfort
Protection from physical harm	To prevent physical injury
Increased learning	To achieve awareness of needs

NURSING INTERVENTIONS

Nursing Treatments
Administer heated humidified oxygen (ET)
OR
Administer intermittent positive pressure breathing (ET)
Encourage coughing
AND
Encourage deep breathing (in a clean environment)
Elevate the head
OR
Place in the sitting position
Place in postural drainage (intermittently)
Encourage adequate rest
Maintain adequate atmospheric humidity
Maintain adequate room ventilation
Discourage smoking
Provide standby emergency equipment (oxygen, endotracheal tube)

Nursing Observations
Inspect the chest for respiratory rate and rhythm
Inspect the chest for symmetrical expansion

Auscultate the chest for abnormal breath sounds
Auscultate the chest for abnormal voice sounds
Auscultate the chest for lung aeration
Auscultate the chest for rales and rhonchi
Palpate the chest for abnormal vocal fremitus
Percuss the chest for abnormal resonance
Percuss the posterior chest for decreased diaphragmatic descent
Inspect the nasal turbinates for abnormalities
Monitor the blood pressure
Monitor blood studies for abnormal hematology
Monitor the laboratory findings of sputum analysis
Observe for cyanosis
Observe for dyspnea
Observe for shock

Health Teaching
Advise against exposure to airborne irritants
Describe those symptoms which should be reported (dyspnea)
Explain the reason for and intended effect of the therapy

EVALUATION

See the evaluation criteria for each specific goal in Chapter 2.

Emergency Phase Pulmonary Edema (71,271,391)

ASSESSMENT

Subjective Data
Intense anxiety
Dyspnea
Orthopnea

Objective Data
Cyanosis
Pink-tinged frothy sputum
Coughing
Restlessness
Wheezing breath sounds
Tachycardia
Cold, clammy skin

Related Data
Commonly Related Diseases:
Congestive heart failure
Myocardial infarction
Pulmonary emphysema
Second- or third-degree burn

POSSIBLE ETIOLOGY

Left ventricular failure in which the heart is unable to pump blood away from the lungs into the circulation. Fluid overload. Inhalation of respiratory irritants, especially ammonia.

NURSING DIAGNOSIS

Emergency phase pulmonary edema: the need for immediate health care when excessive amounts of fluid have collected in the lung tissue

PLANNING

Patient Needs	Primary Nurse-Patient Goals
Oxygen, circulation	To maintain oxygen to all cells
Water-salt balance	To maintain fluid and electrolyte balance
Rest	To achieve rest
Comfort	To achieve comfort
Protection from physical harm	To prevent physical injury
Increased learning	To achieve awareness of needs

NURSING INTERVENTIONS

Nursing Treatments

Administer humidified oxygen (ET) (15–30 liters per minute)
   OR
Administer intermittent positive pressure breathing (ET)
Apply rotating tourniquets (ET)
Slow the intravenous infusion flow rate (if an I.V. is being infused)
Place in the sitting position
Place on complete bed rest
Consult with the physician *(immediately)*

Nursing Observations

Inspect the chest for respiratory rate (increased) and rhythm
Inspect the chest for symmetrical expansion
Auscultate the chest for lung aeration
Auscultate the chest for rales and rhonchi
Palpate the chest for abnormal vocal fremitus
Percuss the chest for abnormal resonance
Percuss the posterior chest for decreased diaphragmatic descent
Inspect the sputum for characteristics
Monitor the blood pressure
Palpate the pulse for rate, rhythm, and volume
Observe for cyanosis
Observe for dyspnea

Health Teaching

Explain the causes of the health problem
Explain the reason for and intended effect of the therapy

Medical Treatments Performed by Nurses
Give the prescribed drugs

EVALUATION

See the evaluation criteria for each specific goal in Chapter 2.

Emergency Phase Respiratory Arrest (70,192,271,391)

ASSESSMENT

Objective Data
Absent breath sounds
No visible chest movements
Increased heart rate with gradual slowing
Cyanosis
Cold, clammy skin
Low blood pressure
Eventual coma and death

Related Data
Commonly Related Conditions:
Laryngeal edema
Laryngeal spasm
Electric shock
Drowning
Exposure to toxic gases
Airway obstruction
Chronically elevated carbon dioxide level
Increased intracranial pressure
Morphine intolerance

Commonly Related Diseases:
Subarachnoid hemorrhage
Poliomyelitis
Myasthenia gravis
Guillian-Barre syndrome
Cerebral vascular accident
Cervical spinal cord injury
Pneumonia
Myocardial infarction

POSSIBLE ETIOLOGY

Total obstruction of airway passages. Respiratory brain center damage.

NURSING DIAGNOSIS

Emergency phase respiratory arrest: the need for immediate health care when respiration has ceased completely

PLANNING

Patient Needs	**Primary Nurse-Patient Goals**
Oxygen	To maintain oxygen to all cells
Waste elimination	To maintain regulating mechanisms and functions
Stimulation	To maintain sensory function and stimulation
Protection from physical harm	To prevent physical injury
Increased learning	To achieve awareness of needs

NURSING INTERVENTIONS

Nursing Treatments
Resuscitate breathing (ET) .
Resuscitate mouth-to-neck when the patient has a laryngectomy (ET)
Strike a quick blow on the anterior chest
Suction the airway
Insert an oral airway
Administer humidified oxygen (ET)
   OR
Administer intermittent positive pressure breathing (ET)
Stimulate by movement, touch, sternal pressure, or speech
Withhold the drugs (respiratory depressants such as morphine)
Attend the patient constantly
Make a referral (to a physician)

Nursing Observations
Inspect the chest for respiratory rate and rhythm
Inspect the chest for symmetrical expansion
Auscultate the chest for abnormal breath sounds
Auscultate the chest for abnormal voice sounds
Auscultate the chest for lung aeration
Auscultate the chest for rales or rhonchi
Palpate the chest for abnormal vocal fremitus
Percuss the chest for abnormal resonance
Percuss the posterior chest for decreased diaphragmatic descent
Monitor the blood pressure
Monitor blood studies for abnormal gas exchange
Observe the level of consciousness
Palpate the pulse for rate, rhythm, and volume

Health Teaching
Explain the causes of the health problem
   AND   } (to the family)
Explain the reason for and intended
   effect of the therapy

EVALUATION

See the evaluation criteria for each specific goal in Chapter 2.

EMERGENCY RESPIRATORY CONDITIONS, POTENTIAL

Potential Increased Intrapleural Pressure (71,192)

ASSESSMENT

Subjective Data
Air hunger

Objective Data
Chest wound
Sucking air sound during inspiration

Related Data
Commonly Related Diseases:
None
   OR
Pneumothorax

POSSIBLE ETIOLOGY

Chest trauma

NURSING DIAGNOSIS

Potential increased intrapleural pressure: the probability that air passage from the external environment through a hole in the chest wall will cause increased pressure within the pleural cavity and collapse the lung

PLANNING

Patient Needs	Primary Nurse-Patient Goals
Oxygen	To maintain oxygen to all cells
Rest	To achieve rest
Comfort	To achieve comfort
Cleanliness	To achieve good hygiene
Protection from physical harm	To prevent physical injury, infection
Increased learning	To achieve awareness of needs

NURSING INTERVENTIONS

Nursing Treatments
Cover the sucking wound immediately (with a sterile dressing or the palm of a clean hand)
Encourage deep breathing (forceful inhalation and exhalation as the sterile dressing is applied)
Position comfortably
Place in the slight sitting (semi-Fowler's) position
Place on the affected side
Place on complete bed rest
Attend the patient constantly

Nursing Observations
Inspect the chest for respiratory rate and rhythm
Inspect the chest for symmetrical expansion.
Auscultate the chest for abnormal breath sounds
Auscultate the chest for abnormal voice sounds
Auscultate the chest for lung aeration
Auscultate the chest for rales and rhonchi
Palpate the chest for abnormal vocal fremitus
Percuss the chest for abnormal resonance
Percuss the posterior chest for decreased diaphragmatic descent
Monitor the blood pressure
Palpate the pulse for rate, rhythm, and volume
Observe for complaints of pain
Observe for cyanosis
Observe for dyspnea
Observe for shock

Health Teaching
Describe those symptoms which should be reported (dyspnea)
Explain the causes of the health problem
Explain the reason for and intended effect of the therapy

EVALUATION

See the evaluation criteria for each specific goal in Chapter 2.

Potential Pulmonary Edema (32,71,113)

ASSESSMENT

Objective Data
High fluid intake, especially intravenous fluids
Overweight
Sedentary living
Infrequent or inability to cough
Prolonged bed rest
Exposure to respiratory irritants
Recent anesthesia
Existing pulmonary congestion

Related Data
Probability increases in cardiac conditions, pulmonary infections, burns, and a history of previous pulmonary edema
Commonly Related Conditions:
Cardiac dysrhythmias
Blast injuries
Commonly Related Diseases:
Myocardial infarction
Arteriosclerotic heart disease

Pulmonary emphysema
Congestive heart failure
Second- and third-degree burns between the second and fifth postburn day

POSSIBLE ETIOLOGY

Heart failure in which the right ventricle can adequately pump blood to the lungs but the left ventricle is unable to pump blood away from the lungs into the circulation causing the lungs to become engorged with fluid. Rapid infusion of intravenous fluids. Inhalation of respiratory irritants, especially ammonia. Inability to cough up pulmonary and respiratory secretions.

NURSING DIAGNOSIS

Potential pulmonary edema: the probability that excessive amounts of fluid will collect in the lung tissue

PLANNING

Patient Needs	Primary Nurse-Patient Goals
Water-salt balance	To maintain fluid and electrolyte balance
Rest	To achieve rest
Protection from physical harm	To prevent physical injury
Increased learning	To achieve awareness of needs

NURSING INTERVENTIONS

Nursing Treatments
Change the patient's position frequently
Elevate the head (put head of bed on 10-inch blocks while patient is sleeping)
Encourage adequate rest
Encourage deep breathing
Encourage decreased sodium-food intake
Encourage intake of diuretic fluids (if not on diuretic drugs)
Restrict the fluid intake according to the weight gain
Slow the intravenous infusion flow rate (to prevent overhydration)
Provide standby emergency equipment (oxygen)

Nursing Observations
Auscultate the chest for abnormal breath sounds (wheezing)
Auscultate the chest for rales (bubbling)
Inspect the sputum for characteristics (frothy pink)
Measure the body weight (daily for gain due to fluid retention)
Monitor the blood pressure (for elevation)
Observe for coughing
Observe for cyanosis
Observe for dyspnea
Observe for restlessness
Palpate the pulse for rate (tachycardia), rhythm, and volume

Health Teaching
Explain the need to avoid overexertion
Describe those symptoms which should be reported (dyspnea, coughing, frothy pink sputum, rapid pulse)
Explain the causes of the health problem
Explain the reason for and intended effect of the therapy

Medical Treatments Performed by Nurses
Give the prescribed drugs (diuretics)

EVALUATION

See the evaluation criteria for each specific goal in Chapter 2.

Potential Respiratory Arrest (71,271,391)

ASSESSMENT

Subjective Data
Anxiety
Dyspnea

Objective Data
Restlessness
Irritability
Confusion
Cyanosis
Wheezing
Obstructing airway secretions
Paralysis
Muscle weakness

Related Data
Commonly Related Conditions:
Laryngeal edema
Laryngeal spasm
Electric shock
Drowning
Exposure to toxic gases
Chronically elevated carbon dioxide level
Morphine intolerance
Commonly Related Diseases:
Poliomyelitis
Myasthenia gravis
Subarachnoid hemorrhage
Guillian-Barre syndrome
Cerebral vascular accident
Myocardial infarction
Pulmonary emphysema
Asthma

POSSIBLE ETIOLOGY
Total airway obstruction. Respiratory brain center damage.

NURSING DIAGNOSIS
Potential respiratory arrest: the likelihood that respiration will cease

PLANNING

Patient Needs	Primary Nurse-Patient Goals
Protection from physical harm	To prevent physical injury
Increased learning	To achieve awareness of needs

NURSING INTERVENTIONS

Nursing Treatments
Suction the airway (as needed)
Encourage coughing
   AND
Encourage deep breathing
Withhold the drugs (respiratory depressants such as morphine)
Withhold the oxygen therapy (if the blood O_2 is elevated)
Provide frequent patient contact
Provide standby emergency equipment (suction machine, oxygen, airway
   tube)

Nursing Observations
Inspect the chest for respiratory rate and rhythm
Inspect the chest for symmetrical expansion
Auscultate the chest for abnormal breath sounds
Auscultate the chest for abnormal voice sounds
Auscultate the chest for lung aeration (periodically)
Auscultate the chest for rales and rhonchi
Palpate the chest for abnormal vocal fremitus
Percuss the chest for abnormal resonance
Percuss the posterior chest for decreased diaphragmatic descent
Monitor the blood pressure
Monitor blood studies for abnormal gas exchange
Inspect the abdomen for distention
Observe for complaints of respiratory muscle weakness
Observe for cyanosis
Observe for dyspnea

Health Teaching
Describe those symptoms which should be reported (dyspnea, weakness)
Explain the causes of the health problem
Explain the reason for and intended effect of the therapy

EVALUATION
See the evaluation criteria for each specific goal in Chapter 2.

Potential Sudden Infant Death Syndrome (7,37)

ASSESSMENT

Objective Data

Child tends to bend the head downward toward the chest when sleeping

Previous apnea for more than 20 seconds

Related Data

Most commonly occurs in the premature child or in a child with a respiratory infection. More frequent in males than in females. Most common age is between 1 and 6 months. Occurs more frequently during November, December, January, and February.

Commonly Related Conditions:

Laryngeal obstruction

Commonly Related Diseases:

Viral respiratory infection

POSSIBLE ETIOLOGY

Laryngeal spasms. Respiratory infection. Not caused by parental neglect.

NURSING DIAGNOSIS

Potential sudden infant death syndrome: the possibility that sudden unexplained death might occur to a sleeping child

PLANNING

Patient Needs	Primary Nurse-Patient Goals
Oxygen	To maintain oxygen to all cells
Protection from physical harm	To prevent physical injury
Increased learning	To achieve awareness of needs and/or use of resources

NURSING INTERVENTIONS

Nursing Treatments

Change the patient's position frequently

Maintain adequate atmospheric humidity

Provide frequent patient contact

Nursing Observations

Inspect the chest for respiratory rate and rhythm

Inspect the chest for symmetrical expansion

Auscultate the chest for lung aeration

Monitor the infant for apnea

Observe for cyanosis

Observe for dyspnea

Observe for mouth breathing

Observe for nasal flare

Health Teaching

Describe those symptoms which should be reported (periods of apnea, respiratory infection)

Explain the reason for and intended effect of the therapy
Explain how to observe respirations
Explain that premature infants require at-home supervision
Inform that airway noise indicates obstruction
Instruct to change (the child's) position frequently

EVALUATION

See the evaluation criteria for each specific goal in Chapter 2.

INADEQUATE MANAGEMENT OF ARTIFICIAL AIRWAYS

Inadequate Information Related to Laryngectomy Management (70,391,523,554,573,574,575)

ASSESSMENT

Subjective Data
Person confirms a lack of information

Objective Data
Person's actions indicate a lack of information regarding:
    the purpose of a laryngectomy
    the need for humidification
    how to keep the laryngectomy stoma clean
    the precautions to be taken

Related Data
Commonly Related Diseases:
Laryngeal carcinoma

POSSIBLE ETIOLOGY

Lack of instruction. Removal of the larynx (voice box) as a result of cancer.

NURSING DIAGNOSIS

Inadequate information related to laryngectomy management: lack of information regarding the care of an opening surgically placed in the anterior neck and joined to the trachea following removal of the larynx

PLANNING

Patient Needs	**Primary Nurse-Patient Goals**
Comfort	To achieve comfort
Cleanliness	To achieve good hygiene
Protection from physical harm	To prevent physical injury
Increased learning	To achieve awareness of needs and/or use of resources

NURSING INTERVENTIONS

Nursing Treatments
Approach unhurriedly

Encourage patient questions

Make a referral (to the Lost Chord Club)

Nursing Observations

Evaluate the response to teaching

Health Teaching

Advise against exposure to airborne irritants

Explain how to adjust clothing to meet health needs

Inform that heavy lifting should be avoided

Inform that handwashing is essential before touching the laryngectomy stoma

Inform that the laryngectomy stoma should be protected against sunburning

Instruct that soap should not be used on the laryngectomy stoma

Instruct to apply a warm, moist compress to the laryngectomy stoma for dyspnea

Instruct to maintain a moist laryngectomy bib

Instruct to protect the laryngectomy from water

Instruct to use a water-base lubricant around the laryngectomy stoma

Recommend the use of a laryngectomy bib

Recommend that the tongue be brushed

Teach how to give vaporized air inhalation

Explain the importance of wearing a Medic Alert tag

Describe those symptoms which should be reported (respiratory distress)

EVALUATION

See the evaluation criteria for each specific goal in Chapter 2.

Inadequate Information Related to Tracheostomy Management (71,391)

ASSESSMENT

Subjective Data

Person confirms a lack of information

Objective Data

Person's actions indicate a lack of information regarding:
the purpose of a tracheostomy
how to suction
how to maintain aseptic technique
humidification of the tracheostomy
the precautions which should be taken

Related Data

Commonly Related Conditions:
Airway obstruction

Commonly Related Diseases:
Laryngeal carcinoma

POSSIBLE ETIOLOGY

Lack of instruction. Need for a permanent tracheostomy.

NURSING DIAGNOSIS

Inadequate information related to tracheostomy management: lack of information regarding the care of a tracheostomy

PLANNING

Patient Needs	Primary Nurse-Patient Goals
Comfort	To achieve comfort
Cleanliness	To achieve good hygiene
Protection from physical harm	To prevent physical injury
Increased learning	To achieve awareness of needs

NURSING INTERVENTIONS

Nursing Treatments
Approach unhurriedly
Encourage patient questions
Encourage deep breathing
Discourage smoking

Nursing Observations
Evaluate the response to teaching

Health Teaching
Advise against exposure to airborne irritants
Advise against exposure to inclement weather
Describe those symptoms which should be reported (dyspnea, severe coughing, bleeding around the tracheostomy site)
Emphasize the danger of breathing cold air
Inform that the tracheostomy must be covered in order to speak
Inform that airway noise indicates obstruction
Instruct to protect the tracheostomy from water
Teach how to clean a tracheostomy
Teach how to inflate and deflate an airway cuff
Teach how to suction an airway
Teach how to give vaporized air inhalation
Explain the reason for and intended effect of the therapy

EVALUATION

See the evaluation criteria for each specific goal in Chapter 2.

INADEQUATE MANAGEMENT OF RESPIRATORY DEVICES

Inadequate Information Related to Respiratory Therapy Devices (70,391)

ASSESSMENT

Subjective Data
Person confirms a lack of information

Objective Data

Person's actions indicate a lack of information regarding:

the purpose of humidifiers, oxygenators, inhalators, positive pressure machines, etc.

when or for how long treatments should be taken

how to operate the machines

how to maintain machine cleanliness

Related Data

Commonly Related Diseases:

Emphysema

Asthma

Pneumonia

POSSIBLE ETIOLOGY

Lack of instruction

NURSING DIAGNOSIS

Inadequate information related to respiratory therapy devices: lack of information regarding the use and care of devices that support improved respirations or respiratory hygiene

PLANNING

Patient Needs	**Primary Nurse-Patient Goals**
Comfort	To achieve comfort
Protection from physical harm	To prevent physical injury
Increased learning	To achieve awareness of needs and/or use of resources

NURSING INTERVENTIONS

Nursing Treatments

Approach unhurriedly

Encourage patient questions

Involve the family

Make a referral (to a respiratory therapist if necessary)

Nursing Observations

Evaluate the response to teaching

Health Teaching

Inform that cleanliness is basic to health

Teach how to clean respiratory equipment

Teach how to give vaporized air inhalation

Teach how to give oxygen therapy

Teach how to give positive pressure breathing

Explain the reason for and intended effect of the therapy

EVALUATION

See the evaluation criteria for each specific goal in Chapter 2.

INADEQUATE INFORMATION RELATED TO RESPIRATORY SYSTEM CANCER

Inadequate Information Related to Lung Cancer (288,333,412)

ASSESSMENT

Subjective Data

Person confirms a lack of information
Anxiety
Concern
Fear

Objective Data

Person's actions indicate a lack of information regarding:
   the early signs and symptoms of lung cancer
   smoking as a primary cause of lung cancer
   the fact that despite prolonged smoking, cessation of smoking greatly
      reduces the possibility of lung cancer
   the need for periodic chest x-rays
   how lung cancer is treated

Related Data

Commonly Related Diseases:
Pulmonary carcinoma

POSSIBLE ETIOLOGY

Lack of instruction

NURSING DIAGNOSIS

Inadequate information related to lung cancer: lack of information regarding the cause and treatment of lung cancer

PLANNING

Patient Needs	**Primary Nurse-Patient Goals**
Comfort	To achieve comfort
Protection from physical harm	To prevent physical injury
Increased learning	To achieve awareness of needs

NURSING INTERVENTIONS

Nursing Treatments

Approach unhurriedly
Encourage patient questions
Involve the family
Discuss the anticipated procedure (associated with treatment of lung cancer)

Nursing Observations
Inspect the chest for respiratory rate and rhythm
Monitor the blood pressure
Evaluate the response to teaching
Health Teaching
Describe the early manifestations of lung cancer
Instruct to immediately report serious symptoms
Explain the causes of the health problem
Recommend a periodic chest x-ray

EVALUATION

See the evaluation criteria for each specific goal in Chapter 2.

28.
NURSING DIAGNOSES RELATED TO
Sensory Perception

HEARING: ALTERED SOUND PERCEPTION

Dependence on Communication Assistance Related to Impaired Hearing, p. 474

Sound Sensitivity (97)

ASSESSMENT

Subjective Data
Person associates noise with confusion

Objective Data
Person seldom turns on radio, T.V., etc.
Is irritable in response to noise
Shows startle reflex

Related Data
Commonly Related Diseases:
None

POSSIBLE ETIOLOGY

Auditory nerve disorders. Nervousness. Being unaccustomed to noise.

NURSING DIAGNOSIS

Sound sensitivity: an intolerance for loud sounds

PLANNING

Patient Needs	Primary Nurse-Patient Goals
Comfort	To achieve comfort
Protection from physical harm	To prevent physical injury
Increased learning	To achieve awareness of needs

NURSING INTERVENTIONS

Nursing Treatments
Place in a private room
Place in a heavily-draped, carpeted room to reduce noise
Provide quiet

Nursing Observations
Observe for evidence of a favorable response to therapy

Health Teaching
Recommend methods for noise reduction
Explain the causes of the health problem
Explain the reason for and intended effect of the therapy

EVALUATION

See the evaluation criteria for each specific goal in Chapter 2.

HEARING: POTENTIAL ALTERED SOUND PERCEPTION

Potential Hearing Loss Related to Trauma (70,113,391)

ASSESSMENT

Objective Data
Pushing earwax further into the eardrum
Placing objects like beads and hair pins into the ear
Swimming and diving while having an ear infection
Flying in an airplane while having a cold or allergy
Being exposed to intense noise in work areas
Playing sports in which balls, bats, etc., can traumatize the ear

POSSIBLE ETIOLOGY

Eustachian tube obstruction by cerumen or mucous secretions. Tympanic membrane rupture. Trauma from foreign objects. Water pressure from diving which destroys eustachian tube tissue.

NURSING DIAGNOSIS

Potential hearing loss related to trauma: the possibility that hearing loss could result from injury

PLANNING

Patient Needs
Protection from physical harm

Increased learning

Primary Nurse-Patient Goals
To prevent physical injury

To achieve awareness of needs

NURSING INTERVENTIONS

Nursing Treatments
Minimize environmental dangers

Nursing Observations
Test the ears for impaired hearing (periodically)

Health Teaching
Explain that yawning and swallowing will equalize ear pressure
Emphasize the need to fly in pressurized airplanes
Emphasize the danger of excessive exposure to noise
Recommend the use of ear mufflers
Recommend methods for noise reduction
Inform that water should be kept out of infected ears
Explain how to remove earwax
Instruct not to insert foreign objects into body orifices
Recommend strict adherence to safety rules (regarding contact sports)
Explain the reason for and intended effect of the therapy

EVALUATION

See the evaluation criteria for each specific goal in Chapter 2.

HEARING: EAR DISCOMFORT

Ear Foreign Body (70,391)

ASSESSMENT

Subjective Data
Earache
Complaints of diminished hearing
Buzzing in the ear when an insect is present

Objective Data
Ear canal swelling
Purulent and bloody ear drainage
Object or insect visible inside the ear

Related Data
Commonly Related Diseases:
None
   OR
Tympanic membrane rupture

POSSIBLE ETIOLOGY

Accidental or intentional insertion of objects into the ear. Accidental flying or crawling of an insect into the ear.

NURSING DIAGNOSIS

Ear foreign body: the presence of an alien object in the ear

PLANNING

Patient Needs	Primary Nurse-Patient Goals
Comfort	To achieve comfort
Protection from physical harm	To prevent physical injury

Increased learning   To achieve awareness of needs

NURSING INTERVENTIONS

Nursing Treatments
Irrigate the foreign particle with alcohol (if it is a bean or such that will expand)
Remove foreign object
Insert an oil cotton pledget into the ear
  OR
Instill warm oil into the ear
Make a referral (to a physician if ear trauma has occurred)

Nursing Observations
Inspect the ears with an otoscope (for inflammation or edema)
Observe for complaints of pain

Health Teaching
Instruct not to insert foreign objects into body orifices
Explain the reason for and intended effect of the therapy

EVALUATION

See the evaluation criteria for each specific goal in Chapter 2.

Eustachian Tube Obstruction Related to Atmospheric Pressure Changes (113,225)

ASSESSMENT

Subjective Data
Feeling of fullness in the ear
Mild, intermittent pain
Internal popping sound when swallowing
Temporary impaired hearing
Sound of own voice echoing in the involved ear

Objective Data
Retracted eardrum without redness or tumor

Related Data
Commonly Related Diseases:
None

POSSIBLE ETIOLOGY

Altitude changes in which the altered atmospheric pressure causes air to be trapped inside the middle ear. Atmospheric pressure changes resulting from weather conditions.

NURSING DIAGNOSIS

Eustachian tube obstruction related to atmospheric pressure changes: a closing off of the auditory canal as a result of changes in the pressure of the atmosphere

PLANNING

Patient Needs	**Primary Nurse-Patient Goals**
Comfort	To achieve comfort
Protection from physical harm	To prevent physical injury
Increased learning	To achieve awareness of needs

NURSING INTERVENTIONS

Nursing Treatments
Change the patient's position gradually
Discourage smoking

Nursing Observations
Inspect the ears with an otoscope (for inflammation or edema)
Test the ears for impaired hearing (if the condition is persistent)

Health Teaching
Describe those symptoms which should be reported (persistent ear fullness
    or impaired hearing)
Explain that yawning and swallowing will equalize ear pressure
Advise gentle nose blowing
Instruct to change position gradually

EVALUATION

See the evaluation criteria for each specific goal in Chapter 2.

Impacted Cerumen (70,391)

ASSESSMENT

Subjective Data
Itching
Complaints of diminished hearing
Tinnitus
Dizziness

Objective Data
Brown, hard earwax
Oily skin

Related Data
Commonly Related Diseases:
None

POSSIBLE ETIOLOGY

Excessive secretion of the ceruminous glands. Narrowed ear meatal canal.

NURSING DIAGNOSIS

Impacted cerumen: an excessive collection of earwax

PLANNING

Patient Needs	**Primary Nurse-Patient Goals**
Comfort	To achieve comfort

Cleanliness	To achieve good hygiene
Protection from physical harm	To prevent physical injury
Increased learning	To achieve awareness of needs

NURSING INTERVENTIONS

Nursing Treatments
Soften and remove the earwax

Nursing Observations
Inspect the ears with an otoscope

Health Teaching
Explain how to remove earwax
Instruct not to insert foreign objects into body orifices (to remove earwax)
Explain the causes of the health problem
Explain the reason for and intended effect of the therapy

EVALUATION

See the evaluation criteria for each specific goal in Chapter 2.

Tinnitus Discomfort (113,453)

ASSESSMENT

Subjective Data
Complains of buzzing, clicking, rumbling, ringing, thumping, hissing, rushing water, whistling, or roaring ear sounds heard in one or both ears
Sounds seem louder at night
Sounds may pulsate with the heartbeat

Related Data
Commonly Related Diseases:
Otitis media
Otosclerosis
Syphilis
Basal skull fracture
Acoustic nerve tumor
Labryinthitis
Meningitis
Hypertension
Arteriosclerosis
Meniere's disease
Acute nonsuppurative labyrinthitis
Aortic coarctation
Polycythemia vera
Diabetes mellitus
Aortic regurgitation

POSSIBLE ETIOLOGY

Impacted cerumen. Foreign body. Infection. Emotional tension. Pressure within the ear. Quinine, streptomycin or salicylate overdose. Auditory canal or eustachian tube obstruction. Allergic response. Endocrine imbalance. Hysteria. Jaw malocclusion. Eardrum perforation. Alcohol ingestion.

NURSING DIAGNOSIS

Tinnitus discomfort: the annoyance of hearing abnormal noises in the ear

PLANNING

Patient Needs	Primary Nurse-Patient Goals
Comfort	To achieve comfort
Protection from physical harm	To prevent physical injury
Increased learning	To achieve awareness of needs

NURSING INTERVENTIONS

Nursing Treatments
Place on the unaffected side
Provide radio and television for diversion (especially radio at night)
Withhold the drugs (salicylates, quinine, streptomycin)
Make a referral (to a physician if there is pathology)

Nursing Observations
Inspect the ears with an otoscope (for impacted cerumen, infection, perforated eardrum)
Inspect the teeth for abnormalities (poor alignment of upper and lower teeth)
Monitor the blood pressure (for elevation)

Health Teaching
Explain the causes of the health problem
Explain the reason for and intended effect of the therapy

EVALUATION

See the evaluation criteria for each specific goal in Chapter 2.

SIGHT: ALTERED VISION

Dependence Related to Partial Vision Loss (10,126,165,347)

ASSESSMENT

Subjective Data
Person relies on nurses for:
    placement of objects in appropriate places
    the provision of devices that support better vision
    assistance with mobility
    maintenance of an environment conducive to ease of mobility
Complains of difficulty seeing objects at either a far or close distance
Vision is blurred or doubled
Impaired central vision
Diminished nighttime vision
Impaired peripheral vision

Objective Data

Person has a visual acuity of 20/70 to 20/200 in the best eye with the help of visual aid

Holds objects either close up or far off when reading

Throws his head backward to see beyond eyelid ptosis

One eye is bandaged

One eyelid is sutured

Therapeutic positioning reduces head movements for adequate vision

Related Data

Commonly Related Conditions:

Aging

Farsightedness

Nearsightedness

Diplopia

Commonly Related Diseases:

Glaucoma

Retinal detachment

Iritis

Conjunctivitis

Horner's syndrome

Myasthenia gravis

Hypertension

Cataract

Glomerulonephritis

Diabetes mellitus

Myopia

Hyperopia

Cerebral vascular accident

Trochlear nerve paralysis

Cerebral contusion

Multiple sclerosis

POSSIBLE ETIOLOGY

Hardening of the lens in middle life. Paralysis or weakness of the third cranial nerve or levator muscle in eyelid ptosis. Retinal degeneration, or the absence of rods or cones at the point of nerve conjunction in central blind spots. Lack of equal eye focus in diplopia. Eyeball elongation causing light rays to focus in the vitreous humor before reaching the retina in nearsightedness. A shortened eyeball causing light rays to focus behind the retina in farsightedness. A refractive error in which light rays are not properly bent to converge on the retina in blurred vision. Optic nerve severence which prevents nerve stimulation from the retina from reaching the brain in impaired peripheral vision. Drug side effects.

NURSING DIAGNOSIS

Dependence related to partial vision loss: reliance on nurses to assist with and facilitate ease of movement about the environment and the maintenance of self-activity when there is partial loss of vision

PLANNING

Patient Needs	**Primary Nurse-Patient Goals**
Comfort	To achieve comfort
Protection from physical harm	To prevent accident, physical injury
Dependence	To achieve comfort
Mastery and competence in skills, Independence	To achieve optimum function
Increased learning	To achieve awareness of needs

NURSING INTERVENTIONS

Nursing Treatments
Anticipate needs
Approach unhurriedly
Reassure verbally
Arrange geographic placement
Place in an uncrowded area
Illuminate the room adequately
Provide a nightlight
Minimize environmental barriers
Place the call light within reach
Place objects within reach
Place objects within sight
Provide a low-height bed
Provide frequent patient contact
Provide large-print reading material
Provide a magnifying glass
Provide prism glasses (when patient is therapeutically positioned flat on his back)
Read to the patient (if the patient desires)
Refrain from performing nonessential procedures

Nursing Observations
Observe for readiness to assume activities of daily living

Health Teaching
Explain that objects should be consistently placed in the same location for the visually impaired
Explain the reason for and intended effect of the therapy

EVALUATION

See the evaluation criteria for each specific goal in Chapter 2.

Dependence Related to Total Vision Loss (10,126,165,347)

ASSESSMENT

Subjective Data
Person relies on nurses for:
    placement of objects in appropriate places

guidance in the use of special methods used for the visually impaired
assistance with mobility
maintenance of an environment conducive to ease of mobility

Objective Data

Person is unable to see at 20 feet what normal-sighted persons can see at
  200 feet
Visual field may be restricted to 20 feet or less
Unable to locate objects by sight
Collides with objects

Related Data

Commonly Related Diseases:
Glaucoma
Gonorrhea
Multiple sclerosis
Diabetes mellitus
Nephritis uveitis
Arteriosclerosis

POSSIBLE ETIOLOGY

Sudden eye trauma or disease. Bandaged eyes or sutured eyelids resulting
from surgical procedure.

NURSING DIAGNOSIS

Dependence related to total vision loss: reliance on nurses to assist with and
facilitate ease of movement about the environment and the maintenance of
self-activity when there is complete loss of vision

PLANNING

Patient Needs	Primary Nurse-Patient Goals
Comfort	To achieve comfort
Protection from physical harm	To prevent accident, physical injury
Dependence	To achieve comfort
Mastery and competence in skills, Independence	To achieve optimum function
Increased learning	To achieve awareness of needs and/or use of resources

NURSING INTERVENTIONS

Nursing Treatments

Anticipate needs
Approach unhurriedly
Reassure verbally
Arrange geographic placement
Place in an uncrowded area
Minimize environmental barriers
Place the call light within reach
Place objects within reach

Provide a low-height bed
Provide frequent patient contact
Read to the patient (if the patient desires)
Refrain from performing nonessential procedures
Make a referral (to the Association for the Blind, if visual impairment is
    permanent)

Nursing Observations
Observe for readiness to assume activities of daily living

Health Teaching
Explain that objects should be consistently placed in the same location for
    the visually impaired
Recommend methods for eating suggested for the visually impaired
Recommend the use of knots to distinguish clothing color for the visually
    impaired
Explain the reason for and intended effect of the therapy

EVALUATION

See the evaluation criteria for each specific goal in Chapter 2.

SIGHT: POTENTIAL
ALTERED VISION

Potential Vision Loss Related to
Eye Abuse (10,126,165,347)

ASSESSMENT

Subjective Data
Considers wearing eyeglasses a weakness
Believes that there is no visual problem unless accompanied by pain

Objective Data
Person does not have regular eye examinations
Has untreated eye disorders
Continues to work despite eye fatigue
Works with poor illumination

Related Data
Commonly Related Conditions:
Aging
Commonly Related Diseases:
None

POSSIBLE ETIOLOGY

Lack of instruction. Apathy.

NURSING DIAGNOSIS

Potential vision loss related to eye abuse: the possibility that vision loss
could occur as a result of inadequate eye care

PLANNING

Patient Needs

Protection from physical harm

Increased learning

Primary Nurse-Patient Goals

To prevent physical injury

To achieve awareness of needs
and/or use of resources

NURSING INTERVENTIONS

Nursing Treatments

Encourage adequate rest

Illuminate the room adequately

Make a referral (to a physician for eye disorders)

Nursing Observations

Observe for complaints of visual disturbance

Test the eyes for impaired vision (periodically)

Evaluate the response to teaching

Health Teaching

Advise against letting light shine directly into the eyes

Advise against wearing unprescribed eyeglasses

Advise proper focusing of the television picture

Advise that the television be viewed from the front, not from side angles

Explain that a light is needed in the television viewing room

Inform that television should be viewed at a moderate distance

Explain how to illuminate a room correctly

Inform that large-print reading material is available

Instruct to avoid rubbing the eyes

Explain the reason for and intended effect of the therapy

EVALUATION

See the evaluation criteria for each specific goal in Chapter 2.

Potential Vision Loss Related to Eye Exposure (113,391)

ASSESSMENT

Subjective Data

Eye irritation

Objective Data

Exopthalmic eye bulging

Incomplete eyelid closure from lid lag

Inability to blink normally

Decreased tear production

Opened eyes when in a coma

Related Data

Commonly Related Conditions:

Coma

Commonly Related Diseases:
Thyrotoxicosis
Cerebral tumor
Cerebral vascular accident
Ocular motor nerve tumor

POSSIBLE ETIOLOGY

Lack of instruction in eye care. Inadequate eye care. Inability to close the eyelids resulting in eye tissue dryness and injury.

NURSING DIAGNOSIS

Potential vision loss related to eye exposure: the possibility that vision loss will occur as a result of eye exposure to the environment

PLANNING

Patient Needs	Primary Nurse-Patient Goals
Sleep, rest	To achieve sleep, rest
Cleanliness	To achieve good hygiene
Protection from physical harm	To prevent physical injury, infection
Increased learning	To achieve awareness of needs

NURSING INTERVENTIONS

Nursing Treatments
Encourage adequate rest
Lubricate the eye
Apply a sterile dressing (over the eye)

Nursing Observations
Observe for complaints of visual disturbance
Evaluate the response to teaching

Health Teaching
Describe those symptoms which should be reported (any eye irritation)
Inform that cleanliness is basic to health
Instruct to avoid rubbing the eyes
Explain the reason for and intended effect of the therapy

EVALUATION

See the evaluation criteria for each specific goal in Chapter 2.

Potential Vision Loss Related to Oxygen Therapy (325)

ASSESSMENT

Subjective Data
Complaints of slightly decreased vision, which gradually becomes more impaired during prolonged oxygen therapy

Related Data

Age:

Premature infants receiving oxygen concentrations above 40%

Children and adults receiving oxygen concentrations above 50%

Commonly Related Diseases:

Any disease in which the person receives O_2 therapy

Retinitis

POSSIBLE ETIOLOGY

Oxygen acts on the eye vessels, causing retinal vessel spasms. This leads to the filtration of blood and serum through vessel walls into retinal tissue with resulting retinal damage and blindness.

NURSING DIAGNOSIS

Potential vision loss related to oxygen therapy: the possibility that prolonged inhalation of concentrated oxygen over 40% or 50% will cause retinal damage and blindness

PLANNING

Patient Needs

Protection from physical harm

Increased learning

Primary Nurse-Patient Goals

To prevent physical injury

To achieve awareness of needs

NURSING INTERVENTIONS

Nursing Treatments

Limit therapeutic oxygen concentrations to below 40%

Nursing Observations

Observe for complaints of visual disturbance

Health Teaching

Explain the causes of the health problem

Explain the reason for and intended effect of the therapy

EVALUATION

See the evaluation criteria for each specific goal in Chapter 2.

Potential Vision Loss Related to Trauma (277,391)

ASSESSMENT

Objective Data

Failure to use protective eye guards

Looking directly at the sun or sun eclipse

Carelessness when using chemicals

Allowing children to play with BB guns, bows and arrows, darts, javelins, hard balls, slingshots, etc.

Sustaining blows to the head or face

Wearing contact lens while sleeping, during eye infections and disorders, or for prolonged periods

Failure to seek medical treatment of an inverted eyelid

POSSIBLE ETIOLOGY

Lack of instruction. Lack of compliance with safety rules. Inadequate eye care.

NURSING DIAGNOSIS

Potential vision loss related to trauma: the possibility that vision loss will occur as a result of activities which lead to eye trauma

PLANNING

Patient Needs

Protection from physical harm

Increased learning

Primary Nurse-Patient Goals

To prevent physical injury

To achieve awareness of needs

NURSING INTERVENTIONS

Nursing Treatments
Minimize environmental dangers
Remove the contact lens (during sleep and eye infection)
Make a referral (to a physician as needed)

Nursing Observations
Observe for complaints of visual disturbance
Evaluate the response to teaching

Health Teaching
Advise against giving toys likely to cause eye injury
Advise precaution when using chemicals
Emphasize the importance of wearing safety goggles
Instruct that sungazing be avoided even when wearing sunglasses
Instruct that contact lens should not be worn beyond the prescribed time,
    during an eye disorder, or while sleeping
Instruct that the eyes should not be wiped with soiled towels
Instruct to avoid rubbing the eyes
Recommend the use of eyeglass safety lens
Recommend strict adherence to safety rules

EVALUATION

See the evaluation criteria for each specific goal in Chapter 2.

Minimal Intraocular Pressure Requirement (113,225,325)

ASSESSMENT

Subjective Data
Eye pain

Objective Data
Eye hemorrhage
Eye trauma
Postcorneal transplant
Postsurgical eye repair

Related Data

Commonly Related Conditions:
Eye contusion

Commonly Related Diseases:
Glaucoma

POSSIBLE ETIOLOGY

Increased intraocular bulk from bleeding, edema, tumor, or abscess. Healing following therapeutic eye surgery.

NURSING DIAGNOSIS

Minimal intraocular pressure requirement: a need to keep the tension within the eyeball at a minimum level

PLANNING

Patient Needs	Primary Nurse-Patient Goals
Sleep, rest	To achieve sleep, rest
Comfort	To achieve comfort
Protection from physical harm	To prevent physical injury
Freedom from pain	To achieve comfort
Increased learning	To achieve awareness of needs

NURSING INTERVENTIONS

Nursing Treatments
Change the patient's position gradually
Elevate the head (slightly)
Do not place in the flat position
Refrain from jarring the bed
Encourage adequate rest
Subdue the room lighting
Discourage oral stimulants
Discourage smoking

Nursing Observations
Observe for complaints of pain
Evaluate the response to teaching

Health Teaching
Advise gentle nose blowing
Inform that coughing should be avoided
Inform that elimination straining should be avoided
Inform that stooping or lowering the head should be avoided
Inform that heavy lifting should be avoided
Instruct to avoid rubbing the eyes
Instruct to change position gradually
Explain the causes of the health problem
Explain the reason for and intended effect of the therapy

EVALUATION

See the evaluation criteria for each specific goal in Chapter 2.

SIGHT: EYE DISCOMFORTS

Light Intolerance Discomfort (325,453)

ASSESSMENT

Subjective Data
Inability to see in bright sunlight
Complaints of eye irritation or pain

Objective Data
Squinting
Excessive tearing

Related Data
Commonly Related Conditions:
Sinus congestion

Commonly Related Diseases:
Measles
Meningitis
Albinism
Colorado tick fever
Yellow fever
Rickettsialpox
Weil's disease
Hypoparathyroidism

POSSIBLE ETIOLOGY

Vitamin A deficiency. Eye tissue inflammation. Systemic disease.

NURSING DIAGNOSIS

Light intolerance discomfort: eye irritation and discomfort occurring on exposure to light

PLANNING

Patient Needs	**Primary Nurse-Patient Goals**
Comfort	To achieve comfort
Protection from physical harm	To prevent physical injury
Increased learning	To achieve awareness of needs

NURSING INTERVENTIONS

Nursing Treatments
Subdue the room lighting
Provide sunglasses (when exposed to bright light)

Nursing Observations
Observe for complaints of pain

Health Teaching
Advise against letting light shine directly into the eyes
Explain the causes of the health problem
Explain the reason for and intended effect of the therapy

EVALUATION

See the evaluation criteria for each specific goal in Chapter 2.

SIGHT: EMERGENCY EYE CONDITIONS

Emergency Phase Eye Foreign Body (192)

ASSESSMENT

Subjective Data
Pain
Diminished vision

Objective Data
Redness
Inflammation
Excessive tearing
Visible foreign object

Related Data
Commonly Related Diseases:
None

POSSIBLE ETIOLOGY

Accidental injury

NURSING DIAGNOSIS

Emergency phase eye foreign body: the need for immediate health care as a result of a foreign body in the eye

PLANNING

Patient Needs
Comfort
Protection from physical harm
Increased learning

Primary Nurse-Patient Goals
To achieve comfort
To prevent physical injury
To achieve awareness of needs

NURSING INTERVENTIONS

Nursing Treatments
Evert the eyelid (to facilitate visualization of the foreign body)
Remove foreign object (with moistened, sterile gauze)
Irrigate the eye (with saline or plain water)
Handle gently
Make a referral (to a physician if there is any eye damage)

Nursing Observations
Inspect for edema
Observe for complaints of pain
Observe for complaints of visual disturbance

Health Teaching
Instruct to avoid rubbing the eyes
Describe those symptoms which should be reported (continued pain, inflammation, visual disturbance)
Explain the reason for and intended effect of the therapy

EVALUATION

See the evaluation criteria for each specific goal in Chapter 2.

SMELL: IMPAIRED OLFACTORY SENSE

Potential Accidental Burn, p. 572

Potential Accidental Suffocation, p. 575

TASTE: IMPAIRED TASTE SENSE

Impaired Ability to Taste Food, p. 928

TOUCH: IMPAIRED TOUCH SENSE

Potential Accidental Burn, p. 572

Potential Decubitus Ulcer, p. 796

SENSORY STIMULATION, ALTERED

Inadequate Pleasant Sensory Stimulation (12,13,94)

ASSESSMENT

Subjective Data
Person spends most hours of the day performing activities perceived as giving little or no satisfaction
Is preoccupied with suffering or frustration
Is chronically fatigued
Person's wishes or desires are seldom gratified

Objective Data
Little or no participation in activities that the person enjoys
Person seldom laughs
Chronically complains
Is seldom exposed to happy people, or a pleasant, cheerful environment

Related Data

Commonly Related Diseases:
None
   OR
Psychoneurosis
Schizophrenia

POSSIBLE ETIOLOGY

Burdensome responsibilities. Inability of the person to identify his own pleasure values. Nonrecognition of the need for pleasurable feelings. Poorly learned activity and socialization skills. Work restrictions.

NURSING DIAGNOSIS

Inadequate pleasant sensory stimulation: the presence of more frequent feelings of unpleasantness than pleasantness

PLANNING

Patient Needs	Primary Nurse-Patient Goals
Comfort	To achieve comfort
Protection from psychologic threat	To prevent emotional injury
Warm, communicating relationships	To achieve effective verbal and nonverbal communications
Endurance	To achieve positive expression, feelings, reactions
Personal growth and maturity	To achieve optimum function
Increased learning	To achieve awareness of needs
Full development of potential	To achieve optimum function
Increased pleasantness	To achieve positive expressions, feelings, reactions

NURSING INTERVENTIONS

Nursing Treatments
Approach unhurriedly
Arrange pleasant surroundings
Assist the patient in restructuring his lifestyle
Assist the patient in setting standards of a meaningful existence
Encourage acceptance of the right to pleasure
Encourage creative activities and play
Encourage laughter
Encourage the enjoyment of life's simple things
Encourage renewal of former interests
Provide gratifying experiences

Nursing Observations
Observe for evidence of a favorable response to therapy

Health Teaching
Explain the causes of the health problem
Explain the reason for and intended effect of the therapy

Advise occasional respite from responsibility
Explain that recreation aids total health

EVALUATION

See the evaluation criteria for each specific goal in Chapter 2.

Increased Physical Stimulation Requirement (70,71,391)

ASSESSMENT

Subjective Data
Annoyance at being aroused

Objective Data
Comatose
Semicomatose
Lethargic
Stuporous
Delirious
Responsive for only short periods to external stimuli

Related Data
Commonly Related Conditions:
Poisoning
Metabolic acidosis
Commonly Related Diseases:
Cerebral concussion
Alcoholism
Subdural hematoma
Cerebral vascular accident

POSSIBLE ETIOLOGY

Drug side effects. Brain cell damage. Metabolic disturbances.

NURSING DIAGNOSIS

Increased physical stimulation requirement: a need for periodic, deliberate arousal to an awareness of the environment

PLANNING

Patient Needs
Stimulation

Protection from physical harm
Increased learning

Primary Nurse-Patient Goals
To maintain sensory function and
stimulation
To prevent physical injury
To achieve awareness of needs

NURSING INTERVENTIONS

Nursing Treatments
Provide frequent patient contact
Stimulate by movement, touch, sternal pressure, or speech (periodically)
Place by a window

Nursing Observations
Observe for evidence of a favorable response to therapy

Health Teaching
Explain the reason for and intended effect of the therapy

EVALUATION

See the evaluation criteria for each specific goal in Chapter 2.

Sensory Deprivation (12,13,378,462)

ASSESSMENT

Subjective Data
Boredom
Depression
Heightened anxiety
Exaggerated emotional reactions
Brooding about imagined injustices
Fatigue
Apathy

Objective Data
Little variation in daily routine
Little or no change in physical surroundings
Few social contacts
Irritability
Complaints of physical discomforts
Little or no display of affection
Little verbal expression of feelings
Restlessness
Passiveness
Poor appetite

Related Data
Commonly Related Conditions:
Failure to thrive
Commonly Related Diseases:
None
   OR
Any prolonged disease or injury

POSSIBLE ETIOLOGY

Little or no touch contact with other humans. Living in a poorly illumi-
nated area. Absence of windows in a room. Prolonged, excessive quiet. Dull
colors in the environment. Little movement of persons or objects in the environment. Prolonged confinement to one area. Constant exposure to plain,
poorly seasoned food. Lack of exposure to a variety of smells. Lack of exercise.

NURSING DIAGNOSIS

Sensory deprivation: lack of sufficient sensory stimulus in the environment surrounding the person to maintain an adequate sensory input

PLANNING

Patient Needs	Primary Nurse-Patient Goals
Activity	To achieve activity
Comfort	To achieve comfort
Stimulation	To maintain sensory function and stimulation
Protection from psychologic threat	To prevent emotional injury
Warm, communicating relationships	To achieve effective verbal and nonverbal communications
Sense of value, usefulness	To achieve positive expressions, feelings, reactions
Increased learning	To achieve awareness of needs
Less of the familiar, more of the novel	To achieve a therapeutic environment
Increased pleasantness	To achieve positive expressions, feelings, reactions

NURSING INTERVENTIONS

Nursing Treatments
Allow unlimited visiting
Assist the patient in restructuring his lifestyle
Dress in colorful clothing
Illuminate the room adequately
Keep the patient's door open
Place by a window
Place in an infant seat
Provide an attractive meal tray
Provide radio and television for diversion
Provide reading material for diversion
Encourage active diversional activities
Sit with the patient
Talk with the patient
Provide frequent patient contact
Touch the patient judiciously

Nursing Observations
Observe for an excessive stress level
Observe for evidence of a favorable response to therapy

Health Teaching
Recommend methods for increasing sensory stimulation
Explain the causes of the health problem
Explain the reason for and intended effect of the therapy

EVALUATION

See the evaluation criteria for each specific goal in Chapter 2.

Sensory Overload (12,13,94)

ASSESSMENT

Subjective Data
Verbal expressions of anxiety
Desire for escape from the situation
Fatigue
Nervousness

Objective Data
Irritability
Startle reflex

Related Data
Commonly Related Diseases:
None

POSSIBLE ETIOLOGY

Overexposure to environmental stimuli such as noise, crowding, etc. Involvement in too many activities above the person's comfort level. The occurrence of multiple stress situations within a short period which require exhaustive coping or adaptation.

NURSING DIAGNOSIS

Sensory overload: excessive stimulation of the senses

PLANNING

Patient Needs	**Primary Nurse-Patient Goals**
Rest	To achieve rest
Comfort	To achieve comfort
Protection from physical harm	To prevent physical injury
Protection from psychologic threat	To prevent emotional injury
Increased learning	To achieve awareness of needs

NURSING INTERVENTIONS

Nursing Treatments
Arrange orderly surroundings
Arrange pleasant surroundings
Arrange a structured environment
Avoid causing intense emotional situations
Encourage adequate rest
Encourage quiet diversional activities
Handle gently
Keep the patient's door closed
Plan undisturbed periods for the patient
Provide frequent patient contact
Provide quiet

Reduce the demands placed upon the patient
Refrain from performing nonessential procedures
Refrain from sudden, stimulating movements
Restrict unwanted visitors

Nursing Observations
Observe for an excessive stress level
Observe for evidence of a favorable response to therapy

Health Teaching
Recommend methods for reducing sensory stimulation
Describe the behavior pattern indicating overstimulation
Explain the causes of the health problem
Explain the reason for and intended effect of the therapy

EVALUATION

See the evaluation criteria for each specific goal in Chapter 2.

Unpleasant Sensory Stimulation

ASSESSMENT

Subjective Data
Verbal expressions of displeasure
Nausea

Objective Data
Disgusted facial expression
Withdrawal from the stimuli

Related Data
Commonly Related Conditions:
Decubitus ulcers
Deformities

Commonly Related Diseases:
Carcinoma
Leprosy
Severe first-, second-, or third-degree burns

POSSIBLE ETIOLOGY

Poor environmental control of odors and sights. A situation that is in conflict with esthetic values. A health condition of the body that no longer meets socializing standards.

NURSING DIAGNOSIS

Unpleasant sensory stimulation: feelings of intense offense of displeasure resulting from unfavorable external stimuli

PLANNING

Patient Needs	**Primary Nurse-Patient Goals**
Comfort	To achieve comfort
Protection from physical harm	To prevent physical injury

Protection from psychologic threat	To prevent emotional injury
Warm, communicating relationships	To achieve effective verbal and nonverbal communications
Increased pleasantness	To achieve positive expressions, feelings, reactions

NURSING INTERVENTIONS

Nursing Treatments
Arrange pleasant surroundings
Encourage the expression of feelings
Remove the stimulus for the emotion

Nursing Observations
Observe for an excessive stress level
Observe for evidence of a favorable response to therapy

Health Teaching
Advise that the precipitating factor be avoided

EVALUATION

See the evaluation criteria for each specific goal in Chapter 2.

INADEQUATE SENSORY ASSISTANCE DEVICE USE

Inadequate Information Related to Artificial Eye Use (391)

ASSESSMENT

Subjective Data
Person confirms a lack of information

Objective Data
Person's actions indicate a lack of information regarding:
   how to insert or remove an artificial eye
   how to clean it
   how to handle it with care

Related Data
Commonly Related Diseases:
None
   OR
Carcinoma
Traumatic injury

POSSIBLE ETIOLOGY

Lack of instruction. No previous experience with the artificial eye.

NURSING DIAGNOSIS

Inadequate information related to artificial eye use: lack of information regarding how to use and care for an artificial eye

PLANNING

Patient Needs	**Primary Nurse-Patient Goals**
Comfort	To achieve comfort
Protection from physical harm	To prevent physical injury, infection
Mastery and competence in skills	To achieve optimum function
Increased learning	To achieve awareness of needs

NURSING INTERVENTIONS

Nursing Treatments
Approach unhurriedly
Encourage patient questions

Nursing Observations
Evaluate the response to teaching

Health Teaching
Describe those symptoms which should be reported (eye irritation from the
  artificial eye)
Inform that cleanliness is basic to health
Teach how to care for an artificial eye
Teach how to insert and remove an artificial eye
Recommend the use of eyeglass safety lens (for the natural eye)

EVALUATION

See the evaluation criteria for each specific goal in Chapter 2.

Inadequate Information Related to Contact Lens Use (277,391)

ASSESSMENT

Subjective Data
Person confirms a lack of information

Objective Data
Person's actions indicate a lack of information regarding:
  how to insert or remove contact lenses
  how to clean them in the proper fluid or container
  the fact that contact lenses are affected by extreme cold or heat
  the dangers associated with wearing contact lenses

Related Data
Commonly Related Diseases:
None
  OR
Myopia
Hyperopia
Astigmatism

POSSIBLE ETIOLOGY

Lack of instruction

NURSING DIAGNOSIS

Inadequate information related to contact lens use: lack of information regarding how to care for and use corrective, curved lenses placed directly over the cornea

PLANNING

Patient Needs

Protection from physical harm

Mastery and competence in skills

Increased learning

Primary Nurse-Patient Goals

To prevent physical injury, infection

To achieve optimum function

To achieve awareness of needs

NURSING INTERVENTIONS

Nursing Treatments
Approach unhurriedly
Encourage patient questions

Nursing Observations
Evaluate the response to teaching

Health Teaching
Advise that contact lenses not be used for eye color change
Describe the discomforts of contact lens adjustment
Describe those symptoms which should be reported (eye inflammation, visual difficulty)
Explain that care should be taken to prevent scratching of the contact lenses
Explain that extreme cold cracks contact lenses
Explain that heat warps contact lenses
Instruct that contact lenses should not be worn beyond the prescribed time, during an eye disorder, or while sleeping
Instruct to avoid rubbing the eyes (especially when wearing contact lenses)
Inform that cleanliness is basic to health
Teach how to clean contact lenses
Teach how to insert and remove contact lenses

EVALUATION

See the evaluation criteria for each specific goal in Chapter 2.

Inadequate Information Related to Eyeglass Use (70,391)

ASSESSMENT

Subjective Data
Person confirms a lack of information

Objective Data
Person's actions indicate a lack of information regarding:
    the fact that broken or scratched glasses should not be worn
    the dangers of wearing someone else's glasses
    how to clean eyeglasses
    how to protect eyeglasses from damage

the fact that eyeglass lenses must be intermittently changed to support vision changes

Related Data

Commonly Related Diseases:
Astigmatism
Myopia
Hyperopia
Strabismus

POSSIBLE ETIOLOGY

Lack of instruction

NURSING DIAGNOSIS

Inadequate information related to eyeglass use: lack of information regarding the care and use of eyeglasses

PLANNING

Patient Needs	**Primary Nurse-Patient Goals**
Comfort	To achieve comfort
Protection from physical harm	To prevent accident, physical injury
Increased learning	To achieve awareness of needs

NURSING INTERVENTIONS

Nursing Treatments
Approach unhurriedly
Encourage patient questions

Nursing Observations
Evaluate the response to teaching

Health Teaching
Advise against wearing unprescribed eyeglasses
Describe those symptoms which should be reported (vision changes)
Inform that eyeglasses should be kept clean, rested on their rims to prevent lens scratching, and placed in a case when unused
Explain that corrective eye lenses require periodic adjustment
Recommend the use of eyeglass safety lens

EVALUATION

See the evaluation criteria for each specific goal in Chapter 2.

Inadequate Information Related to Hearing Aid Use (71,391)

ASSESSMENT

Subjective Data
Person confirms a lack of information

Objective Data
Person's actions indicate a lack of information regarding:

how to adjust the hearing aid amplification
the fact that hearing aid batteries must be intermittently changed
how to properly store a hearing aid

Related Data

Commonly Related Diseases:
Otosclerosis

POSSIBLE ETIOLOGY

Lack of instruction

NURSING DIAGNOSIS

Inadequate information related to hearing aid use: lack of information regarding the care and use of a hearing aid

PLANNING

Patient Needs

Comfort

Protection from physical harm

Increased learning

Primary Nurse-Patient Goals

To achieve comfort

To prevent physical injury

To achieve awareness of needs

NURSING INTERVENTIONS

Nursing Treatments
Approach unhurriedly
Encourage patient questions

Nursing Observations
Evaluate the response to teaching

Health Teaching
Teach how to care for a hearing aid

EVALUATION

See the evaluation criteria for each specific goal in Chapter 2.

29.
NURSING DIAGNOSES RELATED TO
Sleep and Rest

SLEEP AND REST

Additional Rest Requirement
(70,381,391)

ASSESSMENT

Subjective Data
Weakness
Fatigue
Malaise
Dyspnea

Objective Data
Underweight
Irritability
Fever
Rapid pulse
Increased or decreased blood pressure
Person is not easily aroused from sleep
Falls asleep in a chair or riding in a car

Related Data
Commonly Related Conditions:
Oxygen deprivation
Malnutrition
Pregnancy
Aging
Commonly Related Diseases:
Myocardial infarction
Thyrotoxicosis
Pneumonia
Addison's disease
Arteriosclerosis

POSSIBLE ETIOLOGY

Need to restore cell energy depleted by activity, healing, or stress

NURSING DIAGNOSIS

Additional rest requirement: the body's need to obtain an additional amount of rest in excess of the normal requirement

PLANNING

Patient Needs

Sleep, rest

Energy

Comfort

Protection from physical harm

Protection from psychologic threat

Increased learning

Primary Nurse-Patient Goals

To achieve sleep, rest

To maintain regulating mechanisms and functions

To achieve comfort

To prevent physical injury

To prevent emotional injury

To achieve awareness of needs

NURSING INTERVENTIONS

Nursing Treatments
Do not disturb while resting
Encourage adequate rest
Encourage alternate rest and activity
Plan undisturbed periods for the patient
Provide quiet

Nursing Observations
Observe for quality of sleep
Observe the pattern of sleep
Observe for the quantity and inquire about the quality of sleep

Health Teaching
Explain the causes of the health problem
Explain the reason for and intended effect of the therapy

EVALUATION

See the evaluation criteria for each specific goal in Chapter 2.

Disrupted Normal Sleeping Pattern

ASSESSMENT

Subjective Data
Annoyance if disturbed while sleeping at odd hours

Objective Data
Person sleeps when one normally would be awake
Is awake and active when one would normally be asleep
Sleeps during the day and stays awake at night
Eats irregularly because of the reversed sleeping pattern

Related Data

Commonly Related Diseases:
Any disease or injury which interrupts the daily sleep routine

POSSIBLE ETIOLOGY

Need for sleep during the daytime because of illness. Distant travel to areas of time change. May be initiated by daytime, surgical anesthesia followed by a wakeful night. Being aroused for therapeutic interventions at night.

NURSING DIAGNOSIS

Disrupted normal sleeping pattern: altering one's pattern of sleep so it is variant from one's normal pattern

PLANNING

Patient Needs	**Primary Nurse-Patient Goals**
Sleep, rest	To achieve sleep, rest
Protection from physical harm	To prevent physical injury
Increased learning	To achieve awareness of needs

NURSING INTERVENTIONS

Nursing Treatments
Maintain patient wakefulness during the day (until the normal sleep pattern is reestablished)

Nursing Observations
Observe the pattern of sleep

Health Teaching
Recommend a regular sleeping schedule
Explain the causes of the health problem
Explain the reason for and intended effect of the therapy

EVALUATION

See the evaluation criteria for each specific goal in Chapter 2.

Inability to Relax (219,232,379)

ASSESSMENT

Subjective Data
Person experiences physical discomfort
Is often fatigued

Objective Data
Inability to remain quiet for a time
Thrashing about in the bed
Frequent position change while asleep
Concern with trivial things while up and about
Preference for activity rather than inactivity
Diminished attention span
Irritability
Increased pulse and respirations

Related Data

Commonly Related Conditions:
Anoxia
Respiratory acidosis
Threatening respiratory arrest
Hypoglycemia

Commonly Related Diseases:
Any disease or injury, but especially:
Myocardial infarction
Anxiety psychoneurosis
Manic-depressive psychosis
Rocky Mountain spotted fever
Rabies
Sydenham's chorea
Hyperthryoidism

POSSIBLE ETIOLOGY

Emotional distress. Oxygen insufficiency. Discomfort. Pain. Endocrine imbalance. Gastric hyperactivity. Steroid therapy drug side effects. Excessive stimulation from overwork. Uncomfortable environment. Late evening meal.

NURSING DIAGNOSIS

Inability to relax (restlessness): an unquiet, uneasy, continually moving state of the person

PLANNING

Patient Needs	**Primary Nurse-Patient Goals**
Sleep, rest, relaxation	To achieve sleep, rest, relaxation
Comfort	To achieve comfort
Protection from physical harm	To prevent physical injury
Protection from psychologic threat	To prevent emotional injury
Increased learning	To achieve awareness of needs

NURSING INTERVENTIONS

Nursing Treatments
Approach unhurriedly
Administer a warm bath (prior to sleep)
Cover with warm blankets
Massage gently
Position comfortably
Darken the room for sleep
Provide quiet
Discourage oral stimulants
Give nonprescription drugs (ExR) (for pain)

Nursing Observations
Monitor blood studies for abnormal gas exchange
Observe for an excessive stress level

Health Teaching
Recommend methods for achieving total relaxation
Explain the causes of the health problem
Explain the reason for and intended effect of the therapy

Medical Treatments Performed by Nurses
Give the prescribed drugs

EVALUATION

See the evaluation criteria for each specific goal in Chapter 2.

Inability to Sleep (269,404)

ASSESSMENT

Subjective Data
Person thinks about unsettling events while lying awake
Is fatigued on rising

Objective Data
Person falls asleep and suddenly awakens
Lies awake for hours prior to renewed sleep
Falls asleep shortly before awakening time

Related Data
Commonly Related Diseases:
None
   OR
Psychoneurosis
Manic-depressive psychosis
Hypertension

POSSIBLE ETIOLOGY

Ingested stimulants. Overtiredness. Mental fatigue. Tension. Excitement.
Fear of being unable to sleep. Stressful daytime activity causing muscle
tension. Stress from thinking about the day's unaccomplished tasks.
Anxiety-producing conflicts. Fear associated with illness.

NURSING DIAGNOSIS

Inability to sleep: the inability to go to sleep despite physical and mental
efforts to do so

PLANNING

Patient Needs	**Primary Nurse-Patient Goals**
Sleep, rest, relaxation	To achieve sleep, rest, relaxation
Comfort	To achieve comfort
Protection from physical harm	To prevent physical injury
Increased learning	To achieve awareness of needs

NURSING INTERVENTIONS

Nursing Treatments
Anticipate needs

Arrange pleasant surroundings
Administer a warm bath (prior to sleep)
Change the patient's clothes at bedtime
Refresh the patient before sleep
Cover with warm blankets
Give warm liquids (preferably milk)
Discourage oral stimulants
Encourage bladder emptying before rest
Encourage indifference toward sleep
Encourage light reading before sleep
Maintain the usual bedtime rituals
Massage gently (prior to sleep)
Position comfortably
Position on the left side
Darken the room for sleep
Provide quiet
Place in a private room
Do not disturb while resting
Plan undisturbed periods for the patient

Nursing Observations
Observe for an excessive stress level
Observe for restlessness
Observe for the quantity and inquire about the quality of sleep

Health Teaching
Recommend a regular sleeping schedule
Advise against participation in emotional situations before sleep
Recommend methods for achieving total relaxation
Explain the causes of the health problem
Explain the reason for and intended effect of the therapy

Medical Treatments Performed by Nurses
Give the prescribed drugs

EVALUATION

See the evaluation criteria for each specific goal in Chapter 2.

Insufficient Sleep and Rest (326)
ASSESSMENT

Subjective Data
Dizziness
Fatigue
Nervousness

Objective Data
Irritability
Restlessness
Yawning
Dark circles under the eyes
Puffy eyelids

Poor coordination
Use of stimulants

Related Data

Commonly Related Conditions:
Child-rearing
Adolescence
Attending to an ill family member

Commonly Related Diseases:
None
   OR
Manic-depressive psychosis
Catatonic schizophrenia

POSSIBLE ETIOLOGY

Preoccupation with other matters. Sleep interruption because of responsibility. Pain. Poor sleep habits. Worry. Difficulty with the digestive process.

NURSING DIAGNOSIS

Insufficient sleep and rest: the time spent sleeping or resting is below normal requirements for health

PLANNING

Patient Needs	**Primary Nurse-Patient Goals**
Sleep, rest, relaxation	To achieve sleep, rest, relaxation
Protection from physical harm	To prevent physical injury, infection
Protection from psychologic threat	To prevent emotional injury
Increased learning	To achieve awareness of needs

NURSING INTERVENTIONS

Nursing Treatments
Assist the patient in restructuring his lifestyle
Encourage adequate rest
Discourage oral stimulants

Nursing Observations
Observe for the quantity and inquire about the quality of sleep
Observe for restlessness
Observe for the pattern of sleep

Health Teaching
Recommend a regular sleeping schedule
Recommend adherence to a moderate pace of living
Advise against participation in emotional situations prior to sleep
Recommend methods for achieving total relaxation
Explain the causes of the health problem

EVALUATION

See the evaluation criteria for each specific goal in Chapter 2.

SLEEP AND REST THERAPY DISCOMFORTS

Bed-Rest Discomfort

ASSESSMENT

Subjective Data
Confinement heightens anxiety

Objective Data
Person is confined to bed
Is restless
Complains about being in bed
Sometimes gets up when unobserved

Related Data
Commonly Related Conditions:
Aging
Surgery
Shock
Hemorrhage
Cardiac arrythmias
Commonly Related Diseases:
Pulmonary edema
Congestive heart failure
Bone fractures
Myocardial infarction
Pneumonia

POSSIBLE ETIOLOGY

A therapeutic measure intended to prevent energy depletion and to promote healing. Misinformation as to the reason for the therapeutic bed rest.

NURSING DIAGNOSIS

Bed-rest discomfort: discomfort resulting from confinement of the person to bed

PLANNING

Patient Needs	**Primary Nurse-Patient Goals**
Sleep, rest, relaxation	To achieve sleep, rest, relaxation
Comfort	To achieve comfort
Protection from physical harm	To prevent physical injury
Increased learning	To achieve awareness of needs

NURSING INTERVENTIONS

Nursing Treatments
Anticipate needs
Approach unhurriedly
Arrange geographic placement (so the patient can see the nurses)

Arrange pleasant surroundings
Encourage passive diversional activities
Massage gently (periodically for the relaxing effect)
Place by a window
Provide a clean, comfortable bed
Provide a compatible room companion
Position comfortably
Provide frequent patient contact
Provide quiet
Sit with the patient (whenever possible)

Nursing Observations
Observe for restlessness

Health Teaching
Recommend methods for achieving total relaxation
Explain the reason for and intended effect of the therapy

Medical Treatments Performed by Nurses
Give the prescribed drugs

EVALUATION

See the evaluation criteria for each specific goal in Chapter 2.

ANESTHESIA RECOVERY DEPENDENCE

Dependence on Nursing Supervision of Postanesthesia Recovery (70,391)

ASSESSMENT

Subjective Data
Person relies on nurses for:
  smooth transition from unconsciousness to consciousness
  observation for postanesthesia complications
  pain or discomfort relief while regaining consciousness
  protection against injury during postanesthesia period
  the initiation of postoperative treatments
  information regarding the outcome of the surgical procedure
  informing and reassuring his family of his current status

Objective Data
Person has received some form of anesthesia
Is unconscious or in the process of regaining consciousness

Related Data
Commonly Related Diseases:
Any disease or injury requiring anesthesia

POSSIBLE ETIOLOGY

Need for anesthesia in the performance of surgical or diagnostic procedures

NURSING DIAGNOSIS

Dependence on nursing supervision of postanesthesia recovery: reliance on nurses for care and protection during the period of recovery from anesthesia

PLANNING

Patient Needs	**Primary Nurse-Patient Goals**
Oxygen, circulation	To maintain oxygen to all cells
Rest	To achieve rest
Comfort	To achieve comfort
Stimulation	To maintain sensory function and stimulation
Protection from physical harm	To prevent accident, physical injury
Protection from psychologic threat	To prevent emotional injury
Freedom from pain	To achieve comfort
Dependence	To achieve comfort

NURSING INTERVENTIONS

Nursing Treatments
Attend the patient constantly
Approach unhurriedly
Reassure verbally (when conscious)
Anticipate needs
Administer humidified oxygen (ET) (until fully conscious)
Apply a cool, damp cloth to the face (to stimulate the patient)
    OR
Stimulate by movement, touch, sternal pressure or speech
Use the patient's name frequently
Place in the side-lying (Sim's) position (to prevent aspiration)
Change the patient's position frequently
Position comfortably
Maintain body alignment
Cover with lightweight blankets
Safeguard with siderails
Minimize environmental dangers
Encourage deep breathing
Ask the patient what makes him/her comfortable (once consciousness is regained)
Provide standby emergency equipment and drugs
Provide reliable information (regarding the surgical outcome)
Provide emotional support for persons significant to the patient

Nursing Observations
Observe for airway obstruction
Auscultate the chest for lung aeration
Inspect the chest for respiratory rate and rhythm ⎫
Palpate the pulse for rate, rhythm, and volume ⎬ (every 15 minutes)
Monitor the blood pressure ⎭

Observe the level of consciousness (frequently)
Determine the state of orientation (frequently)
Observe for confusion
Observe the preoperative and postoperative response level
Inspect for hemorrhage
Observe for shock
Inspect the abdomen for distention
Observe for vomiting
Inspect the throat for an impaired swallowing reflex (as consciousness is regained)
Inspect the wound dressing frequently
Observe for complaints of pain
Observe for evidence that the patient is reaching out for emotional support (as consciousness is regained)

Medical Treatments Performed by Nurses
Administer a blood transfusion
Administer intravenous fluids
Attach the gastric tube to suction
Give the prescribed drugs

EVALUATION

See the evaluation criteria for each specific goal in Chapter 2.

INADEQUATE REST MANAGEMENT

Inadequate Information Related to Healthy Rest Patterns (89,325,404)

ASSESSMENT

Subjective Data
Person confirms a lack of information

Objective Data
Person's actions indicate a lack of information regarding:
    how many daily hours of sleep are needed for the health of their children, aging or sick relatives, or themselves
    how to promote rest for the body
    why adequate rest is important to health

Related Data

Commonly Related Diseases:
None
    OR
Any disease or injury

POSSIBLE ETIOLOGY

Lack of instruction

NURSING DIAGNOSIS

Inadequate information related to healthy rest patterns: lack of information regarding rest and its role in good health

PLANNING

Patient Needs

Sleep, rest, relaxation

Protection from physical harm

Protection from psychologic threat

Increased learning

Primary Nurse-Patient Goals

To achieve sleep, rest, relaxation

To prevent physical injury

To prevent emotional injury

To achieve awareness of needs

NURSING INTERVENTIONS

Nursing Treatments

Approach unhurriedly

Encourage patient questions

Nursing Observations

Evaluate the response to teaching

Health Teaching

Recommend a regular sleeping schedule

Recommend adherence to a moderate pace of living

Explain that fatigue should be recognized as a stress factor

Explain that parental attitudes (toward sleep, rest) affect child development

Describe the characteristics of fatigue

Describe the specific dangerous effects of poor health practices

Inform of the recommended minimum hours of sleep

Recommend methods for achieving total relaxation

EVALUATION

See the evaluation criteria for each specific goal in Chapter 2.

30.
NURSING DIAGNOSES RELATED TO
Spiritual Distress

SPIRITUAL DISTRESS

Difficulty Maintaining
a Religious Diet (309,320)

ASSESSMENT

Subjective Data
Anxiety
Guilt feelings

Objective Data
If of the Jewish faith, patient is:
 unable to obtain kosher meat or have chicken for the sabbath meal
 unable to use barley and buckwheat cereals as vegetables
 unable to avoid eating milk and meat or fish and milk together
 unable to avoid eating pork or pork products, birds of prey, scavengers,
  or shellfish
 unable to obtain broiled chops and steaks, rye and whole wheat breads,
  dried fruits and noodles, salmon, white, smoked or salted fish
If of the Baptist faith, patient is unable to avoid alcohol in medications
If of the Catholic faith, patient is unable to obtain fish on Friday or days
 prior to special holy days
If of the Seventh Day Adventist faith, patient is:
 unable to maintain a vegetarian diet with no meat, coffee, or tea
 unable to have a large variety of fruits and vegetables
If of the Mormon faith (Latter Day Saints), patient is:
 unable to obtain high proportions of fruit, vegetables, and grain with
  small amounts of meat or unable to avoid coffee or tea

Related Data
Commonly Related Diseases:
Any disease or injury

POSSIBLE ETIOLOGY

Illness dependence on others who are not of the same religious belief. The need for a specific therapeutic diet. Hospitalization.

NURSING DIAGNOSIS

Difficulty maintaining a religious diet: the inability to adhere to the religious requirements of special or limited foods associated with a specific faith

PLANNING

Patient Needs	Primary Nurse-Patient Goals
Comfort	To achieve comfort
Protection from psychologic threat	To prevent emotional injury
Warm, communicating relationships	To achieve effective verbal and nonverbal communications
Religious-philosophic satisfaction	To achieve spiritual goals

NURSING INTERVENTIONS

Nursing Treatments
Encourage the expression of feelings
Honor religious dietary regulations
Listen attentively
Provide an atmosphere of acceptance

Nursing Observations
Observe for an excessive stress level

EVALUATION

See the evaluation criteria for each specific goal in Chapter 2.

Disrupted Spiritual Rituals (134,396,509)

ASSESSMENT

Subjective Data
Sense of loss
Depression
Guilt feelings

Objective Data
Person cannot go to church
Is unable to say daily prayers
Attempts to substitute simplified rituals in place of usual worship

Related Data
Commonly Related Conditions:
Immobility
Isolation and reverse isolation
Commonly Related Diseases:
None

OR

Any disease or injury

POSSIBLE ETIOLOGY

Physical limitations imposed by illness. Illness confinement.

NURSING DIAGNOSIS

Disrupted spiritual rituals: the inability to perform normal ritual activities in honor and respect of the Supreme Being as a result of illness

PLANNING

Patient Needs	**Primary Nurse-Patient Goals**
Comfort	To achieve comfort
Warm, communicating relationships	To achieve effective verbal and nonverbal communications
Increased learning	To achieve awareness of needs and/or use of resources
Religious-philosophic satisfaction	To achieve spiritual goals

NURSING INTERVENTIONS

Nursing Treatments

Assist with bedside religious observances
Encourage the chaplain's visit
Encourage discussion of the patient's spiritual values
Encourage the expression of feelings
Encourage spiritually uplifting conversations
Guide the patient in simple prayer
Pray with the patient
Provide desired religious articles
Provide information about spiritual programs (on radio and television or in the chapel)
Provide religious reading material
Listen attentively

Nursing Observations

Observe for evidence of a favorable response to therapy

EVALUATION

See the evaluation criteria for each specific goal in Chapter 2.

Disrupted Spiritual Trust (134,383,396)

ASSESSMENT

Subjective Data

Doubts the compassion of the Supreme Being
Worries about loss of trust
Heightened anxiety
Ambivalence
Resentment
Guilt feelings

Objective Data

Openly discusses a loss of confidence in God

Decreased attendance at prayer and religious services

Negative verbalization on spiritual matters

Related Data

Commonly Related Conditions:

Sustained unresolved grief

Poor prognosis

Prolonged convalescence

Commonly Related Diseases:

None

　OR

Any disease or injury

POSSIBLE ETIOLOGY

Projected blame. Refusal to accept illness. Diminished positive self-image causing a sense of decreased significance in one's relationship with God. Overwhelming stress from multiple major crises occurring within a short period of time. Inability to find satisfactory reasons for illness, disease, crisis, or disaster. Loss of significant other relationship.

NURSING DIAGNOSIS

Disrupted spiritual trust: loss of confident expectation that the Supreme Being will meet one's needs

PLANNING

Patient Needs	**Primary Nurse-Patient Goals**
Comfort	To achieve comfort
Warm, communicating relationships	To achieve effective verbal and nonverbal communications
Increased learning	To achieve awareness of needs and/or use of resources
Religious-philosophic satisfaction	To achieve spiritual goals

NURSING INTERVENTIONS

Nursing Treatments

Encourage acceptance of unpleasantness

Encourage the chaplain's visit

Encourage discussion of the patient's spiritual values

Encourage the expression of feelings

Provide an atmosphere of acceptance

Listen attentively

Nursing Observations

Evaluate the significance of spirituality in the patient's life

Observe for evidence of a favorable response to therapy

EVALUATION

See the evaluation criteria for each specific goal in Chapter 2.

Difficulty Achieving Desired
Spiritual Dependence (383,396,509)

ASSESSMENT

Subjective Data
An intense in-depth reaching toward God
Person wants to experience the comfort of dependence on God
Feels weak by himself, but strong and safe with God

Objective Data
Person requests spiritual books or articles
More frequently attends spiritual services or listens to spiritual programs
    on television

Related Data
Commonly Related Conditions:
Poor prognosis
Impending death
Commonly Related Diseases:
Cancer
Severe trauma injury

POSSIBLE ETIOLOGY

Illness that decreases one's capacity for independence. Enhanced awareness
of human limitations. Cultural and subcultural norms.

NURSING DIAGNOSIS

Difficulty achieving desired spiritual dependence: a need for assistance in
seeking increased reliance and submission to the direction and support of a
Supreme Being

PLANNING

Patient Needs	Primary Nurse-Patient Goals
Comfort	To achieve comfort
Warm, communicating relationships	To achieve effective verbal and nonverbal communications
Increased learning	To achieve awareness of needs and/or use of resources
Religious-philosophic satisfaction	To achieve spiritual goals

NURSING INTERVENTIONS

Nursing Treatments
Encourage chapel service attendance
Encourage the chaplain's visit
Encourage spiritually uplifting conversation
Guide the patient in simple prayer
Pray with the patient
Provide an atmosphere of acceptance
Provide desired religious articles
Provide information about spiritual programs

Provide religious reading material

Nursing Observations
Determine the level of participation in spiritual rituals

EVALUATION

See the evaluation criteria for each specific goal in Chapter 2.

Spiritually Restricted Health Maintenance (396,509)

ASSESSMENT

Subjective Data
Intense emotions regarding the situation

Objective Data
Person refuses to accept assistance with health problems
Logic does not change his mind
Person verbalizes his basic religious beliefs regarding health care

Related Data
Commonly Related Diseases:
Any disease or injury

POSSIBLE ETIOLOGY

Specific religious beliefs

NURSING DIAGNOSIS

Spiritually restricted health maintenance: the inability to accept certain health treatments which are opposed to one's religious beliefs

PLANNING

Patient Needs	**Primary Nurse-Patient Goals**
Comfort	To achieve comfort
Warm, communicating relationships	To achieve effective verbal and nonverbal communications
Increased learning	To achieve awareness of needs
Religious-philosophic satisfaction	To achieve spiritual goals

NURSING INTERVENTIONS

Nursing Treatments
Encourage the expression of feelings
Listen attentively
Provide an atmosphere of acceptance
Refrain from forcing the treatment
Support a realistic assessment of the situation

Nursing Observations
Evaluate the significance of spirituality in the patient's life
Observe for an excessive stress level

EVALUATION

See the evaluation criteria for each specific goal in Chapter 2.

Part 3.

Nursing Interventions

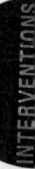

31.
Nursing Treatments

Accept and attempt to relieve unexplainable body complaints When the patient persists in complaining of physical ailments that cannot be diagnosed medically, do not indicate that the ailment is imaginary or of psychic origin. Accept the complaint and take measures to relieve it.

Rationale: The attention and love derived as a result of functional complaints tend to alleviate the functional discomfort or pain. Comfort is promoted through effective communication with others. Nonacceptance of body complaints heightens anxiety or psychologic threat and increases adaptation stress, with resulting energy depletion. Complaints are the most reliable guide to nonhealth conditions.

Resolved Needs: Comfort. Protection from physical harm. Protection from psychologic threat.

Acknowledge dependency For a limited period of time, permit the person to rely on others to meet basic physiologic and psychologic needs.

Rationale: Any physiologic or psychologic disequilibrium is potentially threatening. Regressive behavior is a defensive reaction to threatening situations and a temporary adaptive mechanism toward future equilibrium.

Resolved Needs: Comfort. Protection from physical harm. Protection from psychologic threat. Dependence.

Acknowledge emotional concealment Recognize the patient's right to withhold feelings until such time as emotional expression will bring comfort.

Rationale: The development and use of adaptive psychologic mechanisms foster safety and psychologic equilibrium. The privacy and safety of the person's internal thoughts and feelings are basic human rights deserving respect.

Resolved Needs: Comfort. Protection from psychologic threat. Dignity.

Administer a drug sensitivity test   Before administering any highly antigenic drug, subcutaneously inject a few drops and note any reaction.

Rationale: Sensitivity tests indicate potentially allergic or toxic responses to serum injections.

Resolved Needs: Protection from physical harm.

Administer a hot foot bath   Place the feet in a tub or pan of plain or saline water at about 110°F, and soak for 20–30 minutes.

Rationale: Hot foot soaks promote comfort by drawing excess fluid from congested body parts and by stimulating circulation.

Resolved Needs: Circulation. Comfort. Protection from physical harm.

Contraindications: Hypotension. Dizziness. Impaired peripheral circulation of the lower extremity.

Administer a vaginal douche   Gently insert an irrigating nozzle into the vagina after cleansing the external genitalia with surgical soap and water. Allow an irrigating solution at approximately 105°F to flow in and out of the vagina slowly by careful nozzle rotation.

Rationale: Vaginal irrigations cleanse, discourage bacterial growth, remove foul and irritating discharges, and provide heat or cold therapy.

Resolved Needs: Comfort. Cleanliness. Protection from physical harm.

Contraindications: Pregnancy. Vaginal bleeding. Recent vaginal surgery.

Administer a warm bath   Place the patient in a tub of moderately warm water.

Rationale: Warmth promotes vasodilatation and muscle relaxation, which promotes sleep and relief of pain and fatigue.

Resolved Needs: Sleep, rest, relaxation. Comfort. Protection from physical harm. Freedom from pain.

Administer an enema   Dispense an enema into the colon. Select the amount, type, and temperature of the solution according to the desired result.

Rationale: One quart of fluid (less than 500 cc for a small child) distends the colon sufficiently to stimulate peristalsis. The addition of heat (105°F) and irritants (mild soap solution) further increases peristalsis. A 0.85% sodium chloride solution is isotonic with the blood and does not irritate the colon; tap water is hypotonic and may disrupt water balance. Soap causes the feces to absorb water, but it also irritates the colonic mucosa. A hot soap solution enema will stimulate uterine contractions. A hypertonic saline solution (100 cc sodium phosphate and biphosphate) pulls fluid by

osmotic attraction into the colon, stimulating peristalsis by colonic distention. The urinary (micturition) reflex also is stimulated. A small amount of
oil (100–200 cc) given as a retention enema softens hard fecal masses.
(Especially effective when given 2–3 hours before a cleansing enema.)

Resolved Needs: Waste elimination. Comfort. Stimulation. Cleanliness.
Protection from physical harm.

Contraindications: *Any enema:* Hypokalemia. Intestinal spasms. Uterine
or rectal bleeding. After-birth pains. During peritoneal dialysis. Nausea.
Vomiting. Acute abdominal pain. Premature onset of labor. The presence of
a ureterosigmoidostomy.
  Soap solution enema: Ulcerative or inflammatory intestinal conditions.
  Saline and sodium phosphate enema: Hypernatremia.
  Tap water enema: Hyponatremia. Edema. Ascites. Where there is poten-
tial for water intoxication as in small children or infants.

Administer heated humidified oxygen (ET) Dispense water-
vaporized oxygen by bubbling oxygen down a stem immersed in electrically
heated sterile water.

Rationale: Normally, 40% of body humidity is breathed in from external
air. The internal respiratory tract supplies 60% of the nearly 100% humidity
required. Heating water to 100°–150°F and diffusing oxygen gas out of the
water increases the capacity of the oxygen in external air to hold water
(humidity) at 90% humidity. Therefore, the internal respiratory tract needs
to supply only 10% humidity instead of the normal 60%. This decreases
respiratory tissue dryness, prevents tissue friction during respirations, and
loosens and thins mucus secretions. Normally, a person breathes in 97% of
the 20.95% oxygen in ordinary air, or 20.32% oxygen. Oxygen therapy
builds up a slightly higher oxygen intake by elevating the oxygen concentration of ordinary air from 20.32% to 22.31–33.95%. This increased oxygen
intake eases breathing and promotes comfort.

Resolved Needs: Oxygen. Waste elimination. Comfort. Protection from
physical harm.

Contraindications: High fever. Oxygen toxicity. Increased metabolic rate.

Administer humidified oxygen (ET) Dispense water-vaporized ox-
ygen by bubbling oxygen down a stem immersed in sterile water at room
temperature.

Rationale: When oxygen is humidified, the dry gas is converted to approximately the same moisture level as the humidity of room air. The vapor
thus created decreases the drying effect of oxygen on the respiratory mucosa. Oxygen therapy builds up a higher oxygen intake than provided by
ordinary air. This increased oxygen intake eases breathing and promotes
comfort. When blood volume is low, administering oxygen saturates the

hemoglobin of the remaining blood cells. In conditions of increased metabolic rate, administered oxygen helps ease excessive oxygen consumption. Cool vapor is preferable because heated mist further accelerates the metabolic rate.

Resolved Needs: Oxygen. Comfort. Protection from physical harm.

Contraindications: Oxygen toxicity. Severe chronic obstructive pulmonary disease in which relief of hypoxia with oxygen therapy could precipitate apnea.

Administer intermittent positive pressure breathing (ET)   Give
pressurized air into the lungs during inhalation by mechanically induced intermittent positive pressure.

Rationale: Intermittent positive pressure breathing provides inhalation of air having above-normal atmospheric pressure. This pressure, applied by mouthpiece or mask, inflates the lungs. It pushes pressurized air past mucus and stimulates coughing, which eliminates secretions. On exhalation, the pressure returns to normal atmospheric pressure. Intermittent positive pressure expands alveoli and promotes diffusion of oxygen, increasing the oxygen saturation level of the blood.

Resolved Needs: Oxygen. Waste elimination. Protection from physical harm.

Contraindications: Pulmonary embolus. Pulmonary hemorrhage. Impaired cardiac output such as myocardial infarction.

Administer intravenous fluids (ET)   Infuse physiologic saline solution, glucose, or other intravenous solutions into the vein.

Rationale: Intravenous infusions provide an immediate source of water, electrolytes, and nutrients for the purpose of maintenance, replacement, or as an avenue for drug administration. The basic composition of I.V. fluid is isotonic, but hypotonic fluid may be given (to correct hypertonic dehydration) and hypertonic fluid may be given (to reduce cerebral edema). I.V. fluids increase the vascular pressure, especially when administered rapidly, when, during shock, there is a disproportion between the blood volume and the vascular space. I.V. fluids stimulate urine production during decreased output associated with shock, and when there is fever replaces fluid lost from dehydration so that the body can perspire and cool itself.

Resolved Needs: Water-salt balance. Normal temperature. Stimulation. Protection from physical harm.

Contraindications: Circulatory overload evidenced by venous distention, etc. Thrombophlebitis. Suspected air embolism. Dextrose solutions above 10% and solutions containing alcohol are given only if ordered by a physician.

Administer isotonic saline intravenous fluid between the blood transfusion and glucose infusion   When a blood transfu-

sion has been completed and a glucose solution is ordered to follow, flush the tubing with normal saline I.V. fluid first, or use new tubing.

Rationale: Isotonic saline is compatible with blood and will not cause blood clotting within the tubing. Glucose solution causes hemolysis of the red blood cells in the tubing, resulting in microemboli.

Resolved Needs: Protection from physical harm.

Administer vaporized air   Dispense water vapor through a bubble or diffuse humidifier or vaporizer. Electrically heat the water to 100–105°F. The use of a vaporizer decreases respiratory tissue dryness, prevents friction during respirations, loosens and thins mucus, decongests sinuses, prevents mouth dryness, and promotes comfort.

Resolved Needs: Waste elimination. Comfort. Protection from physical harm.

Contraindications: High fever.

Allow time for thought comprehension   After delivery of a verbal message, allow sufficient time for the person to receive and interpret the message.

Rationale: Rapidity of message reception and interpretation depends on the degree of physiologic and psychologic equilibrium. Psychologic comfort is promoted through effective communication with others.

Resolved Needs: Comfort. Warm, communicating relationships.

Allow unlimited visiting   Permit visitors freedom to come and go as the patient desires and at their own discretion.

Rationale: Psychologic equilibrium is fostered by an awareness that one is not threatened with aloneness. Human contact relieves fear and anxiety. The physical presence and involvement of loved ones reassures the person that he will be cared for.

Resolved Needs: Protection from psychologic threat. Warm, communicating relationships. Unity with loved ones.

Ambulate the patient   Walk the patient as much as possible, especially after surgery or an immobilizing illness or disease. Use assistive equipment such as canes and walkers as needed.

Rationale: Ambulation promotes and helps restore normal physiologic function, stimulates circulation, increases pulmonary ventilation and movement of secretions, stimulates peristalsis, empties renal pelves, promotes the passage of stones, and increases muscle strength and endurance. Improved physiologic function reduces the dependency of illness. During labor, ambulation promotes fetal head descent by placing pressure on the lower uterus and stimulating contractions.

Resolved Needs: Circulation. Waste elimination. Activity, exercise. Energy. Comfort. Stimulation. Protection from physical harm. Dependence.

Contraindications: Temperature elevation above 103°F. Head or spinal cord injury. Internal hemorrhage. Coma or semicoma. Severe energy depletion. Life-threatening situations.

Anchor the tubing securely   When the patient has an intravenous infusion or a urinary, gastric, chest, or any other type of tube, anchor the tubing so that the patient's movements will not displace the tubing. Loop a section of the tubing, then secure it in place with adhesive tape or a bandage.

Rationale: Anchoring tubing provides comfort by minimizing the replacement of dislodged tubes.

Resolved Needs: Comfort. Protection from physical harm.

Anticipate needs   Supply the person's requirements before they are sought or asked for.

Rationale: Physical or psychologic needs unknown to or unmet by the patient could be potentially threatening to health equilibrium. Meeting unsolicited needs offers security, attention, recognition, and acceptance, promotes comfort, restores physical strength, allows for necessary dependency, and nonverbally recognizes the person's value and dignity.

Resolved Needs: Energy. Comfort. Protection from physical harm. Protection from psychologic threat. Dependence. Acceptance. Sense of value. High evaluation of self. Recognition. Dignity. Attention.

Apply a bandana to the unamputated breast   When one breast has been removed, support the remaining breast with a triangular folded fabric kerchief or cloth and fit the breast into the triangle portion of the material.

Rationale: The absence of one breast tends to pull body balance to one side. Support of the remaining breast brings body balance into normal alignment and promotes comfort.

Resolved Needs: Comfort. Protection from physical harm.

Apply a bed cradle   Place a metal or plastic frame over the body, between the sheets and the patient, and cover the cradle with bed linens.

Rationale: Bed cradles prevent bedding from touching the body, yet maintain warmth around the body. A cradle prevents skin irritation and promotes comfort. In paralysis, sheets touching the skin can stimulate the reflex arc or lower motor neurons and cause severe muscle spasm.

Resolved Needs: Comfort. Protection from physical harm.

Apply a brassiere   Apply or have the patient apply a brassiere to the breasts, especially during pregnancy and lactation. The brassiere should have a sufficiently large cup, cover all breast tissue in the underarm area, and have wide supportive straps.

Rationale: The application of a supportive brassiere during pregnancy or to an engorged or lactating breast aids in preventing fluid congestion, shields the breast for cleanliness, relieves discomfort from breast weight by offering support, and prevents backache by enhancing good posture.

Resolved Needs: Comfort. Cleanliness. Protection from physical harm.

Apply a breast binder   Apply a wide binder and encircle it around the breasts. Hold the breasts in the normal position while the binder is being applied snugly but not too tightly. Pin the binder from the bottom up.

Rationale: The application of a breast binder to an engorged or lactating breast aids in preventing fluid congestion, shields the breast for cleanliness, relieves discomfort from breast weight by offering support, and prevents backache by enhancing good posture.

Resolved Needs: Comfort. Cleanliness. Protection from physical harm.

Apply a cold, moist compress   Apply a cold, wet, absorbent cloth by soaking a towel or wool cloth in cold water. Wring it out thoroughly and place it on the skin surface.

Rationale: Cold causes vasoconstriction, which decreases bleeding, pain, and pressure from tissue fluid and gas. Cold especially reduces pain due to burns.

Resolved Needs: Comfort. Protection from physical harm. Freedom from pain.

Contraindications: Avoid cold applications to decubitus ulcers, gangrenous tissue, skin graft areas, varicose veins, areas of paralysis or sensation loss, and aged or debilitated skin.

Apply a cool, damp cloth to the face   Gently touch the face with a cool damp cloth when the patient experiences such discomforts as dizziness, nausea or vomiting, faintness, etc.

Rationale: Coolness constricts blood vessels, sending the blood supply away from the skin to vital organs. It refreshes the face, thus promoting comfort.

Resolved Needs: Comfort. Stimulation.

Apply a greasy substance over the tick   If a tick imbeds itself in the skin or hair, cover the tick with petrolatum, cold cream, lard, margarine, or another greasy substance. Nail polish also may be used.

Rationale: Grease or nail polish smothers the tick, facilitating easy removal.

Resolved Needs: Protection from physical harm.

Apply a heat cradle   Expose the body or body part to dry heat from an electric light bulb. Suspend the bulb from a frame over the body and enclose with a sheet for concentrated warmth.

Rationale: Dry heat increases circulation through mild vasodilatation, relieves pain and congestion, promotes muscle relaxation, and draws pus to the skin surface. With skin burns, peripheral vessels cannot contract to retain body heat. External heat helps maintain normal body temperature.

Resolved Needs: Circulation. Normal temperature. Comfort. Protection from physical harm. Freedom from pain.

Contraindications: Avoid applying heat to areas of paralysis or sensation loss, edema, vasodilatation, or allergic responses, to any body part after heart surgery, to areas of hemorrhage or trauma, to febrile patients, and to persons who are unable to cooperate with safety instructions such as children or confused persons.

Apply a heating pad   Expose the body to dry heat by using an electric heating pad.

Rationale: Dry heat increases circulation through mild vasodilatation, relieves pain and congestion, promotes muscle relaxation, and draws pus to the skin surface. Heat on the bladder stimulates voiding and relieves bladder spasms.

Resolved Needs: Circulation. Relaxation. Comfort. Protection from physical harm. Freedom from pain.

Contraindications: Avoid applying a heating pad on a child or a confused or comatose patient, to areas of paralysis or sensation loss, edema, vasodilatation, or allergic responses, to any body part after heart surgery, to areas of hemorrhage or trauma, and to febrile patients.

Apply a hernia support   Assist the patient in wearing a hernia support garment in the inguinal area.

Rationale: Supportive pressure decreases stress on abdominal muscles and organs, promotes comfort, and reduces pain.

Resolved Needs: Comfort. Protection from physical harm. Freedom from pain.

Apply a hot water bottle   On the affected body part, place a rubber or plastic bag filled with temperature-tested hot water and covered with linen.

Rationale: Dry heat increases circulation through vasodilatation, relieves pain and congestion, promotes muscle relaxation, and draws pus to the skin surface. Heat applied to the bladder stimulates voiding and relieves bladder spasms.

Resolved Needs: Circulation. Relaxation. Comfort. Protection from physical harm. Freedom from pain.

Contraindications: Never use a hot water bottle on a child or a confused or comatose patient. Avoid heat application to areas of paralysis or sensation loss, edema, vasodilatation, or allergic responses, to any body part after heart surgery, to areas of hemorrhage or trauma, and in conditions where fever exists.

Apply a parasiticide   Wet the hair and scalp with warm water. Apply a parasiticide on the affected area and rub vigorously for several minutes. Repeat in 24 hours.

Rationale: A parasiticide reduces head lice and nits, which cause scalp inflammation and potential bacterial infection.

Resolved Needs: Comfort. Cleanliness. Protection from physical harm.

Apply a precordial blow (ET)   In cases where the onset of cardiac arrest is witnessed by the nurse, administer a sharp blow to the midsternum from a height of 8–12 inches, using the soft side of the fist.

Rationale: The shock force from a sternal blow should stimulate heart muscle contractions if administered very soon after a cardiac arrest.

Resolved Needs: Oxygen. Circulation. Stimulation. Protection from physical harm.

Contraindications: Do not use this therapy on children. Do not administer if faint heartbeats can be detected or if the heartbeat has ceased for longer than one minute because the hypoxic heart will not respond to the blow, but instead there will be tissue damage.

Apply a pressure dressing   Apply a firmly anchored sterile bandage or binder. Apply the binder snugly but prevent tightness that may interrupt blood flow.

Rationale: Pressure application prevents bleeding and wound seepage and promotes comfort.

Resolved Needs: Circulation. Comfort. Protection from physical harm.

Apply a safety helmet to the head   Whenever there is danger of head trauma during ambulation, apply a football helmet to the head.

Rationale: Head trauma can damage the vital life centers of the brain.

Resolved Needs: Protection from physical harm.

Apply a saline compress   Apply a sterile dressing, dampened with warm or cool isotonic (0.85%) saline solution.

Rationale: A wet, saline compress is nonirritating to open wounds, promotes growth of granulation tissue, cleans wounds by debridement, softens wound discharges, promotes drainage, and localizes area infection.

Resolved Needs: Comfort. Cleanliness. Protection from physical harm.

Apply a scrotal support   Support the scrotum with a suspensory garment or by proper pillow placement.

Rationale: Scrotal support prevents organ injury and promotes comfort.

Resolved Needs: Comfort. Protection from physical harm.

Apply a sterile dressing   Apply a dry, sterile bandage over a wound.

Rationale: Sterile wound coverings enhance cleanliness, prevent infection and trauma, restrict motion, and absorb secretions.

Resolved Needs: Comfort. Cleanliness. Protection from physical harm.

Apply a stump sock   Snugly apply a soft, absorbent, cone-shaped sock to the amputated stump.

Rationale: The stump sock's porous material allows good stump ventilation. Pressure application reduces edema. The sock protects the skin from prosthesis pressure and irritation.

Resolved Needs: Comfort. Protection from physical harm.

Apply a supportive splint   When the body has been traumatized and is in danger of further injury if moved, immobilize the body part with a supporting splint.

Rationale: Immobilization and support prevents further injury and provides physiologic rest and comfort.

Resolved Needs: Rest. Comfort. Protection from physical harm.

Apply a tourniquet between the extremity wound and the body   Apply a tourniquet 2–4 inches above the injury site on the extremity, between the wound and the body torso. The tourniquet should be loose enough so your finger will fit under it and the arterial pulses can still be felt. Some oozing of the wound will also occur. If there is swelling above the tourniquet, apply another tourniquet a few inches above the first one, leaving the first one in place. Maintain the tourniquet application until medical care is obtained.

Rationale: The application of a tourniquet minimizes the amount of snake venom absorbed into the circulatory system. In trauma, it reduces the degree of hemorrhage.

Resolved Needs: Protection from physical harm.

Apply a warm, moist compress   Apply warm, wet heat by soaking a towel or wool cloth in hot water, wringing it almost dry, and placing it on the skin surface. Unsterile compresses may be used on intact skin, but sterile normal saline compresses are essential over open lesions.

Rationale: Moist heat increases circulation through intense vasodilatation, relieves pain and congestion, promotes muscle relaxation, enhances drainage, localizes infection, and draws pus to the skin surface.

Resolved Needs: Circulation. Comfort. Cleanliness. Protection from physical harm. Freedom from pain.

Contraindications: Avoid applying heat to areas of paralysis or sensation loss, edema, vasodilatation, or allergic responses, to any body part after heart surgery, to areas of hemorrhage or trauma, and to febrile patients.

Apply after-bath powder   Apply a thin layer of powder, usually talcum or zinc oxide, to the skin. Use it sparingly in the winter because of its drying effect. Do not powder the skin folds or between the toes, or apply only a thin film in these areas.

Rationale: Powder has a drying action, permits movement of skin against skin, allows for good air circulation over the skin, reduces friction, and promotes cooling and drying of inflamed skin.

Resolved Needs: Comfort. Protection from physical harm.

Contraindications: Dry skin. Allergic reactions. Do not apply powders containing zinc on the skin of patients receiving radiation therapy.

Apply alcohol to the skin   Rub the body with full-strength alcohol or sponge with alcohol mixed with tepid water.

Rationale: Rubbing the body surface with alcohol stimulates circulation and inhibits bacterial growth on the skin. Alcohol evaporates at a relatively low temperature, rapidly removing heat and cooling the body surface.

Resolved Needs: Normal temperature. Comfort. Cleanliness.

Contraindications: Dry skin. Respiratory distress in which the alcohol fumes might irritate the respiratory mucosa. During oxygen administration in which alcohol fumes might precipitate an explosion.

Apply aluminum paste to the skin   Cover the skin surrounding the colostomy stoma or a ureterostomy with a thin layer of a mixture of half aluminum powder and half oil.

Rationale: Aluminum paste neutralizes the acidity of digestive enzymes found in bowel content. It minimizes skin irritation and excoriation by preventing exudates from coming in contact with the skin.

Resolved Needs: Comfort. Protection from physical harm.

Apply an abdominal support garment   Apply to the abdomen, or suggest that the person wear, clothing articles that uphold the abdominal wall, its contents, and healing tissue. Such garments would include binders and girdles.

Rationale: Supportive pressure decreases stress on abdominal muscles and organs, promotes comfort, and reduces pain.

Resolved Needs: Comfort. Protection from physical harm. Freedom from pain.

Apply an analgesic ointment   Apply an anesthetizing ointment to the skin in order to reduce pain or itching.

Rationale: Decreased pain promotes comfort and rest.

Resolved Needs: Rest. Comfort.

Apply an antibiotic ointment (or Spray)   Locally apply a salve or spray containing an antibiotic drug. Use it on mildly inflamed areas and on nonbleeding or crusted eruptions. Use on open skin areas rather than in skin folds.

Rationale: Antibiotic ointments and sprays reduce or prevent bacterial growth and infection. Ointments retard water evaporation from the skin, soften scabs and scales, and promote comfort.

Resolved Needs: Comfort. Protection from physical harm.

Contraindications: Known drug allergy.

Apply an antiperspirant   After cleansing the skin of the axilla, apply a chemical product under the axilla to control skin odor and inhibit sweating.

Rationale: Body odor is controlled by oxidizing odoriferous material or by inhibiting bacterial growth and decaying putrefaction. Control of body odor promotes comfort. It offers aid in illness dependency.

Resolved Needs: Comfort. Dependence.

Contraindications: Axillary irritation or inflammation.

Apply an arm sling   Support the arm, elbow, hand, and shoulder by application of a triangular sling for temporary use or a commercial sling for long-term use.

Rationale: Support of a traumatized body part prevents further injury and promotes rest for that part.

Resolved Needs: Rest. Comfort. Protection from physical harm.

Apply an elastic bandage   Wrap a rubberized stretch bandage around the affected body area.

Rationale: The gentle, supportive pressure of an elastic bandage around a body part reduces venous stasis and fluid accumulation by increasing circulation.

Resolved Needs: Circulation. Comfort. Stimulation. Protection from physical harm.

Apply an external urinary catheter   Apply an external collection device to the urinary orifice.

Rationale: A urinary collection apparatus promotes accurate output measurement, maintains dryness, cleanliness, and comfort, and improves sleep and rest by decreasing frequent bathroom visits.

Resolved Needs: Sleep, rest. Comfort. Cleanliness. Protection from physical harm.

Contraindications: Irritation or inflammation of the external genitalia.

Apply an ice bag   On the affected body part, place a rubber or plastic bag filled with ice and wrapped with a linen cover. Apply ice bags to the breast for about 48 hours after delivery while the breasts are engorged with milk. When the body temperature is severely elevated, place ice bags along the torso and extremities but stop the treatment when the temperature drops to 101°F, or shock may occur. Interrupt ice applications for a few minutes every hour to insure adequate skin circulation.

Rationale: Dry cold decreases circulation through mild vasoconstriction, relieves pain and congestion, and reduces pus formation, swelling, and bleeding.

Resolved Needs: Normal temperature. Comfort. Protection from physical harm. Freedom from pain.

Contraindications: Avoid cold applications to decubitus ulcers, gangrenous tissue, skin graft areas, varicose veins, areas of paralysis or sensation loss, and aged or debilitated skin.

Apply an ice collar   On the neck, place a collar-shaped rubber or plastic bag filled with ice and wrapped with a linen cover.

Rationale: Dry cold decreases circulation through mild vasoconstriction, relieves pain and congestion, and reduces pus formation, swelling, and bleeding. Coldness around the neck depresses nerve fiber activity and produces vasoconstriction in the carotid vessels, reducing tachycardia.

Resolved Needs: Normal temperature. Comfort. Protection from physical harm. Freedom from pain.

Contraindications: Avoid cold applications to areas of decubitus ulcer, gangrenous tissue, skin graft areas, areas of paralysis or sensation loss, and aged or debilitated skin.

Apply an occlusive dressing   Apply a dressing in which the outer covering is a plastic wrap placed around the dressing.

Rationale: An occlusive dressing prevents the evaporation of the medication being applied by the dressing, assuring more effective use of the medication, which promotes the comfort of healing. It also offers the protection of cleanliness.

Resolved Needs: Comfort. Cleanliness.

Apply an ostomy appliance   Apply an external collection device for a colostomy, ileostomy, ileal conduit, ureterostomy, etc.

Rationale: An ostomy collection apparatus prevents skin irritation from fecal and digestive enzymes or urine. It promotes dryness, cleanliness, comfort, and accurate output measurement.

Resolved Needs: Comfort. Cleanliness. Protection from physical harm.

Apply calamine lotion   Apply a solution of zinc oxide and ferric oxide to the skin. Cover the skin surrounding an ileostomy stoma or a ureterileostomy with a thin layer of calamine. Since it has a drying effect, it is best used in skin folds and where two skin surfaces come together.

Rationale: Calamine lotion soothes the skin's surface. It hardens and contracts superficial skin cells by coagulating cell albumin and forming a thin coating over the cells. It protects against skin irritation and promotes heal-ing. The lotion dries up weeping, oozing areas and reduces skin inflamma-tion. Evaporation of the moisture in the lotion causes cooling and drying. The powder in the lotion absorbs oozing and weeping serum.

Resolved Needs: Comfort. Protection from physical harm.

Apply cornstarch to the skin   Using a powder puff for even skin dis-tribution, apply cornstarch. Prevent starch from collecting in skin folds.

Rationale: The powdery consistency of cornstarch is absorbent, soothes irritated skin, relieves itching, and cleanses the skin. It should be used spar-ingly because as starch absorbs water, the starch granules swell and, when' placed in skin folds, cakes and irritates the skin.

Resolved Needs: Comfort. Cleanliness. Protection from physical harm.

Apply elastic stockings   Put properly measured rubberized stretch stockings (elastic hose) on the lower limbs.

Rationale: The application of supportive pressure to the lower limbs re-duces blood stagnation, speeding up the flow of deeper venous blood back to the heart.

Resolved Needs: Circulation. Comfort. Stimulation. Protection from physical harm.

Contraindications: Circulatory embolus or thrombus.

Apply heat by a gooseneck lamp   Expose the body or body part to dry heat from an electric light bulb suspended in a gooseneck lamp.

Rationale: Dry heat increases circulation through mild vasodilatation, re-lieves pain and congestion, promotes muscle relaxation, and draws pus to the skin surface.

Resolved Needs: Circulation. Relaxation. Comfort. Protection from phys-ical harm. Freedom from pain.

Contraindications: Avoid heat application to areas of paralysis or sensa-tion loss, edema, vasodilatation, or allergic responses, to any body part after heart surgery, to areas of hemorrhage or trauma, to febrile patients, and to persons who are unable to cooperate with safety instructions such as children or confused persons.

Apply hot packs to the breast before breast feeding   Apply a hot water bottle or other heat to the breast 15–20 minutes before breast feeding.

Rationale: Vasodilatation of blood vessels of the breast promotes lactat-ing milk flow and comfort.

Resolved Needs: Comfort.

Apply lemon-milk solution to the skin   Mix the juice of one lemon with a small amount of milk and apply to the skin overnight.

Rationale: Lemon-milk bleaches freckles, bringing about the comfort of clear skin.

Resolved Needs: Comfort.

Contraindications: Skin irritation.

Apply manual pressure over the bleeding area   Apply pressure with the hand over a specific bleeding structure, organ, or area.

Rationale: Pressure application prevents blood and body fluid from escaping outside the circulatory system or tissue structures. It promotes comfort when used to reduce pain.

Resolved Needs: Comfort. Protection from physical harm.

Apply mentholated ointment   Lubricate the skin with cream containing oil of peppermint or mint oils (camphor). Rub deep into the skin.

Rationale: Mentholated ointment produces deep, penetrating warmth that relieves mild pain, muscle spasm, and irritation of deeper structures.

Resolved Needs: Comfort. Freedom from pain.

Contraindications: Skin irritation.

Apply milk of magnesia to the skin   Cover the skin surrounding an ileostomy stoma or a ureterileostomy with a thin layer of milk of magnesia.

Rationale: Milk of magnesia neutralizes the acidity of digestive enzymes found in ileostomy bowel content. It prevents skin irritation and excoriation.

Resolved Needs: Comfort. Protection from physical harm.

Apply rotating tourniquets (ET)   Place a tourniquet above the elbow or above the knee on three extremities. At 15-minute intervals, alternate the application and removal of the tourniquets. Remove one tourniquet every 15 minutes and place it on the extremity that has no tourniquet. Follow a clockwise or counterclockwise pattern.

7:00 AM	off right leg	on right arm, left arm, left leg
7:15	off right arm	on left arm, left leg, right leg
7:30	off left arm	on left leg, right leg, right arm
7:45	off left leg	on right leg, right arm, left leg

Place padding, such as 4'' × 4'' gauze squares, under each tourniquet to protect the underlying tissue. If tourniquets are not available, blood pressure cuffs may be used and inflated to a pressure between the systolic and diastolic blood pressure. To remove all tourniquets, remove them one at a time at 15-minute intervals.

Rationale: The application of tourniquets interferes with venous return by trapping blood in the extremities. This reduces the volume of blood reaching the lungs and prevents excessive fluid collection in the lungs.

Resolved Needs: Oxygen. Protection from physical harm.

Apply sodium bicarbonate to the skin Cover a local, moistened skin area with household baking soda.

Rationale: Soda bicarbonate relieves the discomfort of stinging pain from insects.

Resolved Needs: Comfort. Protection from physical harm. Freedom from pain.

Apply sterile petrolatum gauze Apply sterile gauze covered with transparent, sterile petrolatum.

Rationale: Petrolatum lubricates and smoothes skin, has a neutral (neither acid or alkaline) effect on the skin, prevents skin drying and cracking, promotes comfort, and maintains cleanliness by covering the skin.

Resolved Needs: Comfort. Cleanliness. Protection from physical harm.

Apply the Heimlich maneuver When a person is choking on a foreign object, make a fist with one hand. Place that hand with the thumb side against the abdomen slightly above the navel but below the sternum. Quickly press or thrust the fist into the abdomen above the umbilicus and below the sternum to move the diaphragm upward. Or, press the patient's abdomen against the back of a chair, stair railing, table edge, or similar object.

Rationale: Thrusting movements in the diaphragmatic area force air from the lungs into the throat. The air pressure dislodges the foreign object.

Resolved Needs: Protection from physical harm.

Apply tincture of benzoin Apply tincture of benzoin (a balsic resin from various trees) over areas of potential or acute skin breakdown. To remove the stickiness associated with benzoin, apply a fine film of powder over the dried benzoin.

Rationale: Tincture of benzoin provides a tough protective coating for threatening or impending decubitus ulcers or other skin surfaces threatened by excess pressure. A sticky benzoin surface adheres to linen and clothing and pulls off skin, causing further tissue trauma.

Resolved Needs: Protection from physical harm.

Contraindications: Do not use on deep, raw (granulating) wounds.

Apply zinc oxide to the skin Cover the skin surrounding a colostomy stoma or ureterostomy with a thin layer of zinc oxide paste. This mixture is half zinc powder and half oil.

Rationale: Zinc oxide paste inhibits bacterial growth. It hardens and contracts superficial skin cells by coagulating cell albumin and forming a thin coating over the cells. It protects against skin irritation and promotes healing by preventing exudates from coming in contact with the skin.

Resolved Needs: Comfort. Protection from physical harm.

Approach face to face   When approaching, move forward toward the person's face and refrain from approaching him from the back.

Rationale: The visible approach of one person to another allows preparation for the upcoming interpersonal contact and decreases the anxiety of surprise. A direct face-to-face approach nonverbally indicates directness and honesty.

Resolved Needs: Comfort. Protection from psychologic threat. Warm, communicating relationships.

Approach unhurriedly   Communicate concern through a leisurely, unrushed attitude.

Rationale: When there are physical or psychologic limitations to performance, an unhurried approach eliminates additional tension, especially if tension already exists. An unhurried approach communicates sufficient recognition and respect for the person to warrant the use of another's valuable time.

Resolved Needs: Comfort. Protection from physical harm. Protection from psychologic threat. Warm, communicating relationships. High evaluation of self. Recognition. Dignity. Attention.

Arrange a predischarge planning conference   Bring health team members together to help the patient evaluate his health situation and contribute to problem solving.

Rationale: Comprehensive health planning reduces potential physical and psychologic problems and offers the patient the comfort of a predictable future.

Resolved Needs: Comfort. Protection from physical harm. Protection from psychologic threat. Predictable, orderly world. Increased learning. Increased reality perception and problem-solving ability.

Arrange a structured environment   Offer a routine that is basically the same each day.

Rationale: A structured environment offers security in that the happenings of the day are predictable.

Resolved Needs: Comfort. Protection from psychologic threat. Predictable, orderly world.

Arrange geographic placement   Locate the patient in a room accessible to maximum physical and emotional care, observation, socialization, etc. Assure him that he is close to available nursing care.

Rationale: Close supervision facilitates recognition of health disorders. Human contact relieves fear and anxiety. Psychologic comfort is promoted

through a sense of nearness to others. Placement in an environment conducive to activity increases sensory stimulation.

Resolved Needs: Comfort. Stimulation. Protection from physical harm.
Protection from psychologic threat. Warm, communicating relationships.
Attention.

Arrange orderly surroundings
Provide surroundings in which the
furniture and accessories are so placed as to give a neat, uniform appearance.

Rationale: An orderly environment establishes the whereabouts of objects, decreasing potential injury. It reduces misperceptions and promotes
safety feelings in a familiar and predictable situation. Orderliness reduces
the anxiety of environmental confusion.

Resolved Needs: Comfort. Protection from physical harm. Protection
from psychologic threat. Predictable, orderly world.

Arrange pillows comfortably
Place pillows under the head and body
parts so they support but in no way impair circulation.

Rationale: Pressure prevention and support of a body area promote comfort and assist in illness dependency.

Resolved Needs: Comfort. Dependence.

Arrange pleasant surroundings
Provide surroundings in which the
decor lends a cheerful and attractive atmosphere.

Rationale: The perception of a pleasant environment promotes comfort
which has a positive physiologic and psychologic effect.

Resolved Needs: Comfort. Protection from physical harm. Protection
from psychologic threat. Increased pleasantness.

Arrange situations which encourage patient autonomy
Offer
the patient a choice of experiences therapeutically selected to encourage
him to control the situation. Suggest that he choose his own food, arrange
his furniture, pick companions, decide which activities to attend, etc.

Rationale: Independence evolves from making choices. Comfort and
safety evolve from an awareness that one can cope successfully with life and
can exert sufficient control to prevent harm to oneself.

Resolved Needs: Comfort. Protection from psychologic threat. Adequacy.
Self-reliance. Independence. Dominance over others.

Ask questions which encourage answers that reflect reality perception
Ask the dying patient straightforward questions such as "Do
you feel sick today? How much progress do you think you are making? Do
you think your treatments are doing you any good?" Ask patients experiencing guilt, conflict, etc., questions appropriate to their situation.

Rationale: Straightforward questions offer an opportunity for greater reality perception while still providing the safety of denial answers if there is psychologic threat.

Resolved Needs: Protection from psychologic threat. Increased reality perception and problem-solving ability.

Ask simple, direct questions   When speaking to persons having impaired message reception or delivery, ask only simple, direct questions that are easily understood and answered.

Rationale: Simple and direct communication enhances perception and reduces frustration and anxiety. Psychologic comfort is promoted through effective communication with others.

Resolved Needs: Comfort. Warm, communicating relationships.

Ask the patient what makes him/her comfortable   Discover the particular situations or conditions that make the patient comfortable. Then, provide these comforts.

Rationale: Comfort evolves from an awareness that comfort needs will be met and that previously experienced comforts will be repeated.

Resolved Needs: Comfort.

Assist the dying person with detachment from life (248)   When the dying person reaches total acceptance and indicates his readiness to detach himself from the world, help him do so. Detachment clues include turning the television off, especially at news time, wanting visitor limitations with gradual restriction to family members only, and lack of concern with environmental events.

Rationale: Detachment from the world eases the pain of losses anticipated by the dying person. Awareness that others support detachment brings comfort and rest.

Resolved Needs: Rest. Comfort. Protection from psychologic threat.

Assist the dying person with unfinished business (248)   When a patient says that he cannot allow his death to occur because of commitments such as caring for a sick relative, paying debts, etc., offer assistance in the resolution of these problems whenever possible. It is preferable that these matters be attended to when the patient is still feeling reasonably well.

Rationale: The threatening responsibilities of unfinished business prevent the dying person from experiencing the peace of total acceptance.

Resolved Needs: Comfort. Protection from psychologic threat.

Assist the family in preparing for life changes which will occur after the loved one's death (248)   Discuss with family members their plans for daily living after their loved one has died. This includes housing, finances, changes in social life, etc.

Rationale: Preparation for the future reduces the adaptive stress through recognition of predictable problems. Discussion of what life will be like without a loved one promotes adaptation to the reality that the time is approaching when the loved one will no longer be a part of one's life.

Resolved Needs: Protection from psychologic threat. Increased reality perception and problem-solving ability.

Assist the patient in defining consistent life standards
Assist the person in defining for himself a set of values that can be applied consistently to the broad scope of general living. Discourage different value systems for varying life situations.

Rationale: An accepted value system significantly influences behavioral responses.

Resolved Needs: Comfort. Protection from psychologic threat. Improved values.

Assist the patient in restructuring his lifestyle
Motivate and help the person to plan changes in his daily living habits.

Rationale: To restructure a lifestyle for the benefit of health requires mature reality perception. It includes behavior changes that specifically meet situational demands and individual needs. When the person is able to restructure a new pattern of daily living, he is providing himself with a reasonably predictable world.

Resolved Needs: Protection from physical harm. Predictable, orderly world. Personal growth and maturity. Awareness of potential. Full development of potential. Increased reality perception and problem-solving ability.

Assist the patient in setting standards of a meaningful existence
Help the patient set standards that give significant meaning to his life. In our affluent society, meaningfulness must be more than the basic needs of food, shelter, and clothing.

Rationale: In a society where basic needs have been met, working toward meeting survival needs offers little meaning. Therefore, activities must be developed that are time consuming and give people a sense of value, motivation, and satisfying ideals.

Resolved Needs: Comfort. Protection from psychologic threat.

Assist with bedside religious observances
When bedside prayers or services are being held, assist in any way possible. Directions from the clergymen, patient, or family are excellent sources for knowing how to offer proper and needed assistance.

Rationale: Religious observances help man to spiritually express his relationship with God and to outwardly recognize the Supreme Being.

Resolved Needs: Comfort. Dignity. Dependence. Religious, philosophic satisfaction.

Assist with dressing   Help the patient put his clothes on.

Rationale: Clothing maintains body warmth and promotes comfort. Assistance with dressing meets dependency needs.

Resolved Needs: Comfort. Protection from physical harm. Dependence.

Assist with eating   Help the patient eat and help prepare food and utensils for eating.

Rationale: Balanced nutritional intake is essential to body cell activity and energy production. Relief of visceral hunger promotes comfort. Assistance with eating meets dependency needs.

Resolved Needs: Food balance. Energy. Comfort. Protection from physical harm. Dependence.

Assist with hygiene   Help with hygiene and grooming activities such as bathing and care of hair, nails, teeth, and skin.

Rationale: Assistance with personal hygiene and cleanliness meets dependency needs and provides the comfort of being refreshed and of knowing that one's appearance is pleasing.

Resolved Needs: Comfort. Cleanliness. Protection from physical harm. Dependence.

Assist with mobility   Help the patient to walk, sit, stand, and move about.

Rationale: Mobility is necessary for meeting one's daily needs and for the maintenance of health. Assistance with mobility meets dependency needs.

Resolved Needs: Comfort. Protection from physical harm. Dependence.

Assist with skilled hand activities   Help the person who is having difficulty using his fingers for precise functions. Assist him by strategically placing objects and providing assistive tools.

Rationale: Skilled voluntary movements are dependent on an intact corticospinal tract, and such movements are essential for precise finger movements needed to accomplish daily living skills. Comfort arises from an awareness of one's ability to cope successfully with situations.

Resolved Needs: Activity. Comfort. Dependence.

Attach the chest tube to a water-seal drainage   Attach the chest tube to the tubing that leads to chest bottles or a plastic (Pleur-Evac) water-seal drainage system. The apparatus should be sterile and contain sufficient sterile water so the long tube within the closed system is about one inch below the surface of the sterile water. When using chest bottles, to prevent the tube from kinking, tape a tongue blade to the tubing located at the entry site to the bottle. Tape all connectors to prevent leakage.

Rationale: Water-seal drainage prevents additional air from entering the pleural space while fluid and blood drain from the pleural space. It facilitates reexpansion of a collapsed lung.

Resolved Needs: Oxygen. Protection from physical harm.

Attach the collection appliance (or tube) to straight drainage and a collection container   Connect the collection appliance of an ileal conduit, a ureterostomy, an indwelling urinary catheter, etc., to a closed system of tubing and a collection container.

Rationale: A closed system of straight drainage and a collection container help control the hazards of infection, promote accurate output measurement, prevent skin irritation and promote dryness, cleanliness, and comfort.

Resolved Needs: Comfort. Cleanliness. Protection from physical harm.

Attach the tube to a leg urinal   Connect a plastic or waterproof bag to the urinary drainage tube and attach the bag to the patient's leg.

Rationale: A urinary collection bag promotes accurate output measurement, maintains dryness, cleanliness, and comfort, allows for unlimited mobility, and reduces the threat of social embarrassment.

Resolved Needs: Waste elimination. Comfort. Cleanliness. Protection from physical harm. Protection from psychologic threat.

Attend the patient constantly   Remain with the patient constantly.

Rationale: Constant attendance facilitates recognition of health disorders. Psychologic equilibrium is fostered by an awareness that one is not threatened with aloneness. Human contact relieves fear and anxiety. Comfort is promoted through a sense of adequate communication with others.

Resolved Needs: Comfort. Protection from physical harm. Protection from psychologic threat. Warm, communicating relationships.

Avoid causing embarrassing situations   Do not create situations that will cause uncomfortable or shameful feelings in the patient. If such situations exist, take measures to alter them.

Rationale: Feelings of safety evolve from an awareness that one can cope successfully with the life situation.

Resolved Needs: Comfort. Protection from psychologic threat. Dignity.

Avoid causing intense emotional situations   Do not create circumstances that arouse highly excitable or emotional responses in the patient.

Rationale: Highly emotional responses deplete body energy and may stimulate irritating regulatory secretions. Emotional situations reduce sleep and rest and increase already existing fear and anxiety.

Resolved Needs: Sleep, rest. Energy. Comfort. Protection from physical harm. Protection from psychologic threat.

Avoid causing painful emotional situations   Do not create circumstances that arouse undesirable or painful feelings in the patient.

Rationale: The perception of painful situations results in a defensive response to threat. Emotionally charged interaction interferes with effective communication.

Resolved Needs: Comfort. Protection from psychologic threat. Warm, communicating relationships.

Avoid disconnecting the urinary catheter   Do not pull apart the connecting tubes of a urinary catheter and the attached drainage bag unless it is absolutely necessary.

Rationale: A closed drainage system prevents the entrance of infectious microorganisms into the internal catheter and eliminates their spread from the catheter to the urinary tract. Disconnection of the urinary catheter in tidal drainage alters the established pressure within the system.

Resolved Needs: Cleanliness. Protection from physical harm.

Avoid placing tension on the wound   Do not allow pulling or stretching of tissue to occur around a wound site.

Rationale: Stress around a wound site heightens pain, increases the time needed for healing, and usually distorts tissue replacement.

Resolved Needs: Comfort. Protection from physical harm.

Avoid placing the patient on enforced inactivity   Do not allow the patient to be totally restricted or to restrict himself from all activity.

Rationale: Enforced inactivity increases stress by requiring adaptation to the threat of frustration. Adaptation and adjustment require energy that, in illness, is needed for healing.

Resolved Needs: Energy. Comfort. Protection from physical harm. Protection from psychologic threat.

Avoid reinforcing hope after predeath acceptance (248)   Once the patient has accepted death, do not offer words of encouragement that life will be extended. Instead, offer support that each remaining day be lived to its fullest.

Rationale: Once the reality of death has been accepted, gestures intended to reinforce hope offer no consolation and may temporarily reverse acceptance.

Resolved Needs: Comfort. Protection from psychologic threat. Dignity.

Avoid simultaneously touching electrical equipment and a patient with a pacemaker

Since the patient with a pacemaker is predisposed to electrical shock, do not touch him and adjacent electrical equipment at the same time.

Rationale: A leaking electrical current can pass from one person to another if they are touching and result in electrocution.

Resolved Needs: Protection from physical harm.

Avoid simultaneous use of multiple electrical machines around pacemakers

Since the patient with a pacemaker is predisposed to electrical shock, use only one electrical machine on him at a time, if at all possible.

Rationale: Minimizing the amount of electrical equipment used reduces the potential for electrical current leakage.

Resolved Needs: Protection from physical harm.

Avoid using extension cords around pacemakers

Do not allow the use of extension cords in areas where there is a patient with a pacemaker.

Rationale: Extension cords are a source of current leakage, which increases the potential danger of electrocution.

Resolved Needs: Protection from physical harm.

Avoid using rough-textured bed linens

Do not allow use of bed linens made from coarse materials such as muslin or rough-textured cotton. Use only soft cotton (if possible, percale) sheets.

Rationale: Rough-textured linens cause friction irritation and skin breakdown.

Resolved Needs: Comfort. Protection from physical harm.

Avoid using worn electrical cords, plugs, or outlets around pacemakers

Do not allow the use of electrical cords that are frayed or plugs or outlets that become warm when in use.

Rationale: When electrical cords are frayed and plugs or outlets become warm after use, it indicates poor insulation and offers the potential for electrical current leakage.

Resolved Needs: Protection from physical harm.

Avoid verbal communication   When there are sudden changes in the patient's voice pitch and quality, temporarily avoid communication that necessitates a verbal response. When, in an emotional situation, the patient prefers not to communicate verbally, delay the verbal exchange until later.

Rationale: Speech places stress and discomfort on irritated vocal cords. Avoiding verbal communication at inappropriate times reduces psychologic threat.

Resolved Needs: Comfort. Protection from physical harm. Protection from psychologic threat.

Avoid written communications   Do not give the patient printed or written material that requires his interpretation through reading.

Rationale: Ill persons are hypersensitive to their weaknesses. Awareness of severe health impairment increases feelings of threat.

Resolved Needs: Comfort. Protection from psychologic threat.

Await patient-initiated conversation   When there is impaired message reception and delivery, allow the person time to start the conversation instead of initiating it for him.

Rationale: Persons with aphasic conditions speak better and more comfortably if they initiate the conversation rather than respond to the conversation of others.

Resolved Needs: Comfort. Protection from psychologic threat.

Await placenta delivery (ExR)   Wait 10–20 minutes until the placenta delivers itself through the vulva. Do not under any circumstances force the delivery.

Rationale: Assisting with placenta expulsion promotes maternal safety.

Resolved Needs: Protection from physical harm.

Balance fluid intake to equal output   Maintain a daily balanced fluid intake by offering the patient the same amount of fluid that is put out. Normally, older children and adults need a fluid intake of 1500–3600 cc/day due to 1500 cc urine loss, 500–1000 cc sweat loss, 400 cc loss through respirations, and 500 cc fecal loss. Normally, infants and small children need 125 cc of water for every 2.2 lb of body weight per day. In nonhealth states, the output may be above or below normal. The intake should be balanced accordingly so both are equal.

Rationale: Balanced fluid intake and output are essential to cell functioning. Fluid alterations damage and impair cell activity. Adequate intake is essential for glomerular filtration of nitrogen waste products. Balanced fluid intake reduces the number of foreign particles, such as fat, in the circulation.

Resolved Needs: Water-salt balance. Waste elimination. Comfort. Protection from physical harm.

Balance nutritional intake
Maintain a balanced diet by providing the four basic food groups daily. These include meat, milk and milk products, bread and cereal, and fruits and vegetables.

Rationale: Balanced nutritional intake is essential to body cell activity and energy production from foods. Relief of visceral hunger promotes comfort.

Resolved Needs: Food balance. Energy. Comfort. Protection from physical harm.

Bandage with a draining-wound dressing
Apply a fluffed and loosely packed sterile dressing to the draining wound.

Rationale: Loosely packed gauze draws drainage away from its source. It promotes air circulation, resulting in moisture evaporation and area heat reduction. It maintains cleanliness and comfort.

Resolved Needs: Comfort. Cleanliness. Protection from physical harm.

Bathe daily
Cleanse the patient's body daily by bed bath, sponge bath, shower, or tub.

Rationale: Cleanliness prevents bacterial growth and promotes comfort. It assists in illness dependency. Gently touching the patient's skin during bathing can express concern and relatedness toward the person.

Resolved Needs: Comfort. Cleanliness. Protection from physical harm. Dependence.

Contraindications: Partial baths should be substituted several times a week for persons with very dry skin.

Bathe in a shower
Wash the body with soap and rinse it with water in spray form.

Rationale: The gentle pressure of sprayed water cleanses the skin of infecting microorganisms, promotes comfort, and stimulates peripheral circulation. Steam from a shower helps moisten the lungs of persons with a laryngectomy. It assists in illness dependency.

Resolved Needs: Circulation. Comfort. Cleanliness. Protection from physical harm. Dependence.

Bathe in a tub
Immerse the body in a tub of clean water. Wash with soap and rinse with water.

Rationale: Tub bathing cleanses the skin of infecting microorganisms, promotes comfort, facilitates musculoskeletal movement, and stimulates peripheral circulation. Tub bathing does not pose the threat of water entering the vagina and so is safe during early pregnancy. It assists in illness dependency.

Resolved Needs: Circulation. Comfort. Cleanliness. Protection from physical harm. Dependence.

Contraindications: Avoid tub bathing once the membrane has ruptured, the mucous plug appears, or if there is vaginal bleeding during pregnancy.

Bathe in bed   Wash the body with soap and water during patient confinement to bed.

Rationale: Bathing cleanses the skin of infecting microorganisms, promotes comfort, stimulates peripheral circulation, and offers assistance in illness dependency. Being bathed by someone else reduces energy consumption needed for healing.

Resolved Needs: Energy. Comfort. Cleanliness. Protection from physical harm. Dependence.

Bathe in cool water   Apply cool water to the skin either in a bath or by local sponge application.

Rationale: Liquid solutions in contact with heat change into vapor. When water comes in contact with excessively warm skin, the liquid vaporizes and reduces body temperature. Cooling the body surface promotes comfort.

Resolved Needs: Normal temperature. Comfort.

Bathe in vinegar water   Place the patient in a tub or bathe with a washcloth, using a vinegar-water solution of 2 tablespoons vinegar to 1 pint water.

Rationale: Vinegar-water solution reduces uremic itching by dissolving and removing uremic urate salts from the skin.

Resolved Needs: Comfort. Cleanliness. Protection from physical harm.

Bathe in warm water   Apply warm water (90–100°F) to the skin either by bath or local sponge application.

Rationale: Bathing in warm water increases body temperature, relaxes muscles, promotes comfort, increases extremity circulation through vessel dilatation, stimulates voiding, and relieves bladder spasms.

Resolved Needs: Circulation. Waste elimination. Normal temperature. Relaxation. Comfort. Protection from physical harm.

Bathe locally   Using soap and water, cleanse any body area that frequently becomes soiled. Include areas of drainage, incontinence, and prolonged bleeding.

Rationale: Irritating body discharges promote skin breakdown. Bathing removes skin irritating substances, cleanses infecting microorganisms, and promotes comfort. It assists in illness dependency.

Resolved Needs: Comfort. Cleanliness. Protection from physical harm. Dependence.

Bathe with oil   Use mild oil to bathe a premature infant. Do not use soap and water.

Rationale: Soap and water may irritate the fragile skin of premature infants. Oil cleanses the skin.

Resolved Needs: Cleanliness. Protection from physical harm.

Bathe with water only   Wash the skin with nothing but clear, clean water.

Rationale: Chemical substances on sensitive skin irritate cutaneous tissue and promote skin breakdown. Bathing in clean water cleanses the skin, refreshes, and promotes comfort.

Resolved Needs: Comfort. Cleanliness. Protection from physical harm.

Bivalve and spread the cast to relieve pressure (ET)   When evidence of severe tissue edema or circulatory impairment exists in a casted limb and medical assistance is not available, the cast should be split along both sides. The anterior and posterior cast is then adjusted to allow for the problem and taped or bandaged in place so it still fulfills its function of maintaining immobility.

Rationale: Pressure on edematous tissues could puncture the skin, and prolonged, impaired circulation could cause tissue necrosis and nerve damage.

Resolved Needs: Circulation. Comfort. Protection from physical harm.

Boil the milk   When an allergy or intolerance to milk exists, cook the milk to boiling, cool, and serve.

Rationale: In milk intolerance, boiling milk destroys bacteria, producing a finer, softer curd. Boiling milk supports easier and more rapid digestion and absorption, and, in milk allergy, breaks down protein, reducing allergy responses.

Resolved Needs: Food balance. Comfort. Protection from physical harm.

Brush and comb the hair   Stroke the hair with a brush and comb several times a day.

Rationale: Brushing the hair removes dirt particles and dead scalp cells, promotes comfort, and conserves energy in weak persons.

Resolved Needs: Energy. Comfort. Cleanliness. Dependence.

Brush the infant's hair with a soft hairbrush   Stroke the infant's hair with a soft-bristled brush several times a day.

Rationale: A soft hairbrush prevents irritation to tender skin, removes dirt particles, and promotes comfort.

Resolved Needs: Comfort. Cleanliness. Protection from physical harm. Dependence.

Brush the teeth   Use a toothbrush and abrasive agent to cleanse the patient's teeth and surrounding tissues.

Rationale: Since illness predisposes mouth tissue to infection, cleanliness reduces bacterial action and promotes comfort. Brushing the patient's teeth for him conserves energy needed for healing and aids in illness dependency.

Resolved Needs: Energy. Comfort. Cleanliness. Protection from physical harm. Dependence.

Brush the teeth with a soft toothbrush   When brushing the teeth of a person with injured, degenerating, or bleeding gums, use a soft toothbrush.

Rationale: Using a soft toothbrush prevents trauma to gums and oral mucosa, while maintaining gum stimulation and clean teeth.

Resolved Needs: Comfort. Protection from physical harm.

Brush the tongue   Apply the stroking action of a toothbrush to the tongue surface.

Rationale: Friction from brushing removes coatings or food accumulations from mucous membrane surfaces, reduces irritation, and promotes comfort. Persons having a laryngectomy need an exceptionally clean mouth because of impaired taste and smell.

Resolved Needs: Comfort. Cleanliness. Protection from physical harm.

Call the patient's family to the bedside   Contact the patient's loved ones by telephone, inform them of the patient's condition, and ask that they come and stay with the patient.

Rationale: The presence of loved ones during illness promotes comfort and emotional support. Early notification of a relative's serious illness gives family members time to adapt to the stressful situation.

Resolved Needs: Comfort. Unity with loved ones.

Catheterize one time only   Introduce a sterile catheter through the urethra into the bladder and withdraw the urine. Then, remove the catheter.

Rationale: Catheterization facilitates urine flow from the bladder, maintains normal elimination of nitrogenous and other toxic wastes, and promotes comfort by relieving bladder pressure. Analysis of body wastes reveals potentially harmful physiologic disequilibrium.

Resolved Needs: Waste elimination. Comfort. Protection from physical harm.

Contraindications: Susceptibility to or existing genitourinary infection. Hematuria. Urethral obstruction.

Catheterize with an indwelling urinary catheter   Introduce a sterile catheter through the urethra into the bladder. Inflate the catheter and leave it in place.

Rationale: An indwelling catheter facilitates urine flow from the bladder, maintains normal elimination of nitrogenous and other toxic wastes, promotes comfort by relieving bladder pressure, and prevents skin irritation from incontinence.

Resolved Needs: Waste elimination. Comfort. Cleanliness. Protection from physical harm.

Contraindications: Susceptibility to or existing genitourinary infection. Hematuria. Urethral obstruction.

Caution about breast feeding   When there is breast inflammation or possible nipple cracking, allow the mother to breast feed but caution her against allowing extreme sucking pressure or prolonged feeding.

Rationale: Infant sucking irritates breast tissue.

Resolved Needs: Comfort. Protection from physical harm.

Contraindications: During severe breast tissue irritation or infection, breast feeding is to be avoided.

Change the catheter each time the airway is suctioned   Dispose of the airway suctioning catheter immediately after use and obtain a new, sterile catheter, especially when suctioning tracheostomy and endotracheal tubes. Wear sterile gloves.

Rationale: Airway suctioning with sterile catheters minimizes the introduction of microorganisms into the respiratory system.

Resolved Needs: Cleanliness. Protection from physical harm.

Change the dressing frequently   Check the wound dressing for drainage at least every 4 hours and apply a clean, dry, sterile dressing immediately when soiled.

Rationale: Dry, sterile wound coverings minimize bacterial growth and promote cleanliness and comfort.

Resolved Needs: Comfort. Cleanliness. Protection from physical harm.

Change the hyperalimentation tubing with each dressing change   Remove all the used hyperalimentation tubing, except the subclavian Intracath, and replace with new sterile tubing at each dressing change. Maintain absolute sterile technique, especially at the tubing tips.

Rationale: Clean therapeutic equipment minimizes infection.

Resolved Needs: Cleanliness. Protection from physical harm.

Change the nasal oxygen catheter every eight hours   Remove the oxygen nasal catheter every 8 hours and replace with a new one. Lubricate the catheter with sterile water or normal saline before replacing.

Rationale: Nasal catheters dry out and adhere to nasal mucosa, causing cracking and bleeding of nasal tissue. Cleanliness minimizes infection and promotes comfort.

Resolved Needs: Comfort. Cleanliness. Protection from physical harm.

Change the ostomy appliance as needed   If the patient has a colostomy, an ileostomy, a ureterostomy, or a ureteroilestomy, etc., change the drainage receptacle as often as needed to maintain patient cleanliness and comfort. Appliances attached with adhesive are changed less frequently but require intermittent emptying.

Rationale: Frequently changing the ostomy appliance promotes comfort. It maintains cleanliness, reducing the possibility of infection and skin irritation.

Resolved Needs: Comfort. Cleanliness. Protection from physical harm.

Change the patient's clothes at bedtime   Before bedtime, change the clothes that the patient has been wearing all day. Provide a clean gown.

Rationale: Clean clothes are refreshing, promote comfort, and assist in illness dependency.

Resolved Needs: Comfort. Cleanliness. Dependence.

Change the patient's position frequently   At least every two hours both day and night, move the patient's body from one position to another, from side to side and back to abdomen. Turn frequently.

Rationale: Body position changes prevent respiratory congestion, prolonged pressure on body areas, and contractures. They promote circulation and expectoration, reduce fatigue, and stimulate voiding. Position change assists in illness dependency.

Resolved Needs: Circulation. Waste elimination. Comfort. Protection from physical harm. Dependence.

Contraindications: Spinal cord injuries or bone fractures requiring complete body immobilization.

Change the patient's position gradually   Slowly raise the patient from a lying or sitting position to a step-by-step elevated position.

Rationale: Gradual position change reduces severe arterial and venous blood pressure adaptations, promotes uniform circulation, prevents sudden eye pressure changes, decreases pressure on bones, and in hyperalimentation decreases possible catheter clogging.

Resolved Needs: Circulation. Comfort. Protection from physical harm. Freedom from pain.

Change the sanitary pads frequently   Replace the saturated sanitary pad with a clean one as often as needed.

Rationale: Cleanliness prevents infection and promotes comfort. Changing pads assists in illness dependency.

Resolved Needs: Comfort. Cleanliness. Protection from physical harm. Dependence.

Change the tracheostomy tube   When the inserted tracheostomy tube becomes encrusted with secretions and cannot be cleaned properly while in place, gently remove the tube, use forceps to hold the stoma open, and insert a new tube.

Rationale: A patent airway is essential to normal oxygen and carbon dioxide exchange. Cleanliness prevents respiratory tract infection and promotes comfort.

Resolved Needs: Oxygen. Comfort. Cleanliness. Protection from physical harm.

Contraindications: Delay changing the tube if secretions are too copious for the patient to tolerate being without a tube for a few moments.

Change the urinary catheter   Replace the indwelling urinary catheter when the present catheter is no longer aseptically clean or patent.

Rationale: A sterile catheter minimizes bacterial spread from catheter to urinary tract. A patent catheter facilitates urine flow, maintaining normal elimination of nitrogenous and other toxic wastes, and promotes comfort.

Resolved Needs: Waste elimination. Comfort. Cleanliness. Protection from physical harm.

Change the urinary drainage apparatus   Replace the urinary drainage bag every 24 hours if urinary infection exists. Change it at least every 3 days if no infection exists and if it serves as a receptacle for urine from an indwelling catheter.

Rationale: Urinary drainage bag cleanliness prevents infection.

Resolved Needs: Cleanliness. Protection from physical harm.

Change the wet diaper immediately   Check often to determine when diapers are wet and replace them with dry diapers immediately.

Rationale: Urine ammonia causes skin irritation. Skin dryness promotes cleanliness and comfort.

Resolved Needs: Comfort. Cleanliness. Protection from physical harm.

Clamp the chest tube but for only a short time (559)   If the closed-chest-drainage system breaks, clamp off the chest tube as quickly as possible with a rubberized hemostat. Limit the clamping of the tube to the least possible time, preferably no more than several minutes. Immediately release the clamp if signs of tension pneumothorax (tracheal deviation, severe cyanosis and dyspnea, shock) occur.

Rationale: When a patient has had lung surgery or has a large pneumothorax, if there is leakage of air from the lung, clamping the chest tube will cause air to build up in the chest, increasing the pleural pressure resulting in lung collapse (tension pneumothorax). A clamped chest tube prevents air from being sucked into the thoracic cavity when the closed-chest-drainage system has been interrupted.

Resolved Needs: Comfort. Protection from physical harm.

Clamp the indwelling urinary catheter intermittently
When retraining is essential to maintain bladder control, intermittently clamp the catheter to prevent urinary flow. At first the catheter should be clamped for periods of 1–2 hours, gradually working up to 4-hour periods.

Rationale: Catheter clamping increases urine volume in the bladder. The increased pressure on bladder tissues and nerves improves bladder muscle tone and stimulates the voiding reflex. Bladder control is essential to the removal of body wastes, the maintenance of dryness to prevent skin irritation, and comfort.

Resolved Needs: Waste elimination. Comfort. Protection from physical harm.

Clean the artificial eye
Use normal saline or tap water to remove unclean particles from an artificial eye.

Rationale: Cleansing the artificial eye prevents infection and promotes comfort. It offers assistance during illness dependency.

Resolved Needs: Comfort. Cleanliness. Protection from physical harm. Dependence.

Clean the contact lenses
Using the appropriate cleaning fluid, remove all dirt and smudge from the contact lenses.

Rationale: Clean contact lenses reduce the potential for eye infection and aid good vision.

Resolved Needs: Comfort. Cleanliness. Protection from physical harm. Dependence.

Clean the dentures
Place the patient's artificial teeth in cleansing solution. Brush the teeth with a toothbrush, rinse them with cool water, and then soak them in mouthwash for a short period. Table salt or sodium bicarbonate may be used as a cleansing agent.

Rationale: Since illness predisposes mouth tissue to infection, cleanliness reduces bacterial action and promotes comfort. Cleansing the patient's dentures helps conserve energy and offers assistance during illness dependency.

Resolved Needs: Energy. Comfort. Cleanliness. Protection from physical harm.

Clean the eye(s)
Use sterile gauze to remove accumulated secretions from the eye.

Rationale: Eye cleansing prevents tissue irritation and infection. It promotes comfort and visual acuity.

Resolved Needs: Comfort. Cleanliness. Protection from physical harm.

Clean the eyeglasses   Remove soil, dirt, lint, or cloudiness from the eyeglasses before the patient wears them.

Rationale: Cleaning eyeglasses promotes visual acuity essential to physical safety and comfort and offers assistance during illness dependency.

Resolved Needs: Comfort. Cleanliness. Protection from physical harm. Dependence.

Clean the nails   Soak the finger- and toenails, then use an orange stick to remove dirt from under and around the nails.

Rationale: Cleanliness minimizes microorganism transfer into and onto body areas that have finger contact. It promotes comfort and offers assistance during illness dependency.

Resolved Needs: Comfort. Cleanliness. Protection from physical harm. Dependence.

Clean the skin with a drying soap   Wash the skin with an oil-removing soap that causes skin dryness. Such soaps include Fels Naptha and Kirkman's soap.

Rationale: Drying soaps remove oils that obstruct sebaceous glands, causing inflammation.

Resolved Needs: Cleanliness. Protection from physical harm.

Contraindications: Avoid using on dry skin.

Clean the skin with an astringent   Wash the skin with an astringent, metallic salt solution such as zinc oxide or aluminum acetate.

Rationale: Astringent chemicals cause vasoconstriction in superficial tissues, and their drying effect on the skin reduces skin oiliness. Cleanliness promotes comfort.

Resolved Needs: Comfort. Cleanliness. Protection from physical harm.

Contraindications: Avoid using on dry skin.

Clean the tracheostomy (or laryngectomy) tube inner cannula   Remove and wash the tracheostomy (or laryngectomy) tube inner cannula with hydrogen peroxide and clean it with pipe cleaners or sterile gauze. After cleaning the cannula, soak it for a few moments in sterile water to remove any cleansing agents that might irritate tracheal tissue.

Rationale: Oxygen and carbon dioxide exchange through respirations is essential to life. Cleanliness inhibits the growth of infecting microorganisms into the respiratory tract.

Resolved Needs: Oxygen. Waste elimination. Cleanliness. Protection from physical harm.

Clean the urinary catheter externally at the meatus   Using benzalkonium (Zephiran) chloride, hydrogen peroxide, or surgical soap, clean the outside of the urinary catheter, especially in the area surrounding the meatus.

Rationale: Cleanliness minimizes the number of infecting microorganisms entering the urinary meatus and promotes comfort.

Resolved Needs: Comfort. Cleanliness. Protection from physical harm.

Clean with alcohol Remove skin dirt and bacteria through a friction application of alcohol.

Rationale: Alcohol in 70% solution stops bacterial growth. Cleanliness promotes comfort.

Resolved Needs: Comfort. Cleanliness. Protection from physical harm.

Contraindications: Avoid using alcohol on an open wound since it causes severe pain. Do not use if it causes chilling of the skin.

Clean with antiseptic solution Clean the skin or wound with a chemical agent that prevents microorganism growth, such as the skin antiseptic ethyl alcohol or wound antiseptic potassium permanganate.

Rationale: Antiseptics inhibit bacterial growth, preventing infection and promoting cleanliness and comfort.

Resolved Needs: Comfort. Cleanliness. Protection from physical harm.

Clean with castile or lanolin soap Wash dirt and bacteria from the skin using castile soap (made from olive oil and caustic soda) or lanolin soap (made from wool fat or grease).

Rationale: Castile and lanolin soap oils soothe the skin and prevent epidermal irritation. Soap friction promotes the comfort of cleanliness.

Resolved Needs: Comfort. Cleanliness. Protection from physical harm.

Clean with hydrogen peroxide Wash the wound or skin with a 3% hydrogen peroxide solution.

Rationale: Hydrogen peroxide destroys bacteria through oxidation and removes adhered exudates and debris from areas where microorganisms might grow. Cleanliness promotes comfort.

Resolved Needs: Comfort. Cleanliness. Protection from physical harm.

Contraindications: Avoid using in closed body cavities (bladder, chest tubes, open wounds into cavities) because excess pressure will result when the gas produced by the hydrogen peroxide becomes trapped in the cavity.

Clean with surgical soap Remove skin dirt and bacteria through the use of antibacterial soap and sterile water.

Rationale: Antibacterial soap removes skin bacteria, preventing infection. Soap friction promotes the comfort of cleanliness.

Resolved Needs: Comfort. Cleanliness. Protection from physical harm.

Clear nasal secretions   Free the internal nares of dirt and secretions by gently inserting a moistened cotton-tipped applicator or folded tissue into the nares and removing undesirable substances.

Rationale: Cleaning the internal nares allows for free passage of respiratory gases. It promotes comfort and offers assistance during illness dependency.

Resolved Needs: Oxygen. Waste elimination. Comfort. Cleanliness. Protection from physical harm. Dependence.

Clothe in flannel pajamas at night   Cover the body with soft woolen clothing during nighttime sleeping hours.

Rationale: Flannel fabric absorbs excessive moisture on the skin from sweating and prevents the discomfort of chilling.

Resolved Needs: Normal temperature. Comfort.

Collect radiation-contaminated linen in a special laundry bag   Place in a special laundry bag, linens used by a person receiving radium implants or other radioactive substances producing gamma rays. Label the bag for special handling.

Rationale: Radiation causes physical harm to exposed persons.

Resolved Needs: Protection from physical harm.

Collect radiation-contaminated urine in a lead-lined container   Place in jugs inside lead-lined boxes, urine excreted by a person receiving radium implants or other radioactive substances producing gamma rays. Do not remove the urine until radioactivity has decreased to 30 millicuries.

Rationale: Radiation causes physical harm to exposed persons.

Resolved Needs: Protection from physical harm.

Comb dandruff from the scalp   Press the teeth of the comb against the scalp and comb the dandruff away from the scalp.

Rationale: Removal of dead scalp tissue promotes cleanliness and reduces the discomfort of itching. When sebaceous gland inflammation exists, dandruff accumulation promotes hair loss or thinning.

Resolved Needs: Comfort. Cleanliness. Protection from physical harm.

Communicate by gesture   Send messages by expressing ideas through the use of motions related to significant objects.

Rationale: Nonverbal gesturing clarifies the meaning of words. Psychologic comfort is promoted through a sense of adequate communication with others. Increased external stimuli enhance perception and response to stimuli.

Resolved Needs: Comfort. Stimulation. Warm, communicating relationships.

Communicate nurse sensitivity to the person's pain Verbally and nonverbally communicate that the nurse experiences feelings for the patient's suffering and will make every effort to perceive the suffering as the patient sees it.

Rationale: Feelings of comfort evolve from an awareness that one is not threatened with aloneness. Relief measures, in terms of the patient's perception of pain, result from the nurse's sensitivity to the patient's situation.

Resolved Needs: Comfort. Protection from psychologic threat.

Communicate recent news events to the disoriented patient Acquaint the patient with the environment by telling him or her important current happenings going on in the world and in the local community.

Rationale: The ability to comprehend one's environment in regard to time, place, and person identity prevents confusion and anxiety.

Resolved Needs: Protection from psychologic threat. Increased reality perception.

Communicate that the nurse feels comfortable with the patient's discussions of death (248) Express to the dying patient that you are comfortable and not threatened with discussions of death. Let the patient know that when he wants to talk, he need only call for you to listen and comfort. Do not run off, change the subject, or deal in trivial conversation when death is mentioned.

Rationale: The dying patient, who senses that health personnel are threatened by the discussion of death, feels isolated and unable to resolve conflicts. Dying patients sometimes pretend denial in order to maintain the comfort of health personnel. Discussion of death at the patient's pace promotes comfort and reduces threat.

Resolved Needs: Comfort. Protection from psychologic threat. Warm, communicating relationships.

Compress the wound edges together Press the two wound edges together and hold them in a closed position when the opening of a wound threatens life.

Rationale: Manually closing an open wound stops hemorrhage, prevents air entry into the pleural spaces, prevents escape of the abdominal viscera, diminishes interruption of normal function, and promotes cleanliness.

Resolved Needs: Cleanliness. Protection from physical harm.

Confine suspected infected animals If an animal has inflicted injury on a person, lock the animal in a specific area where he can be observed.

Rationale: Confining an animal offers opportunity to observe it for the presence of disease and prevents the animal from inflicting further injury on others.

Resolved Needs: Protection from physical harm.

Consult with the physician   On behalf of the patient, discuss with the physician the patient's problem and the alternatives available for solving the problem.

Rationale: Nursing consultation with the patient's physician provides patient safety and comfort.

Resolved Needs: Comfort. Protection from physical harm.

Control excessive spasticity with firm hand pressure   When excessive muscular convulsive movements and rigidity result from upper motor neuron lesions, exert pressure over the spastic muscle with your hand, using firm but gentle pressure.

Rationale: Applied pressure to an extremely tense muscle reduces tension and promotes relaxation, which enhances comfort and decreases pain.

Resolved Needs: Relaxation. Comfort. Freedom from pain.

Control ileostomy-colostomy odor by deodorization   Disagreeable odors from an ileostomy or colostomy can be controlled by keeping the patient, his clothes, and the appliance clean; by inserting deodorant tablets such as charcoal, chlorophyll, and aspirin into the bag following each emptying; by placing an alcohol-saturated cloth or tissue in the bag; by using spray deodorant; or by applying an extra plastic covering such as kitchen wrap over the bag.

Rationale: Freedom from body odor promotes comfort.

Resolved Needs: Comfort.

Control offensive odors by removing the source   When odors are disagreeable, remove the source from which the odors come, such as urinals, bedpans, soiled sheets, genitorurinary collection bags, soiled dressings, or soiled ostomy bags.

Rationale: Offensive odors irritate olfactory senses, causing severe discomfort. Illness produces hypersensitive olfactory sensory perception which heightens the irritation.

Resolved Needs: Comfort.

Correct misinterpreted messages immediately   If there is evidence that a message has been interpreted incorrectly, immediately correct this misinterpretation.

Rationale: Message reception and interpretation is influenced by physiologic and psychologic disequilibrium. Psychologic comfort is promoted through a sense of adequate communication with others.

Resolved Needs: Protection from physical harm. Protection from psychologic threat. Warm, communicating relationships.

Cover the bed with netting   Put fine netting over the bed when there are flying insects in the environment or when there is potential for a child to fall out of bed.

Rationale: Insects transmit viral and bacterial disease, and their bites reduce human comfort. Netting prevents children from climbing over the sides of beds.

Resolved Needs: Comfort. Protection from physical harm.

Cover the hands with mittens   Place the patient's hand in a mitten or mitten substitute to restrict finger movements of a small child or an incoherent adult.

Rationale: Limiting finger movements decreases the ability to cause skin irritation and infection through scratching.

Resolved Needs: Protection from physical harm.

Cover the head   Whenever hair loss is severe, the patient's head should be covered with a nightcap, scarf, etc.

Rationale: An applied covering to a hairless scalp or head promotes warmth and comfort normally supplied by the hair. It protects the patient from embarrassment in social situations.

Resolved Needs: Normal temperature. Comfort. Protection from physical harm. Protection from psychologic threat.

Cover the sucking wound immediately   Cover a sudden, open chest wound immediately so that air cannot be sucked into the pleural cavity. Use available dressings, clothes, or even the palm of your hand.

Rationale: Air entering the pleural space increases intrapleural pressure and causes lung collapse.

Resolved Needs: Protection from physical harm.

Cover with lightweight blankets   Place lightweight sheets and blankets over the patient.

Rationale: Lightweight blankets maintain body heat with a minimum of pressure and weight. They prevent excessive warming of the body, thereby supporting a normal metabolic rate and lessening the burden on an ailing cardiac or respiratory system. In shock, lightweight covers maintain peripheral coolness so the circulating blood can meet the needs of vital internal organs.

Resolved Needs: Normal temperature. Comfort. Protection from physical harm.

Contraindications: Very low body temperature.

Cover with warm blankets   Place warm sheets and blankets over the patient.

Rationale: Warm bed covering promotes comfort by increasing environmental heat surrounding the body and maintaining normal temperature. It decreases body heat loss to the environment.

Resolved Needs: Normal temperature. Comfort. Protection from physical harm.

Contraindications: Avoid warm blankets during shock and increased metabolic rate.

Create giving situations   Create circumstances in which the person has the opportunity to give emotionally to others without receiving a reward. Usually, this situation occurs between loved ones and friends. However, if a patient lacks affection from significant persons, nursing personnel can offer warmth and friendship as a temporary substitute.

Rationale: Love given unconditionally requires a high degree of maturity. Self-esteem is nourished by the development of interpersonal skills and from positive responses from others.

Resolved Needs: Comfort. Love and affection. Warm, communicating relationships. Approval from others. Sense of value, usefulness. High evaluation of self. Personal growth and maturity. Increased pleasantness.

Cut off the electrical power source causing the injury   Stop the flow of electricity into a person by curtailing the source of power. Use insulated wire cutters or gloves if it is necessary to come in direct contact with the electrical source.

Rationale: The disruption of the electrical power source terminates the injuring force.

Resolved Needs: Protection from physical harm.

Cut the food into small bites   Slice the food into small pieces so it can be handled easily when placed in the mouth.

Rationale: The intake of food determines the nutritional state. With involuntary or absent tongue movements, food cannot be properly masticated. Cutting food into small bites aids the digestive process and meets dependency needs. It promotes the comfort of ease in chewing or swallowing, and it prevents choking and aspiration.

Resolved Needs: Food balance. Comfort. Protection from physical harm. Dependence.

Damp-dust the room of allergy-prone persons daily   With a slightly damp cloth, dust the room and furniture surfaces daily.

Rationale: Dust removal prevents allergic and asthmatic responses.

Resolved Needs: Comfort. Protection from physical harm.

Dangle the legs   Gradually bring the patient to a sitting position and slowly move his feet and legs off the side of the bed. Provide foot support with a chair.

Rationale: Dangling, the first step in reestablishing activity, supports strength renewal. The downward gravitational force improves the vascular tone of the muscles, which, in turn, improves circulation. Assistance with activity meets illness dependency needs.

Resolved Needs: Circulation. Activity. Protection from physical harm. Dependence.

Contraindications: Avoid dangling when there is leg edema or impaired peripheral circulation.

Darken the room for sleep Turn off or remove all light sources within the immediate environment.

Rationale: Light stimuli promote wakefulness. Adequate sleep is essential in that the decreased metabolic rate occurring during sleep restores depleted cell energy reserves that result from body adaptation requirements.

Resolved Needs: Sleep, rest, relaxation. Energy. Comfort. Protection from physical harm.

Decrease drafts Reduce the volume of air currents in the environment.

Rationale: Decreasing drafts allows low body temperature to return to normal by reducing the evaporation of perspiration. It prevents itching of irritated skin and reduces body chilling. Drafts over a wet cast cause coldness, which may result in the discomfort of a chill. Drafts stimulate open nerve endings of an open stump and cause pain or phantom sensation. Drafts stimulate the reflex arc or lower motor neurons in paralyzed muscles, causing severe muscle spasm.

Resolved Needs: Normal temperature. Comfort. Protection from physical harm.

Decrease the time interval between infant feedings Feed the infant more often than the present schedule. If he has been eating every 4 hours, feed him every 3 hours. This applies to both bottle and breast feeding.

Rationale: More frequent feedings satisfy the infant's desire for prolonged sucking, provide a greater quantity of food, and promote comfort.

Resolved Needs: Food balance. Comfort.

Defer speech communication for 72 hours after a partial laryngectomy Following a partial laryngectomy, suggest that the patient not attempt to make any sound for at least 72 hours.

Rationale: Vibrations made when attempting to speak can traumatize healing tissue.

Resolved Needs: Protection from physical harm.

Defibrillate the heart muscle (ET) Discharge an electrical current into the heart muscle just after the R wave of the QRS complex, if cardiac arrythmia exists. If ventricular fibrillation occurs, no QRS complex will

exist, so timing the electrical shock is not dependent on the R wave, and the procedure should be performed immediately.

Rationale: The discharge of an electrical current into the heart muscle promotes simultaneous contraction and relaxation of all cardiac muscles at appropriate intervals, thus facilitating the flow of oxygen saturated blood to body tissues. Inadequate oxygenation causes damage or death to body tissue.

Resolved Needs: Oxygen, circulation. Protection from physical harm.

Deflate the airway-tube cuff periodically   Release air from the endotracheal or tracheostomy tube cuff. Suction during cuff deflation. Usually the cuff is deflated for 5–15 minutes every 1 to 4 hours. The cuff often is deflated immediately after intermittent positive pressure breathing and meals and is not inflated again until the next treatment or meal.

Rationale: Deflation of an airway tube cuff relieves pressure on the tracheal and laryngeal mucosa. It decreases potential tissue necrosis from inflation pressure.

Resolved Needs: Protection from physical harm.

Delay bathing   Temporarily put off bathing.

Rationale: Water, upon evaporation, tends to cool the body. A chilled body may already be too cool and uncomfortable for bathing. In severe illness, the activity of bathing may further deplete energy reserves.

Resolved Needs: Energy. Comfort. Protection from physical harm.

Delay communication   Put off communicating until the patient is ready to express his thoughts and feelings.

Rationale: Thoughts and feelings are the person's internal world, the privacy of which should be respected until there is a desire for external expression. Information is poorly communicated when a person is emotionally disturbed, distracted, or preoccupied.

Resolved Needs: Protection from psychologic threat. Dignity.

Demonstrate attitudes consistent with the child's parents' attitudes   Maintain the same behavioral approach as parents display toward their child provided the parental attitude is healthy.

Rationale: Feelings of safety arise from familiar and predictable situations that have been handled successfully in the past.

Resolved Needs: Comfort. Protection from psychologic threat. Predictable, orderly world.

Demonstrate calmness   Assume a calm, although concerned, attitude about the patient's problem. Display confidence, knowledge, and decisive judgment in helping the patient.

Rationale: Identification with the positive attitudes of other people reduces fear and anxiety and promotes positive attitudes in oneself.

Resolved Needs: Comfort. Protection from psychologic threat.

Detect communicable disease cases   Find persons who have been exposed to or have contracted a communicable disease. Report such findings to the health department.

Rationale: Persons who have contracted or have been exposed to a communicable disease can potentially transmit that disease to others.

Resolved Needs: Protection from physical harm.

Dilute the medication   Thin the medication consistency with water or syrup, giving the same dosage but in a larger volume.

Rationale: Dilution of medications reduces gastric irritation, damage to teeth, and unpleasant taste.

Resolved Needs: Comfort. Protection from physical harm.

Dilute the milk   Mix milk with water to decrease the concentration of the milk.

Rationale: The gastrointestinal system tolerates diluted milk more easily. The kidneys of infants under 4 months of age have difficulty handling cow's milk since it contains four times the solute content of breast milk. Therefore, infants can handle diluted milk more easily.

Resolved Needs: Comfort. Protection from physical harm.

Disconnect unused electrical equipment around pacemakers   All electrical equipment not in use should be unplugged from its power source and not just turned off.

Rationale: When a piece of electrical equipment having a three-prong plug is turned off at the switch, current is interrupted in only one wire, leaving current in the other two wires available for possible current leakage and shock.

Resolved Needs: Protection from physical harm.

Discontinue the blood transfusion   Stop the infusion of typed and crossmatched blood by clamping off the blood flow or removing the injection needle.

Rationale: Circulatory overload, infusion-transmitted infection, severe allergic reactions, or hemolytic reactions to incompatible blood pose a serious threat to life.

Resolved Needs: Protection from physical harm.

Discontinue the intravenous infusion   When intravenous fluids have infiltrated tissues, have become contaminated, or have been completed, remove the needle immediately.

Rationale: Edema pressure within the tissues causes tissue trauma. Certain drugs intended for intravascular use may cause severe damage when they come in contact with extravascular tissue. Contaminated fluids can cause serious infection. Removal of a needle upon fluid completion supports comfort.

Resolved Needs: Comfort. Protection from physical harm.

Discourage decision-making when one is under severe stress
Point out that it is not wise to make important decisions while one is under severe stress. Such decisions should be withheld until there has been time for adjustment to crisis situations and reality perception has been reestablished. A widow should not sell her home immediately after the death of her husband. A divorced daughter should not move back home until she has had time to adjust and realistically consider the situation.

Rationale: Decisions made during times of severe stress often reflect distorted thinking or the opinions of others and often are regretted at a later date. Important decisions require one's full attention to problem solving and are best made when stress is not an influencing factor.

Resolved Needs: Protection from psychologic threat. Increased reality perception and problem-solving ability.

Discourage goal seeking during confused thinking
Support attempts at goal achievement only when the person is capable of well-organized thinking.

Rationale: Confusion of thought increases frustration because of reduced ability to decisively overcome barriers to goals. Successful achievement in overcoming barriers to a goal enhances the ability to cope and results in increased adequacy feelings.

Resolved Needs: Comfort. Protection from psychologic threat. Adequacy. Goal achievement.

Discourage oral stimulants
Suggest restraint from using coffee, tea, amphetamines, or alcohol.

Rationale: Oral stimulants can alter cardiac patterns being recorded by monitor. Alcohol and coffee increase peristaltic activity, increase bladder irritability, and stimulate voiding. Alcohol causes skin vasodilatation with decreased vasoconstriction. Alcohol depresses the central nervous system even though initially it appears to stimulate it. Caffeine causes vasodilatation and has a temporary stimulative effect. Caffeine, in both coffee and tea, heightens fever. Caffeine stimulates the adrenal cortex to produce adrenalin, causing the liver to change glycogen into glucose and raising the blood glucose. Stimulants produce a temporary increase in metabolic rate, cause excitement of nerve and muscle tissue, and increase the general level of body activity, ultimately decreasing energy reserves and threatening the healing process.

Resolved Needs: Sleep, rest, relaxation. Comfort. Protection from physical harm.

Discourage smoking   Suggest restraint from smoking tobacco products.

Rationale: Tobacco fumes irritate nasal and pulmonary tissue, causing increased secretions. The fumes paralyze tracheobronchial cilia with the resulting danger of secretion retention. The constriction of circulatory blood vessels by tobacco's chemical irritants results in decreased tissue oxygenation, in impaired extremity circulation, and in a decrease of 1–2°F in skin temperature. Tobacco smoke moves from the throat to the eustachian canal and irritates the inner ear. Smoking discolors teeth and irritates gums. During pregnancy, smoking causes a high carbon monoxide blood level in the fetus. This, and the nicotine vasoconstrictive effect, is suspected of causing cardiac anomalies in infants. Breast milk from heavy smoking mothers contains nicotine, which can be harmful to the child. Smoking inhibits peristaltic activity, which contributes to constipation. It delays gastric emptying, which inhibits normal digestion. It decreases the hunger sensation by deadening the taste receptors. Smoking stimulates the heart rate 8–10 beats faster per minute and, by doing so, often makes sleeping difficult. Its stimulative effect can alter cardiac patterns being recorded by a monitor.

Resolved Needs: Oxygen, circulation. Comfort. Cleanliness. Protection from physical harm.

Discourage strenuous activities   Suggest that the patient not participate in activities that greatly increase the metabolic rate and body energy requirements.

Rationale: Fatigue results from activity or energy-depleting responses to physiologic stress stimuli.

Resolved Needs: Energy. Comfort. Protection from physical harm.

Discourage talking while eating   Suggest that the person refrain from talking while eating.

Rationale: Avoiding talking while eating reduces the possibility of aspirating food or swallowing air into the stomach. Since all activity requires energy, refraint from talking provides the extremely fatigued patient with a little more energy to direct toward food consumption.

Resolved Needs: Protection from physical harm.

Discourage the setting of time limits   Suggest that the patient not set a specific date or a specific time for reaching a goal.

Rationale: Failure to meet self-expectations results in the threat of frustration. The stimulus of needing to hurry causes muscular tension requiring the use of energy, which, in illness, is vital to healing.

Resolved Needs: Energy. Comfort. Protection from physical harm. Protection from psychologic threat.

Discuss possible pain-reducing measures   Mention all possible measures available for pain relief. Emphasize measures other than drugs.

Let the patient make his own choice of pain relief. Offer such measures as heat and cold applications, repositioning, relief of pressure or constriction, relaxation measures, attention diversion, and subdued lighting.

Rationale: Awareness that pain relief measures other than drugs are available reduces the anxiety of potential drug addiction. Comfort feelings are enhanced by awareness that one has choices and has sufficient independent control to prevent harm and bring comfort to oneself.

Resolved Needs: Comfort. Protection from psychologic threat. Freedom from pain. Warm, communicating relationships.

Discuss the anticipated procedure
Provide a clear description of the procedure confronting the patient and verbally illustrate what can be expected to occur. In addition, use drawings, pictures, models of organs, toys, and sensory information for clarification.

Rationale: Positive preparation before an occurrence promotes psychologic safety by reducing fear and anxiety of the unknown. Safety feelings arise from familiar and predictable situations.

Resolved Needs: Comfort. Protection from psychologic threat. Predictable, orderly world. Increased learning.

Disguise drugs with fruit-flavored syrup
Mix a distasteful drug with syrup that is the flavor of a favorite fruit.

Rationale: Enhancing the favorable taste of drugs increases the probability of the drug being taken.

Resolved Needs: Comfort.

Disinfect contaminated articles
Cleanse objects or materials that have been exposed to infecting microorganisms with disinfectant solution. Whenever possible, expose the objects or materials to open air and sunlight for 12 to 24 hours.

Rationale: Removal of infectious microorganisms from surfaces decreases the potential for transfer of disease from one person to another.

Resolved Needs: Cleanliness. Protection from physical harm.

Disinfect the bathtub after each use
Each time the bathtub is used, cleanse it with disinfecting solution.

Rationale: Cleanliness prevents the spread of infection.

Resolved Needs: Cleanliness. Protection from physical harm.

Distribute the fluid intake over 24 hours
When fluids are restricted, divide the intake of allowable fluids so they are available over the entire 24 hours. Give three-fourths during waking hours and save one-fourth for thirst during sleeping hours. If possible, have the patient divide the intake as it most pleases him.

Rationale: Awareness that fluids are available to quench thirst 24 hours a day provides comfort.

Resolved Needs: Comfort.

Distribute the intravenous fluid infusion over 12 to 24 hours
When administering intravenous fluids, distribute the total volume over a 12- to 24-hour period instead of administering fluids over a few short hours.

Rationale: Fluids infused over a long period provide a more balanced fluid and electrolyte level than those given over a short time.

Resolved Needs: Water-salt balance. Protection from physical harm.

Divert attention from preoccupation with guilt
Divert the patient's attention away from concentrated thinking about the wrongdoing in which he was involved. Focus his attention on the reality activities of the day and on activities that can bring social approval.

Rationale: Focusing attention on external stimuli temporarily relieves the tension of internal stress and enhances involvement with reality. Self-esteem requires that a person experience positive response from others.

Resolved Needs: Comfort. Protection from psychologic threat. High evaluation of self. Increased reality perception and problem-solving ability.

Do not add potassium to fluids given by hypodermoclysis
When fluids are given by hypodermoclysis, avoid adding potassium to the infusion.

Rationale: Potassium infused directly into subcutaneous tissues causes tissue irritation.

Resolved Needs: Protection from physical harm.

Do not allow air into the dialysis instillation tubing
Do not allow air to enter the tubing through which the dialysis fluid flows into the peritoneum. Clamp the tubing when the fluid level reaches the neck of the bottle.

Rationale: Air flowing into the peritoneal cavity increases pressure and causes pain.

Resolved Needs: Comfort. Protection from physical harm.

Do not allow foreign objects into the intravenous solution
Do not allow any foreign substance such as air, blood clots, or oils to enter the vascular system.

Rationale: Foreign substances within the vascular system obstruct normal blood flow with resulting cardiac impairment and inadequate tissue oxygenation.

Resolved Needs: Protection from physical harm.

Do not allow skin surfaces to touch   Do not allow body surfaces to touch one another. Separate fingers, toes, legs, skin folds, and the area under the breasts. Place gauze between burned fingers to keep them separated during healing. Under the breasts and between the buttocks, apply a gauze padding to keep the skin apart, absorb moisture, and allow air to pass over the skin.

Rationale: Body surfaces that touch produce friction irritation.

Resolved Needs: Protection from physical harm.

Do not allow unpleasant surprise situations   Reduce fear by preventing elements of surprise and confusion in stressful or fearful situations.

Rationale: The threat of fear is reduced when there is time to prepare for the threat and adapt with appropriate defenses.

Resolved Needs: Comfort. Protection from psychologic threat.

Do not disguise drugs in food   Do not attempt to hide bad-tasting drugs by mixing the drug in food.

Rationale: Drugs mixed in food frequently make food distasteful, causing dislike or rejection of that food. When drugs are disguised in food, unless all the food is eaten, an undetermined portion of the drug is not taken.

Resolved Needs: Protection from physical harm.

Do not disturb while resting   Do not allow persons to enter the room of the resting patient or to awaken him for any reason.

Rationale: The stimulus of the presence of other persons promotes wakefulness. Adequate sleep is essential in that the decreased metabolic rate occurring during sleep restores depleted energy reserves of cells.

Resolved Needs: Sleep, rest, relaxation. Energy. Comfort. Protection from physical harm.

Do not give a blood transfusion via a subclavian Intracath   Do not give a blood transfusion or allow blood to be given through the subclavian Intracath being used for hyperalimentation.

Rationale: Blood cells will coat the internal catheter surface and obstruct the catheter, altering the flow rate of the hyperalimentation solution.

Resolved Needs: Protection from physical harm.

Do not give blood unrefrigerated for more than one hour   If blood for transfusion has been left unrefrigerated for 1 hour or more, it should not be administered. Blood should never be allowed to warm up, be recooled, and then be administered.

Rationale: Blood that has been kept under proper refrigeration, when left unrefrigerated, will increase in temperature 10° in 1 hour's time. This 10° temperature increase allows for bacterial growth.

Resolved Needs: Protection from physical harm.

Do not give blood which is over three weeks old   Do not administer blood by transfusion if it is more than 3 weeks old.

Rationale: The oxygen-carrying capacity of blood decreases with age.

Resolved Needs: Protection from physical harm.

Do not give electrolyte-free solutions by hypodermoclysis   Do not give by hypodermoclysis fluids that do not contain electrolytes. Such fluids include hypertonic solutions such as 10% dextrose in water, 10% invert sugar in water, 10% fructose in water, and gastric replacement, fat emulsion, alcohol, and amino acid or glucose solutions.

Rationale: Solutions that are electrolyte-free and contain glucose decrease plasma volume by drawing electrolytes from the plasma, with a resulting hypotension or peripheral vascular collapse.

Resolved Needs: Water-salt balance. Protection from physical harm.

Do not give medications via a subclavian Intracath   Do not give medications through the subclavian Intracath being used for hyperalimentation.

Rationale: Medications may coat the Intracath surface and obstruct the catheter, altering the flow rate of hyperalimentation solution.

Resolved Needs: Protection from physical harm.

Do not induce vomiting   Do not perform any procedure that would cause vomiting.

Rationale: Vomiting ingested caustic poisons further traumatizes intestinal mucosa as the highly irritating chemicals pass over the tissue a second time.

Resolved Needs: Protection from physical harm.

Do not inject drugs into a blood transfusion   Drugs should never be injected into blood being transfused intravenously.

Rationale: Many drugs, especially calcium, are incompatible with blood and cause blood clotting.

Resolved Needs: Protection from physical harm.

Do not massage   Do not rub any body area where circulatory impairment, thrombus, or frostbite exists.

Rationale: Massage may dislodge a thrombus, sending it into the bloodstream where it might occlude the blood supply to a vital organ. Massaging an area of impaired circulation or frostbite may cause gangrene because massage increases the tissue's need for blood that cannot be provided when blood vessels are severely damaged or diseased.

Resolved Needs: Protection from physical harm.

Do not neutralize the chemical injuring the eye   Do not attempt
to counteract chemical reactions in the eye by using an alkali on an acid or
an acid on an alkali. Instead, flush the eye with clean water from the nasal
corner to the outer corner of the eye.

Rationale: Neutralization of chemicals brings about a chemical heat reaction that can further damage the eye.

Resolved Needs: Protection from physical harm.

Do not place in the flat position   Do not allow the patient to lie flat
who is in respiratory distress, who has potential for increased intracranial
pressure, who has severe hypertension or any other condition in which the
flat position would contribute to discomfort.

Rationale: The flat position inhibits air flow during respiratory distress,
increases intracranial pressure when there is potential for pressure elevation, and increases the blood pressure within the brain to an abnormally
high degree if the blood pressure is already elevated.

Resolved Needs: Comfort. Protection from physical harm.

Do not place the amputation stump in the flexion position   Do
not allow the person with a below-knee amputation stump to bend (flex) the
stump backward. Instead, the stump should be kept straight (extended) and
in alignment with the rest of the body. Do not place a pillow under the
thigh or knee.

Rationale: Extension alignment of an amputated stump prevents flexion
contractures and promotes positioning conducive to successful prosthesis
walking.

Resolved Needs: Protection from physical harm.

Do not pump the breasts   Do not pump or attempt to express milk
from the breasts.

Rationale: Pumping milk from the breasts stimulates increased milk secretion, which causes fullness discomfort.

Resolved Needs: Comfort. Protection from physical harm.

Do not start I.V.s or draw blood in the affected extremity   When the extremity is severely swollen or tissue has been
traumatized, do not start intravenous fluids or draw blood from the veins in
the affected extremity.

Rationale: Needle punctures in edematous or traumatized tissue further
injure the tissue.

Resolved Needs: Protection from physical harm.

Do not withdraw by catheter more than 1000 cc of urine at
one time   When voiding is not possible and a catheter is inserted to pro-

mote urinary flow, do not allow more than 1000 cc of urine to be drained at one time. If it appears that the bladder contains more than 1000 cc of fluid, clamp the catheter after the first 1000 cc of urine have been withdrawn. Wait 30–40 minutes and then allow up to another 1000 cc of urine to be withdrawn.

Rationale: The sudden pressure changes created by emptying an overdistended bladder can cause hypotension and will retard the return of muscle tone of the bladder.

Resolved Needs: Protection from physical harm.

Do surgical (or perineal) prep   Before surgery or delivery, prepare the skin by thoroughly cleansing and removing all hair from the appropriate skin area.

Rationale: Cleansing and removing bacteria and hair from the skin decreases the potential for infection.

Resolved Needs: Cleanliness. Protection from physical harm.

Drain condensation from the nebulizer tubing periodically   When giving aerosol nebulization, drain the accumulated water or liquid from the aerosol tubing into a waste container every 1 or 2 hours. The accumulation is evident by a bubbling sound.

Rationale: Heated condensation in an aerosol tubing may splash and burn the skin or be sucked into the airway, causing death from drowning.

Resolved Needs: Protection from physical harm.

Drape for warmth   When covering the patient for bathing or examinations, make certain that the drape is sufficient and properly placed to insure comfortable body warmth.

Rationale: Normal body warmth promotes comfort and prevents chilling, which often stimulates muscle spasms.

Resolved Needs: Comfort. Protection from physical harm.

Drape modestly   Keep the patient's body covered at all times and prevent the unnecessary display of the uncovered body, especially during examinations and procedures.

Rationale: Comfort and safety feelings are increased when normal sociocultural values are upheld, despite dependency on others. Awareness of esteem from others results from satisfactory and respectful relationships with others.

Resolved Needs: Comfort. Protection from psychologic threat. Dignity.

Dress in colorful clothing   When there is evidence that the person's spirit or mood is low, suggest that brightly colored clothing be worn.

Rationale: Bright colors often promote comforting sensory stimulation.

Resolved Needs: Comfort. Stimulation.

Dress in lightweight clothing   Clothe the person in garments made of light material.

Rationale: Lightweight clothing increases heat lost to the environment, causing a reduction in body temperature and increased comfort. Such clothing reduces pressure on skin lesions and decreases fatigue by preventing strain or pull on shoulder muscles. Lightweight socks lessen foot perspiration.

Resolved Needs: Normal temperature. Energy. Comfort. Protection from physical harm.

Contraindications: Subnormal temperature. Tendency to chill.

Dress in minimum clothing   Dress the person in the least amount of clothing essential to modesty.

Rationale: Minimum clothing, by increasing the amount of heat lost to the environment, helps to decrease an elevated body temperature to within normal limits. Minimum clothing gives persons bothered by incontinence the comfort of being able to easily remove garments. In peritoneal dialysis and ascites, a minimum of clothing reduces the sensation of pressure within the peritoneum and promotes comfort.

Resolved Needs: Normal temperature. Energy. Comfort. Protection from physical harm.

Contraindications: Subnormal temperature. Reduced metabolic rate. Low environmental temperature.

Dress in personal clothing   Have the patient wear his own clothing each day.

Rationale: Safety feelings are promoted by objects that represent past pleasure and security. Certain material objects provide symbolic identification of the self.

Resolved Needs: Comfort. Protection from psychologic threat.

Dress in warm clothing   Clothe the person in garments made of wool, fur, etc., which protect the body against exposure to severe temperature changes.

Rationale: Warm clothing increases environmental heat surrounding the body. It decreases heat lost to the environment and promotes the comfort of the normal body temperature.

Resolved Needs: Normal temperature. Comfort. Protection from physical harm.

Contraindications: Fever. Increased metabolic rate. Allergic reactions.

Dress the patient   Clothe the patient completely without his assistance.

Rationale: When the patient is unable to clothe himself, meeting such needs offers comfort and allows for dignified dependency.

Resolved Needs: Comfort. Dependence. Dignity.

Dust the skin with antiperspirant powder   Apply powder to the feet or under the arms to reduce sweat gland secretion. Do not powder skin folds or between the toes, or apply only a thin film in these areas.

Rationale: Inhibiting sweat gland secretion reduces skin odor and promotes comfort. Powder has a drying action, permits movement of the skin against skin, allows good air circulation over the skin, reduces friction, and promotes cooling and drying of inflamed skin.

Resolved Needs: Comfort. Protection from physical harm.

Dust the skin with medicated powder   Apply a medicated powder to the skin. Do not powder skin folds or between the toes, or apply only a thin film to these areas. Apply fairly heavy amounts to open, inflamed skin.

Rationale: Medicated powder soothes the skin surface and absorbs moisture. Powder has a drying action, permits movement of skin against skin, allows good air circulation over the skin, reduces friction, and promotes cooling and drying of inflamed skin. An antibacterial powder minimizes bacterial growth on the skin and inhibits skin odor.

Resolved Needs: Comfort. Protection from physical harm.

Contraindications: Known medication allergy.

Elevate the affected body part   Raise the body part by placing a pillow comfortably beneath it.

Rationale: Body part elevation promotes circulation and decreases edema by reducing pressure in veins and capillaries, thus facilitating fluid reabsorption.

Resolved Needs: Circulation. Comfort. Protection from physical harm.

Elevate the extremity   Lift or raise the limb above the normal flat level to either a 20- or 30-degree angle. When elevating the arm, be sure the hand is higher than the elbow, and the elbow is higher than the shoulder. Extremity elevation can be done by using a pillow or by using a sling made from a stockinette slipped over the extremity and attached to an I.V. pole.

Rationale: Decreasing the pulling effect of gravity reduces or prevents fluid accumulation in interstitial spaces. Excessive fluid accumulation in body tissues results in discomfort.

Resolved Needs: Circulation. Rest. Comfort. Protection from physical harm. Freedom from pain.

Elevate the foot of the bed   Raise the foot of the bed and then raise the knee gatch until the knees are no longer in hyperextension (stretched out).

Rationale: Foot elevation enhances circulation, reduces pressure on the injured limb, and prevents the patient from slipping down in bed.

Resolved Needs: Circulation. Comfort. Protection from physical harm.

Contraindications: Hypertension. Increased intracranial or intraoccular pressure. Respiratory distress. Ascites. Congestive heart failure. Severe peripheral arterial disease.

Elevate the head   Lift or raise the head above the level of the heart.

Rationale: Head elevation decreases intracranial pressure, promotes venous blood flow from the brain to the heart, reduces potential damage to brain centers controlling the vital signs, increases peripheral blood flow, and clears the airway for improved respiratory ventilation. Raising the head decreases pain from intracranial pressure when the pain results from the inability of the skull to expand. During peritoneal dialysis, pressure placed on the diaphragm from the dialysis fluid in the peritoneal cavity can cause respiratory difficulty. Elevating the head reduces the pressure on the diaphragm, facilitating ease of respirations. Elevation of the body after death prevents discoloration of the exposed body and gives an appearance of sleep.

Resolved Needs: Oxygen. Circulation. Comfort. Protection from physical harm. Freedom from pain.

Contraindications: Shock. Labrynthitis vomiting. Potential fainting. Meningitis and cerebral conditions (especially tumors) in which gravity will pull the brain further downward into the cranium (tentorium), causing increased pressure on the medulla breathing center, resulting in respiratory failure.

Emphasize the importance of fair play in competition   Promote the idea that fair play in competition is more important than winning so when the person loses he can still take pride in having played well.

Rationale: Rivalry and competition promote the threat of frustration and hostility, which results in aggression. Self-esteem is maintained when a person perceives himself as living up to cultural expectations. Safety and comfort feelings evolve from an awareness that one can cope successfully with life. Maturity and growth involve reality perception and behavioral changes that appropriately meet situational demands and individual needs.

Resolved Needs: Comfort. Protection from psychologic threat. High evaluation of self. Self-reliance. Personal growth and maturity. Increased reality perception and problem-solving ability.

Emphasize the person's normal characteristics   Frequently point out to the person those personal qualities that he shares with the majority of others.

Rationale: An awareness of one's normal characteristics fosters a sense of adequacy and comfort.

Resolved Needs: Comfort. Adequacy.

Emphasize the person's value as an individual   Make the person aware that he is contributing something worthwhile and that his ideas and feelings are valuable. Emphasize that he has something to give to others.

Rationale: A positive response from others indicates acceptance and promotes self-esteem.

Resolved Needs: Comfort. Acceptance. Approval from others. Sense of value, usefulness. High evaluation of self. Adequacy.

Empty the collection appliance (or container)   Remove from the collection appliance or container the fluid or substance that has drained into the container. Measure the amount emptied.

Rationale: Emptying collection appliances or containers removes disagreeable sights and odors, promotes cleanliness, and provides for observation of new drainage that may have changed character from previous drainage.

Resolved Needs: Comfort. Cleanliness. Protection from physical harm.

Encourage a full day of activities   Involve the person in external activity for the entire day, beginning at the time of arising and ending at bedtime.

Rationale: Focusing attention on external stimuli temporarily relieves the tension of internal stress, enhances involvement with reality, and promotes comfort.

Resolved Needs: Comfort. Stimulation. Protection from psychologic threat. Increased reality perception.

Encourage a positive life approach   Encourage the patient to think mostly positive thoughts and to converse habitually on cheerful, positive subjects.

Rationale: Positive attitudes motivate positive behavior and self-perception because of the affirmative responses they elicit from others.

Resolved Needs: Comfort. Protection from psychologic threat. High evaluation of self. Personal growth and maturity. Increased reality perception and problem-solving ability. Increased pleasantness.

Encourage ability testing   Sustain the patient by encouraging him to test those abilities that he is capable of attaining. Discourage him from attempting goals that are doomed to failure.

Rationale: Mastering abilities and developing potential supports a comforting sense of adequacy that evolves from an awareness that one can cope successfully with life.

Resolved Needs: Comfort. Stimulation. Adequacy. Self-reliance. Mastery and competence in skills. Full development of potential.

Encourage   acceptance   of   forgiveness   offered   by others   Assist the patient in reappraising his relationship with God and other people and help him recognize that forgiveness is available from both, if only he will accept it.

Rationale: The healing of guilt comes not in erasing it, but in the ability to see oneself as worthy of accepting the forgiveness offered. Safety feelings require that a person experience awareness of acceptance by others.

Resolved Needs: Comfort. Protection from psychologic threat. Acceptance. High evaluation of self.

Encourage acceptance of interdependency
Verbally reinforce the truth that people must be interdependent if they are to enjoy a rich, full life. Stress the fact that at times we must be willing to help one another and at other times be able to accept help from others without shame.

Rationale: When a person is forced into dependency, he needs care that is physically and emotionally reminiscent of the safe mother-child relationship. Psychologic comfort is promoted through a sense of relatedness to others and the ability to communicate one's needs. Self-esteem requires that a person experience positive responses from others.

Resolved Needs: Comfort. Protection from psychologic threat. Dependence. Warm, communicating relationships. High evaluation of self.

Encourage acceptance of limitations in others
Teach that all human beings have weaknesses of one sort or another. Suggest that it is best to look upon other human beings favorably despite human frailties and not to expect perfection from others.

Rationale: Safety and comfort are promoted through a sense of adequate communication with others. Sound health approaches to behavioral problems promote safety and comfort, enhance the natural tendency to organize perceptual data into relationships and selections, and promote growth and maturity.

Resolved Needs: Protection from psychologic threat. Warm, communicating relationships. Personal growth and maturity. Increased reality perception and problem-solving ability.

Encourage acceptance of partial goal satisfaction
When the person attempts to totally withdraw from goals that he cannot accomplish, suggest ways he can gain satisfaction through partial accomplishment of those same goals.

Rationale: Withdrawal removes the person from perceived threat. Negative perception can be altered through identification with the positive perceptions of another and result in reduced threat. Comfort and safety feelings evolve from an awareness that one can cope successfully with life. The anticipation of satisfying achievement leads to activity.

Resolved Needs: Comfort. Protection from psychologic threat. Adequacy. Goal achievement. Increased reality perception and problem-solving ability.

Encourage acceptance of responsibility
Assist the person in accepting tasks or duties and in fulfilling the obligation assumed.

Rationale: The acceptance of responsibility results from a sense of clear self-identity, competencies, and adult values. The ability to overcome the ambivalence of dependency-independency needs is essential to growth and maturity.

Resolved Needs: High evaluation of self. Adequacy. Self-reliance. Mastery and competence in skills. Independence. Personal growth and maturity. Full development of potential. Improved values.

Encourage acceptance of self-limitations
Assist the person in recognizing that all human beings have weaknesses and that limitations are not unique. Suggest that the person look upon himself favorably despite human frailties.

Rationale: A positive self can be developed only when self-expectations are in harmony with the realistic self. Comfort and adequacy are fostered by an awareness that one's weaknesses are not unique.

Resolved Needs: Comfort. Protection from psychologic threat. High evaluation of self. Personal growth and maturity. Increased reality perception.

Encourage acceptance of the right to pleasure
Assist the person in realizing that he has a right to enjoy pleasure.

Rationale: A positive self results from positive responses from others. Persons receiving reasonable amounts of pleasure experience a more positive approach to life and more successfully tolerate unpleasant experiences.

Resolved Needs: Protection from psychologic threat. High evaluation of self. Increased pleasantness.

Encourage acceptance of unpleasantness
Suggest that the person recognize and be willing to accept limited amounts of pain, unhappiness, dissatisfaction, and delayed gratification. Help him to live objectively in the real world and not merely in the fantasy of ideas.

Rationale: Facing life's realities includes the maturity of accommodating to the inevitable stress of unmet or delayed pleasure.

Resolved Needs: Personal growth and maturity. Increased reality perception and problem-solving ability.

Encourage active diversional activities
Suggest that the person participate in an activity in which something is produced; for example, fishing, doing crossword puzzles, woodburning, making jewelry, making crepe paper flowers, lettering, crayoning, clay modeling, weather forecasting, box gardening, photography, creative writing, stamp collecting, coin collecting, stuffing toys, painting pictures, knitting, potting, basket weaving.

Rationale: Focusing attention on external stimuli temporarily relieves the tension of internal stress by promoting temporary escape from conscious perception of threats of fear, anxiety, and pain. Creativity enhances self-actualization and healthy human functioning.

Resolved Needs: Comfort. Stimulation. Protection from psychologic threat. Freedom from pain. Full development of potential. Increased pleasantness.

Encourage adequate rest Encourage a minimum of 6–8 hours rest a day for persons who are well. Encourage about 9–12 hours of partial rest a day for persons who have a localized infection, who only a few days previously had an elevated temperature that is now normal, who feel weak and are gradually attempting to restore energy, who are gradually increasing mobility activities, who are convalescing, or who have a slight illness. Encourage about 13–17 hours of moderate rest a day for persons with a slight temperature elevation of 99–101°F, who have conditions in which energy is depleted fairly quickly, who are moderately ill, or who are slowly restoring mobility activities. Encourage about 18–23 hours of intensive rest a day for persons who have a moderate temperature of 101–103°F, who have a moderate blood pressure elevation, who have conditions in which there is severe energy depletion, or who have a serious illness. Since travel is stressful, encourage persons going on trips to rest adequately during the days before the trip to minimize the degree of stress placed on the body.

Rationale: Rest is essential to the maintenance of body function. Rest replenishes cell energy, which the body uses for the maintenance of life and physical and emotional activity, and promotes healing and comfort.

Resolved Needs: Sleep, rest. Energy. Comfort. Protection from physical harm. Protection from psychologic threat.

Encourage admission of wrongdoing Assist the person to verbally express the details of the wrongdoing.

Rationale: Confession relieves the anxiety of anticipated detection and punishment, reestablishes an inner sense of love-worthiness, and can divert punishment and gain approval. Self-esteem requires that a person experience positive responses from others.

Resolved Needs: Comfort. Protection from psychologic threat. Acceptance. Approval from others.

Encourage alternate rest and activity For each hour of activity, have the patient rest for 10 minutes. As fatigue is reduced, increase the length of activity with less frequent rest periods.

Rationale: Fatigue, feelings of tiredness, and weariness result from activity or energy requiring responses to physiologic and psychologic stress stimuli. Fatigue conditions are decreased by reducing stress stimuli or by restoring energy by means of reducing metabolic requirements during rest. The accomplishment of activity without fatigue promotes comfort.

Resolved Needs: Rest. Energy. Comfort. Protection from physical harm. Protection from psychologic threat.

Encourage attentive patient listening Call to the person's attention the need to listen carefully to what others are saying before drawing conclusions about the meaning of the message being sent. Also, suggest he listen carefully to his own spoken messages.

Rationale: Message reception is influenced by the person's current needs and interests and can result in pleasurable or threatening interpretation. Preoccupation and emotionally charged thinking interfere with correct delivery, reception, and interpretation of messages.

Resolved Needs: Protection from psychologic threat. Warm, communicating relationships.

Encourage awareness of positive responses from others   Suggest that the person consciously make mental notes each time someone responds favorably to him. At the end of the day, have the person enumerate those responses.

Rationale: Positive feelings regarding one's self result from positive responses from others.

Resolved Needs: Comfort. Protection from psychologic threat. Acceptance. Approval from others. High evaluation of self.

Encourage balanced long- and short-range goals   While long-range goals are being attempted, suggest short-term objectives that can be accomplished intermittently along with the extended goal.

Rationale: The accomplishment of short-term goals reduces the adaptation to frustration that accompanies long-range goals. Adaptation and adjustment require energy that, in illness, is needed for healing. Successful achievement in overcoming barriers to a goal enhances the ability to cope, with a resulting increased sense of adequacy.

Resolved Needs: Energy. Comfort. Protection from physical harm. Protection from psychologic threat. Adequacy. Goal achievement.

Encourage bladder emptying before rest   Suggest to the person that he empty his bladder just before resting.

Rationale: A full bladder produces a certain degree of bladder tension as the muscles stretch to contain urine. The relief of this muscular tension through bladder emptying promotes relaxation.

Resolved Needs: Relaxation. Comfort.

Encourage chapel-service attendance   While the patient is hospitalized, inform him of available chapel services and provide transportation to the chapel.

Rationale: Religious observances help people to spiritually express their relationship with God and outwardly to recognize the Supreme Being.

Resolved Needs: Comfort. Religious, philosophic satisfaction.

Encourage continuation of education   Assist the patient in realizing that continuing one's education through the usual years of formal learning gives a person increased knowledge with which to meet life's problems

and enhances his chances of obtaining and keeping desired and well-paying employment.

Rationale: Sound approaches to problems promote increased reality perception.

Resolved Needs: Increased reality perception and problem-solving ability.

Encourage coughing   Place the patient in a sitting position. Have him inhale deeply, then forcefully exhale with a cough.

Rationale: The forceful movement of air from the lower to the upper respiratory tract propels thick mucus from the tracheobronchial tree, improving respirations and removing infectious material.

Resolved Needs: Oxygen. Waste elimination. Protection from physical harm.

Contraindications: Increased intrathoracic, intraocular, intraabdominal, or intracranial pressure. Pulmonary hemorrhage.

Encourage creative activities and play   Suggest that the person participate in activities in which something is produced. Provide a friendly, stimulating climate for creativity.

Rationale: Focusing attention on external stimuli temporarily relieves the tension of internal stress by promoting temporary escape from conscious perception of threats of fear, anxiety, and pain. Creativity enhances growth toward self-actualization and healthy human functioning. Self-expression through creativity preserves mental and physical well-being by fostering inner peace and harmony.

Resolved Needs: Comfort. Stimulation. Protection from psychologic threat. Personal growth and maturity. Increased creativity. Increased reality perception. Increased pleasantness.

Encourage crying   In anxiety states or depression resulting from loss, suggest accepting that the person cry. Bring up tear-producing subjects if necessary.

Rationale: Weeping promotes internal tension reduction and is a psychologic mechanism for reestablishing stability in a threatened equilibrium. The reduction of internal tension promotes comfort.

Resolved Needs: Comfort. Protection from psychologic threat.

Encourage decision-making   Assist the person in making decisions by himself regarding situations, problems, or matters affecting him and his future.

Rationale: The ability to maintain self-direction and be free from control of others requires clear self-identity, knowledge, competencies, and adult values. The ability to overcome the ambivalence of dependency-independency needs is essential to growth and maturity. Feelings of safety evolve from an awareness that one can cope successfully with life. Vulnerability to the outcome of decisions made by others produces anxiety.

Resolved Needs: Comfort. Protection from psychologic threat. Adequacy. Self-reliance. Independence. Personal growth and maturity.

Contraindications: Confusion states.

Encourage decreased acid-ash-food intake

Suggest that the person decrease the intake of highly acid-ash food. Foods to avoid include meat, fish, poultry, eggs, cheese, plums, cranberries, prunes, all breads, cakes, cookies, cereals, crackers, macaroni, spaghetti, noodles, brazil nuts, peanuts, walnuts, corn, and lentils.

Rationale: A reduced acid-ash diet will cause a more alkaline urine, resulting in less uric acid and cystine stone formation.

Resolved Needs: Protection from physical harm.

Contraindications: Potential calcium or phosphate calculi.

Encourage decreased acid-food intake

Suggest that the person decrease the intake of highly acid foods. Foods to avoid include citrus fruits and juices, pickles, vinegar, sauerkraut.

Rationale: Decreased intake of highly acid foods reduces saliva stimulation, irritation of the intestinal tract, and promotes a neutral acid-base balance.

Resolved Needs: Acid-base balance. Comfort. Protection from physical harm. Freedom from pain.

Contraindications: Reduced saliva secretion. Alkalosis.

Encourage decreased calcium-food intake

Suggest that the person decrease the intake of high calcium food. Foods to avoid include milk and milk products; meat and poultry; dark green leafy vegetables such as mustard greens, turnip greens, and broccoli; sardines, clams, oysters; and yogurt.

Rationale: Decreased calcium intake reduces potential formation of calcium urinary stones, especially in existing kidney disease and illness-enforced immobility. It helps maintain normal acid-base balance.

Resolved Needs: Water-salt balance. Acid-base balance. Protection from physical harm.

Contraindications: Blood clotting abnormalities. Poor lactation. Impaired bone growth. When patients are receiving large volumes of citrated blood by transfusion.

Encourage decreased calorie intake

Suggest that the person reduce the intake of foods having high fuel and energy value. Foods to avoid include potatoes, bread, butter, cream, sugar, sweets, greasy foods, and alcoholic beverages. Low-calorie foods are recognized by their thin, watery dilutions, high fiber content, and crispness due to excess water.

Rationale: Lowered calorie intake decreases body weight by forcing the body to use stored energy resources. Since the calorie intake available for fuel and energy does not meet daily requirements, decreased body weight reduces the cardiac workload and improves tissue oxygenation.

Resolved Needs: Food balance. Protection from physical harm.

Contraindications: Increased metabolic rate. Excessive weight loss. When persons are underweight.

Encourage decreased carbohydrate intake

Suggest that the person decrease the intake of foods having high sugar and starch value. Foods to avoid include breads, cereals, sugar, candy, cakes with icing, pies, pastry, milk, ice cream, sauces, gravies, chocolate, syrups, honey, puddings, and cocktails. Food to eat include meat, poultry, fish, eggs, butter, margarine, limited vegetables and fruits.

Rationale: Lowered carbohydrate intake decreases body weight by forcing the body to use stored energy resources since the carbohydrates available for fuel and energy do not meet daily requirements. The decreased body weight reduces the cardiac workload and improves tissue oxygenation. Low carbohydrate intake is compatible with steroid (cortisone) therapy since steroids cause increased blood and urine sugar with diminished carbohydrate tolerance. The physician orders a low-carbohydrate diet for diabetics in whom insulin secretion is inadequate to metabolize normal carbohydrate intake.

Resolved Needs: Food balance. Protection from physical harm.

Contraindications: Increased metabolic rate. Renal failure. Excessive weight loss. When persons are underweight.

Encourage decreased cholesterol-food intake

Suggest that the person decrease the intake of foods more highly composed of unsaturated than saturated fats. Foods to avoid include egg yolks; butter; cream cheese; shellfish such as lobster, crab, and shrimp; organ meats such as liver, brains, heart, kidney, and sweet breads.

Rationale: Lowered cholesterol intake decreases fat deposits in arterial tissue, reducing the threat of arterial degeneration.

Resolved Needs: Protection from physical harm.

Encourage decreased fatty-food intake

Suggest that the person decrease the intake of foods high in triglyceride or lipid content. Foods to avoid include fatty meat; gravy; salad dressings; rich and heavy desserts; fried foods; highly flavored vegetables such as legumes and melons; packaged, canned, or frozen foods and dinners; and poultry skin. Foods to eat include meat, gravy from meat drippings that have been chilled and the fat removed, vegetable oils, whole or skim milk, eggs, cottage cheese, bread and vegetables, fruits and cereals.

Rationale: Fatty foods increase abnormal bile secretion in the liver and bile volume stored in the gallbladder. They stimulate pancreatic secretions.

Decreased fat intake reduces organ activity, allowing for tissue healing and reduced tissue trauma. The physician orders a low-fat diet in gallbladder and pancreatic disease.

Resolved Needs: Comfort. Protection from physical harm. Freedom from pain.

Contraindications: Gastric hyperacidity. Hypoglycemia.

Encourage decreased gas-forming-food intake   Suggest that the person decrease the intake of foods causing stomach or intestinal gas. Foods to avoid include kidney, lima, and navy beans, broccoli, brussels sprouts, cabbage, cauliflower, corn, cucumbers, kohlrabi, leeks, lentils, onions, black-eyed and split peas, green peppers, pimento, radishes, rutabagas, sauerkraut, scallions, shallots, turnips, soybeans, cantaloupe, honeydew melon, raw apples, avocados, and watermelon.

Rationale: Flatulence results from fermentation (oxidative decomposition by microorganisms) or putrefaction (decomposition by bacteria or fungi). The ingestion of foods causing decreased fermentation and putrefaction reduces flatulence. Flatulence causes pressure within the intestinal walls, resulting in severe, sharp pain and discomfort.

Resolved Needs: Comfort. Protection from physical harm. Freedom from pain.

Encourage decreased potassium-food intake   Suggest that the person decrease the intake of foods high in potassium. Foods to avoid include cereals, dried peas and beans, nuts, molasses, fresh fish and poultry, cocoa, fresh vegetables such as spinach, unstrained orange juice, prunes, tangerines, grapefruit and tomatoes, coffee, milk, cream, eggs, bananas, raisins, dried apricots.

Rationale: Normal blood potassium is essential to intracellular fluid balance, osmotic pressure regulation, acid-base balance, and the conduction of nerve impulses in muscle tissue. The physician orders a low-potassium diet in kidney failure because kidney failure inhibits the normal elimination of potassium.

Resolved Needs: Water-salt balance. Acid-base balance. Protection from physical harm.

Contraindications: Diarrhea. Vomiting. Diuresis. Impaired muscle function. Profuse colostomy, ileostomy, ileal conduit or T-tube drainage. When patients are on steroid therapy or receiving large volumes of I.V. dextrose or saline.

Encourage decreased protein-food intake   Suggest that the person decrease the intake of foods high in nitrogenous compounds. Foods to avoid include cheese, meat, fish, poultry, bread, cereals, legumes, nuts, and gelatin. Use protein-foods of high biologic value (milk and eggs or commercial formulas of essential amino acids) to provide the limited amount of protein allowed. Protein-free foods include pure carbohydrates (sugar, honey, jelly, hard candy) and pure fats (butter and margarine).

Rationale: The liver breaks down amino acids into keto acid and ammonia, and coverts the ammonia into urea which is excreted by the kidneys. In severe liver disease, ammonia is formed more rapidly than it can be converted to urea, and high ammonia blood levels result, contributing to hepatic coma. In kidney failure, urea is not eliminated as rapidly as it is formed, and high blood urea levels result, contributing to uremia. Decreasing the intake of protein, and limiting the protein to essential amino acids, results in a decreased amount of ammonia and/or urea accumulation, and provides the essential amino acids needed for maintenance and repair of tissue. In liver and renal failure, the physician orders specific amounts of dietary protein.

Resolved Needs: Protection from physical harm.

Contraindications: Edema not associated with liver or renal failure. During the growth years. When persons are burned.

Encourage decreased residue-food intake
Suggest that the person decrease the intake of foods containing considerable bulk and fat. Increase foods that are almost completely absorbed, leaving little or no intestinal waste. Foods to avoid include milk, cheese, vegetables, fruits, coarse breads and cereals, relishes, sweets, fried foods, tough meats, and condiments. Foods to eat include tender meat, fish, poultry, refined bread and cereals, fat-free clear soup, plain gelatin, coffee, tea, sugar, butter, and margarine.

Rationale: Reduced residual waste matter decreases intestinal irritation, lessens gastrointestinal spasms, prevents contamination of a ureterosigmoidostomy site, and promotes the comfort of reduced bowel elimination.

Resolved Needs: Comfort. Protection from physical harm.

Contraindications: Constipation.

Encourage decreased sodium-food intake
Suggest that the person decrease the intake of foods containing sodium. Low-sodium foods include up to 1 pint of milk a day, fresh or frozen meat or poultry, low-sodium canned tuna and salmon, asparagus, green, lima, or navy beans, broccoli, brussel sprouts, cabbage, cauliflower, chicory, corn, cucumbers, eggplant, lentils, mushrooms, lettuce, okra, onions, yellow and green peas, red and green peppers, sweet and white potatoes, pumpkin, radishes, yellow turnips, tomatoes, squash, turnip greens, fresh fruits, low-sodium bread, salt-free cakes and cookies, rice, hominy grits, oatmeal, noodles, spaghetti, flour, and unsalted butter and oils.

Rationale: A normal level of sodium salts is essential for electrolyte balance, regulation of osmotic pressure in cells and fluid, and acid-base balance. In severe cardiac damage, venous stasis and increased pressure prevent sodium and water from returning from interstitial tissues to the bloodstream to be excreted by the kidneys. When kidney excretion of sodium is reduced, restricted sodium intake decreases the blood sodium. Osmotic pressure then pulls sodium and water from the interstitial spaces into the bloodstream, relieving tissue edema. In cardiac and renal disorders, the physician orders specific amounts of dietary sodium.

Resolved Needs: Water-salt balance. Acid-base balance. Protection from physical harm.

Contraindications: Diarrhea. Vomiting. Excessive sweating. Diuresis. Second- or third-degree burns. Repetitive paracentesis. Fever. Profuse colostomy, ileostomy, ileal conduit, fistula or T-tube drainage. When patients are receiving large volumes of I.V. dextrose.

Encourage decreased yellow fruit and vegetable intake
Suggest that the patient lower the intake of yellow fruits and vegetables. Suggest a balanced intake of yellow, green, white, and other vegetables.

Rationale: Excessive ingestion of yellow fruits and vegetables discolors the skin.

Resolved Needs: Food balance. Protection from physical harm.

Encourage deep breathing
Have the patient slowly inhale air to maximum chest expansion and then slowly exhale. Have him deep breathe for a 10- to 15-minute period three to four times a day.

Rationale: Lung expansion increases arterial oxygen concentrations, facilitates gas exchange within the lungs, increases negative pressure in the thorax, promotes emptying of large veins, stimulates the cough reflex by placing pressure on mucous secretions, and promotes muscle relaxation. Forceful inhalation and exhalation when covering a chest wound helps to reexpand the collapsed lung.

Resolved Needs: Oxygen, circulation. Waste elimination. Relaxation. Protection from physical harm.

Contraindications: Pulmonary hemorrhage. Respiratory alkalosis.

Encourage differentiation between self-ideal and actual self
Help the person evaluate the difference between the self he sees as ideal and the actual functioning self. Help him incorporate into his frame of reference realism and harmony between the two.

Rationale: A poorly organized self-concept leads to disorganized behavior because behavior is consistent with the self-concept. Increased and accurate information about one's self leads to mature reality perception, awareness of potential, value clarification, and enhanced adequacy in solving problems and making decisions.

Resolved Needs: Sense of value. Adequacy. Personal growth and maturity. Awareness of potential. Improved values. Increased reality perception and problem-solving ability.

Encourage discussion of the patient's spiritual values
Initiate conversation about the patient's spiritual life and its value to him. Help him clarify his values and renew his spiritual goals.

Rationale: Spiritual goals assist in developing an understanding of the essential meaning of life.

Resolved Needs: Personal growth and maturity. Improved values. Religious, philosophic satisfaction.

Encourage early replacement of dwindling therapeutic supplies
Suggest that the patient procure additional supplies approximately 1 week before they are needed.

Rationale: Anticipating the need for and acquiring therapeutic supplies in advance supports uninterrupted therapeutic treatment.

Resolved Needs: Protection from physical harm.

Encourage enhanced involvement in already established relationships
Contribute to involving one person in the feelings of another. Direct activities that will increase feeling intensity between persons with established relationships.

Rationale: Sensitivity responses are more frequent in established friendships and group situations than in newly developed relationships. Awareness of feelings in another arouses a corresponding emotional effect and promotes a more realistic perception of another's emotional world.

Resolved Needs: Warm, communicating relationships. Personal growth and maturity.

Encourage exploration of the dark when fearful of the dark
Suggest that fear of the dark can be prevented or reduced by accompanying the person into the darkened area and allowing him to search for his fear with a flashlight.

Rationale: Since fear stems from a sense of helplessness in the face of danger, a sense of adequacy in confronting the danger reduces fear. Adequacy evolves from an awareness of one's ability to cope with life. Sound health approaches to behavioral problems bring about safety, comfort, growth, and maturity.

Resolved Needs: Comfort. Protection from psychologic threat. Adequacy. Personal growth and maturity. Increased reality perception.

Encourage families to seek the opinions of elders
Suggest to family members that they sincerely seek the opinions of the older, more experienced family members.

Rationale: Awareness that one's opinion is valuable increases self-esteem. The availability of experienced knowledge provides the recipient of the knowledge with increased assurance of success.

Resolved Needs: Comfort. Sense of value, usefulness. High evaluation of self. Importance and influence. Increased learning.

Encourage family-shared pleasures
Discover those activities en-

joyable to all family members and suggest mutual participation in the events.

Rationale: Sharing pleasurable events promotes positive interpersonal relationships between the persons involved.

Resolved Needs: Comfort. Unity with loved ones. Increased pleasantness.

Encourage family-shared responsibility
Suggest that all family members be included in the patient's direct or indirect care and that relatives divide the responsibility so no one family member is burdened.

Rationale: Mutually shared responsibility promotes feelings of safety, adequacy, and comfort. Involvement in meeting the needs of others promotes self-esteem.

Resolved Needs: Comfort. Protection from psychologic threat. Unity with loved ones. Sense of value, usefulness. Adequacy. Endurance. Personal growth and maturity. Increased reality perception and problem-solving ability.

Encourage family support of the patient's acceptance of death
Offer the family of a dying patient, who has reached the acceptance stage, an understanding of the feelings of the patient. Show them how they can comfort their loved one by sharing in his acceptance of the approaching death.

Rationale: When a dying person reaches the acceptance stage but perceives that loved ones cannot accept the inevitable, he experiences intense inner conflict until his family also reaches the point of acceptance.

Resolved Needs: Comfort. Protection from psychologic threat. Acceptance. Unity with loved ones. Personal growth and maturity.

Encourage goals leading to self-enhancement
Arouse positive behavior in which the person will pursue goals leading to deep, inner feelings of importance and personal status.

Rationale: Genuine status results from accomplishments that bring deep inner satisfaction rather than from successes achieved to please others.

Resolved Needs: High evaluation of self. Goal achievement. Importance and influence. Status. Increased pleasantness.

Encourage gradual mastery of a situation
Assist the person to gradually move into an emotionally disturbing situation. Encourage him to overcome the problem slowly, gaining increased confidence with each success. For instance, if he is afraid of heights, have him go one story higher in a building each day.

Rationale: Unpleasant situations can be less threatening when experienced in small doses. Feelings of adequacy arise from an awareness of one's ability to cope with life. Gradual success supports gradual recognition of one's strengths.

Resolved Needs: Comfort. Protection from psychologic threat. Adequacy. Endurance.

Encourage habitual peaceful thinking   Suggest that anxiety can be reduced by habitually imagining serene experiences.

Rationale: Confusion and excitable thoughts support anxiety. Mental orderliness results in physiologic and psychologic tension reduction and in a more realistic approach to problem solving.

Resolved Needs: Comfort. Protection from psychologic threat. Personal growth and maturity. Increased reality perception and problem-solving ability.

Encourage honesty in presenting oneself to others   Suggest that when a person presents himself to others as he really is, he has greater assurance of being loved for what he is.

Rationale: Honesty relieves the anxiety of anticipated detection of dishonesty. Self-esteem is maintained as long as a person sees himself as living up to cultural expectations. Sound health approaches to behavioral problems promote safety, comfort, growth, and maturity.

Resolved Needs: Comfort. Protection from psychologic threat. Acceptance. High evaluation of self. Personal growth and maturity. Increased reality perception.

Encourage identification of specific life values   Help the person to define for himself specific values for successful living and to avoid situations in which intense value conflict exists.

Rationale: The threat of anxiety results when there is a value conflict, when one does not trust his own valuing process, or when there is a breakdown of cultural values. Feelings of adequacy and comfort evolve from an awareness that one can cope successfully with life within a framework of well-defined values.

Resolved Needs: Comfort. Protection from psychologic threat. Adequacy. Improved values.

Encourage identification of success standards   Assist the person in clearly identifying those qualities that he sees as associated with success.

Rationale: A positive self can be enhanced by identifying and behaving in accordance with qualities compatible to a person's perception of success.

Resolved Needs: High evaluation of self.

Encourage identification of values acquired from one's own culture   Help the person identify, in detail, those values imposed by his own culture. Promote an awareness of why those values exist and, if possible, their origin.

Rationale: Culture is a principal element in human development. Each society teaches concepts, values, and desired behavior in an effort to meet needs and perpetuate the society. The realization of how cultural values affect one's self leads to greater self-insight, acceptance, and problem solving. It provides the basis for improved values when current cultural values are unacceptable.

Resolved Needs: Comfort. Acceptance. Personal growth and maturity. Improved values. Increased reality perception and problem-solving ability.

Encourage identification of values in common with the values of others

Help the person to exchange verbally and to define those standards that he has in common with others.

Rationale: Psychologic comfort is promoted through a sense of commonality between persons. An accepted value system significantly influences behavioral responses.

Resolved Needs: Comfort. Protection from psychologic threat. Acceptance. Approval from others. Increased reality perception and problem-solving ability.

Encourage increased acid-ash-food intake

Suggest that the person raise the intake of foods that promote an acid state. Foods to increase include meat, fish, poultry, eggs, cheese, plums, cranberries, prunes, all breads, cakes, cookies, cereals, crackers, macaroni, spaghetti, noodles, brazil nuts, peanuts, walnuts, corn, and lentils.

Rationale: An increased acid-ash diet will cause a more acid urine, resulting in a diminished potential for infection and calcium and phosphate stone formation.

Resolved Needs: Protection from physical harm.

Contraindications: Potential uric acid or cystine stones.

Encourage increased acid-food intake

Suggest that the person increase the intake of highly acid foods. Foods to increase include citrus fruits and juices, pickles, vinegar, sauerkraut.

Rationale: Increased intake of acid foods will stimulate salivation.

Resolved Needs: Acid-base balance. Protection from physical harm.

Contraindications: Excessive salivary flow. Gastric hyperacidity.

Encourage increased calcium-food intake

Suggest that the person raise the intake of high-calcium foods such as milk; milk products; meat and poultry; dark green leafy vegetables like mustard greens, turnip greens, and broccoli; sardines, clams, oysters; and yogurt.

Rationale: A high-calcium diet provides calcium for normal bone growth and function, assists in blood clotting, promotes lactation, enhances nerve and muscle functioning, and activates enzymes.

Resolved Needs: Water-salt balance. Protection from physical harm.

Contraindications: Potential calcium urinary calculi. Illness-enforced immobility. Potential cardiac arrythmia. When the patient has a high alkali intake.

Encourage increased calorie intake   Suggest that the person raise the intake of foods having high fuel and energy value. Include all regular foods plus additional amounts of cereals, potatoes, bread, butter, cream, sugars, and sweets.

Rationale: Increased metabolic rate and illness causing weight loss require added energy and fuel resources to promote oxidation and provide nutrition to body tissue.

Resolved Needs: Food balance. Energy. Protection from physical harm.

Contraindications: Obesity. Severe cardiac damage with impaired circulation. Diabetes mellitus.

Encourage increased carbohydrate intake   Suggest that the person raise the intake of foods having high sugar and starch value. Include syrups and jellies; fine cereals and breads; starch puddings; high carbohydrate vegetables like potatoes, beets, carrots, peas, beans, lentils, turnips, and parsnips; high carbohydrate fruits such as bananas, raisins, prunes, dried dates, and figs; ice cream, fruit pies, and cakes.

Rationale: Increased metabolic rate and illness causing weight loss require high carbohydrate intake that will yield sufficient calories to produce adequate energy and fuel resources to promote oxidation and provide nutrition to body tissue. In renal failure, the physician orders a high carbohydrate diet to reduce the conversion of tissue protein into urea, since the failing kidneys cannot excrete the urea.

Resolved Needs: Food balance. Energy. Protection from physical harm.

Contraindications: Obesity. Severe cardiac damage with impaired circulation. Diabetic states. When the patient is receiving steroid therapy.

Encourage increased fatty-food intake   Suggest that the person increase the intake of foods with triglyceride or lipid content. Include cream, butter, bacon, salad oils and dressings, meat, eggs, and cheese.

Rationale: Fats combine with oxygen and release energy for tissue cell oxidation and nutrition. Fatty foods are digested slowly and remain in the stomach longer than other foods. The prolonged digestion reduces and neutralizes acidity, decreases pain, and defers hunger. The physician orders a high-fat diet in hypoglycemia because fatty foods depress Isle of Langerhans activity, causing reduced insulin production.

Resolved Needs: Food balance. Comfort.

Contraindications: Cholecystitis. Cholelithiasis. Cholangitis. Pancreatitis.

Encourage increased high-vitamin-food intake   Suggest that the person increase the intake of foods having high vitamin content.

Vitamin A: milk, cod liver oil, egg yolks, leafy green and yellow vegetables, limes, oranges, liver, pineapple, cantaloupe, and prunes.

Vitamin B: egg yolks, fruits and vegetables, whole grain breads and cereals, nuts, legumes, and yeast, poultry and meat, rice, and bran.

Vitamin C: oranges, strawberries, pears, apricots, plums, peaches, pineapple, tomatoes, raw cabbage, carrots, lettuce, celery, onions, green peppers, radishes, and rutabagas.

Vitamin D: egg yolk, butter, fat, cod liver oil, and milk.

Vitamin K: oats, wheat, rye, alfalfa, and fats.

Rationale: Vitamins increase the conversion of food into energy although they are not an energy source in themselves. Vitamins prevent deficiency diseases that occur from poor nutritional intake.

Resolved Needs: Food balance. Energy. Protection from physical harm.

Contraindications: Avoid an excessively high intake of any high-vitamin food.

Encourage increased iron-food intake   Suggest that the person increase the intake of foods having a high iron content. Include sardines, lobster, clams, liver, oysters, shellfish, kidney, heart, lean meat, tongue, leafy vegetables, egg yolks, dried peas and beans, dried fruits, dark molasses, enriched breads and cereals.

Rationale: The liver must store sufficient iron for the manufacture of hemoglobin in new red blood cells. Hemoglobin is necessary to form oxyhemoglobin, which provides tissue oxidation and nutrition.

Resolved Needs: Food balance. Energy. Protection from physical harm.

Encourage increased potassium-food intake   Suggest that potassium be replaced following episodes of diarrhea, vomiting, or diuresis by eating foods high in potassium, such as tea, coffee, chocolate or cocoa drinks; meat, poultry, or fish; fresh or dried nuts; spinach; whole-grain cereals; milk solids such as ice cream; dried peas and beans; fresh fruits, especially grapefruit, tangerines, oranges, bananas, prunes, and tomatoes.

Rationale: In diarrhea, potassium is lost in the feces. In vomiting, potassium is lost in the gastric juices. In diuresis, fluid reabsorption from the renal tubules is prevented with a resulting loss of potassium in the urine. A normal potassium level is essential to salt balance, acid-base balance, normal osmotic pressure, and nerve impulse conduction, especially to muscle and cardiac tissue.

Resolved Needs: Water-salt balance. Acid-base balance. Protection from physical harm.

Contraindications: Hyperkalemia. Renal failure with oliguria or anuria. During the shock stage of severe second- or third-degree burns or crushing injuries. Adrenal insufficiency. Ventricular fibrillation. When the patient is receiving I.V. infusions containing potassium.

Encourage increased protein-food intake

Suggest that the person increase the intake of foods high in protein content. Include milk, cheese, eggs, lean meats, fish, poultry, wheat bread and cereals, wheat germ, yeast, legumes, nuts, gelatin, chicken breasts, tuna fish, leg of lamb, beef, and loin pork.

Rationale: Proteins are essential for tissue growth and repair. Proteins increase immunity, resistance to infection, and body heat production. They provide cell oxidation and nutrition, and decrease negative nitrogen balance caused by steroid therapy. Normally, the protein level is higher in the blood than it is in interstitial fluid. When the blood protein level is low, the return of fluid from the interstitial tissues to the blood is decreased, contributing to edema and ascites. If the protein intake increases, the elevated blood protein level reestablishes the normal return of the fluid from the interstitial tissues to the blood supporting fluid balance. In cirrhosis, hypertension exists within the portal vein, forcing fluid and albumin from the blood into the tissues with resulting ascites. With increased protein intake, a balanced colloid osmotic pressure is established between the blood and the tissues allowing the blood to retain fluid at its normal level and decrease fluid (ascites) in the tissues. Increased protein intake is especially important in prolonged starvation, burns, and proteinuria. The physician orders a high-protein diet when there is liver damage without liver failure, after the shock stage of burns, and for hypoproteinuria when there is no kidney failure.

Resolved Needs: Water-salt balance. Food balance. Normal temperature. Energy. Protection from physical harm.

Contraindications: Impending hepatic coma. Renal insufficiency or failure.

Encourage increased residue-food intake

Suggest that the person raise the intake of foods containing considerable bulk. Include long-fibered vegetables such as greens, cabbage, and celery, raw vegetables and fruits, cooked fruits, and whole-grain bread and cereals.

Rationale: An increased quantity of residue waste matter after food is digested and absorbed improves intestinal muscle tone, promoting comfortable intestinal elimination.

Resolved Needs: Waste elimination. Comfort. Protection from physical harm.

Contraindications: Intestinal irritation. Gastrointestinal spasm. Ureterosigmoidostomy. Rectal bleeding, irritation, or inflammation.

Encourage increased sodium-food intake

Suggest that sodium be replaced after episodes of diarrhea, vomiting, diuresis, profuse drainage or excessive sweating from high environmental temperatures, fever, or heavy exercising. Sodium can be replaced by eating ham, bacon, salted nuts, salted or frozen fish, potato chips, salted crackers, pretzels, peanut butter, ketchup, mustard, bread, butter, milk, frozen peas, lima beans, cake, cookies, artichokes, sauerkraut, beets, carrots, celery, hominy, mustard greens, spinach, white turnips, cheese, or table salt.

Rationale: Sodium is the principal electrolyte of the plasma and other body fluids and is essential to fluid balance, electrolyte balance, normal osmotic pressure, and acid-base balance. Normal sodium loss occurs in the urine, but abnormal amounts are lost when there is profuse perspiration and when reabsorption of intestinal secretions is hindered, as in vomiting, diarrhea, or drainage from a tube, sinus, or wound. Profuse losses of sodium and water result in circulatory failure unless replacement is maintained. Replacement of water and sodium losses with low sodium fluids (water, Coca Cola, 7-Up, apple juice, orange juice, etc.) may result in water intoxication.

Resolved Needs: Water-salt balance. Acid-base balance. Protection from physical harm.

Contraindications: Impaired renal function. Edema. Ascites. Cardiac damage with impaired circulation. Dehydration. When the patient is on steroid therapy, is receiving large volumes of I.V. saline, or is on a low sodium diet.

Encourage indifference toward sleep   Suggest that the person assume an "I don't care" attitude about whether or not he falls asleep.

Rationale: When one does not consciously try to go to sleep, the body relaxes and sleep occurs. Adequate sleep is essential in that the decreased metabolic rate occurring during sleep restores the depleted cell energy reserves.

Resolved Needs: Sleep, rest, relaxation. Energy. Comfort. Protection from physical harm.

Encourage intake of diuretic fluids   Suggest that drinks having a diuretic effect be taken rather than regular fluids. These include coffee, tea, beer, apple cider, lemonade.

Rationale: Fluids having a diuretic effect are less likely to contribute to fluid retention than are regular fluids.

Resolved Needs: Water-salt balance. Comfort. Protection from physical harm.

Contraindications: When patients are on prescription diuretics. Hypokalemia. If there are prescribed dietary limitations that exclude the use of any of the diuretic fluids.

Encourage involvement in community affairs   Suggest that a retired person become involved in at least one group activity and preferably something that has meaning in the community.

Rationale: Group activities after retirement are a substitute for the socialization that normally occurs in business. Sound health practices promote comfort.

Resolved Needs: Comfort. Warm, communicating relationships. Group companionship.

Encourage involvement in helping others
Suggest that by helping to lighten the burdens of others, we also lighten our own burdens. Becoming involved in the problems of others reduces our troubles to their proper perspective.

Rationale: Involvement in meeting the needs of another promotes a sense of self-esteem, maturity, and increased reality perception.

Resolved Needs: Protection from psychologic threat. Sense of value, usefulness. Personal growth and maturity. Increased reality perception.

Encourage involvement in totally new interests
Help the person to participate in interesting and stimulating activities in which he has had no previous involvement. Promote interests from which satisfaction and pleasure can be experienced.

Rationale: Involvement in totally new interests fosters growth and development of potential. Novel interests prevent boredom.

Resolved Needs: Comfort. Stimulation. Personal growth and maturity. Awareness of potential. Full development of potential. Less of the familiar, more of the novel.

Encourage laughter
Help the person view the problem with a sense of humor.

Rationale: Laughter brings problems into realistic perspective and assists in reducing tension.

Resolved Needs: Comfort. Protection from psychologic threat. Increased reality perception.

Encourage light reading before sleep
Suggest that the person read unemotional and preferably boring material while in bed, just before sleep.

Rationale: Lack of stimulation from boredom promotes sleep. Adequate sleep is essential in that the decreased metabolic rate occurring during sleep restores depleted cell energy reserves.

Resolved Needs: Sleep, rest, relaxation. Energy. Comfort. Protection from physical harm.

Encourage maintenance of an established favorable reputation
Arouse positive behavior by verbalizing those qualities of character highly regarded in the person and expected to be maintained in the future.

Rationale: The need for esteem from others promotes acceptance of and conformity to the expectations of others.

Resolved Needs: Sense of value. High evaluation of self. Goal achievement. Reputation of good character.

Encourage meaningful activity   Involve the person in some activity that he sees as having value and importance.

Rationale: The perception of an activity as being important supports motivation toward accomplishing the activity, which in turn supports a positive self-image since the achievement has a positive value.

Resolved Needs: Comfort. Sense of value, usefulness. High evaluation of self.

Encourage moderate activity   Suggest that the person set for himself a schedule of reasonable, nonstrenuous activity.

Rationale: Moderate activity supports normal functioning of body systems and reduces internal tension. During impaired health, it is preferable to excessive activity, in that it provides a reduction in the amount of energy expended for adaptation, making available more energy for healing.

Resolved Needs: Activity. Energy. Comfort. Protection from physical harm. Protection from psychologic threat.

Encourage moderate physical exercise   Promote muscular and joint activity through the performance of daily chores.

Rationale: Muscular exertion through exercise enhances free joint mobility, strengthens muscle tone, develops coordination, prevents nonfunctional contractures, and promotes increased blood circulation. Exercise uses up excessive body calories. Exercise improves pelvic circulation and stretches pelvic ligaments, reducing menstrual pain.

Resolved Needs: Circulation. Activity, exercise. Protection from physical harm.

Contraindications: Fever. States of severe energy depletion. Any nonhealth condition in which the performance of daily chores is incompatible with health maintenance.

Encourage modes of travel other than flying   Recommend to persons for whom air travel is unsuitable that they travel by bus, car, train, or boat.

Rationale: Human safety and comfort are promoted when there is exposure to lesser atmospheric pressure changes in a bus, car, train, or boat, as compared to greater pressure changes in an airplane.

Resolved Needs: Comfort. Protection from physical harm.

Encourage mutual problem solving   Interact with and help the

person to identify problems and discover methods for solving them. Assist the patient in dealing objectively with the difficulty.

Rationale: Knowledge of one's self and situation, plus the pursuit of realistic goals, promotes growth, maturity, increased adequacy, and reduced anxiety. Comfort arises from a sense of effective communication with others.

Resolved Needs: Comfort. Protection from physical harm. Protection from psychologic threat. Warm, communicating relationships. Adequacy. Goal achievement. Mastery and competence in skills. Personal growth and maturity. Increased learning. Increased reality perception and problem-solving ability.

Encourage new goals at past goal achievement As the person achieves one goal successfully, immediately present a new goal to be accomplished.

Rationale: A positive self-image is supported when new and important goals are anticipated in the near future.

Resolved Needs: Comfort. Protection from psychologic threat. Sense of value, usefulness. High evaluation of self.

Encourage new skill development Suggest new skills that the person might enjoy performing. Assist, if possible, with the learning of these previously unknown abilities.

Rationale: The ability to maintain self-direction through one's own competencies supports feelings of adequacy and self-esteem. The ability to maintain independence is essential to growth and maturity.

Resolved Needs: High evaluation of self. Adequacy. Self-reliance. Mastery and competence in skills. Independence. Personal growth and maturity. Full development of potential.

Encourage noncompetitive activities Involve the person in activities and relationships in which there is minimum or no competition.

Rationale: Competition is a stimulus for aggressive behavior and can result in regrettable conduct when there is difficulty maintaining emotional control. Suspicious people strive to prove their superiority through competition but are highly threatened on losing, which often results in heightened distrust.

Resolved Needs: Comfort. Protection from psychologic threat. Warm, communicating relationships.

Encourage normal use of the involved limb Have the patient use the remaining strength in a limb as frequently as possible in everyday activities even if at first the use is limited.

Rationale: The exertion of muscular activity through exercise promotes circulation and free joint mobility, strengthens muscle tone, develops coordination, and prevents nonfunctional contractures.

Resolved Needs: Circulation. Exercise. Comfort. Protection from physical harm.

Encourage participation in activities of the young   Suggest involvement in the gaiety of childhood experiences, such as attending birthday parties of favorite children, taking children to the circus or sporting events, and chaperoning teenage dances.

Rationale: Identifying with the positive attitudes of others (especially the young) promotes positive self-attitudes, comfort, and helps to bring one's problems into perspective.

Resolved Needs: Comfort. Protection from psychologic threat. Personal growth and maturity. Increased reality perception.

Encourage participation in safe, thrilling experiences   When a person seeks the stimulation of thrill, suggest participation in safe but thrilling experiences, such as inventive and research activities, travel to distant and exciting places, seeing horror movies, attending amusement parks.

Rationale: Novel experiences provide stimulation and thrill. Confining thrilling experiences to safe experiences reduces the potential for injury.

Resolved Needs: Stimulation. Protection from physical harm. Less of the familiar, more of the novel. Less of the simple, more of the complex.

Encourage participation in therapeutic group interaction   Suggest that the person become involved in interaction between a number of group members for a period of several weeks or months.

Rationale: Group interaction protects against threatening individual involvement and promotes interpersonal satisfaction when the relationships prove to be nonthreatening. Behavioral insight gained through group interaction promotes emotional growth.

Resolved Needs: Comfort. Protection from psychologic threat. Warm, communicating relationships. Personal growth and maturity.

Encourage part-time employment   Suggest that part-time employment is possible and profitable. Some part-time endeavors include typing, babysitting, running a mail-order business, and creating artistic works or crafts.

Rationale: Part-time employment provides socialization and a sense of meaningfulness, maintains status, and offers financial security.

Resolved Needs: Comfort. Protection from psychologic threat. Sense of value, usefulness. High evaluation of self.

Encourage passive diversional activities   Suggest that the person participate in nonphysical activities in which there is sensory intake but little or no productivity. These include watching television or movies; listening to records, tapes, and radio; reading newspapers, magazines, or books; bird-watching; star-gazing; riding in a car or wheelchair.

Rationale: Focusing attention on external stimuli temporarily relieves the tension of internal stress. It promotes temporary escape from conscious perception of threats of fear, anxiety, and pain and decreases energy consumption.

Resolved Needs: Comfort. Protection from physical harm. Protection from psychologic threat. Freedom from pain.

Encourage patience in illness adjustment   Reassure both the patient and his family that adjustment to illness can be very slow and painstaking, and that these adaptations require endurance on the part of all concerned and are vital to regaining health.

Rationale: In severe physiologic or psychologic disequillibrium, the healing process requires considerable time. Knowing what to expect supports endurance, promotes comfort, and increases reality perception.

Resolved Needs: Comfort. Protection from physical harm. Protection from psychologic threat. Endurance. Increased reality perception.

Encourage patient (parent or family) questions   Offer the patient every opportunity to ask questions and emphasize the importance of his inquiring to better understand the health problem.

Rationale: Adequate health knowledge increases a person's ability to protect his health and prevent harm to himself.

Resolved Needs: Comfort. Protection from physical harm. Protection from psychologic threat. Increased learning. Increased reality perception and problem-solving ability.

Encourage patient to make a verbal no-suicide contract   Encourage the patient to make a verbal commitment in which he states that he will not take his life accidentally or intentionally without calling the nurse first. Set a time limit of 1 day, 1 week, 1 month, or whatever is suitable to the patient. When the time limit expires, have the patient renew the contract for another length of time. Give the patient your phone number and be available to him 24 hours a day. When the therapeutic relationship is terminated, encourage the patient to give you a long-term commitment.

Rationale: Encouraging the patient to make a no-suicide contract makes him feel that he is important to someone, and therefore, he feels important to himself.

Resolved Needs: Protection from physical harm. Protection from psychologic threat. Warm, communicating relationships. Sense of value, usefulness. Dignity. Appreciation from others.

Encourage planned, one-day-at-a-time living   In the morning, help the person to look no further ahead than today. In the evening, if the patient desires, help him to look no further than tomorrow.

Rationale: Stress is reduced by limiting the demands on oneself to a single day's responsibilities. This reduction in stress enhances clear perception and allows concentrated use of powers to meet demands adequately. When the threat of death appears relatively imminent, concentration on the immediate future promotes realistic goals and gives a feeling of the extension of a meaningful life. Planning for the next day promotes the safety of a predictable future.

Resolved Needs: Comfort. Protection from psychologic threat. Predictable, orderly world. Adequacy. Endurance.

Encourage pride in appearance
Direct the person toward good grooming and appropriate dress so his appearance will be satisfying to himself and to others.

Rationale: Self-esteem requires that a person experience positive feelings about one's self and positive response from others.

Resolved Needs: Comfort. Approval from others. High evaluation of self.

Encourage quiet diversional activities
Offer activities that can be performed noiselessly and in a relatively noise-free environment.

Rationale: Quiet makes the body's adaptation to stress easier.

Resolved Needs: Comfort. Protection from physical harm.

Encourage reaching activities
Place objects just far enough away so that the person will have to reach for them.

Rationale: Muscular exertion through exercise promotes circulation and free joint mobility, strengthens muscle tone, and develops coordination.

Resolved Needs: Circulation. Activity, exercise. Protection from physical harm.

Contraindications: Severe cardiac damage.

Encourage realistic perception of others
Help the person to perceive in others a balance of good and bad qualities and to avoid extremes in acceptance or rejection of others.

Rationale: Positive human relationships are acquired through the perception of interpersonal relationships as safe and beneficial. Viewing others realistically promotes honest evaluation of one's relationships with others, clarity of perception, growth, and maturity.

Resolved Needs: Protection from psychologic threat. Warm, communicating relationships. High evaluation of self. Personal growth and maturity. Increased reality perception and problem-solving ability.

Encourage recognition of one's various roles in life
Help the person to identify clearly how he sees himself in the role most important to him.

Rationale: A positive self-image is fostered by behavior compatible with a person's perception of his significant roles.

Resolved Needs: Comfort. Sense of value, usefulness. High evaluation of self.

Encourage relationships between persons with common interests and goals   Foster a pleasant relationship between persons who have similar interests and goals.

Rationale: Psychologic comfort is promoted through a sense of effective communication with others. When group goals are clearly perceived, group unity tends to increase because of participation in reaching those goals.

Resolved Needs: Comfort. Warm, communicating relationships. Group companionship.

Encourage renewal of former interests   Help the person reestablish past behaviors and activities from which pleasure and satisfaction were gained.

Rationale: Pleasurable pursuit of goals promotes growth in self-actualization. Interest in external stimuli temporarily relieves the tension of internal stress and enhances involvement with reality. Renewed interest in former successful endeavors promotes self-esteem.

Resolved Needs: Comfort. High evaluation of self. Personal growth and maturity. Full development of potential. Increased reality perception. Increased pleasantness.

Encourage respect for the rights of others   Help the person to fulfill his own needs. At the same time, help him recognize that his needs can be met only as long as they do not infringe on the rights of others.

Rationale: Properly managed aggression contributes to strength of character by control of self-assertion, which in turn reduces the threat of social disapproval. Self-esteem is maintained when a person perceives himself as living up to cultural expectations and receiving the approval of others. Maturity and growth involve reality perception and behavioral changes which appropriately meet situational demands and individual needs.

Resolved Needs: Protection from psychologic threat. Approval from others. High evaluation of self. Personal growth and maturity. Increased reality perception and problem-solving ability.

Encourage rest periods while eating   While the person is eating, have him stop and rest periodically for 3 or 4 minutes before he starts to eat again.

Rationale: Fatigue is decreased by reducing stress stimuli or by restoring energy through rest. The accomplishment of activity without fatigue promotes comfort.

Resolved Needs: Energy. Comfort. Protection from physical harm.

Encourage role-playing to develop sensitivity   Suggest that the person act out the situation of another as if he were that person.

Rationale: The ability to assume the role of another person promotes sensitivity feelings for the behavior of others.

Resolved Needs: Personal growth and maturity. Increased reality perception.

Encourage self-explanation of the causes of pain (248)   When someone with a terminal illness asks the cause of pain, do not name the specific disease. Instead, ask the patient what he thinks is the cause. If he says he doesn't know, direct the conversation so that eventually he will answer his own question. Even if the answer is not the total truth, the degree of truth which the patient states is usually the level at which he can presently tolerate the reality.

Rationale: Self-definition of the cause of pain offers an opportunity for greater reality perception but still provides the safety of denial, if a person is highly threatened.

Resolved Needs: Protection from psychologic threat. Increased reality perception.

Encourage self-performance   Suggest that the patient do as much as possible for himself, and that he rely on his own capabilities.

Rationale: The ability to maintain self-direction and be free from control of others requires clear self-identity, knowledge, and competencies. The ability to overcome the ambivalence of dependency-independency needs is essential to growth and maturity. Independence is built on successful past experience.

Resolved Needs: High evaluation of self. Adequacy. Self-reliance. Mastery and competence in skills. Independence. Dignity. Personal growth and maturity. Full development of potential.

Encourage simple signal language during impaired communication   When attempting to communicate with a person who cannot relay messages verbally, encourage the use of simple signals for yes and no, such as blinking the eyes or moving the fingertip up and down. Avoid using complex symbols or signals that the patient may find difficult to understand.

Rationale: Simple signal language supports improved communication when there is communication impairment.

Resolved Needs: Comfort. Warm, communicating relationships.

Encourage single goal seeking   Suggest that only one objective be attempted at a time. After one goal has been accomplished, then another can be sought.

Rationale: Multiple goal seeking requires intense diversion of thought, which often results in mental confusion and nonachievement of any goal. Successfully overcoming barriers to a goal enhances the ability to cope and results in increased adequacy feelings.

Resolved Needs: Comfort. Protection from psychologic threat. Adequacy. Goal achievement.

Encourage social activities

Promote activities in which there is contact with other people and in which the patient can relate to others. Such activities include sewing together, dancing, playing music and games, choral groups, talent shows, and discussion groups.

Rationale: Comfort and safety feelings evolve from an awareness that one is not threatened with aloneness.

Resolved Needs: Comfort. Protection from psychologic threat. Warm, communicating relationships. Group companionship.

Encourage spiritually uplifting conversation

Encourage the patient to discuss spiritual thoughts that he has experienced as bringing about feelings of joy and peace.

Rationale: Conversation about the love of God and the beauty of His creations can have an uplifting effect and fosters closer God-human relationships.

Resolved Needs: Comfort. Improved values. Religious, philosophic satisfaction.

Encourage strivings toward realistic goals

Assist the person in choosing and striving toward realistic objectives. Initially support attempts at small goal achievements that most likely will be accomplished with success. Gradually support more difficult goals as the minor aims are overcome.

Rationale: Safety feelings and adequacy evolve from an awareness that one can cope successfully with life. Self-esteem is enhanced by the development of new competencies and the achievement of important goals. Honest evaluation of one's self and one's situation, plus the pursuit of realistic goals, promotes growth and maturity.

Resolved Needs: Comfort. Protection from psychologic threat. High evaluation of self. Adequacy. Self-reliance. Goal achievement. Personal growth and maturity. Increased reality perception and problem-solving ability.

Encourage telephone calls between significant persons

Suggest that the patient and his distant family speak to each other by telephone as frequently as possible.

Rationale: Comfort is promoted through a sense of effective communication with others. Unity with loved ones reduces stress and strengthens the capacity to cope with it.

Resolved Needs: Comfort. Protection from physical harm. Warm, communicating relationships. Unity with loved ones.

Encourage the bringing in of outside food   Suggest to families and friends that they bring the patient food prepared outside the hospital.

Rationale: Balanced nutritional intake and comfort are enhanced by the availability of familiar and desired foods.

Resolved Needs: Food balance. Comfort.

Contraindications: Special diet restrictions.

Encourage the chaplain's visit   Call the chaplain or a clergyman to bring spiritual aid to the ill person.

Rationale: Clergy provide spiritual guidance designed to bring spiritual peace and understanding.

Resolved Needs: Comfort. Religious, philosophic satisfaction.

Encourage the desire for satisfactory achievement   Suggest that specific goals be sought for the purpose of realizing a sense of satisfaction and reward that accompanies achievement.

Rationale: Anticipation of satisfying achievement leads to activity.

Resolved Needs: Goal achievement. Increased pleasantness.

Encourage the enjoyment of life's simple things   Suggest that in the search for pleasure, life can be enriched by simple joys such as a cool breeze, the blue sky, or a refreshing rain.

Rationale: Habitually enjoying the simple things in life brings more joy because these things are more available than complex pleasures. Sound health practices promote growth, maturity, and increased reality perception.

Resolved Needs: Comfort. Personal growth and maturity. Increased reality perception. Increased pleasantness.

Encourage the expression of feelings   Foster communication with the nurse or between significant persons in which emotional feelings are revealed. Communicate to the person that the verbal expression of feelings, ideas, hopes, and doubts will be received favorably, and that there need be no fear of humiliation, embarrassment, or punishment.

Rationale: Feeling ventilation supports honesty and objectivity of the situation in which the people are involved. Awareness of another's feelings arouses a corresponding emotional effect and promotes a more realistic perception of another's emotional world. When differences can be accepted, people feel free to look at themselves fearlessly and no longer feel restricted in growth.

Resolved Needs: Comfort. Protection from psychologic threat. Warm, communicating relationships. Acceptance. High evaluation of self. Personal growth and maturity. Increased reality perception and problem-solving ability.

Encourage the person to face fear (anxiety or grief)   Suggest that the person face the unknown that is causing his fear or anxiety, and to face painful emotions such as grief.

Rationale: Fear is reduced when the safe reality of a situation is confronted. Facing fear promotes comfort, growth, and maturity. Painful emotions tend to diminish when realistically dealt with.

Resolved Needs: Comfort. Protection from psychologic threat. Personal growth and maturity. Increased reality perception and problem-solving ability.

Encourage the practical application of the accepted value system   Help the person who has objectively assessed his situation to fit the situation into his value system. Help him to state in detail how his values can be applied to successful living.

Rationale: Maturity and growth involve the ability to perceive and cope with the demands and limitations of the real world and to organize perceptions into a meaningful whole.

Resolved Needs: Personal growth and maturity. Improved values. Increased reality perception and problem-solving ability.

Encourage the reduction of generalizations to specifics   Help the person to explain his views in detail whenever there is a tendency to speak in indefinite terms or to make general assumptions.

Rationale: Detailed verbalization clarifies mental imagery and enhances growth toward total perception of the situation.

Resolved Needs: Protection from psychologic threat. Personal growth and maturity. Increased reality perception and problem-solving ability.

Encourage the sharing of common problems with others   Suggest that persons having similar difficulties verbally share their problems and methods for solving the problems.

Rationale: Psychologic comfort is promoted through a sense of effective communications. The exchange of common problems enhances realistic perception, the solution of one's own problems and growth and maturity.

Resolved Needs: Comfort. Personal growth and maturity. Increased reality perception and problem-solving ability.

Encourage the substitution of real-life endeavors for fantasized endeavors   When a person fantasizes about accomplishments, substitute goals that can be applied to the real world and that will bring satisfaction. Offer the person assistance in fulfilling those goals.

Rationale: Fantasy is stimulated by frustrated desires and need gratification. Maturity and growth involve reality perception and goal seeking which meets situational demands and individual needs.

Resolved Needs: Personal growth and maturity. Increased reality perception and problem-solving ability.

Encourage the substitution of undesirable habits with favorable habits   Suggest that injurious habits can be changed by substituting a pleasant habit in its place. Nail biting can be replaced with gum chewing. Smoking can be substituted with sucking on hard candy.

Rationale: Sound health approaches promote safety, growth, maturity, and increased problem-solving ability.

Resolved Needs: Protection from physical harm. Protection from psychologic threat. Personal growth and maturity. Increased reality perception and problem-solving ability.

Encourage the use of a warm, saline gargle   Suggest that a warm, salt solution gargle be used two to four times a day.

Rationale: A warm saline gargle promotes soothing comfort to irritated mucosa and minimizes infection through cleansing.

Resolved Needs: Cleanliness. Comfort.

Contraindications: Hypernatremia. When on a low-sodium diet.

Encourage the use of an artificial larynx (or esophageal speech) as directed by the speech therapist   Encourage the patient to follow the directions of the speech therapist in using either an artificial larynx or esophageal speech. In using an artificial larynx, the vibrator is placed either externally against the side of the neck or internally toward the side and back of the mouth. In using esophageal speech, air is taken into the mouth, the lips are brought together tightly and air is forced into the esophagus. As pressure increases in the upper esophagus, a tonal vibration is produced.

Rationale: An artificial larynx and/or esophageal speech offer methods for verbal communication when such communication has been interrupted by a laryngectomy.

Resolved Needs: Comfort. Warm, communicating relationships.

Encourage the use of normal coping mechanisms   Encourage the use of normal adaptive methods for dealing with emotions.

Rationale: The development and use of adaptive psychologic mechanisms fosters safety, comfort, and psychologic equilibrium. External attempts to remove psychologic defenses increase anxiety.

Resolved Needs: Comfort. Protection from psychologic threats.

Encourage the use of spiritual resources   Suggest that spiritual assistance can give direction and purpose to a floundering life and that feelings of helplessness or fear can be reduced through the development of internal strength drawn from the unlimited strength of an Almighty Power.

Rationale: Awareness of the value of spirituality leads to closer God-human relationships, which bring about the satisfaction of strength, comfort, and maturity.

Resolved Needs: Comfort. Protection from psychologic threat. Endurance. Personal growth and maturity. Improved values. Religious, philosophic satisfaction. Increased pleasantness.

Encourage the use of the bathroom   If at all possible, encourage the patient to get out of bed and use the bathroom facilities.

Rationale: Use of the bathroom promotes relaxation, comfort, and normal body function.

Resolved Needs: Waste elimination. Comfort. Cleanliness.

Contraindications: Maximum 24-hour bed rest.

Encourage vacationing   Suggest that the person change his surroundings by taking a pleasant trip.

Rationale: A change of scene and carefree distraction promotes temporary escape from threatening situations and supports emotional healing. Involvement in new interests interrupts habitual patterns of thought.

Resolved Needs: Comfort. Protection from psychologic threat. Less of the familiar, more of the novel.

Encourage visiting by significant others   Suggest that persons significant to the patient visit as frequently as possible.

Rationale: The presence of significant persons promotes comfort and assurance that one will be cared for properly.

Resolved Needs: Comfort. Protection from psychologic threat. Unity with loved ones.

Encourage visits with friends when lonely   Suggest that the lonely person become involved in activities with friends.

Rationale: Safety and comfort feelings are fostered by an awareness that one is not threatened with aloneness and can communicate with others. Positive response from others promotes positive self-attitudes.

Resolved Needs: Protection from psychologic threat. Warm, communicating relationships. High evaluation of self

Encourage volunteers to visit the sick   Encourage volunteers from churches or social organizations to visit sick persons routinely.

Rationale: Positive feelings about one's self result from positive responses from others and an awareness that one is not threatened with aloneness.

Resolved Needs: Comfort. Warm, communicating relationships.

Encourage youths toward goal achievement to please significant others   Arouse positive behavior by suggesting that goals be achieved for loved ones or for persons with whom there is close identification.

Rationale: When youths earn awards, etc., their self-esteem is enhanced as a result of the esteem they receive from significant others.

Resolved Needs: Love and affection. Unity with loved ones. Sense of value, usefulness. Goal achievement.

Ensure the patient's feelings of safety before introducing unpleasantness   Choose a time when the person is under little or no tension or threat to convey to him any unpleasantness or bad news.

Rationale: When a person feels secure, threatening situations are less frightening than at times when he feels less secure. When a person feels well, he has greater strength for adaptation to bad news. When a state of psychologic safety exists, perception tends to identify associated objects and situations as nonthreatening.

Resolved Needs: Comfort. Protection from psychologic threat.

Escort the patient during off-ward activities   When the patient goes off the nursing unit for therapeutic or other reasons, provide constant accompaniment by a responsible staff member.

Rationale: Aloneness offers a person with self-destructive tendencies an opportunity to harm himself physically. Recognition of potentially harmful physical threats promotes safety. Respect for the basic worth of human beings promotes the support of life whenever possible.

Resolved Needs: Protection from physical harm.

Establish routines familiar to the patient   Discover the person's previous routines and make every effort to reestablish the same daily habits in relation to time and detail.

Rationale: Feelings of threat result from the disruption of established behavior patterns by illness. Feelings of safety arise from familiar and predictable situations that have been handled successfully in the past.

Resolved Needs: Comfort. Protection from psychologic threat. Predictable, orderly world.

Estimate the required daily calories
Determine the approximate number of daily calories required by an adult involved in normal daily activity. Base this estimate on average daily requirements of 9 calories per pound of body weight. To maintain a constant weight base, the calorie estimate is determined by the present weight. To bring about weight loss or gain, determine the desired weight and multiply that by 9 calories per pound.

Rationale: Normal body weight enhances normal body function. Calorie intake should approximate caloric output.

Resolved Needs: Food balance. Protection from physical harm.

Evert the eyelid
Lay a cotton-tipped applicator across the eyelid edge. Gently grasp the eyelashes with the fingers of the other hand. Pull the lid outward from the eye and turn it upward.

Rationale: Eyelid eversion facilitates visualization of foreign bodies in the eye and prevents eye tissue irritation caused by eyelid inversion.

Resolved Needs: Comfort. Protection from physical harm.

Exercise in range of motion
Promote muscular and joint activity by carrying out the total exercising of muscles and joints. This may be done solely by the patient, or with nursing assistance.

Rationale: Muscular exertion through exercise promotes circulation and free joint mobility, strengthens muscle tone, develops coordination, and prevents nonfunctional contractures.

Resolved Needs: Circulation. Exercise. Protection from physical harm.

Contraindications: Circulatory embolus-thrombus. Severe inflammation or pain. Fracture. Recent surgery on or near the joint.

Exercise the fingers with a ball
Have the patient squeeze a rubber ball tightly with his fingers as often as possible. Include an equal amount of time for full extension of the fingers.

Rationale: Muscular exertion through exercise promotes circulation and free joint mobility, strengthens muscle tone, develops coordination, and prevents nonfunctional contractures.

Resolved Needs: Circulation. Exercise. Protection from physical harm.

Expand the patient's mobility distance
Increase the distance that the patient can cover within the confines of the setting. If he has been limited to one or two rooms, allow him to visit the coffee shop, lobby, etc. thereby gradually expanding his world.

Rationale: A gradual increase in environmental contacts promotes independence, self-confidence, and a sense of adequacy through an awareness that one can cope successfully with an expanded world. It provides a change of environment and a larger area for exercise.

Resolved Needs: Activity, exercise. Stimulation. Adequacy. Self-reliance. Independence.

Explore superficial topics and reasons for avoiding in-depth feelings
Help the patient to examine why he avoids discussing his feelings. Let him know that feelings are natural and should be experienced. Discuss happy, sad, angry feelings and explain that feelings are good in themselves.

Rationale: Exploring provides an opportunity to perceive and express one's own deep feelings regarding an emotional topic. Persons who are aware that they are understood by another will continue to communicate freely.

Resolved Needs: Protection from psychologic threat. Warm, communicating relationships. Personal growth and maturity.

Explore with the patient his strengths and resources
Help the person to give a verbal, detailed account of his resources and capabilities. Include such areas as physical, intellectual, emotional, financial, social, and specific ability resources. Help the person become aware that he has great physical and emotional reserves that will support him during times of stress.

Rationale: A positive attitude toward oneself promotes positive behavior. Increased and accurate information about oneself leads to mature reality perception, awareness of potential, value clarification, increased meaningfulness, and enhanced adequacy in solving problems and making decisions. An awareness of man's enduring strength builds confidence in oneself which reduces fear and promotes comfort, growth, and maturity.

Resolved Needs: Comfort. Protection from psychologic threat. Adequacy. Personal growth and maturity. Awareness of potential. Increased reality perception and problem-solving ability.

Explore with the patient how he would feel in situations experienced by others
Help the patient to imagine himself in the same situation as another person. Have him give the details of the situation and the feelings he might experience if he were in the same situation.

Rationale: Awareness of feelings in another arouses a corresponding emotional effect and promotes a more realistic perception of another's emotional world.

Resolved Needs: Personal growth and maturity. Increased reality perception and problem-solving ability.

Explore with the patient previous achievements of success
Help the person to enumerate verbally past life experiences in detail that in his perception have been successful.

Rationale: Memories of past success promote positive self-attitudes toward present tasks.

Resolved Needs: Comfort. Protection from psychologic threat. Sense of value. High evaluation of self. Adequacy.

Explore with the patient previous displays of courage Help the person to recall those life experiences in which he displayed courage and to enumerate the details of that courage.

Rationale: A positive, detailed image of one's qualities, capabilities and strengths promotes a positive self.

Resolved Needs: Comfort. Protection from psychologic threat. Sense of value. High evaluation of self.

Explore with the patient reasons for criticism by others Help the person to identify, in detail, reasons why other persons criticize him.

Rationale: Increased and accurate information about oneself leads to mature reality perception and enhanced adequacy in solving problems and making decisions.

Resolved Needs: Adequacy. Personal growth and maturity. Increased reality perception and problem-solving ability.

Explore with the patient reasons for criticisms of others Help the person to identify, in detail, his motives for criticizing other persons.

Rationale: Increased and accurate information about one's self leads to mature reality perception and enhanced adequacy in solving problems and making decisions.

Resolved Needs: Adequacy. Personal growth and maturity. Increased reality perception and problem-solving ability.

Explore with the patient reasons for likes and dislikes Help the person to identify, in detail, his motives and reasons for personal likes and dislikes of objects, places, situations, and specific persons.

Rationale: Increased and accurate information about oneself leads to mature reality perception and enhanced adequacy in solving problems and making decisions.

Resolved Needs: Adequacy. Personal growth and maturity. Increased reality perception and problem-solving ability.

Explore with the patient reasons for recurring problems Help the person to identify, in detail, motives, reasons, and circumstances that evolve around a frequently recurring emotional reaction.

Rationale: Increased and accurate information about one's self leads to mature reality perception and enhanced adequacy in solving problems and making decisions.

Resolved Needs: Adequacy. Personal growth and maturity. Increased reality perception and problem-solving ability.

Explore with the patient reasons for self-criticism Help the person to identify, in detail, his motives for looking negatively at himself. Such reasons would include a poorly developed self-image and lack of positive feedback from others.

Rationale: Increased and accurate information about one's self leads to mature reality perception and enhanced adequacy in solving problems and making decisions.

Resolved Needs: Adequacy. Personal growth and maturity. Increased reality perception and problem-solving ability.

Explore with the patient the difference between his child and adult conscience Help the person to distinguish between the childhood conscience based on fear of punishment and the adult conscience based on one's self-ideal. Indicate the need to use self-judgment rather than parentally imposed judgments of what is right or wrong. Help the person develop an adult conscience based on an evaluation of what he ought to do as related to his feelings of individual obligation, and not based on blind rigidity to society's standards and values.

Rationale: The rigid conscience results from painful human relations with early authorities and, when maintained in adulthood, perpetuates similar relationships. Modifying the rigid conscience allows for internal self-direction based on realistic values. The capacity to make moral judgments and justify actions enhances self-esteem.

Resolved Needs: Comfort. Protection from psychologic threat. High evaluation of self. Improved values. Increased reality perception and problem-solving ability.

Explore with the patient the effects of his behavior on others Help the patient to recognize that his behavior is a stimulus that causes responses in other persons. These responses may be favorable or unfavorable in the life of the person responding.

Rationale: Awareness that one's behavior has an effect on others promotes greater consideration for others with resulting increased harmony in interpersonal relationships.

Resolved Needs: Personal growth and maturity. Increased reality perception and problem-solving ability.

Explore with the patient the need for approval Help the person to determine the extent of his need for positive regard from others and if that need is so great as to thwart personal growth and freedom.

Rationale: The need for approval stems from man's interdependency and from the realization that assistance from others is acquired through socially

approved behavior. Increased self-insight leads to mature reality perception.

Resolved Needs: Personal growth and maturity. Increased reality perception and problem-solving ability.

Explore with the patient the need for attention   Help the person
to determine motives behind his attempts to bring attention to himself.

Rationale: An awareness of one's own need for attention reveals underlying feelings of inferiority and lack of sensitivity to others' needs. It promotes
growth, maturity, and reality perception.

Resolved Needs: Personal growth and maturity. Increased reality perception and problem-solving ability.

Explore with the patient the need for dominance   Help the person to determine the extent of his need to control others, the reasons for it,
and responses that dominating behavior elicits from others.

Rationale: The need to exert control stems from perceived threat. Increased and accurate information about one's self leads to mature reality
perception and enhanced adequacy in solving problems and making decisions.

Resolved Needs: Adequacy. Personal growth and maturity. Increased reality perception and problem-solving ability.

Expose the draining wound (burn or decubitus) to air   Expose
an injured, burned, infected, degenerating, or ulcerated body area to the air
without a protective dressing.

Rationale: Wound exposure to air promotes exudate drying and crusting
which supports skin regeneration beneath the crust and protects the wound
from bacterial invasion.

Resolved Needs: Protection from physical harm.

Expose the drying cast to air   When an orthopedic cast has been
applied, expose it to the circulating air and protect it from dampness for at
least 24 hours. A wet cast will be gray, dull, feel damp, and have a musty
odor. When dry, it will be shiny white and firm. Normally, it takes 24 to 48
hours for complete drying.

Rationale: A therapeutic cast provides immobility and support to injured
limbs, preventing further injury and enhancing healing.

Resolved Needs: Protection from physical harm.

Expose the skin to sunlight   Place the patient in the outdoor sun for
short periods several times a day or by an open window or door through
which the sun rays can come.

Rationale: Ultraviolet sun rays reduce the yellowness in jaundiced skin.

Resolved Needs: Comfort. Protection from physical harm.

Express approval Display favorable attitudes toward the person's behavior and actions. This is accomplished through favorable comments and nonverbal expressions of approval.

Rationale: Feelings of comfort require that the person experience approval from others.

Resolved Needs: Comfort. Approval from others.

Express breast milk manually Gently massage the breast for a few moments. Place one hand on top of the other above the breast. Bring the hands down over the breast, turn the fingers downward as the hands are drawn apart and encircle the breast. Use three fingers to cup and support under the breast as well as bring the breast forward and upward. Place the forefinger below and the thumb above the alveoli and apply gentle pressure until the milk flows in a stream. Gently rotate the fingers around the alveoli until all milk is expressed. The opposite hand should be used for holding a sterile container. Hand-washing is essential prior to expressing breast milk.

Rationale: When breast feeding is temporarily curtailed, breast milk must be removed artificially or lactation will be inhibited permanently. The expression of milk from the lactating breast promotes comfort.

Resolved Needs: Comfort. Protection from physical harm.

Contraindications: Intentional lactation suppression.

Express breast milk mechanically Breast milk may be expressed by either a hand or electric pump. When a hand pump is used, apply the suction cup to the nipple and alternately squeeze and release the suction bulb. When an electric pump is used, apply the suction cup to the nipple with a low degree of vacuum. Breast suctioning should be gradual, intermittent, continued for no more than 15 minutes, and stopped earlier if the breast is empty. The milk is measured and saved in a sterile container for later infant feeding. Hand-washing is essential prior to expressing breast milk.

Rationale: When breast feeding is temporarily curtailed, breast milk must be removed artificially or lactation will be inhibited permanently. The expression of milk from the lactating breast promotes comfort.

Resolved Needs: Comfort. Protection from physical harm.

Contraindication: Intentional lactation suppression.

Express empathy Display feeling and understanding of the person's emotions, problems, desires, and goals. This is accomplished by relating similar self-experiences and emotions.

Rationale: An awareness that one is understood by others decreases anxiety and aloneness.

Resolved Needs: Comfort. Protection from psychologic threat. Warm, communicating relationships.

Express warmth and friendliness Display attitudes of kindness, interest, cheerfulness, and peaceful coexistence as you move toward another person. Indicate that you are receptive to knowing and interacting with him.

Rationale: Comfort is promoted through the ability to relate to others and to communicate one's needs.

Resolved Needs:· Comfort. Protection from psychologic threat. Warm, communicating relationships.

Facilitate delivery by gently guiding the infant through the vulva (ExR) As the infant presents himself at the vulva opening, gently lift his chin up through the vulva. To assist in delivering the anterior (upper) shoulder, gently guide the infant's head downward. Gently turn the head upward to deliver the lower shoulder.

Rationale: Assisting with childbirth promotes maternal and infant safety.

Resolved Needs: Protection from physical harm.

Feed by bottle Nourish an infant with liquids by means of a bottle and artificial nipple.

Rationale: Balanced nutritional intake is essential to body cell activity and energy production from food. Relief of the visceral hunger sensation promotes comfort. Feeding meets dependency needs.

Resolved Needs: Water-salt balance. Food balance. Energy. Comfort. Protection from physical harm. Dependence.

Feed by cup Offer the child a drink with a cup.

Rationale: Eating, being a social event, requires learning socially acceptable conduct. A child's use of a cup supports independence.

Resolved Needs: Comfort. Independence.

Feed by medicine dropper Provide liquid food for the premature infant by using a medicine dropper.

Rationale: A medicine dropper provides sufficiently small amounts of food so premature infants may swallow safely without choking. Feeding meets dependency needs.

Resolved Needs: Water-salt balance. Food balance. Protection from physical harm. Dependence.

Feed by syringe Administer oral fluids or pureed foods with a syringe.

Rationale: Balanced nutritional intake is essential to body cell activity and energy production from food. Relief of the visceral hunger sensation promotes comfort. Feeding meets dependency needs.

Resolved Needs: Water-salt balance. Food balance. Comfort. Protection from physical harm. Dependence.

Feed slowly   Unhurriedly nourish the patient with food and fluids. Allow adequate time for chewing, swallowing, and pauses between food bites.

Rationale: The stress of hurrying causes intestinal spasms with reduced digestive functioning. Relaxed eating promotes comfort.

Resolved Needs: Relaxation. Comfort. Protection from physical harm.

Feed the patient   Place food and drink into the patient's mouth when he cannot do so himself.

Rationale: Food is essential to life maintenance. Feeding meets dependency needs.

Resolved Needs: Water-salt balance. Food balance. Protection from physical harm. Dependence.

File the nails in one direction and only on the underside   File the nails in one direction, not back and forth. File on the under surface of the nail and not on the upper or side surface. Use a metal file for shaping long, hard nails. Use the coarse side of an emery board for shaping normal nails and the fine side to finish the shaping.

Rationale: Filing the nails in one direction and only on the underside prevents nail splitting. Ragged or excessively long fingernails are prone to catch on objects with which they come in contact causing nail injury.

Resolved Needs: Protection from physical harm.

Fold a towel between the legs during incontinence   Fold a towel into a 6-inch wide roll. Tuck between the patient's legs, covering the perineal area. Change immediately when soiled.

Rationale: Collecting urine or fecal wastes in absorbent material reduces skin wetness, decreasing potential skin irritation from waste products. Cleanliness promotes comfort.

Resolved Needs: Comfort. Cleanliness. Protection from physical harm.

Follow distasteful drugs with fruit juice   When drugs taste bad, and the taste cannot be disguised, give a favorite fruit juice immediately after the drug is taken.

Rationale: Fruit juice following distasteful drug ingestion provides the comfort of a desirable flavor in the mouth.

Resolved Needs: Comfort.

Follow quick-acting glucose with long-acting carbohydrates

After the patient with hypoglycemia has received a quick-acting glucose source (orange juice or candy), follow this with long-acting carbohydrates such as bread or crackers.

Rationale: A quick-acting glucose source immediately raises the blood sugar, but only for a short period. When a long-acting carbohydrate is given to follow the quick-acting glucose source, the blood sugar will be maintained at a normal level for a longer period.

Resolved Needs: Food balance. Protection from physical harm.

Follow through on promises

When you give your word that you will do something for a patient, be absolutely certain that the commitment is fulfilled in the alloted time. If, for some reason, the promise cannot be carried out, give a thorough explanation as to why and offer a substitute commitment.

Rationale: Trust is enhanced when important matters pertaining to the person are considered matters of concern by others.

Resolved Needs: Comfort. Protection from psychologic threat. Warm, communicating relationships.

Give a pacifier to the infant

Place a plastic or rubber nipple or teething ring in the baby's mouth.

Rationale: Use of a pacifier during tube feeding promotes digestion and speeds the development of the infant's sucking ability. It promotes sucking contentment when contentment from human contact is limited or when adequate sucking is not sufficient during feeding.

Resolved Needs: Comfort. Stimulation.

Contraindications: Avoid using a pacifier to keep the child quiet.

Give a whole-milk substitute

When an allergy or intolerance to milk exists, milk substitutes such as skim milk, soybean formula, evaporated milk, or protein hydrolysate formulas can be given. Milk also can be diluted with water.

Rationale: A milk substitute provides an alternate to milk, maintains the nutrition of whole milk, and minimizes undesirable physical responses.

Resolved Needs: Food balance. Comfort. Protection from physical harm.

Give an antidote as recommended on the poison container label

Read the container label of the ingested product and use the suggested antidote for that particular product as stated on the label.

Rationale: A proper antidote will neutralize the harmful effects of a poison.

Resolved Needs: Protection from physical harm.

Give bland foods Give foods low in residue, acid, and spice content. These include milk, eggs, cream, butter, mild cheese, tender meat, poultry and fish, low residue and low acid fruits and vegetables, white bread, refined cereals, plain desserts, and starches like potatoes, rice, and macaroni. Avoid giving foods containing seeds, coarse fibers and skins, heavy seasoning, caffeine and alcohol.

Rationale: Bland foods neutralize acids, reduce gastric juice secretion and peristalsis and will not stimulate salivation to the degree that seasoned foods will.

Resolved Needs: Food balance. Energy. Comfort. Protection from physical harm.

Give buttermilk or yogurt Give a glass of buttermilk or a serving of yogurt.

Rationale: Buttermilk and yogurt contain lactobacilli that increase the absorption of nutritional substances such as vitamins. During and following antibiotic therapy or diarrhea, buttermilk or yogurt restore normal intestinal bacteria which improves digestion and promotes comfort. Yogurt is a good source of calcium, riboflavin, and protein.

Resolved Needs: Comfort. Protection from physical harm.

Give carbonated beverages Dispense an effervescent drink.

Rationale: Vomiting removes hydrochloric acid from the stomach causing alkalosis. The carbon dioxide (effervesence) in carbonated beverages is acid. When alkalosis exists, it helps restore normal pH and increases fluid intake. Carbonated beverages cause air in the stomach to bubble and move up the esophagus relieving the discomfort of trapped air. Carbonated beverages produce alkaline urine. The ginger root, a basic ingredient in ginger ale, soothes the intestinal mucosa.

Resolved Needs: Water-salt balance. Acid-base balance. Comfort.

Contraindications: Acidosis. High susceptibility to tooth decay. Gastric hyperacidity. Potential or existing calcium renal calculi. Abdominal distention from intestinal disorders. Respiratory disorders in which there is carbon dioxide retention.

Give charcoal solution orally Give between 100 and 200 cc of activated charcoal orally.

Rationale: Charcoal absorbs poisons, reducing tissue damage.

Resolved Needs: Protection from physical harm.

Give citrus fruit juice Give citrus fruit juice to the patient who has swallowed a corrosive alkali poison. If a child is 1–5 years old, give 1–2 cups of juice. If he is over 5 years of age, give up to 1 quart (1000 cc) of juice. Citrus fruit juices include orange and grapefruit. If a patient is in shock, give citrus fruit juice only if he is able to swallow.

Rationale: The high acid content of citrus fruit juices neutralizes the alkali in alkali poisons and in alkalosis. The high glucose content of citrus fruit juices tends to offset shock.

Resolved Needs: Water-salt balance. Acid-base balance. Protection from physical harm.

Give clear liquid foods   Give water and nutritional liquids including tea with lemon and sugar, coffee, carbonated beverages, fat-free broth, flavored gelatin, fruit ices, and strained or clear fruit juices.

Rationale: Clear liquid foods replace lost fluids. Their nonirritating effect reduces flatulence and excessive peristaltic stimulation. Relief of visceral hunger promotes comfort.

Resolved Needs: Water-salt balance. Food balance. Comfort. Protection from physical harm.

Give cough drops   Dispense a lozenge or troche having a demulcent effect.

Rationale: Cough drops soothe and comfort inflamed or irritated mucous membrane.

Resolved Needs: Comfort.

Contraindications: Do not give to small children, the aged, persons with cerebral vascular accident who have impaired oral control, or persons whose sugar intake is restricted. Do not give after procedures such as bronchoscopy until the effects of local anesthesia have worn off completely.

Give distilled water orally   Give water orally that has been purified by distillation and is free of sodium.

Rationale: Distilled water helps maintain water balance without increasing the blood sodium level.

Resolved Needs: Water-salt balance. Protection from physical harm.

Contraindications: Hyponatremia.

Give drugs judiciously for emotional repression   Recognize that drugs can be given appropriately for the repression of emotions during times of crisis, but that the drugs should no longer be given when the crisis is over.

Rationale: Drugs during a time of crisis help to repress intense emotions and assist the patient in coping with the situation. Once the crisis is over, drugs should no longer be given since the patient needs to face his emotions in the now less stressful situation. If emotions are repressed constantly, they will surface at a later time, causing a painful, inappropriate experience. Honest confrontation with one's emotions promotes growth, maturity, and reality perception.

Resolved Needs: Comfort. Protection from psychologic threat. Personal growth and maturity. Increased reality perception and problem-solving ability.

Give dry crackers   Give the person experiencing nausea or vomiting dry, preferably salted, crackers to eat.

Rationale: Dry crackers absorb and neutralize intestinal acids and promote comfort.

Resolved Needs: Acid-base balance. Comfort. Protection from physical harm.

Contraindications: Avoid salted crackers in salt- or sodium-restricted diets.

Give enteric-coated medications or enclose the medication in a gelatin capsule   Give medications coated with or enclosed in a substance that prevents their destruction until after they pass through the stomach.

Rationale: Enteric-coated medications or drugs enclosed in a gelatin capsule do not disintegrate and are not absorbed until they reach the small intestine. They protect the stomach against irritation from the drug and protect the drug from exposure to gastric acid.

Resolved Needs: Comfort. Protection from physical harm.

Contraindications: Restricted sugar intake.

Give explicit directions   Give firm, simple directions that can be understood and acted on easily.

Rationale: Simple, direct communications enhance perception and reduce threats of frustration and anxiety. Lengthy directions reduce available time for thinking and deciphering messages and result in confusion and discomfort. When a patient cannot make decisions because of overtaxed adaptation needs, direction from a person uninvolved in the crisis reduces threat and promotes comfort.

Resolved Needs: Comfort. Protection from physical harm. Protection from psychologic threat. Dependence.

Give flavor-intensified food   Give foods whose flavor has been accentuated by adding monosodium glutamate.

Rationale: Monosodium glutamate intensifies food flavor without adding new flavor. When taste is physiologically impaired, improved flavor promotes comfort and the desire to eat.

Resolved Needs: Food balance. Comfort.

Contraindications: Sodium-restricted diet. Intolerance to monosodium glutamate.

Give fresh fruits   Dispense nonprocessed fruits that are in the natural state, such as apples, oranges, plums, grapes, pineapple.

Rationale: Fresh fruits contain indigestible cellulose that supplies bulk for normal comfortable elimination. Fresh fruits supply nutritional vitamins.

Resolved Needs: Food balance. Waste elimination. Comfort.

Contraindications: Diarrhea. Hyperperistalsis. Gastric ulceration.

Give full-liquid foods   Give liquid or semiliquid foods that are free of cellulose and spices. Include carbonated beverages, milk, coffee, tea, cocoa, strained or fine whole grain cereals, custards, plain gelatin, ice cream, sherbert, junket, cornstarch puddings, raw or softly cooked eggs, strained juices, strained or creamed meat and vegetable soups, butter, sugar, salt, and egg nog.

Rationale: When food is tolerated poorly, a full liquid diet supplies nourishment and facilitates easy digestion. Relief of visceral hunger promotes comfort. Salivation is increased by mechanical stimulation of taste buds with full-liquid foods.

Resolved Needs: Water-salt balance. Food balance. Comfort. Protection from physical harm.

Give hard candy   Dispense hard candy for sucking.

Rationale: Sucking on hard candy (especially lemon and peppermint) promotes comfort and hygiene by refreshing the mouth and sour breath. It prevents mouth dryness and is a quick source of glucose. Candy is a substitute for less desirable oral satisfactions such as smoking, chewing tobacco, etc. Lemon candy increases salivation.

Resolved Needs: Energy. Comfort. Protection from physical harm.

Contraindications: Do not give when sugar intake is restricted, except in emergency insulin shock. Susceptibility to tooth decay.

Give high-calcium fluids orally   Give milk or liquids such as milk shakes, malts, milk sodas, melted ice cream, cocoa, milk punch.

Rationale: High-calcium fluids increase a low-calcium blood level and help maintain acid-base and fluid balance.

Resolved Needs: Water-salt balance. Acid-base balance. Protection from physical harm.

Contraindications: Potential or existing calcium urinary calculi. High alkali intake. Prolonged illness enforced immobility or bed rest. Nausea. Vomiting. Diarrhea. Respiratory infection. High fever.

Give high-glucose fluids orally   Give liquids such as lemonade, orange juice, or tea or coffee with sugar, honey, or corn syrup.

Rationale: Glucose ingestion raises a low blood sugar to normal, produces energy from food, balances fluid intake and body acid-base.

Resolved Needs: Water-salt balance. Acid-base balance. Energy. Protection from physical harm.

Contraindications: Do not give when sugar intake is restricted, except in emergency insulin shock. Susceptibility to tooth decay.

Give high-magnesium fluids orally   Raise the intake of high magnesium liquids. Include milk, cocoa, chocolate, prune juice.

Rationale: A normal magnesium level is essential to osmotic pressure balance, enzyme activation, nerve and muscular activity, normal bone development, and acid-base balance.

Resolved Needs: Water-salt balance. Protection from physical harm.

Contraindications: Hypermagnesemia. Diabetic acidosis. Dehydration. Profuse sweating.

Give high-potassium fluids orally   Dispense fluids containing high levels of potassium. Include grape, grapefruit, orange, prune, tangerine, or tomato juice and tea, coffee, chocolate, and meat broth.

Rationale: Normal blood potassium is essential to intracellular fluid balance, osmotic pressure regulation, acid-base balance, and the conduction of nerve impulses in muscle tissue. High potassium intake offsets the tendency of steroid therapy to cause negative nitrogen balance and replaces potassium lost through diarrhea and vomiting.

Resolved Needs: Water-salt balance. Acid-base balance. Protection from physical harm.

Contraindications: Hyperkalemia. Renal failure with oliguria or anuria. Adrenal insufficiency. Ventricular fibrillation. During the shock stage of severe second- or third-degree burns or crushing injuries. When the patient is receiving I.V. infusions containing potassium.

Give high-sodium fluids orally   Dispense liquids having a high sodium content, such as milk, root beer, instant, dry coffee, Dutch chocolate.

Rationale: A normal sodium level is essential to fluid and electrolyte balance, normal osmotic pressure, and acid-base balance. It replaces sodium lost through diarrhea and vomiting.

Resolved Needs: Water-salt balance. Acid-base balance. Protection from physical harm.

Contraindications: Impaired renal function. Edema. Ascites. Cardiac damage with impaired circulation. If the patient is receiving steroid therapy, large volumes of intravenous saline, or is on a low sodium diet.

Give hot coffee   Offer a cup of hot coffee, preferably without sugar or cream.

Rationale: Hot coffee reduces fatigue through its stimulative effect. It increases circulation, counteracts overdoses of barbiturates and sleeping pills, increases fluid intake, and promotes bowel and bladder elimination.

Resolved Needs: Circulation. Water-salt balance. Waste elimination. Comfort. Stimulation. Protection from physical harm.

Contraindications: Impaired blood supply to the cardiac muscle. Poisonous snake bites. Electrical shock. Excessive peristalsis. Urinary frequency. Vasodilatation. Nervousness or irritability. Hypoglycemia. Increased metabolic rate. Cracked or sensitive teeth. Sensitive gums or oral mucous membranes.

Give hot tea　Offer a cup of hot tea, preferably without sugar and cream.

Rationale: Vomiting removes hydrochloric acid from the stomach, causing alkalosis. The tannic acid in tea helps reestablish normal pH, and the fluid increases liquid intake. Theine in tea makes it mildly stimulating, causing temporarily improved circulation, fatigue reduction, and ease of fatigue headaches. It counteracts overdoses of barbiturates and sleeping pills.

Resolved Needs: Circulation. Water-salt balance. Acid-base balance. Comfort. Stimulation. Protection from physical harm. Freedom from pain.

Contraindications: Impaired blood supply to the cardiac muscle. Poisonous snake bites. Electrical shock. Excessive peristalsis. Urinary frequency. Vasodilatation. Nervousness or irritability. Hypoglycemia. Increased metabolic rate. Cracked or sensitive teeth. Sensitive gums or oral mucous membranes.

Give iced liquids　Give fluids that are chilled or iced, such as ice water or fruit juices.

Rationale: Cold liquids in the stomach and duodenum stimulate the gastrocolic reflex, causing colon contractions and peristalsis. Iced liquids reduce elevated body temperature and stimulate the vagus nerve to slow the heart. Cool liquids cause vasoconstriction which prevents mouth bleeding.

Resolved Needs: Water-salt balance. Waste elimination. Normal temperature. Comfort. Protection from physical harm.

Contraindications: Low body temperature. Impaired blood circulation. Bladder or intestinal spasms. Diarrhea or hyperperistalsis. Cracked or sensitive teeth. Sensitive or receding gums.

Give important messages only when the patient is receptive　Convey thoughts and ideas of importance only in a nondistracting environment when the person's attention can be focused on the message.

Rationale: The quality of message reception and interpretation is reduced by distracting environmental influences and events. Comfort is promoted through a sense of effective communication with others.

Resolved Needs: Comfort. Protection from psychologic threat. Warm, communicating relationships.

Give iodized salt   Dispense salt fortified with either sodium or potassium iodide.

Rationale: The use of iodized salt prior to or during the early stages of iodine deficiency usually will correct the problem. Iodine is essential to thyroxin production necessary for normal thyroid function.

Resolved Needs: Protection from physical harm.

Contraindications: Hypernatremia. Hyperkalemia.

Give isotonic drinks orally   Dispense liquid drinks containing a 0.9% water solution of sodium chloride. These drinks can be individually prepared or obtained from commercial manufacturers.

Rationale: Sodium and chloride are essential to fluid and acid-base balance. When large amounts of sodium chloride are lost through urine, sweating, vomiting, and diarrhea, body cells become overhydrated because of failure to maintain equal concentrations of water and solute (osmosis) within the cells. Isotonic drinks reestablish normal osmotic pressure so water can pass to and from the cells equalizing the solute and water concentration. Isotonic drinks maintain fluid, salt, and acid-base balance.

Resolved Needs: Water-salt balance. Acid-base balance. Protection from physical harm.

Contraindications: Hypernatremia. Hyperchloremia.

Give light foods before sleep   Give a light snack of easily digestible foods just prior to bedtime.

Rationale: The stimulus of discomforting hunger promotes wakefulness. Adequate sleep is essential in that the decreased metabolic rate occurring during sleep restores depleted cell energy reserves.

Resolved Needs: Sleep, rest, relaxation. Energy. Comfort. Protection from physical harm.

Give low-calcium fluids orally   Dispense fluids containing little or no milk.

Rationale: Decreased calcium intake reduces the potential formation of calcium urinary stones especially in existing kidney disease and illness enforced immobility. It increases fluid intake and helps restore electrolyte balance when the blood calcium level is elevated.

Resolved Needs: Water-salt balance. Protection from physical harm.

Contraindications: Blood clotting abnormalities. Poor lactation. Impaired bone growth. If the patient is receiving large volumes of citrated blood by transfusion.

Give low-magnesium fluids orally   Decrease the intake of high magnesium liquids, such as milk, fruit juice, cocoa, and chocolate.

Rationale: A normal magnesium level is essential for osmotic pressure balance, enzyme activation, nerve and muscular activity, normal bone development, and acid-base balance.

Resolved Needs: Water-salt balance. Protection from physical harm.

Contraindications: Hypomagnesemia. Impaired bone development.

Give low-potassium fluids orally Dispense liquids having little potassium content such as apple, pear, peach, pineapple, and cranberry juice.

Rationale: In kidney failure, potassium cannot be eliminated causing an elevated blood potassium level. A normal blood potassium level is essential to intracellular fluid balance, osmotic pressure regulation, acid-base balance, and the conduction of nerve impulses in muscle tissue.

Resolved Needs: Water-salt balance. Acid-base balance. Protection from physical harm.

Contraindications: Diarrhea. Vomiting. Diuresis. Impaired muscle function. Profuse colostomy, ileostomy, ileal conduit, or T-tube drainage. If the patient is on steroid therapy or receiving large volumes of I.V. dextrose or saline.

Give low-sodium fluids orally Dispense liquids having little sodium content. Salt-free tomato juice, dry roasted coffee, orange, pineapple, apple, cranberry, prune and tangerine juice, cola drinks, Kool-Aid, lemonade, tea, and ginger ale are recommended.

Rationale: A normal blood sodium level is essential for electrolyte balance, osmotic pressure regulation in cells, and fluid and acid-base balance. In severe cardiac damage, venous stasis and increased venous pressure prevent the return of sodium and water from interstitial tissues into the bloodstream for excretion by the kidneys. When kidney excretion of sodium is reduced, restricted sodium intake decreases the blood sodium level. Osmotic pressure then pulls sodium and water from the interstitial spaces into the bloodstream relieving tissue edema.

Resolved Needs: Water-salt balance. Acid-base balance. Protection from physical harm.

Contraindications: Diarrhea. Vomiting. Excessive sweating. Diuresis. Second- or third-degree burns. Repetitive paracentesis. Fever. Profuse colostomy, ileostomy, illeal conduit, fistula, or T-tube drainage. If the patient is receiving a large volume of I.V. dextrose.

Give magnesium sulfate solution orally Give 2 tablespoons of magnesium sulfate in two glasses of water. In bichloride of mercury poisoning, give one ounce of magnesium sulfate in a pint of water.

Rationale: Magnesium sulfate has a neutralizing effect on specific poisons which include overdoses of codeine, paregoric, bromides, sleeping pills and barbiturates It also neutralizes poisoning by the ingestion of food. bichloride of mercury, DDT, and mushrooms.

Resolved Needs: Protection from physical harm.

Give mechanically soft foods   Give mechanically soft foods that can
be chewed easily. Such foods include ground or minced meats, soft breads, chopped or diced cooked vegetables, soft raw vegetables such as tomatoes and lettuce, soft fruits such as apricots, peaches, bananas, oranges, grapefruit, berries, pears, and finely chopped dried fruits and nuts, mashed potatoes, ice cream, custards and gelatin.

Rationale: The normal digestive process includes the reduction of food to small particles by the teeth. The edentulous diet allows for the omission of mastication in the digestive process when teeth are missing. Balanced nutritional intake is essential to body cell activity and energy production from food. Relief of the visceral hunger sensation promotes comfort.

Resolved Needs: Food balance. Energy. Comfort. Protection from physical harm.

Give medication by injection or in liquid form instead of pills   When medication in pill form causes gastric irritation, give the
same medication either by injection or as a liquid.

Rationale: Liquid medications are absorbed more easily by the gastric mucosa, and medication by injection has no contact with the gastric mucosa.

Resolved Needs: Comfort. Protection from physical harm.

Contraindications: Drugs that require a different dosage when given parenterally instead of orally must be reordered by the physician.

Give milk   Give homogenized milk.

Rationale: Milk neutralizes the harmful effects of acids and promotes comfort. It dilutes the effects of overdoses of pep pills, iron compounds, alcohol, aspirin, headache and cold drugs, paregoric, codeine, and belladonna. It offsets the corrosive effects of poisons such as sodium fluoride, arsenic, strychnine, iodine, bichloride of mercury, chlorine bleach and disinfectant, oil of Wintergreen, rubbing alcohol, carbolic acid disinfectant, furniture polish, gasoline, kerosene, pine oil, and turpentine.

Resolved Needs: Comfort. Protection from physical harm.

Contraindications: Milk intolerance. Infants younger than 4-6 months of age.

Give milk with medications   Dispense milk when administering oral
medications that irritate the stomach lining.

Rationale: The soothing effect of milk on the stomach lining promotes comfort and reduces irritation.

Resolved Needs: Comfort. Protection from physical harm.

Contraindications: Milk intolerance. When giving medications that have adverse reactions with milk. Conditions of decreased gastric absorption.

Give nonprescription drugs (ExR)   Give medical substances readily available to the public that do not require a prescription to be obtained.

Rationale: Drugs consist of chemicals that combine with body processes to either alter or improve body function, to promote comfort or elimination, to regulate body temperature, and to protect from inflammatory or infectious conditions.

Resolved Needs: Waste elimination. Normal temperature. Comfort. Protection from physical harm. Freedom from pain.

Contraindications: Hypersensitivity to the drug. Presence of diseased conditions that may be affected adversely. If the patient is taking a prescription drug that is incompatible with the nonprescription drug.

Give olive oil orally   Give 2 ounces of olive oil orally.

Rationale: Olive oil has a neutralizing effect on specific poisons.

Resolved Needs: Protection from physical harm.

Give only physiologic electrolyte fluids by hypodermoclysis   When administering a hypodermoclysis, give only those fluids whose electrolyte content is nearly the same as that of extracellular fluid. Such fluids include Darrow's solution, 2.5% dextrose in half-strength Ringer's lactate solution, 2.5% dextrose in half-strength Ringer's solution. Ringer's lactage solution, Ringer's solution, hypotonic solutions, 2.5% dextrose in half-isotonic (0.45%) saline.

Rationale: Solutions containing normal electrolyte content, when given by hypodermoclysis, do not irritate tissue or alter electrolyte balance.

Resolved Needs: Water-salt balance. Protection from physical harm.

Give one direction at a time   Direct the person toward accomplishing one activity at a time. Avoid giving further directions until that activity has been completed.

Rationale: Impaired cerebral function limits the accomplishment of more than one activity at a time.

Resolved Needs: Comfort. Protection from psychologic threat.

Give perineal care   Give perineal care by cleansing the vulva and perineum and pouring water over the external female genitalia.

Rationale: Cleanliness minimizes bacterial growth leading to infection and reduces tissue irritation from diseased conditions.

Resolved Needs: Comfort. Cleanliness. Protection from physical harm.

Give prune juice   Dispense a glass of prune juice at least once a day.

Rationale: Prune juice promotes intestinal mobility through the by-product of the prune called dihydroxyphenylisatin. Normal elimination promotes comfort.

Resolved Needs: Waste elimination. Comfort.

Contraindications: Diarrhea. Hyperperistalsis. Hypercalcemia.

Give pureed foods   Give foods boiled to a pulp consistency and strained through a sieve.

Rationale: Pureed foods are swallowed and digested easily because of their pulp consistency and minimal cellulose. Salivation is increased by mechanical stimulation of the taste buds with pureed foods. Balanced nutritional intake is essential to body cell activity and energy production from food. Relief of visceral hunger promotes comfort.

Resolved Needs: Food balance. Energy. Comfort. Protection from physical harm.

Give raw egg white orally   Give two raw egg whites beaten up or mixed with water.

Rationale: Raw egg whites have a neutralizing effect on specific poisons such as household ammonia, washing soda, and carbolic acid disinfectant.

Resolved Needs: Protection from physical harm.

Give raw vegetables   When small children reject soft, mushy food such as cooked vegetables, give raw, firm vegetables.

Rationale: The ability to grasp food firmly makes eating easier and more pleasurable for the child whose small muscle coordination is not developed fully.

Resolved Needs: Comfort.

Give salt-soda solution orally   Give a salt-soda solution made up of 1 teaspoon of salt and 1/2 teaspoon of baking soda added to 1 quart of water. Adults should be given 4 ounces every 15 minutes; children age 1–12 years, 2 ounces; and infants less than 1 year, 1 ounce. If not contraindicated, lemon or lime may be added for flavor.

Rationale: A salt-soda solution provides adequate fluid and electrolyte replacement to assist in reversing shock.

Resolved Needs: Water-salt balance. Protection from physical harm.

Give salt solution orally   Give a mixture of 1 teaspoon of salt in a glass of water. Give one-half glass every 15 minutes for 1 hour.

Rationale: Salt solution provides adequate electrolyte replacement to assist in reversing acidosis.

Resolved Needs: Water-salt balance. Protection from physical harm.

Give small, frequent drinks   Give small amounts of fluid, but give it at frequent intervals such as every 1–2 hours.

Rationale: Small amounts of fluids given at frequent intervals can provide adequate fluid intake, promote comfort, and meet dependency needs.

Resolved Needs: Water-salt balance. Comfort. Protection from physical harm. Dependence.

Contraindications: Restricted oral intake.

Give small, frequent feedings   Give nourishing food in small amounts at least six times a day.

Rationale: Small food amounts at frequent intervals are easily digested, prevent fatigue and abdominal distention, and maintain balanced nutritional intake. Relief of visceral hunger promotes comfort. The intake of small, frequent feedings requires less physical exertion, which reduces oxygen consumption in severe cardiac and pulmonary disorders.

Resolved Needs: Food balance. Energy. Comfort. Protection from physical harm.

Give snacks   Between meals give foods that add to the nutrients of the day. Include foods like milk products, fruits and sandwiches instead of non-nutritious foods such as concentrated sweets and carbonated beverages.

Rationale: Balanced nutritional intake is essential to body cell activity and energy production from food. Relief of visceral hunger promotes comfort.

Resolved Needs: Food balance. Energy. Comfort.

Contraindications: Obesity.

Give sodium bicarbonate solution orally   Orally, give a solution of 1 tablespoon sodium bicarbonate in 1 quart water. For the ingestion of iron compounds, mix two teaspoons of sodium bicarbonate in a glass of warm water.

Rationale: Sodium bicarbonate has a neutralizing effect on overdoses of iron compounds, alcohol, aspirin, headache and cold drugs. It counteracts poisoning from phosphorous, oil of Wintergreen, and rubbing alcohol. It assists in reversing acidosis.

Resolved Needs: Acid-base balance. Protection from physical harm.

Give soft foods   Give foods that are soft, easily digested, not highly seasoned, and contain no harsh fibers. Such foods include bread, dry or cooked cereals, mild cheese, angel food and sponge cakes, custards, gelatin salads with fruit, sherbert, ice creams and pudding, creamed soups, cookies, tender meats, vegetables without skins, all beverages, eggs except when fried, canned or cooked fruit.

Rationale: Soft foods decrease intestinal irritation and bowel spasm and promote comfort. Balanced nutritional intake is essential to body cell activity and energy production from food.

Resolved Needs: Food balance. Energy. Comfort. Protection from physical harm.

Give starch paste orally   Give a drinkable, pastelike mixture of cornstarch and water.

Rationale: A starch antidote neutralizes ingested tincture of benzoin and reduces the harmful effects.

Resolved Needs: Protection from physical harm.

Give strongly seasoned foods   Give foods highly seasoned with herbs, spices, and salts that enhance food tastes.

Rationale: Strong seasoning increases taste when taste has been physiologically impaired and promotes a greater desire to eat.

Resolved Needs: Food balance. Comfort.

Contraindications: Avoid in oral tissue injury, gastric or intestinal irritation.

Give sugar   During persistent hiccoughs, give several teaspoons of table sugar orally.

Rationale: Swallowing sugar crystals stops hiccoughs by stimulating the vagus and phrenic nerves.

Resolved Needs: Comfort.

Contraindications: Restricted sugar intake.

Give tetanus toxoid (ET)   If the patient has received a severe wound, especially a burn, puncture, or deep wound, he should receive tetanus immunization. If he has been immunized fully with tetanus toxoid and has received a booster within the last 5 years, no additional tetanus toxoid is needed. If the last booster is older than 5 years, he should receive a booster dose of toxoid. If the patient has never received tetanus toxoid, he should receive tetanus immune globulin (human) for immediate protection and begin tetanus toxoid immunization as soon as his condition permits. Use tetanus antitoxin (animal serum) only if human globulin is not available because of the dangerous sensitivity reactions possible.

Rationale: The injection of antigens into the body produces antibodies that react against the infectious organisms that attack the body.

Resolved Needs: Protection from physical harm.

Contraindications: Known hypersensitivity reactions to tetanus immunization.

Give the universal antidote orally   Give a mixture of two parts

charcoal, one part tannic acid, and one part magnesium oxide. Put 5 teaspoonfuls of this mixture in a half glass of warm water.

Rationale: Charcoal has an absorbing effect on poisons. Tannic acid separates metals and alkaloids from solution. Magnesium neutralizes the acid in poisons.

Resolved Needs: Protection from physical harm.

Give urine-acidifying juices orally   Give acid-ash juices of apple, cranberry, plum, or prune juice.

Rationale: Increased urine acidity decreases the formation of calcium urinary stones. Effective urinary tract hydration prevents the separation of potential calculi particles from solution and decreases stone formation. Following digestion and oxidation, acid-ash juices alter the bladder pH toward an acid level that deters bacterial growth.

Resolved Needs: Water-salt balance. Acid-base balance. Protection from physical harm.

Contraindications: Hyperuricemia. Cystine renal stones.

Give urine-alkalinizing juices orally   Give carbonated beverages, orange juice, and other fruit juices except cranberry, apple, prune, and plum.

Rationale: Increased alkaline in the urine decreases uric acid and cystine urinary stone formation. Effective urinary tract hydration prevents the separation of potential calculi particles from solution and decreases stone formation.

Resolved Needs: Water-salt balance. Acid-base balance. Protection from physical harm.

Contraindications: Calcium renal stones. Urinary tract infection.

Give vegetable oil orally   Give 2 ounces of salad or vegetable oil by mouth.

Rationale: Vegetable oil neutralizes the harmful effects of specific poisons such as furniture polish, gasoline, kerosene, pine oil, and turpentine.

Resolved Needs: Protection from physical harm.

Contraindications: Do not give vegetable oil antidote for the ingestion of insect or rat poisons that contain phosphorous.

Give vinegar solution orally   Give a solution of 2 tablespoons of vinegar in two glasses of water by mouth.

Rationale: Dilute vinegar solution neutralizes the harmful effects of specific poisons such as household ammonia and washing soda.

Resolved Needs: Protection from physical harm.

Give warm liquids   Offer heated liquids.

Rationale: Warm liquids increase body temperature, promote relaxation, enhance circulation which decreases pain, reduce bladder spasms, promote comfort, increase fluid intake, and promote elimination.

Resolved Needs: Circulation. Water-salt balance. Waste elimination. Normal temperature. Sleep, rest, relaxation. Comfort. Protection from physical harm. Freedom from pain.

Give warm liquids after meals   Suggest that fluids not be taken with meals and then offer a warm drink at the end of the meal.

Rationale: Warm fluids after a meal reduce flatulence.

Resolved Needs: Comfort.

Give water in the infant's bottle at bedtime   When a child needs a bottle to suck on to go to sleep, fill the bottle with plain water only.

Rationale: Water, a noncarbohydrate, when sucked on for a prolonged period, will not cause tooth decay.

Resolved Needs: Protection from physical harm.

Give water orally   Give water orally to the patient who has swallowed a poison or is in impending or early shock. If a child is 1–5 years of age, give 1–2 cups. If he is over 5 years, give up to 1 quart (1000 cc).

Rationale: Water dilutes poisons, reducing their irritating effect on mucous membranes. Water increases the circulating blood volume and thereby assists in reversing shock.

Resolved Needs: Water-salt balance. Protection from physical harm.

Contraindications: Do not give oral fluids if the patient is well into shock because the existing hypoxia generally stops peristalsis and oral fluids would result in abdominal distention and vomiting.

Give wine before meals   Offer a small glass of wine 30 minutes before meals.

Rationale: The alcohol content of wine causes vasodilatation which enhances peripheral circulation, relieves internal congestion, and increases appetite.

Resolved Needs: Circulation. Comfort. Protection from physical harm.

Gradually increase the amount of feedings   Initially, offer small amounts of food and liquids. As the small amounts are tolerated, add a little more with each feeding until normal nutritional quantity is established.

Rationale: Small food amounts in the stomach prevent pressure against the cardiac sphincter and reduce possible regurgitation. Gradually increasing nutritional intake promotes slow stomach filling and thorough digestion by gastric juices. Infants require a gradual increase in feedings as the child makes the transition from liquids to solids.

Resolved Needs: Comfort. Protection from physical harm.

Gradually increase the amount of ventilator pressure   When artificial ventilation disturbs the person, use a very low pressure setting at first. After the patient is comfortable with that pressure, gradually increase it, keeping in mind individual pressure tolerances.

Rationale: Low-pressure ventilation offers comfort and slow adjustment to greater pressure settings.

Resolved Needs: Comfort.

Grant special requests   If the person wishes to have a particular favor granted, willingly offer to do it.

Rationale: Positive self-attitudes are reinforced by positive responses from others. Granting requests meets dependency needs.

Resolved Needs: Comfort. Dependency. High evaluation of self. Recognition. Dignity. Attention.

Guide the patient in simple prayer   If the patient is unable to pray, guide him in short meaningful prayer, such as: "My God, I offer You all my suffering," or "Thank you, Lord, for all your blessings," or "My God, I love you."

Rationale: Communication with God promotes comfort and understanding and fosters closer God-human relationships.

Resolved Needs: Comfort. Religious-philosophic satisfaction.

Handle gently   Move the patient's body slowly and carefully. Avoid jarring or sudden movements.

Rationale: Nerve fibers throughout skin layers convey pain impulses. The greater the external stimuli on nerve fibers, the greater the pain potential. Respect for the human body promotes dignity.

Resolved Needs: Comfort. Protection from physical harm. Freedom from pain. Dignity.

Hold the infant while feeding   While feeding, hold the infant in your arms so he feels contact with another human body. Elevate his head above his stomach.

Rationale: Head elevation above the stomach during feeding prevents food aspiration into the lungs. Human contact during infant feeding supports an association of love with food and promotes comfort.

Resolved Needs: Comfort. Protection from physical harm. Love and affection.

Hold the jaw forward to maintain an airway   Place three fingers behind the angle of the jaw and apply pressure upward on the jaw.

Rationale: Upward jaw movement brings the tongue forward and maintains an open airway.

Resolved Needs: Oxygen. Protection from physical harm.

Honor religious dietary regulations   Be certain that the patient's religious dietary regulations are met. Seek patient and family guidance in this matter.

Rationale: Religious observances assist man in spiritually expressing and outwardly recognizing his relationship with God.

Resolved Needs: Comfort. Dignity. Religious-philosophic satisfaction.

Ignore undesirable behavior   Refuse to take notice of undesirable behavior by acting as if it never occurred. Instead, satisfy the need for attention by noticing favorable behaviors.

Rationale: Self-esteem is acquired through acceptable sociocultural behavior. Ignoring undesirable behavior prevents diminished self-esteem which would result from social disapproval. It supports increased perception that attention cannot be acquired by socially unacceptable behavior.

Resolved Needs: Protection from psychologic threat. Increased reality perception.

Illuminate the room adequately   Provide suitable room lighting according to individual needs.

Rationale: Adequate lighting supports maximum visual acuity, decreases sensory misinterpretation, and promotes comfort. It meets dependency needs.

Resolved Needs: Comfort. Protection from physical harm. Protection from psychologic threat. Dependence.

Immobilize the affected body part   Stabilize the injured body area and the joints above and below the injury. Place the patient in the injury assumed position or in a comfortable position. When there is an existing or suspected spinal cord injury, place the patient on a firm board before transporting to medical services.

Rationale: Immobilization and support of a traumatized body area prevents further injury, possible circulation loss through vascular damage and decreases fluid loss in burns. It promotes rest and comfort.

Resolved Needs: Circulation. Rest. Comfort. Protection from physical harm.

Immunize against infectious disease (ExR)   Inject immunizing drugs into the body to bring about resistance to disease.

Rationale: Resistance against disease prevents needless suffering and maintains a healthier society.

Resolved Needs: Protection from physical harm.

Contraindications: Viral infections. Pregnancy. Special situations as stated in the drug brochures.

Incise and drain the wound (ExR)   Cut into the wound and drain infectious material from the tissue. Do so only after a well-defined area of pus has formed in the center of the lesion.

Rationale: Incision and drainage remove infected material from tissue which enhances the potential for healing and promotes comfort by relieving the pressure that caused the pain. If wounds are opened before the inflammatory process has walled off the infectious substance, drainage will increase the potential for the spread of infection.

Resolved Needs: Comfort. Cleanliness. Protection from physical harm.

Increase drafts   Increase the volume of air currents in the environment.

Rationale: Increased drafts decrease elevated body temperature by perspiration vaporization and promote comfort.

Resolved Needs: Normal temperature. Comfort.

Increase fluid intake according to weight loss   Weigh the person and increase his fluid intake 500 cc for each pound of weight lost on the previous day.

Rationale: A 1-pound weight loss in 24 hours is considered a 500 cc fluid loss.

Resolved Needs: Water-salt balance. Protection from physical harm.

Increase fluid intake to about 2000 cc daily   Increase the daily fluid intake to 2000 cc (eight 8-ounce glasses) or 500 cc above the normal daily requirement of 1500 cc. Fluids include water, fruit juice, Jello, Kool-Aid, tea, ginger ale, etc.

Rationale: Conditions of fever, excessive perspiration, dehydration due to vomiting or diarrhea require large fluid intake to replace fluid loss. Increased fluid intake moistens mucous membranes, dilutes chemical materials within the body which cause itching, distends a prolapsed bladder by helping to reestablish muscle tone, dilutes alcohol in the blood, reducing its effect, and promotes comfort.

Resolved Needs: Water-salt balance. Waste elimination. Normal temperature. Comfort. Protection from physical harm.

Contraindications: Edema. Ascites. Renal insufficiency or failure. Congestive heart failure.

Increase fluid intake to about 3000 cc daily   Increase the daily fluid intake to 3000 cc (twelve 8-ounce glasses of liquid). Fluids can include water, fruit juice, Jello, Kool-Aid, tea, ginger ale, etc.

Rationale: Effective urinary tract hydration prevents separation of calculi particles from solution, decreasing stone formation. Increased fluid intake assists in moving urinary calculi through and out of the urinary tract. It prevents burning on urination, dilutes ingested poisons, and reduces their effects. Fluid balance promotes comfort.

Resolved Needs: Water-salt balance. Waste elimination. Comfort. Protection from physical harm.

Contraindications: Edema. Ascites. Renal insufficiency or failure. Congestive heart failure.

Increase fluids at mealtime   Give an increased quantity of liquids with each meal.

Rationale: Saliva moistens food and aids swallowing. When saliva production is low, liquids can be substituted to moisten foods.

Resolved Needs: Comfort. Protection from physical harm.

Contraindications: Excessive flatulence. Postmeal diarrhea resulting from the dumping syndrome.

Increase the intravenous infusion flow rate   Raise the intravenous flow rate above the maintenance rate until the blood pressure reaches normal. Then return the flow rate to 60 drops per minute.

Rationale: When the blood volume is less than the volume of vascular space available for blood, circulation becomes inadequate, causing arteries to loose normal tone with resulting blood pressure drop and cardiac failure. Rapid replacement of fluid volume increases arterial tone, and the blood pressure returns to normal, supplying the heart with an adequate blood volume for tissue oxygenation. An output of less than 15–20 cc of urine per hour indicates more rapid fluid loss than replacement, and that normal fluid requirements are not being met.

Resolved Needs: Water-salt balance. Protection from physical harm.

Contraindications: Circulatory overload. When the output is more than 80 cc of urine per hour because of overhydration. Neurogenic or vasogenic shock. Renal failure.

Increase the physical distance between persons   Increase the physical distance between persons until nonverbal behavior (relaxation and decreased body motion) indicates comfort between them.

Rationale: Close physical proximity often makes interaction less effective because of tension produced by crowding. Satisfactory and respectful relationships with others promote comfort.

Resolved Needs: Comfort. Protection from psychologic threat. Dignity.

Increase the weaning time off therapeutic devices gradually   Gradually increase the time during which a patient is free of life-supporting measures or machines.

Rationale: Awareness that one can sustain his own life without supportive measures promotes comfort. Professional recognition of potential danger resulting from sudden, complete withdrawal of life-supporting measures promotes safety. Gradually increased self-dependency enhances self-reliance and adequacy, while reducing stress and anxiety.

Resolved Needs: Comfort. Protection from physical harm. Protection from psychologic threat. Adequacy. Self-reliance.

Indicate that difference is desirable Indicate both verbally and nonverbally that differences in persons and in opinions are good. Reveal that to be realistically unique and original shows maturity.

Rationale: A positive response from others indicates acceptance and promotes self-esteem. When differences are accepted, the person feels free to look at himself fearlessly and no longer feels restricted in growth.

Resolved Needs: Comfort. Acceptance. Sense of value. High evaluation of self. Personal growth and maturity. Less rigid conventiality.

Induce vomiting immediately Give an oral solution that causes vomiting, such as warm tap water, warm salt water (1 teaspoon salt to one-half glass water), mustard water (1 teaspoon mustard to one-half glass water), syrup of ipecac (15–20 cc given once and then repeated once 15 minutes later), or induce vomiting by inserting the finger down the throat. Note: If syrup of ipecac does not produce vomiting within 30 minutes, wash it out of the stomach.

Rationale: Vomiting removes poisons from the stomach.

Resolved Needs: Protection from physical harm.

Contraindications: Avoid inducing vomiting when caustic poisons have been ingested such as household ammonia, lye, washing soda or when oily preparations such as pine oil, kerosene, or gasoline are taken.

Inflate the airway tube cuff Inject air into the endotracheal or tracheostomy tube cuff until no breath escapes around the cuff. Then release the air slowly until a small leak occurs. Leave the cuff at this pressure or put enough air back into the cuff to stop the leak.

Rationale: Airway cuff inflation prevents air leakage during ventilation procedures and food aspiration during meals.

Resolved Needs: Protection from physical harm.

Initiate external cardiac massage (ET) Rhythmically compress the heart between the lower sternum and thoracic vertebrae.

Rationale: Rhythmic pressure over the sternum compresses the heart and reestablishes arterial circulation bringing oxygen to tissue cells.

Resolved Needs: Oxygen, Circulation. Protection from physical harm.

Insert a colon tube Place a short rectal tube into the colon through the anus about 4–5 inches.

Rationale: Colon tubes promote removal of irritating flatulence and prevent abdominal distention. When a ureterosigmoidostomy tube is in place, a colon tube keeps the rectosigmoid area empty, decreasing urinary leakage that may occur through anastomosis.

Resolved Needs: Waste elimination. Comfort. Protection from physical harm.

Contraindications: Rectal bleeding. Severe rectal irritation or pain. Do not insert a colon tube earlier than 1 week after perineal surgery. Fecal impaction. Diarrhea. Rectal stricture. Bradycardia. Cardiac arrythmias.

Insert a gastric tube and attach to suction (ET)

Pass a gastric tube through the nose, down the esophagus, and into the stomach. Anchor the tube at the nasal orifice to prevent tube movement or displacement. Attach to a suction machine.

Rationale: The insertion of a patent tube into the stomach permits withdrawal and analysis of stomach contents and relieves distention discomfort.

Resolved Needs: Waste elimination. Comfort. Protection from physical harm.

Insert a nasal airway

Place a soft, rubber nasal airway into the nostril. This is often used for comatose patients or conscious persons with facial trauma in whom ventilation is impaired.

Rationale: A nasal airway provides a patent airway into the pharynx and is tolerated more easily than the oral airway by conscious persons.

Resolved Needs: Oxygen. Comfort.

Insert a padded tongue blade

Place a wooden tongue blade, padded to a thickness equal to or greater than the tongue, between the upper and lower teeth on one side of the mouth. If a tongue blade is unavailable, use a substitute.

Rationale: Tongue blade insertion between the teeth prevents tongue tissue trauma when the teeth are involuntarily brought together.

Resolved Needs: Protection from physical harm.

Contraindications: When teeth are diseased and very fragile. When missing teeth reduce the stability of the remaining teeth so that tongue blade pressure might loosen the existing teeth. During a convulsive seizure while the jaw muscles already are contracted.

Insert an oiled cotton pledget into the ear

When an insect ventures into an ear, soak a cotton ball with a drop of oil and place it in the ear for a few seconds. Then, remove both the cotton and the immobilized insect. Chloroform may be used instead of oil.

Rationale: Oil prevents insect movement.

Resolved Needs: Comfort. Protection from physical harm.

Insert an oral airway Place an artificial airway device in the mouth, above the tongue, to maintain a clear air passage for respiratory gas exchange. If the patient has fragile teeth, use a rubber airway instead of the standard plastic type.

Rationale: Oxygen and carbon dioxide exchange through respirations is essential to tissue cell life. Oral airways frequently prevent biting on an endotracheal tube. A rubber airway prevents damage to fragile teeth.

Resolved Needs: Oxygen. Circulation. Waste elimination. Protection from physical harm.

Insert and remove the artificial eye To insert an artificial eye, pull down on the lower eyelid or use a suction cup and gently slip the eye into position. To remove an artificial eye, place gentle pressure below the eye, with the finger or suction cup, until the prosthesis slips out of its socket.

Rationale: Artificial eye insertion promotes comfort, prevents eye socket shrinkage, supports positive body image, and aids in dependency. Removal of the artificial eye permits prosthesis cleansing, offers protection against infection, and reduces eye orbit irritation.

Resolved Needs: Comfort. Cleanliness. Protection from physical harm. Dependence.

Contraindications (for Insertion): Eye socket irritation, inflammation, or infection.

Insert and remove the contact lens To insert a contact lens, pull the upper lid up and the lower lid down with the index finger and thumb of one hand. Moisten the contact lens with wetting solution. Place the outer surface of the lens on the tip of the index finger of the other hand and gently put the left lens on the left cornea and the right lens on the right cornea. Most right contact lens are identified by a black dot. In order to remove a contact lens from the cornea, open the person's eye. Pull the side of the eye (near the ear) outward with one hand. With the other hand, gently pull the lids together and the lens should pop out. Before attempting to remove a lens, be sure it is over the cornea. If it is not, gently close the eyelid and with very gentle pressure, move the lens toward the cornea. After removing the lens, be careful to place them in the lens case or in a safe container. Do not mix the right and left lens.

Rationale: Contact lens insertion promotes visual acuity essential to safety and comfort and aids in illness dependency. Prolonged wearing of contact lens may cause corneal injury.

Resolved Needs: Comfort. Cleanliness. Protection from physical harm. Dependence.

Contraindications (for Insertion): Eye irritation, inflammation, or infection. Do not insert if the person is confused, sedated, or likely to have his eyes closed for a prolonged period.

Insert and remove the dentures   Place the person's artificial teeth in his mouth if he is unable to do so. Take the patient's artificial teeth out of his mouth at appropriate times.

Rationale: Artificial teeth aid in chewing and digestion, maintain natural jaw contour, promote comfort and dignity through a pleasant appearance, and aid in illness dependency. Removal of artificial teeth allows for denture cleansing and oral hygiene.

Resolved Needs: Food balance. Comfort. Cleanliness. Protection from physical harm. Dependence. Dignity.

Contraindications (for Insertion):   Oral mucosa irritation. Gum inflammation and infection. When persons are comatose, confused, or helpless. When there is the possibility of vomiting.

Instill warm oil into the ear   Drop a small amount of warm olive oil or mineral oil into the ear.

Rationale: Warm oil relieves ear dryness, soothes ear pain, softens hardened earwax, and smothers insects that fly into the ear.

Resolved Needs: Comfort. Protection from physical harm.

Contraindications: Perforated eardrum. Evidence of ear infection.

Insulate exposed pacemaker electrodes   Insulate bare pacemaker wires by holding them with a rubber-gloved hand or placing the generator box in a rubber glove.

Rationale: Rubber insulates electric current and promotes safety.

Resolved Needs: Protection from physical harm.

Introduce irrigating solutions slowly   When introducing solution into a body opening, minimize the pressure of solution flow by maintaining a slow flow rate.

Rationale: Pressure prevention promotes comfort and reduces the potential for tissue injury from rapid organ distention.

Resolved Needs: Comfort. Protection from physical harm.

Introduce one anxiety situation at a time   When the patient is facing several stressful situations, assist in scheduling them one at a time. If x-ray studies are scheduled for one day, delay instructions on colostomy care until the next day. If the patient is in pain, withhold unfavorable news until the pain subsides.

Rationale: Meeting one stressful situation at a time reduces the degree of physical and emotional adaptation and promotes comfort.

Resolved Needs: Comfort. Protection from physical harm. Protection from psychologic threat.

Introduce the patient to replacement personnel before an impending separation   Gradually bring the therapeutic relationship to a close by notifying the patient of the impending separation and by introducing him to the person who will take your place.

Rationale: Gradual changes decrease adaptation stress. Psychologic comfort is promoted from predictable situations.

Resolved Needs: Comfort. Protection from psychologic threat. Predictable, orderly world.

Introduce to persons who have successfully undergone the same experience   Acquaint the person who is threatened with an unsafe situation with someone who successfully encountered the same experience.

Rationale: Feelings of safety increase through identification with persons who have successfully met the same situation.

Resolved Needs: Comfort. Protection from psychologic threat.

Involve multiple staff members in limited patient contact   Involve all staff members in limited contact with the patient while still maintaining an attitude of concern.

Rationale: Limited contact with a number of persons promotes safety through emotional noninvolvement with each. When many people attend to one person's needs, that person gains a feeling of importance.

Resolved Needs: Comfort. Protection from psychologic threat. Importance.

Involve the family   Include the patient's family or other significant persons in as much planning and care as possible. Keep them continuously informed of all happenings. Verbalize to the patient their participation in his care.

Rationale: Family members experience fear and anxiety from lack of factual information and noninvolvement in the care of their loved ones. The involvement of loved ones reassures the patient that he will be cared for. Encouraging families to care for their own provides the opportunity for expressions of love. When guilt exists, it helps the family member make amends for past misdeeds or omissions.

Resolved Needs: Comfort. Protection from physical harm. Protection from psychologic threat. Unity with loved ones.

Irrigate the eye   Instill isotonic sterile saline at body temperature into the eye and allow it to flow gently over the eye tissue, escaping from the outer canthus.

Rationale: Irrigations have cleansing and antiseptic effects which minimize infection. They promote comfort by reducing pain through solution warmth.

Resolved Needs: Comfort. Cleanliness. Protection from physical harm.

Irrigate the foreign particle with alcohol   Instill an alcohol solution, warmed to body temperature, into the ear containing a foreign object.

Rationale: Objects that absorb water swell and, when located in a small body orifice, obstruct the opening. Alcohol prevents swelling.

Resolved Needs: Comfort. Protection from physical harm.

Contraindications: Perforated eardrum.

Irrigate the gastric tube with saline   Introduce 10–30 cc of normal saline into the gastric tube after releasing it from the suction apparatus. Gently inject the solution and aspirate the same amount.

Rationale: Gastric tube irrigation assures patency, facilitates removal of gastric contents by suction, and prevents abdominal distention. Irrigation of a gastric tube with saline prevents chloride loss that would occur from the use of hypotonic fluid (water).

Resolved Needs: Water-salt balance. Protection from physical harm.

Irrigate the nose   Gently introduce small amounts of warm sodium bicarbonate, normal saline, or other solution into one nostril. Have the patient open his mouth, allowing the return fluid to flow out.

Rationale: Nasal irrigation cleanses infected tissue while the warm solution promotes comfort.

Resolved Needs: Comfort. Cleanliness. Protection from physical harm.

Irrigate the urinary catheter   Introduce 50 cc of sterile saline or other solution into an indwelling urinary catheter at periodic intervals. Allow the solution to return by gravity flow.

Rationale: A patent catheter facilitates urine flow from the bladder and promotes comfort.

Resolved Needs: Waste elimination. Comfort. Protection from physical harm.

Contraindications: It is not necessary to irrigate a Silastic catheter since they are designed to prevent residue from attaching itself to the catheter.

Irrigate the wound   Flush a wound with a sterile saline or other solution until the tissue appears clean and free from harmful debris.

Rationale: Wound irrigations promote comfort and healing by cleansing tissue and removing foreign particles.

Resolved Needs: Comfort. Cleanliness. Protection from physical harm.

Isolate infected persons   When a person is infected with a contagious disease, restrict him to the confines of his home or, if traveling, detain him from entering the country.

Rationale: Pathogen transfer from person to person is decreased through limited human contact.

Resolved Needs: Protection from physical harm.

Isolate persons exposed to communicable disease
When a person has been exposed to a communicable disease, but has not contracted the disease, restrict him to the confines of his home or, if traveling, detain him from entering the country.

Rationale: Pathogen transfer from person to person is decreased through limited human contact.

Resolved Needs: Protection from physical harm.

Keep the drainage container below bladder (chest, stomach, nephrostomy, or t-tube) level
Keep the drainage container below the level of the tube insertion site. If the container must be moved to a level higher than the tube insertion site, the drainage tubing should be clamped off securely so fluid cannot flow backward.

Rationale: The backflow of drainage into an internal organ site would cause pressure on the organ resulting in tissue drainage or organ collapse. The backflow of drainage contaminated with bacteria poses the threat of infection.

Resolved Needs: Protection from physical harm.

Keep the hyperalimentation tube patent with 5% dextrose in water
If the hyperalimentation infusion runs dry, add 5% dextrose in water to keep the subclavian catheter patent. Remove all air bubbles and run the D5W until another bottle of hyperalimentation solution is available.

Rationale: A clotted subclavian Intracath has to be replaced, causing the patient unnecessary pain. Air embolus allowed to flow into the subclavian vein can prove fatal.

Resolved Needs: Comfort. Protection from physical harm.

Keep the patient's door closed
Protect the person from environmental stimuli and exposure to other persons by keeping the door to his room closed.

Rationale: Comfort and safety feelings are increased when privacy is respected. Doors act as barriers to noise and reduce noise level.

Resolved Needs: Comfort. Protection from physical harm. Protection from psychologic threat. Dignity.

Keep the patient's door open
Keep the door to the person's room open to increase exposure to external stimuli and to afford the patient an opportunity to investigate the world outside his room.

Rationale: External stimuli increases sensory perception.

Resolved Needs: Stimulation. Increased reality perception.

Keep the patient's windows closed Protect the person from environmental discomforts and stimuli by keeping the windows in his area closed.

Rationale: Closed windows keep out pollen that causes hypersensitivity reactions or weather elements that cause discomfort. Windows act as a barrier to noise and reduce the noise level.

Resolved Needs: Rest. Comfort. Protection from physical harm.

Keep treatment equipment out of sight Keep treatment equipment out of sight of the person on whom it has been or will be used. Also keep it out of sight of visitors if the presence of the equipment causes embarrassment for the patient. Genitourinary bags can be covered with a sheet, etc.

Rationale: Equipment previously associated with pain or discomfort can serve as emotional stimuli for anxiety. Equipment kept out of sight of visitors protects the patient from the embarrassment of being exposed when in a position of social disadvantage.

Resolved Needs: Comfort. Protection from psychologic threat.

Lavage the stomach (ET) Insert a nasogastric tube into the stomach, and wash out the stomach contents with water or normal saline. Instill no more than 300 cc of the solution in an adult stomach at one time.

Rationale: Gastric lavage removes substances harmful to the gastric mucosa or general body systems.

Resolved Needs: Protection from physical harm.

Lay the drying cast on pillows While the cast is wet, do not lay it on a hard bed surface. Instead, place soft, fluffy pillows under the wet cast.

Rationale: A wet cast placed on a hard surface will become flattened over bony prominences with the resulting pressure causing decreased circulation to tissues enclosed in the cast.

Resolved Needs: Comfort. Protection from physical harm.

Lift the drying cast with the palms of the hand When raising a wet cast off a flat surface, pull upward with the entire palm of your hand, not with your fingers.

Rationale: Finger indentations in soft plaster change the cast's shape and, through pressure, decrease circulation to tissues enclosed in the cast.

Resolved Needs: Protection from physical harm.

Lift with a hydraulic hoist Raise the patient off a flat surface using a hydraulic hoist.

Rationale: The use of a hydraulic hoist for lifting provides even body distribution, limited pressure on cutaneous nerves, and aids in illness dependency.

Resolved Needs: Comfort. Protection from physical harm. Dependence.

Limit blood pressure cuff inflation to a few moments   As soon as the blood pressure cuff is inflated, immediately read the monometer and release the cuff pressure. If the reading needs rechecking, wait until the cuff is completely depressurized and wait for a period of 2 minutes before repeating the procedure.

Rationale: Pressure prevention in any body area promotes comfort. Keeping the blood pressure cuff inflated or reinflating the cuff before completely emptying it causes vasomotor changes that give a false blood pressure reading.

Resolved Needs: Comfort. Protection from physical harm.

Limit communication to one person at a time   When a patient has impaired message reception or delivery, allow only one person at a time to communicate verbally with the patient.

Rationale: The reception and interpretation of messages is enhanced by nondistracting environmental influences. Psychologic comfort is promoted through a sense of effective communications with others.

Resolved Needs: Comfort. Warm, communicating relationships.

Limit conversation to short discussions   When speaking to a person who has impaired message reception or delivery, limit the conversation to short uninvolved discussions.

Rationale: Simple and direct communications enhance perception and reduce the threat of frustration and anxiety. Comfort is promoted through effective communications with others.

Resolved Needs: Comfort. Warm, communicating relationships.

Limit excessive demands   Curtail the requirements the patient places on the nursing staff. Explain that staff assistance is available, but that demands must be reasonable. Explore with the patient his reasons for excessive demands and respond appropriately.

Rationale: External control of behavior supports internal control when the latter cannot be maintained independently. Comfort is promoted through the ability to effectively communicate one's needs. Limitations protect against future shame resulting from presently uncontrolled behavior.

Resolved Needs: Comfort. Protection from psychologic threat. Increased reality perception and problem-solving ability.

Limit infant crying by feeding on schedule and immediately changing soiled diapers   Reduce the infant's crying to an absolute

minimum by providing food on or before the schedule and by changing the diaper just as soon as it is soiled.

Rationale: Infant crying increases intracranial pressure, depletes energy needed for healing, and places a strain on already painful areas.

Resolved Needs: Energy. Comfort. Protection from physical harm.

Limit IPPB treatments to short periods   If artificial ventilation disturbs the person, refrain from lengthy treatments. Administer the first few treatments only so long as the patient is comfortable and remove the ventilator during patient discomfort.

Rationale: Short treatment periods promote comfort and support adjustment to longer treatments.

Resolved Needs: Comfort.

Contraindications: Acute or life-threatening respiratory distress.

Limit patient use of the telephone   Do not allow persons who have difficulty with message reception or delivery to use the telephone.

Rationale: Persons experiencing asphasic conditions only can understand tone over the telephone and receive little of the message being delivered. The inability to see the other person also impairs message reception and heightens anxiety. Fear that others will hang up if silence occurs on the telephone causes excitement and confusion in the asphasic person.

Resolved Needs: Comfort. Protection from psychologic threat.

Limit the amount of time visitors are exposed to radiation   When a patient receives radium implants or other radioactive substances emitting gamma rays, limit the time that relatives and friends stay with the patient. Exposure to radiation over a year should not exceed 5 rads or 5000 millirads. In 1 hour of contact, the exposed person will receive 20 millirads. It is recommended that a person receive no more than 10 millirads a day. This means that radiation exposure should not exceed 30 minutes a day.

Rationale: Body exposure to radioactive substances results in blood cell disturbances, sterility, internal burns, genetic changes, gastrointestinal upsets, and altered tissue cell structure.

Resolved Needs: Protection from physical harm.

Limit the distance from which visitors approach the radiated patient   When a patient receives radium implants or other radioactive substances emitting gamma rays, limit relatives and friends to a distance of at least 3 feet from the patient, but as far away as possible. Each time the distance is doubled (from 2 to 4 feet, 4 to 8 feet, 8 to 16 feet), the radiation intensity is cut by one-quarter.

Rationale: The rate of radiation exposure decreases as the square of the distance from the radiated patient increases. Body exposure to radioactive substances results in blood cell disturbances, sterility, internal burns, genetic changes, gastrointestinal upsets, and altered tissue cell structure.

Resolved Needs: Protection from physical harm.

Limit the patient's mobility distance
Limit the area in which the patient moves about to one in which nursing supervision is possible.

Rationale: Supervision of health disorders promotes safety.

Resolved Needs: Protection from physical harm.

Limit the therapeutic oxygen concentration to below 40%
Do not allow patients, especially premature infants, to receive oxygen concentrations above 40% over prolonged periods.

Rationale: High oxygen concentrations cause spasms of the retinal vessels. This leads to blood and serum filtration through the vessel walls into the retinal tissue with resulting blindness.

Resolved Needs: Protection from physical harm.

Limit the touching of suspicious persons
Avoid close physical contact with the person, especially skin contact.

Rationale: Suspicious persons frequently feel threatened by touch because of misinterpretations of the social meaning of personal contact. They may feel that touch is an invasion of privacy, or that it has evil connotations.

Resolved Needs: Protection from psychologic threat.

Limit visitors
Control the persons and number of persons who visit, especially during acute illness.

Rationale: Visitor limitations provide rest and comfort, reduce stress, and conserve energy for healing which would be used for socialization. Infected visitors should stay away from other ill persons.

Resolved Needs: Rest. Energy. Comfort. Protection from physical harm. Protection from psychologic threat.

Listen attentively
Listen with full attention to the message being communicated and observe for the full meaning of the message.

Rationale: Attentive listening conveys sufficient recognition and respect for a person to warrant the use of another's valuable time. It also supports feeling ventilation.

Resolved Needs: Comfort. Warm, communicating relationships. Sense of value. Recognition. Dignity. Attention. Increased reality perception and problem-solving ability.

Lubricate the external nares
Moisten the external nares with small amounts of petrolatum, mineral oil, baby oil, or lotion.

Rationale: External nares lubrication softens crusted exudate, prevents nasal irritation from intubation, and promotes comfort.

Resolved Needs: Comfort. Cleanliness. Protection from physical harm.

Contraindications: Do not use when there is danger that the patient might aspirate the oils.

Lubricate the eye(s)
Instill one drop of sterile mineral oil into each eye.

Rationale: Mineral oil instillation into the eye prevents loss of visual acuity due to eye tissue dryness.

Resolved Needs: Comfort. Protection from physical harm.

Lubricate the lips
Apply petrolatum, cocoa butter, mineral oil, baby oil, or lanolin to the lips.

Rationale: The emollient effect of lubrication promotes comfort by softening and soothing the skin and preventing cracking and drying.

Resolved Needs: Comfort. Protection from physical harm.

Lubricate the skin with baby oil, bath oil, or body lotion
Apply a thin coating of baby oil, bath oil, or body lotion to the skin. Use only on intact skin.

Rationale: The lubricating effect of baby oil, bath oil, or body lotion promotes comfort by soothing the skin and preventing cracking and drying.

Resolved Needs: Comfort. Protection from physical harm.

Contraindications: Do not use on skin that remains wet from perspiration, such as when the patient is lying on a bed covered with a plastic mattress cover. Do not use in skin folds, such as under the breast. Avoid using when there is a known allergic response.

Lubricate the skin with cocoa butter, glycerine, lanolin, mineral oil, or olive oil
Apply a thin coating of cocoa butter, glycerine, lanolin, mineral oil, or olive oil to the skin. Use moderately on inflamed eruptions or in areas of poor circulation such as the skin over varicose veins. Glycerine is most effective when diluted with water or applied after the skin has been moistened with water.

Rationale: Emollients promote comfort by softening and soothing the skin. They are less drying than lotions because they retard water evaporation from the skin, while preventing cracking and drying. When applied following removal of a cast, they loosen crusting and dead skin residue.

Resolved Needs: Comfort. Protection from physical harm.

Contraindications: Avoid using on oozing or weeping eruptions. Do not use in skin folds or when there is a known allergic response.

Lubricate the skin with petrolatum Apply to the skin a transparent, fatlike substance obtained from petroleum (petrolatum). Use on areas of long-term, mild inflammation or eruption, and on scaling skin. It is more effective on open skin than on skin folds.

Rationale: Petrolatum produces a soothing, comforting effect. It has a neutral (neither acid or alkaline) effect and prevents skin drying or cracking. It softens scales by retarding moisture evaporation from the skin.

Resolved Needs: Comfort. Protection from physical harm.

Maintain a clean environment Remove all dust and dirt particles from the immediate surroundings.

Rationale: Dust and dirt particles irritate mucous membranes and carry microorganisms. The reduction of irritating environmental factors promotes comfort and assists in illness dependency.

Resolved Needs: Comfort. Cleanliness. Protection from physical harm. Dependence.

Maintain a cool room temperature Keep the room temperature at about 65°F.

Rationale: A cool room temperature decreases environmental heat surrounding the body and increases heat loss to the environment, promoting decreased or normal body temperature. It assists in maintaining fluid and electrolyte balance because of the reduced need for perspiration cooling. It decreases oxygen and energy consumption since the body's metabolic requirements are lower than in warm surroundings. In states of shock, a cool environment helps maintain peripheral vasoconstriction which supports adequate blood supply to vital organs.

Resolved Needs: Water-salt balance. Normal temperature. Energy. Comfort. Protection from physical harm.

Maintain a normal room temperature Keep the room temperature between 68–72°F.

Rationale: Normal environmental temperature promotes comfort by reducing the body's stress and adaptation requirements to temperature extremes. It prevents burn crusts from softening and separating as would occur in an excessively warm room.

Resolved Needs: Normal temperature. Comfort. Protection from physical harm.

Maintain a warm room temperature Keep the room temperature between 75–78°F. In premature nurseries, maintain the temperature at 80°F.

Rationale: A warm room temperature increases environmental heat surrounding the body, decreases heat lost to the environment and raises the body temperature. Premature infants require warmth because they cannot maintain body heat due to lack of insulating skin fat, poor reflex control of skin capillaries, and small muscle inactivity. A warm room reduces chilling, often responsible for urinary frequency, bedwetting or muscle spasm.

Resolved Needs: Normal temperature. Comfort. Protection from physical harm.

Contraindications: Fever. Oxygen deficiency. Shock. Increased metabolic rate.

Maintain adequate atmospheric humidity Keep the air moisture
between 40–50% by regulating the room humidifier. In premature nurseries, maintain the humidity at between 55–65%.

Rationale: Normal air humidity supports normal lung production of moisture. A higher than normal humidity for premature infants decreases their tendency toward dehydration which is often responsible for weight loss and body temperature instability. Atmospheric humidity at 40–50% prevents burn crusts from cracking. Adequate atmospheric humidity reduces crusting of nasal mucosa, especially in perforated nasal septum.

Resolved Needs: Water-salt balance. Normal temperature. Comfort. Protection from physical harm.

Maintain adequate room ventilation Inquire as to the amount of
fresh air preferred by the person and maintain the desired ventilation. Provide sufficient air movement to remove stagnant air.

Rationale: Pleasant environmental factors promote comfort. Cool room ventilation helps maintain normal body temperature and refreshes the air. Adequate air currents ventilating a room remove discomforting odors and infectious agents. Attending to room ventilation offers assistance in illness dependency.

Resolved Needs: Normal temperature. Comfort. Protection from physical harm. Dependence.

Maintain alignment of the drying cast through positioning While a newly applied cast is still wet, turn the patient on the
uncasted body side to decrease the pressure placed on the cast.

Rationale: Lack of pressure on a drying cast prevents misshaping of the cast that could constrict circulation to tissues enclosed in the cast.

Resolved Needs: Protection from physical harm.

Maintain body alignment Position and support the extremities, head,
and other body parts in a normal line of function or in a therapeutic position. For example: When a person is lying on his back (supine), support his knees in a slightly flexed position to prevent hyperextension of the knees. When he is lying on his abdomen (prone), support his ankles and shins to prevent plantar flexion of his feet. When he is lying on his side, support the upper leg and arm with pillows to prevent internal rotation of the hip and shoulder joints. When a fracture of the neck is known or suspected, main-

tain the neck in a straight line (neither flexed nor extended) while transporting to the hospital. When an extremity is in traction, maintain the same alignment that was established when the traction was applied (or adjusted).

Rationale: Functional body alignment promotes circulation and comfort, helps prevent joint deformities, painful stretching or shortening of tendons, and further damage to vital tissues by fractured bones. Nonfunctional or therapeutic alignment of extremities in traction may be necessary to hold the fractured bone pieces in position for healing.

Resolved Needs: Circulation. Comfort. Protection from physical harm.

Maintain consistent staff behavior Demonstrate staff behavior that remains constant in attitude and performance. Avoid discrepancy between the spoken word and actions.

Rationale: Safety feelings and confidence in others increase when consistent and predictable attitudes and behaviors are demonstrated by others.

Resolved Needs: Comfort. Protection from psychologic threat. Predictable, orderly world.

Maintain countertraction force Maintain a constant equal pull in two opposing directions while the patient is in traction. When there is an upper extremity fracture, the countertraction force is maintained by the patient's body weight and friction against the bed. When there is a lower extremity fracture, the countertraction is maintained by the patient's body weight and may be increased by elevating the foot of the bed.

Rationale: Countertraction helps maintain proper direction and force of the applied traction.

Resolved Needs: Protection from physical harm.

Maintain dry, clean linen Immediately change wet linen and replace with clean, dry linen. Frequently check for wet linens where there is incontinence or profuse drainage.

Rationale: Any wet substance in prolonged contact with the skin may damage or irritate the skin. Maintaining clean, dry linens promotes comfort and aids in illness dependency.

Resolved Needs: Comfort. Cleanliness. Protection from physical harm. Dependence.

Maintain dry skin When the skin becomes wet from perspiration, discharges, or excretions, remove such substances with mild soap and water, and dry the skin thoroughly. Frequently check for wet skin where there is incontinence or profuse drainage. Immediately after hot pack or ice bag applications, dry the wet or damp skin.

Rationale: Any wet substance in prolonged contact with the skin may damage or irritate the skin. Maintaining a dry skin surface promotes cleanliness and comfort and aids in illness dependency.

Resolved Needs: Comfort. Cleanliness. Protection from physical harm. Dependence.

Maintain honesty   Maintain truthfulness at all times in interpersonal relationships.

Rationale: Psychologic threat results from dishonest interpersonal relationships. When a person is viewed as trustworthy, satisfying interpersonal relationships are enhanced.

Resolved Needs: Comfort. Protection from psychologic threat. Warm, communicating relationships.

Maintain hot bath water   While a bed bath is in progress, check the bath water every 10 minutes. If it becomes cool, replace with warm water.

Rationale: Coldness disturbs skin receptors while warmth promotes comfort. Providing bath water assists in illness dependency.

Resolved Needs: Comfort. Dependence.

Maintain isolation technique   Carry out precautionary measures to prevent the spread of infectious conditions. These include wearing a gown and mask, maintaining room cleanliness, disinfecting clothing, linens, dishes, etc.

Rationale: Isolation technique minimizes the contact of noninfected persons with the bacteria present in infected persons, reducing infection transmission.

Resolved Needs: Protection from physical harm.

Maintain patient wakefulness during the day   During the day, periodically awaken the patient despite a possible annoyance response from him. Keep him awake until his normal bedtime hour.

Rationale: Reestablishing normal sleeping hours promotes the comfort of sound nighttime sleep. Maintaining wakefulness throughout the day maintains stimulation and reduces withdrawal.

Resolved Needs: Sleep, rest. Comfort. Stimulation.

Maintain reverse isolation   Approach persons highly susceptible to infection only when wearing a mask and gown and after thorough hand-washing.

Rationale: Pathogen transfer from person to person decreases through the protective shield of a gown, mask, and hand-washing. During periods of high infection susceptibility, resistance is very low and could result in severe or fatal infectious conditions. Reverse isolation protects the ill person from exposure to bacteria carried by the health staff, family, and visitors.

Resolved Needs: Protection from physical harm.

Maintain silence Maintain a state of silence when the person indicates the need or when attempting to promote conversation in another.

Rationale: When the patient indicates a need for silence as an adaptive mechanism, maintaining such fosters feelings of safety. When attempting to promote therapeutic conversation, remaining silent often makes the person so uncomfortable that he will initiate conversation to relieve the discomfort.

Resolved Needs: Comfort. Protection from psychologic threat. Warm, communicating relationships.

Maintain social formality Contribute attitudes toward an interpersonal relationship that indicate respectful, psychologic distance and restraint.

Rationale: External attempts to remove psychologic defenses increases anxiety. Awareness of esteem from others results from satisfactory and respectful relationships with others.

Resolved Needs: Protection from psychologic threat. Dignity.

Maintain social informality Contribute attitudes toward an interpersonal relationship that indicate freedom and ease in communication.

Rationale: Relief of rigid social standards decreases fear and anxiety by reducing tension. Comfort is promoted through effective communication with others.

Resolved Needs: Comfort. Protection from psychologic threat. Warm, communicating relationships. Less rigid conventionality.

Maintain the usual bedtime rituals Ask the person about the rituals he performs before going to sleep and see that these rituals are carried out. Presleep rituals include such activities as drinking a glass of milk, tucking sheets a certain way, using special blankets or pillows, saying nighttime prayers.

Rationale: Customary rituals before sleep promote relaxation. Adequate sleep is essential to restore depleted cell energy.

Resolved Needs: Sleep, rest, relaxation. Energy. Comfort. Protection from physical harm.

Maintain wrinkle-free sheets Keep the bed sheets smooth, flat, and without wrinkles.

Rationale: Wrinkled sheets cause pressure on and irritation of skin surfaces with resulting tissue trauma and discomfort. Providing wrinkle-free sheets offers assistance in illness dependency.

Resolved Needs: Comfort. Protection from physical harm. Dependence.

Make a referral When certain needs can be met by an allied health agency or individual, write or call the agency or individual and make arrangements for the patient to benefit from the services offered.

Rationale: Community resources often provide health care not available in other health agencies. They often support sound approaches to problem solving and may be a resource for developing potential, independence, and self-reliance.

Resolved Needs: Comfort. Protection from physical harm. Protection from psychologic threat. Self-reliance. Independence. Increased reality perception and problem-solving ability. Full development of potential.

Contraindications: Medical referrals are the prerogative of the physician.

Massage bony prominences   Rhythmically stimulate and manipulate body areas having prominent bony structures. Such areas include the heels, ankles, knees, iliac crest, scapula and clavicle, wrists, elbows, chin, nose, ear pinna, and sacrum.

Rationale: Prolonged pressure of bone against skin results in decreased area circulation with increased susceptibility to irritation, necrosis, and discomfort. Stimulation of these areas promotes circulation which prevents tissue damage.

Resolved Needs: Circulation. Comfort. Stimulation. Protection from physical harm.

Contraindications: Circulatory thrombus. Severe circulatory impairment.

Massage gently   With rhythmic gentle stroking, manipulate the body muscles in appropriate areas, producing a soothing effect. Use either alcohol or an emollient preparation.

Rationale: Gentle massage promotes muscle relaxation, stimulates circulation, conditions the skin, relieves muscle tension, and produces relaxation of nerve fibers which relieves pain. Gentle massage stimulates flow of breast milk. During labor, gentle circular strokes over the abdomen are used as a diversional method to ease labor pain.

Resolved Needs: Circulation. Sleep, rest, relaxation. Comfort. Protection from physical harm. Freedom from pain.

Contraindications: Do not massage extremities (especially calves) in the presence of thrombi and any tissue with seriously impaired circulation. Avoid massaging where there is spinal cord injury with the potential for nerve damage.

Massage the infant's gums   With one finger, gently rub the infant's gum surface.

Rationale: Gum massage promotes circulation and reduces pain.

Resolved Needs: Circulation. Comfort.

Massage the uterine fundus   Place your hand on the patient's ab-

domen, grasp the body of the uterus and externally massage by applying moderate pressure.

Rationale: Uterine fundus massage reduces hemorrhage.

Resolved Needs: Protection from physical harm.

Contraindications: Avoid uterine massage if the fundus is firm.

Massage vigorously   Using rhythmic, strong strokes, manipulate muscular tissue to produce an invigorating effect.

Rationale: Vigorous muscular stroking greatly increases circulation and promotes comfort and stimulation.

Resolved Needs: Circulation. Comfort. Stimulation. Protection from physical harm.

Contraindications: Circulatory thrombus. Severe circulatory impairment. Emotional overstimulation.

Minimize environmental barriers   Decrease to a minimum objects in the way of the person attempting mobility. This entails moving furniture to its most efficient and nonobstructive position.

Rationale: The removal of mobility barriers enhances freedom of movement, reduces injury potential, aids in illness dependency, and promotes the comfort of successful coping. Short or tall persons frequently are confronted with environmental barriers unknown to average height persons.

Resolved Needs: Energy. Comfort. Protection from physical harm. Dependence.

Minimize environmental dangers   Keep harmful objects out of the patient's reach. These include objects such as knives, cleaning fluids, matches, glass objects.

Rationale: The removal of potential danger prevents illness, injury, and disease. It aids in safeguarding dependent persons.

Resolved Needs: Protection from physical harm. Dependence.

Mobilize by invalid chair   Help the person to move about by placing him in a high-back padded chair with wheels. The invalid chair can be folded out like a stretcher should the person become tired.

Rationale: Moving about reduces pulmonary fluid congestion, stimulates circulation, restores normal physiologic function, promotes comfort and independence, and aids in illness dependency.

Resolved Needs: Circulation. Activity, exercise. Comfort. Protection from physical harm. Dependence. Independence.

Contraindications: Unstabilized head or spinal cord injury. Internal hemorrhage. Coma or semicoma. Temperature above 103°F. Any life-threatening situation.

Mobilize by stretcher   Help the person to move about by placing him in a prone position on a stretcher and have him propel himself about using the wheels of the stretcher.

Rationale: Moving about reduces pulmonary fluid congestion, stimulates circulation, restores normal physiologic function, promotes comfort and independence, and aids in illness dependency.

Resolved Needs: Circulation. Activity, exercise. Comfort. Protection from physical harm. Dependence. Independence.

Contraindications: Severe energy depletion.

Mobilize by walker   Help the person to move about by providing a supportive frame within which he can walk.

Rationale: Moving about reduces pulmonary fluid congestion, stimulates circulation, restores normal physiologic function, promotes comfort and independence, and aids in illness dependency.

Resolved Needs: Circulation. Activity, exercise. Comfort. Protection from physical harm. Dependence. Independence.

Contraindications: Severe energy depletion.

Mobilize by wheelchair   Help the person to move about by placing him in a wheelchair. When able, encourage him to propel himself about.

Rationale: Moving about reduces pulmonary fluid congestion, stimulates circulation, restores normal physiologic function, promotes comfort and independence, and aids in illness dependency.

Resolved Needs: Circulation. Activity, exercise. Comfort. Protection from physical harm. Dependence. Independence.

Contraindications: Unstabilized head or spinal cord injury. Internal hemorrhage. Coma or semicoma. Temperature above 103°F. Any life-threatening situation.

Mobilize with a cane   Help the person to move about by providing a cane while walking.

Rationale: Moving about reduces pulmonary fluid congestion, stimulates circulation, restores normal physiologic function, promotes comfort and independence, and aids in illness dependency.

Resolved Needs: Circulation. Activity, exercise. Comfort. Protection from physical harm. Dependence. Independence.

Contraindications: Severe energy depletion. Impaired body balance.

Moisten the dressing before removal   When a dressing becomes dried onto or encrusted around a wound, soak the dressing with sterile normal saline before removing.

Rationale: Moistening a dressing before removal minimizes tissue trauma and bleeding and reduces pain and discomfort.

Resolved Needs: Comfort. Protection from physical harm. Freedom from pain.

Moisten the hair with conditioning formula
Use conditioner on the hair shafts following shampoo.

Rationale: Conditioning solutions replace hair oils for maintenance of healthy, untraumatized hair shafts.

Resolved Needs: Comfort. Protection from physical harm. Dependence.

Moisten the mouth with cracked ice
Moisten the lips and mouth with ice chips. Do so according to fluid intake allowance and restrictions. Include ice chips on the fluid intake record.

Rationale: The coolness and wetness of ice refreshes, soothes, and comforts the lips and mouth without significantly increasing fluid intake.

Resolved Needs: Comfort.

Move the entire body as a single unit
When turning or moving the patient's body, use four persons to move the body as a whole unit. Maintain complete support of the total body area.

Rationale: Moving the body as a single unit prevents pressure on any particular body area and reduces the potential for injury.

Resolved Needs: Protection from physical harm.

Move the entire cast as a single unit
When turning or moving a casted body part, move the cast and the body part involved as one whole unit. Maintain complete support of the total area.

Rationale: Complete support of a traumatized body part prevents further injury and maintains a healing position. It prevents sudden, uncontrollable movements of the part caused by excessive cast weight.

Resolved Needs: Comfort. Protection from physical harm.

Name the patient's present location frequently during periods of disorientation
Acquaint the person with the environment by telling him where he is presently located. Specifically include the state, city, street, and name and location of the building.

Rationale: The ability to comprehend one's environment with regard to time, place, and person identity helps restore orientation.

Resolved Needs: Protection from psychologic threat. Increased reality perception.

Notify the family of the patient's room change
When a patient is moved from one room to another, immediately notify the family of the change.

Rationale: Fear and anxiety result from lack of information. Families coming into a loved one's empty room often think the worst.

Resolved Needs: Comfort. Protection from psychologic threat.

Obtain feedback of the communicated message   Have the listener repeat the message he received.

Rationale: Feedback of messages clarifies the extent to which the original idea was correctly received. Comfort is promoted through effective communications with others.

Resolved Needs: Protection from physical harm. Protection from psychologic threat. Warm, communicating relationships.

Obtain permission for procedures   Before performing a therapeutic procedure or nursing care, ask the patient or family if such activities are favorable with them.

Rationale: Comfort and independence are enhanced by having sufficient control to prevent harm to one's self and through respectful relationships with others.

Resolved Needs: Comfort. Protection from psychologic threat. Independence. Dignity.

Offer assurance of other measures if the pain-relief method fails   After administering pain relief, assure the patient that if the present measure fails, other measures are available.

Rationale: An awareness that pain can be terminated decreases pain intensity by relieving tension produced by the anxiety of pain anticipation.

Resolved Needs: Comfort. Protection from psychologic threat.

Offer assurance that decisions are revokable   Point out that a decision is not necessarily a final, unchangeable determination. Decisions can be altered by the person, and at times, external forces alter decisions.

Rationale: Awareness that decisions are revokable reduces anxiety and promotes comfort.

Resolved Needs: Comfort. Protection from psychologic threat.

Offer assurance that return visits are acceptable despite termination of the therapeutic relationship   Gradually bring the therapeutic relationship to a close by notifying the patient of the impending separation and favorably suggest that he come back to visit whenever he so desires.

Rationale: Gradual changes decrease adaptation stress. Comfort is promoted through relatedness to others, predictable situations, and having sufficient control of a situation.

Resolved Needs: Comfort. Protection from psychologic threat. Predictable, orderly world. Warm, communicating relationships.

Offer environmental stimulation through contact with varied personnel, environmental change, and variety in daily routine   When a person is confined to the hospital for a prolonged period, offer environmental stimulation by frequently changing familiar personnel who care for him, moving the patient to a new room, rearranging the room, taking him outside for short periods, and adding variety to his daily routine.

Rationale: Perception of the external environment is enhanced by the degree of external stimuli.

Resolved Needs: Stimulation.

Offer feedback of the patient's expressed feelings   Restate what the patient has said in such a way as to emphasize those words that carry emotional significance.

Rationale: Reflected feelings promote insight into emotional responses, which in turn supports growth and maturity.

Resolved Needs: Personal growth and maturity. Increased reality perception and problem-solving ability.

Offer hope   Offer the dying, or permanently ill patient, the anticipated trust that new drugs, treatments, techniques, and research will extend or improve life. Offer this hope with a genuine belief that all things are possible.

Rationale: Hopelessness brings feelings of isolation that result in depression. Hope reestablishes confidence in the future.

Resolved Needs: Comfort. Protection from psychologic threat.

Contraindications: Once predeath acceptance has occurred, avoid reinforcing hope.

Offer praise   Verbally express praise for the efforts that the person puts forth regardless of success or failure.

Rationale: A high self-esteem results from positive responses from others. Rewards transform the threat of frustration into motivation by giving ego satisfaction.

Resolved Needs: Comfort. Approval from others. Sense of value, usefulness. High evaluation of self. Adequacy. Appreciation from others.

Offer reading material with familiar content   When a person has impaired message reception, give him only reading material with contents that are familiar to him.

Rationale: Safety and comfort feelings arise from familiar situations that have been handled successfully in the past.

Resolved Needs: Comfort. Warm, communicating relationships.

Offer to write letters   Suggest to the person that you will write letters for him if he will dictate the message.

Rationale: Comfort is promoted through the ability to communicate needs through a second person, when first-person messages are restricted because of health disorders. Such communication fosters unity with loved ones, which lessens stress and strengthens the capacity to cope.

Resolved Needs: Comfort. Protection from psychologic threat. Warm, communicating relationships. Unity with loved ones.

Open packaged foods   Open cereal boxes, milk cartons, salt and pepper shakers, packaged utensils, and peel fresh fruit.

Rationale: Assistance in making food easily available promotes comfort and aids in illness dependency.

Resolved Needs: Comfort. Dependence.

Pack sterile cotton between the ingrown nail and the skin   Gently pack sterile cotton under the ingrown nail so it no longer touches the skin.

Rationale: Packing cotton between an ingrown nail and the skin takes the pressure off the skin area and promotes normal nail growth.

Resolved Needs: Comfort. Protection from physical harm.

Pack the draining wound with gauze   Gently insert sterile, fine mesh gauze into a wound cavity until that cavity is filled.

Rationale: Fine mesh gauze inserted into a wound promotes cleanliness, soaks up drainage, protects the wound from injury, and prevents the wound from sealing off at the skin surface before granulation tissue fills the wound.

Resolved Needs: Comfort. Cleanliness. Protection from physical harm.

Pad the bedpan   Before offering a bedpan to a patient with potential or existing skin breakdown, pad the top surface of the bedpan with a folded towel or foam rubber.

Rationale: Soft padding reduces pressure and irritation on the skin surface and promotes comfort.

Resolved Needs: Comfort. Protection from physical harm.

Pad the bony prominences   Apply gauze, elastic bandages, polystyrene foam blocks, fitted sheepskin, or similar substances to prominent bony structures. Include the heels, ankles, knees, iliac crest, scapula and clavicle, wrists, elbows, chin, nose, and ears.

Rationale: Prolonged pressure of bone against skin results in decreased area circulation with increased susceptibility to irritation and potential necrosis. Soft padding reduces pressure and irritation of the skin surface and promotes comfort.

Resolved Needs: Comfort. Protection from physical harm.

Pad the rough cast edges   Cover hard cast edges with stockinette. If however, the cast edges are rough or sharp, add felt padding, soft gauze, or other protective material.

Rationale: Pressure from cast edges causes irritation and discomfort and could puncture the skin.

Resolved Needs: Comfort. Protection from physical harm.

Patch the eye(s)   Place a protective sterile covering over the eye.

Rationale: Protective eye coverings reduce injury or strain and maintain cleanliness which prevents infection. Eye tissue exposed to air for prolonged periods will become traumatized from tissue drying, dust, and dirt.

Resolved Needs: Rest. Comfort. Cleanliness. Protection from physical harm.

Percuss the amputation stump to increase firmness   Begin by gently tapping the stump of an amputated limb against a soft pillow or the hand. Gradually increase the pressure by tapping on firmer surfaces until a hard surface can be used. Percussion must be done in relation to gradual decrease in stump pain sensitivity.

Rationale: Percussion of an amputated stump toughens the skin by gradually decreasing nerve sensitivity. It prepares the stump for the pressure of a prosthesis.

Resolved Needs: Protection from physical harm.

Contraindications: Stump bleeding or nonhealing.

Perform a tracheostomy (ET)   Make a vertical incision through the tracheal cartilage. Insert a tracheostomy tube if it is available, or any clean tubing as a temporary measure.

Rationale: An emergency tracheostomy provides an airway through which gas exchange is possible and life is sustained.

Resolved Needs: Oxygen. Waste elimination. Protection from physical harm.

Place a bed board under the mattress   Put a plywood board between the mattress and bedsprings. Have the board cover as many of the springs as possible.

Rationale: A firm mattress prevents body sagging, maintains body alignment, and promotes comfort. A sagging mattress causes flexion contractures of an amputated stump.

Resolved Needs: Comfort. Protection from physical harm. Freedom from pain.

Place a blanket directly against the skin   Place a woolen blanket beneath the sheet directly next to the person's body

Rationale: Warmth promotes vasodilatation which results in relaxation, sleep, pain, and fatigue relief.

Resolved Needs: Sleep, rest, relaxation. Energy. Comfort. Protection from physical harm.

Contraindications: Increased metabolic rate. Sensitivity to wool.

Place a footboard at the feet   Put a board at the foot of the bed and position the soles of the feet against the board.

Rationale: Foot placement against a board maintains dorsal flexion, keeps pressure from bed covers off the feet, and promotes foot circulation through pressing exercises against the board.

Resolved Needs: Protection from physical harm.

Place a footstool at the bedside   Put a footstool at the bedside if the bed is too high for the patient to reach the floor easily.

Rationale: A stepping stool diminishes potential injury from falling and allows for comfortable movement into and out of bed.

Resolved Needs: Comfort. Protection from physical harm.

Place a hand roll under the fingers   In the palm of the hand and under the fingers, place a hand roll.

Rationale: A hand roll helps maintain proper hand positioning which prevents contractures and assures further functional hand use.

Resolved Needs: Protection from physical harm.

Place a kneerest under the knees   Roll a blanket or pillow and place it under the knees.

Rationale: Kneerests promote comfort by relieving strain on abdominal muscles and on tendons beneath the knees.

Resolved Needs: Comfort. Protection from physical harm.

Contraindications: Circulatory thrombus. Under a below-knee amputation stump.

Place a pillow between the knees   Place a soft pillow lengthwise between the patient's knees when he is lying flat or turned with knees flexed.

Rationale: A pillow between the knees prevents friction irritation, discomfort, and pressure. It aligns the knees, reducing internal rotation.

Resolved Needs: Comfort. Protection from physical harm.

Place a pillow on the affected side   If a person complains of pain, place a pillow adjacent to the body part affected with pain.

Rationale: Pillow placement gives support to the injured body area and relieves strain and tension that cause pain.

Resolved Needs: Comfort. Protection from physical harm. Freedom from pain.

Place a shield over the breast nipple   When breast nipples are cracked or irritated, place a soft protective shield over the nipple, especially while the infant is nursing.

Rationale: A nipple shield prevents irritation and pressure to nipple tissue, allows time for healing, and promotes continued infant breast feeding.

Resolved Needs: Comfort. Protection from physical harm.

Place a smoldering match on the imbedded tick   Light a match and blow out the flame. While the match is still smoking and hot, apply it to the tick imbedded in the skin. Be extremely careful not to touch the patient's skin with the match.

Rationale: When an embedded tick is touched with a smoldering match, the tick will back out of his entrenched position and then can be removed easily.

Resolved Needs: Protection from physical harm.

Place a trochanter roll for positioning   Fold a sheet or blanket to one-fourth its size lengthwise. Place the narrow dimension tight against the outer thigh and slightly under the hip line.

Rationale: Trochanter roll support holds the legs in good alignment, prevents outward leg rotation, and reduces contractures.

Resolved Needs: Protection from physical harm.

Place a urinal at the perineum   Keep the urinal placed at the perineum so that the container will catch involuntary urine flow. An emesis basin also may be used.

Rationale: Urine collection in a container reduces the area of skin wetness, decreasing potential skin irritation. Cleanliness promotes comfort.

Resolved Needs: Comfort. Cleanliness. Protection from physical harm.

Place by a window   Locate the person next to a window with a pleasurable view. In case of depression, be certain the window is tightly secured.

Rationale: Outside activities perceived through a window divert attention from internal stress, promoting comfort. Light from a window stimulates persons in mild coma.

Resolved Needs: Comfort. Stimulation. Protection from physical harm. Increased pleasantness.

Place in a heavily draped, carpeted room to reduce noise
Decrease the person's exposure to noise by placing him in a heavily draped, thickly carpeted room.

Rationale: Heavy drapes and carpeting absorb noise, reducing the noise level. Certain levels of quiet are essential to normal physical and emotional function.

Resolved Needs: Comfort. Protection from physical harm. Protection from psychologic threat.

Place in a playpen   Put a child who is learning to walk in a playpen.

Rationale: Playpens allow children to experiment with walking while maintaining safety through restricted wandering.

Resolved Needs: Protection from physical harm.

Place in a private room   Arrange for the person to be in a room by himself.

Rationale: A private room provides quiet, reduces the stress of environmental stimuli, allows for individual regulation of room temperature, and provides the comfort of privacy.

Resolved Needs: Sleep, rest, relaxation. Comfort. Protection from physical harm. Protection from psychologic threat. Dignity.

Place in a room with a patient having a favorable prognosis
When a person is aware that death is approaching, do not place him in a room with someone who is likely to die before he does or who is dying a painful death. Put him in a room with someone who probably will get well.

Rationale: The presence of death heightens anxiety even in well persons. Awareness that an experience can be very painful decreases the potential for a satisfactory experience.

Resolved Needs: Comfort. Protection from psychologic threat.

Place in a whirlpool bath   Put the patient in a bath of swirling water.

Rationale: Swirling warm water dilates blood vessels, stimulates circulation, promotes muscle relaxation which relieves spasticity, and promotes comfort and cleanliness.

Resolved Needs: Relaxation. Comfort. Cleanliness. Protection from physical harm.

Place in an Infant seat   Place the infant in a vertical position in an infant seat.

Rationale: The vertical position prevents aspiration after eating and promotes comfort through greater awareness and visualization of the surroundings.

Resolved Needs: Comfort. Stimulation. Protection from physical harm.

Place in an uncrowded area   Arrange for the person to be in an area where there is considerable space between persons and where there are few persons.

Rationale: Decreased sensory input reduces stress and promotes comfort. Stress reduction decreases energy consumption for the diseased body. Uncrowded areas allow for maximum mobility when motor function is impaired. An uncrowded area is cooler and offers comfort to persons with heat intolerance.

Resolved Needs: Oxygen. Rest. Comfort. Protection from physical harm. Protection from psychologic threat.

Place in postural drainage   Determine the lobe of the lung that needs drainage and position the patient accordingly for 5 to 15 minutes.

Right or left upper lobes: Place in a sitting position.

Right or left anterior upper lobes: Lean backward 30°.

Right or left posterior upper lobes: Lean forward 30°.

Right or left anterior lower lobes: Place the patient on his back with two pillows under the hips so his head is 30–45° downward.

Right or left posterior lower lobes: Place the patient on his abdomen with two pillows under his hips so his head is 30–45° downward.

Right upper lateral (side) lobe: Place on the right side.

Left lower lateral (side) lobe: Place on the left side.

Rationale: Postural drainage facilitates secretion removal from the lung through the pull of gravity.

Resolved Needs: Waste elimination. Protection from physical harm.

Contraindications: Hypertension. Increased intracranial or intraocular pressure. Ascites. Esophageal bleeding. If dyspnea is increased or if traction is disrupted by the position.

Place in the face-down (prone) position   Lay the patient flat on his abdomen with face turned to the side, palms turned downward, and feet extended.

Rationale: The prone position relieves sacral area pressure. It promotes hip joint hyperextension which preserves the normal gait, provides secretion drainage, and promotes comfort.

Resolved Needs: Comfort. Protection from physical harm.

Contraindications: Respiratory distress.

Place in the face-upward (supine) position   Place the head, face up, in a neutral, straight position so it is in perfect alignment with the rest of the body.

Rationale: The neutral position is less likely to cause further spinal cord injury when cervical vertebrae are fractured.

Resolved Needs: Protection from physical harm.

Place in the flat position   Lay the person horizontally on his back (supine or dorsal position) so the body is level.

Rationale: General blood circulation is most adequate and the heart's workload is least when the body is flat. The flat position reduces enlarged hemorrhoids, increases blood flow to the brain during shock, and when the head is turned to the side, prevents aspiration of emesis into the lungs. The flat position is preferred during peritoneal dialysis; otherwise, intraperitoneal pressure may become too great, causing pain and injury.

Resolved Needs: Circulation. Rest. Comfort. Protection from physical harm. Freedom from pain.

Contraindications: Hypertension. Increased intracranial pressure. Ascites. Severe respiratory distress.

Place in the foot-elevated, head-lowered (Trendelenburg) position   Raise the foot of the bed, elevating the legs and feet at a 45° angle, with the head lower than the hips.

Rationale: The Trendelenburg position facilitates drainage by gravity, pushes abdominal contents into the upper abdomen near the diaphragm, increases cerebral blood flow, holds back the presenting infant from the birth canal, and prevents pressure from cutting off an infant's oxygen supply in case of a prolapsed cord.

Resolved Needs: Circulation. Comfort. Protection from physical harm.

Contraindications: Hypertension. Increased intracranial or intraocular pressure. Ascites. Respiratory distress.

Place in the functional position   Place the hands, feet, and knees in the natural position of function. Position the hand so that the wrist is slightly hyperextended (slight upward position), the fingers slightly flexed (bent), the thumb flexed and adducted (rotated inwardly) toward the first finger. Position the feet in the neutral position at a right angle with the leg, and avoid outward rotation. Position the knee in a slightly flexed (bent) position.

Rationale: Placing the hands or feet in the functional position increases the potential for normal use after the current injury is healed.

Resolved Needs: Protection from physical injury.

Place in the knee-chest position   Have the patient rest her chest and knees on the bed, keeping the thighs erect and the abdomen off the bed. Place her arms above and on either side of her head. Encourage the patient to empty her bladder before assuming this position.

Rationale: The knee-chest position corrects uterus or ovary displacement, causes the fetal head to move away from the pelvis, reducing pressure on a prolapsed cord, and relieves lower pelvic pain.

Resolved Needs: Comfort. Protection from physical harm.

Contraindications: Do not place a mother in the knee-chest position until 3 weeks after delivery.

Place in the lithotomy (dorsosacral) position   Have the patient lie on her back with legs and thighs flexed and knees held widely apart.

Rationale: The lithotomy position facilitates exposure of the perineal, rectal and vaginal areas for examination and for the administration of therapeutic procedures.

Resolved Needs: Protection from physical harm.

Place in the side-lying (Sims', lateral, semiprone) position   Place the patient on his left side with the upper arm forward, the under leg slightly flexed, and the upper leg flexed at the thigh and knee. Support the knee and head with a pillow.

Rationale: The side-lying position aids drainage of body cavities, helps prevent postoperative pulmonary and circulatory complications, minimizes aspiration of regurgitated food, prevents the tongue from falling backward, causing airway obstruction, is favorable for examination of the female pelvis and the administration of enemas.

Resolved Needs: Comfort. Protection from physical harm.

Contraindications: Pulmonary hemorrhage. Atelectasis. Pneumonitis (pneumonia). Pleural effusion.

Place in the sitting position   Put in a sitting position with the back resting comfortably against a firm surface. Place a pillow under each arm for comfortable support.

Rationale: The sitting position facilitates abdominal drainage, supports improved respirations, reduces tracheal edema and abdominal pressure on the diaphragm during ascites, provides room for pulmonary expansion by lowering the diaphragm, and promotes comfort.

Resolved Needs: Oxygen. Comfort. Protection from physical harm.

Contraindications: Shock. Potential fainting. Labrinythitis vomiting.

Place in the slight foot-elevated head-lowered (semi-Trendelenburg) position   Raise the foot of the bed, elevating the legs and feet at a 20° angle. Place the head lower than the hips.

Rationale: The semi-Trendelenburg position facilitates drainage by gravity, displaces intestines into the upper abdomen, and increases cerebral blood flow. It holds back the presenting infant from the birth canal by exerting mild pressure against the presenting part and prevents pressure from cutting off an infant's oxygen supply in the case of prolapsed cord. In shock resulting from blood loss, this position increases arterial blood flow to the brain and promotes venous blood flow from the lower extremities to the right atrium.

Resolved Needs: Circulation. Comfort. Protection from physical harm.

Contraindications: Hypertension. Increased intracranial or intraocular pressure. Ascites. Respiratory distress.

Place in the slight sitting (semi-Fowler's, semirecumbent) position   Raise the head of the bed approximately 12 inches above normal bed level and elevate the knees.

Rationale: The slight sitting position improves respiratory ventilation, lessens fluid accumulation in the lungs, relieves painful tension on surgical incisions, minimizes the liver's pressure on the diaphragm, and promotes pelvic drainage.

Resolved Needs: Oxygen. Comfort. Protection from physical harm.

Contraindications: Shock. Potential fainting.

Place objects out of reach   Place objects so the person cannot reach them or so they cannot be reached by persons who should not have access to them. This is especially true of harmful objects such as alcohol, drugs, cleaning fluid, etc.

Rationale: The elimination of potentially harmful threats promotes safety.

Resolved Needs: Protection from physical harm.

Place objects within reach   Place objects to facilitate their easiest possible use in meeting the needs of the particular person.

Rationale: Easy access to needed objects promotes independence, prevents unnecessary use of energy, and aids in illness dependency.

Resolved Needs: Energy. Comfort. Protection from physical harm. Dependence. Independence.

Place objects (or equipment) within sight   Keep within visual range, objects or equipment that the person uses to meet hygienic and other basic needs. Also keep within sight pictures of loved ones, as well as flowers and cards from family and friends.

Rationale: Seeing familiar objects or equipment that represents safety promotes comfort.

Resolved Needs: Comfort.

Place on a bedpan at the first sign of full-bladder clues
Response to signs of a full bladder when normal bladder sensations are absent promotes control. Such signs include perspiration, headache, goose pimples, feelings of abdominal fullness, and restlessness. When these signs occur during bladder retraining, the patient should be given the urinal immediately or placed on the bedpan.

Rationale: Bladder control is essential to the maintenance of skin dryness, cleanliness, comfort, and socialization.

Resolved Needs: Comfort. Cleanliness. Protection from physical harm.

Place on a CircOlectric bed
Put the person on a frame and canvas bed in which position change can be electrically controlled.

Rationale: The CircOlectric bed allows for position change while maintaining immobility, for gradual head elevation, gradually increased standing tolerance, and aids in maintaining circulation.

Resolved Needs: Protection from physical harm.

Place on a flotation mattress
Place the patient on a water bed. Periodically, observe the mattress for holes that might allow leakage, for proper positioning of the mattress on the bed, and appropriate water temperature.

Rationale: A flotation mattress relieves pressure against the skin and improves tissue oxygenation. It reduces surface tension and decreases body weight through partial submergence in water.

Resolved Needs: Protection from physical harm.

Place on a nonelectric bed if wearing a pacemaker
Do not put patients with pacemakers on an electric bed. Electric beds may be safe when doubly insulated, but mechanical beds are the safest.

Rationale: Electric beds increase the potential for electrical current leakage.

Resolved Needs: Protection from physical harm.

Place on a polyurethane foam pad
Put a pad made of porous, resilient, easily compressible polyurethane between the patient and the mattress.

Rationale: Polyurethane foam prevents friction irritation against cutaneous tissue, reducing pressure on tissue and promoting comfort.

Resolved Needs: Comfort. Protection from physical harm.

Place on a rocking bed
Lay the patient on a motorized bed that alternately raises and lowers the head and feet in a seesaw motion.

Rationale: Alternately elevating and lowering the body improves circulation and assists respiration through diaphragmatic movement.

Resolved Needs: Oxygen. Circulation. Protection from physical harm.

Contraindications: Increased intracranial or intraocular pressure. Hypertension. Ascites.

Place on a sheepskin   Lay sheep's wool under the person who must lie or sit for prolonged periods.

Rationale: Air spaces in the sheepskin keep the skin area dry. Sheepskin softness eases pressure on the skin, preventing decubitus formation, while the oil from the lamb's wool lubricates the skin.

Resolved Needs: Comfort. Protection from physical harm.

Place on a silicone pad   Place a gel foam pad, which has the consistency of human fat, under the person who must lie or sit for prolonged periods.

Rationale: Gel foam pads support body weight and, by preventing friction between the pad and the patient, reduce the potential for decubitus formation. Its softness promotes comfort.

Resolved Needs: Comfort. Protection from physical harm.

Place on a split-foam mattress   Place a thick foam mattress, split so that the buttocks are suspended in mid-air, under the patient who must lie in bed for prolonged periods.

Rationale: The suspension of bony prominences in air reduces pressure and maintains normal skin circulation.

Resolved Needs: Protection from physical harm.

Place on a Stryker frame   Put the person on a frame and canvas bed that can be turned anteriorly and posteriorly.

Rationale: A Stryker frame allows for position change while maintaining immobility.

Resolved Needs: Protection from physical harm.

Place on an alternating pressure mattress   Place the person on a mattress that alternately fills and empties with air.

Rationale: The reduction of constant pressure on any body area by alternately changing the pressure point increases blood circulation to tissues, preventing tissue degeneration.

Resolved Needs: Protection from physical harm.

Place on an orthopedic bed   Put the patient on a fracture bed with an overhead frame to which can be added traction and assistive moving devices. These beds are usually 3–6 inches longer than ordinary beds.

Rationale: The orthopedic bed provides a flat, firm surface for fractured limbs and facilitates the use of devices such as traction and overhead bars. It provides comfort for very tall persons.

Resolved Needs: Comfort. Protection from physical harm.

Place on complete bed rest   Place the patient on 24-hour bed rest. This applies to instances such as sudden cardiac episodes, during high or severe temperature elevations of 103–108°, in head or spinal cord injuries, hemorrhage, coma or semicoma, during severe energy depletion, very high blood pressure elevations, or in any life-threatening situation.

Rationale: Complete bed rest prevents further tissue injury and reduces the probability of complications associated with activity. It replenishes cell energy that the body uses for the maintenance of life and activity and promotes healing and comfort.

Resolved Needs: Sleep, rest. Energy. Comfort. Protection from physical harm.

Place on nonadherent sheeting   For burns use a special sheeting that will not stick to the open wound.

Rationale: Nonadherent sheeting reduces pain and trauma by preventing sheeting from sticking to and pulling against injured tissue.

Resolved Needs: Comfort. Protection from physical harm.

Place on sterile linens   When there are severe burns or open wounds or when the patient is highly susceptible to infection, cover the bed and the patient with linens that have been sterilized.

Rationale: Reduced exposure to microorganisms minimizes infection.

Resolved Needs: Cleanliness. Protection from physical harm.

Place on the affected side   When there is evidence of pulmonary hemorrhage, pleural fluid or inflammation, or when one lung is not ventilating adequately, position the patient on the affected side.

Rationale: Pressure applied to a bleeding area reduces and localizes blood flow. When applied to the chest in pleura inflammation, it stabilizes the chest wall and reduces pain. Placement on the affected side localizes fluid accumulation and prevents compression of the other lung. When one lung has diminished ventilation, it supports maximum ventilation of the other lung.

Resolved Needs: Oxygen. Comfort. Protection from physical harm. Freedom from pain.

Contraindications: Atelectasis.

Place on the unaffected side   Place the person on the body side that is free of the troublesome symptom. If there is pain, position on the pain-free side. If there is tinnitus, position on the side of the quiet ear. If the heart is pounding, place the patient on the right side so the pounding is less perceptible.

Rationale: Positioning on the unaffected side decreases the amount of pressure in the body area of a troublesome symptom, resulting in a reduction of the intensity of the symptom.

Resolved Needs: Comfort.

Place only warm hands and objects on the patient   Do not
touch the patient with anything that is cold. Run warm water over the surface of the bedpan before it is used. Prior to touching the patient, rub your hands together so they will be warm. Rub the stethoscope between your hands to warm it.

Rationale: Sudden coldness disturbs skin receptors while warmth promotes comfort. Warmth prevents chilling, which often stimulates muscle spasms.

Resolved Needs: Comfort. Protection from physical harm.

Place the amputation stump in the extension position   Have
the person with a below-knee amputation turn from side to side or lie on his abdomen so that the amputated stump is extended and maintained in alignment with the rest of the body.

Rationale: Extension alignment of an amputated stump prevents contractures and promotes positioning conducive to successful prosthesis walking.

Resolved Needs: Protection from physical harm.

Place the call light within reach   Arrange the call light so it is easily
accessible and can be reached without difficulty.

Rationale: Awareness that help can be easily obtained reduces anxiety and meets dependency needs.

Resolved Needs: Comfort. Protection from physical harm. Protection from psychologic threat. Dependence.

Place the feet in hard-soled ankle-top shoes   Place the feet in
bootlike high-ankle shoes. Pad the inside of the shoe to prevent skin breakdown. Place the shoe soles against a footboard.

Rationale: Ankle-top shoes prevent plantar flexion by maintaining ankle alignment.

Resolved Needs: Protection from physical harm.

Place the foot in the dorsiflexion position   Bend the foot and toes
up toward the knee.

Rationale: Dorsiflexion position inhibits the transmission of motor nerve impulses to a spastic muscle. This decreases muscle tension and relieves the pain and discomfort of foot and leg spasms.

Resolved Needs: Comfort. Freedom from pain.

Place the head below the knees   Place the person's head below the level of his knees by bending his body forward at the waist.

Rationale: Lowering the head increases brain circulation during syncope (fainting).

Resolved Needs: Circulation. Protection from physical harm.

Contraindications: Hypertension. Increased intracranial or intraocular pressure. Spinal cord injury.

Place the newborn in an incubator   Place the newborn or premature infant in a temperature-regulated incubator.

Rationale: Newborn infants cannot regulate their own temperature for 8–36 hours following birth. Premature infants cannot regulate their body temperature until they reach considerable maturity. The incubator maintains a stable environmental temperature.

Resolved Needs: Normal temperature. Protection from physical harm.

Place the work at a comfortable level   Put the work and work tools at a level where muscle strain is decreased to a minimum.

Rationale: Fatigue conditions are decreased by reducing stress stimuli that require energy depleting responses. The accomplishment of activity without fatigue promotes comfort.

Resolved Needs: Energy. Comfort. Protection from physical harm.

Plan undisturbed periods for the patient   Adjust nursing activities and visiting schedules so there will be a period during the day when the person will be undisturbed.

Rationale: Undisturbed periods support rest, relaxation, and renewal of energy resources needed for healing.

Resolved Needs: Rest, relaxation. Energy. Comfort.

Position comfortably   Place the body in a position suitable and comforting to the person. Be sure the position supports body areas without applying pressure. When restfully positioning an infant for breast feeding, place the child in the mother's arms so he can grasp the whole nipple and not just the end. Avoid pressing the infant's nose against the breast. When bottle feeding, restfully position the infant's head slightly to one side.

Rationale: Restful positioning, with lack of pressure on any body surface, promotes comfort. Comfort arises through association with positions previously experienced as comforting. Proper positioning meets illness dependency needs.

Resolved Needs: Sleep, rest, relaxation. Comfort. Freedom from pain. Dependence.

Contraindications: Avoid any positioning that will cause or increase body injury.

Position on the left side   Suggest that the person lie on his left side when ready to go to sleep.

Rationale: Lying on the left side causes slowed heart action and reduces circulation which promotes sleep.

Resolved Needs: Sleep, rest, relaxation. Comfort. Protection from physical harm.

Contraindications: Right-sided pulmonary hemorrhage or inflammation. Pleural fluid. Left-sided atelectasis.

Position the affected limb lower than the rest of the body   Place the limb wounded by a poisonous snake or spider at a level lower than the rest of the body.

Rationale: Lowering the limb wounded by a snake or spider decreases the rapidity with which the venom circulates through the blood.

Resolved Needs: Protection from physical harm.

Position the infant with the head elevated for burping   Bubble the infant by raising his head and gently rubbing or patting the posterior chest after bottle feeding.

Rationale: External stimulation brings stomach air up the esophagus with resulting pressure and pain relief.

Resolved Needs: Comfort. Protection from physical harm. Freedom from pain.

Contraindications: Meningitis.

Position the pacemaker generator box comfortably   While the patient is in bed, place the generator box so there is neither strain on the wires nor any discomfort.

Rationale: Proper positioning of the pacemaker generator box safeguards against the wires being accidentally pulled out and provides comfort.

Resolved Needs: Comfort. Protection from physical harm.

Position to promote drainage of the infected area   If a draining infection exists, position that body area so the pull of gravity will exert pressure and increase drainage flow. For instance, if the left ear is draining, raise the right side of the head with a pillow so the left ear is the lowest part of the head.

Rationale: Drainage of infected material promotes healing, prevents infection spread to adjacent body parts, reduces pressure, and decreases pain.

Resolved Needs: Comfort. Protection from physical harm. Freedom from pain.

Position with pillows Assist with the maintenance of a desired body position by propping the body with pillows.

Rationale: Pillows will support the body in alignment without placing undue pressure against body tissue.

Resolved Needs: Comfort. Protection from physical harm.

Position with sandbags Place canvas bags filled with sand around the body part after proper positioning.

Rationale: Sandbag weight promotes immobilization and protects against poor alignment and contractures.

Resolved Needs: Protection from physical harm.

Postpone feeding when the patient is fatigued If the patient is fatigued, withhold food until he is well rested, usually after having slept.

Rationale: Fatigue reduces appetite.

Resolved Needs: Comfort.

Pray with the patient If the patient wishes to pray, stand beside him and offer to pray with him.

Rationale: The turning of heart and mind toward God promotes spiritual growth.

Resolved Needs: Comfort. Religious, philosophic satisfaction.

Prepare the patient for a painful experience When a person is to be faced with a painful experience, calmly tell him what can be expected and that every effort will be made to minimize the pain as much as possible.

Rationale: Anxious anticipation of pain increases tension which enhances the painfulness of the actual experience. Preparation before a painful experience decreases tension which reduces pain.

Resolved Needs: Comfort. Protection from psychologic threat.

Prepare the patient for the clergy's visit In anticipation of a clergy member's visit, refresh the patient and dress him in clothing respectful of the clergyman. Provide a clean, neat environment and privacy so the patient may feel free to discuss religious or other problems.

Rationale: Preparation for a clergyman's visit promotes patient comfort.

Resolved Needs: Comfort.

Present change gradually Slowly present for acceptance alterations and substitutions for that which presently exists.

Rationale: Gradual change decreases adaptation stress. Safety feelings arise from predictable situations.

Resolved Needs: Comfort. Protection from psychologic threat. Predictable, orderly world. Adequacy. Self-reliance.

Prop with a back rest   Provide a supportive back rest for comfortable sitting.

Rationale: Back support promotes relaxation and comfort.

Resolved Needs: Relaxation. Comfort.

Protect the water-seal drainage apparatus from damage   If chest bottles are used for water-seal drainage, place them in a wooden cradle or holder so the bottles will not be broken accidentally. If a plastic apparatus is used, position it so it is not subject to puncture or tearing.

Rationale: Water-seal drainage systems must be protected from damage because if the system is interrupted, the atmospheric pressure will cause air to enter the chest cavity and collapse the lung.

Resolved Needs: Protection from physical harm.

Protect with a plastic bib   Place a water-repellent bib over the neck and chest.

Rationale: Cleanliness promotes comfort.

Resolved Needs: Comfort. Cleanliness.

Protect with absorbent padding   Lay padding that will soak up liquid excretions and drainage under the patient and around draining wounds.

Rationale: Absorbent materials draw wetness that otherwise would lay in contact with the skin. This lessens skin irritation and promotes cleanliness and comfort.

Resolved Needs: Comfort. Cleanliness. Protection from physical harm.

Protect with plastic pants   When the person is incontinent, but up and about, have him wear plastic pants.

Rationale: Plastic pants prevent skin irritation by limiting the skin area exposed to wetness, preventing soiled clothes, promoting comfort, and reducing the potential for embarrassment.

Resolved Needs: Comfort. Cleanliness. Protection from physical harm. Protection from psychologic threat.

Contraindications: Diaper rash or severe skin irritation.

Provide a bedpan   Supply a shallow vessel for elimination purposes for persons confined to bed.

Rationale: Less energy is required to use a bedpan than to walk to the bathroom for elimination purposes. Limited mobility often requires the use of a bedpan. Adequate elimination facilities promote comfort and cleanliness.

Resolved Needs: Energy. Comfort. Cleanliness. Protection from physical harm.

Provide a bedside commode   Place a portable commode at the patient's bedside for elimination purposes.

Rationale: Less energy is required to use a bedside commode than to use a bedpan or to walk to the bathroom for elimination purposes. Adequate elimination facilities promote comfort and cleanliness.

Resolved Needs: Energy. Comfort. Protection from physical harm.

Contraindications: Maximum 24-hour bed rest.

Provide a calendar   Acquaint the person with the environment by providing a large, single-day calendar and placing it on the wall where it is easily seen.

Rationale: The ability to comprehend one's environment with regard to time, place, and person identity prevents confusion and anxiety.

Resolved Needs: Protection from psychologic threat. Increased reality perception.

Provide a clean, comfortable bed   Provide freshly washed bed linen on a bed with a firm mattress.

Rationale: Clean bed linen refreshes the skin, promotes comfort and rest, protects against bacterial infection, and assists in illness dependency.

Resolved Needs: Sleep, rest. Comfort. Cleanliness. Protection from physical harm. Dependence.

Provide a clock   Acquaint the person with the environment by providing a large clock and placing it where it can be seen easily.

Rationale: The ability to comprehend one's environment with regard to time, place, and person identity prevents confusion and anxiety.

Resolved Needs: Protection from psychologic threat. Increased reality perception.

Provide a compatible room companion   Place the patient in a room with someone having a compatible personality and whose length of stay approximates that of the patient.

Rationale: Persons with compatible personalities associate comfortably and support positive feelings between each other.

Resolved Needs: Comfort. Warm, communicating relationships.

Provide a convenient bed (or meal) tray   Furnish an over-the-bed or meal tray within easy reach and adjust to proper height.

Rationale: Accessibility to needed objects promotes comfort and supports independence when there is illness dependency.

Resolved Needs: Comfort. Dependence. Independence.

Provide a drinking straw   Furnish a straw through which liquids may be sucked into the mouth.

Rationale: A straw facilitates easy ingestion of liquids, especially during limited range of motion or muscular weakness. It prevents staining or injury by allowing liquids to bypass the teeth and keeps glass pressure from traumatizing lip blisters and pustules.

Resolved Needs: Comfort. Protection from physical harm.

Contraindications: Traumatized, bleeding, or sutured oral mucosa. Excessive flatulence.

Provide a firm mattress   Furnish a mattress that has a solid compact surface and does not sag under body weight.

Rationale: A firm mattress offers a smooth, level lying surface that results in good back support and body alignment. It provides comfort, distributes body weight, and promotes even distribution of circulation.

Resolved Needs: Circulation. Comfort. Protection from physical harm. Freedom from pain.

Provide a fracture bedpan   For persons confined to bed, provide an extremely shallow, almost flat vessel for elimination purposes. Have them use the fracture pan instead of the standard size bedpan.

Rationale: Less energy is required to raise the body over a nearly flat surface than over an elevated surface for elimination purposes. A flat surface under the body provides minimal disturbance of body alignment and minimizes movement pain and discomfort.

Resolved Needs: Energy. Comfort. Protection from physical harm.

Provide a home visit   Go to the patient's home, observe the total situation, identify needs, and provide nursing care.

Rationale: The home situation indicates the person's overall lifestyle, physical and emotional needs, and resources. A home visit communicates caring.

Resolved Needs: Comfort. Protection from physical harm. Protection from psychologic threat. Warm, communicating relationships.

Provide a language interpreter   When attempting to communicate with a person who does not speak the same language, furnish an interpreter.

Rationale: Comfort is promoted through a sense of effective communication with others.

Resolved Needs: Comfort. Protection from psychologic threat. Warm, communicating relationships.

Provide a low-height bed Furnish a bed low enough for the patient to place his feet on the floor while sitting on the side of the bed.

Rationale: A low-height bed diminishes the potential for injury from falling and allows for comfortable movement out of and into the bed.

Resolved Needs: Comfort. Protection from physical harm. Independence.

Provide a magnifying glass Furnish a magnifying glass which enlarges objects many times.

Rationale: Enlarged objects promote visual acuity, reduce eyestrain, and promote comfort.

Resolved Needs: Comfort. Protection from physical harm.

Provide a mirror for reflection of the self Give the patient a mirror so that he can see himself frequently or place the patient's bed in a position facing a mirror.

Rationale: Frequent visualization of one's physical appearance helps establish self-image. The new mother viewing herself and her newborn child in the mirror receives reinforcement for the realization of her new role. When death is approaching, the reflection of oneself in the mirror may promote acceptance.

Resolved Needs: Increased reality perception.

Contraindications: It is sometimes best not to let a person see himself in the mirror after severe trauma such as burns, contusions with swelling, and mutilations until the severity of the situation has lessened. Jaundiced persons often do better not viewing themselves in the mirror.

Provide a night light Furnish a night light so there is a sufficient amount of illumination for seeing in the dark.

Rationale: Illumination of the dark prevents accidents, allows minimal disturbance of sleep, and prevents distorted perception.

Resolved Needs: Comfort. Protection from physical harm. Protection from psychologic threat. Increased reality perception.

Provide a nontempting environment Remove objects from the environment that entice the person to perform unhealthy actions from which restraint is difficult. This includes keeping candy out of sight of a diabetic and cigarettes away from a heavy smoker.

Rationale: Decreased sensory perception of desired but harmful objects or situations reduces internal conflict or threat and the harm the object or situation can produce.

Resolved Needs: Comfort. Protection from physical harm. Protection from psychologic threat.

Provide a pain-relief measure of the patient's choice Give the person a choice as to the pain-relief measure preferred and administer the one indicated.

Rationale: Comfort is enhanced by the availability of choices and having sufficient control to bring comfort or prevent harm to oneself.

Resolved Needs: Comfort. Protection from psychologic threat.

Provide a paper bag for breathing Furnish a paper bag into which the person may breathe and rebreathe his own exhaled air.

Rationale: Rebreathing accumulations of excessively exhaled carbon dioxide collected within a paper bag raises the blood level of carbon dioxide to normal and reestablishes respiratory acid-base balance.

Resolved Needs: Acid-base balance. Protection from physical harm.

Contraindications: Increased blood carbon dioxide level. Emphysema.

Provide a paper bag for tissue disposal Pin a paper bag on the side of the bed so used tissues may be discarded easily and will not be touched by persons other than the patient.

Rationale: Proper disposal of infectious material prevents the spread of infection from one person to another.

Resolved Needs: Comfort. Cleanliness. Protection from physical harm.

Provide a scratching device Furnish a thin, long, dull piece of wood or plastic to be inserted between the skin and the cast for scratching areas that itch. Covering the device with gauze and dipping it in alcohol may cool the irritated areas.

Rationale: Scratching relieves itching discomfort.

Resolved Needs: Comfort.

Contraindications: An incisional or other wound under the cast.

Provide a short drinking straw Furnish a short, 4- or 5-inch, drinking straw.

Rationale: A short drinking straw reduces fatigue because less energy is required for sucking.

Resolved Needs: Energy. Comfort.

Contraindications: Traumatized, bleeding, or sutured oral mucosa. Excessive flatulence.

Provide a sputum container Make available a clean, covered container for sputum collection.

Rationale: Placing specimens in a container prevents infection spread from one person to another.

Resolved Needs: Comfort. Cleanliness. Protection from physical harm.

Provide a sugar substitute   When the dietary intake of sugar is restricted, furnish artificial sugar.

Rationale: Sugar substitutes prevent the metabolic imbalances caused by natural sugar in certain disorders, and their sweet taste promotes comfort.

Resolved Needs: Comfort. Protection from physical harm.

Provide a transfer board   Provide a wide, flat, firm board to bridge the gap and support the patient's weight as he moves from the bed to the wheelchair. Take extra care that the patient does not slide across the board and produce friction against tender skin.

Rationale: A transfer board allows for independent transfer from bed to wheelchair and back to bed.

Resolved Needs: Activity, exercise. Independence.

Provide a trapeze bar   Furnish a swinging, overhead bar immediately above the patient's head.

Rationale: Pulling exercises performed on a trapeze bar promote muscle strength. A trapeze bar allows for easier in-bed movement and increases in and out of bed mobility.

Resolved Needs: Activity, exercise. Comfort. Independence.

Provide alphabet letters for word composition   Make available letters of the alphabet which are printed, painted, cut out, or magnetic. Help the patient use them for word or sentence composition.

Rationale: When there is impaired communication ability, alternate methods of word composition promote comfort.

Resolved Needs: Comfort. Warm, communicating relationships.

Provide an atmosphere of acceptance   Display accepting attitudes that create an environment in which the patient feels that he is favorably received as a person. Acceptance involves communicating the worth of the person because he is a person. It does not indicate approval of unacceptable behavior.

Rationale: Psychologic safety requires that a person experience awareness of acceptance by others. Acceptance allows for testing reality and the reactions of others. Acceptance is acquired through cultural roles and relationships with others and promotes mutual respect.

Resolved Needs: Comfort. Protection from psychologic threat. Acceptance. High evaluation of self. Dignity. Personal growth and maturity.

Provide an attractive meal tray   Furnish a colorful, nicely set meal tray.

Rationale: Attractive meal trays enhance the appearance of food which promotes appetite.

Resolved Needs: Comfort. Protection from physical harm.

Provide an emesis basin Supply a basin for collecting emesis.

Rationale: Available facilities for cleanliness promote comfort.

Resolved Needs: Comfort. Cleanliness.

Provide an over-the-bed table for the leaning-forward position Make available an over-the-bed table with a soft pillow on top of it so that the orthopneic patient may lean forward and ease difficult breathing.

Rationale: Proper positioning in respiratory difficulty promotes comfort and improves ventilation.

Resolved Needs: Oxygen. Comfort.

Provide braille reading material Make available reading material that has been printed with raised dots representing language symbols.

Rationale: Braille allows those who cannot see the printed words to read by touch.

Resolved Needs: Comfort. Mastery and competence in skills. Independence.

Provide clean clothing Provide freshly washed or cleaned clothing.

Rationale: Clean clothing refreshes the skin, promotes comfort, reduces bacterial entrance into wounds, and assists in illness dependency.

Resolved Needs: Comfort. Cleanliness. Protection from physical harm. Dependence.

Provide cold water for mouth rinsing but not swallowing Give the patient a small amount of cold water with which he can rinse his mouth. Be sure that the water is not swallowed but discarded after the rinsing.

Rationale: Cold water moistens dry oral mucosa and refreshes the mouth, temporarily relieving thirst.

Resolved Needs: Comfort.

Provide conditions which the patient desires for peaceful dying Provide whatever conditions the person requires for a peaceful death. These usually include dying at home, dying surrounded by family, visits from dear friends, the company of a faithful pet, the beauty of flowers in the room, having a chance to communicate with God, quiet surroundings, favorite drinks and food, or any other individual preferences.

Rationale: Recognition of a person's wishes indicates attitudes of value and dignity toward him.

Resolved Needs: Comfort. Protection from psychologic threat. Unity with loved ones. Dignity.

Provide desired personal articles Furnish personal articles that the patient may desire such as clothing, knick-knacks, a special blanket.

Rationale: Familiar articles promote safety and comfort feelings.

Resolved Needs: Comfort. Protection from psychologic threat.

Provide desired religious articles Furnish religious articles that the patient may desire such as a Bible, statues, crucifix, rosary, prayerbook, religious candles.

Rationale: Religious articles assist man to spiritually express his relationship with God.

Resolved Needs: Comfort. Religious, philosophic satisfaction.

Provide disposable tissue Provide paper handkerchiefs that can be discarded after use.

Rationale: Disposable handkerchiefs prevent the transfer of infectious respiratory conditions from one person to another.

Resolved Needs: Comfort. Cleanliness.

Provide emotionally safe experiences Set up situations in which the person feels free from all threat. These should be situations in which he previously experienced comfort and success.

Rationale: Safety feelings arise from familiar and predictable situations successfully handled in the past and from an awareness that one can cope successfully with life.

Resolved Needs: Comfort. Protection from psychologic threat. Predictable, orderly world. Adequacy.

Provide emotional support for persons significant to the patient Sustain persons who are important to the patient by meeting their needs as they become evident.

Rationale: Awareness that there is concern for one's loved ones promotes comfort. Support from others promotes feelings of strength, reducing fear and anxiety.

Resolved Needs: Comfort. Protection from psychologic threat. Endurance.

Provide extra food helpings at mealtimes Furnish extra food in addition to the regular meal whenever there is a request for it.

Rationale: Increased metabolic rate and illness that causes weight loss require additional energy and fuel resources to provide tissue oxidation and nutritior. Relief of visceral hunger promotes comfort.

Resolved Needs: Food balance. Energy. Comfort.

Contraindications: Obesity. Special diet restrictions.

Provide finger food   Offer foods that can be eaten with the fingers, such as celery, carrot and bread sticks, crackers, apple slices, crisp bacon, raw vegetables, fruits.

Rationale: The consistency of finger foods gives pleasure when taste is undeveloped. Finger foods are helpful in chewing and swallowing problems, and are good for children who have difficulty holding up their head. They are a substitute for such behaviors as thumb sucking and nail biting. When persons are hyperactive and cannot sit still to eat, or are slow eaters, finger foods can be caried about.

Resolved Needs: Food balance. Comfort.

Provide firm eating utensils   Supply knives, forks, spoons, glasses, and dishes made of hard material that does not bend.

Rationale: During limited hand motion, muscular weakness, and developing coordination of the small child, manipulation of objects is often difficult. Utensils that do not bend against pressure are easiest to manipulate.

Resolved Needs: Comfort. Mastery and competence in skills.

Provide fluid selection   Furnish a number of liquids and juices to choose from.

Rationale: Balanced fluid intake is enhanced by the availability of familiar and desired liquids. Fluid selection promotes comfort.

Resolved Needs: Water-salt balance. Comfort.

Contraindications: Dietary restrictions such as salt and potassium.

Provide foam-rubber pillows   Make available pillows made of foam rubber. Avoid using cotton or down-filled pillows.

Rationale: Foam-rubber pillows are nonirritating to hypersensitive respiratory systems.

Resolved Needs: Comfort. Protection from physical harm.

Provide foods and toys for chewing   When a small child needs to bite, supply the child with apples, crackers, cookies, or chewing toys.

Rationale: Biting and chewing meet the oral activity needs of a developing child. Providing appropriate objects for biting reduces the potential for inappropriate biting of humans and animals by children.

Resolved Needs: Comfort.

Provide foods at their most appetizing temperature   Give foods that are heated or cooled to their most desirable temperature. Be certain that the coffee is hot and the ice cream is cold when the patient receives it.

Rationale: Proper food temperature offers the comfort of improved taste and oral palatability and assists in illness dependency.

Resolved Needs: Comfort. Dependence.

Provide food selection   Furnish a choice of foods, particularly those especially liked and desired. When introducing a child to new foods, place the foods on a plate. Leave the child alone and let him select what he wants.

Rationale: Balanced nutritional intake is enhanced by the availability of familiar and desired foods. The privilege of being able to select foods promotes comfort.

Resolved Needs: Food balance. Comfort.

Contraindications: Special diet restrictions reduce the amount of selection.

Provide frequent patient contact   Attend to the person for short periods at frequent intervals and be certain that the patient is aware of your presence.

Rationale: Fear and anxiety are reduced by an awareness that one is not threatened with aloneness. Frequent patient contact enhances the probability of detecting abnormal physical conditions.

Resolved Needs: Comfort. Protection from physical harm. Protection from psychologic threat. Attention.

Provide fresh drinking water   Furnish and frequently replace cool, fresh water at the bedside.

Rationale: Cool water relieves thirst, promotes comfort, and assists in illness dependency.

Resolved Needs: Comfort. Dependence.

Provide glucose ice chips   Make available ice cubes made from 20–50% glucose.

Rationale: When fluid intake is restricted but caloric intake needs to be maintained, glucose ice cubes can fill both needs.

Resolved Needs: Food balance. Protection from physical harm.

Contraindications: Caloric dietary restrictions.

Provide gratifying experiences   Create circumstances in which the person can obtain pleasure and satisfaction from the experience.

Rationale: Perception of an experience as pleasurable reduces all threat and enhances renewal of that experience. When rewarding and gratifying conditions are seen as an end result, behavioral growth changes are more easily accomplished.

Resolved Needs: Comfort. Protection from psychologic threat. Warm, communicating relationships. Personal growth and maturity. Increased pleasantness.

Provide hearing-aid care Properly care for the patient's hearing aid by removing the batteries when the aid is not in use, cleaning the ear inserts, and safeguarding it against damage.

Rationale: A well-maintained hearing aid promotes improved auditory function.

Resolved Needs: Comfort. Dependence.

Provide heavyweight utensils Make available eating utensils, pencils, etc., made of heavyweight material. Avoid lightweight plastic objects.

Rationale: In impaired proprioception, the position of heavily weighted objects is most easily determined.

Resolved Needs: Comfort.

Contraindications: Muscle or motor impairment. Severe weakness.

Provide information about spiritual programs Inform the patient of the religious or spiritual programs available within the institution and on television or radio.

Rationale: Religious or spiritual programs that serve as a substitute for attendance at one's own church are comforting.

Resolved Needs: Comfort. Religious, philosophic satisfaction.

Provide large-print reading material Furnish reading matter printed in very large type and found in most public libraries.

Rationale: As eye muscle tone decreases, large print is more easily read and its use prevents eyestrain. Reading promotes focused attention on external stimuli which temporarily relieves internal stress.

Resolved Needs: Comfort. Protection from physical harm.

Provide lightweight utensils Supply knives, forks, spoons, glasses, and dishes made of lightweight plastic material.

Rationale: Lightweight utensils are easily held when there is muscle or motor impairment or fatigue.

Resolved Needs: Comfort. Independence.

Contraindications: Impaired proprioception.

Provide loose bedding with toe pleats Avoid tightly tucked bed sheets over the toes by putting toe pleats in the top sheet at the bottom of the bed.

Rationale: Pressure from tight bedding holds the foot in plantar flexion. Such prolonged pressure could tighten the heel cord and eventually prevent the patient from placing his heel flat on the floor when standing. Toe pleats prevent pressure, yet allow for neatly tucked linen.

Resolved Needs: Comfort. Protection from physical harm.

Provide needed supplies   Furnish equipment needed to perform a desired function.

Rationale: Providing task tools promotes the comfort of independent action.

Resolved Needs: Comfort. Independence.

Provide nursing availability   Reassure the patient that a professional nurse is easily attainable and readily accessible whenever the need arises.

Rationale: Illness often presents a situation where some needs cannot be met by independent action, causing the person to rely on others to meet those needs. Safety feelings arise from the assurance that help is available for need satisfaction.

Resolved Needs: Comfort. Protection from physical harm. Protection from psychologic threat. Dependence. Warm, communicating relationships. Attention.

Provide objects related to the message   When speaking to a person who has impaired message reception, give the person the object about which you are speaking. For instance, if you want him to scrub his teeth, tell him so and give him a toothbrush.

Rationale: Visual perception enhances reception of verbal messages. Comfort is promoted through effective communications with others.

Resolved Needs: Comfort. Warm, communicating relationships.

Provide objects which symbolize safeness   Furnish the person with material objects identified with past pleasure and safety, such as a child's blanket, an adult's favorite book.

Rationale: Feelings of safety arise from the presence of objects representing past pleasure and security. Stability evolves from the possession of objects perceived as permanent.

Resolved Needs: Comfort. Protection from psychologic threat. Stability.

Provide objects which symbolize sex identity   Provide the patient with objects symbolically identified with his or her particular sex. Male objects would include a pipe, objects associated with male sports, pictures of rugged scenes, work tools, model ships, boats, cars. Females would enjoy feminine clothes, perfumes, beauty products, recipes, needlework, dainty wall decorations. In order to meet the patient's needs, these objects must be highly individualized.

Rationale: Objects that are strongly identified with one's sexuality clarify the self-image and promote comfort.

Resolved Needs: Comfort. Sexuality. High evaluation of self.

Provide objects which symbolize status   At a time of status loss, the patient may find comfort in objects that represent status in his life. Such objects may include a uniform, a badge, the key to the executive washroom, framed diplomas.

Rationale: Objects strongly identified with one's status tend to clarify self-image and bring comfort.

Resolved Needs: Comfort. Status.

Provide pleasant experiences with feared objects   Associate a pleasurable sensation or event with the feared object.

Rationale: The threat of fear is reduced when a pleasurable emotion can be associated with the fear.

Resolved Needs: Comfort. Protection from psychologic threat.

Provide picture cards of objects   When attempting to communicate with a person who has impaired reception of verbal messages, furnish picture cards of objects in order to convey the message. If possible, include written descriptions of the object on the card.

Rationale: Comfort is promoted through effective communications with others.

Resolved Needs: Comfort. Warm, communicating relationships.

Provide prior notification of an impending separation
Gradually bring the therapeutic relationship to a close by notifying the patient of the impending separation ahead of time.

Rationale: Gradual change decreases adaptation stress. Safety feelings arise from predictable situations.

Resolved Needs: Comfort. Protection from physical harm. Protection from psychologic threat. Predictable, orderly world.

Provide prism eyeglasses   When a patient must continuously lie flat and is unable to hold a book for reading, furnish prism eyeglasses.

Rationale: The cut of glass into prisms allows for the upward reflection of objects. The ability to read promotes focused attention on external stimuli which temporarily relieves internal stress.

Resolved Needs: Comfort.

Provide quiet   Offer peaceful and tranquil surroundings.

Rationale: A quiet environment reduces the need for adaptation to stress.

Resolved Needs: Sleep, rest, relaxation. Comfort. Protection from physical harm.

Provide radio and television for diversion Turn on the radio or television to subjects which do not relate to the patient's problem. Periodically check to be sure that the radio or television topic has not changed to one that could disturb the patient.

Rationale: Focusing attention on external stimuli relieves internal stress by promoting temporary escape from conscious perception of threats such as fear, anxiety, and pain.

Resolved Needs: Comfort. Stimulation. Protection from physical harm. Protection from psychologic threat. Freedom from pain.

Provide reading material for diversion Furnish books and magazines whose topics do not relate to the patient's problem. Be certain that the topics satisfy the patient's interest.

Rationale: Focusing attention on external stimuli relieves internal stress by promoting temporary escape from conscious perception of threats such as fear, anxiety, and pain.

Resolved Needs: Comfort. Stimulation. Protection from physical harm. Protection from psychologic threat. Freedom from pain.

Provide receiving situations Create circumstances in which the person may be the recipient of positive and pleasant experiences fostered by others.

Rationale: Normal growth and maturity are dependent on the ability to give and receive love. A positive response from others indicates acceptance and promotes self-esteem and a sense of relatedness to others.

Resolved Needs: Comfort. Love and affection. Acceptance. Warm, communicating relationships. Approval from others. Sense of value. High evaluation of self. Attention. Personal growth and maturity. Increased pleasantness.

Provide reliable information Provide factual information regarding any situation.

Rationale: Fear and anxiety result from misperceptions due to lack of factual information. Adequacy and comfort evolve from factually analyzing situations and coping with them.

Resolved Needs: Comfort. Protection from psychologic threat. Adequacy.

Provide religious reading material Provide reading material having a spiritual theme.

Rationale: Spiritual reading elevates man's thoughts to higher resources.

Resolved Needs: Comfort. Religious, philosophic satisfaction.

Provide safe banging objects   Offer such objects as pots, rag dolls, old boards, and punching bags that can be banged on without injury to the person or object.

Rationale: Release of emotion in nonharmful ways prevents injury. Since banging is a normal developmental activity of children, safe banging objects should be provided.

Resolved Needs: Comfort. Protection from physical harm. Protection from psychologic threat.

Provide safe play equipment for children   Provide play equipment that is safe and suitable to the age of the child. Furnish the infant with such playthings as rattles, balls, rings to chew on, soft dolls and animals, noisemakers, bathtub toys, large blocks, pull toys, linen books. Furnish the preschool child with blocks, a sandbox with shovel and pail, a wagon, kiddy car, bicycle, rocking horse, boxes, balls, toys for playing house or store, dolls, trains, trucks, automobiles, airplanes, fire engines, stuffed animals, crayons and coloring books, chalk and blackboard, clay paints, mallets and hammers, picture books of all types, and large-piece puzzles. Furnish the school-age child with roller and ice skates, baseballs, footballs, jumping rope, croquet, tennis, complicated puzzles, nondangerous tools, games of all kinds, and books of adventure, suspense, and heros.

Rationale: Infant play should stimulate manipulation and investigation, gradually increase motor skills, lay the foundation for learning about size, shape, and texture, and promote development of large muscles. Preschool play should promote motor skills, sensory perception, physical development, creative imagination, and social relations with peers. School-age play should develop special interests and promote perfection of already learned skills, and skill competition between peers. All play should be safe.

Resolved Needs: Comfort. Protection from physical harm.

Provide seclusion   Place the emotionally disturbed person in an area or room totally away from contact with others.

Rationale: External control of behavior supports internal control when the latter cannot be maintained. Limitations protect against future shame resulting from presently uncontrolled behavior.

Resolved Needs: Comfort. Protection from physical harm. Protection from psychologic threat. High evaluation of self.

Provide standby emergency equipment (and/or drugs)
Furnish equipment or drugs that may be needed in an emergency. Keep it close to the patient as long as the possibility of an emergency exists. This includes oxygen, airways, tongue blades, rubber-tipped hemostats, tracheostomy tubes and trays, tourniquets, wire cutters, endotracheal tubes, defibrillators, suction machines, etc.

Rationale: Readily available emergency equipment and drugs can save a life when time is of the utmost importance.

Resolved Needs: Protection from physical harm.

Provide sufficiently long tubing to allow freedom of movement
Whenever tubing is inserted into the body, make certain it is long enough for the patient to freely turn and move about.

Rationale: Freedom of movement is essential to good circulation, general comfort and care.

Resolved Needs: Comfort. Protection from physical harm.

Provide sunglasses
Furnish eyeglasses containing colored lenses.

Rationale: Glare reduction prevents damage to optic tissue and nerves.

Resolved Needs: Comfort. Protection from physical harm.

Contraindications: Impaired vision where reduced illumination will raise the potential that the person might fall.

Provide unbreakable objects
Supply articles made of materials that will not break when dropped.

Rationale: Unbreakable objects, when dropped, will not result in physical injury.

Resolved Needs: Comfort. Protection from physical harm.

Provide words-and-phrases cards
When attempting to communicate with a person having impaired reception of verbal messages, furnish cards that have words and phrases written on them. If possible, supply pictures above the words and phrases.

Rationale: Comfort and competence are promoted through effective communications with others.

Resolved Needs: Comfort. Warm, communicating relationships.

Provide writing pad and pencil
When attempting to communicate with a person who is unable to speak, furnish a writing pad and pencil for his use.

Rationale: Comfort is promoted through effective communications with others.

Resolved Needs: Comfort. Warm, communicating relationships.

Read to the patient
When a person is unable to read due to visual impairment, brain damage, or position, offer to do it for him.

Rationale: Reading is a major source of comfort in communication of ideas and thoughts.

Resolved Needs: Comfort.

Reassure that pain will subside
While offering some measure for pain relief, verbally assure the person that the pain will soon be alleviated.

Rationale: Awareness that pain relief has been initiated promotes relaxation, which, in itself, decreases pain and promotes comfort.

Resolved Needs: Relaxation. Comfort. Protection from psychologic threat.

Contraindications: In intractable pain, it is better to reassure the person that pain will be reduced rather than alleviated.

Reassure verbally   Place the patient's mind at ease by verbal assurance that problems can be solved, and that the nurse will help solve these problems.

Rationale: Identification with the positive attitudes of other persons reduces fear and anxiety and promotes comfort.

Resolved Needs: Comfort. Protection from psychologic threat. Warm, communicating relationships.

Recognize the need for superstition   Permit belief in superstition but do not agree with such beliefs.

Rationale: Interference with deeply accepted superstitions causes feelings of threat and heightened anxiety.

Resolved Needs: Protection from psychologic threat.

Recognize the need for the use of appropriate defense mechanisms   Recognize the person's need for denial when acceptance of the situation is too difficult for adaptation within a short period of time. Recognize that reality sometimes must be presented in small doses so it can be accepted over a prolonged period of time.

Rationale: Denial is a therapeutic step toward future acceptance, supports normal coping, and temporarily fosters safety from threat. Temporary psychologic disequilibrium requires the utilization of protective mechanisms to decrease fear and anxiety and reestablish equilibrium.

Resolved Needs: Protection from psychologic threat. Personal growth and maturity. Increased reality perception and problem-solving ability.

Recognize the need for unique personal adjustments to change   Acknowledge that the patient must adapt to changes in life situations according to his or her age, stage of development, past life experiences, and physical and psychologic health. Support adjustment at the person's own pace.

Rationale: When there are physical or psychologic limitations in performance, an unhurried approach eliminates additional tension to the already tension-filled threat of inadequacy. Reduced tension provides more energy for physical healing and psychologic coping.

Resolved Needs: Comfort. Protection from physical harm. Protection from psychologic threat.

Record the battery-change date on the pacemaker generator box
Whenever the battery is changed in a pacemaker, place the date of change on the box where it is clearly visible.

Rationale: Since pacemaker batteries have a potential 3-year life, it is essential to know the replacement date to maintain a functional pacemaker.

Resolved Needs: Protection from physical harm.

Reduce infant handling to a minimum
Handle the infant (especially the irritable child) only when it is absolutely necessary. At all other times, leave him undisturbed.

Rationale: Decreased external stimuli reduces the need for adaptive responses, promotes sleep, and decreased energy depletion.

Resolved Needs: Sleep, rest, relaxation. Energy. Comfort. Protection from physical harm.

Reduce the demands placed upon the patient
Decrease the requirements placed upon the person and include only those that are essential.

Rationale: Adaptation and adjustment to demands require energy that, in illness, is needed for healing. Safety feelings evolve from an awareness that one can cope successfully with life.

Resolved Needs: Comfort. Protection from physical harm. Protection from psychologic threat. Adequacy.

Refocus on a safe conversational subject
When a person is obviously anxious regarding a particular subject of conversation, change the topic to a safe subject.

Rationale: External attempts to remove psychologic defenses increase anxiety. Refocusing on a safe conversational subject removes the discomfort and fosters psychologic equilibrium.

Resolved Needs: Comfort. Protection from psychologic threat.

Refrain from administering gastric lavage
Do not insert a nasogastric tube into the stomach for the purpose of washing out stomach contents.

Rationale: A gastric lavage performed after the ingestion of strong caustic poisons could cause perforation of the injured tissue.

Resolved Needs: Protection from physical harm.

Refrain from arguing
Avoid all verbal disputes despite the attempt of another to coax you into an argument.

Rationale: Emotionally charged interaction interferes with effective communications and is perceived as threatening.

Resolved Needs: Protection from psychologic threat. Warm, communicating relationships.

Refrain from asking the patient to repeat the message too often
When attempting to communicate with a person having an impaired ability to send messages, do not ask him to repeat the message over and over again. If the message is not understood on the first attempt, stop all other activity, ask the person to repeat the message, and concentrate fully on interpreting what is being said. If the message is still not understood, come to an agreement with the person on a more effective method of communication.

Rationale: Loss of the ability to communicate causes anxiety. Effective communication promotes comfort.

Resolved Needs: Comfort. Protection from psychologic threat.

Refrain from cleansing with alcohol
Do not clean the wound or injured body area with alcohol.

Rationale: Alcohol causes pain on burned areas and severely irritates some wounds.

Resolved Needs: Comfort. Protection from physical harm. Freedom from pain.

Refrain from dislodging blood clots
Do not touch a blood clot formed to seal off hemorrhage. Do not force a blood clot lodged in a needle into the vein.

Rationale: The disruption of blood clots formed to prevent hemorrhage can cause renewed hemorrhage. Dislodging clots from a needle into a vein can result in circulatory obstruction with tissue damage or death.

Resolved Needs: Protection from physical harm.

Refrain from distracting the patient while he swallows
Do not take the person's attention away from the task of swallowing. Avoid conversation and laughing.

Rationale: Pharyngeal or esophageal trauma, obstruction, impaired nerve or muscle function, inflammation, or congenital defects can make swallowing sufficiently difficult to require total concentration. Difficulty swallowing poses the potential threat of food aspiration into the lungs.

Resolved Needs: Protection from physical harm.

Refrain from doing a rectal examination
Do not insert a finger into the rectum for examination purposes.

Rationale: A foreign object inserted into the rectum causes mechanical stimulation of the defecation reflex and increases tissue injury, infection potential, and discomfort. Rectal stimulation results in vagus nerve stimulation which decreases the heart rate.

Resolved Needs: Comfort. Protection from physical harm.

Refrain from drawing blood studies via the subclavian Intracath   Do not draw blood or allow blood to be drawn for laboratory analysis through the subclavian Intracath being used for hyperalimentation.

Rationale: Blood cells will coat the internal catheter surface and obstruct the catheter, altering the flow rate of the hyperalimentation solution.

Resolved Needs: Protection from physical harm.

Refrain from elevating the bed at the knee gatch   Do not raise the bed under the patient's knee when there is venous stasis in the lower extremity.

Rationale: Elevating the bed at the knee gatch places pressure behind the knee, decreasing blood circulation.

Resolved Needs: Circulation. Protection from physical harm.

Refrain from equating sleep with the absence of pain   Do not assume that pain has subsided because the patient has fallen asleep.

Rationale: Pain can cause exhaustion that induces sleep during which pain is still felt.

Resolved Needs: Comfort. Protection from physical harm.

Refrain from forcing distasteful drugs   Do not forcibly insist that bad tasting medicine be taken. Instead, attempt to promote free choice regarding how the medication will be taken.

Rationale: Forcing bad tasting drugs may cause aspiration and decreases the chance of future voluntary medication ingestion.

Resolved Needs: Comfort. Protection from physical harm.

Refrain from forcing the treatment   Avoid insisting or physically forcing a person to accept unwanted health treatment.

Rationale: Forcing treatments causes intense anxiety and feelings of threat. The realization that one has sufficient control to prevent harm to oneself promotes comfort. Awareness that others respect one's wishes reinforces human dignity.

Resolved Needs: Comfort. Protection from psychologic threat. Dignity.

Contraindications: When persons are incapable of making appropriate decisions, some force may be required, but it should be kept at an absolute minimum.

Refrain from giving an alcohol rub   Do not apply friction to the skin by means of an alcohol rub.

Rationale: Alcohol has a drying effect on the skin. Alcohol fumes irritate respiratory mucosa. Since alcohol is highly volatile, it is never used on patients receiving oxygen.

Resolved Needs: Protection from physical harm.

Refrain from giving animal or vegetable oil orally   Do not give a poison antidote that contains animal or vegetable oil.

Rationale: Animal or vegetable oils are not soluble in insect or rat poisons that contain phosphorous and are therefore ineffective.

Resolved Needs: Protection from physical harm.

Refrain from giving between-meal feedings   Do not allow the patient with gastric ulceration to eat between meals. Provide three well-balanced meals a day with antacids between meals. Do not give food between meals to obese persons.

Rationale: Each time food is placed in the stomach, gastric secretions are stimulated, causing further irritation of ulcerated mucosa. When gastric secretions are stimulated only three times a day, there is less irritation and more time for healing. Between-meal feedings increase the caloric intake, compounding the problem of obesity.

Resolved Needs: Protection from physical harm.

Refrain from giving bicarbonates   Do not give any foods or drugs that contain carbonic acid.

Rationale: Low serum potassium can result in metabolic alkalosis, and bicarbonate ingestion will speed this complication.

Resolved Needs: Water-salt balance. Acid-base balance. Protection from physical harm.

Contraindications: Severe acidosis.

Refrain from giving carbonated beverages   Do not give effervescent drinks. If they must be given, vigorously stir the drink and let it stand until the effervescence is gone.

Rationale: The carbon dioxide (effervescence) in carbonated beverages is acid and can irritate sensitive gastrointestinal tissue, damage tooth enamel, and enhance acidosis by increasing the blood's carbon dioxide content. Carbonated beverages cause an alkaline urine which enhances the chance of calcium calculi formation and forms a carbon gas in the stomach which increases abdominal distention.

Resolved Needs: Acid-base balance. Comfort. Protection from physical harm.

Refrain from giving continuous positive pressure breathing   Do not allow continuous inhalation and exhalation of air into the lungs through mechanically induced positive pressure.

Rationale: Continuous inhalation and exhalation under positive pressure impairs normal cardiac output and increases intrathoracic pressure which decreases venous return. It is especially threatening when the blood volume has been lowered due to excessive fluid or blood loss.

Resolved Needs: Protection from physical harm.

Refrain from giving crumbling, flaking foods   Do not give foods that crumble and flake, such as cookies, crackers, cakes, coconut, dry cereals, hard biscuits.

Rationale: Crumbling or flaking foods can enter a tracheostomy and cause airway irritation or obstruction.

Resolved Needs: Protection from physical harm.

Refrain from giving enemas   Do not administer fluid into the rectum and colon.

Rationale: Enemas deplete body potassium and will further decrease low blood potassium levels. They increase peristalsis and intestinal spasm as a result of colon distention and, by stimulating peristalsis increase uterine contractions, causing severe after-birth pains or uterine bleeding. When a ureterosigmoidostomy is performed, the pressure of an enema may force feces into the ureters. During peritoneal dialysis, the intraabdominal pressure from the simultaneous instillation of enema fluid and dialysis fluid could rupture a visceral organ. When there is an inflamed appendix, the increased pressure from an enema may rupture the organ and cause peritonitis. Any time nausea, vomiting, or abdominal pain are present, enemas should not be given.

Resolved Needs: Water-salt balance. Protection from physical harm.

Refrain from giving hot liquids   Do not give very hot liquids such as coffee, tea, or soup.

Rationale: Hot liquids increase body temperature, injure oral mucous membranes or gums, increase the metabolic rate, cause vasodilatation which in severe cardiac impairment results in stagnation of the blood flow with reduced tissue oxygenation, increases peristalsis which is undesirable in diarrhea, may cause expansion of a cracked tooth, or pain in a cracked or sensitive tooth.

Resolved Needs: Normal temperature. Comfort. Protection from physical harm.

Refrain from giving iced liquids   Do not give extremely cold liquids.

Rationale: Iced liquids decrease body temperature, promote muscular and bladder spasm, cause vasoconstriction with resulting decreased blood supply to tissues, stimulate peristalsis which is undesirable during diarrhea, can cause retraction of a cracked tooth, or pain in a cracked or sensitive tooth.

Resolved Needs: Normal temperature. Comfort. Protection from physical harm.

Refrain from giving insulin   Do not allow the patient to receive insulin.

Rationale: Persons with Addison's disease have a chronically low blood glucose level. The administration of insulin will further lower the blood glucose level, causing death.

Resolved Needs: Protection from physical harm.

Refrain from giving intravenous or intramuscular injections
Do not give intravenous or intramuscular injections for at least 4–6 hours immediately after hemodialysis.

Rationale: Heparinization during hemodialysis enhances the bleeding tendency.

Resolved Needs: Protection from physical harm.

Refrain from giving laxatives   Do not give purgative and cathartic medications.

Rationale: Laxatives stimulate peristalsis, contractions, and cramping that can further damage irritated, traumatized, or poison-corroded intestinal mucosa. Harsh laxation causes dehydration. When laxatives are given during uterine bleeding, the heightened peristalsis increases uterine contractions causing more severe bleeding.

Resolved Needs: Comfort. Protection from physical harm.

Refrain from giving local cold applications   Do not apply cold to decubitus ulcers, gangrenous tissue, varicose veins, areas of vascular grafts, paralysis or sensation loss, or to age debilitated skin. Cold is usually not applied to skin grafts.

Rationale: Cold applications decrease body temperature, can stimulate chills, and can cause vasoconstriction which reduces tissue circulation.

Resolved Needs: Comfort. Protection from physical harm.

Refrain from giving local heat applications   Do not apply heat to areas of paralysis or sensation loss, edema, hemorrhage or trauma, the right lower abdomen in suspected appendicitis, the head following injury, or any body part after heart surgery.

Rationale: Heat applied to areas of diminished or absent sensation may result in a burn. When applied to enclosed tissues where the vasodilating effect expands tissue fluids or gases, it may cause increased pain, swelling, or rupture of tissues. Applications of heat increase tissue metabolism which in turn increases the cardiac workload. Warmth promotes the itching and discomfort of allergic reactions. Heat applied to the scrotum will destroy spermatozoa.

Resolved Needs: Protection from physical harm.

Refrain from giving magnesium laxatives and antacids   Do not give laxatives or antacids that contain a magnesium compound.

Rationale: The ingestion of magnesium salts increases the magnesium blood level.

Resolved Needs: Water-salt balance. Protection from physical harm.

Refrain from giving milk or juice in the infant's bottle at bedtime   Do not give the child a bottle of milk or juice to suck on while in bed.

Rationale: Carbohydrates sucked on for prolonged periods or allowed to remain in the mouth cause tooth decay.

Resolved Needs: Protection from physical harm.

Refrain from giving milk or milk products   Do not give milk, milk shakes, malts, ice cream, cream soups, etc.

Rationale: After digestion, milk produces a large amount of solid wastes that must be eliminated through the kidneys. In any condition where there is an increased need for fluids (fever, upper respiratory infection, etc.) milk will further increase the need for fluid resulting in dehydration and thickening of secretions.

Resolved Needs: Comfort. Protection from physical harm.

Refrain from giving oral analgesics   Do not administer oral analgesics immediately after surgery.

Rationale: Disturbances in gastrointestinal function following surgery result in unpredictable drug absorption.

Resolved Needs: Protection from physical harm.

Refrain from giving oral stimulants   Do not give coffee, tea, amphetamines, or alcohol.

Rationale: During electrical shock or when the myocardial blood supply is impaired, oral stimulants can cause ventricular fibrillation resulting in death. After a snake bite, oral stimulants increase circulation thereby hastening the flow of venom throughout the body.

Resolved Needs: Protection from physical harm.

Refrain from giving positive pressure breathing   Do not introduce air into the lungs during inhalation by mechanically induced intermittent positive pressure.

Rationale: When the patient already has an inadequate cardiac output such as myocardial infarction, IPPB reduces filling of the right side of the heart and thereby further reduces cardiac output. When the lung has been ruptured, the pressure from IPPB causes air to enter the pleural space building up pressure which results in shock. IPPB spreads active tuberculosis and increases pulmonary hemorrhage.

Resolved Needs: Protection from physical harm.

Refrain from giving potassium-containing drugs and solutions   Do not give drugs such as penicillin G potassium or whole blood containing potassium to persons with an elevated blood potassium level.

Rationale: Potassium drugs and solutions further elevate an already increased potassium blood level.

Resolved Needs: Water-salt balance. Protection from physical harm.

Refrain from giving saline laxatives   Do not give purgative or cathartic medications containing sodium. Such laxatives include magnesium citrate, magnesium sulfate, sodium potassium tartrate, sodium sulfate, sodium phosphate.

Rationale: Saline laxatives, by the process of osmosis, cause fluid withdrawal from body tissues and circulation into the intestines. If saline laxatives are given frequently, fluid loss will result in dehydration.

Resolved Needs: Water-salt balance. Protection from physical harm.

Refrain from giving table salt   Do not give iodized sodium chloride traditionally used as table salt.

Rationale: Decreasing sodium intake reduces the blood sodium level. Osmotic pressure then pulls sodium and water from the interstitial spaces into the blood, relieving tissue edema. In renal failure, bicarbonate loss due to increased urine excretion causes an increase in the blood's chloride level.

Resolved Needs: Water-salt balance. Protection from physical harm.

Refrain from giving tap water   When there are severe burns or sodium intake is restricted, do not give tap water.

Rationale: Tap water does not contain the balanced electrolyte factor needed in fluid replacement for burns. The large volume of tap water needed to quench the burned person's thirst would cause water intoxication. There is sufficient sodium in tap water to interfere with the maintenance of a specific restricted sodium intake.

Resolved Needs: Water-salt balance. Protection from physical harm.

Refrain from inserting a rectal tube   Do not insert a rectal tube into the colon.

Rationale: A foreign object inserted into the rectum causes mechanical stimulation of the defecation reflex and increases tissue injury, infection potential, and discomfort. Rectal stimulation results in vagal nerve stimulation which decreases the heart rate.

Resolved Needs: Comfort. Protection from physical harm.

Refrain from inserting objects into a bleeding orifice   Tubes or other objects should not be inserted into any bleeding orifice until the exact cause of bleeding has been determined.

Rationale: Irritating objects placed into a bleeding orifice promote further bleeding or cause increased tissue damage.

Resolved Needs: Protection from physical harm.

Refrain from jarring the bed   Do not allow the bed to be shaken or vibrated.

Rationale: Jarring can stimulate muscle spasms, severe pain, drainage of wounds and fistulas, and in hyperparathyroidism, can cause bone breakage.

Resolved Needs: Comfort. Protection from physical harm.

Refrain from lubricating the internal nares   Do not lubricate the nasal mucous membrane if there is difficulty breathing or evidence of past nasal allergies.

Rationale: Dust particles, when inhaled, cling to lubricated mucous membranes making breathing more difficult.

Resolved Needs: Protection from physical harm.

Refrain from making a specific length-of-life estimate (248)   When a person asks how long he will live, do not answer in months or days. Explain that there are many variables such as individual strength, disease progression, and treatments. An exception should be considered when the anticipated life span is short and the patient has significant responsibilities. Even in these cases the time should be expressed as "not very long" or "a very short time."

Rationale: Setting specific anticipated death dates heightens anxiety and increases hopelessness.

Resolved Needs: Comfort. Protection from psychologic threat.

Refrain from making promises   Avoid making promises and commitments that are difficult to keep.

Rationale: Refraint from making promises reduces the potential for distrust when promises cannot be met.

Resolved Needs: Protection from psychologic threat.

Refrain from making sudden, stimulating movements   Do not make sudden movements that will cause a startle reaction or lead to misinterpreted perception.

Rationale: Startle reactions cause temporary discomfort, accelerate physiologic activity, and require a response to perceived threat.

Resolved Needs: Comfort. Protection from physical harm. Protection from psychologic threat.

Refrain from negatively criticizing Do not make destructive remarks regarding a person's personality or character.

Rationale: Negative responses from others usually are perceived as threatening, while positive responses enhance positive self-evaluation.

Resolved Needs: Comfort. Protection from psychologic threat. Acceptance. Warm, communicating relationships. High evaluation of self.

Refrain from performing nonessential procedures Avoid doing treatments and procedures that are not absolutely necessary.

Rationale: Therapeutic procedures often present irritating external stimuli frequently perceived as threatening. They require adaptations that drain energy needed for the healing process. Many procedures cause patient embarrassment or increase anxiety if the patient feels his privacy is invaded.

Resolved Needs: Sleep, rest, relaxation. Energy. Comfort. Protection from physical harm. Protection from psychologic threat.

Refrain from personality comparing Do not verbally compare the qualities of one person with another. If evaluation is necessary, confine it to one person.

Rationale: Comparison with others promotes the threat of inadequacy. Comfort feelings require that a person experience acceptance from and relatedness to others.

Resolved Needs: Comfort. Protection from psychologic threat. Acceptance.

Refrain from placing a pillow under the knee Do not put a pillow or rolled blanket under the knee when there is venous stasis.

Rationale: Pressure applied under the knee decreases circulation.

Resolved Needs: Circulation. Protection from physical harm.

Refrain from placing fresh flowers in the room Do not put fresh flowers in the room. Suggest that family and friends bring artificial flowers.

Rationale: Fresh flowers often cause allergic or asthmatic responses.

Resolved Needs: Comfort. Protection from physical harm.

Refrain from placing in the chin-downward flexion position Do not allow the patient's head to bend forward, down toward the chest.

Rationale: The flexion head position causes fractured cervical vertebrae to injure or sever spinal cord nerves.

Rationale: Protection from physical harm.

Refrain from pulling the patient across the sheets   Do not pull the patient's body across the sheet surface. Instead, lift the body from one position to another.

Rationale: Pulling the body across a sheet causes friction irritation of the skin.

Resolved Needs: Comfort. Protection from physical harm.

Refrain from pulling the umbilical cord during placenta expulsion   Never attempt removal of the placenta by pulling the umbilical cord.

Rationale: Pulling the umbilical cord before the placenta is expelled can turn the uterus inside out.

Resolved Needs: Protection from physical harm.

Refrain from rapidly replacing lagging hyperalimentation solution   Do not rapidly increase the flow rate of hyperalimentation solution in an effort to make up for a slowed rate. Instead, reassess the desired fluid intake and readjust the flow rate at a moderate pace.

Rationale: The excessive metabolic stress caused by the rapid infusion of hyperalimentation solution can cause shock.

Resolved Needs: Protection from physical harm.

Refrain from relocating the patient in another room   Once the person is assigned and located in a room, do not move him to another room.

Rationale: A stable environment decreases tension by reducing frequent, forced adaptation.

Resolved Needs: Comfort. Protection from psychologic threat. Stability. Predictable, orderly world.

Refrain from removing the placenta except during uterine contraction   Never attempt to remove the placenta when the uterus is not firmly contracted.

Rationale: Removing the placenta from a relaxed uterus will turn the uterus inside out.

Resolved Needs: Protection from physical harm.

Refrain from restricting fluids   Do not limit the intake of fluids.

Rationale: During pregnancy, it is the high salt intake, not the fluid intake, that causes edema. Fluids are essential to the maintenance of normal body function during pregnancy. In diabetes insipidus, limiting fluids will not reduce the output of urine since the cause is not the amount of fluid intake but failure of the body to produce adequate antidiuretic hormone.

Resolved Needs: Protection from physical harm.

Refrain from saying anything you would not want the patient to hear   Avoid speaking in a whisper in the presence of the patient, or discussing any topic that would be distressing or disturbing to him.

Rationale: During illness, comments made by others often are misinterpreted. The illness may be such that clarification of the message is impossible. If the message reveals unpleasantness, the additional stress may increase anxiety and inhibit rest needed for healing.

Resolved Needs: Protection from physical harm. Protection from psychologic threat.

Refrain from sealing the tube with a heavy clamp   Do not close off tubes with large heavy metal clamps. Use lightweight small clamps.

Rationale: Heavy clamps pull tubing out of place and add the discomfort of having the tube reinserted.

Resolved Needs: Protection from physical harm.

Refrain from shouting at persons with communication disorders   Do not use a loud voice when speaking to persons with aphasic disorders, partial deafness, a stroke, in a coma, or who speak a foreign language. Changing one's voice to a higher or lower tone, rather than making it louder, often facilitates communications.

Rationale: Loud voice sounds frequently cause mental confusion and emotional stress. Voice tone changes are more readily perceptible.

Resolved Needs: Comfort. Protection from psychologic threat.

Refrain from simultaneously powdering and lubricating the skin   Do not powder and oil the skin at the same time. It is preferable not to powder until all oils have soaked into the skin, to powder without applying oil, or to oil without applying powder.

Rationale: A mixture of oil and powder on the skin causes caking and irritation.

Resolved Needs: Comfort. Cleanliness. Protection from physical harm.

Refrain from strapping the ventilator mask in place   When artificial ventilation disturbs the person, refrain from strapping the mask onto his face. Instead, have him hold the mask tightly against the face with his hand or use a mouthpiece.

Rationale: The ability to control an undesirable or frightening object that affects respirations, promotes comfort.

Resolved Needs: Comfort.

Refrain from supporting the patient's delusions (illusions or hallucinations) Do not participate actively in the patient's delusions, illusions, or hallucinations. If he says that he is a king and asks for a crown, do not pretend to give him one. If, when hallucinating, he sees snakes, do not agree with him. If he thinks a lace curtain is a spider web, do not support the illusion.

Rationale: Other person's noninvolvement in delusional, hallucinatory, or illusional behavior enhances reality perception.

Resolved Needs: Increased reality perception.

Refrain from taking rectal temperatures Do not take the temperature rectally. Instead use the oral or axillary method.

Rationale: Thermometer insertion into the rectum may cause pain, bleeding, stimulation of the defecation reflex, or vagal nerve stimulation which decreases the heart rate. It increases existing tissue injury and, when worm lavae come in contact with the rectal thermometer, causes further contamination thereby increasing the potential for infection.

Resolved Needs: Protection from physical harm.

Refrain from taping the intestinal tube until it is fully advanced When gastrointestinal tubes are to be advanced at specific times, do not tape the tubing with each advancement. Wait until the tube has reached its final desired location before taping.

Rationale: A taped tube will not advance naturally in response to peristaltic movements. Frequent application and removal of tape damages the skin.

Resolved Needs: Comfort. Protection from physical harm.

Refrain from teasing Do not verbally jest or make satirical remarks.

Rationale: Persons with sensitive perception may interpret teasing as a negative and threatening response from others.

Resolved Needs: Comfort. Protection from psychologic threat.

Refrain from tight bandaging Do not apply bandages so tightly that they will constrict blood flow. Do not apply tape so it completely encircles an extremity.

Rationale: Injured tissues require unimpaired circulation for healing. Swelling following an injury may cause a snug bandage to impair circulation with resulting tissue damage.

Resolved Needs: Comfort. Protection from physical harm.

Refrain from using a cotton-filled gauze tracheostomy dressing Do not use cotton-filled gauze when changing a tracheostomy dressing. Nonwoven or premade molded gauze is preferable.

Rationale: Cotton gauze shreds. When pieces of cotton are sucked into the tracheostomy on inhalation, respiratory obstruction can occur.

Resolved Needs: Protection from physical harm.

Refrain from using a cream-based soap
Do not use soap having a base of cream such as cold cream.

Rationale: Cream-based soaps add oil to the skin and further obstruct overactive sebaceous glands.

Resolved Needs: Protection from physical harm.

Contraindications: Very dry skin.

Refrain from using a ventilator nose clip
When artificial ventilation disturbs the person, refrain from placing a ventilator clip on the nose. Instead, have the patient hold his nose with his fingers.

Rationale: The ability to control an undesirable or frightening object that affects respirations promotes comfort.

Resolved Needs: Comfort.

Refrain from using an alkaline soap on the skin
Use soaps that are combined with oils and do not have a high percentage of alkali. Inexpensive soaps are usually alkaline.

Rationale: Excessive alkali in soap is a potential source of skin irritation.

Resolved Needs: Protection from physical harm.

Refrain from using punitive measures in exercising authority
Exercise authority in a quiet, unassuming, firm manner that cannot be interpreted as punishment. Avoid the use of punitive measures.

Rationale: Punishment is associated with dependency which poses the threat of loss of control.

Resolved Needs: Comfort. Protection from psychologic threat. Warm, communicating relationships.

Refresh the patient before sleep
Use hygienic measures to refresh the body before sleep.

Rationale: Cleanliness promotes comfort and relaxation which supports rest and sleep.

Resolved Needs: Sleep, rest, relaxation. Comfort.

Refresh with a mouth freshener
Spray a chemically refreshing solution into the mouth.

Rationale: Mouth freshener promotes the comfort of a clean, fresh mouth.

Resolved Needs: Comfort. Cleanliness.

Refresh with a mouthwash   Offer a refreshing and cleansing solution to swirl in the mouth. If oral tissues are inflamed or irritated, dilute the mouthwash with water.

Rationale: The removal of decaying food by bubbling action and the reduction of bacteria controls bad breath and promotes cleanliness. Alkaline mouthwashes cause less saliva stimulation than acid mouthwashes. Alkaline mouthwashes contain calcium, magnesium, potassium, or sodium hydroxide.

Resolved Needs: Comfort. Cleanliness. Protection from physical harm. Dependence.

Contraindications: Avoid using alkaline mouthwashes in hypernatremia, hyperkalemia, hypercalcemia, and sodium-restricted diets.

Regulate the hypodermoclysis rate to prevent painful swelling   When giving a hypodermoclysis, maintain a rate sufficiently slow to prevent painful tissue swelling and skin blanching.

Rationale: Since blood will absorb only the amount of fluid needed for fluid balance, when painful edema exists at the hypodermoclysis site, it indicates that fluid absorption is slower than fluid administration, and that the flow rate should be decreased.

Resolved Needs: Comfort. Protection from physical harm.

Reinforce concern throughout the entire illness   Frequently assure the person that every possible thing will be done for him in the way of treatment and comforting measures. Throughout the entire illness, assure him that all health personnel are available and sincerely concerned for his welfare.

Rationale: Awareness that others are supportive prevents feelings of isolation, anxiety, and hopelessness.

Resolved Needs: Comfort. Protection from psychologic threat. High evaluation of self. Endurance. Dignity.

Release restraints and walk the patient periodically   Remove the patient's restraints at least every 6 hours. If possible, ambulate or sit the patient up. Maintain constant nursing supervision during this time.

Rationale: Long-term restraint impairs tissue circulation because of limited motion. Release from restraints reduces anxiety associated with forced immobility.

Resolved Needs: Circulation. Comfort. Protection from psychologic threat.

Contraindications: Extreme agitation.

Remove adhesive tape and adhesive debris   Gently remove the adhesive tape from the skin. Remove the adhesive debris by applying baby oil, cold cream, acetone, or peanut butter to the area and then wiping it clean.

Rationale: Removing adhesive tape and the remaining adhesive debris promotes skin cleanliness and reduces irritation.

Resolved Needs: Comfort. Cleanliness. Protection from physical harm.

Remove blisters from the burned area (47)   If a large skin area is burned, use mild pressure applied with sterile gauze, a sterile scapel, or sterile scissors to break the blisters. If the burned area is small, leave the blisters intact.

Rationale: When blisters cover a large burned area, they cannot be protected from breaking. Breaking the blisters under sterile conditions facilitates the maintenance of a clean skin area.

Resolved Needs: Cleanliness. Protection from physical harm.

Remove constrictive clothing   Remove clothing that causes tightness around the patient's body or that limits free, normal body movements.

Rationale: Constriction that prevents venous return will impair circulation and result in tissue damage. Limitations placed on body movements prevent normal mobility.

Resolved Needs: Circulation. Comfort. Protection from physical harm. Freedom from pain.

Remove food from the mouth   When a person is choking, manually remove unchewed food from his mouth or have him spit the food out.

Rationale: Foreign objects in the mouth can be aspirated into the lung during a choking episode, causing impaired pulmonary ventilation.

Resolved Needs: Oxygen. Cleanliness. Protection from physical harm.

Remove foreign object(s)   Remove any object from the skin or body orifice that does not normally belong there. This may require the use of forceps, irrigations, and so forth. When removing foreign objects from the eye, use moistened sterile gauze. Never use cotton in the eye. Remove foreign objects with great care so further injury does not occur.

Rationale: Foreign particles may cause mucosal irritation, infection, or obstruction of passages.

Resolved Needs: Oxygen. Comfort. Protection from physical harm.

Remove hair with a depilatory cream   Use a chemical cream compound that will remove hair.

Rationale: Hair removal with a depilatory cream minimizes the potential for being cut with a razor and promotes thorough cleansing of the body part.

Resolved Needs: Comfort. Protection from physical harm.

Contraindications: Any evidence of skin irritation before or after using the cream.

Remove harmful objects from the environment
Watch for and remove all objects that could cause physical harm such as knives, razors, sheets, belts, cleaning fluids, electric sockets, utensils, glasses, dishes.

Rationale: Certain common objects, when possessed by persons with self-destructive tendencies, can be used to carry out physical self-harm. Recognition of potential physical threats promotes safety. Respect for the basic worth of man promotes the support of life whenever possible.

Resolved Needs: Protection from physical harm. Dignity.

Remove immediately to a safe area
When a person has been harmed by some environmental condition, move the person away from the area of danger.

Rationale: An unsafe environment increases the potential for health impairment.

Resolved Needs: Protection from physical harm.

Remove loose burned skin with a gauze pad and slight pressure (47)
In the early stage of burn, while the skin is still soft, gently rub the skin with a gauze pad and, with slight pressure, gently remove the burned tissue from the living tissue.

Rationale: The removal of loose burned skin minimizes infection by eliminating areas under which bacteria prefer to collect.

Resolved Needs: Cleanliness. Protection from physical harm.

Remove the arteriovenous shunt clot
Shunt clots can be removed by aspirating them with a piece of sterile gauze, with a sterile syringe after a heparinized, normal saline solution has been injected, or by inserting a thin plastic tube into the cannula and aspirating with a syringe.

Rationale: Removal of an arteriovenous shunt clot prevents the clot from entering the circulatory system. It minimizes clogging of the shunt that would require tube removal and replacement.

Resolved Needs: Protection from physical harm.

Remove the bedpan immediately following its use
Remove the bedpan immediately after it has been used and wash and dry it.

Rationale: Quickly removing the bedpan reduces pressure on the skin, decreases tissue irritation, and offers assistance in illness dependency.

Resolved Needs: Comfort. Protection from physical harm. Dependence.

Remove the colon tube for bowel elimination and then reinsert about 4 inches   When the patient has a ureterosigmoidostomy, a rectal tube is kept in place for the first 10 postoperative days. When the patient needs to have a bowel elimination, gently remove the tube. Following elimination, reinsert it 4 inches into the rectum.

Rationale: With a ureterosigmoidostomy, a colon tube is placed in the rectum for urine drainage. Since feces cannot pass through the tube, it is removed for bowel elimination.

Resolved Needs: Waste elimination.

Remove the contact lens   If the patient has an eye infection or is going to sleep, remove his contact lenses if he is unable to do so. In order to remove a contact lens from the cornea, open the person's eye. Pull the side of the eye (near the ear) outward with one hand. With the other hand, gently pull the lids together and the lens should pop out. Before attempting to remove a lens, be sure it is over the cornea. If it is not, gently close the eyelid and, with very gentle pressure, move the lens toward the cornea. After removing the lenses, be careful to place them in a case or a safe container. Do not mixup the right and left lens.

Rationale: Wearing contact lenses during sleep or eye infection may cause corneal injury.

Resolved Needs: Comfort. Cleanliness. Protection from physical harm. Dependence.

Remove the dentures   Take the patient's artificial teeth out of his mouth.

Rationale: The removal of artificial dentures prevents respiratory obstruction in unconscious or confused states. When the dentures are irritating the oral mucosa, their removal prevents tissue trauma.

Resolved Needs: Protection from physical harm.

Remove the fecal impaction manually   With a slightly lubricated gloved finger, gently remove accumulated feces tightly wedged in the colon.

Rationale: Removal of hard fecal material promotes comfort and elimination. It prevents loss of rectal muscle tone from prolonged distention.

Resolved Needs: Waste elimination. Comfort. Protection from physical harm.

Remove the insect stinger   When a person is bitten by an insect with a stinger, remove the stinger by pulling it out of the skin.

Rationale: Removing an insect stinger eliminates the source of pain.

Resolved Needs: Comfort. Freedom from pain.

Remove the person from the electrocuting source with a non-conducting material   Use dry objects made of wood, rubber, or rope to remove the person from the source of electrical shock.

Rationale: Rubber, wood, and rope do not conduct electricity and will prevent the electrical current from harming the rescuer.

Resolved Needs: Protection from physical harm.

Remove the stimuli which support the misperception   When the environment contains stimuli that the patient perceives as disturbing, remove those stimuli whenever possible. Example: If a statue of a kitten is perceived to be a dangerous tiger, remove it from the room. Replace the object when the patient's condition improves.

Rationale: The removal of objects misperceived as threatening promotes rest and comfort.

Resolved Needs: Sleep, rest, relaxation. Comfort. Protection from psychologic threat.

Remove the stimulus for the emotion   Remove persons, objects, or situations that arouse severely unpleasant or disturbing feelings.

Rationale: An awareness that controls exist to prevent harm to oneself promote comfort and safety feelings.

Resolved Needs: Comfort. Protection from physical harm. Protection from psychologic threat.

Remove the sutures (ExR)   When healing appears to have occurred, about the fifth or sixth day after suturing, remove the sutures. Using forceps to lift each suture, cut the suture near the skin with surgical scissors and pull them out one by one.

Rationale: Once healing has occurred, sutures are no longer needed. Removing them reduces their potential for causing a wound infection.

Resolved Needs: Comfort. Protection from physical harm.

Remove the therapeutic tube when the treatment is terminated   Gently remove such tubes as gastric, hyperalimentation, colon, or T-tubes, urinary or venous catheters, etc., when they are no longer needed for treatment.

Rationale: The removal of unneeded tubes increases comfort and reduces the injury and infection potential.

Resolved Needs: Comfort. Cleanliness. Protection from physical harm.

Remove the tick with tweezers   If a tick has imbedded itself in the skin or hair, use tweezers rather than your fingers to remove it.

Rationale: Removal of the tick with tweezers enhances the chance of complete removal and prevents the tick from striking the person attempting to remove it with his fingers.

Resolved Needs: Protection from physical harm.

Repeat the message until it is understood   Repeat messages not properly interpreted until they are correctly understood.

Rationale: Message repetition enhances communication by reinforcing perception of the intended ideas and thoughts.

Resolved Needs: Warm, communicating relationships.

Replace the pacemaker batteries   Between 30 and 36 months after batteries have been installed in a pacemaker, exchange them for new batteries.

Rationale: Proper pacemaker function is essential to life. Awareness that such a device is functioning properly supports patient comfort.

Resolved Needs: Comfort. Protection from physical harm.

Replace the prolapsed umbilical cord into the vagina   When the physician is not immediately available, wash the protruding portion of the umbilical cord with a sterile soap solution and, using sterile gloves, replace the cord into the vagina.

Rationale: A sterile umbilical cord must be maintained to prevent infection of the birth canal.

Resolved Needs: Protection from physical harm.

Respond immediately to the patient's call   When a person signals for help, provide immediate attention and effective measures to resolve the difficulty.

Rationale: Early recognition of abnormalities by health personnel promotes safety. Psychologic comfort is fostered by an awareness that one is not alone when threatened with pain, fear, or anxiety.

Resolved Needs: Comfort. Protection from physical harm. Protection from psychologic threat. Attention.

Restrain the patient   Limit the person's freedom of movement with restraining devices only after due consideration of patient safety and the legal factors involved.

Rationale: Gentle restraint protects the person from accidental injury.

Resolved Needs: Protection from physical harm.

Contraindications: When the use of physical force threatens the person's integrity, promotes distrust or aggressive behavior. When restraint benefits institutional routine and not patient safety.

Restrict fluids at mealtime   Do not give fluids with the meal, though warm fluids may be sipped after the meal.

Rationale: In the dumping syndrome, fluid ingestion during meals causes the production of a hypertonic solution in the small intestine. This hypertonic solution pulls fluid from the blood into the intestine, causing intestinal distention and irritation, which results in diarrhea.

Resolved Needs: Protection from physical harm.

Restrict head movements with sandbags and pillows   Place sandbags or pillows snugly against the side of the face to prevent sudden turning or movement of the head.

Rationale: Sudden head movements may increase pressure within the eye, causing visual damage in eye disorders. In trauma, sudden head movements frequently cause further injury.

Resolved Needs: Protection from physical harm.

Restrict the blood transfusion rate to 500 cc every two to four hours   Regulate the rate of blood being transfused to no more than 500 cc over a 2- to 4-hour period. In cases of severe emergency and blood depletion, up to 100 cc/minute may be given.

Rationale: A rapid increase in circulating fluid volume can cause pulmonary edema or fluid and electrolyte imbalance.

Resolved Needs: Water-salt balance. Protection from physical harm.

Restrict the fluid intake according to the weight gain   Limit the amount of fluid taken in a 24-hour period to the amount of weight gained in the past 24 hours. For every pound of weight gained, limit fluid intake 500 cc.

Rationale: When water balance is maintained, the body weight remains unchanged if the person is in nutritional balance and not in negative nitrogen balance. A loss or gain of solid tissue is accompanied by a loss or gain of water. A 1-pound weight gain in 24 hours is considered to be a 500 cc accumulation of excess fluid.

Resolved Needs: Water-salt balance. Protection from physical harm.

Contraindications: Pregnancy.

Restrict the fluid intake to 600 cc plus the output   Maintain the person's fluid intake at 600 cc plus the amount of output lost through urine, gastric secretions, profuse perspiration, wound drainage, etc.

Rationale: 600 cc fluid intake is essential for normal renal function under conditions of normal body and environmental temperature. The additional intake of other output losses prevents dehydration.

Resolved Needs: Water-salt balance. Protection from physical harm.

Contraindications: Pregnancy. Diabetes insipidus.

Restrict the glucose intravenous solution rate according to the weight   Intravenous solutions of glucose should be given at a calculated hourly rate of 0.5 g of glucose per kilogram of body weight.

Rationale: Rapid intravenous glucose infusions can cause glucosuria or potassium depletion.

Resolved Needs: Water-salt balance. Protection from physical harm.

Restrict the hypertonic intravenous solution rate to 200 cc per hour   Regulate the rate of a hypertonic intravenous solution containing more than 0.9% salt or over 5% sugar in water so it does not exceed 200 cc/hr. Check bottle labels indicating which fluids are hypertonic.

Rationale: When hypertonic solutions are introduced into the circulatory system, the fact that they contain more salt or sugar and less water (increased osmotic pressure) than the blood causes them to pull fluid from the blood cells to equalize the pressure differences between the fluid and the cell contents. This physiologic change results in shrinkage of the blood cells and should not be allowed to occur at a rapid rate.

Resolved Needs: Water-salt balance. Protection from physical harm.

Restrict the hypotonic intravenous solution rate to 400 cc per hour   Regulate the rate of a hypotonic intravenous solution containing less than 0.9% salt or less than 5% sugar in water so it does not exceed 400 cc/hr. Check bottle labels indicating which fluids are hypotonic.

Rationale: When hypotonic solutions are introduced into the circulatory system, the fact that they contain less salt or sugar and more water (decreased osmotic pressure) than the blood causes fluid to be pulled from the solution into the blood cells to equalize the pressure differences between the fluid and the cell contents. This physiologic change results in swelling of the blood cells and should not be allowed to occur at a rapid rate.

Resolved Needs: Water-salt balance. Protection from physical harm.

Restrict the intake to nothing by mouth   Do not allow the intake of any food or fluid.

Rationale: Withholding food and fluids decreases gastric juice secretion, irritation of intestinal mucosa, and stimulation of peristalsis. A clean intestinal tract is necessary for many diagnostic studies.

Resolved Needs: Comfort. Protection from physical harm.

Contraindications: In severe debilitation and in very young children, limit the NPO restriction to as short a time as possible.

Restrict the intravenous potassium to 20 mEq per hour or 200 mEq per 24 hours   When administering potassium containing intravenous infusions, regulate the potassium so that the adult patient receives no more than 20 mEq each hour.

Rationale: Potassium, given too rapidly, causes cardiac irritability with resulting arrythmia and potential cardiac standstill.

Resolved Needs: Water-salt balance. Protection from physical harm.

Restrict the isotonic intravenous solution rate to 600 cc per hour
Regulate the rate of an isotonic intravenous solution containing 0.9% salt or 5% sugar in water so it does not exceed 600 cc/hr. Preferably it is given at a much slower rate. However, in cases of severe emergency and fluid depletion, as much as 2000 cc may be given per hour. Check bottle labels indicating which fluids are isotonic.

Rationale: When isotonic solutions are introduced into the circulatory system, the fact that they contain a concentration of salt or sugar (osmotic pressure) equal to that of the blood makes them safe to give at a fairly rapid rate. Isotonic solutions maintain the blood cells in a relatively normal state and do not produce the shrinkage effect of hypertonic solutions or the swelling effect of hypotonic solutions on cells.

Resolved Needs: Water-salt balance. Protection from physical harm.

Restrict unwanted visitors
Prevent specifically named persons from visiting the patient when it is evident that these persons are a disturbing influence. Limits should be enforced when the patient expresses negative feelings toward persons but is himself unable to control the visiting without a breakdown in interpersonal relationships.

Rationale: Highly emotional conditions deplete body energy and stimulate irritating regulatory secretions. Safety feelings evolve from an awareness that sufficient control can be exerted to prevent harm to oneself.

Resolved Needs: Comfort. Protection from physical harm. Protection from psychologic threat.

Resuscitate breathing (ET)
When respirations have ceased as a result of accident or a cardiopulmonary pathologic state, immediately administer artificial ventilation. Remove foreign matter from the mouth and pharynx. Bend the head backward. Push the jaw outward to move the tongue from the back of the throat. Pinch the nostrils closed. Open the patient's mouth wide. Take a deep breath. Place your mouth on his and blow vigorously into his airway. Remove your mouth and watch for chest movement and returned air through the mouth and nose. Repeat the procedure approximately 12 times a minute until respirations are spontaneous or mechanical respirator assistance is available. If the patient is a child, place your mouth over the child's nose and mouth and promote shallow breaths about 20 times a minute. Moderate intermittent pressure on the diaphragm also will stimulate respirations. The pressure should be applied only for inspiration and omitted momentarily for expiration.

Rationale: Oxygen and carbon dioxide exchange is essential to life and the prevention of brain tissue damage.

Resolved Needs: Oxygen. Waste elimination. Protection from physical harm.

Resuscitate mouth-to-neck when the patient has a laryngectomy (ET)   When a person who has had a laryngectomy requires resuscitation, place the patient on his back. Place your mouth around the stoma (or tracheostomy tube) and blow air into the trachea until the chest rises. Allow time for the chest to fall and repeat the procedure. If the chest fails to rise, place the palm of the hand over the lips and mouth. Hold the jaw upward and pinch the nose closed before resuscitation.

Rationale: When a person has a total laryngectomy, air cannot reach the lungs by way of the mouth or nose and must be administered through the stoma.

Resolved Needs: Oxygen. Waste elimination. Protection from physical harm.

Retract and clean the foreskin   Each time the male infant is bathed, gently pull back the penal foreskin and clean the head of the penis. Gently pull the skin back in place once cleansing is completed.

Rationale: Cleanliness prevents infection.

Resolved Needs: Cleanliness. Protection from physical harm.

Return the blood to the blood bank after a reaction   When a blood transfusion reaction occurs, return the remaining blood to the blood bank.

Rationale: Checking for blood incompatibility or bacterial contamination reduces the potential for further harm to the patient.

Resolved Needs: Protection from physical harm.

Reveal the patient's ambivalent feelings   Bring to the person's attention opposing feelings that his behavior indicates he is experiencing.

Rationale: Insight into one's own feelings promotes growth, maturity, and problem solving.

Resolved Needs: Personal growth and maturity. Increased reality perception and problem-solving ability.

Rinse the mouth with dilute hydrogen peroxide   Using a solution of half water and half hydrogen peroxide, have the patient rinse his mouth several times a day.

Rationale: The oxidizing action of hydrogen peroxide acts as a cleansing agent and discourages the growth of certain microorganisms.

Resolved Needs: Cleanliness. Protection from physical harm.

Safeguard the patient's artificial eye   Protect the patient's artificial eye by placing it in a case or container.

Rationale: Protecting the artificial eye prevents scratches on it which could cause socket irritation, minimizes breakage, and maintains cleanliness which prevents infection.

Resolved Needs: Comfort. Cleanliness. Protection from physical harm.

Safeguard the patient's contact lenses Protect the patient's contact lenses by placing them in a lens wetting solution or plain water. Keep the lenses in a protective case.

Rationale: Protection of contact lenses assures their availability as an aid to better vision.

Resolved Needs: Comfort. Protection from physical harm.

Safeguard the patient's dentures Protect dentures from damage and from being lost by placing them in a safe container and location. Be certain to inform the patient of their whereabouts.

Rationale: Artificial teeth aid in the chewing and digestion of food, maintain a natural jaw contour, and promote comfort.

Resolved Needs: Comfort. Protection from physical harm.

Safeguard the patient's eyeglasses Protect eyeglasses from cracking, breaking, and scratching.

Rationale: Eyeglass safety supports visual acuity and reduces the economic stress of having to replace them.

Resolved Needs: Comfort. Protection from physical harm.

Safeguard the patient's hearing aid Protect the hearing aid by placing it where it cannot be damaged or broken.

Rationale: Protection of the hearing aid assures its availability to improve hearing.

Resolved Needs: Comfort. Protection from physical harm.

Safeguard the patient's personal belongings Keep articles belonging to the person in a secure place and properly labeled with adequate identification.

Rationale: Respect for a patient's personal belongings indicates respect for the person.

Resolved Needs: Comfort. Protection from psychologic threat. Dignity.

Safeguard with a crib dome Protect the child from falling or getting out of bed by applying a plastic crib dome over the bed.

Rationale: Adequate safety measures prevent severe injury.

Resolved Needs: Protection from physical harm.

Safeguard with accurate identification   Protect the patient with a corrent identification band.

Rationale: Accurate patient identification promotes safety and exhibits dignity through concern for the patient.

Resolved Needs: Protection from physical harm. Dignity.

Safeguard with siderail padding   Place cushioned bed rails on either side of the bed.

Rationale: Adequate safety measures prevent severe injury.

Resolved Needs: Protection from physical harm.

Safeguard with siderails   Place bed rails on either side of the bed.

Rationale: Adequate safety measures prevent severe injury.

Resolved Needs: Protection from physical harm.

Save the poison container for content analysis   If a poisonous substance has been ingested and the identification of the product is unknown, keep the container and send it with the patient when he seeks medical care.

Rationale: Knowledge of the substance ingested allows for effective treatment with appropriate antidotes.

Resolved Needs: Protection from physical harm.

Schedule toileting   Take the patient to the bathroom or place him on the bedpan or bedside commode at specific times, periodically throughout the day or night. Select a time compatible with the person's prior elimination schedule and his present daily activities.

Rationale: Offering the opportunity for elimination prevents accidents and promotes elimination. When bowel or bladder retraining is essential to maintain elimination control, the body systems adapt more readily to routine functioning than to unscheduled activity.

Resolved Needs: Waste elimination. Comfort. Cleanliness. Protection from physical harm. Dependence.

Screen the patient for privacy   Protect the person from the observation of others by means of a curtain or screen.

Rationale: Comfort is increased when normal sociocultural values are upheld, despite dependency on others. Awareness of esteem from others results from satisfactory and respectful relationships with others.

Resolved Needs: Comfort. Protection from psychologic threat. Dignity.

Scrub the skin with Betadine   Cover the skin area with the iodine preparation, Betadine.

Rationale: Betadine has a prolonged antiseptic effect. It kills skin bacteria, fungus, viruses, yeasts, and protozoa. It is used to treat chronic skin infection (pyoderma), fresh lacerations, and beginning decubitus.

Resolved Needs: Cleanliness. Protection from physical harm.

Contraindications: Known Betadine allergy.

Season the food for individual taste   Add salt and pepper to already prepared foods in amounts preferred by the person.

Rationale: Seasoning food enhances flavor and promotes a greater desire to eat.

Resolved Needs: Comfort.

Contraindications: Salt-restricted diets.

Set limits on unacceptable behavior   Request cooperation in curtailing unacceptable behavior by clearly defining roles, responsibilities, routines, and what the person can and cannot do. Limits may be set by verbal comments or judicious restraint.

Rationale: External control of behavior supports internal control when the latter cannot be maintained. Limitations protect against future shame resulting from presently uncontrolled behavior. Esteem needs from others promote acceptance of and conformity to expectations of others.

Resolved Needs: Comfort. Protection from psychologic threat. Personal growth and maturity. Increased reality perception and problem-solving ability.

Shampoo the hair (scalp)   Clean the hair with soap and water or shampoo.

Rationale: Cleanliness prevents infection and promotes comfort.

Resolved Needs: Comfort. Cleanliness. Protection from physical harm.

Contraindications: Skull fracture. Potential or existing intracranial hemorrhage. Extra caution should be taken when there are skull tongs for cervical traction.

Shave the hair surrounding the burned area (47)   Using shaving cream and a safety razor or Weck blade, remove the hair on the uninjured skin around a burned area. Heat from the burn usually removes the hair from the burned area. If some hair still remains, it too should be shaved gently.

Rationale: Hair around or on a burn collects bacteria which heightens the potential for infection.

Resolved Needs: Cleanliness. Protection from physical harm.

Shield the tracheostomy (or laryngectomy stoma) from water   Cover a tracheostomy or laryngectomy stoma with a protective

shield such as a folded washcloth or the hand whenever the patient takes a shower. Never use a plastic bag as a covering.

Rationale: Water in a tracheostomy tube or laryngectomy stoma obstructs the airway.

Resolved Needs: Protection from physical harm.

Shield visitors from exposure to radiation   When a visitor stays with a patient receiving radiation therapy, protect that person through radiation shielding. Have him wear a lead-lined apron and sit behind lead-lined drapes or a thick concrete wall.

Rationale: Certain materials decrease the spread of radiation rays. Body exposure to radioactive substances results in blood cell disturbances, sterility, internal burns, genetic changes, gastrointestinal upsets, and altered tissue cell structure.

Resolved Needs: Protection from physical harm.

Sit the patient in an armchair   Assist the patient into a well-supported sitting position in a comfortable armchair.

Rationale: Sitting up prevents fluid congestion in the lungs, stimulates circulation, restores normal physiologic function, and promotes comfort. An armchair provides the safety of a supportive structure against which the weakened patient may lean.

Resolved Needs: Rest, relaxation. Activity, exercise. Comfort. Stimulation. Protection from physical harm.

Contraindications: Temperature elevation above 103°F. Head or spinal cord injury. Internal hemorrhage. Coma or semicoma. Severe energy depletion. Life-threatening situations.

Sit with the patient   Sit in a chair beside the patient either silently or engaging in activity and conversation.

Rationale: Psychologic comfort results from an awareness that one is not alone. The presence of another person is stimulative, provides attention, and supports interpersonal communications.

Resolved Needs: Comfort. Stimulation. Protection from psychologic threat. Warm, communicating relationships. Attention.

Slow the intravenous infusion flow rate   Decrease the intravenous flow rate to 20–40 drops per minute. If the blood pressure rises, further decrease the drops per minute.

Rationale: Excessive fluid entering the circulation increases arterial pressure, which results in a loss of fluid into tissue spaces, causing edema. Slowing the intravenous infusion prevents edema and blood pressure elevation because it reduces circulatory overload. The excretion of more than 80 cc of urine per hour indicates that fluid intake is far more rapid than fluid output and that fluid imbalance or circulatory overload exists.

Resolved Needs: Water-salt balance. Protection from physical harm.

Contraindications: Circulatory failure. Hypotension.

Soak in a colloidal bath   Immerse the body in an oatmeal or corn starch bath, taking care not to allow large amounts of starch to gather in skin folds.

Rationale: Starch or oatmeal have an emollient effect, relieving irritation and itching and cleansing the skin. As starch absorbs water, the starch granules swell in skin folds and cause irritation.

Resolved Needs: Comfort. Cleanliness. Protection from physical harm.

Soak in a sitz bath   Apply hot (96°–106°F) water to the pelvic area by having the person sit in a tub filled with water to the umbilical level.

Rationale: Moist heat promotes relaxation and healing by cleansing. It relieves pain through local vasodilatation of the pelvic area.

Resolved Needs: Comfort. Cleanliness. Freedom from pain.

Contraindications: Persons subject to episodes of hypotension must be observed closely, especially when getting out of the tub.

Soak in Betadine solution   Place the injured body area in an iodine solution and allow it to soak for some time.

Rationale: Betadine has a prolonged antiseptic effect, killing skin bacteria, fungus, viruses, yeasts, and protozoa. It is used to treat chronic skin infections (pyoderma), fresh lacerations, and beginning decubitus.

Resolved Needs: Cleanliness. Protection from physical harm.

Contraindications: Known Betadine allergy.

Soak in cold water   Submerge the burned skin area in cold, clean water, not ice water.

Rationale: Cold water reduces the pain of burns.

Resolved Needs: Comfort. Protection from physical harm. Freedom from pain.

Contraindications: Avoid on areas of decubitus ulcers, gangrenous tissue, skin graft, varicose veins, paralysis or sensation loss, or with aged, debilitated skin.

Soak in saline solution   Immerse the arm, hand, fingers, leg, foot, or toes in a warm hypertonic (2 teaspoons of salt to 500 cc of water) saline solution for approximately 20–30 minutes, three to four times a day. Apply only to intact skin.

Rationale: The local application of a warm saline solution supports cleanliness and has an astringent effect that promotes the relief of pain and edema of inflamed tissues by improving circulation to the area.

Resolved Needs: Comfort. Cleanliness. Protection from physical harm.

Contraindications: Open wounds should be soaked in isotonic solutions since plain water or a hypertonic saline solution causes a burning sensation.

Soak the nails in warm oil   When the nails are brittle or the cuticle ragged, soak them in warm olive oil or liquid lanolin for 15–20 minutes.

Rationale: Soaking the nails in warm oil loosens dead cuticle and replaces the natural oils and moisture of the dried nails.

Resolved Needs: Comfort. Protection from physical harm.

Socialize gradually   Bring the patient into gradual contact with other persons. Begin by having one person sit silently beside the patient and later introduce conversation. Increase the exposure to nonthreatening persons, one at a time, until there is comfort in socialization.

Rationale: Decreased stimuli offers less threat to adaptation than intense stimuli. Comfort is promoted through a sense of effective communication with others.

Resolved Needs: Comfort. Protection from psychologic threat. Warm, communicating relationships.

Soften and remove the earwax   Place a few drops of mineral oil into the ear for 30 minutes to 1 hour or put two drops of liquid stool softner (Colace) into the ear. Compress the ear opening several times to push the softening agent into the ear. Wait 2–5 minutes. Then, wash the wax out with a bulb syringe.

Rationale: Removal of earwax improves hearing when hearing loss is due to wax accumulations. It promotes comfort and offers assistance during illness dependency.

Resolved Needs: Comfort. Cleanliness. Protection from physical harm. Dependence.

Contraindications: Earache. Ear infection.

Soften the hair with a cream rinse   After shampooing the hair, rinse with a mild, oily hair cream.

Rationale: Cream rinse softens the hair shafts, prevents tangling, and promotes comfort.

Resolved Needs: Comfort. Protection from physical harm.

Solicit the family's assistance in understanding the patient's speech   When attempting to communicate with a person having impaired communication ability, seek the assistance of family members to interpret the person's message.

Rationale: Familiarity with a person's nonverbal methods of communication facilitates clarity of message interpretation. Comfort is promoted through effective communication with others.

Resolved Needs: Comfort. Warm, communicating relationships.

Splint the incisional area   Hold a pillow firmly against the area of a fresh abdominal or chest incision while the patient coughs, turns in bed, or gets up to a sitting position.

Rationale: Supportive pressure decreases stress on incisional areas, promotes comfort, and reduces pain.

Resolved Needs: Comfort. Freedom from pain.

Sponge the wound clean: Soak up wound drainage by gently inserting sterile, absorbent, gauze into the wound. Immediately remove after it has become saturated and replace it with clean gauze.

Rationale: Removal of wound drainage promotes cleanliness and rapid healing.

Resolved Needs: Comfort. Cleanliness. Protection from physical harm.

Stand the patient for urination   When a man has difficulty voiding while in bed, allow him to assume the standing position for a brief period.

Rationale: The standing position increases gravity pull within the bladder, promoting urine flow, and is the natural voiding position for men.

Resolved Needs: Waste elimination. Comfort.

Contraindications: Temperature elevations above 103°F. Head or spinal cord injury. Internal hemorrhage. Coma or semicoma. Severe energy depletion. Life-threatening situations.

Sterilize the bedpan after each use   Each time the bedpan is used, sterilize it thoroughly before it is used again.

Rationale: Cleanliness prevents the spread of infection.

Resolved Needs: Cleanliness. Protection from physical harm.

Stimulate by movement, touch, sternal pressure, or speech   Arouse a response by repeatedly speaking to the person, touching him, applying sternal pressure, or moving him about.

Rationale: Stimuli promote full orientation of the person with impaired cerebral activity, bring attention to current needs, and promote realistic perception of objects and situations.

Resolved Needs: Stimulation. Protection from physical harm. Protection from psychologic threat. Increased reality perception and problem-solving ability.

Contraindications: Avoid sternal pressure when there is a chest injury.

Stimulate gagging with a tongue blade   Place a tongue blade at the back of the mouth to cause gagging.

Rationale: Gagging stimulates the vagus nerve which slows the heart rate.

Resolved Needs: Protection from physical harm.

Stimulate salivation with sour-flavored foods   Stimulate the salivary glands by offering bitter or sour foods such as lemons, limes, pickles, or sour-ball candies.

Rationale: Saliva is essential for food digestion and absorption, and oral comfort. Stimulation of salivation decreases the chance for parotitis when the patient is NPO for long periods.

Resolved Needs: Comfort. Protection from physical harm.

Stimulate the infant with back stroking or foot thumping   Arouse the infant by lightly rubbing his back with your hand, or thumping the bottom of his feet with your finger.

Rationale: Infant stimulation brings about crying which acrates the lungs. It enhances perception of available food and the surrounding environment.

Resolved Needs: Oxygen. Stimulation. Protection from physical harm.

Stimulate the infant with a mobile   Arouse the infant's perception by placing, above and in front of him, a structure whose parts move by air currents.

Rationale: A moving mobile enhances perception of shapes, sizes, motion, and color.

Resolved Needs: Stimulation.

Stimulate the memory by repeating the patient's last expressed thought   When there is difficulty in recall, repeat the last few words or sentences that the person spoke or mention the general trend of thought.

Rationale: Repetition of recent verbally expressed thoughts reinforces thought content and reduces the threat and anxiety of memory failure.

Resolved Needs: Stimulation. Protection from psychologic threat.

Stimulate the reflex bladder by applying cold to the abdomen, stroking the inner thigh, or running water   When retraining for bladder control, the reflex bladder may be stimulated by applying a cold towel to the abdomen, stroking the inner thigh, turning on the water faucet, or pulling public hair.

Rationale: External stimulation triggers the bladder's spastic reflex.

Bladder control is essential to the maintenance of dryness, comfort, cleanliness, and to the prevention of skin irritation.

Resolved Needs: Comfort. Cleanliness. Protection from physical harm.

Contraindications: Do not apply cold to the abdomen if the patient has bladder spasms.

Stimulate the reflex bowel by abdominal stroking and anal stimulation   When retraining for bowel control, the reflex bowel can be stimulated by stroking downward on the abdomen, applying pressure in front of, in back of, and to the side of the anus, inserting the finger into the anus and manually stimulating it.

Rationale: External stimulation triggers the bowel's spastic reflex. Bowel control is essential to the maintenance of dryness, comfort, cleanliness, and to the prevention of skin irritation.

Resolved Needs: Comfort. Cleanliness. Protection from physical harm.

Contraindications: If there is any anal tissue injury.

Stimulate the sucking reflex through jaw or lip pressure   Promote the sucking reflex in an infant during feeding by placing gentle finger pressure on each side of the jaw or below and to the side of the lips.

Rationale: The stimulation of infant sucking is essential to food and fluid intake.

Resolved Needs: Stimulation.

Strike a quick blow on the anterior chest   For respiratory depression, slap the anterior chest near the diaphragm with the palm of the hand. Take care that the force of the slap does not cause air already in the lungs to be expelled.

Rationale: A quick blow in the diaphragmatic area will stimulate respirations.

Resolved Needs: Oxygen. Protection from physical harm.

Contraindications: Known chest injury.

Strip the chest tubing   Hold the chest tube securely with the fingers of one hand. Lubricate the fingers of the other hand and clamp them below those of the first hand, pulling the clamped fingers down the tubing to empty it of fluid and air.

Rationale: Chest-tube stripping maintains chest tube patency since the negative pressure created by the stripping dislodges clots and sediment in the tubing.

Resolved Needs: Protection from physical harm.

Subdue the room lighting   Prevent glare from windows or artificial

lamps from reaching the patient. Tilt or close blinds or shades. Use only soft room lighting.

Rationale: In conditions such as cerebral edema, measles, meningitis, or drug reactions, light glare irritates nerves and tissue, causing pain. Subdued lighting decreases external stimuli and promotes sleep and comfort.

Resolved Needs: Sleep, rest, relaxation. Comfort. Protection from physical harm.

Contraindications: Impaired vision where poor lighting might cause injury.

Substitute artificial salt   When natural sodium chloride is restricted from the diet, offer an artificial salt substitute.

Rationale: Seasoning food enhances flavor and increases the desire to eat.

Resolved Needs: Comfort. Protection from physical harm.

Contraindications: Conditions in which increased potassium intake is not advisable, such as hyperkalemia.

Substitute caffeine-free coffee   When regular coffee is restricted from the diet, offer a noncaffeine substitute.

Rationale: Noncaffeine coffee does not cause the gastric acidity, cardiac and respiratory stimulation, and diuretic effects of regular coffee.

Resolved Needs: Comfort. Protection from physical harm.

Suction the airway   Using a catheter or bulb syringe, suction the mouth, nose, pharynx, or trachea and remove obstructing secretions.

Rationale: Secretion removal maintains a patent airway, allowing for respiratory gas exchange.

Resolved Needs: Oxygen. Waste elimination. Protection from physical harm.

Suction the snake (or spider) venom   When a poisonous snake or spider bite has occurred, incise the site of the bite and, with a suction cup or your mouth, draw out the venom. Do not use your mouth for suctioning if there are mouth ulcers or lacerations, and take care not to swallow the venom.

Rationale: Removal of venom prevents its toxic effects from harming the body.

Resolved Needs: Protection from physical harm.

Suggest home adaptations appropriate to the health problem   Offer ideas as to how home adjustments may be made to fit the health problem. Suggest methods that support independence of the ill person and reduced stress on those caring for him.

Rationale: Home adaptations to health problems support independent and comfortable living.

Resolved Needs: Comfort. Independence. Increased problem-solving ability.

Suggest more appropriate means of emotional expression

Suggest that emotional energy by diverted into acceptable and rewarding endeavors.

Rationale: Behavioral changes are more easily accomplished when they result in reward and gratification.

Resolved Needs: Protection from psychologic threat. Personal growth and maturity.

Suggest more appropriate means of need gratification

When a person is gaining need satisfaction through demands or impositions on others, suggest less damaging and more fulfilling ways in which those needs can be met.

Rationale: Gratification of one's needs without imposition on others results in more favorable response from others which in itself heightens need gratification.

Resolved Needs: Protection from psychologic threat. Personal growth and maturity.

Suggest nursing home care

Suggest that the person consider going to a nursing home where care can be given 24 hours a day.

Rationale: Nursing homes provide continuous custodial care, companionship, and activity for lonely persons.

Resolved Needs: Comfort. Dependence. Increased reality perception and problem-solving. Ability.

Suggest possible child adoption

When a couple cannot have children of their own, suggest they consider adoption.

Rationale: Adopted children provide the same need gratification as one's own children.

Resolved Needs: Comfort. Sexuality. Love and affection. Sense of value, usefulness. High evaluation of self.

Contraindications: Avoid if there is a high potential for rejection by the adoption agency.

Suggest private nurse care

Suggest that the person might consider employing a private nurse to come into the home and administer care.

Rationale: Private nursing care allows a person to remain in the security of his home despite illness.

Resolved Needs: Comfort. Dependence. Increased reality perception and problem-solving ability.

Suggest that one relative remain with the dying person When death is fast approaching and all family members cannot remain at the bedside because of other commitments, suggest that the family member who feels most comfortable in the stressful situation remain at the bedside.

Rationale: The presence of one relative with a dying family member assures the others who must leave that death was not met with loneliness. This reduces the potential for guilt feelings.

Resolved Needs: Comfort. Unity with loved ones.

Suggest that reparation will diminish guilt Suggest that guilt will diminish when one makes amends for damage done to another.

Rationale: When a guilty person makes reparation, the injured party usually responds in a positive manner, offering acceptance and approval.

Resolved Needs: Comfort. Protection from psychologic threat.

Suggest that volunteers might offer assistance with home care Suggest that the sick person consider obtaining assistance from volunteers. This service sometimes is offered by church organizations or close friends.

Rationale: Assistance with daily care aids in illness dependency and allows the person to remain in his desired environment.

Resolved Needs: Comfort. Dependence. Increased problem-solving ability.

Suggest substitute means of goal attainment Suggest alternate means by which anticipated goals can be reached when the present approach seems ineffective.

Rationale: Successful achievement in overcoming barriers to a goal enhances the ability to cope and results in increased adequacy feelings.

Resolved Needs: Comfort. Protection from physical harm. Protection from psychologic threat. Adequacy. Goal achievement. Increased reality perception and problem-solving ability.

Supplement inadequate breast feeding with bottle feeding Give the infant bottle feedings in addition to breast feedings if lactation deficiency exists.

Rationale: Adequate nutrition is essential to life and health.

Resolved Needs: Food balance. Protection from physical harm.

Supplement protein intake Offer high protein drinks and snacks between meals. Include milk and gelatin drinks, nuts, tunafish and meat sandwiches, and specially prepared protein formulas.

Rationale: A higher than normal protein intake is needed for healing (replacement) during major tissue loss such as burns, hepatitis, and major surgery. A high protein intake increases immunity, resistance to infection, and body heat production.

Resolved Needs: Food balance. Energy. Protection from physical harm.

Contraindications: Renal failure. Liver failure.

Support a realistic assessment of the situation   Help the person evaluate the situation not from assumption but from factual data. Have him explain the situation in detail and draw conclusions from his explanation. Assist in the reevaluation of the situation.

Rationale: Growth and maturity involve the ability to perceive and cope with the demands and limitations of the real world and to organize perceptions into a meaningful whole.

Resolved Needs: Protection from psychologic threat. Personal growth and maturity. Increased reality perception and problem-solving ability.

Support the affected body part   When moving the person, support the body part that is injured, infected, inflamed, or traumatized.

Rationale: Support of a traumatized body area prevents further injury and promotes comfort.

Resolved Needs: Comfort. Protection from physical harm. Freedom from pain.

Support with a binder   Offer support to the pelvic area by applying a single-tailed or T-binder, to the torso by applying a straight binder, and to any body area needing support by applying a many-tailed or Scultetus' binder.

Rationale: Binders provide a firm support against uncomfortable movement and the painful or tiring gravity pull on tissues.

Resolved Needs: Comfort. Protection from physical harm.

Suture the wound (ExR)   After thorough cleansing, stitch together the skin and tissue that have been separated by an injury.

Rationale: Suturing promotes the healing of separated skin and tissue and reduces the potential for infection of internal tissue.

Resolved Needs: Comfort. Protection from physical harm.

Contraindications: When wound infection is highly probable, the wound should be left open for drainage.

Swab the mouth with diluted glycerine   Soak a cotton-tipped applicator or a gauze-tipped tongue blade in a 50% water-glycerine solution and cleanse the oral mucous membranes. For flavor, add a little lemon.

Rationale: Diluted glycerine breaks down mucous collections in the mouth and removes it from teeth and gums. It cleanses and lubricates the mouth.

Resolved Needs: Comfort. Cleanliness.

Contraindications: Do not add the lemon flavor if there is excessive salivation or mucosal ulcerations.

Take nasal and oral secretion precautions   Dispose of nasal and oral secretions in approved sanitation facilities. Be careful not to have hand contact with the secretions.

Rationale: Pathogen transfer from person to person is decreased by control and precaution when handling pathogens.

Resolved Needs: Cleanliness. Protection from physical harm.

Take needle-syringe precautions   Carefully dispose of all needles and plastic syringes so they cannot be reused accidentally. If glass syringes are being used instead of the disposable ones, soak the needles and syringes in strong disinfecting solution then autoclave them.

Rationale: Pathogens, especially for hepatitis and malaria, are readily transferred by contaminated needles and syringes.

Resolved Needs: Cleanliness. Protection from physical harm.

Take skin-contact precautions   Wear gloves to prevent direct contact with communicable skin lesions.

Rationale: Pathogen transfer from person to person can be decreased by avoiding contact with the pathogens.

Resolved Needs: Cleanliness. Protection from physical harm.

Take sputum precautions   Dispose of infective sputum in approved sanitation facilities. Avoid hand contact with secretions.

Rationale: Pathogen transfer from person to person is decreased by control and precaution in handling pathogens.

Resolved Needs: Cleanliness. Protection from physical harm.

Take stool precautions   Dispose of stools in approved sanitation facilities. Avoid hand contact with the stool.

Rationale: Pathogen transfer from person to person is decreased by control and precaution when handling the pathogens. In typhoid fever, flies and hands carry organisms from feces to food, and the food, when eaten, transmits the organisms.

Resolved Needs: Cleanliness. Protection from physical harm.

Take urine precautions   Dispose of urine contaminated with infectious organisms or radioactive isotopes in approved sanitation facilities. Avoid hand contact with the urine.

Rationale: Pathogen transfer from person to person is decreased by control and precaution when handling pathogens.

Resolved Needs: Cleanliness. Protection from physical harm.

Talk with the patient (family, visitor, or significant others)
Converse with the person(s) for as long as necessary to meet his needs.

Rationale: The exchange of verbal responses assures the person of one's concern, reduces loneliness, supports positive interpersonal relationships, and is stimulating.

Resolved Needs: Comfort. Protection from psychologic threat. Stimulation. Warm, communicating relationships.

Tape implements to the bandaged hands   When a burned patient has both hands bandaged, tape or strap eating implements and other assistive tools to the bandages. This will allow for some self-care.

Rationale: Comfort feelings arise from independent activity despite limitations.

Resolved Needs: Comfort. Independence.

Contraindications: Do not bandage implements to the hands if skin has been grafted on them.

Tape the pacemaker wire to the patient   Position the pacemaker wire so that it does not fall under the patient. Coil it to the proper length and tape it to the chest.

Rationale: Proper positioning of the pacemaker wire provides safety and comfort.

Resolved Needs: Comfort. Protection from physical harm.

Tape the urinary catheter onto the abdomen   When a male patient has prolonged insertion of an indwelling catheter, tape the end of the catheter onto the abdomen.

Rationale: Taping the urinary catheter onto the abdomen prevents ulceration on the penal-scrotal junction by keeping pressure off the glans and urethra.

Resolved Needs: Protection from physical harm.

Contraindications: Abdominal surgical incision.

Terminate emotionally threatening conversation immediately   Whenever the person indicates a desire to talk about death or an incurable disease, support such discussions. However, the moment the person changes the subject to a life topic, the previous discussion should no longer be pursued.

Rationale: When truth can no longer be tolerated, denial becomes essential to prevent intense psychologic threat. Respectful attitudes toward a person's limitations support dignity.

Resolved Needs: Protection from psychologic threat. Dignity.

Test the bath water temperature When a person has decreased skin sensation, test the temperature of the bath water making sure it is no hotter than 96°F. If a bath thermometer is not available, expose your wrist to the water's heat. If the heat feels comfortable to the wrist, then the water temperature should be safe.

Rationale: Testing water before exposing the body to its heat prevents skin burns.

Resolved Needs: Protection from physical harm.

Tie off and cut the umbilical cord (ExR) Tie umbilical tape around the umbilical cord about 4–5 inches from the infant's umbilicus, making sure the cord is completely obstructed. Tie a second knot about 2 inches away from the original knot toward the mother. Then cut the cord between the two knots with sterile scissors.

Rationale: Tying off the umbilical cord prevents hemorrhage. Cutting the umbilical cord frees the infant from its mother so it may assume independent life.

Resolved Needs: Protection from physical harm.

Toilet frequently Offer the bedpan or urinal or take the patient to the bathroom at consistently close intervals.

Rationale: Frequently emptying the bladder promotes elimination, prevents the embarrassment of elimination accidents, promotes comfort and cleanliness, and helps relieve intraabdominal pressure during labor.

Resolved Needs: Comfort. Cleanliness. Protection from physical harm. Protection from psychologic threat.

Touch the patient judiciously Express concern and human relatedness by touching the patient's skin. This can be done in one of many ways: cuddling a child, playing touch games such as patti-cake and ring-around-the-rosey, holding the patient's hand, rocking the child, placing a hand on the patient's shoulder, or an arm around the waist, patting or stroking, or squeezing the patient's arm, and touching the patient when dressing or bathing him.

Rationale: The expression and perception of emotional feelings can be activated through stimulation of skin nerves. Touch meets man's most basic need for relatedness to others. The feel of the body is basic to self-perception.

Resolved Needs: Comfort. Stimulation. Warm, communicating relationships.

Contraindications: Avoid touch communications in nearness tension or when working with suspicious persons.

Tour the patient through the health care facility   When a person experiences anxiety associated with health care, escort him through the facility and introduce him to the personnel.

Rationale: Safety and comfort arise from familiar and predictable situations.

Resolved Needs: Comfort. Protection from psychologic threat. Predictable, orderly world.

Contraindications: Delay if the tour heightens anxiety.

Trim the hangnail   When there is evidence of broken skin at the nail edge, the skin should be trimmed with a nail scissors or clipper.

Rationale: Trimming hangnails prevents the pulling of them and injury to epidermal tissue.

Resolved Needs: Comfort. Protection from physical harm.

Turn the mattress frequently   Turn the bed mattress end-over-end and side-over-side alternately every day if possible and not less than once a week.

Rationale: Mattress rotation prevents the formation of weakened, sagging mattress areas. It provides a smooth, level lying surface for good back support, body alignment, comfort, and provides assistance in dependency needs.

Resolved Needs: Comfort. Protection from physical harm. Dependence.

Turn off the radio and television to reduce noise   Decrease the amount of environmental stimuli by eliminating the sound of radio and television.

Rationale: Certain levels of quiet are essential to normal physical and emotional function.

Resolved Needs: Comfort. Protection from physical harm.

Unplug the electrical monitor during a bath   When an electrical monitor is plugged into an wall outlet, the plug should be pulled during the daily bath. The plug is reinserted as soon as the patient's skin is dry.

Rationale: When water comes in contact with electrical equipment, the possibility of electrical shock is highly probable.

Resolved Needs: Protection from physical harm.

Use a chest restraint   Use chest restraints so that free movement of the limbs is still possible. Be sure that the restraint is tied to the bed, with

the patient close enough to the head of the bed, so that he cannot slip down or off the side of the bed and strangle himself.

Rationale: Limb restraints result in the discomfort of arm and leg immobility, increased pressure on skin tissue, and heightened anxiety when loss of mobility is realized. Chest restraints allow arm and leg mobility, and promote comfort in the knowledge that body integrity is in no way threatened.

Resolved Needs: Comfort. Protection from physical harm. Protection from psychologic threat.

Use a large-holed nipple for feeding
When an infant is struggling to obtain liquid through a nipple or when the infant is in a weakened condition and will have to expend large amounts of energy to obtain milk, use a nipple with a larger than usual hole.

Rationale: When the amount of energy expended to obtain nourishment approaches the amount of energy produced by the nutrients, the infant will fail to thrive.

Resolved Needs: Water-salt balance. Food balance. Comfort.

Contraindications: Swallowing difficulty.

Use a small-holed nipple for feeding
When feeding the infant a bottle, use a nipple with a small hole.

Rationale: A small-holed nipple increases the length of feeding time and satisfies the infant's desire for prolonged sucking.

Resolved Needs: Comfort.

Contraindications: Infant weakness. Intense infant hunger.

Use a waist safety strap during mobility
When a person is relearning to walk or is very weak when walking, place a safety strap around his waist. Hold the strap and stand behind the patient during his relearning efforts.

Rationale: Safety straps allow for mobility freedom, protect against potential falling, and assist in illness dependency.

Resolved Needs: Protection from physical harm. Dependence.

Use an aromatic spray
When odors are disagreeable, spray a pleasant artificial odor that is stronger than the unpleasant odor. Avoid overuse of the spray and keep it well away from the patient's face.

Rationale: Offensive odors irritate olfactory senses, causing discomfort.

Resolved Needs: Comfort.

Use direct eye contact to terminate excessive crying
When a depressed person cries excessively, sit directly in front of him. Hold his

hand and ask him to look into your eyes. This technique usually stops crying.

Rationale: The termination of exhaustive crying reduces energy consumption and promotes comfort.

Resolved Needs: Comfort. Protection from physical harm.

Use only clean artificial ventilation equipment

Use only ventilation equipment that has been thoroughly washed with antibacterial solution.

Rationale: Unclean artificial ventilation equipment directly transmits microorganisms into the respiratory tract.

Resolved Needs: Cleanliness. Protection from physical harm.

Use only three-prong electrical plugs in the patient area

When a patient has a pacemaker, do not allow the use of any electrical equipment in the patient area that does not have a three-prong plug. Adaptors that provide for the insertion of a two-prong plug into a three-prong wall adaptor should not be used.

Rationale: The use of a third grounding wire in electrical plugs allows for correct polarization of electrical current and prevents electrocution.

Resolved Needs: Protection from physical harm.

Use paper or transparent tape instead of adhesive on the skin

Instead of using adhesive tape on the skin, use paper or transparent tape.

Rationale: Paper or transparent tape is nonirritating, prevents tissue trauma, and promotes comfort.

Resolved Needs: Protection from physical harm.

Use positive suggestion in pain relief

While administering pain relief medications, make positive statements regarding their effectiveness.

Rationale: Anticipated pain relief causes muscle and emotional relaxation which facilitates the analgesic effect of drugs.

Resolved Needs: Comfort. Freedom from pain.

Use separate hyperalimentation infusion sets for incompatible solutions

When administering hyperalimentation solutions of fat, carbohydrates, and amino acids, use different infusion sets.

Rationale: Incompatible solutions clump, cause tube clogging, and change the rate of infusion.

Resolved Needs: Protection from physical harm.

Use simple words and short sentences

When persons have impaired communication ability, use short sentences composed of simple, common words.

Rationale: The use of simple words and sentences facilitates ease in understanding messages.

Resolved Needs: Comfort. Warm, communicating relationships.

Use single-word communication Communicate with single words, avoiding the use of sentences or phrases.

Rationale: Persons with auditory and sensory aphasia frequently can understand single words but not phrases or sentences.

Resolved Needs: Comfort. Warm, communicating relationships.

Use small-gauge injection needles When injecting a person who bleeds easily, use the smallest possible needle gauge.

Rationale: The smaller the needle puncture, the lower the probability of severe bleeding.

Resolved Needs: Protection from physical harm.

Use sterile adhesive strips for wound closure Place an adhesive strip on one side of an open wound. Pull the wound edges together. Bring the tape over and to the other side of the wound. When the wound edges appear aligned, anchor the tape to the skin. Several adhesive strips sometimes are required to hold one incisional line closed.

Rationale: Alignment of wound edges promotes healing, comfort, and cleanliness.

Resolved Needs: Comfort. Cleanliness. Protection from physical harm.

Use sterile technique Maintain sterile technique when doing procedures that involve sterile equipment, sterile body cavities (bladder, trachea), or wounds.

Rationale: Sterile technique minimizes microorganism entrance into the catheters, wounds, etc.

Resolved Needs: Cleanliness. Protection from physical harm.

Use the patient's name frequently Whenever the opportunity arises, call the person by name.

Rationale: The comprehension of one's identity minimizes disorientation. A person's name is his most basic core of identity.

Resolved Needs: Comfort. Protection from psychologic threat. Recognition.

Verbalize daily the patient's successful progress At the end of each day, assist the patient to enumerate verbally the success and progress made since the previous day, no matter how small that progress may be.

Rationale: Focusing attention on success promotes positive self-attitudes.

Resolved Needs: Comfort. Protection from psychologic threat. High evaluation of self. Adequacy.

Wait for a response to one message before delivering another
When a person has communication difficulties, wait until there is clear evidence that the first message has been received and interpreted before going on to the second message.

Rationale: The reception and interpretation of messages is reduced by perceptual overload. Comfort is promoted through effective communication with others.

Resolved Needs: Comfort. Warm, communicating relationships.

Walk with the patient
When a person indicates a need to move about to decrease internal stress, is in need of companionship, or requires close supervision, walk with the person.

Rationale: Comfort and safety are promoted through relatedness to others, the ability to communicate one's needs, and protection associated with physical limitations.

Resolved Needs: Comfort. Protection from physical harm. Protection from psychologic threat. Warm, communicating relationships.

Warm the dialysis fluid before instillation
Warm the dialysis fluid to body temperature (98–99°F) before instilling it into the peritoneal cavity.

Rationale: Warming dialysis fluid prevents abdominal cramping and helps maintain normal body temperature.

Resolved Needs: Normal temperature. Comfort.

Wash the brush and comb with a parasiticide
Make a water and parasiticide solution. Soak the comb and brush of a patient with hair infestations in the solution.

Rationale: A parasiticide kills lice or nits transferred to the comb and brush from infected hair.

Resolved Needs: Cleanliness. Protection from physical harm.

Wash the patient's hands
Wash the patient's hands before meals and after elimination.

Rationale: Cleanliness, through hand-washing, prevents infection and promotes comfort.

Resolved Needs: Comfort. Cleanliness. Protection from physical harm.

Wash with a germicidal solution
Wash the skin with a solution that will destroy germs. Such solutions include Betadine and iodine.

Rationale: The destruction of germs by germicidal solutions prevents or reduces infection.

Resolved Needs: Cleanliness. Protection from physical harm.

Wash your hands between contacts Wash your hands thoroughly with water, soap, friction rubbing, and rinsing. Repeat after each contact with a patient or contaminated articles.

Rationale: Surface removal of infectious microorganisms decreases the potential for the transfer of disease from one person to another.

Resolved Needs: Cleanliness. Protection from physical harm.

Waterproof the cast surface Tuck cloth-lined plastic or a Chux-like product around the edges of a cast so the plastic will keep the cast dry and the cloth will protect the skin from the plastic. A waterproofing lacquer may be applied by brush or spray, especially when the cast edges tend to crumble or are exposed to excessive moisture. The cast site will determine the advisability of using coating products that give off fumes.

Rationale: Protection against moisture prevents weakening and deterioration of the cast. Protection against soiling by urine and fecal material also helps prevent unpleasant odors and skin breakdown.

Resolved Needs: Comfort. Cleanliness. Protection from physical harm.

Contraindications: Do not use lacquers or sprays on casts located near the respiratory system, if the patient has allergies, or in a closed room.

Wear a clean gown and mask Wear a fresh gown and mask with each patient contact and discard them afterward.

Rationale: A clean gown and mask prevent the transfer of pathogen from person to person. Reuse of gowns and masks reduces the safety factor because of bacteria accumulation.

Resolved Needs: Cleanliness. Protection from physical harm.

Wear a mask when suctioning When suctioning a patient with a tracheostomy, wear a mask.

Rationale: Since suctioning requires close proximity with the patient, wearing a mask prevents the spread of bacteria into the trachea by the person suctioning.

Resolved Needs: Cleanliness. Protection from physical harm.

Wear sterile gloves Wear sterile gloves when doing sterile procedures such as suctioning a tracheostomy, dressing changes, sterile soaks, packing a wound, and catheterizations.

Rationale: Sterile gloves prevent the transfer of bacteria from one person to another.

Resolved Needs: Cleanliness. Protection from physical harm.

Withhold food until the patient requests it   Inform the patient that his food will not be served until he asks for it.

Rationale: The availability of choice enhances the person's control over a situation. When there is gastric distress, food will be most comforting when the patient feels hungry or desires food.

Resolved Needs: Comfort.

Contraindications: Prolonged periods of no food intake.

Withhold the drug(s)   Refrain from giving drugs that cause toxic, allergic, or other harmful side effects in the person.

Rationale: Harmful effects from drugs may increase in severity with each dose taken, even causing death. Some drugs cause insidious effects such as electrolyte imbalance.

Resolved Needs: Protection from physical harm.

Contraindications: When drugs are essential to the maintenance of life, consult with the physician before withholding them.

Withhold the oxygen therapy   Remove the oxygen equipment when the person who has received large and prolonged doses of oxygen therapy suddenly develops decreased respirations.

Rationale: Excessive oxygenation of the blood reduces the respiratory stimulating effect of carbon dioxide resulting in depressed respirations.

Resolved Needs: Protection from physical harm.

Wrap the amputation stump   Wrap an elastic bandage around the amputation stump. Begin at the mid-anterior thigh, bringing one length of bandage down to the stump, under the stump, and up over the anterior stump and thigh. A crisscross or figure eight pattern is used, never a circular pattern. Apply the bandage with even pressure and change in the morning, afternoon, and before bedtime.

Rationale: Wrapping the stump shrinks and shapes it in preparation for a prosthesis, gives support to soft tissue, decreases edema, and promotes comfort.

Resolved Needs: Comfort. Protection from physical harm.

Write messages   Communicate the desired message by writing it down and letting the patient read it.

Rationale: Persons with only auditory agnosia can understand written messages.

Resolved Needs: Comfort. Protection from psychologic threat. Warm, communicating relationships.

32.
Nursing Observations

Auscultate and palpate the arteriovenous shunt for patency Place the stethoscope on the venous side of the shunt and listen for a bruit. Place your fingers over the shunt and feel for a thrill.

Rationale: Absence of a bruit or a palpable thrill indicates inadequate blood flow or pressure within the vein due to clotting within the arteriovenous shunt.

Resolved Needs: Protection from physical harm.

Auscultate the abdomen for abnormal bowel sounds (113,225) Place the stethoscope bell over each abdominal quadrant and listen for absent, diminished, gurgling, or rushing bowel sounds, succussion splash, bruit, and peritoneal friction rub.

Rationale: Absent or diminished bowel sounds indicate peritoneal irritation or intestinal obstruction. Gurgling bowel sounds, which sound like broken, noisy current, are associated with partial pyloric or intestinal obstruction and excessive intestinal contraction as in diarrhea or colic. Rushing bowel sounds, which sound like rushing water, indicate obstruction. Succussion splash, which sounds like fluid striking or dashing about, is associated with excessive abdominal fluid, gastric dilatation, and obstruction of the stomach. This sound is normal following the intake of large amounts of fluid. A bruit is heard as a whish-whish, blowing sound over the abdominal aorta. It indicates arterial occlusion or dilatation and is associated with an aneurysm. Peritoneal friction rub, which sounds like two pieces of leather being rubbed together, suggests peritoneal inflammation and is most commonly associated with splenic infarction.

Resolved Needs: Protection from physical harm.

Auscultate the abdomen for renewed bowel sounds When abdominal bowel sounds have been absent, listen periodically for the return of normal bowel sounds.

Rationale: Renewed bowel sounds indicate that an intestinal obstruction has been cleared or that bowel function has returned following gastrointestinal surgery.

Resolved Needs: Protection from physical harm.

Auscultate the apical and palpate the radial pulses for a pulse deficit   Simultaneously have one person count the radial pulse rate and another person listen to the heartbeat. If the rates differ, a pulse deficit exists.

Rationale: A pulse deficit indicates the presence of atrial fibrillation, during which some of the ventricular contractions do not produce enough blood to result in a radial pulse.

Resolved Needs: Protection from physical harm.

Auscultate the apical heartbeat for rate and rhythm   Place the stethoscope diaphragm alternately over the entire precordium and listen for normal heart rate and rhythm.

Rationale: Auscultation of the apical heartbeat allows for accurate counting of the pulse of infants, young children, and critically ill persons. It also indicates the adequacy of cardiac function since abnormalities are readily recognized.

Resolved Needs: Protection from physical harm.

Auscultate the bone for crepitation (113)   Listen with the stethoscope for a crackling, wrinkled cellophane sound heard when the body part is cautiously moved.

Rationale: Crepitus bone sounds indicate bone fracture.

Resolved Needs: Protection from physical harm.

Auscultate the carotid arteries for bruit (113)   With the stethoscope, listen over the carotid artery for the whish-whish blowing sound of a bruit (murmur).

Rationale: A bruit over the carotid artery indicates arterial constriction or dilatation and is associated with aneurysm, arteriosclerosis, and thyroid artery dilatation in thyrotoxicosis.

Resolved Needs: Protection from physical harm.

Auscultate the chest for abnormal breath sounds (113,225)   In a quiet place, have the patient sit upright and breathe deeply through his mouth. With a stethoscope, proceed from the chest top downward and from right to left. Listen for and identify duration of breath sounds. Normally, there is a long inspiratory phase and a short expiratory phase with a "whishing" sound over the lung surface. Listen for the quality of sound such as absent, diminished, bronchial, bronchovesicular, asthmatic, and amphoric breath sounds.

Rationale: Absent and diminished breath sounds indicate airflow obstruction. They are associated with atelectasis, pleural effusion, emphysema, airway obstruction, pneumothorax, or consolidation. Bronchial (tubular) breath sounds are short inspiratory and prolonged expiratory breath sounds. On expiration, there is a harsh, high-pitched lung sound like wind going through a hollow tube or breathing through a clay pipe. They are associated with pulmonary consolidation or compression of pulmonary tissue. Bronchovesicular breathing is normal except when heard in areas other than the manubrium sterni and upper interscapular region. In such cases, it indicates pulmonary consolidation or compression of pulmonary tissue. Asthmatic (wheezing) breath sounds have a hissing, whistling sound. They indicate airflow obstruction and are associated with atelectasis, pulmonary edema, and airway obstruction. Amphoric (cavernous) breath sounds, which sound like air being blown over the mouth of a bottle, indicate a pulmonary cavity.

Resolved Needs: Protection from physical harm.

Auscultate the chest for abnormal heart sounds

(113,225)   Use the stethoscope diaphragm to hear high-frequency first heart sounds. Have the patient lie on his back. Listen over the precordium for a normal "lubb" systolic sound. Place the stethoscope over the aortic (second right intercostal space) and the apical area (fifth left intercostal space at the midclavicular line). Listen for the faint first heart sounds "lubb" that are less intense than the normal "lubb" sound. This will occur at the end of atrial contraction when the valves are almost closed. Then, listen for a loud first heart sound "lubb" that is more intense or louder than the normal "lubb" sound. This occurs during atrial contraction when the valves are wide open and sounds like sheets snapping in the wind.

Place the stethoscope over the lower left sternal border (xiphoid area). Listen for splitting of the first heart sound "lubb" into two sounds "lubb-lubb." It is a reduplication or doubling sound.

Move the stethoscope to the aortic area (second right intercostal space) and the pulmonic area (second left intercostal space) and listen for a very faint second heart sound. If very faint, the sound may be disguised by a murmur sound. Then, listen for a louder than normal "dubb" sound which follows the first heart sound "lubb." If the second heart sound "dubb" is louder in the aortic area than in the pulmonic area, and if the patient is under 25 years of age, then loud aortic second heart sounds exist.

Move the stethoscope to the pulmonic area (second left intercostal space). During inspiration and expiration, listen for a splitting of the second heart sound "dubb" into two sounds "dubb-dubb." Listen for a louder than normal "dubb" sound which follows the first heart sound "lubb." If the second heart sound "dubb" is louder in the pulmonic area than in the aortic area, and if the patient is over 25 years of age, then loud pulmonic second heart sounds exist.

Using the stethoscope bell, have the patient lie on his left side. Place the stethoscope over the xiphoid area (left lower sternal border). Listen for third heart sounds occurring after second heart sounds "dubb" but before the first heart sounds "lubb." It is a weak, low-pitched dull sound.

Place the stethoscope over the apical area (fifth left intercostal space in midclavicular line). At the beginning of expiration, listen for the same weak, low-pitched dull sound.

Have the patient lie on his back. Place the stethoscope over the apical area (fifth intercostal space in midclavicular line) or in the xiphoid area (lower left sternal border). Then, listen for very faint first heart sounds (gallops) which may occur when the normal first heart sound "lubb" is delayed after the normal second heart sound "dubb" of the previous contraction. These sounds occur when the PR interval is prolonged and is prior to the first heart sound.

Using the stethoscope diaphragm or bell, have the patient sit up and lean forward slightly. Place the stethoscope over the apical area (fifth left intercostal space at the midclavicular line). Listen for a soft blowing or rasping second heart sound (diastolic murmur) slight at beginning diastole and clear at the end of diastole.

Place the stethoscope over the aortic area (second right intercostal space) and the pulmonic area (second left intercostal space). Listen for a loud booming or rumbling second heart sound (diastolic regurgitant murmur) heard from the beginning to the end of diastole. Then, listen for a soft, blowing sound (systolic murmur) occurring during the systolic interval between the first and second heart sounds. Systolic murmurs are best heard in the pulmonic area along the left sternal border, or at the apex. Listen for a medium-pitched blowing first heart sound (systolic ejection murmur), inaudible at the beginning and end of systole but audible at midsystole. The sound disappears before the second heart sound.

Place the stethoscope over the pulmonic area (second left intercostal space) and apical area (fifth left intercostal space at the midclavicular line). Listen for a loud booming or rumbling first heart sound (systolic regurgitant murmur) heard from the beginning to the end of systole.

Rationale: Faint first heart sounds indicate the presence of pericardial or pleural fluid, weak ventricular contraction, lung tissue distention, or arterial thickening or plugging. Loud first heart sounds indicate valve narrowing or thickening, increased atrial pressure causing increased force of the valve opening, or atrial systole occurring before ventricular contraction. First heart sound splitting indicates unsynchronized ventricular contraction.

Loud aortic second heart sounds indicate increased back pressure on the aortic valve which causes forceful valve closure and accentuated sound. Inspiratory second heart sound splitting (paradoxical splitting) indicates delayed pulmonic valve closure or early aortic valve closure with diminished left ventricle pressure. During expiration, second heart sound splitting indicates delayed aortic valve closure, poor ventricle contraction with delayed emptying, delayed left ventricular excitation, or prolonged emptying of the left ventricle. Loud pulmonic second heart sounds indicate increased back pressure on the pulmonic valve causing forceful closure and accentuated sound.

The third heart sound is normal in children and young adults. In older persons, when heard in the apical area, it indicates overfilling of a failing ventricle.

Fourth heart sounds indicate unsynchronized ventricular beats or forceful atrial contractions from left ventricular hypertrophy.

A diastolic murmur indicates valve narrowing or thickening. Diastolic regurgitant murmurs indicate incomplete valve closure with blood backflow. Systolic murmurs indicate an accelerated blood flow, pulmonary artery dilatation, or impaired circulatory flow, any of which cause turbulent currents which result in the murmur sound. Systolic regurgitant murmurs indicate blood backflow from ventricle to atrium.

Resolved Needs: Protection from physical harm.

Auscultate the chest for abnormal voice sounds (pectoriloquy, bronchophony, or egophony) (113,225)

In a quiet place, have the patient sit upright. With a stethoscope, proceed from the chest top downward and from right to left, while the patient repeatedly says out loud "ninety-nine" or "one-two-three." Listen for pectoriloquy, in which these sounds are transmitted abnormally through the lung and are especially audible when whispered. Listen for bronchophony, in which the voice sounds are greatly increased. Then, have the patient say "e" out loud. Listen for egophony, in which the "e" sounds like an "a."

Rationale: Pectoriloquy indicates increased lung volume and is associated with pulmonary consolidation, embolus, or atelectasis. Bronchophony indicates a hollow lung space or increased lung volume and is associated with pulmonary consolidation. Egophony indicates increased lung volume or the presence of pleural fluid and is associated with pulmonary consolidation or pleural effusion.

Resolved Needs: Protection from physical harm.

Auscultate the chest for crepitation (113,225)

In a quiet place, have the patient sit upright and breathe deeply through his mouth. With a stethoscope, proceed from the chest top downward and from right to left. Listen for a grating sound.

Rationale: Crepitus rib sounds indicate rubbing fractured rib ends and are associated with rib fracture.

Resolved Needs: Protection from physical harm.

Auscultate the chest for lung aeration (113,225)

Using the stethoscope diaphragm or bell, listen for the sound of air moving through the lungs on inspiration and expiration.

Rationale: Proper lung aeration is essential to normal body function and gas exchange.

Resolved Needs: Protection from physical harm.

Auscultate the chest for pleural friction rub (113,225) In a quiet place, have the patient sit upright and breathe deeply through his mouth. With a stethoscope, proceed from the chest top downward and from right to left. Listen with each inspiration and expiration for a sound like rubbing sandpaper or a leather creaking sound.

Rationale: Friction rub sounds indicate pulmonary inflammation or rubbing pulmonary membranes. They are associated with pulmonary embolus and pleurisy.

Resolved Needs: Protection from physical harm.

Auscultate the chest for rales and/or rhonchi (113,225)   In a quiet place, have the patient sit upright and breathe deeply through his mouth. With a stethoscope, proceed from the chest top downward and from right to left. Listen for gurgling, bubbling and crackling rales, and musical or sonorous rhonchi.

Rationale: Gurgling rales are loud, low-pitched, intermittent noisy current sounds best heard at the beginning of inspiration. They indicate fluid in the large bronchi and are associated with pulmonary edema and airway obstruction. Bubbling rales sound like bubbles being blown underwater or fizzling carbonated beverages. They are best heard halfway through inspiration. Bubbling rales indicate thin fluid moving in small bronchi and are associated with pulmonary congestion, edema, consolidation, embolus, cavity, and infection. Crackling rales sound like crackling cellophane and are heard either at the end of inspiration or on both inspiration and expiration. They indicate thick exudate or inflamed edematous lung alveoli. They are associated with pulmonary consolidation, congestion, cavity, embolus, and infection. Musical rhonchi have a high-pitched, tinkling sound. Sonorous rhonchi have a snoring sound. They indicate pulmonary inflammation, bronchial or pulmonary fluid, or thick exudate. Both are associated with pulmonary congestion or edema.

Resolved Needs: Protection from physical harm.

Auscultate the head for cranial bruit (113,225)   Place the stethoscope bell over the cranium and listen for a blowing sound over the mastoid process, the temples, or each closed eye.

Rationale: Cranial bruit sounds indicate dilatation or constriction of cranial vessels. They are associated with aneurysms.

Resolved Needs: Protection from physical harm.

Auscultate the head for cranial crepitation sounds (113,225)   Place the stethoscope bell over the cranium and listen over the mastoid process, the temples, and each closed eye. Listen for small crisp, sudden repeated sounds like wrinkled cellophane.

Rationale: Cranial crepitus sounds indicate air or fluid in tissue. They are associated with intracranial bleeding or cranial bone fracture.

Resolved Needs: Protection from physical harm.

Auscultate the head for cranial friction sounds (113,225)

Place the stethoscope bell over the cranium and listen over the mastoid process, the temples, and each closed eye for sounds like sandpaper being rubbed or leather creaking during bone movement.

Rationale: Cranial friction sounds indicate bone fracture.

Resolved Needs: Protection from physical harm.

Auscultate the thyroid for bruit (113,225)

Place the stethoscope over the thyroid and listen for a hum sometimes accompanied by a palpable tremor. It is heard near the center of the thyroid gland.

Rationale: As the thyroid gland enlarges, accelerated blood flow through the thyroid arteries causes the hum. Thyroid bruits are associated with thyroidtoxicosis.

Resolved Needs: Protection from physical harm.

Check for fluctuation of the fluid level in the water-seal container

Periodically check to see that the level of the water in the long tubing inside the chest drainage container goes up and down simultaneously with respiratory inspiration and expiration.

Rationale: Proper fluctuation of fluid within the water-seal drainage system indicates that the system is functioning properly. When fluctuation stops, the tubing is either obstructed or the lung has reexpanded.

Resolved Needs: Protection from physical harm.

Check for infiltration of the solution

Watch for signs that the solution may have leaked into the subcutaneous tissue, evident by swelling at the injection site.

Rationale: Solution infiltration into tissues could cause tissue damage.

Resolved Needs: Protection from physical harm.

Check that the traction weights are hanging free

Periodically check that the traction weights are hanging free, have not fallen to the floor, and are not caught in the bed grooves or chairs.

Rationale: Free-hanging traction weights allow for constant pulling pressure against specific bones so the healing position may be maintained.

Resolved Needs: Protection from physical harm.

Check the cane for correct length

Have the patient stand erect and hold the cane head. Place the cane tip a few inches in front of and to the side of the patient's foot. If the cane is the proper height, the patient's arm will be at a 30-degree angle. If the cane is too long, remove its rubber tip and saw it to the correct length.

Rationale: Proper cane length is essential for correct body alignment, weight bearing, comfort, and mobility.

Resolved Needs: Protection from physical harm.

Check the chest-bottle drainage for quality and quantity

Check the chest bottle content for bright bloody drainage. Each hour determine the amount of drainage and report an excess of 125 cc/hour.

Rationale: Bright red blood or copious chest drainage indicates blood loss, tissue damage, or imbalanced thoracic pressure.

Resolved Needs: Protection from physical harm.

Check the crutches for correct length

Have the patient lay supine. Measure from the anterior fold of the axilla to a point 6 inches out from the patient's heel. This is the length which the crutch should measure and be adjusted to if it is an inaccurate length.

Rationale: Proper crutch length is essential for correct body alignment, weight bearing, and mobility.

Resolved Needs: Protection from physical harm.

Check the crutches for intact rubber tips

Periodically check the rubber tips on crutches for adequate width, for wearing on one side, and for secure attachment to the crutch.

Rationale: A firm, stable base is essential to safe ambulation and prevention of falling.

Resolved Needs: Protection from physical harm.

Check the crutch handbar for position

Check that the crutch handbar is positioned properly so when the patient places weight on the bar, his arm is completely extended.

Rationale: A properly positioned crutch handbar is essential for correct body alignment, weight bearing, and mobility.

Resolved Needs: Protection from physical harm.

Check the dialysis circuit for leakage

Watch for a leak in either the peritoneal or hemodialysis setup.

Rationale: Leakage within the dialysis circuit causes fluid loss and heightens the infection potential.

Resolved Needs: Protection from physical harm.

Check the drainage system for leakage

Intermittently, look over the chest, genitourinary, gastrointestinal, etc., drainage system for any sign of leakage around connection sites.

Rationale: A closed drainage system minimizes the potential for bacterial invasion into the tubing insertion site. The water-seal system, which is closed to atmospheric pressure, prevents air from replacing drainage and allows the return of the normal intrapleural negative pressure.

Resolved Needs: Protection from physical harm.

Check the environmental controls on the incubator periodically
Check that the premature infant's incubator is being controlled at an environmental temperature of between 32–36°C, oxygen concentrations individualized according to blood gases, and a humidity around 40–60%.

Rationale: Warm environmental temperature is essential to the life of the premature infant because the child is unable to maintain body heat, due to lack of insulating skin fat, poor reflex control of skin capillaries, and inactive small muscles. High air humidity is essential because of the infant's tendency toward dehydration which results in weight loss and temperature instability. Oxygen concentrations must meet his individualized needs.

Resolved Needs: Protection from physical harm.

Check the hemodialysis AV shunt for cleanliness and patency
Check the hemodialysis U-shaped tube by watching for blood clotting, tube kinking, and infection.

Rationale: The arterial tube of the dialysis shunt carries toxic blood to be filtered into the dialysis machine and the venous tube carries the detoxified blood back to the patient. Recognition and correction of nonfunctioning, inefficient therapeutic devices promote safety and assure their therapeutic effect.

Resolved Needs: Protection from physical harm.

Check the hemodialysis equipment for mechanical breakdown
Watch for signs that the artificial kidney is not mechanically sound. These include clotting in the shunt or coils, rupture of the cellophane membrane, or decreased blood flow through the machine.

Rationale: Proper artificial kidney functioning is essential to patient safety and successful removal of body wastes.

Resolved Needs: Protection from physical harm.

Check the hyperalimentation solution for cloudiness and precipitation
Check that the hyperalimentation fluid is not cloudy and that no precipitation of particles exists.

Rationale: The administration of therapeutically safe hyperalimentation solution is essential to patient safety.

Resolved Needs: Protection from physical harm.

Check the label on the blood container for correct patient identification
Check the patient's hospital identification number, his name, blood type, and Rh factor against the same data on the blood container.

Rationale: The infusion of blood intended for another person could lead to a serious blood transfusion reaction and even death.

Resolved Needs: Protection from physical harm.

Check the monitor electrodes for placement periodically   Periodically check the placement and attachment of monitor electrodes on the skin. Placement should be:#1 and #2 negative, beneath the right clavicle; lead #1 positive, beneath the left clavicle; lead #2 positive, on the left upper thigh; ground electrode on the right chest side.

Rationale: Recognition and correction of nonfunctioning, inefficient therapeutic devices promote safety and assure the intended effect of the device.

Resolved Needs: Protection from physical harm.

Check the oxygen flow rate on the nonrebreathing mask   When administering oxygen with a nonrebreathing mask, watch the bag as the patient inspires. If the bag completely collapses on inspiration, the oxygen flow rate is too low. If the bag collapses only partially on inspiration, the oxygen flow rate is sufficient.

Rationale: An adequate volume of oxygen is essential for blood and tissue oxygenation and life maintenance.

Resolved Needs: Protection from physical harm.

Check the pacemaker for pacing rate   Verify pacemaker effectiveness. Count the apical pulse. Determine if the generator light flashes and the dial needle moves immediately before the pulse beat. Run an EKG strip and determine if a long or short straight line exists before each QRS complex.

Rationale: In a well functioning pacemaker, one electrical stimulus coincides with each single heartbeat. If pacing occurs intermittently or if the straight line "blip" does not appear before each QRS complex on the EKG strip, it indicates an altered catheter position, dislodged or broken catheter, or some failure of the monitor equipment. If the pacing occurs more often than one electrical stimulus to one heartbeat, then it may indicate a tissue reaction to the catheter or possible infection.

Resolved Needs: Protection from physical harm.

Check the peritoneal dialysis catheter for leakage or displacement   Continuously check the peritoneal catheter for leakage around or displacement from the abdominal site of insertion.

Rationale: The normal flow of dialysate solution into and out of the peritoneal cavity removes diffusible toxins, urea, and electrolytes through the peritoneal membrane from the blood.

Resolved Needs: Protection from physical harm.

Check the peritoneal dialysis fluid for bloody or cloudy return
Watch for blood or milkiness in the dialysis fluid being withdrawn from the peritoneum.

Rationale: Heparin placed in the dialysis fluid could precipitate bleeding. Cloudy dialysis fluid return indicates protein loss.

Resolved Needs: Protection from physical harm.

Check the peritoneal dialysis fluid for retention or drainage in excess of 500 cc
Continuously check to determine if there is an excess of 500 cc of dialysate solution retained or drained from the peritoneal cavity.

Rationale: An excessive amount of fluid lost through peritoneal drainage will result in excessive electrolyte loss. When large amounts of dialysate fluid are not returned during peritoneal drainage, it indicates that an excess amount has been absorbed and could lead to circulatory overload.

Resolved Needs: Protection from physical harm.

Check the respirator for proper functioning
Check how well the respirator is functioning especially if changes in the patient's respirations alter the respirator's cycling.

Rationale: The proper exchange of oxygen and carbon dioxide through respirations is essential to life.

Resolved Needs: Protection from physical harm.

Check the solution for flow rate
Check that fluids are not flowing at either excessively slow or rapid rates. This includes such fluids as intravenous, hypodermoclysis, tidal drainage, tube feeding, dialysis, hyperalimentation, etc.

Rationale: Excessively slow flow rates may contribute to inadequate hydration or nutrition and ineffective therapy. Excessively rapid flow rates can contribute to circulatory overload, shock, or gastric dilatation.

Resolved Needs: Protection from physical harm.

Check the tracheostomy (or laryngectomy) tube for patency and cleanliness
Check that there is no purulent or infectious drainage, bleeding, tissue trauma, or crusting in or around the tracheostomy or laryngectomy tube. Listen for noisy, obstructed respirations. Hold your palm 4–6 inches away from the tube and feel for sufficient air on exhalation.

Rationale: Tracheostomy and laryngectomy patency is essential to adequate respiratory gas exchange, and cleanliness reduces infection potential.

Resolved Needs: Protection from physical harm.

Check the traction ropes and pulleys for alignment
Periodically check if the traction ropes are secure in the pulley wheel grooves, the support-

ing apparatus is free of the pulleys, and good alignment exists. Watch for frayed cords and loosened knots.

Rationale: Properly aligned traction ropes and pulleys allow for constant pulling pressure against specific bones so the healing position is uninterrupted.

Resolved Needs: Protection from physical harm.

Check the tube for patency   Check that tubes are not obstructed by kinking, secretions, or other collected material. Watch for free-flowing drainage or fluids. This includes intravenous, genitourinary, gastric, airway, chest, local drainage tubes, etc.

Rationale: Recognition and correction of nonfunctioning tubes associated with therapeutic procedures promote safety and assure the therapeutic effect of the treatment.

Resolved Needs: Protection from physical harm.

Check the tube's placement before giving tube feeding   Before giving tube feeding, check that the tube is located in the stomach by aspirating for gastric contents with a syringe. Place the open end of the tube in water. If bubbles appear on exhalation, the tube is in the respiratory tract and the feeding should not be given. If there are no bubbles, the tube is in the stomach and feeding may proceed.

Rationale: The introduction of liquids or food into a feeding tube that is accidentally located in or approximal to the lungs can cause death.

Resolved Needs: Protection from physical harm.

Check the walker for proper height   Have the patient grasp the top of the walker frame. If the walker height is correct, the patient's elbow will be bent at a 30-degree angle. If the height is incorrect, a new walker should be provided.

Rationale: Proper walker height is essential for correct body alignment, weight bearing, and mobility.

Resolved Needs: Protection from physical harm.

Count the number of sanitary pads used   Count the number of saturated sanitary pads used within an 8-hour period. Determine the amount of saturation by one-fourth, one-half, three-fourths, or totally saturated.

Rationale: If more than four sanitary pads are saturated in an 8-hour period, it indicates excessive vaginal bleeding.

Resolved Needs: Protection from physical harm.

Determine if the message is correctly received   Having given a person a message, listen to his verbal response and watch his activities to determine if he has correctly received the intended communication.

Rationale: Correct message reception is essential for healthy interpersonal relationships.

Resolved Needs: Protection from psychologic threat.

Determine if the prosthesis is effective   Determine if the patient is getting effective usefulness from the prosthesis and if it is causing any undesirable effects.

Rationale: A prosthesis assists the person in carrying out normal daily activities. Proper fit and quality are essential for safety.

Resolved Needs: Protection from physical harm.

Determine the degree of insight   Watch for verbal and nonverbal clues as to the person's understanding of the problem. Observe if he recognizes its existence, knows why and how it occurred, and how it might be resolved.

Rationale: The degree of insight greatly affects the recognition and resolution of problems.

Resolved Needs: Protection from physical harm. Protection from psychologic threat.

Determine the extent of behavioral suggestibility   Watch for the person's response to the expressed thoughts of others. Determine if these thoughts are considered and weighed before acceptance or if they are immediately incorporated into the listener's thinking.

Rationale: Unhealthy levels of suggestibility exist when a person feels controlled by other persons' thoughts and ideas.

Resolved Needs: Protection from psychologic threat.

Determine the extent of emotional flexibility   Watch for the acceptance of new ideas and situational changes. Determine if the person is adequately flexible, changes with some difficulty, or rigidly adheres to set thoughts and situations.

Rationale: Any interruption of rigidly held patterns or challenges to rigid thinking may prove threatening.

Resolved Needs: Protection from psychologic threat.

Determine the extent of group pressure conformity   Watch for the person's strength or weakness in conforming to group pressure.

Rationale: Self-confidence and well-defined values are compatible with strong resistance to group pressure. Persons lacking self-confidence and well-defined values perceive group pressure as threatening and submit to that pressure by conforming.

Resolved Needs: Protection from psychologic threat.

Determine the extent of lack of information Determine the person's overall general level of knowledge.

Rationale: The person's general level of knowledge usually indicates interests, the extent of formal education, and the capacity to recognize and solve problems.

Resolved Needs: Protection from physical harm. Protection from psychologic threat.

Determine the extent of the child's comprehension of death Watch for verbal and nonverbal clues as to the child's concept of what death is and of how he copes with it.

Rationale: At different levels of growth and development, a child's perception of death and his adaptation responses to stress vary.

Resolved Needs: Protection from psychologic threat.

Determine the extent of the person's comprehension of a poor prognosis Watch for clues as to what the person knows, what he wants to know, and what his needs are regarding the diagnosis of a terminal illness.

Rationale: The extent to which a person can comprehend a poor prognosis and still feel safe determines the nursing approach to the patient.

Resolved Needs: Protection from psychologic threat.

Determine the infant's Apgar Determine the status of the newborn during the first 10 minutes of life. Score the following conditions as 0, 1, or a high of 2:heart rate, respiratory effort, muscle tone, reflex irritability, and color. Total the score of all the conditions. An Apgar score of 7–10 indicates a good infant condition; 4–6 is fair; 0–3 is very poor.

Rationale: The infant's Apgar score serves as a baseline of information from which to plan patient care.

Resolved Needs: Protection from physical harm.

Determine the influence of culture on the pain reaction After discovering the patient's cultural background, watch for pain reactions frequently associated with that culture, such as: Italians react with fear of pain and need quick relief; Jewish persons become anxious over the source of pain and its meaning as it relates to family responsibility; persons from pioneer, American families minimize pain and seldom complain.

Rationale: Awareness that persons react to pain according to cultural standards affects the nursing approach to the treatment of pain.

Resolved Needs: Protection from physical harm. Protection from psychologic threat.

Determine the level of participation in spiritual rituals Determine which spiritual rituals are a part of the patient's daily life, such as when and if he goes to church, which prayers he prefers to say, if he is an active or passive participant.

Rationale: Spiritual rituals important in health should be made available during illness.

Resolved Needs: Protection from psychologic threat.

Determine the precipitating factors   Watch for and identify those factors that bring about pain, cyanosis, weakness, rapid pulse, etc.

Rationale: Awareness of those factors that contribute to distress supports prevention of their future occurrence.

Resolved Needs: Protection from physical harm.

Determine the relieving factors   Watch for and identify those situations and therapies that bring about cessation of the specific abnormality such as pain, dizziness, etc.

Rationale: Awareness of factors that relieve impaired health is valuable in initiating therapy to relieve the condition.

Resolved Needs: Protection from physical harm.

Determine the state of orientation   Determine the person's awareness of time, place, environment, who he is, who others are, and what is happening.

Rationale: Disorientation is associated with toxic states, brain trauma, psychic disturbances, and social isolation.

Resolved Needs: Protection from physical harm. Protection from psychologic threat.

Determine the urgency of pain relief   Determine how quickly pain relief needs to be given. If the cause of pain is life threatening, as in myocardial infarction, then the relief should be immediate. When a person has endured pain for a prolonged period, his tolerance for pain is decreased, and he requires immediate relief. If moderate pain exists, then perhaps some delay may be tolerated. In all painful conditions, relief should be given as quickly as possible.

Rationale: Pain is a signal of threat or disruption of body integrity. Its degree reveals the severity of the threat and the rapidity with which relief must be given.

Resolved Needs: Protection from physical harm. Protection from psychologic threat.

Estimate the amount of feeding the baby will need   Determine the approximate amount of milk or similar feeding the child will need at different age levels.

1–2 months	3–4 oz feeding (24 oz total)
2–3 months	4–5 oz feeding (25 oz total)
3–4 months	6–8 oz feeding (24–28 oz total)
4–5 months	7–8 oz feeding (32 oz total)
5–6 months	1 quart of milk a day

Rationale: Adequate nutrition is essential to healthy growth and development.

Resolved Needs: Protection from physical harm.

Estimate the blood volume loss
Visually inspect for and estimate the amount of blood lost.

Rationale: A blood loss of 1500 cc or more in an adult threatens life because a severely decreased circulating blood volume results in inadequate tissue oxygenation.

Resolved Needs: Protection from physical harm.

Estimate the degree of pain experienced (619)
Determine the approximate level of pain that the person is experiencing. Use the pain assessment tool developed by Kuempel, based on ratings from one to 10.

Childbirth	10
Passing kidney stones	10
Postsurgical coughing	10
Gallbladder attack	10
Spinal headache	10
Immediate postsurgical pain	10
Bone pain	8
Burn pain	7–8
Coronary thrombosis	4–6
Hand contractions	5
Migraine headache	5
Back pain	2–4
48 hour postsurgical pain	1–4
Stomach ulcer	2–3.5
Postsurgical walking	2
Toothache	2
Ordinary headache	0.5–1.5

Rationale: Although pain brings about highly individualized reactions in different persons and in the same person under different circumstances, the threshold for recognition of pain stimuli remains approximately equal from one person to another in whom the nervous system is functionally normal.

Resolved Needs: Protection from physical harm.

Estimate the degree of stress experienced   Using the Social Readjustment Rating Scale of Holmes and Rohe, estimate how much stress the person is experiencing in his present situation.

LIFE EVENT	MEAN VALUE
1. Death of spouse	100
2. Divorce	73
3. Marital separation	65
4. Jail term	63
5. Death of close family member	63
6. Personal injury or illness	53
7. Marriage	50
8. Fired at work	47
9. Marital reconciliation	45
10. Retirement	45
11. Change in health of family member	44
12. Pregnancy	40
13. Sex difficulties	39
14. Gain of new family member	39
15. Business readjustment	39
16. Change in financial state	38
17. Death of close friend	37
18. Change to different line of work.	36
19. Change in number of arguments with spouse	35
20. Mortgage over $10,000	31
21. Foreclosure of mortgage or loan	30
22. Change in responsibilities at work	29
23. Son or daughter leaving home	29
24. Trouble with in-laws	29
25. Outstanding personal achievement	28
26. Wife begin or stop work	26
27. Begin or end school	26
28. Change in living conditions.	25
29. Revision of personal habits	24
30. Trouble with boss	23
31. Change in work hours or conditions	20
32. Change in residence	20
33. Change in schools	20
34. Change in recreation	19
35. Change in church activities	19
36. Change in social activities	18
37. Mortgage or loan less than $10,000	17
38. Change in sleeping habits	16
39. Change in number of family get-togethers	15
40. Change in eating habits	15

41. Vacation   13
42. Christmas   12
43. Minor violations of the law   11

Reprinted with permission from T. H. Holmes and R. H. Rohe and from the Pergamon Press Ltd. The Social Readjustment Scale, *Journal of Psychosomatic Research* 11:213–218, 1967.

Rationale: Awareness of the amount of stress being experienced by the person supports a more realistic approach to therapeutic care.

Resolved Needs: Protection from psychologic threat.

Evaluate pain for intensity and quality

Watch for the severity and nature of the experienced pain. Pain intensity includes intractable, severe, moderate, or mild pain. Pain quality includes aching, burning, constrictive, cramping, gnawing, neuralgic, pleuritic, stabbing, stinging, tenderness, throbbing, and tingling pain.

Rationale: Pain intensity and quality signals the degree of body threat and determines the relief approach.

Resolved Needs: Protection from physical harm. Protection from psychologic threat.

Evaluate the adequacy of the housing

Determine if the facilities in which the person is housed have sufficient room, adequate sanitation, ventilation, lighting, heating, and furnishings, and if they are safe and well kept.

Rationale: Adequate shelter is essential to protect man from the environment and for the maintenance of health.

Resolved Needs: Protection from physical harm.

Evaluate the effectiveness of the pain-relief measures

Look for clues that the pain-relief measures have been effective. Observe for verbalization of pain relief, relaxation of tense facial expressions, freedom of movement when movement was previously restricted, decreased restlessness, and a return of normal skin color.

Rationale: Evaluating the effectiveness of pain-relief measures determines if comfort has been provided or if another relief approach should be tried.

Resolved Needs: Protection from physical threat.

Evaluate the message for emotional content

Listen to words used in verbal or written communications and consider the emotions that those words express.

Rationale: Psychologic distress can be revealed through the use of words having emotional or inferred meaning.

Resolved Needs: Protection from psychologic threat.

Evaluate the person's relatedness with others

Determine the person's ability to interact with others. This includes communication abilities, acceptance of role and place in the life situation, and the ability to form meaningful relationships with skill and success.

Rationale: Psychologic comfort is promoted through the ability to relate to others.

Resolved Needs: Protection from psychologic threat.

Evaluate the response to teaching (or suggestions)   Watch and listen for verbal and nonverbal responses that reveal if learning has taken place and if it is meaningful to the person.

Rationale: Information that has not been learned needs to be retaught to prevent physical or psychologic threat.

Resolved Needs: Protection from physical harm. Protection from psychologic threat.

Evaluate the safety of the environment   Watch for existing and potential safety hazards within the environment. These include high beds, spills on floors, belongings placed too far out of reach, fire hazards, poorly placed furniture, ineffective call buttons, inadequate lighting, and any other situation deemed unsafe for the patient.

Rationale: A safe environment is essential to health.

Resolved Needs: Protection from physical harm.

Evaluate the significance of emotional distress mannerisms   Watch for nonverbal indications of emotional upset such as crying, hand-wringing, floor-pacing, chain-smoking, lip and nail biting, fidgeting.

Rationale: When psychologic defenses are threatened, mannerisms give evidence of that threat.

Resolved Needs: Protection from psychologic threat.

Evaluate the significance of nonverbal communication   Watch for facial expressions, hand gestures, body postures and movements, clothing attire, associations with other persons, and preferences in life style peculiar to the person.

Rationale: Nonverbal communications reveal much about and promote understanding of the person.

Resolved Needs: Protection from psychologic threat.

Evaluate the significance of spirituality in the patient's life   Determine how important the spiritual aspects of life are to the patient by listening to his conversation and noticing his involvement in spiritual affairs.

Rationale: When spiritual involvement is important in health, it should be recognized as significant during illness.

Resolved Needs: Protection from psychologic threat.

Examine the rectum for a fecal impaction   Using a lubricated gloved finger, check the rectum for hard fecal masses. Additional signs of fecal impaction include rectal pain and fullness, inability to eliminate feces, and seepage of liquid stool around the impaction.

Rationale: Waste elimination is essential to normal body functioning.

Resolved Needs: Protection from physical harm.

Identify abnormal perceptions   Watch for indications that the person is receiving abnormal sensory input. Note any inability to discriminate between persons, distortion of one's self-image or the image of others, illusions in which one misperceives the identity of persons or objects, or hallucinations of an auditory, visual, olfactory, or tactile nature.

Rationale: Persons react to situations as they perceive them. Faulty perceptions are often the cause of abnormal behavior.

Resolved Needs: Protection from psychologic threat.

Identify abnormal thought content   Watch for indications that the person thinks about false beliefs, delusions regarding self or others, involuntary and unsuppressible obsessive thoughts, irrational phobias, autistic thinking, or prolonged fixed ideas.

Rationale: The thought process is impaired by physiologic or psychologic disequilibrium.

Resolved Needs: Protection from physical harm. Protection from psychologic threat.

Identify appropriate use of defense mechanisms (363)   Recognize those unconscious mental mechanisms that the patient is using appropriately in an effort to maintain psychologic equilibrium. Appropriate defense mechanisms are as follows:

Identification that contributes to growth of conscience, gives the child a model for patterns of success, provides parental approval, reinforces the parents' positive attitudes toward the child, and develops the characteristic of empathy within the person.

Sublimation of sexual and aggressive impulses that is directed into socially acceptable behavior.

Repression that can involuntarily exclude from the consciousness unacceptable internal impulses and ideas, thus reducing anxiety and allowing the remaining tensions to be used constructively.

Denial that blocks out the occurrence of intolerable thoughts and situations only long enough to give the person time to adjust to that which is intolerable and move on to acceptance.

Reaction formation that denies the consciousness of unacceptable thoughts and feelings through the expression of directly opposite, but acceptable, thoughts and feelings.

Compensation that results in increasing self-esteem and feelings of security that occur from the person's strivings to overcome the sources of insecurity.

Rationalization that conceals the person's real motives with the result that self-esteem is maintained and guilt feeling resolved.

Substitution that provides an alternate but satisfactory goal in place of the original goal is always appropriate.

Displacement that allows the individual to avoid recognizing unacceptable feelings toward a person by displacing those same feelings toward another person or objects that represent that person.

Projection that provides comfort by recognizing in others those unfavorable characteristics in ourselves that we prefer not to admit exist.

Symbolism that results in merely transferring an emotional value to an object.

Regression that maintains some adult behavior along with the regressed behavior and that is used to support the process of adjustment.

Fixation and dissociation are not appropriate.

Rationale: Defense mechanisms are essential for the maintenance of psychologic equilibrium. Recognition of their appropriate use offers assurance that the patient is coping adequately and making a satisfactory adjustment. It is a clue to the nurse to support such coping mechanisms.

Resolved Needs: Protection from psychologic threat. Personal growth and maturity.

Identify attention span abnormalities   Watch for an inability to focus attention for any length of time or the concentration of attention on a single subject.

Rationale: The ability to function is impaired by attention span abnormalities.

Resolved Needs: Protection from physical harm. Protection from psychologic threat.

Identify disturbing conversation topics   Listen for discussion of topics that cause tension or emotional upset.

Rationale: When psychologic defenses are threatened, emotional responses give evidence of that threat.

Resolved Needs: Protection from psychologic threat.

Identify emotion-stimulating events   Identify those environmental stimuli and situations that arouse undesirable feelings and cause stressful emotional reactions.

Rationale: Emotional comfort and safety are influenced by environmental stimuli.

Resolved Needs: Protection from psychologic threat.

Identify environmental discomfort Identify existing or potential environmental discomforts, such as room overheating or underheating, excessive noise, unpleasant odors, and dust.

Rationale: Environmental discomforts often threaten the body integrity.

Resolved Needs: Protection from physical harm. Protection from psychologic threat.

Identify former pleasurable interests Watch for clues of interests from which the person gained pleasure before his present health problem.

Rationale: The pursuit of pleasurable interests promotes both physical and psychologic health.

Resolved Needs: Protection from physical harm. Protection from psychologic threat.

Identify inappropriate emotional responses Determine if the person's emotional responses are appropriate to the situation. Does he laugh in a happy situation, or does he inappropriately cry when laughter is in order? Take into account cultural influences.

Rationale: When stress becomes so threatening that normal defenses become inadequate, response through inappropriate emotions becomes evident.

Resolved Needs: Protection from psychologic threat.

Identify inappropriate use of defense mechanisms (363) Recognize those unconscious mental mechanisms that the patient is using inappropriately in an effort to maintain psychologic equilibrium. Inappropriate defense mechanisms are as follows:

Identification that causes the child to assume undesirable characteristics of the parent or when one transfers the identification of one person to another similar person.

Repression that is insufficient to reduce anxiety, and that impairs the capacity for reality perception, often resulting in hallucinations or delusions.

Denial that permanently blocks out the occurrence of intolerable thoughts and situations and does not lead to later acceptance, or denial that results in malingering.

Reaction formation that becomes exaggerated or inappropriate or when it interferes with adjustment.

Compensation that results in unrealistic self-esteem such as delusions of grandeur that occur from the excessive strivings to overcome the insecurity.

Rationalization that conceals one's true motives and is based on such false causes as to prevent goal-seeking, causes self-depreciation, or results in delusions.

Displacement that uses symbols to avoid recognizing unacceptable feelings, such as a phobia.

Projection that results in the unrealistic perception of oneself, disrupts favorable interpersonal relationships through excessive criticism, hostility, and prejudice, promotes the suspiciousness of paranoia, causes ideas of reference, illusions, hallucinations, and delusions.

Symbolism that results in forbidden impulses being expressed by acceptable physical symptoms, obsessive thoughts, compulsive acts, phobias, or undoing behavior.

Fixation that prevents mature and independent personality development by limiting personality growth to a past era of satisfaction.

Regression that brings about disorganization of the personality such as in schizophrenia.

Dissociation that results in loss of control over the integration of the personality and is expressed in automatic writing, sleep-walking, fugue states, dual or multiple personalities, and conversion reactions.

Rationale: Defense mechanisms that are used inappropriately are failing to maintain psychologic equilibrium. Recognition of their inappropriateness can serve as a guide to direct the patient toward the appropriate use of defense mechanisms and the reestablishment of psychologic balance.

Resolved Needs: Protection from psychologic threat. Personal growth and maturity.

Identify life values significant to the person   Identify those moral values that are important to the person.

Rationale: Man's value codes are essential to his safety and comfort.

Resolved Needs: Protection from psychologic threat.

Identify potentially destructive behavior   Watch for potential suicide, assaultive, or threatening behavior.

Rationale: Potentially destructive behavior must be curtailed to preserve the safety of persons involved.

Resolved Needs: Protection from physical harm. Protection from psychologic threat.

Identify reality-acceptance clues   Listen for clues of the person's ability to accept the reality of the situation. In health situations, such clues would include statements such as "I'm dying bit by bit," "I'm half dead," "I'm almost 6 feet under," "I'm a peg-legged sailor," etc. There are times when the person has not been told of a poor prognosis, yet he exhibits these clues because he has nonverbally perceived the truth.

Rationale: Ill persons frequently come to accept the reality of situations through the nonverbal communications of others. They quickly perceive changes in the amount of attention they receive, new approaches by health personnel, and saddened family members who cannot hide their feelings. The ill person frequently returns the communication through indirect inferences. An awareness of the patient's level of perception and acceptance highly influences the course of treatment.

Resolved Needs: Protection from psychologic threat.

Identify the current dominant emotion   Identify the person's prevailing mood. Through verbal and nonverbal communications, discover present emotions such as depression, anger, anxiety, joy, hatred, ambivalence, grief, and the like.

Rationale: Current emotional states affect experiences of perception, thinking, motivation, and internal safety feelings.

Resolved Needs: Protection from physical harm. Protection from psychologic threat.

Inspect and palpate the painful site   Look for inflammation, edema, brusing, bone distortion, distention, etc., of the painful area. Palpate for rigidity, tenderness, subcutaneous swelling, skin warmth, etc. If the area itself is not painful, look for foreign objects in the bed linen or clothing (pins, splinters, etc.) that may be the source of pain.

Rationale: Inspection of the painful site offers clues as to the cause of pain and supports action to reduce pain.

Resolved Needs: Protection from physical harm.

Inspect for abnormal body movements   Look for unusual body movements such as irregular jerking, purposeless, spastic twitching, wormlike movements, and tremors.

Rationale: Abnormal body movements occur with nervous system degeneration or organic brain disease.

Resolved Needs: Protection from physical harm.

Inspect for an abnormal body discharge   With the aid of a light, look for abnormal excretions through normal body orifices, including the eyes, ears, nose, mouth, vagina, anus, and urethra.

Rationale: Purulent and odoriferous discharges indicate infection. Hardened discharges may cause obstruction. Bloody discharges indicate tissue injury.

Resolved Needs: Protection from physical harm.

Inspect for bleeding   Remove the patient's clothing and look for small amounts of bloody discharge from wounds or body orifices. A light may facilitate visualization. Observe for the amount, color, flow rapidity, and source.

Rationale: Bleeding can lead to reduced circulating blood volume which, if prolonged, can threaten life.

Resolved Needs: Protection from physical harm.

Inspect for deformity   Look for abnormal structural formation in any or all body areas.

Rationale: Recognition and correction of deformities often improves body function.

Resolved Needs: Protection from physical harm.

Inspect for dehydration   Watch for signs of insufficient body fluid, including thinness, sunken eyes, parched or cracked lips, dry-thick tongue coating, hollow cheeks, gray skin discoloration, poor skin turgor, sunken fontanels, lethargy, or irritability.

Rationale: Altered fluid balance damages and impairs cell activity.

Resolved Needs: Protection from physical harm.

Inspect for drainage   Look for oozing or flow of fluid or pus from a cavity, wound, or other area. Note the color, consistency, amount, and odor.

Rationale: Purulent drainage indicates the presence of infection. Excessive drainage indicates delayed healing. Inadequate drainage indicates obstruction.

Resolved Needs: Protection from physical harm.

Inspect for edema   Look for swollen body areas. Press those areas and watch for deep impressions resulting from finger pressure. Such swelling usually occurs in the feet, ankles, fingers, eyelids, or sacral area.

Rationale: Edema is an abnormal accumulation of fluid in the interstitial spaces and may be the result of many disorders including increased permeability of capillary walls, increased capillary pressure (venous obstruction, CHF), lymphatic obstruction, impaired kidney function, inadequate plasma protein, fluid and electrolyte imbalance, inflammatory reactions, and hormone imbalance.

Resolved Needs: Protection from physical harm.

Inspect for foreign bodies   Look for small objects in any body opening.

Rationale: Foreign objects cause irritation, inflammation, infection, and respiratory obstruction.

Resolved Needs: Protection from physical harm.

Inspect for hemorrhage   Remove the patient's clothing and look for any evidence of severe blood loss. Observe for the amount, color, rapidity of flow, and the source. After delivery, watch the mother for vaginal bleeding of 500 cc or more. Especially watch mothers with large babies, large amounts of amniotic fluid, premature placenta separation, or multiple births.

Rationale: Hemorrhage decreases the circulating blood volume, resulting in circulatory impairment or collapse. Even though approximately 5000 cc of blood normally circulates through the adult body, the rapid loss of more than 500 cc of blood seriously threatens life.

Resolved Needs: Protection from physical harm.

Inspect for inflammation   Look for redness, heat, swelling, pain, and loss of function (especially if a joint is involved).

Rationale: An inflammatory response is a natural body defense indicating a tissue reaction to irritation from toxic, bacterial, chemical, or mechanical injury.

Resolved Needs: Protection from physical harm.

Inspect for renewed bleeding   Once bleeding has stopped, check every 15 minutes to 1 hour for resumed bleeding.

Rationale: Renewed bleeding can cause decreased circulating blood volume or shock.

Resolved Needs: Protection from physical harm.

Inspect for signs of infection   Look for signs indicating an infection such as pain, redness, swelling, heat, and impaired function.

Rationale: The recognition of infection supports the initiation of treatment to reduce the infection.

Resolved Needs: Protection from physical harm.

Inspect for stool abnormalities   Look for watery or hard feces, abnormal shapes such as ribbon or cylinder stool, abnormal color such as clay or tarry stools, and obvious abnormal content such as undigested food, blood, or mucus. Note the time of occurrence, frequency, and accompanying discomforts.

Rationale: Abnormal stools indicate gastrointestinal disorders.

Resolved Needs: Protection from physical harm.

Inspect for the percentage of burned area   Look over the burned adult body surface and estimate the percentage of injury. The entire head is considered 9%, each arm 9%, each leg 18%, the front torso 18%, the back torso 18%, and the genital area 1%.

Rationale: Therapy and prognosis are determined by the percentage of burned body surface.

Resolved Needs: Protection from physical harm.

Inspect the abdomen for ascites: Watch for a single curved profile of the abdomen, an inverted umbilicus, and bulging flanks.

Rationale: Ascites indicates an excessive fluid accumulation in the peritoneal cavity.

Resolved Needs: Protection from physical harm.

Inspect the abdomen for distention   Inspect for taut, abdominal wall stretching with umbilical protrusion and thin, glossy abdominal skin.

Rationale: Gas or fluid accumulation in the intestines or peritoneal cavity results in abdominal distention and severe pain.

Resolved Needs: Protection from physical harm.

Inspect the abdomen for vein engorgement (113,225)   Look for abnormal, prominent veins (venation) over the abdominal walls. If present, inspect the direction of blood flow in the following manner. Place both the right and left index fingertips over the vein and compress it. Maintaining the same pressure, slide the fingers apart in opposite directions. Release the right finger and watch for venous filling from that side. Repeat the same test, releasing the left finger instead of the right.

Rationale: An upward, venous blood flow from the lower abdomen indicates inferior vena cava obstruction. An upward flow from the upper abdomen indicates portal obstruction. A downward flow from the upper abdomen indicates superior vena cava obstruction.

Resolved Needs: Protection from physical harm.

Inspect the abdomen for visible peristalsis (113,225)   Inspect the upper abdomen for waves of intestinal contractions that begin at the upper left quadrant and slant downward toward the right lower quadrant.

Rationale: Visible peristalsis indicates excessive intestinal contraction or obstruction.

Resolved Needs: Protection from physical harm.

Inspect the adenoids for enlargement (113,225)   With a small light, look into the open mouth. Inspect the tonsil area for oversized adenoids.

Rationale: Enlarged adenoids affect speech sounds, cause mouth breathing, respiratory obstruction, and allow infectious agents to pass from the throat to the eustachian tube and infect the ear.

Resolved Needs: Protection from physical harm.

Inspect the amniotic fluid for meconium   During the labor process, watch for a greenish stool substance in the amniotic fluid, especially at the time of uterine membrane rupture.

Rationale: Meconium in amniotic fluid indicates fetal distress or breech presentation.

Resolved Needs: Protection from physical harm.

Inspect the arms and hands for venous distention
(113,225) Watch for arm and hand veins that appear swollen or are pulsating with a bounding thrust when the hands and arms are held at heart level.

Rationale: Distention of arm and hand veins indicates circulatory fluid overload or the presence of a trauma-related or congenital arteriovenous fistula.

Resolved Needs: Protection from physical harm.

Inspect the bones for alignment
Inspect the body for straight alignment of the bones.

Rationale: Nonalignment of bone can indicate disease, deformity, or cause of illness.

Resolved Needs: Protection from physical harm.

Inspect the breasts for abnormalities
Inspect the breasts for symmetry, vein distention, flat, depressed, or inverted nipples, excessive or diminished lactation, bloody nipple discharge, dimpling, engorgement, lumps, inflammation, or cracked nipples.

Rationale: Breast irregularities indicate abnormal conditions or diseases.

Resolved Needs: Protection from physical harm.

Inspect the cast for tightness
Watch for evidence that a cast is too tight on a limb. Such evidence includes swelling, toe or finger pallor or cyanosis, pain, numbness, and inadequate capillary filling. Check the skin at the edges of the cast for evidence of excessive pressure, including redness, pain, and abrasion.

Rationale: A tight cast can impair tissue circulation, cause tissue necrosis, and produce severe pain.

Resolved Needs: Protection from physical harm.

Inspect the chest for precordial bulge (113,225)
Inspect for a chest swelling or protrusion, especially in the right ventricle and upper sternal area.

Rationale: Precordial bulge indicates cardiac enlargement or aortic aneurysm.

Resolved Needs: Protection from physical harm.

Inspect the chest for respiratory rate and rhythm
Count the number of respirations that occur each minute. Watch for abnormal respiratory patterns such as abdominal, Cheyne-Stokes, Dyspneic, orthopneic,

rapid, shallow, slow, noisy, jerky, wheezing, mouth breathing, and sighing respirations. Watch for deviations from the normal newborn respirations of 30–50/minute and normal adult respirations of 16–20/minute.

Rationale: Normal respirations are essential to blood and tissue oxygenation.

Resolved Needs: Protection from physical harm.

Inspect the chest for symmetrical expansion   Inspect for chest movements in which both sides of the chest move up and down at the same time.

Rationale: Asymmetrical chest expansion indicates that both lungs are not receiving the same amount of air at the same time.

Resolved Needs: Protection from physical harm.

Inspect the ears and nose for cerebral spinal fluid leakage   Watch for a yellowish fluid leaking from the nose, ear, or head wound. Spinal fluid feels slick or oily and will give a positive glucose reaction on Tes-Tape.

Rationale: Spinal fluid loss indicates a skull fracture.

Resolved Needs: Protection from physical harm.

Inspect the ears with an otoscope (113,225)   Use a lighted speculum to visualize the inner canal of the ear and the tympanic membrane. When examining adults, gently pull the ear upward and backward. With infants and children, gently pull the ear downward. Inspect for a normal, shiny, pearl-gray membrane.

Rationale: A blue internal ear membrane indicates blood in the middle ear. A chalky white membrane indicates pus. An amber or yellow membrane indicates serum. A dull membrane indicates fibrosis. An amber membrane with air bubbles indicates fluid accumulation.

Resolved Needs: Protection from physical harm.

Inspect the extremity (or extremities) for adequate circulation   Inspect the extremities for pallor or cyanosis. Touch the extremity skin, feeling for normal body warmth, and check for capillary filling.

Rationale: Diminished tissue oxygenation results from impaired circulation, which increases the potential for tissue necrosis.

Resolved Needs: Protection from physical harm.

Inspect the eyelids for drooping   Watch for an inability to voluntarily keep the eyelid open or for the lid to involuntarily fall lower than normal when the eye is open.

Rationale: Poor control of the eyelid indicates an oculomotor nerve disturbance.

Resolved Needs: Protection from physical harm.

Inspect the eyelids for incomplete closure   Watch for indications that the person is unable to tightly close his eyes or eye.

Rationale: Eyelid closure protects the eye from foreign particle trauma.

Resolved Needs: Protection from physical harm.

Inspect the eyes for discoloration   With a light, look for yellow or red color changes in the normally white sclera.

Rationale: Scleral jaundice indicates that red blood cell pigments are not being normally excreted through the bile. Scleral redness indicates eyestrain or infection.

Resolved Needs: Protection from physical harm.

Inspect the eyes for exophthalmia   Examine the eyes for lid retraction, a widened opening between the eyelids, lid lag, a staring expression, forward displacement of a swollen eye, and a limited upward gaze.

Rationale: Exophthalmia most often indicates thyrotoxicosis.

Resolved Needs: Protection from physical harm.

Inspect the eyes for papilledema (113,225)   Examine the eye with an ophthalmoscope and look for blurring of the upper and lower nasal disk margins with extended blurring to diverging vessels. The eye veins appear distended and pulseless and may appear to bend sharply over the edge of the disk.

Rationale: Papilledema indicates increased intracranial pressure. The central retinal vein is compressed and the return of blood from the eye is obstructed, causing edema and potential blindness.

Resolved Needs: Protection from physical harm.

Inspect the eyes for pupil equality and response changes   Examine the pupils for equal size. Shine a light into each eye and determine if the pupil constricts quickly and if both constrict with equal rapidity.

Rationale: The third cranial nerve controls pupillary response, and because of the nerves location, it provides an accurate sign of increased intracranial pressure.

Resolved Needs: Protection from physical harm.

Contraindications: Conditions that cause photophobia such as meningitis and measles.

Inspect the fingers for clubbing (113,225)   Determine if the fingernail sets at a 10-degree or 20-degree angle to the finger. Press the skin near the cuticle with your fingertip. In finger clubbing, you can feel the nail plate move toward the bone and then spring back when your finger pressure is released. The fingers may have a stub or stunted shape.

Rationale: Finger clubbing is associated with blood disorders, thyroid enlargement, cardiac inflammation, tuberculous, pulmonary infection, pulmonary tumor, and liver cirrhosis.

Resolved Needs: Protection from physical harm.

Inspect the genitalia for abnormalities   Look for edema, irritation, inflammation, loss of pubic hair, and abnormal organ development of the genitalia.

Rationale: Genitalia abnormalities may reveal disorders of the reproductive organs.

Resolved Needs: Protection from physical harm.

Inspect the gums for abnormalities   Inspect the fleshy tissue at the base of the teeth for bleeding, inflammation, ulceration, receding, tenderness, discoloration, paleness, swelling, and hyperplasia.

Rationale: Poor gum conditions reflect basic health disorders. Sore gums indicate niacin deficiency. Bleeding gums occur in leukemia, vitamin C deficiency, excessive tartar deposits, and gum infection. Gum inflammation occurs with vitamin C deficiency. Gum hyperplasia may occur during prolonged Dilantin therapy.

Resolved Needs: Protection from physical harm.

Inspect the hair for abnormalities   Watch for unusual hair conditions such as excessive dryness or oiliness, thinning, matting, hair loss, parasites, bleeding onto the hair, or abnormal hair distribution.

Rationale: Hair abnormalities indicate poor hygiene or physiologic disorders.

Resolved Needs: Protection from physical harm.

Inspect the hands for impaired grasp   Have the patient squeeze your hand and determine if the strength of the squeeze is normal. Determine the person's grasping ability. Notice if he's able to close safety pins, button clothing, pick up coins, and perform other activities requiring precise finger movements.

Rationale: The inability to firmly grasp objects is indicative of brain or nerve cell damage. Skilled voluntary movements are dependent on an intact corticospinal tract. The inability to perform daily living skills usually is perceived as threatening.

Resolved Needs: Protection from physical harm.

Inspect the hands for tremors   Look for mild shaking in the head and hands. Flapping tremors are evident when the hand is outstretched and it flaps like a wing.

Rationale: Tremors indicate disorders affecting the nervous system. Flapping tremors result from impending hepatic coma.

Resolved Needs: Protection from physical harm.

Inspect the head for Battle's sign Inspect for a spongy area on the temple and behind the ear, which may appear bruised.

Rationale: A positive Battle's sign indicates skull fracture.

Resolved Needs: Protection from physical harm.

Inspect the joints for abnormalities Look for joint disorders such as limited joint movement, muscle atrophy around a joint, swelling, tenderness, pain, increased joint size, and heat.

Rationale: Normal fibrous connective tissue and cartilage are essential for freely moveable joints.

Resolved Needs: Protection from physical harm.

Inspect the joints for impending contractures Look for a drooping hand or foot, chronically bent knees or elbows, turning of the neck toward one side, flexed fingers, or decreased finger movement.

Rationale: Muscle shortening prevents normal functional use of the joints. Early treatment of contractures maintains normal joint movement.

Resolved Needs: Protection from physical harm.

Inspect the mouth for abnormal salivation Look for excessive accumulation or production of saliva or decreased salivation.

Rationale: Excessive saliva can cause choking. Excessive production of saliva is evident in poisonous spider bites and epileptic seizures. Decreased saliva occurs with salivary gland obstruction.

Resolved Needs: Protection from physical harm.

Inspect the mucous membranes for abnormalities Look for abnormalities of the mucous membranes of the mouth, nose, throat, and vagina. These include inflammation, edema, exudates, irritation, trauma, allergy responses, pallor, yellow discoloration of the hard palate, rashes, lesions, and dryness.

Rationale: Healthy mucous membranes are moist and well lubricated and protect the underlying tissue. Traumatized oral mucosa impairs eating and drinking and reduces comfort. Abnormal mucous membranes may indicate other underlying disorders.

Resolved Needs: Protection from physical harm.

Inspect the muscles for impaired tone Look for muscle size reduction, weakened muscular capabilities, paralysis, spasms, and clumsy movements.

Rationale: Decreased muscle tone results from interrupted nerve supply, immobilization disuse, and inadequate tissue nutrition.

Resolved Needs: Protection from physical harm.

Inspect the nails for abnormalities Inspect the finger- and toenails for cleanliness, excessive length, ragged edges, hangnails, abnormal nail formation, thickness, discoloration, splitting, or ulcers appearing around the nail.

Rationale: Nail changes occur in nutritional deficiencies, systemic illnesses, and local infection.

Resolved Needs: Protection from physical harm.

Inspect the nasal turbinates for abnormalities Using a light, gently inspect the inner nasal tissue for redness, paleness, or swelling.

Rationale: Pale, swollen nasal turbinates occur with hay fever and allergies. Red, swollen nasal turbinates occur with the common cold.

Resolved Needs: Protection from physical harm.

Inspect the neck veins for distention Determine if the neck veins appear swollen or if they pulsate with a bounding thrust.

Rationale: Distended neck veins of a person resting with the head elevated at a 45° angle indicate venous congestion that may be the result of left ventricular failure, severe pulmonary obstructive disease, or vascular overload.

Resolved Needs: Protection from physical harm.

Inspect the nose for asymmetry With a light, examine the nasal septum, externally and internally, for marked deviation to one side of the face. If the nasal passages are not of equal size, then the septum is not straight.

Rationale: Asymmetrical nasal passages can cause nasal obstruction or inadequate sinus drainage.

Resolved Needs: Protection from physical harm.

Inspect the nose for epistaxis Look for nose bleeding, especially serious bleeding.

Rationale: Rapid loss of more than 1 pint (500 cc) of blood in an adult poses a threat to life.

Resolved Needs: Protection from physical harm.

Inspect the nose for polyps With a light, look for small growths protruding from the nasal lining.

Rationale: Nasal polyps obstruct normal air flow.

Resolved Needs: Protection from physical harm.

Inspect the nose, mouth, and throat for evidence of burns With a light, look for scorched hairs in the nose and abnormal coloration and drying.of the mucous membrane.

Rationale: Nose, mouth, or throat burns may indicate burns extending into the lungs.

Resolved Needs: Protection from physical harm.

Inspect the orthopedic pin for position and for cleanliness Periodically check the entrance site of the orthopedic pin into the skin. Look for infection, crusting, and drainage.

Rationale: Exudate at a wound opening promotes bacterial growth causing wound and bone infection. If the pin slips out of position, it pulls the contaminated pin into the tissue.

Resolved Needs: Protection from physical harm.

Inspect the palms for coloration With the fingers stretched, look for white, pink, or red coloring in the lines of the hand or yellow pigment on the palm.

Rationale: White or no coloring in the lines of the hands indicates anemia. Bright red coloring indicates polycythemia vera. Yellow palm discoloration indicates liver disease or myxedema.

Resolved Needs: Protection from physical harm.

Inspect the patient's mouth for concealed medications When giving oral medications, check the mouth carefully for medications that have not been swallowed.

Rationale: Small, therapeutic doses of drugs can be collected and, when taken in large doses, cause death.

Resolved Needs: Protection from physical harm.

Inspect the placenta for abnormalities Look for separation of the placenta into two parts, atrophy, incomplete placenta, and umbilical cord attachment at the margins.

Rationale: Placental abnormalities indicate potential uterine or hemorrhage disorders. When portions of the placenta are missing, it indicates that some of the placenta has been retained in the uterus.

Resolved Needs: Protection from physical harm.

Inspect the skin for breakdown Look for redness, irritation, duskiness, blistering, and broken skin.

Rationale: Skin breakdown supports infection and reduces circulation which furthers tissue necrosis.

Resolved Needs: Protection from physical harm.

Inspect the skin for discoloration   Look for redness, blueness, blanching, bronzing, yellow, purple, or other skin discoloration.

Rationale: Red or red-blue pinpoint skin discolorations indicate blood dyscrasias or capillary fragility. Blanching or blue discoloration indicates inadequate oxygen supply. Jaundice indicates biliary obstruction. Bronzing is evident in adrenal disorders.

Resolved Needs: Protection from physical harm.

Inspect the skin for impaired feeling perception   Have the patient close his eyes. With a pin, touch the skin and watch for a decreased pain response. Touch the patient with heat or cold and determine if the response is normal.

Rationale: Impaired feeling perception indicates nerve or circulatory damage, and increases the potential for tissue trauma.

Resolved Needs: Protection from physical harm.

Inspect the skin for infectious lesions   Look for open sores, fever, swelling, redness, crusting, ulceration, warts, rashes, pain, chains or clusters of blisters, vesicles, discolored lumps, gummas, chancre, or thick, leathery, nodular skin lesions.

Rationale: Invasion of the skin by viruses, bacteria, and fungus causes infection and discomfort.

Resolved Needs: Protection from physical harm.

Inspect the skin for irritation   Look over the skin for signs of redness.

Rationale: Signs of skin irritation when heeded can prevent skin breakdown.

Resolved Needs: Protection from physical harm.

Inspect the skin for pallor   Look for lack of color and whiteness of the skin.

Rationale: Localized pallor results from peripheral blood vessel constriction, localized edema, or obstructed arterial flow. Generalized pallor indicates shock.

Resolved Needs: Protection from physical harm.

Inspect the skin for perspiration abnormality   Look for discolored perspiration, excessive sweating at night, absent perspiration, profuse sweating, frosty or snowlike perspiration, or excessively salty sweating.

Rationale: Excessive perspiration may lead to dehydration or may indicate the need for body temperature regulation. Frosty, snowlike perspiration indicates uremia. Discolored sweat indicates toxicity. Excessive salty sweating may lead to electrolyte imbalance. Absent perspiration indicates an inability of the body to cool itself.

Resolved Needs: Protection from physical harm.

Inspect the skin for petechiae Look for small, purplish, hemorrhagic spots on the skin.

Rationale: Petechiae indicate a blood clotting disorder, capillary fragility, or a severe systemic disorder such as meningococcal septicemia or bacterial endocarditis.

Resolved Needs: Protection from physical harm.

Inspect the skin for skin spiders Look over the face, neck, upper trunk, and arms for small, reddened spiderlike vascular abnormalities. They may pulsate enough for the pulsation to be seen and felt.

Rationale: Most vascular spiders are arterioles, and although they are associated with cirrhosis, their specific cause is not known.

Resolved Needs: Protection from physical harm.

Inspect the sputum for characteristics Look for the amount, consistency, and appearance of the sputum.

Rationale: Blood-tinged sputum indicates respiratory tract inflammation. Pink sputum is evident in pneumonia and pulmonary edema. Very bloody sputum occurs with tuberculosis, embolism, and carcinoma. Rusty sputum is seen in pneumococcal pneumonia. Stringy sputum is associated with asthma, and frothy sputum with pulmonary edema. Yellow, green, or dirty gray (purulent) sputum indicates lung infection. Gelatinous sputum suggests pneumonia. Soot in the sputum may indicate that burns have extended into the respiratory system.

Resolved Needs: Protection from physical harm.

Inspect the teeth for abnormalities Inspect the teeth for caries, chipping, cracking, discoloration, and alignment.

Rationale: Teeth are essential to chewing and digestion, maintenance of natural jaw contour, and comfort.

Resolved Needs: Protection from physical harm.

Inspect the throat for an impaired swallowing reflex Touch the posterior pharyngeal wall with an applicator stick and note if gagging occurs. If there is question as to the ability to swallow, have the patient suck a piece of ice or drink small sips of water and note how well he swallows.

Rationale: Swallowing is necessary for the passage of food and fluid into the digestive system. An impaired swallowing reflex indicates soft palate paralysis, stroke, head injury or trauma and may result in choking.

Resolved Needs: Protection from physical harm.

Inspect the tongue for abnormalities Inspect the tongue for scars, tremors, sharp pointedness, protrusion, enlargement, atrophy, bleeding, inflammation, cracking, dryness, longitudinal furrows, tenderness, ulceration, rashes, discoloration, coatings, paleness, swelling, and deviations from the midline.

Rationale: A normal tongue is essential to food manipulation when chewing, taste perception, and speech. An abnormal tongue may indicate other underlying disorders.

Resolved Needs: Protection from physical harm.

Inspect the umbilical cord for abnormalities   At childbirth, inspect the umbilical cord for the presence of two arteries and one vein. During the infant's first few weeks of life, inspect the umbilical cord area for a weeping discharge, excessive bulging, or hemorrhage.

Rationale: The absence of umbilical cord arteries or vein indicates a congenital abnormality. Other abnormalities indicate poor healing, infection, or herniation.

Resolved Needs: Protection from physical harm.

Inspect the vagina for a prolapsed umbilical cord   Following membrane rupture and the gush of amniotic fluid, look for protrusion of the umbilical cord through the vagina.

Rationale: An umbilical cord visible at the vagina indicates umbilical cord prolapse. A prolapsed umbilical cord, compressed between the fetal head and pelvis, can cause fetal strangulation or fatal circulatory impairment.

Resolved Needs: Protection from physical harm.

Inspect the vagina for discharge   Inspect for normal and abnormal vaginal discharges.

Normal vaginal discharges include:

A clear, mucoid discharge occurring with normal ovulation.

Lochia, which is a moderate, bloody, mucus flow during the first 3 days; decreases and becomes watery and pink from about the fourth to the ninth day; becomes thin, colorless, and scant after the tenth day; and usually disappears or is just a slight brownish, mucoid discharge at 21 days post partum. Lochia should never have an offensive odor.

Menstruation of moderate flow and duration.

A bright red or red-brown discharge or spotting lasting 3–6 weeks after a hysterectomy.

A red-brown discharge lasting for several days after a dilatation and curettage (D&C).

Abnormal vaginal discharges include:

A brown or chocolate discharge associated with endometriosis or uterine carcinoma.

A cheesy discharge occurring with Monilia infection.

A creamy, white discharge occurring with streptococcal or staphyloc-
cal infection or radiation therapy.

A frothy white discharge indicating Trichomonas infection or radiation therapy.

A mucoid, yellow discharge associated with streptococcal or
staphylococcal infection.

A thick, yellow discharge occurring with Gonococcus infection.

Rationale: Early detection and treatment of reproductive disorders prevent progression to serious disease.

Resolved Needs: Protection from physical harm.

Inspect the vocal cords for lesions   With a small light, a tongue
depressor, and a dental mirror, look through the open mouth into the lower
pharynx for vocal cord tumors.

Rationale: Vocal cord tumors affect the ability to speak and to communicate. When large enough, such tumors cause respiratory obstruction or difficulty swallowing food.

Resolved Needs: Protection from physical harm.

Inspect the wound dressing frequently   Inspect the wound dressing at least every 4 hours, and more often if necessary. Look for wetness,
cleanliness, adequate wound coverage, bleeding, and drainage. Inspect the
bed and clothing underneath the wound since drainage sometimes seeps out
from under the dressing instead of being absorbed by it.

Rationale: Frequent observation of wound dressings supports detection of
abnormalities and the need for dressing change.

Resolved Needs: Protection from physical harm.

Inspect the wound for evisceration   Determine if a surgically
closed wound has broken open and area organs are exposed.

Rationale: Wound evisceration poses the threat of infection and shock.

Resolved Needs: Protection from physical harm.

Keep a dialysis flow sheet   Record the time that each dialysis treatment is begun and when each drainage period is concluded. Also, include
the amount of fluid instilled, the volume drained, and any medications
given.

Rationale: An accurate record of the dialysis process assists the physician
in evaluating the treatment being given and promotes patient safety.

Resolved Needs: Protection from physical harm.

Measure the body weight   Determine the body weight by using a
standard scale that gives body weight in pounds or kilograms or a

metabolic scale that records weight in kilograms only (each kilogram equals 2.2 pounds).

Rationale: Body weight changes indicate loss or retention of fluids, food intake changes, food absorption abnormalities, or increased adaptation requirements on body processes. Kilograms are used for measuring body weight when accuracy is essential for computing drug dosage, fluids, and nutrient intake.

Resolved Needs: Protection from physical harm.

Measure the chest drainage after clamping the chest tube, and attaching a new drainage system

Clamp the chest tube close to the insertion site. Remove the present water-seal drainage system and immediately replace it with a new, sterile system. Remove the clamp from the chest tube and check that it is patent. Then measure the amount of drainage in the old container by measuring the total volume and subtracting from it the amount of sterile water originally placed in the water-seal drainage system.

Rationale: Measuring the chest drainage gives an estimate of the amount of blood lost and facilitates equivalent blood or fluid replacement.

Resolved Needs: Protection from physical harm.

Measure the girth of the (specific body part)

Measure the circumference of a body area with a tape measure as often as necessary.

Rationale: The abdominal or extremity girth increases with fluid accumulation in tissues. A child's head circumference increases abnormally with increased intracranial pressure.

Resolved Needs: Protection from physical harm.

Measure the head for abnormal size

Measure the infant's head and chest. Normally, they are approximately equal in size.

Rationale: An enlarged infant's head indicates skull expansion from internal pressure.

Resolved Needs: Protection from physical harm.

Measure the height

Measure in feet and inches (meters and cm) the distance between the person's feet and the top of his head.

Rationale: Measuring height allows for determination of normal and abnormal growth patterns and proportional body development between height and weight. Normal child growth is 3–5 inches a year.

Resolved Needs: Protection from physical harm.

Measure the intake

Measure the volume of fluids taken in over a 24-hour period. This includes all liquids such as water, milk, soups, soft drinks, intravenous fluids, ice cream, Jello, juices, ice, ice chips and irrigating fluids which have not been withdrawn.

Rationale: Accurate intake and output measurement is essential for correct fluid replacement therapy. Balanced fluid intake and output is essential to cell functioning. Severely altered fluid balance damages and impairs cell activity.

Resolved Needs: Protection from physical harm.

Measure the output   Measure and record the fluid volume and wastes excreted from the body in a 24-hour period. Include urine, liquid feces, approximate plasma loss from burns, gastrointestinal drainage, T-tube bile drainage, excessive wound drainage, chest drainage, etc.

Rationale: Accurate intake and output measurement is essential for correct fluid replacement therapy. Balanced fluid intake and output are essential to cell functioning. Severely altered fluid balance damages and impairs cell activity.

Resolved Needs: Protection from physical harm.

Measure the pelvic size   Using a pelvimeter, determine if the pelvic diameter size is large enough for normal delivery. Normal measurements should be: Externally, 26 cm between the iliac spines, 29 cm between the iliac crests, 31 cm between the great trochanters, 20 cm between the last lumbar spine and the pubic front surface. Internally, 12.5 cm from the pubic outer edge to the sacral promontory (diagonal conjugate), 11 cm from the inner symphysis pubis to the sacral promontory (true conjugate), 11.5 cm between the ischial spines, 11 cm between the ischial tuberosities, 11.5 cm between the sacrum and pubis.

Rationale: The birth canal must be sufficiently large for the infant to pass safely through without harm.

Resolved Needs: Protection from physical harm.

Measure the residual urine   Measure the urine volume that remains in the bladder after voiding. Have the patient void, then insert a catheter into the bladder to remove the remaining urine and measure the volume.

Rationale: Retained urine of 50 cc or more after voiding indicates decreased bladder efficiency.

Resolved Needs: Protection from physical harm.

Measure the urine output hourly   Measure the urine volume excreted within 1 hour. Normal adult urine excretion is approximately 60 cc/hr with a minimum of 30 cc/hr.

Rationale: The excretion of less than 15–20 cc of urine per hour indicates failure of the kidneys to excrete, inadequate fluid intake, excessive salt intake, overproduction of antidiuretic hormones, shock, transfusion reaction, or excess fluid loss through burns or diarrhea. The excretion of more than 80 cc of urine per hour indicates failure of the kidneys to concentrate the urine, deficient production of antidiuretic hormones, or excessive intravenous or oral fluid intake.

Resolved Needs: Protection from physical harm.

Monitor blood studies for abnormal acid-base
(154,254)   Watch for laboratory analysis reports indicating abnormal acid-base levels. These include alkali reserve, base excess, bicarbonate, pH, and carbon dioxide.

Rationale: *Alkali reserve:*   A normal blood alkali is essential to neutralize blood acids. Increased blood alkali reserve occurs with metabolic alkalosis or respiratory acidosis. Decreased blood alkali reserve occurs with metabolic acidosis or respiratory alkalosis.

   Base excess: A normal blood base is essential for neutralizing acids. An abnormality indicates a change in the blood buffer base at a given level of hemoglobin concentration. It reveals the amount of nonvolatile acid or base accumulated in the blood. Elevated base excess occurs with metabolic alkalosis or respiratory acidosis.

   Bicarbonate: This study reveals the amount of salt that results when carbonic acid is not completely neutralized or when carbon dioxide mixes in excessive amounts with a base. Increased blood bicarbonate occurs with metabolic alkalosis or respiratory acidosis. Decreased blood bicarbonate occurs with metabolic acidosis, renal acidosis, or respiratory alkalosis.

   pH: This study reveals the blood's hydrogen ion concentration by indicating the ratio between bicarbonate and carbonic acid blood levels. It shows the blood's acid-alkaline concentration. Increased blood pH occurs with respiratory and metabolic alkalosis. Decreased blood pH occurs with metabolic, respiratory, and renal acidosis.

   Carbon dioxide: This test reveals the amount of carbon dioxide present in the blood. Increased blood carbon dioxide occurs with respiratory acidosis and metabolic alkalosis. Decreased blood carbon dioxide occurs with respiratory alkalosis and metabolic acidosis.

Resolved Needs: Protection from physical harm.

Monitor blood studies for abnormal adrenal function
(154,254)   Watch for laboratory analysis reports indicating adrenal hyperactivity or insufficiency. These include cortisol, sodium, and glucose.

Rationale: *Cortisol:*   Increased blood cortisol indicates adrenal hyperactivity (Cushing's syndrome). Decreased blood cortisol indicates adrenal insufficiency (Addison's disease).

   Sodium: Increased blood sodium indicates adrenal hyperactivity. Decreased blood sodium reveals adrenal insufficiency and is the result of impaired sodium reabsorption by the kidneys.

   Glucose: Increased blood glucose indicates adrenal hyperactivity. Decreased blood glucose indicates adrenal insufficiency.

Resolved Needs: Protection from physical harm.

Monitor blood studies for abnormal carbohydrate metabolism

(154,254)   Watch for laboratory analysis reports indicating the ability of the body to metabolize carbohydrates. These include glucose tolerance, glucose, acetone, fatty acids.

Rationale: *Glucose tolerance:*   This test reveals the body's ability to metabolize glucose over a 4- to 5-hour period. Increased blood glucose tolerance can occur with diabetes mellitus.

Glucose: Increased blood levels can indicate diabetes mellitus and decreased levels are associated with hypoglycemia.

Acetone: When increased, this test indicates an elevation in the ketone end products of fat metabolism that occurs with impaired carbohydrate metabolism.

Fatty acids: Fatty acids are hydrocarbons resulting from fat digestion. They are increased with impaired carbohydrate metabolism.

Resolved Needs: Protection from physical harm.

Monitor blood studies for abnormal cardiac enzymes

(154,254)   Watch for laboratory analysis reports indicating cardiac tissue necrosis. These include aldolase, CPK (creatine phosphokinase), LDH (lactate dehydrogenase), SGOT and SGPT (transaminase).

Aldolase: Aldolase is a muscle enzyme necessary for conversion of glycogen into lactic acid. Increased blood aldolase occurs with myocardial ischemia and necrosis.

CPK: Increased blood CPK occurs with myocardial ischemia and necrosis.

LHD: Lactate dehydrogenase is an enzyme causing lactic acid to lose hydrogen through oxidation. The numbers of hydrogens (H) lost help determine the organ in which the disorder exists. Elevated LDH occurs with tissue necrosis.

SGOT and SGPT: These enzymes are generally present in tissues. When tissue injury occurs, the enzymes are released into the bloodstream. Increased SGOT and SGPT occurs with myocardial ischemia and necrosis.

Resolved Needs: Protection from physical harm.

Monitor blood studies for abnormal cholesterol (254)   Watch

for laboratory results indicating an increased blood cholesterol (lipids).

Rationale: Increased blood cholesterol is associated with familiar hypercholesterolemia which is believed to predispose to arteriosclerotic disease.

Resolved Needs: Protection from physical harm.

Monitor blood studies for abnormal clotting mechanism

(154,254)   Watch for laboratory analysis reports indicating an abnormality in blood coagulation. These include bleeding time, clotting time, prothrombin time, PTT (partial thromboplastin time), fibrinogen, and the antihemophilic factor.

Rationale: *Bleeding time:*   This test reveals how long it takes blood to cease flowing following a small wound puncture. An increased bleeding time occurs with prolonged small blood vessel nonconstriction, or anticoagulant therapy.

Clotting time: An increased blood clotting time occurs with a clotting factor deficiency or anticoagulant therapy.

Prothrombin time: This study reveals the level of the prothrombin protein essential to coagulation. Prothrombin is formed in the liver in the presence of vitamin K. When there is impaired liver function, the liver cannot adequately absorb vitamin K from the intestines and so prothrombin cannot be adequately formed. Prothrombin formation is also dependent on fibrinogen, calcium, and factors V, VIII, and X. If any of these essentials are missing, there will be a tendency toward bleeding. The number of seconds in which prothrombin forms and coagulation occurs is increased when there is liver cell damage or necrosis, a deficiency of a clotting factor, or during anticoagulant therapy.

PTT: This test reveals deficiencies of essential coagulation factors. Increased blood PTT occurs when there are deficiencies in clotting factors VIII, IX, and X.

Antihemophilic factor: Decreased blood antihemophilic factor occurs with a deficiency of clotting factor VIII and indicates potential abnormal bleeding.

Fibrinogen: A normal fibrinogen level is essential for conversion of thrombin into fibrin for normal blood clotting. Increased blood fibrinogen occurs with noninflammatory kidney degeneration, acute infection, hemoconcentration, lung inflammation, and pregnancy.

Resolved Needs: Protection from physical harm.

Monitor blood studies for abnormal electrolytes
(154,254)   Watch for laboratory analysis reports indicating an abnormality in blood sodium, potassium, chloride, calcium, and magnesium levels.

Sodium: A normal blood sodium level is essential for fluid and electrolyte balance, normal osmotic pressure, and acid-base balance. Increased blood sodium levels occur with kidney inflammation, diuresis caused by insufficient antidiuretic hormone, dehydration, adrenal hyperactivity, hemoconcentration, aldosterone hypersecretion, obstructed intestines, excessive sodium intake, and as a side effect of steroid therapy. Decreased blood sodium levels occur with overhydration, renal acidosis, adrenal and pituitary insufficiency, diarrhea and vomiting, metabolic acidosis, and diminished cardiac output.

Potassium: This mineral is essential to fluid balance, acid-base balance, normal osmotic pressure, and nerve impulse conduction, especially to muscle and cardiac tissue. Potassium is found in large amounts in cells and in small amounts in serum. Increased blood potassium levels occur with kidney failure, adrenal insufficiency, excessive potassium intake, impaired carbohydrate metabolism, renal acidosis, and diminished myocardial excitability and conduction rate in diastole. Decreased blood potassium levels occur with kidney inflammation, upper and lower gastrointestinal fluid loss, diuretic fluid loss, adrenal hyperactivity, aldosterone hypersecretion, impaired carbohydrate metabolism, diminished cardiac output, overhydration, as a side effect of steroid therapy, and with diminished myocardial excitability and conduction rate in systole.

Chloride: This salt is essential to balanced osmotic pressure and electrolytes. Increased blood chloride levels occur with metabolic acidosis, respiratory alkalosis, insufficient antidiuretic hormone causing diuresis and dehydration, kidney inflammation, genitourinary obstruction, and dehydration. Decreased blood chloride levels occur with metabolic alkalosis, respiratory acidosis, loss of plasma, obstructed intestines, adrenal hyperactivity, lung inflammation, diminished cardiac output, vomiting and diarrhea.

Calcium: Calcium is a metallic element essential to blood coagulation. normal bone and tooth development, lactation, muscle, nerve, and enzyme activity, and electrolyte balance. Increased blood calcium levels occur with metabolic alkalosis, parathyroid hypersecretion, kidney inflammation, and excessive cardiac muscle contraction. The intake of alkali impairs the renal excretion of calcium. Calcium is then excessively absorbed from cow's milk, elevating the blood level. Decreased blood calcium levels occur with diminished cardiac contraction, excessive neuromuscular irritability, renal acidosis, noninflammatory kidney degeneration, parathyroid hyposecretion, small intestine malabsorption, diarrhea, and as a steroid therapy side effect.

Magnesium: The mineral magnesium maintains osmotic pressure, electrolyte balance, muscle and nerve activity, and enzyme functioning. An increased blood magnesium level occurs with kidney failure. Decreased blood magnesium levels occur with pregnancy toxicity, vomiting, excessive neuromuscular irritability, aldosterone hypersecretion, and kidney failure.

Resolved Needs: Protection from physical harm.

Monitor blood studies for abnormal gas exchange (154,254)
Watch for laboratory study reports indicating an abnormality in blood gas exchange. These include O_2 saturation, PaO_2, CO_2 combining power, CO_2 content, $PaCO_2$, and hemoglobin.

Rationale: *CO_2 combining power:* This study reveals the amount of carbon dioxide that is absorbed by or combines with the blood at a specific temperature and pressure. Increased blood CO_2 combining power occurs with respiratory acidosis, metabolic alkalosis, and upper gastrointestinal fluid loss. Decreased blood CO_2 combining power occurs with metabolic acidosis, obstructed intestines, traumatic shock, and diarrhea.

CO_2 content: This test reveals the amount of carbon dioxide present in

the blood. Increased blood carbon dioxide content occurs with upper gastrointestinal fluid loss, impaired pulmonary gas exchange, and obstructed intestines. A decreased blood carbon dioxide content occurs with respiratory alkalosis, diarrhea, renal acidosis, kidney inflammation, and pregnancy toxicity.

O_2 *saturation:* This study indicates the ratio of oxygen in the blood in relation to the amount of oxygen the blood is capable of holding. Increased blood O_2 saturation occurs with excessive blood oxygenation caused by oxygen therapy. Decreased blood O_2 saturation occurs with decreased red blood cell oxygenation, diminished cardiac output, and impaired pulmonary gas exchange.

PaO₂: This study shows the partial pressure of oxygen in the arteries. It reveals the amount of pressure being exerted against the artery by oxygen. Decreased blood PaO_2 occurs with impaired pulmonary gas exchange or diminished cardiac output.

PaCO₂: This study indicates the partial pressure of carbon dioxide in the arteries. It reveals the amount of pressure being exerted against the artery by carbon and oxygen gases when chemically combined. The blood level is in proportion to the amount of carbon dioxide produced by the cells and the rate of gas exchange in alveolar ventilation. Increased blood $PaCO_2$ occurs with metabolic alkalosis, respiratory acidosis, and impaired pulmonary gas exchange. Decreased blood $PaCO_2$ occurs with metabolic acidosis or respiratory alkalosis.

Hemoglobin: A normal hemoglobin is essential for carrying oxygen from the lungs to body tissues. An increased blood hemoglobin occurs with impaired pulmonary gas exchange. A decreased hemoglobin predisposes red blood cells to carry less oxygen.

Resolved Needs: Protection from physical harm.

Monitor blood studies for abnormal glucose (154,254) Watch
for laboratory results indicating an elevated or decreased blood glucose.

Rationale: *Glucose:* Glucose results from carbohydrate metabolism. Glucose is essential to the maintenance of body energy, especially in muscles and nerves. Increased blood glucose levels occur with adrenal hyperactivity, impaired glucose metabolism, early stage pituitary hypersecretion, excessive thyroid production, kidney inflammation or failure, pregnancy, and as a side effect of steroid therapy. Decreased blood glucose levels occur with impaired carbohydrate metabolism, adrenal insufficiency, insulin excess, prolonged pituitary hypersecretion, thyroid insufficiency, and liver cell necrosis.

Resolved Needs: Protection from physical harm.

Monitor blood studies for abnormal hematology
(154,254) Watch for laboratory analysis reports indicating an abnormality in blood gas exchange. These include erythrocyte count (RBC), hematocrit, hemoglobin, MCH (mean corpuscular hemoglobin), MCV (mean corpus-

cular volume), MCHC. (mean corpuscular hemoglobin concentration), plasma total volume, platelet count, reticulocytes, sedimentation rate.

Rationale: *Erythrocyte count:*   Normal erythrocyte levels are essential for carrying oxygen to and carbon dioxide from tissues, acid-base balance, and the development of bile pigment. Increased erythrocyte count occurs with water deprivation, diminished cardiac output, impaired pulmonary gas exchange, fluid intolerance dehydration, lower gastrointestinal fluid loss, excessive red blood cell production, and as a steroid therapy side effect. Decreased erythrocyte count occurs with vitamin B_6 and B_{12} deficiencies, iron deficiency, chronic infections, chronic renal insufficiency, pathologic conditions, and bone marrow failure.

   Hematocrit: This test indicates the percentage of red blood cells in the total blood volume. Increased blood hematocrit occurs with dehydration, impaired pulmonary gas exchange, increased red blood cell volume, diminished cardiac output, hemoconcentration and adrenal insufficiency. Decreased blood hematocrit occurs with blood loss, malnutrition, decreased red blood cell and plasma volume, anticoagulant therapy, and red blood cell destruction.

   Hemoglobin: A normal hemoglobin is essential for carrying oxygen from the lungs to body tissues. Increased blood hemoglobin occurs with diminished cardiac output, increased red blood cell volume, impaired pulmonary gas exchange, and dehydration. A decreased blood hemoglobin occurs with decreased red blood cell and plasma volume, blood loss, malnutrition, decreased red blood cell oxygenation, and red blood cell destruction.

   MCH: The MCH level indicates the amount of hemoglobin found in each red blood cell. Increased blood MCH occurs with excessive red blood cell hemoglobin.

   MCV: The MCV indicates the volume of red blood cells. Increased blood MCV occurs with excessive red blood cell volume. Decreased blood MCV occurs with a low red blood cell volume.

   MCHC: The MCHC indicates the percentage of hemoglobin concentration in each red blood cell. Decreased blood MCHC occurs with a low red blood cell hemoglobin and with overhydration.

   Plasma total volume: This study reveals the proportion of blood in the body as related to total body weight. Increased blood plasma total volume occurs with a reduced secretion of antidiuretic hormone. Decreased blood plasma total volume occurs with upper and lower gastrointestinal fluid loss or dehydration.

   Platelet count: This study reveals the number of thrombocytes (platelets) in the blood. A normal platelet count is essential, for these cells clump together and form clots to stop bleeding. An increased platelet count occurs with generalized infection and increased red blood cell volume, and after surgery, trauma, and delivery. A decreased platelet count occurs with impaired red blood cell production, acute infection, diminished blood coagulation, excessive white blood cell production, capillary fragility, and bone marrow failure.

Reticulocytes: Reticulocytes are immature red blood cells. Their quantity reveals how rapidly they are being released from bone marrow in relation to the norm. Increased blood reticulocytes occur with excessive bone marrow activity, infection, and hemorrhage. Decreased blood reticulocytes occur with impaired bone marrow activity and excessive white blood cell production.

Sedimentation rate: This test reveals the speed at which red blood cells settle in a test tube after an anticoagulant has been added to the blood. Increased sedimentation rate occurs with infection, tissue cell destruction, and pregnancy.

Resolved Needs: Protection from physical harm.

Monitor blood studies for abnormal liver function (453)   Watch

for laboratory analysis reports indicating impaired liver function. These include alkaline phosphatase, bilirubin, LDH (lactate dehydrogenase), prothrombin time, cephalin flocculation, thymol turbidity, total protein, SGOT and SGPT (transaminase), BSP (bromosulphthalein test).

Rationale: *Alkaline phosphatase:*   In liver disease, increased levels of the alkaline phosphatase enzyme are released into the bloodstream.

Bilirubin: Increased serum bilirubin indicates hepatic jaundice.

LDH: This enzyme causes lactic acid to lose hydrogen through oxidation. The number of hydrogens (H) lost helps determine the organ in which the disorder exists. Elevated LDH occurs with tissue necrosis.

Prothrombin time: This study reveals the level of prothrombin, a protein essential to coagulation. Prothrombin is formed in the liver in the presence of vitamin K. When there is severely impaired liver function, the liver cannot adequately use vitamin K absorbed from the intestines, so prothrombin production is reduced.

Cephalin flocculation: This study reveals changes in globulin protein. These protein changes cause the fatty substance cephalin to collect into small clumps (flocculate). Since protein metabolism occurs in the liver, the clumping of cephalin indicates liver damage which may or may not affect other systems. Increased blood cephalin flocculation occurs with liver cell necrosis, diminished cardiac output, infection and lung inflammation.

Thymol turbidity: Thymol is a gamma globulin protein. When in solution and serum is added to it, the solution becomes cloudy if the proteins are concentrated. Since protein metabolism occurs in the liver, this test reveals liver damage. Increased thymol turbidity occurs with liver cell necrosis.

Total protein: This study reveals the ratio of albumin, globulin, and fibrinogen to total protein. An increased globulin level in the protein occurs with liver disease.

SGOT and SGPT: These enzymes are generally present in tissues. When tissue injury occurs, the enzymes are released into the bloodstream. Increased blood SGOT and SGPT levels occur with liver cell damage, necrosis, or inflammation.

BSP: This test reveals the adequacy of liver cells to remove BSP dye from the blood. Elevated BSP occurs with liver cell damage.

Resolved Needs: Protection from physical harm.

Monitor blood studies for abnormal pancreatic function

(154,254) Watch for laboratory analysis reports indicating impaired pancreatic function. These include amylase, lipase, and SGOT.

Rationale: *Amylase:* Amylase is a digestive enzyme found in pancreatic secretions. An increased blood amylase level occurs with acute pancreatic inflammation or obstruction.

Lipase: Lipase is an enzyme that is secreted by the pancreas and aids in fat digestion. An increased lipase level indicates pancreatic inflammation.

SGOT: This enzyme is generally present in tissues. When tissue injury occurs, the enzyme is released into the bloodstream. An increased SGOT level occurs with pancreatic inflammation.

Resolved Needs: Protection from physical harm.

Monitor blood studies for abnormal parathyroid function

(154,254) These include calcium and phosphate.

Rationale: *Calcium:* Calcium regulation is maintained by the parathyroid hormone. An elevated calcium can indicate hyperactivity of the parathyroid gland. A decreased calcium level may indicate impaired parathyroid function.

Phosphate: This study reveals the blood level of the salt phosphoric acid that maintains acid-base balance through its buffering action. Increased blood phosphate occurs with parathyroid hyposecretion.

Calcium and phosphate have a reciprocal relationship, when one goes up, the other goes down.

Resolved Needs: Protection from physical harm.

Monitor blood studies for abnormal pituitary function

(154,254) Watch for a laboratory analysis report of cortisol indicating impaired pituitary function.

Rationale: A decreased blood cortisol level indicates pituitary insufficiency.

Resolved Needs: Protection from physical harm.

Monitor blood studies for abnormal renal function

(154,254) Watch for laboratory analysis reports indicating impaired kidney function. These include urea, urea nitrogen, creatinine, and albumin.

Rationale: *Urea and urea nitrogen:*   Normally, the kidney excretes urea and urea nitrogen following protein metabolism. When adequate amounts are not excreted, the blood level rises. Increased blood urea levels occur with kidney inflammation, degeneration, or failure.

Creatinine: Creatinine is an alkaline nonprotein blood component and results from creatine metabolism. Normal blood levels are maintained by daily creatinine excretion through the kidneys. An increased blood creatinine level occurs with kidney inflammation or failure and during rejection of kidney transplant.

Albumin: A decreased blood albumin level occurs with the nephrotic syndrome.

Resolved Needs: Protection from physical harm.

Monitor blood studies for abnormal thyroid function (324)   Look for laboratory analysis reports revealing impaired thyroid function. These include T4 (thyroxin), T3 (triiodothyronine), and thyrotropin (TSH) (RIA).

Rationale: *T4 and T3:*   The serum levels of thyroid hormones are increased in hyperthyroidism (thyrotoxicosis and some tumors) and decreased in hypothyroidism (myxedema, cretinism). The T4 level is normally higher during the first few weeks of life. These are the major tests for checking the amount of hormone being produced.

TSH (RIA): The serum level of thyrotropin measured by a radioimmunoassay method (RIA) is a test for hypothyroidism. The normal level is below 10 micro units/ml. Levels elevated over 20 micro units/ml indicate hypothyroidism; levels between 10–20 micro units/ml suggest a decreased thyroid reserve. Levels are low in hyperthyroidism.

Resolved Needs: Protection from physical harm.

Monitor blood studies for biliary obstruction (154,254)   Watch for laboratory analysis reports indicating obstruction of bile flow from either the liver, gallbladder, or biliary ducts. These include direct bilirubin, icterus index, lecine aminopeptidase, cholesterol, lipase, alkaline phosphatase, SGOT, and SGPT.

Rationale: *Direct bilirubin:*   Direct bilirubin is a measurement of how the liver manages the bilirubin and is increased when there is biliary obstruction.

Icterus index: Increased blood icterus index occurs with biliary obstruction and indicates an increased ratio of bilirubin to blood.

Leucine aminopeptidase, cholesterol, lipase, alkaline phosphatase, SGOT, and SGPT: All are elevated when there is biliary obstruction.

Resolved Needs: Protection from physical harm.

Monitor blood studies for blood type   Note the type of blood that

laboratory analysis indicates the patient has. Types include A, B, AB, and O. The blood may be Rh positive or negative.

Rationale: During pregnancy, detecting that the mother has Rh negative blood and could produce antibodies angainst the antigens in the infant's red blood cells causing hemolysis of the infant's cells, supports early treatment for infant safety. When plans are being made for a kidney transplant, both the donor and the recipient must have the same blood types. When a patient is given a blood type incompatible with his type, the results could be fatal.

Resolved Needs: Protection from physical harm.

Monitor blood studies for evidence of gastric ulceration
(154,254) Watch for laboratory analysis reports revealing the presence of gastric ulceration. These include amylase and lipase.

Rationale: *Amylase:* Amylase is a digestive enzyme found in intestinal secretions. An increased blood amylase level occurs with gastric ulceration.

Lipase: A normal lipase level maintains adequate fat digestion. As increased blood lipase level occurs with gastrointestinal ulceration.

Resolved Needs: Protection from physical harm.

Monitor blood studies for evidence of infection
(154,254,324) Watch for laboratory analysis reports revealing infection. These include the leukocyte count, sedimentation rate, and WBC differential.

Rationale: *Leukocyte count:* A normal leukocyte count is essential for body defense and tissue repair. An increased leukocyte count occurs with bacterial infection and excessive white blood cell production. A decreased leukocyte count occurs with viral infection.

Sedimentation rate: An increased sedimentation rate occurs with infection.

WBC differential: This report gives the percentage of each type of white blood cell contained in the blood specimen examined.

Neutrophils normally make up over 60% of the white blood cells. Their primary function is to attack bacteria (phagocytosis) so an increased neutrophil level indicates infection. A decreased neutrophil level indicates either an overwhelming infection because of the excessive destruction of cells or a viral infection. Certain drugs and chemicals also cause a decreased level.

Monocytes make up 2–6% of the WBC count. An elevated number of monocytes indicates recovery from serious infection, subacute bacterial endocarditis, tuberculosis, Rocky Mountain spotted fever, and typhoid fever.

Lymphocytes make up 20–40% of the white blood cells. An increased number of lymphocytes occur in many viral infections such as influenza, mumps, German measles, and infectious mononucleosis. Children and young adolescents have a normally higher percentage of lymphocytes than adults. A decreased lymphocyte count occurs with severe stress as in burns or trauma, and in patients taking drugs such as epinephrine, ACTH, and cortisone.

Eosinophils and basophils comprise only 1–4% of the white blood count. An increased eosinophil count occurs with allergic reactions, parasite infestations, and brucellosis. A decreased count occurs when epinephrine, ACTH, or large doses of insulin are given. Basophils are increased in chronic granulocytic leukemia and hemolytic anemia.

The presence of immature WBCs occurs in leukemia and severe, acute infection.

The WBC may normally vary as much as 2000/cu mm from morning to evening because of such activities as exercise, eating, or emotional stress.

Resolved Needs: Protection from physical harm.

Monitor blood studies for evidence of kidney rejection
(70,391)   Look for blood analysis studies of creatinine, urea nitrogen, protein, and white blood cells indicating that the transplanted kidney is being rejected by the immunological system.

Rationale: Increased levels of these substances indicate kidney rejection.

Resolved Needs: Protection from physical harm.

Monitor blood studies for increased barbiturate level   Look for
a laboratory report indicating an elevated blood barbiturate level.

Rationale: An elevated blood barbiturate level occurs with excessive ingestion of barbiturate drugs.

Resolved Needs: Protection from physical harm.

Monitor blood studies for increased digitalis level   Look for a
laboratory report indicating an elevated blood digitoxin or digoxin level.

Rationale: An increased blood digitalis level occurs with prolonged drug ingestion and may indicate toxicity.

Resolved Needs: Protection from physical harm.

Monitor blood studies for increased lactic acid
(154,254)   Look for laboratory reports indicating elevated lactic acid. Lactic acid results from glycogen breakdown following muscle activity. When in excess, the lactate ion binds the calcium ion. This interferes with the normal calcium function of transmitting nerve impulses causing intense anxiety associated with the increased blood level.

Rationale: An elevated lactic acid level occurs with increased muscular activity, decreased tissue oxygenation, anxiety, and metabolic acidosis.

Resolved Needs: Protection from physical harm.

Monitor blood studies for increased quinidine level   Look for a
laboratory report indicating an elevated blood quinidine level.

Rationale: An increased blood quinidine level occurs with prolonged drug ingestion and may indicate toxicity.

Resolved Needs: Protection from physical harm.

Monitor blood studies for increased salicylate level Look for laboratory findings that reveal an elevated salicylate blood level.

Rationale: An increased blood salicylate level occurs with prolonged drug ingestion and may indicate toxicity.

Resolved Needs: Protection from physical harm.

Monitor blood studies for increased triglycerides (154,254) Look for indications that the blood triglyceride level is elevated. Triglycerides are fatty acids and glycerol. Their concentration in the blood causes the degree of cloudiness seen when the blood is examined.

Rationale: An elevated blood triglycerides level occurs in myocardial ischemia and necrosis.

Resolved Needs: Protection from physical harm.

Monitor blood studies for increased uric acid (154,254) Look for indications that the blood uric acid level is abnormally elevated. Uric acid results from purine metabolism. Normally, sufficient amounts are excreted daily through the urine in order to maintain a balanced blood level.

Rationale: Increased blood uric acid levels occur with kidney inflammation, pregnancy toxicity, excessive white blood cell production, and excessive purine metabolism.

Resolved Needs: Protection from physical harm.

Monitor blood studies for positive VDRL Look for a positive VDRL blood report.

Rationale: This study is a screening test for syphilis. It does not confirm the diagnosis but supports the need for further laboratory studies.

Resolved Needs: Protection from physical harm.

Monitor blood studies for Rh factor (71:143) Look for laboratory reports indicating whether the mother has Rh-positive or Rh-negative blood. If she has Rh-negative blood, then the father's Rh factor must also be checked. If the mother has Rh-negative blood and the father has Rh-positive blood, then referral to a physician should be made.

Rationale: When the mother has Rh-negative blood and the father has Rh-positive blood, the mother will produce antibodies against the antigens in the baby's blood, causing destruction of red blood cells.

Resolved Needs: Protection from physical harm.

Monitor cerebral spinal fluid studies for abnormalities (154,254)
Look for laboratory reports indicating abnormalities in cerebral spinal fluid. These include chloride level, cell count, and protein level.

Rabionale: *Chloride:* Decreased levels of spinal fluid chloride occur with infection.

Cell count: Increased spinal fluid cell count occurs with infection.

Protein: Increased levels of spinal fluid protein occur with meningeal irritation and spinal cord tumor.

Resolved Needs: Protection from physical harm.

Monitor culture for positive evidence of gonorrhea
Look for a culture report on vaginal or urethral secretions indicating the presence of gonorrhea infection.

Rationale: Detection and treatment of gonorrhea prevents the spread of disease and can lower the incidence of blindness in infants.

Resolved Needs: Protection from physical harm.

Monitor gastric analysis studies for abnormalities (154,254)
Look for laboratory reports indicating abnormal gastric analysis studies. These include combined acid and total acid studies.

Rationale: *Combined acid:* A study showing increased combined acid indicates excessive gastric hydrochloric acid. A study showing decreased combined acid indicates gastric inflammation.

Total acid: Increased gastric total acidity occurs with gastrointestinal ulceration. Decreased gastric total acidity occurs in the presence of malignant gastric cells.

Resolved Needs: Protection from physical harm.

Monitor the axillary temperature
Measure body heat by placing a thermometer into the axilla so that the thermometer bulb has good skin contact. Axillary temperatures are taken when oral and rectal temperatures are contraindicated; they are also indicated for premature infants. Normal axillary temperature is 98.1°F (36.7°C).

Rationale: Abnormal body temperatures are caused by the body's protective mechanisms and are indicative of excessive body heat production or loss or poor temperature regulating mechanisms. Axillary temperatures are preferable for patients with self-destructive tendencies, as they lessen the possibility of ingestion of glass.

Resolved Needs: Protection from physical harm.

Monitor the blood pressure
Determine the pressure exerted by the blood on arterial walls by use of a mercury manometer and aircuff. Note abnormalities in blood pressure readings. Normal adult blood pressure con-

sists of a systolic reading of 100–140 mm mercury and a diastolic reading of 60–90 mm mercury. In the infant the normal systolic reading is 55–90 mm mercury and the diastolic is 40–60 mm mercury.

Rationale: Blood pressure is controlled by heartbeat force, vessel tone, and blood volume and viscosity. Systolic blood pressure indicates the circulatory pressure during ventricular contraction. Decreased systolic blood pressure is associated with reduced circulating blood volume and cardiac output. Increased systolic blood pressure is associated with excessive water and sodium in the blood, which causes increased blood volume. It also may involve increased tension in arterial walls, plugging of arterial walls with fat deposits, decreased arterial dimensions caused by scar tissue, or severe stress causing contraction of arterial wall muscles and resulting in increased arterial pressure. Diastolic blood pressure indicates the circulatory pressure during ventricular relaxation. Decreased diastolic blood pressure is associated with reduced peripheral resistance caused by vasodilatation. Increased diastolic blood pressure is associated with increased peripheral resistance caused by vasoconstriction.

Resolved Needs: Protection from physical harm.

Contraindications: When an extremity has a fractured bone, circulatory embolus, AV shunt or fistula, lymphatic obstruction, or IV infusion.

Monitor the body temperature with an electronic thermometer   In adults with fever, insert a rectal probe. For infants, firmly anchor an electronic thermometer (Thermistor) against the abdominal skin, above and beside the umbilicus. Periodically check temperature readings and be certain that the thermometer is securely in place.

Rationale: Electronic thermometers facilitate continuous temperature readings; they are especially valuable when there is high fever or impaired ability to regulate body temperature.

Resolved Needs: Protection from physical harm.

Monitor the cardiogram   Record and interpret signals indicating regular or irregular heart action by using a surveillance device that records electrical discharges from the heart.

Rationale: Electrocardiograph recordings indicate the heart's electrical activity as levels of excitation in the different cardiac chambers. Recognition of inadequate circulation and cardiac inadequacies prevents damage to body tissues and tissue death.

Resolved Needs: Protection from physical harm.

Monitor the central venous pressure (71)   After the central venous pressure (CVP) catheter has been inserted through the arm or neck vein into the superior vena cava, attach the catheter to the water manometer and intermittently monitor and record the CVP reading. Normal CVP is 5–15 cm water. Since CVP readings are influenced by blood pressure, respiratory rate, emotional state, urine output, and intravenous fluids, several readings are desirable; one should not rely on a single abnormal reading.

Rationale: CVP reflects the circulating blood volume, the efficiency of cardiac function, and the vascular tone. Increased CVP indicates increased circulating blood volume and impaired cardiac function. Decreased CVP occurs with blood or fluid loss.

Resolved Needs: Protection from physical harm.

Monitor the fetal heart sounds Place the stethoscope or headscope over the maternal anterior abdominal wall and listen to the heart sounds of the unborn infant. Listen between contractions or at contraction termination. Listen for irregular, rapid, or slow heartbeats and for fetal heart sounds immediately after the uterine membrane has ruptured and again 10 minutes later. If the fetal pulse is greatly accelerated or decreased, also watch for meconium in the amniotic fluid indicating fetal distress.

Rationale: Fetal heart sounds assist in determining if there is fetal life. Movement of fetal heart sounds can give clues to the progress of labor. If umbilical cord prolapse occurs, it will be evidenced by fetal distress immediately after or shortly after membrane rupture. During maternal seizures, fetal circulation is impaired, and fetal heart sounds can warn of fetal distress. When the fetal head is exerting pressure on the umbilical cord, abnormally rapid or abnormally slow fetal heart sounds signal distress.

Resolved Needs: Protection from physical harm.

Monitor the infant for apnea Place a monitor under the crib sheet and place the infant on it with his chest positioned directly over it.

Rationale: Monitoring infants for apnea can facilitate early recognition and treatment of respiratory distress.

Resolved Needs: Protection from physical harm.

Monitor the laboratory findings of sputum analysis (154,254) Look for laboratory reports of sputum analysis.

Rationale: Analysis of sputum specimens can indicate respiratory system disorders. Clear thin (mucoid) sputum occurs with early bronchitis. Thick, frothy, greenish (mucopurulent) sputum indicates late bronchitis, pneumonia, or tuberculosis. Thick yellow (purulent) sputum occurs with lung abscess, bronchiectasis, empyema, or late tuberculosis. Gelatinous rusty sputum indicates pneumonia. Offensive dark brown (prune juice) sputum occurs with pneumonia, pulmonary gangrene, or early lung growth. Jellylike blood-clotted (red currant jelly) sputum indicates early lung growth.

Resolved Needs: Protection from physical harm.

Monitor the oral temperature Measure body heat by inserting a thermometer into the mouth. Wait 30 minutes after intake of hot or cold foods. Oral temperatures are most frequently used to measure body heat and are most valuable when rectal temperatures are contraindicated. Normal oral temperature is 98.6° F (37° C).

Rationale: Abnormal body temperatures are caused by the body's protective mechanisms and are indicative of excessive body heat production or loss or poor temperature regulating mechanisms.

Resolved Needs: Protection from physical harm.

Contraindications: Do not take oral temperatures of infants or unconscious or confused persons or when there is mouth breathing, respiratory congestion, a wired jaw, or a convulsive disorder.

Monitor the pap smear for positive findings Look for laboratory reports of a positive pap smear. Pap smears can be performed on uterine cells and on fluid expressed from the prostate. Pap smear results are classified by Papanicolau as:

Class 1. No abnormal cells.
Class 2. Some abnormal cells, no malignancy.
Class 3. Abnormal cells suggesting possible malignancy.
Class 4. Abnormal cells strongly suggesting malignancy.
Class 5. Definite malignant cells.

Rationale: A positive pap smear supports early detection and treatment of cancer.

Resolved Needs: Protection from physical harm.

Monitor the positional blood pressure Check the blood pressure when the patient is standing, sitting, and lying down. Compare the readings.

Rationale: Normally, blood pressure readings are approximately the same regardless of position. In congestive heart failure the cardiac output is reduced in the standing position, which results in decreased blood pressure.

Resolved Needs: Protection from physical harm.

Contraindications: Patients on 24-hour bed rest.

Monitor the pulse pressure Subtract the diastolic blood pressure reading from the systolic blood pressure reading to obtain pulse pressure. If the pulse pressure is more than 50 points or less than 30 points, it is abnormal.

Rationale: Pulse pressure indicates the tone of the arterial walls. A pulse pressure of more than 50 points indicates decreased arterial elasticity (increased arterial rigidity), which reduces arterial blood flow and impairs normal oxygen transport. A pulse pressure of less than 30 points indicates insufficient circulating blood volume, which results in decreased tissue oxygenation.

Resolved Needs: Protection from physical harm.

Monitor the rectal temperature   Measure body heat by inserting the bulb of a thermometer into the rectum. Rectal temperatures are taken when oral temperatures are contraindicated. The normal range of rectal temperature is 99.1–99.6°F (32.2°C–37.5°C).

Rationale: Abnormal body temperatures are caused by the body's protective mechanisms and are indicative of excessive body heat production or loss or poor temperature regulating mechanisms.

Resolved Needs: Protection from physical harm.

Contraindications: Rectal surgery. Fecal impaction. Diarrhea. Rectal stricture. Rectal pain or bleeding. Bradycardia. Cardiac arrhythmias. Intestinal worms.

Monitor tidal volume studies for decreased lung capacity   Look for laboratory reports indicating a decrease in the total volume of air inspired and expired with each normal breath.

Rationale: Decreased tidal volume indicates decreased pulmonary muscle strength or increased pulmonary tissue or airway resistance.

Resolved Needs: Protection from physical harm.

Monitor urine studies for abnormal adrenal function (154,254)   Look for urinalysis reports that indicate impaired adrenal function. Levels of aldosterone, sodium, 17-hydroxycorticoids, and 17-ketosteroids are monitored.

Rationale: *Aldosterone:*   Aldosterone is a mineralocorticoid that is essential for balanced sodium, potassium, and chloride metabolism. Increased urinary levels of aldosterone occur with adrenal cortex hypersecretion of aldosterone.

Sodium: Increased urinary levels of sodium occur with adrenal insufficiency. Decreased urinary levels of sodium occur with diuresis resulting from insufficient antidiuretic hormone, adrenal hyperactivity, and aldosterone hypersecretion.

17-Hydroxycorticoids: 17-Hydroxycorticoids are involved primarily in regulating carbohydrate and protein metabolism. Their secretion is dependent on ACTH production. Decreased urinary levels of 17-hydroxycorticoids occur with adrenal insufficiency (Addison's disease). Increased urinary levels of 17-hydroxycorticoids indicate adrenal hyperactivity (Cushing's syndrome).

17-Ketosteroids: The alpha and beta 17-ketosteroids are produced in the adrenal cortex and gonads and are normally excreted in the urine. Decreased urinary levels of 17-ketosteroids occur with adrenal insufficiency. Increased urinary levels of 17-ketosteroids occur with adrenal hyperactivity.

Resolved Needs: Protection from physical harm.

Monitor urine studies for abnormal carbohydrate metabolism

(154,254) Look for urinalysis reports indicating impaired carbohydrate metabolism. Levels of acetone, glucose, and ammonia are monitored.

Rationale: *Acetone:* The presence of acetone in the urine indicates that the ketone and other products of fat metabolism have spilled into the urine. The presence of acetone in the urine indicates impaired carbohydrate metabolism that has caused excessive fat metabolism.

Glucose: The sugar glucose results from carbohydrate metabolism. Excesses are spilled into the urine. Increased urinary levels of glucose occur with impaired glucose metabolism.

Ammonia: Ammonia gas results from the metabolism of proteins and amino acids by the liver. Increased urinary levels of ammonia occur with impaired glucose metabolism.

Resolved Needs: Protection from physical harm.

Monitor urine studies for abnormal liver function

(154,254) Look for urinalysis findings indicating impaired liver function. Levels of ammonia, urobilinogen, copper, and porphobilinogen are monitored.

Rationale: *Ammonia:* Ammonia gas results from the metabolism of proteins and amino acids by the liver. The liver then converts the ammonia to urea for excretion by the kidneys. Increased urinary levels of ammonia occur with liver cell damage.

Urobilinogen: Normally, urobilinogen is absorbed by the circulatory system and returned to the liver. Increased urinary levels of urobilinogen indicate that the liver cannot adequately convert urobilinogen to urobilin because of impaired liver function.

Copper: Copper is normally found in the liver and is excreted by the kidneys. Increased urinary levels of copper occur with liver cell damage.

Porphobilinogen: Porphobilinogen is one of several porphyrin compounds that unite with the protein globin to form hemoglobin. A standard test will reveal excessive excretion of porphobilinogen, which occurs with chronic liver disease.

Resolved Needs: Protection from physical harm.

Monitor urine studies for abnormal parathyroid function

(154,254) Look for urinalysis findings indicating impaired thyroid function. Rate of phosphate clearance and level of calcium are monitored.

Rationale: *Phosphate clearance:* A standard test reveals the kidney's ability to excrete phosphate. Increased urinary levels of phosphate occur with parathyroid hypersecretion. Decreased urinary levels of phosphate occur with parathyroid hyposecretion.

Calcium: A standard test reveals the ratio of calcium to phosphorus. If the urinary level of calcium is excessive, the urinary level of phosphorus will be low. Increased urinary levels of calcium occur with parathyroid hypersecretion.

Resolved Needs: Protection from physical harm.

Monitor urine studies for abnormal pituitary function

(154,254) Look for urinalysis studies indicating impaired pituitary function. Levels of 17-hydroxycorticoids, potassium, and pituitary gonadotropin are monitored.

Rationale: *17-Hydroxycorticoids:* 17-Hydroxycorticoids are involved primarily in regulating carbohydrate and protein metabolism. Their secretion is dependent on ACTH production. Decreased urinary levels of 17-hydroxycorticoids occur with pituitary insufficiency.

Potassium: Decreased urinary levels of potassium occur with pituitary insufficiency.

Pituitary gonadotropin: The pituitary gonadotropin hormones are released by the anterior pituitary; they include follicle-stimulating hormone, interstitial-cell-stimulating hormone, luteinizing hormone, and luteotropic hormone. Decreased urinary levels of pituitary gonadotropin occur with pituitary insufficiency.

Resolved Needs: Protection from physical harm.

Monitor urine studies for abnormal renal function

(154,254) Look for urinalysis findings indicating impaired renal function. Rates of creatinine clearance and urea clearance, levels of protein (albumin), phosphorus, urea, uric acid, and phenolsulfonphthalein (PSP), and specific gravity are monitored.

Rationale: *Creatinine clearance:* The rate of creatinine clearance indicates, the kidney's ability to excrete creatinine. A decreased rate of urinary creatinine clearance occurs with kidney glomerular dysfunction.

Protein: Proteins (albumin) appear in the urine when there is impaired renal function caused by inflammation of glomeruli, excessive pressure within renal arteries, or urinary tract infection. Increased urinary levels of protein occur with kidney inflammation.

Phosphorus: Decreased urinary levels of phosphorus occur with kidney inflammation.

Urea and urea clearance: Normally the kidneys excrete a specific amount of urea following protein metabolism. Decreased urinary levels of urea occur with kidney failure.

Uric acid: Uric acid results from purine metabolism and is excreted in normal amounts daily. Decreased urinary levels of uric acid occur with kidney inflammation.

PSP: The level of PSP indicates the quality of the kidney's excretory functioning and its ability to concentrate urine and maintain body fluid and electrolyte balance. Decreased urinary levels of PSP occur with kidney tubule dysfunction and genitourinary infection or obstruction.

Specific gravity: The test for specific gravity reveals the degree of urine concentration. Decreased urinary specific gravity indicates a decreased ability to concentrate urine. Increased specific gravity indicates a decreased ability to reabsorb sodium, etc.

Resolved Needs: Protection from physical harm.

Monitor urine studies for abnormal thyroid function (324)   Look for urinalysis findings indicating impaired thyroid function. These include radioactive iodine uptake.

Rationale: *Radioactive iodine uptake:*   Following oral ingestion of radioactive iodine, the thyroid removes some of the iodide from the blood, and the remainder is excreted by the kidneys within a 24-hour period. In addition to a Geiger counter survey of the neck, the entire 24-hour urine output is checked for radioactivity. Excretion of 40% or less of the radioactive iodine during the 24-hour period indicates thyrotoxicosis.

Resolved Needs: Protection from physical harm.

Monitor urine studies for biliary obstruction (154,254)   Look for urinalysis reports that indicate biliary obstruction. Levels of bilirubin and urobilinogen are monitored.

Rationale: *Bilirubin:*   When an obstruction prevents bile from flowing into the intestines, it goes into the blood and is excreted by the kidneys. With increased urinary levels of bilirubin, the bile pigment colors the urine dark yellow, green yellow, or brown.

Urobilinogen: When the liver excretes bile, it is broken down into bilirubin and goes into the intestines. The intestinal bacteria break it down further into urobilinogen. The intestinal circulation absorbs some of the urobilinogen and returns it to the liver to be converted into urobilin. Normally a specific amount leaves the circulation and is excreted in the urine. If the kidneys excrete large amounts, this may indicate that the liver is unable to convert urobilinogen to urobilin. Increased urinary levels of urobilinogen occur with incomplete biliary obstruction. Decreased urinary levels of urobilinogen occur with complete biliary obstruction.

Resolved Needs: Protection from physical harm.

Monitor urine studies for decreased D-xylose absorption (154,254)   Look for an abnormally low urinary D-xylose level.

Rationale: Decreased urinary levels of D-xylose occur with malabsorption in the small intestine.

Resolved Needs: Protection from physical harm.

Monitor urine studies for evidence of kidney rejection (391)   Look for urinalysis studies indicating that the transplanted kidney

is being rejected by the immunologic system. Level of protein and white blood cell (lymphocyte) counts are monitored.

Rationale: Increased urinary levels of protein and increased white blood cell counts indicate kidney rejection.

Resolved Needs: Protection from physical harm.

Monitor urine studies for evidence of urinary tract infection (154,254)
Look for urinalysis studies indicating infection of the genitourinary system, as indicated by the presence of erythrocystes, hemoglobin, hyaline casts, leukocytes, and tubular casts.

Rationale: *Erythrocytes:* The presence of these red blood cells in the urine indicates urinary tract inflammation or irritation. Increased urinary levels of erythrocytes occur with genitourinary infection and kidney inflammation or failure.

Hemoglobin: The presence of hemoglobin in the urine indicates the abnormal presence of red blood cells. Increased urinary levels of hemoglobin occur with kidney inflammation.

Hyaline casts: The presence of pale, cylinder-shaped hyaline casts indicates kidney irritation. Increased urinary levels of hyaline casts occur with genitourinary infection and kidney inflammation, degeneration, or failure.

Leukocytes: White blood cells in the urine occur with genitourinary infection and kidney inflammation.

Tubular casts: The presence of tube-shaped waxy casts indicates separation of dead epithelial cells from the renal system. Increased urinary levels of tubular casts occur with noninflammatory kidney degeneration, kidney failure, genitourinary infection, and renal acidosis.

Resolved Needs: Protection from physical harm.

Monitor urine studies for increased barbiturate level
Look for urinalysis reports showing an elevated barbiturate level.

Rationale: Increased urinary levels of barbiturates occur with excessive barbiturate drug ingestion.

Resolved Needs: Protection from physical harm.

Monitor urine studies for increased Bence Jones protein (154,254)
Look for the presence of Bence Jones protein in the urine. This protein dissolves when urine is boiled and precipitates when the urine cools.

Rationale: Bence Jones protein occurs in the urine of patients with bone tumors, lymph tissue malignancy and hyperplasia, excessive white blood cell production, brittle bones, and parathyroid hypersecretion.

Resolved Needs: Protection from physical harm.

Monitor urine studies for increased catecholamines (154,254)
Look for urinalysis reports showing elevated urinary levels of

catecholamines. The test reveals the levels of epinephrine and norepinephrine bein excreted by the adrenal medulla.

Rationale: Increased urinary levels of catecholamines occur with adrenal medulla tumor and peripheral vasoconstriction.

Resolved Needs: Protection from physical harm.

Monitor urine studies for increased gonadotropins (154,254) Look for urinalysis reports indicating elevated urinary levels of gonadotropins.

Rationale: Gonadotropins (hormones) stimulate the sex glands, which are responsible for cell formation in human reproduction. During pregnancy the gonadotropin level is elevated.

Resolved Needs: Protection from physical harm.

Monitor urine studies for increased salicylate Look for urinalysis reports showing elevated urinary levels of salicylate.

Rationale: Increased urinary levels of salicylate occur with prolonged drug ingestion and may indicate toxicity.

Resolved Needs: Protection from physical harm.

Monitor urine studies for increased uric acid (154,254) Look for indications that the urinary level of uric acid is abnormally elevated. Uric acid derives from purine metabolism and is excreted in normal amounts daily.

Rationale: Increased urinary levels of uric acid occur with excessive white blood cell production, with excessive purine metabolism, and as a side effect of steroid drugs.

Resolved Needs: Protection from physical harm.

Monitor urine studies for increased VMA (154,254) Look for urinalysis reports showing elevated levels of vanilmandelic acid (VMA). VMA is a product of catecholamine metabolism.

Rationale: Increased urinary levels of VMA occur with adrenal medulla tumor and peripheral vasoconstriction, which causes hypertension.

Resolved Needs: Protection from physical harm.

Observe and record the food intake Record the amounts and kinds of solid and semisolid foods the patient eats for a 24-hour period. Sometimes this record is referred to a dietitian for a calorie count.

Rationale: A record of food intake provides a basis from which to initiate a balanced nutritional intake.

Resolved Needs: Protection from physical harm.

Observe for a blood transfusion reaction Observe the patient for sudden complaints of chest pain or tightness, fever, chills, facial burning,

back pain, bloody urine, absent or decreased urine output, dyspnea, cyanosis, skin rash or hives, decrease in blood pressure, nausea, vomiting, laryngeal edema, wheezing, and distended neck veins.

Rationale: A blood transfusion reaction may result from an excessive increase in blood volume, which causes circulatory overload, or from the transmission of viruses, bacteria, or parasites from a donor to the recipient who usually forms antibodies to the allergens contained in the donor blood. When incompatible blood is administered, the red blood cells received from the donor clump together (agglutinated) in the plasma of the recipient. The red cells are rapidly broken down by enzymes, exceeding the liver's ability to detoxify the products, which results in damage of the kidney tubules when the excess is excreted.

Resolved Needs: Protection from physical harm.

Observe for a hypersensitivity response   Look for an unfavorable antigen-antibody reaction manifested by the symptoms of frequent sneezing, tearing, dyspnea, wheezing, skin rashes and inflammation, nausea, vomiting, diarrhea, local edema, itching, cyanosis, choking, weak and rapid pulse, hypotension, clammy skin, or convulsions.

Rationale: Foreign bodies introduced into the body act as antigens. The antigen reacts with antibodies that respond to the specific antigen. When the antigen-antibody reaction is unfavorable, adjacent cells and tissue are damaged.

Resolved Needs: Protection from physical harm.

Observe for abnormal fluid intake   Look for inadequate fluid intake of less than 1500 cc daily or excessive fluid intake of more than 3500 cc daily.

Rationale: Balanced fluid intake is essential to normal body functioning.

Resolved Needs: Protection from physical harm.

Observe for abnormal fluid loss   Look for unusually large fluid losses occurring from diarrhea, tube drainage, vomiting, or urine output in excess of 1500 cc daily.

Rationale: Balanced fluid intake and output are essential to normal body functioning.

Resolved Needs: Protection from physical harm.

Observe for abnormal gait   Look for unsteadiness, shuffling, staggering, limping, stooped walking, high stepping, propulsion walking, weaving, waddling, spastic gait, scissor gait, chorea gait, or atactic gait.

Rationale: Abnormal gait indicates musculoskeletal, neurologic, or circulatory disorders.

Resolved Needs: Protection from physical harm.

Observe for acute pain onset Look for indications that pain has suddenly occurred.

Rationale: Acute pain is generally associated with inflammatory conditions, coronary artery disease, muscle spasms, and trauma.

Resolved Needs: Protection from physical harm.

Observe for airway obstruction Observe whether the airway is clear for adequate gas exchange. Airway obstruction may be evidenced as respiratory distress, restlessness, airway noise, cyanosis, or anxious behavior.

Rationale: A patent airway is essential for the maintenance of life.

Resolved Needs: Protection from physical harm.

Observe for an excessive stress level Determine whether the patient perceives an extreme threat and feels that it is imposed on him and is beyond his control, whether a great number of adjustive demands are being made within a short time, or whether extremely important needs are not being met.

Rationale: Excessive stress causes severe disequilibrium because adaptive capacities are overtaxed.

Resolved Needs: Protection from physical harm. Protection from psychologic threat.

Observe for behavior modification Look for change from unhealthy behavior patterns to the healthy behavior patterns that have been suggested.

Rationale: A change to healthy behavior patterns will support the development of improved health in the future.

Resolved Needs: Protection from physical harm.

Observe for chewing difficulty Look for signs that the patient cannot chew or is having difficulty chewing.

Rationale: Chewing is essential to food breakdown prior to digestion.

Resolved Needs: Protection from physical harm.

Observe for chills Listen for complaints of intermittent internal coldness. Chills may or may not be accompanied by shaking, pallor, teeth chattering, or external skin coldness. Note the length and severity of the chill.

Rationale: Chills indicate the body's need for increased temperature or the existence of a fever.

Resolved Needs: Protection from physical harm.

Observe for clothing which constricts circulation Look for tight clothing that constricts circulation, such as garters, girdles, purse straps over the arm, hatbands, or belts.

Rationale: Constricting clothing impairs circulation and reduces tissue oxygenation.

Resolved Needs: Protection from physical harm.

Observe for cold, clammy skin Touch the skin and feel for cold or moistness.

Rationale: Cold, clammy skin is caused by activation of sweat glands, with concomitant peripheral blood vessel constriction; it indicates circulatory impairment.

Resolved Needs: Protection from physical harm.

Observe for complaints of constipation Listen for complaints of difficult passage of hard, dry stools.

Rationale: Constipation may be associated with inactivity, pregnancy, gastrointestinal disorders, trauma to the intestinal tract during surgery, or inadequate intake of bulk food or fluid.

Resolved Needs: Protection from physical harm.

Observe for complaints of dizziness Listen for complaints of a whirling sensation in the head, with or without giddiness or confusion. Watch for unstable walking.

Rationale: Dizziness may indicate a circulatory or neurologic disorder.

Resolved Needs: Protection from physical harm.

Observe for complaints of dysuria Listen for complaints of painful or difficult urination.

Rationale: Dysuria may occur with bladder or urethral inflammation, urethral stricture, uterine prolapse, prostate enlargement or ulceration, painful menstruation, or cervical carcinoma.

Resolved Needs: Protection from physical harm.

Observe for complaints of excessive flatulence Listen for complaints of stomach or intestinal gas.

Rationale: Excessive flatulence may occur with liver and gastrointestinal problems. It causes pressure within the stomach or intestines, resulting in severe, sharp pain and discomfort.

Resolved Needs: Protection from physical harm.

Observe for complaints of headache Listen for complaints of pressure or pain within the cranium.

Rationale: Headache indicates a disorder within the head, scalp, sinuses, or other body area.

Resolved Needs: Protection from physical harm.

Observe for complaints of itching   Watch for scratching of any body part as indicative of the itching sensation.

Rationale: Itching may indicate internal or external skin irritation or a sensitivity reaction to a specific agent.

Resolved Needs: Protection from physical harm.

Observe for complaints of malaise   Listen for complaints of a generalized feeling of being barely able to function.

Rationale: Malaise is common during infection and general body dysfunction.

Resolved Needs: Protection from physical harm.

Observe for complaints of nausea   Listen for complaints of the sensation of stomach queasiness.

Rationale: Nausea can indicate gastric irritation, intestinal obstruction, motion sickness, increased intracranial pressure, severe pain, toxic and disease states, or psychogenic disturbances.

Resolved Needs: Protection from physical harm.

Observe for complaints of numbness and tingling   Listen for complaints of loss of sensation or complaints of pinprick sensations in some body area.

Rationale: Numbness and tingling occur when there is inadequate circulation to peripheral nerves or when there is nerve damage.

Resolved Needs: Protection from physical harm.

Observe for complaints of pain   Listen for complaints of distressful hurting anywhere in the body.

Rationale: Pain is the body's signal of impending or existing tissue damage.

Resolved Needs: Protection from physical harm. Protection from psychologic threat.

Observe for complaints of pain duration   Listen for a description of the length of time a patient's pain lasts. Determine its duration (minutes, hours, or days) and whether it is intermittent or continuous.

Rationale: Pain duration assists in determining the cause. Prolonged pain is usually perceived as threatening.

Resolved Needs: Protection from physical harm. Protection from psychologic threat.

Observe for complaints of pain-perceived stimulus   Listen for clues to those stimuli that the patient perceives as being the cause of his pain.

Rationale: Once a stimulus is perceived as painful, it will tend to continue to be perceived as painful. Any recurrence of a pain-perceived stimulus will most likely result in pain.

Resolved Needs: Protection from physical harm. Protection from psychologic threat.

Observe for complaints of pain radiation
Listen for complaints of pain occurring in areas other than the area of its first appearance. This includes radiation to the back, shoulder, arm, hand, jaw, neck, head, or any body area.

Rationale: Pain radiation follows nerve pathways and signals body distress. During the instillation of peritoneal dialysis fluid, pain may occur in the left shoulder. This indicates diaphragmatic irritation from fluid pressure within the peritoneum.

Resolved Needs: Protection from physical harm.

Observe for complaints of respiratory muscle weakness
Listen for complaints of not having sufficient strength to breathe.

Rationale: Respiratory muscle weakness occurs in endocrine, metabolic, and nervous system disorders.

Resolved Needs: Protection from physical harm.

Observe for complaints of thirst
Listen for complaints of a dry, cottony feeling in the mouth.

Rationale: Thirst indicates physiologic body changes related to fluid or electrolyte imbalance. It occurs with dehydration, when it may be associated with fever, vomiting, diarrhea, hemorrhage, shock, or polyuria. Thirst results when there is decreased fluid volume, in which loss of water is disproportionately higher than loss of salt. It also occurs when there is increased fluid volume, in which salt losses are disproportionately higher than water losses. Potassium depletion and drug side effects also cause thirst.

Resolved Needs: Protection from physical harm.

Observe for complaints of tinnitus
Listen for complaints that the patient is hearing ringing or buzzing sounds or the like. These sounds usually seem louder at night.

Rationale: Tinnitus may indicate a hearing disorder, a drug side effect, impacted earwax, tension, a foreign body in the ear, inflammation, or skull fracture.

Resolved Needs: Protection from physical harm.

Observe for complaints of visual disturbance
Listen for complaints of changes in vision, such as blurring, double vision, and light flashes.

Rationale: Visual disturbances are often associated with physiologic disorders such as cerebral pressure, vascular disorders, acid-base imbalance, and respiratory gas-exchange disorders, as well as with digitalis and atropine overdosage.

Resolved Needs: Protection from physical harm.

Observe for complaints of weakness   Listen for complaints of decreased strength, such as weakness on exertion, a desire to lie down, muscle tremors, irritability, nervousness, clumsy movements, rapid breathing, and inability to deal with complex problems. Note any increase or decrease in blood pressure or any increase in pulse pressure.

Rationale: Muscle weakness may result from impaired nerve supply, decreased circulation, muscle disuse, inadequate nutrition, muscle glycogen depletion, or lactic acid accumulation.

Resolved Needs: Protection from physical harm.

Observe for confusion   Determine if the patient is bewildered or perplexed.

Rationale: Confusion may occur with inadequate brain oxygenation or with disorganization of thought or emotion resulting from excessive physiologic or emotional stress.

Resolved Needs: Protection from physical harm.

Observe for convulsions   Look for involuntary muscle contraction and relaxation, often accompanied by loss of consciousness. This includes tonic contractions, which are often seen in infants, jacksonian seizures of localized twitching or jerking, and petit mal seizures, in which there is momentary cessation of activity and thought.

Rationale: Convulsions may indicate brain, nerve, or chemical disorders; they increase the possibility of physical harm from environmental sources and can cause inadequate pulmonary ventilation during and after the episode.

Resolved Needs: Protection from physical harm.

Observe for coughing   Watch to see if the patient begins to cough.

Rationale: Coughing is associated with certain cardiac and respiratory conditions, such as pulmonary edema, asthma, congestive heart failure, the common cold, pneumonia, and lung cancer.

Resolved Needs: Protection from physical harm.

Observe for cyanosis   Look for blue, gray, slate, or dark purple discoloration in the nailbeds and skin and around the lips.

Rationale: Normal oxygen saturation of hemoglobin is 97% or 14.5 grams. Cyanosis indicates oxygen deficiency in the blood. Cyanosis occurs when there are 5 grams or more of reduced hemoglobin in the blood.

Resolved Needs: Protection from physical harm.

Observe for dehiscence   Look for signs that a wound has begun to open, such as serosanguineous fluid at the incision site, complaints of a sharp pulling sensation, and breaking of some but not all sutures.

Rationale: Early detection of dehiscence can prevent wound evisceration.

Resolved Needs: Protection from physical harm.

Observe for delayed healing   Observe wounds that fail to heal within the average 4–7 days or wounds that intermittently heal and reopen.

Rationale: Delayed wound healing may be related to inadequate blood supply, failure to keep wound edges together, serious nutritional deficits, or malignant cells.

Resolved Needs: Protection from physical harm.

Observe for diarrhea   Watch to see if the patient has frequent unformed and liquid stools.

Rationale: Diarrhea is associated with gastrointestinal disorders.

Resolved Needs: Protection from physical harm.

Observe for diet intolerance   Observe the patient for any inability to tolerate food, such as refusal to eat, nausea, vomiting, abdominal distention after eating, and complaints that the food is poorly tolerated.

Rationale: Foods incompatible with the patient's physiologic state irritate the stomach and intestinal mucosa and disrupt the digestive process.

Resolved Needs: Protection from physical harm.

Observe for drug reactions   Look for drug reactions, such as allergic responses (rash, itching, etc.), anaphylactic responses (difficulty in breathing, circulatory failure), and toxic or overdose effects specific to the drug.

Rationale: Early recognition and treatment of drug reactions can reduce their harmful effects on the body.

Resolved Needs: Protection from physical harm.

Observe for dyspnea   Look for signs of difficult breathing, such as gasping, anxiety, rapid and shallow breathing, dilated nostrils, moist and cyanotic skin, and retraction respirations.

Rationale: Respiratory difficulty prevents adequate blood and tissue oxygenation and may threaten life.

Resolved Needs: Protection from physical harm.

Observe for emotional instability   Look for verbal and nonverbal emotional responses that are inconsistent and indicative of instability. Determine whether these are habitual feeling responses or newly adopted responses.

Rationale: Behavior patterns are influenced by physiologic and psychologic disorders.

Resolved Needs: Protection from physical harm. Protection from psychologic threat.

Observe for euphoria   Look for indications of sudden feelings of unusual well-being, such as sudden bursts of energy, unusual cheerfulness, and overactivity.

Rationale: Euphoria, when it appears in a previously depressed patient, may indicate resolved conflict and a decision to commit suicide. While experiencing euphoria, a person tends to minimize danger and indulge in unsafe activities. Persons who are potential drug abusers often become euphoric on drugs given for therapeutic effect. Euphoria should be a clue to prescribe as little drug therapy as possible.

Resolved Needs: Protection from physical harm. Protection from psychologic threat.

Observe for evidence of a favorable response to therapy   Observe whether the patient's therapy is having the effect that was intended. Determine whether it is reducing the fever, blood pressure, or pain, promoting healing, or altering emotional responses.

Rationale: Therapy that does not produce the intended effect should be reevaluated and new therapy initiated.

Resolved Needs: Protection from physical harm.

Observe for evidence of pressure on the skin   Look for areas of redness or indentation on the skin.

Rationale: Pressure on a body area impairs circulation to that area and could result in tissue necrosis.

Resolved Needs: Protection from physical harm.

Observe for evidence that the patient (or family) is reaching out for emotional support   Look for signs indicating that the person is seeking emotional support from others. Such signs include frequently turning on the call light, crying, unwarranted angry outbursts, withdrawal of various degrees, chronic complaining, holding out the arms or hands to reach for others, returning to thumb sucking, holding onto a blanket or toy while sleeping, excessive eating, and excessive talking.

Rationale: Emotional support from others reduces the intensity of suffering. When persons feel unable to directly ask for emotional support, they will reach out by using indirect behavioral methods.

Resolved Needs: Protection from psychologic threat.

Observe for excessive talking Watch for the patient who talks at an excessively rapid rate or who talks consistently without pause.

Rationale: Excessive talking may indicate rapid metabolic rate, intracranial pressure, neurologic or circulatory brain disorders, or anxiety.

Resolved Needs: Protection from physical harm. Protection from psychologic threat.

Observe for fatigue Look for signs of fatigue such as yawning, irritability, dark shadows under the eyes, uncoordinated movements, inability to concentrate, shortness of breath, rapid pulse, and complaints of being tired.

Rationale: Fatigue results when the body cells, because of adaptation requirements, have depleted their energy reserves and require a period of restoration.

Resolved Needs: Protection from physical harm.

Observe for heart failure Look for signs that the heart is unable to deliver adequate oxygenated blood to meet the body's needs. Such signs include dyspnea on exertion, a nonproductive cough, a need to sleep on several pillows, jugular vein distention, nausea, chest pain, dependent edema, gallop heart rhythm, and crackling rales at the base of the lung.

Rationale: Heart failure reduces blood flow, resulting in circulatory impairment.

Resolved Needs: Protection from physical harm.

Observe for hemoptysis Look for evidence that the patient is coughing up blood.

Rationale: Hemoptysis indicates lung hemorrhage.

Resolved Needs: Protection from physical harm.

Observe for hiccoughs Listen for the short, sharp sound of intermittent diaphragmatic spasms.

Rationale: Hiccoughs indicate diaphragmatic irritation, often due to peritoneal inflammation.

Resolved Needs: Protection from physical harm.

Observe for hyperactivity Look for signs of overactivity in which the patient is seldom or never quiet.

Rationale: Hyperactivity may indicate hormone imbalance, emotional stress, drug or chemical side effects, or cerebral dysfunction.

Resolved Needs: Protection from physical harm. Protection from psychologic threat.

Observe for impaired conceptual thinking   Observe the patient's ability to think clearly and rationally and to comprehend the various factors involved in an idea.

Rationale: The thought process is influenced by the physiologic and psychologic states.

Resolved Needs: Protection from physical harm. Protection from psychologic threat.

Observe for impaired judgment   Observe the patient's ability to identify problems and arrive at adequate solutions.

Rationale: An ability to solve problems indicates integration of self, creativity, knowledge, and experience. It is affected by the physiologic and psychologic states.

Resolved Needs: Protection from physical harm. Protection from psychologic threat.

Observe for impaired learning ability   Observe the patient for any impairment of ability to learn. Compare the patient's responses with normal responses or with previous patient responses.

Rationale: Impaired learning ability may indicate central nervous system disorder or psychologic disequilibrium.

Resolved Needs: Protection from physical harm. Protection from psychologic threat.

Observe for impaired self-attitudes   Observe the patient for expressions of self-doubt, distorted self-image, diminished feelings of usefulness, unrealistic levels of aspiration, and other poor attitudes toward the self.

Rationale: An integrated self-concept is essential to emotional maturity and safety feelings.

Resolved Needs: Protection from psychologic threat.

Observe for incoherent thinking   Observe the patient for disorganization and instability of thought processes. This includes conversations and expressions of ideas in which thoughts are loosely connected or totally disconnected.

Rationale: The thought process is influenced by physiologic and psychologic states.

Resolved Needs: Protection from physical harm. Protection from psychologic threat.

Observe for incontinence   Observe the patient for inability to control the urinary sphincter and retain urine.

Rationale: Urinary incontinence may result from cerebral impairment, spinal cord injury or pressure, urinary tract irritation, or nerve or muscle degeneration.

Resolved Needs: Protection from physical harm.

Observe for increased nutritional requirements   Watch for the onset of conditions in which the patient will need additional nourishment, such as endocrine disorders, fever, severe tissue damage, pregnancy, lactation, rapid growth during childhood, or loss of body weight.

Rationale: Meeting increased nutritional needs promotes human safety.

Resolved Needs: Protection from physical harm.

Observe for infant head-rolling   Watch for head movements in which the infant chronically turns his head from side to side, usually accompanied by profuse perspiration on the face and forehead.

Rationale: Infant head-rolling may indicate rickets or an attempt to focus poorly coordinated eyes.

Resolved Needs: Protection from physical harm.

Observe for intestinal obstruction   Look for indications that the intestinal lumen is blocked. Such indications include wavelike abdominal pains, diarrhea or passage of blood or mucus without passage of fecal matter or flatus, fecal vomiting, drowsiness, malaise and aching, intense thirst, abdominal distention, weak and rapid pulse, lowered temperature and blood pressure, cold and clammy skin.

Rationale: Intestinal obstruction prevents the waste elimination that is essential to life.

Resolved Needs: Protection from physical harm.

Observe for irritability   Look for signs of a high level of susceptibility to stimuli, such as quick excitement responses, quickness to anger, impatience, and becoming easily annoyed or frustrated.

Rationale: Irritability may indicate body chemical imbalance or high physical or emotional stress levels.

Resolved Needs: Protection from physical harm. Protection from psychologic threat.

Observe for laryngeal edema   Look for swelling in the laryngeal area, especially after intubation. Signs include hoarseness, difficulty in swallowing, and difficult breathing.

Rationale: Laryngeal swelling obstructs the airway.

Resolved Needs: Protection from physical harm.

Observe for lethargy   Observe the patient for severe drowsiness and sluggishness.

Rationale: Lethargy indicates interference with normal cerebral and sensory function. It is often evident before convulsions or with meningitis.

Resolved Needs: Protection from physical harm.

Observe for memory impairment   Observe the patient for any inability to remember facts and events or difficulty with recall. Notice whether memory gaps begin and end abruptly, whether they are confined to one particular period or are scattered over a lengthy time, whether they are associated with only unpleasant events or with both pleasant and unpleasant events, whether they are related to lack of attention or to poor retention and recall, and whether the patient is aware of the memory problem.

Rationale: Impaired recall is influenced by current physiologic and psychologic states and affects the capacity to function.

Resolved Needs: Protection from physical harm. Protection from psychologic threat.

Observe for menstruation cycle abnormalities   Observe the patient for menstruation occurring more frequently than every 21 days, occurring less frequently than every 35 days, or having a duration of less than 3 days or more than 7 days.

Rationale: Abnormal menstruation is frequently indicative of endocrine or reproductive system disorders.

Resolved Needs: Protection from physical harm.

Observe for mental blocking   During conversations, watch for moments during which the patient is temporarily unable to think. Take into account the topic that is being discussed when the blocking or hesitancy occurs.

Rationale: Anxiety can give rise to hesitant speech patterns and thought disorganization.

Resolved Needs: Protection from psychologic threat.

Observe for mental retardation   Observe the patient for limitations of mental capacity. These may be indicated by an inability to learn at a normal rate, by poor physical development, or by behavior difficulties. Estimate the degree of retardation by observing the patient's abilities in regard to self-care, responses to others, and command of language, as well as by comparing the patient to average children:

At 3–4 months the normal child balances his head, smiles, laughs, reaches, squirms, and turns his head toward sound.

At 6–7 months the normal child reaches, grasps, sits, rolls over, bounces up and down, laughs when laughed at, and makes increasing sounds.

At 9 months the normal child sits without support, creeps, pulls up to stand, feeds himself crackers and a bottle, and copies sounds.

At 12 months the normal child stands alone, takes a few steps, attempts to eat with a spoon, squeals, and imitates familiar words.

At 18 months the normal child begins to run, pulls toys, hugs dolls, cooperates in dressing himself, claims possession of his own things, knows between 5 and 20 single words, and chatters.

The normal 2-year-old child runs well, walks up and down stairs, assists in dressing himself, uses a spoon with some spilling, and combines two to three words to express ideas.

At 3 years of age the normal child rides a tricycle, throws a ball, marks with crayon or pencil, participates in some cooperative play, uses long sentences, and refers to himself as "I."

At 4 years of age the normal child runs, skips, climbs, does simple tricks, uses imaginative play, counts to 10, and is social and talkative.

At 5 years of age the normal child can roller-skate, jump rope, sing and dance, and participate in competitive play. He uses connective words such as "but" and "and."

The normal 6-year-old child plays simple table games, uses a telephone, counts to 30, writes or prints his name, and has become sensitive to others.

If the child's development seems to be between 50% and 75% of that of the normal child, then the exceptional child is educable, and his IQ will range between 50 and 75. If his development seems to be between 25% and 50% of normal, the exceptional child is trainable, and his IQ will range between 25 and 50. If his development seems to be less than 25% of normal, the child is totally dependent, and his IQ will be below 25.

Rationale: Persons with impaired mental capacity need the supervision of more mature persons to insure their safety. Mentally retarded persons require special training in order to meet their own daily needs.

Resolved Needs: Protection from physical harm. Protection from psychologic threat.

Observe for mobility capabilities   Observe the patient's ability to
move about. Determine whether the child can crawl at the age of 9 months, walk with assistance at 12 months, walk alone at 15 months, run successfully at 18 months, and jump at 2 years. Determine whether the adult can walk or run without assistance and, if not, what his mobility capabilities are.

Rationale: Normal mobility is essential to uninhibited activity as well as safety.

Resolved Needs: Protection from physical harm.

Observe for mouth breathing   Note whether the patient consistently
breathes through his mouth.

Rationale: Mouth breathing indicates nasal obstruction.

Resolved Needs: Protection from physical harm.

Observe for muscle twitching   Look for sudden quick jerks of the
muscles.

Rationale: Muscle twitching may indicate increased blood potassium, decreased blood calcium, hypoglycemia, or a neurologic or psychosomatic disorder.

Resolved Needs: Protection from physical harm.

Observe for nasal congestion   Look and listen for evidence of obstructing secretions or swollen tissues in the nose, such as inability to breathe in and out of one or both nostrils, frequent nasal drainage, and noisy breathing when the mouth is closed.

Rationale: Nasal congestion can result in airway obstruction and severe discomfort.

Resolved Needs: Protection from physical harm.

Observe for nasal flare   Determine whether the lower nares are full and expanded outward during respirations. This occurs most frequently during sleep.

Rationale: Nasal flaring is characteristic of dyspnea in infants, especially with atelectasis and other obstructions.

Resolved Needs: Protection from physical harm.

Observe for nervousness   Observe the patient for signs of easy excitability and agitation.

Rationale: Nervousness may indicate that the body's regulatory mechanisms are in a state of disorder or that the nervous system has been overstimulated.

Resolved Needs: Protection from physical harm.

Observe for noise sensitivity   Look for indications that noise greatly disturbs the patient. Such indications include irritability when in a noisy environment, closing oneself off from noise, startle reactions when noises occur, and asking others to turn off radios and televisions.

Rationale: Hypersensitivity causes heightened responses to environmental stimuli and requires increased adaptation to stresses.

Resolved Needs: Protection from physical harm.

Observe for nonverbal communication of pain   Look for nonverbal indications of pain, such as skin redness, pallor, restlessness, excessive perspiration, increased respirations, bedfastness, distorted facial expression (drawn expression, clenched teeth, wrinkled forehead), or fatigue. Note posture variations, such as lying perfectly straight and still, knee flexion, kneeling, and stooping.

Rationale: Swelling and redness occur with inflammatory pain. Pallor is associated with painful circulatory constriction. The severe intensity of colicky pain resulting from intestinal, kidney, or biliary tract disorders causes restlessness and sometimes vomiting. Pain increases perspiration secretion.

Pain stimulates the autonomic nervous system, which controls respirations. Withdrawal from normal activity to bedrest reveals a disruption or threat of disruption in normal body function. Facial grimaces reveal pain. The stress of body adaptation while experiencing pain quickly produces fatigue. Deviations from normal posture indicate efforts at self-protection against pain and discomfort.

Resolved Needs: Protection from physical harm.

Observe for orthopnea   Look for difficulty in breathing, in which the patient elevates his head and thorax while resting.

Rationale: Orthopnea may indicate severe cardiac or respiratory disorder.

Resolved Needs: Protection from physical harm.

Observe for poor communication skills   Look for signs that the patient has difficulty in sending or receiving messages. These include stuttering, stammering, dysarthria, inappropriate emotional responses to messages, disorganization in the message sent, message misinterpretation, lack of interest in communicating, and making inferences not intended.

Rationale: Psychologic comfort and safety are promoted through effective communications with others.

Resolved Needs: Protection from psychologic threat.

Observe for positive skin test   After a small amount of toxin or antigen has been injected under the skin, watch for an area of redness to occur. Depending on the drug, the redness will be evident 24 to 48 hours following injection. This applies to toxins for diphtheria, tuberculosis (Mantoux), and the systemic fungal diseases (histoplasmosis, coccidioidomycosis, etc.).

Rationale: When the blood does not contain enough antitoxin to protect the patient against the toxin of a disease, a positive reaction of redness will occur at the point of injection. In such cases a prophylactic immunization should be given to protect against the disease.

Resolved Needs: Protection from physical harm.

Observe for presuicide calmness   Look for any development of a sense of unusual well-being and serenity in a patient who previously has displayed self-destructive behavior.

Rationale: Once the decision for self-destruction has been made, the patient may perceive his troubles as being resolved and may exhibit a sense of well-being. Recognition of potentially harmful physical threats can promote safety. A sense of the basic worth of the individual supports the continuance of life.

Resolved Needs: Protection from physical harm.

Observe for readiness to assume activities of daily living   Determine those activities of daily living that the patient can perform and is ready to perform. Such activities may include moving about in bed, obtaining objects from a bedside table, grooming and personal hygiene, dressing and undressing, feeding oneself, walking or pushing a wheelchair, and all the activities involving use of the hands and fingers, such as writing, turning on lights, turning book pages, smoking, winding a watch, etc.

Rationale: When a patient cannot carry on the activities of daily living, his needs must be met by others.

Resolved Needs: Protection from physical harm.

Observe for requests for increased drug dosage   Note any requests for drugs at more frequent intervals or at increased dosages.

Rationale: As the body builds up tolerance to a habit-forming drug, the amount and frequency of the drug must be increased in order to obtain the desired effect. This is a clue that the patient may be inclined toward drug habituation.

Resolved Needs: Protection from physical harm.

Observe for required eating assistance   Observe the patient's ability to feed himself and to chew and swallow his food.

Rationale: Recognition of the need for assistance in eating can promote balanced nutritional intake.

Resolved Needs: Protection from physical harm.

Observe for restlessness   Watch for frequent movements when the patient is attempting to rest or sleep.

Rationale: Poor tissue oxygenation, pain, discomfort, internal stress, or tension may cause restlessness.

Resolved Needs: Protection from physical harm.

Observe for shock   Look for signs and symptoms of circulatory collapse. They may include rapid pulse, pallor, cool and clammy skin, increased respirations, restlessness, hypotension, lethargy or anxiety, thirst, decreased urine output by the kidneys, coma or stupor, and dilated pupils.

Rationale: Shock may be the result of depressed cardiac output, severe blood or fluid loss, severe pain, septicemia, or nervous system disorder.

Resolved Needs: Protection from physical harm.

Observe for signs of healing   Look for evidence that the wound is being restored to health by healing. Evidence of healing includes no inflammation or drainage, closure of the edges of the wound, and the formation of granulation tissue to fill the area between the edges of a wound.

Rationale: Healing is essential to good functional use of body areas.

Resolved Needs: Protection from physical harm.

Observe for sneezing Be alert to the onset of sneezing episodes.

Rationale: Sneezing may be an early sign of impending upper respiratory infection. Awareness of its significance can prevent the transmission of infection to other persons. Sneezing also may indicate a hypersensitivity response.

Resolved Needs: Protection from physical harm.

Observe for syncope Observe the patient for weakness, lightheadedness, confusion, or blacking out that lasts for several minutes.

Rationale: Syncope indicates impaired nourishment and oxygenation of the brain as a result of low blood sugar, myocardial insufficiency, abnormal cardiac rhythm, or poor vascular resistance.

Resolved Needs: Protection from physical harm.

Observe for tetany Observe the patient for tonic muscular spasms.

Rationale: Tetany is most often seen with hyperventilation or alkalosis or in the early postoperative period following thyroidectomy.

Resolved Needs: Protection from physical harm.

Observe for the quantity and inquire about the quality of sleep Determine the characteristics and the kind of sleep the patient experiences. This may include light, normal, deep, or interrupted sleep.

Rationale: During sleep, body energy is utilized for healing. Loss of sleep can delay restoration to health and can threaten good health.

Resolved Needs: Protection from physical harm.

Observe for the sudden absence of severe pain Take note when the patient who has been experiencing severe pain states that the pain is suddenly gone.

Rationale: Sudden disappearance of severe pain often indicates rupture of the affected organ or passage of a kidney stone. It also occurs at the onset of shock in peritonitis.

Resolved Needs: Protection from physical harm.

Observe for thought rapidity Observe the speed at which the patient thinks. Determine whether responses are rapid, normal, slow, or retarded and whether they indicate a flight of ideas.

Rationale: The thought process is influenced by physiologic and psychologic states. Slow thinking can lead to physical harm.

Resolved Needs: Protection from physical harm. Protection from psychologic threat.

Observe for urinary frequency Determine whether the adult voids more often than every 5 hours. Normal urine output is 30–60 cc per hour.

Normal bladder capacity is approximately 450 cc before the elimination reflex is activated. Observe the patient for intake of large amounts of liquids, especially tea and coffee. Determine whether the increased intra-abdominal pressure of pregnancy is the cause of frequency.

Rationale: Urinary frequency may result from kidney inflammation, pressure against the bladder, high urea or uric acid concentrations, reflex stimulation of calculi in the ureter, or loss of bladder tone.

Resolved Needs: Protection from physical harm.

Observe for uterine membrane rupture   Be alert for the release of the amniotic and chorionic fluid that surrounds the unborn infant in a membranous sack.

Rationale: Uterine membrane rupture at the normal stage of labor indicates normal progress toward delivery. Delayed or early uterine membrane rupture may require therapeutic intervention. Once the uterine membrane ruptures, the potential for uterine infection exists.

Resolved Needs: Protection from physical harm.

Observe for voice changes   Listen for voice changes, such as hoarseness, loss of voice, whispering, and changes in tone.

Rationale: Marked voice changes indicate pressure on or inflammation of the vocal cord or pharynx. A husky voice during puberty is evidence of the maturing youth.

Resolved Needs: Protection from physical harm.

Observe for vomiting   Determine the quantity of emesis, force of projection, color, consistency, and those factors that precipitate its occurrence.

Rationale: Vomiting may indicate gastric irritation, intestinal obstruction, motion sickness, increased intracranial pressure, severe pain, toxic or disease states, or a psychogenic disturbance.

Resolved Needs: Protection from physical harm.

Observe for water intoxication   Observe the patient for indications of overhydration, such as anxiety, disorientation, confusion, shouting, inattention, convulsions, anorexia, nausea, vomiting, hyperventilation, sudden weight gain and edema, headache, gurgling respirations, pulse irregularity, and tremors.

Rationale: When the patient has received excess fluid and the circulatory system is overloaded with more water than the kidneys can excrete, the potential for shock and pulmonary edema exists.

Resolved Needs: Protection from physical harm.

Observe for writing abnormalities   Observe the patient's work for unreadable writing and inability to relate thoughts and ideas through writing.

Rationale: Writing abnormalities occurring in persons who have been educated to write may indicate neurologic or muscular disorders.

Resolved Needs: Protection from physical harm.

Observe personal hygiene habits   Observe the patient's practice of hygiene, including bath, hair care, nail care, mouth care, and general cleanliness.

Rationale: Cleanliness can have an effect on the growth and transmission of microorganisms that cause illness and disease. Attitudes toward personal hygiene reflect internal self-attitudes.

Resolved Needs: Protection from physical harm. Protection from psychologic threat.

Observe the amputation stump for odor   Note any unpleasant odor coming from an amputated stump.

Rationale: Infection or tissue necrosis may be manifested by an unpleasant odor.

Resolved Needs: Protection from physical harm.

Observe the breath for abnormal odors   Determine whether the patient has abnormal breath odors, such as a mousy, acid-fruit (acetone), fermented, ammonia, fecal, or foul odor. Note any sour or disagreeable breath or the smell of blood.

Rationale: A mousy odor is associated with liver disease; an acid-fruit (acetone) odor is associated with diabetes; a fermented odor is associated with alcohol consumption; an ammonia odor is associated with uremia. Disagreeable breath may be caused by spicy foods, smoking, or a dirty or infected mouth. A fecal odor is associated with lower intestinal obstruction; sour breath is associated with digestive disorders; a foul odor is associated with potential renal acidosis. The smell of blood occurs with gastrointestinal bleeding and esophageal varices.

Resolved Needs: Protection from physical harm.

Observe the cast for an expanding bleeding area   When bleeding appears on a cast, outline the area with pencil or pen and mark the time and date of each outline. Periodically check for bleeding that spreads beyond the marked area.

Rationale: Bleeding reduces circulating blood volume, and a wet cast provides an opening for the entry of infectious organisms.

Resolved Needs: Protection from physical harm.

Observe the cast for odor   Note any unpleasant odor coming from a cast.

Rationale: Unseen tissue necrosis beneath the cast covering can be detected because of an unpleasant odor.

Resolved Needs: Protection from physical harm.

Observe the characteristics of the child's cry Listen for variations in the crying of the infant that may indicate abnormalities or unmet needs.

Rationale: Different qualities of the infant's cry may indicate various types of distress. Pain may be indicated by a shrill, loud cry interrupted by whimpering and groaning, as well as by a short, sharp, piercing cry. Discomfort is evidenced by a low whimpering cry. Hunger is communicated by a loud cry with interrupted sucking motions. Fatigue is indicated by crying accompanied by eye rubbing, yawning, and eyelid drooping. Fear or apprehension may be evidenced by crying, clinging to the mother, and turning away from the frightening situation. Brain damage may be indicated by a weak, infrequent cry. Neurologic infection should be suspected when there is a shrill, weak cry. Nervous tension is indicated by excessive crying when there is no physical problem but when an apprehensive atmosphere exists within the family. Colic may be evidenced by a piercing scream and abdominal distention, with the infant pulling his legs up and stiffening his legs. A spoiled child may cry angrily until someone appears, then suddenly stop crying.

Resolved Needs: Protection from physical harm. Protection from psychologic threat.

Observe the characteristics of the cough Observe the frequency, sound, productiveness, and precipitating factors of a cough.

Rationale: Coughing indicates respiratory tract stimulation caused by irritation.

Resolved Needs: Protection from physical harm.

Observe the eating pattern for abnormality Determine the types of food eaten, how frequently eating occurs, the rate of eating, and whether the amount of food consumed is appropriate for age, height, weight, and health condition.

Rationale: Balanced nutrition is essential to normal cellular function. Anorexia and polyphagia may indicate physiologic or psychologic disorders.

Resolved Needs: Protection from physical harm.

Observe the extremities for motor function Observe the patient's ability to move both arms and legs normally.

Rationale: Abnormal motor function in the extremities indicates a nerve or muscle disorder.

Resolved Needs: Protection from physical harm.

Observe the level of consciousness Determine the patient's level of response. Check for:

alertness or lethargy
ability to cooperate or inability to cooperate
orientation or disorientation as to time, place, other people, oneself
    (does not respond to own name)
response to painful stimuli
  purposeful (tries to pull away from stimulus or push the stimulus
    away)
  purposeless (moves about irrelevantly or hyperventilates)
  no response
corneal and gag reflexes (when these are absent, the patient is com-
    atose)

Rationale: Levels of consciousness are altered by pathologic conditions involving the cerebral cortex and brain stem. Levels of consciousness affect behavior patterns and the capacity to function.

Resolved Needs: Protection from physical harm.

Observe the newborn for drug withdrawal

Observe the newborn for signs of drug withdrawal; these may appear immediately after birth, several hours later, or within 4 days, depending on the quantity of drug taken by the mother and the time of last ingestion. Signs of drug withdrawal include hyperirritability, tremors, shrill and high-pitched crying, sneezing, sweating, vomiting, diarrhea, ravenous appetite, and abrasions caused by the rubbing of skin on sheets. Without treatment, the child will develop convulsions, apnea, fever, and dehydration progressing to circulatory collapse and death.

Rationale: The newborn drug withdrawal syndrome, when untreated, is potentially fatal.

Resolved Needs: Protection from physical harm.

Observe the onset time of infant jaundice

Note the number of hours or days between birth and the appearance of the first signs of infant jaundice.

Rationale: Jaundice beginning within 36 hours of birth indicates erythroblastosis fetalis, which is the excessive formation of erythroblasts in the blood caused by production of maternal antibodies in an Rh-negative mother against an Rh-positive fetus. Jaundice beginning within 48–72 hours of birth indicates physiologic jaundice, in which there is a sudden increase in the destruction rate of red blood cells shortly after birth. Jaundice beginning 3–4 days after birth is usually caused by septicemia. Jaundice beginning about the second week of life indicates bile duct obstruction.

Resolved Needs: Protection from physical harm.

Observe the pattern of sleep

Note the times of day the patient sleeps and how consistently the sleep schedule is followed. Note whether he sleeps at night or during the day, whether he goes to bed at the same time every day, and whether the pattern suddenly changes.

Rationale: A consistent sleep pattern is essential to good health and to normal functioning of the internal clock. Altered sleep patterns should be returned to the normal pattern as soon as possible.

Resolved Needs: Protection from physical harm.

Observe the person's activity pattern   Note the pattern of daily activity the patient pursues. Listen to his discussions of his daily routine and the activities he is involved in.

Rationale: Daily activity patterns give clues to the patient's lifestyle, interests, physical fitness, and capabilities. If his activity pattern is not commensurate with his physical capabilities, the pattern can be adjusted to meet his health needs.

Resolved Needs: Protection from physical harm.

Observe the preoperative and postoperative response level   Determine whether the patient's level of cerebral response is the same as before surgery, especially for patients whose surgery required artificial oxygenation or circulation maintenance by pump.

Rationale: Inadequate oxygenation of cerebral tissues will result in impaired cerebral function.

Resolved Needs: Protection from physical harm.

Observe the seizure characteristics   Monitor the occurrence of any seizure, and determine the circumstances surrounding the seizure. This includes the factors involved in its onset, the areas of body involvement, the severity of muscle twitching, the length of the episode, the level of consciousness, the sequence of movement, and any preseizure and postseizure signs and symptoms.

Rationale: Seizures indicate neurologic disorder.

Resolved Needs: Protection from physical harm.

Observe the time of the first meconium stool   Determine when meconium is passed from the infant's rectum and is replaced by normal yellow stool. This usually occurs within the first 10 hours of life.

Rationale: Anal malformation or bowel obstruction may prevent passage of meconium.

Resolved Needs: Protection from physical harm.

Observe the time of the newborn's first voiding   Determine whether the newborn infant voids within the first 24–36 hours of life.

Rationale: Newborn infants normally void within the first 36 hours of life.

Resolved Needs: Protection from physical harm.

Observe the urine for abnormal color, content, and odor Inspect the urine for pigment (color) other than the normal yellow, orange, or brownish yellow. Inspect the urine for mucus, fat globules, blood, or other visible solids and determine whether there is any unusual urine odor.

Rationale: Bile-colored urine may be associated with jaundice. Black urine may indicate malignant tumors, hemorrhage, or mercury, lead, or phenol poisoning. Blue urine indicates prior use of methylene blue or indigo. Milky white urine is associated with fat globules. Red urine indicates bleeding. Cloudiness is associated with pus and urinary tract infection.

Mucus in the urine is associated with inflammation. Albumin is associated with fever, excessive physical exercise or exertion, Bright's disease, and scoliosis. Fat in the urine indicates kidney degeneration. Sugar indicates faulty carbohydrate metabolism. White precipitate suggests excessive phosphates, while pink precipitate suggests excessive uric acid. Blood in the urine indicates hemorrhage, urinary tract trauma, blood dyscrasias, or renal disease. Foam suggests protein loss and the nephrotic syndrome.

Acetone urine odor is associated with the excessive fat metabolism of diabetes. Ammonia odor indicates uremia. Fecal odor indicates intestinal or urinary fistulas. Fishy odor suggests kidney inflammation.

Resolved Needs: Protection from physical harm.

Obtain a bacterial culture Using sterile technique, collect a specimen of body fluid, drainage, or secretion and have it incubated for bacterial growth.

Rationale: A culture of body secretions may reveal potentially harmful infection.

Resolved Needs: Protection from physical harm.

Obtain standard laboratory studies and evaluate for normal levels Have blood and urine studies done according to the standard procedure of the institution or organization in which practice is being conducted.

Rationale: Laboratory studies help to determine normal and abnormal health status.

Resolved Needs: Protection from physical harm.

Palpate for arterial pulsations (218) Count the expansions of the arterial wall occurring in 1 minute by placing the fingertips over the artery. Determine whether there is soreness, distention, or bounding pulsation and whether right and left pulses are of equal strength. Examine the temporal artery at the temple above and outside the eye, the external maxillary artery (facial), the carotid artery on the side of the neck, the brachial artery on the inner arm above the elbow joint, the radial artery on the thumb side of the wrist, the femoral artery in the groin, the popliteal artery behind the knee, and the arteria dorsalis pedis on the top of the foot near the ankle.

Rationale: Pulsation and expansion of the arterial walls occur with each ventricular contraction. Abnormalities indicate cardiac or circulatory pathology.

Resolved Needs: Protection from physical harm.

Palpate for fetal position   Palpate the maternal abdomen, feeling for the fetal head, buttocks, and extremities. Determine whether the fetus is facing left or right.

Rationale: Palpation for fetal position helps locate the back of the fetus, where fetal heart sounds are most easily heard. Fetal position indicates whether the infant will be delivered in cephalic or breech presentation.

Resolved Needs: Protection from physical harm.

Palpate for tenderness   Feel body areas for soreness or sensitivity to pain when palpation is attempted.

Rationale: Abdominal tenderness may indicate organ distention or inflammation of the abdominal viscera, wall, or peritoneum. Calf tenderness may result from a localized blood clot. Cranial tenderness may occur with trauma, fracture, or abrasions. Thoracic tenderness may indicate injury.

Resolved Needs: Protection from physical harm.

Palpate the abdomen for a fluid wave (113,225)   With the patient flat on his back, sharply tap one side of the flank with one hand. At the same time, have the other hand on the opposite flank waiting to receive the tap impulse on that side.

Rationale: An abdominal fluid wave indicates free fluid in the abdominal cavity.

Resolved Needs: Protection from physical harm.

Palpate the abdomen for tenderness, rigidity, and masses (113,225)   Gently press the hand into each of the four abdominal quadrants. The patient may feel rebound tenderness, in which the sudden release of pressure causes pain. Palpate for rigidity, in which there is a feeling of resistance. Feel for masses.

Rationale: Rebound tenderness occurs with inflammation. Abdominal rigidity may indicate inflammation, peritoneal irritation, or abdominal tissue growth.

Resolved Needs: Protection from physical harm.

Palpate the abdominal aorta for increased pulsation (113,225)   Feel for an increased or bounding epigastric pulsation and for a pulsating mass. Normally there is only slight epigastric pulsation.

Rationale: Very strong pulsation in the abdominal aorta indicates arterial dilatation and may be associated with aneurysm or aortic insufficiency.

Resolved Needs: Protection from physical harm.

Palpate the bladder for distention (113,225)   Feel for an enlarged
bladder by placing the fingers over the lower middle abdomen. Feel for distention and masses. An empty bladder cannot be palpated.

Rationale: Bladder distention indicates urine retention. Abnormal bladder masses can be detected by palpation.

Resolved Needs: Protection from physical harm.

Palpate the breasts for nodules (113,225)   Examine the patient
for breast nodules in the following manner: Ask the patient to raise both her arms. Carefully observe breast tissue for bulging, edema, and dimpling. Compare the sizes and shapes of the breasts. Carefully palpate the tissue in all four quadrants of the breasts for increased heat, tenderness, and masses. Beginning at the breastbone, gently palpate the inner half of the breast. With the flat part of the fingers, palpate the nipple. Ask the patient to place her arm at her side; then feel the tissues that extend to the axilla. Examine the upper and lower outside quadrants of the breast.

Rationale: Breast palpation reveals abnormalities that can be resolved if detected and treated early.

Resolved Needs: Protection from physical harm.

Palpate the cervix for dilatation   With the patient flat on her back
with knees flexed, slowly insert a lubricated index finger into the rectum. Feel for a depression surrounded by a circular ridge, and determine the extent of cervical expansion by the size of the circular ridge. Dilatation begins with 1 cm and ends with 10 cm. The progression is as follows: 1 cm (½-inch circular ridge), 2 cm (¾-inch circular ridge), 3 cm (1 ¼-inch circular ridge), 4 cm (1 ½-inch circular ridge), 5 cm (2-inch circular ridge), 6 cm (2 ¼-inch circular ridge), 8 cm (3-inch circular ridge), 10 cm (3 ¾-inch circular ridge).

Rationale: Cervical dilatation measures the progress of labor and allows for recognition of abnormalities.

Resolved Needs: Protection from physical harm.

Palpate the chest for a precordial heave (113,225)   On the an-
terior chest, look for and then palpate for any pulsation at the left 5th interspace, the right 3rd, 4th, and 5th interspaces, and the lower sternum.

Rationale: A precordial heave may indicate increased myocardial tone (from increased metabolic rate) and right ventricular hypertrophy (from a failing cardiac valve). It may be associated with pulmonary or tricuspid insufficiency, mitral, pulmonary, or tricuspid stenosis, or thyrotoxicosis.

Resolved Needs: Protection from physical harm.

Palpate the chest for a thrill (113,225)   Feel for vibrations over the chest precordium. The feeling is similar to that felt when placing a hand on the chest of a purring cat.

Rationale: A thrill indicates that blood is flowing through an abnormal heart or arteries. It is associated with aortic or mitral stenosis.

Resolved Needs: Protection from physical harm.

Palpate the chest for abnormal vocal fremitus (113,225)   Moving the hand over the anterior thorax from left to right, feel the costal cartilages, ribs, and rib interspaces. Apply the fingers of one hand to the interspaces and ask the patient to say "ninety-nine." Feel for a strong tremor, a diminished tremor, or the absence of a tremor within the chest wall.

Rationale: Increased tremor within the chest wall indicates increased lung volume and is associated with pulmonary consolidation. Decreased tremor within the chest wall occurs with airflow obstruction and is associated with pleural effusion and pneumothorax.

Resolved Needs: Protection from physical harm.

Palpate the chest for an abnormal precordial thrust (113,225)   Feel for the normal cardiac pulsation at the point of maximum impulse (PMI). Determine whether the pulsation is weak or excessively forceful and whether it covers a wider area than normal.

Rationale: An excessively forceful precordial thrust may indicate increased myocardial tone (from increased metabolic rate) or left ventricular hypertrophy (from a failing cardiac valve). It may be associated with hypertension, aortic or mitral insufficiency, aortic stenosis, or thyrotoxicosis.

Resolved Needs: Protection from physical harm.

Palpate the cranial suture line for separation   Feel for nonclosure of the arrow-shaped (sagittal) and long (longitudinal) skull bones that connect the two fontanels. Run a hand over the baby's head and feel the skull bone with the fingertips.

Rationale: A separated infant suture line indicates increased intracranial pressure.

Resolved Needs: Protection from physical harm.

Palpate the eyeballs for tension   Place the tip of the forefinger on the closed eyelid. Gently press the eyeball with the finger. Determine whether the eyeball firmness is approximately the same as that of a normal eye.

Rationale: Increased eyeball tension indicates glaucoma. Decreased eyeball tension indicates severe dehydration.

Resolved Needs: Protection from physical harm.

Palpate the fontanel for abnormality (113,225)   Feel for variations in the soft space between the cranial skull bones of the baby. Such variations may include delayed closure of the posterior fontanel beyond 2 months, delayed closure of the anterior fontanel beyond 18 months, premature fontanel closure before 10 months, or bulging or depression of the anterior fontanel. Palpate by running a hand over the baby's head and feeling the fontanel with the fingertips.

Rationale: Delayed fontanel closure may indicate insufficient intake or absorption of calcium or vitamin D. Premature fontanel closure prevents normal brain growth. Fontanel bulging indicates increased intracranial pressure. Fontanel depression indicates dehydration.

Resolved Needs: Protection from physical harm.

Palpate the head for a cranial bulge   Grasp the infant's head in the fingertips and firmly press over the entire cranial and facial bone surface. Examine for areas of cranial projection or protuberance and for unusually hard or soft areas.

Rationale: Cranial bulge may be indicative of trauma, tumor, or congenital defect.

Resolved Needs: Protection from physical harm.

Palpate the liver for enlargement (113,225)   Examine the liver by placing the palm of the left hand over the lower anterior ribs of the right thorax. Strike the back of the left hand lightly with a right-handed fist and determine whether pain or tenderness is experienced. Feel the liver for enlargement and determine whether it moves with each artificial pulsation.

Rationale: Liver enlargement indicates congestion caused by cardiac failure, poor nutrition, or impaired liver function. It may be associated with an intraabdominal mass, cardiac failure, liver damage, liver failure, or malnutrition.

Resolved Needs: Protection from physical harm.

Palpate the lymph nodes for enlargement (113,225)   Stand behind the patient and gently palpate the entire neck under the jaw and behind and in front of the ears. Determine whether there is tenderness, and feel for heat or swelling in the nodes. Then palpate the axillary area for the same symptoms.

Rationale: Lymph node swelling may indicate obstruction or disease of lymph nodes and lymph vessels or infection.

Resolved Needs: Protection from physical harm.

Palpate the parotid gland for swelling (113,225)   Feel for enlargement of the parotid glands located near each ear.

Rationale: Parotid gland swelling may indicate viral or bacterial infection.

Resolved Needs: Protection from physical harm.

Palpate the pulse for rate, rhythm, and volume Count the expansions of the arterial wall occurring in 1 minute by placing the fingertips over the wrist artery. Normal pulse rate is 70–80 pulses per minute in adults, 85–110 in children, and 130–140 in infants. Rhythm should be consistent, and volume should be moderate.

Rationale: Pulsation of the arterial walls occurs with each left ventricular contraction. Abnormalities indicate cardiac or circulatory pathology.

Resolved Needs: Protection from physical harm.

Palpate the skin for crepitation Feel the skin areas over the chest, neck, extremities, and face for a bubbling, crackling sensation.

Rationale: Skin crepitation indicates air in subcutaneous tissues. It may occur in the neck when there is tracheal or esophageal injury, in the extremities with gas gangrene, and in the face when there is major trauma.

Resolved Needs: Protection from physical harm.

Palpate the spleen for enlargement (113,225) Have the patient lie on his back and place his left fist under his 11th rib, near his waist. Curl the fingers of both your hands around the left costal margin so that they fit up under the ribs. Ask the patient to breathe in deeply. The margin of the spleen can be felt with the fingertips. If it is enlarged, it will be displaced downward from behind the thoracic cage toward the right iliac fossa, or it may extend to the midline.

Rationale: A moderately enlarged, soft spleen with blunt edges may indicate infection or increased red blood cell destruction. A firm, hard spleen with sharp edges may indicate chronic disease. An enlarged spleen also may indicate congestion caused by cardiac failure or circulatory disturbance.

Resolved Needs: Protection from physical harm.

Palpate the thyroid gland for enlargement (113,225) Examine the thyroid gland by standing behind the patient. Place the tips of two or three fingers of each hand on each side of the trachea. Ask the patient to swallow. Feel for nodule fullness, which will glide upward if there is an abnormality.

Rationale: Thyroid nodules and thyroid enlargement may occur with tumorous growth, tissue hyperplasia, or thyroid hyperactivity.

Resolved Needs: Protection from physical harm.

Palpate the trachea for deviation (113,225) Feel the trachea and determine whether it is in the normal midline position with the sternal notch.

Rationale: If there is pressure on the trachea, it may shift its location to the right or left side of the sternal notch. Tracheal deviation may be associated with pulmonary atelectasis, pulmonary cavity, or pleural effusion.

Resolved Needs.   Protection from physical harm.

Palpate the uterus for contraction quality   Place one finger on the abdomen above the uterine area and attempt to indent the finger into the uterine wall when a contraction and pain occur.

Rationale: When an excellent uterine contraction occurs, finger indentation cannot occur. When a moderately good contraction occurs, slight finger indentation is possible. When a poor contraction occurs, finger indentation occurs easily. Contractions cease completely in uterine rupture.

Resolved Needs: Protection from physical harm.

Palpate the uterus for firmness   Feel the uterus and determine whether it is hard or soft.

Rationale: Normally the uterus is hard. A soft or boggy quality indicates internal uterine bleeding.

Resolved Needs: Protection from physical harm.

Palpate the uterus for fundus height   Feel the uterine fundus through the abdominal wall. Immediately after birth the fundus is felt halfway between the umbilicus and the bony prominence under the pubic hair. It gradually rises until about 12 hours after birth, when it lies slightly above the umbilicus. Each day the fundus height should be palpated. It should normally decrease about ½ inch per day until the 10th day, when it is no longer detectable.

Rationale: A uterine fundus that does not descend approximately ½ inch per day may indicate poor uterine muscle tone, retained placental tissue, or endometrium inflammation.

Resolved Needs: Protection from physical harm.

Palpate the uterus for normal enlargement during pregnancy (460)   Feel the uterus during different stages of pregnancy to determine whether it is enlarging appropriately. At the end of the third month the uterus should have enlarged sufficiently that it can be felt at the level of the symphysis pubis. At the end of the fifth month it should be at the level of the umbilicus. At the middle of the eighth month it should be palpable at the xiphoid cartilage located near the lower sternum.

Rationale: Gradual enlargement of the uterus during pregnancy permits estimation of the size of the fetus and determination of whether growth is adequate.

Resolved Needs: Protection from physical harm.

Percuss the abdomen for abnormal resonance (113,225)
Percuss each abdominal quadrant. Normally a resonant, vibrating sound

should be heard. Listen for decreased resonance (dullness) or a hollow, drumlike (tympany) sound.

Rationale: A dull abdominal percussion sound may indicate peritoneal cavity fluid or a full bladder. Tympanic abdominal sounds may indicate air or gas within the stomach, intestines, or peritoneal cavity.

Resolved Needs: Protection from physical harm.

Percuss the chest for abnormal resonance (113,225)   Begin
under the clavicle and work downward from right to left, percussing each symmetric rib interspace. Normally a resonant, vibrating sound should be heard, except in areas of cardiac dullness. Listen for decreased resonance. Have the patient pull his shoulders forward; working down the posterior chest from right to left, percuss each rib interspace. Normally the resonant sounds end about the ninth rib. Listen for dullness (decreased resonance), flatness (absence of resonance), hyperresonance, and tympany (hollow, drumlike sound).

Rationale: Dull thoracic sounds may indicate pulmonary fluid, increased lung volume, or a deflated lung; they are associated with pulmonary atelectasis, pulmonary consolidation, and pulmonary congestion. Flat thoracic sounds may indicate chest fluid and increased lung volume and are associated with pulmonary consolidation, pleural effusion, and pulmonary congestion. Increased resonance sounds may indicate increased lung volume and pleural fluid. When heard over the upper lung, they are associated with emphysema or pleural effusion. Tympanic thoracic sounds indicate a hollow lung space and are associated with a pulmonary cavity.

Resolved Needs: Protection from physical harm.

Percuss the chest for cracked-pot sounds (113,225)   Begin
under the clavicle and work downward from right to left, percussing each symmetric rib interspace. Normally a resonant, vibrating sound should be heard, except in areas of cardiac dullness. Listen for a sound with a clinking quality. Have the patient pull his shoulders forward; working down the posterior chest from right to left, percuss each rib interspace. Normally the resonant sounds end about the ninth rib. Listen for a clinking sound.

Rationale: Cracked-pot thoracic sounds indicate a hollow lung space, often associated with a tuberculosis cavity.

Resolved Needs: Protection from physical harm.

Percuss the chest for widened cardiac dullness
(113,225)   With the patient lying on his back, gently tap his chest. Begin at the patient's side and percuss toward the midline in the fifth, fourth, and third interspaces. While percussing, listen for a change from a resonant lung sound to a cardiac dullness. Make a note of the point of sound change in relationship to the midclavicular line.

Rationale: Cardiac border percussion provides a rough estimate of the heart's contour, which permits estimation of its size. It can reveal cardiac border displacement, which may be associated with hypertension or aortic or mitral stenosis or insufficiency.

Resolved Needs: Protection from physical harm.

Percuss the posterior chest for decreased diaphragmatic descent (113,225)   With the patient in a forward-bent position, percuss the posterior thorax from the scapula downward. Note the point at which dullness is heard. Then ask the patient to take a deep breath and hold it. Continue percussion to a point where a new level of dullness is heard. Measure the distance between the two points; normally it should be 4–6 cm (1½–2½ inches). Compare the two sides of the chest to determine whether the measurements are equal.

Rationale: On inspiration, the diaphragm descends as the lungs fill with air. When one side of the diaphragm does not descent as far as the other, one should suspect atelectasis in that lung.

Resolved Needs: Protection from physical harm.

Perform a physical examination and evaluate if the findings are normal (ExR)   Examine the patient according to the standard procedure followed by the institution or organization in which the practice is being conducted. Include all body systems.

Rationale: By means of a physical examination, it can be determined whether the patient's health status is normal or abnormal.

Resolved Needs: Protection from physical harm.

Review the dietary intake with the patient to determine adherence to the prescribed diet   Have the patient describe his complete dietary intake over a particular period. Determine whether this intake is correct in relation to the diet prescribed for his condition.

Rationale: Adherence to a prescribed diet is essential for maintenance of health.

Resolved Needs: Protection from physical harm.

Strain the urine   Filter all urine output through gauze or a strainer in order to catch renal stones.

Rationale: Filtering out renal stones confirms passage of the stones. Analysis of renal stones provides information which supports the use of preventive measures against future stone formation.

Resolved Needs: Protection from physical harm.

Test for a positive Babinski sign (113)   Using a hard object, stroke the sole of the foot from the heel up along the outer edge and across the ball of the foot. Note any abnormal upward movement (dorsal extension) of the big toe or spreading of the other toes. Normally the great toe should flex downward when the sole of the foot is stroked. A positive Babinski sign is

normally found in the newborn infant, but it should disappear after approximately 1 year.

Rationale: A positive Babinski sign may indicate an immature nervous system or upper motor neuron lesion.

Resolved Needs: Protection from physical harm.

Test for a positive Homans' sign (113,225)   When the patient complains of calf tenderness, bend the foot up toward the knee (dorsiflexion) and observe for complaints of pain in the calf.

Rationale: A positive Homans' sign indicates thrombosis.

Resolved Needs: Protection from physical harm.

Test for a positive Trousseau's sign (113)   Apply pressure to the brachial artery on the inside of the upper arm by inflating a blood pressure cuff above that area. Between the systolic and diastolic readings, determine if the hand bends downward (palmar flexion). If spasmodic contractions of the muscles occur, this is a positive Trousseau's sign.

Rationale: A positive Trousseau's sign indicates tetany caused by decreased blood calcium levels.

Resolved Needs: Protection from physical harm.

Test for abnormal deep-reflex responses (113,225)   Strike a sudden blow with a rubber hammer over the tendon (pectoralis, biceps, brachioradial, pronator, triceps, quadriceps, adductor, Achilles) of a muscle. Look for a highly sensitive response or a weak response of a nerve impulse occurring on external stimulation.

Rationale: An increased deep-reflex response is caused by loss of normal reflex control of the reflex arc as a result of an injury in the spinal cord at a level higher than the reflex arc. A decreased deep-reflex response indicates an interrupted reflex arc.

Resolved Needs: Protection from physical harm.

Test for Chvostek's sign (113)   Lightly tap the face just below the temple and watch for twitching. This sign is normal in infants up to 6 months of age, but otherwise it is abnormal.

Rationale: A positive Chvostek's sign indicates calcium deficit.

Resolved Needs: Protection from physical harm.

Test for impaired coordination (113)   Look for signs that the normally smooth integration of body movements is impaired. This may be done in several ways. Have the patient walk a straight line, placing each foot directly in front of the other. Have the patient bring the tip of his index finger to the tip of his nose, once with his eyes open and once with his eyes closed. With the patient lying flat, have him extend one leg and then run the heel of the other foot from the knee to the foot of the extended leg. Observe

the patient's ability to write, to button and unbutton clothing, to tie shoelaces, and to pick up small objects such as pins and needles.

Rationale: Impaired coordination may indicate a cerebellar lesion or extrapyramidal disorder.

Resolved Needs: Protection from physical harm.

Test for impaired smell perception   Listen for complaints of decreased ability to smell. Watch for lack of response to odor-producing objects such as flowers, food, etc.

Rationale: Impaired smell perception may result from nasal masses, nasal packing, dry nasal mucous membranes, or nerve injury. Smell perception affects taste perception, which in turn affects nutritional intake.

Resolved Needs: Protection from physical harm.

Test for impaired taste perception   Listen for complaints of decreased ability to taste. Watch for lack of response to foods such as pickles and lemons.

Rationale: Impaired taste perception may result from brain or nerve damage, tongue or oral mucosa inflammation, or decreased smell perception. Taste perception affects nutritional intake.

Resolved Needs: Protection from physical harm.

Test for the degree of muscle strength (113)   Have the patient actively move the muscles being tested. Then either pull against the patient's tensed muscles or hold his body area in a stabilized position and have him attempt resistance. The degrees of muscle strength are as follows:

Minimum muscle weakness: Complete joint movement with almost complete muscle contraction when resistance is applied against the joint.

Mild muscle weakness: Complete joint movement with some muscle contraction when resistance is applied against the joint.

Moderate muscle weakness: Complete joint movement with some muscle contraction so long as there is no application of resistance against the joint.

Severe muscle weakness: No joint movement. Some muscle contraction.

Complete muscle weakness: No joint movement. No muscle contraction.

Rationale: Testing the patient's muscle strength gives an indication of his activity capabilities.

Resolved Needs: Protection from physical harm.

Test for urine phenylalanine with ferric chloride   Apply a ferric chloride solution to a freshly saturated diaper and interpret the chemical reaction.

Rationale: A reaction producing a green color indicates phenylketonuria, which indicates the possibility of mental retardation.

Resolved Needs: Protection from physical harm.

Test the abdomen for hyperesthesia (113,225) Using a pin, lightly stroke the abdomen from the umbilicus downward. Have the patient indicate whether the pin feels sharper in any area.

Rationale: Abdominal hyperesthesia may indicate visceral or peritoneal irritation or inflammation.

Resolved Needs: Protection from physical harm.

Test the amniotic fluid pH Using Nitrazine paper, determine the pH level of the amniotic fluid once the membrane has ruptured or if it is suspected that the membrane has ruptured. Normal vaginal secretions have a pH of 4.5 to 5.5, while amniotic fluid pH is 7.0 to 7.5.

Rationale: When fluid is escaping from the vagina, but there is doubt about whether the membrane has ruptured, this test will determine whether the fluid is amniotic or is from another source.

Resolved Needs: Protection from physical harm.

Test the ears for impaired hearing (113,225) To use the whisper test, begin whispering 20 feet from the patient and decrease the distance 5 feet at a time until the patient can hear the whisper. To use the Weber test, hold a tuning fork at the skull midline and have the patient compare the sound intensities in his two ears. To use the Rinne test, place a tuning fork against the patient's mastoid process (bone conduction) and count the number of seconds until he no longer hears the sound. Then hold the tuning fork 1 inch from his ear (air conduction) and time his hearing again.

Rationale: Impaired hearing is said to exist when a person cannot hear a whisper at 10 feet, when there is a higher intensity of sound in one ear with the Weber test, or when the Rinne test indicates that bone-conducted sound is heard as long as or longer than air-conducted sound.

Resolved Needs: Protection from physical harm.

Test the eyes for decreased corneal reflex (225) Test each eye separately and have the patient look to one side while being tested. Gently place a wisp of sterile cotton on the cornea. Normally the eyelids will blink when the cornea is touched. If the corneal reflex is decreased, there will be little or no blinking.

Rationale: A decreased corneal reflex may indicate a lesion of the fifth or seventh cranial nerve.

Resolved Needs: Protection from physical harm.

Test the eyes for impaired coordination (113,225) Hold a light at the level of the patient's eyes, then move the light in a U pattern, from

top to bottom, across, and bottom to top. Ask the patient to follow the light with his eyes.

Rationale: Jerky eye movements indicate impaired eye muscle coordination. If, after the age of six months, an infant cannot coordinate his eyes, there may be impaired neuromuscular development.

Resolved Needs: Protection from physical harm.

Test the eyes for impaired vision (225)   Place a Snellen chart 20 feet in front of the patient. In the visual acuity formula (e.g., 20/20) the first number is the distance the patient is standing from the chart. The first line on the chart is normally read at 200 feet, the second line at 50 feet, the third line at 40 feet, the fourth line at 30 feet, the fifth line at 20 feet, the sixth line at 15 feet, and the seventh line at 10 feet. Ask the patient to read as far down the chart as he can. Identify the number of the line to which he can read (e.g., line 7). Then insert as the second number in the visual acuity formula the normal number of feet for that line (e.g., 10 feet for line 7). Thus the patient has 20/10 vision.

If no chart is available, hold up any number of fingers and ask the patient to identify the number.

Also notice whether the patient bumps into things, refuses to read, requests brighter lights, squints when reading, cannot locate nearby objects, or misidentifies other people.

Rationale: As measured by the Snellen chart, vision of 20/30 or below (20/20 or 20/10) is normal. Any higher rating (20/40, 20/50, etc.) indicates impaired vision.

Resolved Needs: Protection from physical harm.

Test the eyes for light sensitivity   Watch for unusual light intolerance, such as squinting, frowning, wearing sunglasses when others don't need them, and complaints of headache.

Rationale: Light sensitivity may occur with inflammatory conditions, vitamin deficiency, or increased intracranial pressure.

Resolved Needs: Protection from physical harm.

Test the infant for the Moro reflex (225)   Suddenly change the infant's position, and provide jarring or loud noise stimuli. Notice whether the infant appears startled, tenses his muscles, makes a wide embracing motion with his arms, and extends his legs.

Rationale: The Moro reflex is normal in children younger than 8 weeks of age. If it lasts beyond 4 months, it may indicate an inability to walk.

Resolved Needs: Protection from physical harm.

Test the infant for the neck-righting reflex   Place the child on his back and turn his head to one side. Normally he will turn his whole body in an effort to maintain alignment with his head. This reflex is normal up to the age of 5 months, but it should disappear between 6 and 8 months of age.

Rationale: When the neck-righting reflex lasts beyond 8 months of age, it may indicate an inability to walk.

Resolved Needs: Protection from physical harm.

Test the infant for the rooting reflex (225)
Touch the infant on the cheek. Normally he will turn his head in the direction of the touch in an effort to find or root for food. When something is placed in his mouth, normally he will suck on it in an effort to obtain food.

Rationale: When the infant does not respond normally with the rooting reflex, this may indicate central nervous system or intracranial injury.

Resolved Needs: Protection from physical harm.

Test the urine for pH
Determine the urine acidity or alkalinity with litmus or Nitrazine paper or other chemical agents. The first morning urine specimen is usually more acidic than any other sample during the day.

Rationale: The urine pH (acidity or alkalinity) has an influence on the tendency to form renal stones.

Resolved Needs: Protection from physical harm.

Test the urine for protein
Use a commercial product such as Combistix or Urostix to determine the presence of protein in the urine.

Rationale: Protein in the urine may indicate impaired kidney function, impending pregnancy toxemia, impending kidney transplant rejection, prostatitis or epididymitis.

Resolved Needs: Protection from physical harm.

Test the urine for sugar and/or acetone
Use a commercial product such as Clinitest, Diastix, or Tes-Tape to determine the presence of sugar in the urine. Use Acetest or Ketostix to determine the presence of acetone in the urine.

Rationale: Sugar in the urine indicates that insulin secretion is insufficient to break down glucose carbohydrates for storage in the liver as energy. This causes sugars to appear in the urine and brings about an acid state. Acetone in the urine indicates that body fat is being used for energy in place of sugar.

Resolved Needs: Protection from physical harm.

Time uterine contractions
Place a warm hand just above the umbilicus and feel the uterus rise in the abdominal cavity, contract, become very hard, and then relax. Count the number of seconds that the uterus remains very hard; this is the duration of a contraction. Determine the interval between contractions by counting the minutes between the beginning of one contraction and the beginning of the next. The relaxation time is the time between the end of one contraction and the beginning of the next.

Rationale: Timing uterine contractions determines whether the uterus is progressing toward cervical dilatation. Uterine contractions will cease completely if there is uterine rupture.

Resolved Needs: Protection from physical harm.

33.
Health Teaching

Advise a gradual return to activity   Suggest that the patient gradually take on more activities. When one activity has been accomplished successfully several times without fatigue, have him take on another.

Rationale: Feelings of comfort and safety arise from an awareness that one can successfully and independently cope with and master the skills of everyday living. The accomplishment of activities without fatigue promotes comfort.

Resolved Needs: Protection from physical harm. Protection from psychologic threat. Adequacy. Independence. Increased learning.

Advise acceptance of the drug user's return home   When a family member has temporarily left the family to join other drug users, but then suddenly wants to return home, suggest that his return be accepted without bitterness and reproach.

Rationale: On realizing his mistake, the young drug user may wish to return to normal life. Acceptance by loved ones allows for a new beginning.

Resolved Needs: Comfort. Protection from psychologic threat. Unity with loved ones. Increased learning.

Advise adherence to the immunization schedule   Suggest that periodic immunizations be maintained according to the recommended schedule of health officials.

Rationale: Immunizations protect against potentially threatening disease.

Resolved Needs: Protection from physical harm. Increased learning.

Advise against causing defensive responses in others
Suggest that the patient never place another person in such a position that the person feels compelled to protect his sense of pride. This can only result in defensive behavior.

Rationale: Behavior based on defensive attitudes is often socially unacceptable; it can result in shame or guilt at a later time.

Resolved Needs: Protection from psychologic threat. Personal growth and maturity. Increased learning. Increased reality perception and problem-solving ability.

Advise against chewing gum
Suggest that gum chewing be avoided when the patient suffers from excessive flatulence.

Rationale: As gum is chewed, air is swallowed and added to intestinal gases, further increasing flatulence and the associated pressure discomfort.

Resolved Needs: Comfort. Protection from physical harm. Increased learning.

Advise against committing alcoholics to promises of sobriety
Suggest that the family not ask the alcoholic to promise that he will stop drinking.

Rationale: If an alcoholic promises not to drink and then breaks the promise, he suffers guilt feelings and loss of self-respect, which further promote drinking.

Resolved Needs: Comfort. Increased learning.

Advise against communicating double-meaning messages
Suggest that messages that convey conflicts of feeling be avoided. Point out that it is unwise to make such statements as these: "I know you're capable, but I doubt you can meet the challenge." "Your friend is a fine person, but you're not to associate with him."

Rationale: Double-meaning messages cause confusion and doubt. They do not convey a single clear meaning, and they render the receiver unable to determine the real intent of the message and unable to determine an appropriate response.

Resolved Needs: Protection from psychologic threat. Personal growth and maturity. Increased learning. Increased reality perception and problem-solving ability.

Advise against correlating God's love and death to children
Suggest that a child not be told that a family member was taken to heaven because God loved him.

Rationale: Loss of a loved one causes anger; if the loss is associated with God, it can result in anger toward God, with the potential for depression and anxiety over moral conflict.

Resolved Needs: Protection from psychologic threat. Increased learning.

Advise against denouncing erroneous perceptions
When delusional, illusional, or hallucinational ideas are expressed, suggest that they should not be laughed at and that the person expressing them should not be

told he is "crazy" or is mistaken. Instead, it should be made known to him that he has a right to his feelings, but that others may not agree with him.

Rationale: When persons are told that they are mistaken about their perceptions, they are threatened with confusion, anxiety, and fear. Acceptance associated with disagreement supports a return to realistic perception.

Resolved Needs: Protection from psychologic threat. Increased reality perception. Increased learning.

Advise against drawing secretions to the back of the throat   Suggest that nasal secretions not be drawn to the back of the throat, but be removed by blowing the nose.

Rationale: Drawing secretions to the back of the throat causes pressure changes on sinus tissue and pulls fluid into the sinuses. If the secretions are infectious and the material is swallowed into the digestive tract, this increases the potential for generalized infection.

Resolved Needs: Protection from physical harm. Increased learning.

Advise against driving at night   Suggest that persons with night blindness avoid driving after dark, even for short distances.

Rationale: Driving with impaired vision heightens the potential for injury.

Resolved Needs: Protection from physical harm. Increased learning.

Advise against eating dairy products in foreign countries   Suggest that persons traveling to foreign countries avoid milk, ice cream, cream sauces, or soft cheeses.

Rationale: In some foreign countries milk is not pasteurized, and it can cause intestinal distress to persons unaccustomed to raw milk.

Resolved Needs: Protection from physical harm. Increased learning.

Advise against eating in unlicensed restaurants   Suggest that one look for a license from the local health authority on the wall of a restaurant before eating there.

Rationale: To receive a license to operate, a restaurant must meet sanitation standards.

Resolved Needs: Protection from physical harm. Increased learning.

Advise against eating raw fruits and vegetables in foreign countries   Suggest to persons traveling to foreign countries that raw fruits and vegetables not be eaten. Only those that are well cooked are safe.

Rationale: Many foreign countries use human excreta for fertilizing fruits and vegetables; this increases food contamination with dysentery organisms. Hygienic standards for food handling in many foreign countries are low.

Resolved Needs: Protection from physical harm. Increased learning.

Advise against eating sweets   Suggest that sweets be avoided. This includes sugar, candy, honey, jam, jelly, marmalade, syrups, pies, cakes, cookies, pastries, condensed milk, soft drinks, and candy-coated gum.

Rationale: Since the diabetic pancreas fails to produce sufficient insulin to metabolize glucose adequately, foods high in glucose are not converted into energy, but instead disrupt metabolic equilibrium. A sugar environment on the teeth promotes bacterial growth, which leads to decay.

Resolved Needs: Protection from physical harm. Increased learning.

Advise against emphasizing past problems caused by another   Suggest that it is inadvisable to remind another person that he was the cause of past failures or unpleasant experiences.

Rationale: Being reminded of one's past failures reinforces feelings of guilt and shame and supports defensive behavior.

Resolved Needs: Comfort. Protection from psychologic threat. Adequacy. Personal growth and maturity. Increased learning. Increased reality perception and problem-solving ability.

Advise against exposure to airborne irritants   Suggest that persons with allergies or artificial airways avoid environments where dust levels or pollen counts are high. If airborne irritants are unavoidable, suggest that a mask of filtering material be worn over the nose or artificial airway.

Rationale: Respiratory irritation may stimulate coughing, cause bronchial spasm, or injure tissue.

Resolved Needs: Comfort. Protection from physical harm. Increased learning.

Advise against exposure to inclement weather   Suggest that cold, windy, or damp weather be avoided in nonhealth conditions.

Rationale: Cold weather causes vasoconstriction and increases cardiac workload as the heart pumps blood through constricted vessels. Cold decreases the metabolic rate. Cold causes bronchoconstriction causing dyspnea.

Resolved Needs: Comfort. Protection from physical harm. Increased learning.

Advise against exposure to intense heat   Suggest that an effort be made to avoid high environmental temperatures and hot objects.

Rationale: Intense environmental heat causes vasodilatation and sluggish blood flow which, in impaired cardiac function, overtaxes the heart; increases the metabolic rate causing energy consumption and malaise; and alters fluid and electrolyte balance by increasing perspiration. Sunrays and contact with hot objects can cause severe skin burns.

Resolved Needs: Normal temperature. Comfort. Protection from physical harm. Increased learning.

Advise against fighting fear (or anxiety)   Explain that a mental effort to fight fear or anxiety reinforces the emotion and maintains focus on it. Fear is best conquered by facing the cause of the fear and using logic and constructive thinking.

Rationale: Since fear and anxiety stem from a sense of helplessness in the face of danger, fighting fear and anxiety merely reinforces that sense of helplessness, while logical thinking supports adequacy through realistic perception of the danger.

Resolved Needs: Comfort. Protection from psychologic threat. Personal growth and maturity. Increased learning. Increased reality perception and problem-solving ability.

Advise against giving toys likely to cause eye injury   Explain that toys such as pointed sticks, bows and arrows, BB guns, fireworks, and slingshots can cause eye accidents and should be given only to children who are old enough to handle them.

Rationale: Eye injury may cause diminished vision or blindness.

Resolved Needs: Protection from physical harm. Increased learning.

Advise against gulping food and drink   Suggest that food and drink not be swallowed rapidly in large amounts at one time.

Rationale: While gulping food and drink, large amounts of air are carried into the stomach and added to intestinal gases. This further increases flatulence and the associated pressure discomfort. Gulping food and drink heightens the potential for aspiration.

Resolved Needs: Comfort. Protection from physical harm. Increased learning.

Advise against intense surveillance of the drug user   Suggest that parents who suspect their child of using drugs avoid searching through personal possessions, listening in on telephone conversations, and monitoring mail.

Rationale: When persons are aware that they are being watched, they begin to distrust those who are watching them, and communication may be seriously threatened.

Resolved Needs: Protection from psychologic threat. Warm, communicating relationships. Increased learning.

Advise against letting light shine directly into the eyes   Suggest that light never be allowed to shine directly into the eyes and that light bulbs always be shaded.

Rationale: Reduced glare can prevent damage to optic tissue and nerves.

Resolved Needs: Comfort. Protection from physical harm. Increased learning.

Advise against making emotional appeals to the alcoholic
Suggest that the family avoid appeals such as these: "Will you stop drinking out of love for me?" "If you cared for your family, you'd stop drinking."

Rationale: Emotional appeals to the alcoholic who cannot stop drinking increase his sense of guilt, which in turn supports further drinking.

Resolved Needs: Comfort. Increased learning.

Advise against making excuses for the alcoholic
Suggest that the family not try to cover up the real reason why the alcoholic hasn't gone to work or met other commitments.

Rationale: Encouraging the alcoholic to employ readily available excuses fosters behavior disorders.

Resolved Needs: Increased learning. Increased reality perception and problem-solving ability.

Advise against mingling in crowds
Suggest that the patient stay away from crowds and from persons with infections.

Rationale: Exposure to crowds enhances the potential for infection.

Resolved Needs: Protection from physical harm. Increased learning.

Advise against participation in emotional situations before sleep
Suggest that the patient not become involved in emotionally induced tension just before going to bed.

Rationale: The stimulus of emotional tension promotes wakefulness, disrupting needed sleep. Emotional situations that excite the child prior to sleep can cause enuresis.

Resolved Needs: Sleep, rest, relaxation. Comfort. Protection from physical harm. Increased learning.

Advise against piercing lesions
Suggest that skin lesions not be opened with objects such as pins, needles, and the like. If a lesion has come to a head, it should be incised and drained with sterile technique by qualified persons.

Rationale: Opening skin lesions may traumatize underlying tissue, cause bleeding, and result in the introduction of bacteria into the open wound.

Resolved Needs: Protection from physical harm. Increased learning.

Advise against prolonged skin (or scalp) exposure to the sun
Suggest that prolonged body exposure to the sun's rays be avoided.

Rationale: Prolonged exposure to the sun's rays activates melanin pigment and discolors and burns the skin.

Resolved Needs: Comfort. Protection from physical harm. Increased learning.

Advise against prolonged skin (or scalp) exposure to water   Suggest that the skin not be exposed to water, especially salty or chemically treated water, for prolonged periods.

Rationale: Prolonged exposure to water removes natural skin oils and causes skin irritation.

Resolved Needs: Comfort. Protection from physical harm. Increased learning.

Advise against pulling off dead skin (or scabs)   When underlying skin has not adequately healed, or when scabs have formed over a wound, suggest that dead skin or scabs not be pulled off. Skin should be removed only if healing is adequate, and no discomfort or bleeding should result. Scabs should be allowed to fall off.

Rationale: Pulling off dead skin or scabs before they are ready to fall off may traumatize the underlying skin, cause pain and bleeding, and permit the entrance of bacteria into the open wound.

Resolved Needs: Comfort. Protection from physical harm. Increased learning.

Advise against questioning the alcoholic about drinking   Suggest that it is inadvisable to question the alcoholic about whether he has been drinking.

Rationale: If an alcoholic has been drinking, it will soon become evident; the distrust aroused by questioning him will increase his anxiety, thus precipitating further drinking.

Resolved Needs: Protection from psychologic threat. Increased learning. Increased reality perception and problem-solving ability.

Advise against reading or looking out the window while in a moving vehicle   Suggest that reading or looking out the window while riding in a car, airplane, boat, or train be avoided if one is prone to motion sickness.

Rationale: The eye movement that occurs when reading or when watching passing scenery increases motion stimuli to the medulla, thus raising the potential for motion sickness.

Resolved Needs: Protection from physical harm. Increased learning.

Advise against removing the alcoholic's liquor supply   Suggest that the family not throw away or hide liquor from the alcoholic.

Rationale: Once the alcoholic realizes that his liquor supply is threatened, he will resort to deceptive practices to assure an available supply.

Resolved Needs: Protection from psychologic threat. Increased learning. Increased reality perception and problem-solving ability.

Advise against responding to gesture speech Suggest that parents who have children with delayed or impaired speech patterns respond only to verbal communications, not to gesturing or jargon.

Rationale: When children become aware that adults respond only to verbal communications, they will find it essential to develop appropriate speech skills.

Resolved Needs: Warm, communicating relationships. Mastery and competence in skills. Increased learning.

Advise against scratching Suggest that an effort be made to avoid scratching skin that itches; substitute methods such as dabbing the itch with an alcohol sponge or applying a cool cloth or ice cubes.

Rationale: Scratching further irritates already inflamed oversensitive skin. Reduced scratching can diminish skin irritation and promote comfort.

Resolved Needs: Comfort. Protection from physical harm. Increased learning.

Advise against squeezing the skin (or lesion) Suggest that skin pustules not be squeezed. To hasten their removal, the skin should be thoroughly washed and heat should be applied, allowing pustules to dry naturally.

Rationale: Squeezing the skin bruises and traumatizes tissue and may force pathogenic microorganisms into the bloodstream.

Resolved Needs: Protection from physical harm. Increased learning.

Advise against threatening the alcoholic Suggest that the family not threaten, argue with, or put intense pressure on the alcoholic in an effort to stop his drinking.

Rationale: When severely threatened, the alcoholic may respond with violence.

Resolved Needs: Increased learning. Increased reality perception and problem-solving ability.

Advise against using ice cubes made from potentially unsafe water Suggest that ice cubes never be used in drinks if they are made with water that might be contaminated. For cooling, set the glass or container in a bucket of ice with the ice around it, not in it.

Rationale: Freezing contaminated water does not destroy bacteria.

Resolved Needs: Protection from physical harm. Increased learning.

Advise against using mineral oil laxatives Suggest that chronic use of mineral oil laxatives be avoided.

Rationale: Mineral oil in the intestinal tract interferes with absorption of fat-soluble vitamins, especially vitamins A and K.

Resolved Needs: Protection from physical harm. Increased learning.

Advise against using tampons   Suggest that tampons not be used whenever there is an infectious vaginal discharge, when the patient has undergone a hysterectomy, or when there is nonmenstrual vaginal bleeding.

Rationale: Tampons obstruct the flow of an infectious vaginal discharge and prevent proper drainage. Following a hysterectomy, tampons irritate the incised vagina.

Resolved Needs: Protection from physical harm. Increased learning.

Advise against verbally comparing significant persons
Suggest that verbal comparisons of the qualities of significant persons be avoided. If evaluation is necessary, it should be confined to one person.

Rationale: Comparisons with others may promote feelings of inadequacy. Comfort feelings require that a person experience acceptance from others and relatedness to others.

Resolved Needs: Comfort. Protection from psychologic threat. Increased learning. Increased reality perception and problem-solving ability.

Advise against walking barefoot   Explain that bare feet are subject to injury and infection.

Rationale: Walking barefoot subjects one to injury from sharp objects, to the larvae of fecal worms present in the soil, to insect and snake bites, and to poisonous plants and fungus growths.

Resolved Needs: Protection from physical harm. Increased learning.

Advise against wearing constrictive clothing   Suggest that tight clothing such as girdles, hatbands, belts, ties, and garters either not be worn or be fastened loosely.

Rationale: Constriction prevents adequate venous return, and this impairs blood circulation and results in tissue damage.

Resolved Needs: Protection from physical harm. Increased learning.

Advise against wearing unprescribed eyeglasses   Suggest that eyeglasses manufactured for general use or those prescribed for another person not be worn.

Rationale: Unprescribed eyeglasses may cause eye damage because the correction in the glass may be inappropriate to the visual problem.

Resolved Needs: Protection from physical harm. Increased learning.

Advise against whispering around ill persons   Suggest that persons visiting a sick patient refrain from speaking in whispers.

Rationale: Whispering between two visitors can contribute to tension in the patient and lead to misinterpretation. The patient knows that something is being said, but can only guess what it is.

Resolved Needs: Comfort. Increased learning.

Advise an annual gynecologic examination Suggest that a yearly examination of the female reproductive organs and a vaginal smear be done. This is especially important for women who have had children.

Rationale: Annual physical examinations are a means of early disease detection.

Resolved Needs: Protection from physical harm. Increased learning.

Advise daily bathing Suggest that a bath be taken daily to maintain cleanliness.

Rationale: Cleanliness prevents bacterial growth and promotes comfort.

Resolved Needs: Comfort. Cleanliness. Protection from physical harm. Increased learning.

Contraindications: When a person has excessively dry skin, a complete bath and a partial bath should be taken on alternate days.

Advise daily hair brushing Suggest that the hair be brushed each day, preferably with the head down.

Rationale: Hair brushing stimulates circulation and normal secretion of sebaceous glands, removes dirt particles and dead scalp cells, and promotes comfort.

Resolved Needs: Comfort. Cleanliness. Protection from physical harm. Increased learning.

Advise early and consistent use of the toothbrush Suggest that a child be taught to use a toothbrush just as soon as teeth appear.

Rationale: Brushing the teeth removes food particles, reduces the potential for decay, and provides the comfort of a refreshed mouth.

Resolved Needs: Cleanliness. Protection from physical harm. Increased learning.

Advise early correction of problems Suggest that small health problems be corrected as soon as they are noticed.

Rationale: If corrected in their early stages, most problems cause minimal discomfort and never have cumulative effects.

Resolved Needs: Protection from physical harm. Protection from psychologic threat. Increased learning.

Advise early replacement of lost teeth Suggest that natural teeth be replaced as soon as possible after they are lost.

Rationale: When lost teeth are not replaced, the remaining teeth become disarranged and the gum structure changes. Teeth are essential to chewing food and to adequate digestion.

Resolved Needs: Comfort. Protection from physical harm. Increased learning.

Advise frequent and early dental attention   As soon as a child has fully developed teeth, suggest that they receive dental attention at least once a year and preferably every 6 months.

Rationale: Early recognition and treatment of caries can prevent the spread of caries.

Resolved Needs: Protection from physical harm. Increased learning.

Advise frequent nose blowing   Suggest that the patient blow his nose gently and often during the day. Every 2 hours is recommended when there is increased secretion flow.

Rationale: Frequent nose blowing removes excessive secretions before they can drip down the back of the throat.

Resolved Needs: Comfort. Protection from physical harm. Increased learning.

Contraindications: Nasal trauma. Epistaxis.

Advise frequent sanitary pad change   Suggest that clean perineal pads be applied every few hours when there is an infectious vaginal discharge.

Rationale: Cleanliness prevents the spread of infection and promotes comfort.

Resolved Needs: Comfort. Cleanliness. Protection from physical harm. Increased learning.

Advise gentle nose blowing   Suggest that the nose be blown with minimum force or pressure.

Rationale: Harsh nose blowing irritates the nasal mucous membrane and forces infected material into the ears and sinuses.

Resolved Needs: Protection from physical harm. Increased learning.

Advise handwashing after elimination   Suggest that the hands be washed thoroughly with soap and water after each bowel or urinary elimination.

Rationale: Cleanliness through handwashing prevents the spread of infection from one body part to another and from person to person.

Resolved Needs: Cleanliness. Protection from physical harm. Increased learning.

Advise handwashing before meals   Suggest that the hands be washed thoroughly with soap and water before each meal.

Rationale: Cleanliness through handwashing prevents infection and promotes comfort.

Resolved Needs: Cleanliness. Protection from physical harm. Increased learning.

Advise limited talking When the patient's throat is irritated, suggest that he avoid speaking except for essentials. When the patient talks excessively, suggest that he limit his speaking to brief conversation.

Rationale: Excessive talking irritates the vocal cords, and when associated with vocal cord disease, it can permanently damage speech. Excessive talking can irritate other people and reduce favorable social responses.

Resolved Needs: Protection from physical harm. Protection from psychologic threat. Increased learning.

Advise limited use of hair spray Suggest that hair spray be used in small quantities or not at all when scalp and hair problems exist.

Rationale: Hair sprays may irritate scalp tissue, damage hair follicles, and contribute to uncleanliness.

Resolved Needs: Cleanliness. Protection from physical harm. Increased learning.

Advise limited use of powder on the infant's skin When dusting powder is being applied to an infant's skin, suggest that the powder be sprinkled onto the mother's hands; her hands should then be rubbed together lightly, removing excess powder, and rubbed over the baby's skin, leaving only a light film.

Rationale: Heavy layers of dusting powder on the skin tend to cake in skin folds and irritate the skin surface. Sprinkling powder directly on the baby causes inhalation of powder particles, which results in respiratory irritation.

Resolved Needs: Comfort. Protection from physical harm. Increased learning.

Advise minimal infant handling Suggest that irritable infants be handled only when it is absolutely necessary and at other times be left undisturbed.

Rationale: Decreasing the external stimuli reduces the need for adaptive responses, promotes sleep, and decreases energy depletion.

Resolved Needs: Protection from physical harm. Protection from psychologic threat. Increased learning.

Advise moderation in douching Explain that it is not necessary to douche daily, after menstruation, or after sexual intercourse. Douching should be used only for cleanliness and therapeutic purposes.

Rationale: Consistent douching may lead to vaginal irritation. Since douching removes the natural vaginal flora, it increases the potential for vaginal infection from other organisms.

Resolved Needs: Protection from physical harm. Increased learning.

Advise mouth rinsing when brushing is inconvenient When
one is unable to brush his teeth after each meal, suggest that the mouth be
rinsed with water.

Rationale: Removing food particles from the teeth reduces the potential
for decay and provides the comfort of a refreshed mouth.

Resolved Needs: Comfort. Cleanliness. Protection from physical harm.
Increased learning.

Advise not to drive for three hours after two alcoholic
drinks Suggest that one not drive any sooner than 3 hours after ingesting
two alcoholic drinks.

Rationale: Oxidation of alcohol in the blood takes 3 hours to occur. Before
this oxidation is accomplished, the nervous system experiences impaired
perception and motor skills.

Resolved Needs: Protection from physical harm. Increased learning.

Advise not to drive for three months after cardiac illness
onset Suggest that a person not tax his heart with the stress of automobile driving before there has been sufficient time for tissue healing.

Rationale: Maneuvering a car involves considerable physical exertion, as
well as toleration of frustration and stress. During cardiac healing, when
necrotic tissue is being replaced with new scar tissue, the damaged area is
weak, and excessive stress could result in ruptured tissue or development of
an aneurysm.

Resolved Needs: Protection from physical harm. Increased learning.

Advise not to partake of very hot or cold foods and
drinks Suggest that very hot or cold foods and drinks be avoided and
that warm foods and drinks be chosen instead.

Rationale: Extreme temperatures in food and drink can cause injury to
oral and gastric tissue. Very hot food or drink can cause vasodilatation, and
coldness can cause vasoconstriction.

Resolved Needs: Circulation. Normal temperature. Comfort. Protection
from physical harm. Increased learning.

Advise not to stand for prolonged periods Suggest that standing
be limited to short periods or alternated with walking or sitting.

Rationale: Prolonged standing causes blood pooling in the lower extremities, which reduces circulation throughout the body. Prolonged standing puts pressure on the venous system, predisposing to varicosities. Standing puts pressure on hemorrhoids, and if they are severe, standing can precipitate bleeding.

Resolved Needs: Circulation. Comfort. Protection from physical harm. Increased learning.

Advise not to take enemas and laxatives   Suggest that it is inadvisable to take enemas and laxatives habitually for bowel elimination and that they should not be taken when there is abdominal pain or vaginal bleeding.

Rationale: Frequent use of enemas and laxatives gradually makes the intestinal mucosa insensitive to normal elimination stimulation and decreases the normal muscle tone required for elimination. When there is abdominal pain, the pressure caused by enemas and laxatives may precipitate organ rupture; when there is vaginal bleeding, the pressure may precipitate hemorrhage.

Resolved Needs: Protection from physical harm. Increased learning.

Advise not to take hot baths   Suggest that lukewarm baths, not hot baths, be taken. A bath is too hot when it reddens the skin.

Rationale: Hot baths cause vasodilatation, which can reduce blood pressure in persons subject to hypotension and can cause engorgement of scalp vessels, resulting in increased headache pain.

Resolved Needs: Normal temperature. Protection from physical harm. Increased learning.

Advise not to use a harsh dentifrice   Point out that toothpastes and tooth powders should never cause excessive friction and should bear the mark of approval of the American Dental Association.

Rationale: Harsh dentifrices traumatize the gums.

Resolved Needs: Protection from physical harm. Increased learning.

Advise not to use adhesive tape on the skin   Suggest that adhesive tape not be used for prolonged periods and not be used at all on tender skin. Transparent or paper tape is more appropriate.

Rationale: The sticky surface of adhesive tape irritates skin tissue; when it must be removed frequently from tender skin, it pulls off the surface layer of skin.

Resolved Needs: Protection from physical harm. Increased learning.

Advise not to use an electric blanket   Explain that electric blankets should not be used on small children or on anyone who has experienced loss of heat sensation.

Rationale: When the skin cannot perceive heat correctly, serious burns can result from electric blankets.

Resolved Needs: Protection from physical harm. Increased learning.

Advise occasional respite from responsibility Explain that the stress of responsibility can be reduced if a person is relieved of responsibility by others at reasonable intervals.

Rational: Occasional relief from intense stress is essential to physical and emotional health.

Resolved Needs: Comfort. Protection from physical harm. Protection from psychologic threat. Increased learning.

Advise periodic examinations for known hereditary predispositions Suggest that persons whose blood relatives have diabetes, hypertension, and other genetically transmitted diseases have frequent examinations to determine early evidence of disease.

Rationale: Early treatment tends to be more successful than treatment administered after the disease has become serious.

Resolved Needs: Protection from physical harm. Increased learning.

Advise precaution when using chemicals Whenever and for whatever purpose chemicals are used, suggest that they be used with extreme care. This includes strong household cleaning agents such as those containing poison, lye, lime, or ammonia.

Rationale: Exercising caution when using chemicals can prevent physical injury.

Resolved Needs: Protection from physical harm. Increased learning.

Advise proper focusing of the television picture Explain that the television picture should be properly adjusted for visual clarity.

Rationale: An improperly adjusted television picture places strain on the eyes.

Resolved Needs: Comfort. Protection from physical harm. Increased learning.

Advise that a poor prognosis be shared with significant others Suggest that it is best not to keep a poor prognosis secret from the ill person and other family members.

Rationale: Sharing the information that there is a poor prognosis gives family members the satisfaction and consolation of reaching acceptance together and supporting one another.

Resolved Needs: Protection from psychologic threat. Unity with loved ones. Endurance. Increased learning.

Contraindications: Sometimes it is best to delay telling a severely ill family member of the poor prognosis of another family member.

Advise that between-meal snacks be avoided   Explain to over-
weight persons that between-meal snacks add carbohydrates and calories to their daily food intake, thus increasing body weight.

Rationale: Intake of calories should equal energy expenditure if weight gain is to be avoided.

Resolved Needs: Protection from physical harm. Increased learning.

Contraindications: Increased metabolic rate, as with fever, burns, or hyperthyroidism.

Advise that children participate in grief-related activities
Suggest that children be included in activities that occur following the death of a family member. This includes visiting dying relatives.

Rationale: Participation by children in the family's expression of grief reassures them that they are not alone with their feelings; it provides comfort and enhances their perception of death as a part of life.

Resolved Needs: Comfort. Protection from psychologic threat. Unity with loved ones. Personal growth and maturity. Increased learning.

Advise that communication be delayed during fatigue   Suggest
that important messages be delayed whenever an ill person becomes temporarily fatigued.

Rationale: Messages received during a state of fatigue are poorly perceived. If the message is unpleasant, the potential for stress is increased by the fatigue.

Resolved Needs: Protection from physical harm. Protection from psychologic threat. Increased learning.

Advise that contact lenses not be used for eye color
change   Explain that contact lenses should be worn only for therapeutic correction of visual disorders and never for esthetic eye coloring.

Rationale: Whenever an object is placed in the eye, there is risk of corneal injury.

Resolved Needs: Protection from physical harm. Increased learning.

Advise that discipline be consistent   Suggest that discipline be
consistently firm and that it be such that the child can easily relate it to unacceptable behavior. The use of discipline on one occasion, while letting the same behavior go undisciplined on other occasions, is to be discouraged.

Rationale: Familiar and predictable situations support learning, comfort, and safety feelings.

Resolved Needs: Comfort. Protection from psychologic threat. Predictable, orderly world. Personal growth and maturity. Increased learning. Increased reality perception and problem-solving ability.

Advise that fresh foods be thoroughly washed   Explain that raw fruits and vegetables should be soaked in clear water and scrubbed clean.

Rationale: Washing raw fruits and vegetables removes dirt particles and bacteria, thus reducing the potential for intestinal disturbances.

Resolved Needs: Protection from physical harm. Increased learning.

Advise that highly emotional situations be avoided   Suggest that situations that tend to arouse intense emotions be avoided, whenever possible, by those with certain health disorders.

Rationale: Intense emotions stimulate adrenal secretions, which affect cardiovascular, respiratory and gastric activity.

Resolved Needs: Protection from physical harm. Protection from psychologic threat. Increased learning.

Advise that infants be started on solid foods no later than six months   Explain that infants should be on solid foods no later than 6 months of age and that the foods should be rich in iron and protein. Such foods include fruits, vegetables, meats, and eggs.

Rationale: At the age of 6 months an infant's iron reserves are depleted and need nutritional restoration. Protein foods are essential for rapid growth.

Resolved Needs: Food balance. Protection from physical harm. Increased learning.

Advise that lanolin be applied to brittle nails   Suggest that lanolin be applied under the cuticles and around the nail area.

Rationale: Lanolin softens the nail and surrounding area, decreases skin cracking, and facilitates healing.

Resolved Needs: Protection from physical harm. Increased learning.

Advise that mental stimulation be maintained through variety   Suggest that fatigue be reduced by going to new places and seeing and doing new and different things.

Rationale: Fatigue results from energy-depleting responses to stress stimuli. New interests promote temporary escape from stress and interrupt habitual thought patterns.

Resolved Needs: Energy. Comfort. Increased learning. Increased reality perception and problem-solving ability.

Advise that negative responses from others be regarded with minimum significance   Suggest that negative responses from others are relatively unimportant if the person's behavior has satisfied his inner

1576   ADVISE THAT NORMAL, NOT ACCENTUATED, LIP MOVEMENTS BE USED

self and has met personal value commitments. Suggest that such negative responses might sometimes serve as clues to self-improvement but that they should not be dwelled on at length.

Rationale: A positive self-image is nourished by the achievement of goals that the person perceives as important.

Resolved Needs: Comfort. Protection from psychologic threat. High evaluation of self. Adequacy. Increased learning.

Advise that normal, not accentuated, lip movements be used when speaking to deaf persons
Suggest that normal lip movements be used when speaking to a deaf person and that accentuated pronunciations be avoided.

Rationale: Deaf persons are taught to read normal lip movements. Accentuated pronunciations confuse the lip reader and impair message reception.

Resolved Needs: Comfort. Warm, communicating relationships. Increased learning.

Advise that others should not assume the alcoholic's responsibilities
Suggest that, whenever possible, families refrain from performing those duties and obligations that are the responsibility of the alcoholic.

Rationale: When the family assumes the alcoholic's responsibilities, his sense of value and usefulness is diminished.

Resolved Needs: Comfort. Sense of value, usefulness. Increased learning.

Advise that persons attending the sick economize their energies
Suggest that it is better for several persons to stay for short periods with a patient than for one person to remain continuously at the bedside.

Rationale: The capacity to function is most effective when there is a balance between serving others and meeting one's own needs. One cannot function well under the stress of constant awareness of illness.

Resolved Needs: Rest, relaxation. Protection from physical harm. Protection from psychologic threat. Increased learning.

Advise that positions which impair circulation be avoided
Suggest that prolonged knee bending, leg crossing, standing, and pressure behind the knee be avoided.

Rationale: Positions that compress the veins or that decrease muscle activity impair venous flow and promote thrombosis.

Resolved Needs: Circulation. Comfort. Protection from physical harm. Freedom from pain. Increased learning.

Advise that significant persons express acceptance of one another
Suggest that persons who care for each other openly communi-

cate to one another that each perceives the other as a person of worth simply because he is a unique person.

Rationale: Psychologic safety requires that a person be aware that he has worth simply because he is himself and that his worth will continue even when his behavior is unacceptable.

Resolved Needs: Comfort. Protection from psychologic threat. High evaluation of self. Increased learning.

Advise that significant persons express love for one another
Suggest that persons who care for each other communicate their love and affection through words, through loving gestures of touch, through gift giving, and through general respect for one another.

Rationale: Psychologic comfort is promoted through communicated love and affection. Unity with significant others increases one's self-esteem and sense of value.

Resolved Needs: Comfort. Protection from psychologic threat. Love and affection. Warm, communicating relationships. Unity with loved ones. Sense of value, usefulness. High evaluation of self. Personal growth and maturity. Increased learning. Increased reality perception and problem-solving ability.

Advise that the alcoholic's illness be discussed only during sobriety
Suggest that the family of the alcoholic not discuss the problem while the alcoholic is intoxicated. They should discuss it with him only when he is sober.

Rationale: During intoxication the alcoholic cannot respond favorably or decisively to attempts at correcting the situation.

Resolved Needs: Comfort. Increased learning. Increased reality perception and problem-solving ability.

Advise that the precipitating factor be avoided
Suggest that the person stay away from foods, drugs, situations, environments, etc., that bring about disruption of health.

Rationale: By avoiding factors that can cause poor health states, the chance for good health is increased.

Resolved Needs: Protection from physical harm. Increased learning.

Advise that the responsibility for drug abuse be placed on the abuser, not on other persons
Suggest that it be made clear to the drug user that his abuse involves a rational decision that he alone has made, one that can affect the course of his life. Do not allow him to excuse his abuse as an uncontrollable result of life's traumas.

Rationale: Being held responsible for one's decisions usually precipitates careful consideration or reevaluation of those decisions.

Resolved Needs: Protection from psychologic threat. Increased learning. Increased reality perception and problem-solving ability.

Advise that the television be viewed from the front, not from the side angles   Suggest that the television viewer adjust his sitting position so that the set is at eye level and can be viewed directly in front of him.

Rationale: Viewing television at side angles or from heights above or below eye level causes fatigue of eye and neck muscles.

Resolved Needs: Comfort. Protection from physical harm. Increased learning.

Advise that toilet training failures be ignored   Suggest that failure to control elimination during the period of toilet training be overlooked and that punishment and disapproving communications be avoided.

Rationale: Learning is more easily acquired in a positive environment.

Resolved Needs: Comfort. Increased learning.

Correct misinformation regarding breast feeding   Many untruths about breast feeding have been passed down from generation to generation. Whenever possible, correct such misinformation. Explain that breast size does not affect the amount of lactation, that properly supported breasts will maintain good shape, that neither cesarean section nor Rh factor has any effect on breast feeding, that drugs should be avoided during breast feeding, and that balanced nutrition is essential during lactation.

Rationale: Misinformation about breast feeding may deprive the mother and child of the advantages it offers.

Resolved Needs: Comfort. Protection from physical harm. Increased learning.

Describe the behavior pattern indicating affection deprivation   Explain that the signs that indicate a person is, or feels he is, lacking love include verbal expressions of being unloved, withdrawal, seeking affection from insignificant persons, and frequent weeping.

Rationale: Feeling loved is essential to psychologic safety and comfort.

Resolved Needs: Protection from psychologic threat. Increased learning. Increased reality perception and problem-solving ability.

Describe the behavior pattern indicating drug abuse (21)   Explain the general clues that can alert one to drug dependence in another:
   Sudden changes of behavior to patterns that are out of character with previous conduct
   Sudden changes in discipline and job performance
   Unusual activity or inactivity
   Sudden displays of emotion or temper
   Indifference toward personal appearance
   Guarding personal possessions

Wearing sunglasses and long-sleeved clothes at inappropriate times and places

Frequent borrowing of money or stealing when unable to borrow

More specific clues include:

Glue sniffing; odor of glue on breath and clothes; excessive secretion from nasal and oral mucous membranes; red, watering eyes; carrying of plastic or paper bags or handkerchiefs containing plastic cement; intoxicated appearance, poor motor control, double vision, tinnitus, with drowsiness, stupor, or unconsciousness following use of glue

Use of depressants (barbiturates or tranquilizers): staggering or stumbling; falling into a deep sleep; lack of interest; disorientation; no alcohol on breath

Use of stimulants (amphetamines and related drugs): excessive activity, irritability, argumentativeness, nervousness; inability to sit still; dilated pupils; frequent licking of lips to overcome mouth dryness; long periods without sleeping or eating

Use of narcotics (paregoric, heroin, etc.): red, raw nostrils when inhaling powdered narcotics; injection marks along veins in the feet and ankles as well as arms; availability of injection equipment; lethargy or drowsiness; pupil constriction

Use of marijuana (pot): loud, rapid talking with excessive bursts of laughter, followed by stupor or sleep; dilated pupils; odor of burned rope on breath and clothing

Use of hallucinogens (LSD): sitting in a dreamlike or trancelike state; possibly extreme fearfulness

Rationale: Early recognition of behavior patterns indicating drug abuse can lead to early treatment.

Resolved Needs: Protection from physical harm. Protection from psychologic threat. Increased learning.

Describe the behavior pattern indicating early-, intermediate-, and late-stage alcohol abuse

Explain that the early symptoms of alcohol dependence include drinking at regular times each day, eating irregularly, breaking promises, lying about drinking, gulping drinks, drinking before a party starts, and making excuses for drinking. The intermediate symptoms include carrying a secret supply of alcohol, eating irregularly, frequent intoxication, (especially on weekends), nervousness, missing work because of drinking, minimizing drinking, and unusual behavior. The late symptoms include drinking alone, drinking in the morning, irritability, frequent and severe episodes of intoxication, loss of job, substituting alcohol for food, severe family discord, delirium tremens, and deficiency diseases.

Rationale: Recognition of harmful behavior promotes safety and increases reality perception.

Resolved Needs: Protection from physical harm. Protection from psychologic threat. Increased learning. Increased reality perception and problem-solving ability.

Describe the behavior pattern indicating emotional maturity
Explain that emotional maturity is reflected by many factors: being able to give to others without expecting gain; feeling entitled to and being able to accept love; being able to acknowledge that love is important but that it is not the solution to everything; feeling confident when accepting a challenge; being able to admit defeat; being able to lead others without dominating them; feeling comfortable when others receive attention; welcoming responsibility; genuinely enjoying the world; recognizing that one can take care of oneself and others; accepting the fact that everyone can't be expected to like oneself; feeling comfortable when alone; being able to make undelayed, independent decisions; being able to balance work and recreation; commiting oneself to values; being able to work harmoniously with others; being able to save and spend in moderation; being able to accept and learn from criticism; being able to accept parenthood when married; being able to establish close emotional ties and still remain independent.

Rationale: Awareness of normal patterns of behavior promotes comfort and provides motivation toward such behavior.

Resolved Needs: Comfort. Protection from psychologic threat. Personal growth and maturity. Increased learning. Increased reality perception and problem-solving ability.

Describe the behavior pattern indicating overstimulation
Explain that when the nervous system is overstimulated, palpitations, tremors, fatigue, insomnia, confusion, irritability, and panicky feelings occur.

Rationale: Awareness of harmful behavior patterns promotes safety and increased reality perception.

Resolved Needs: Protection from physical harm. Protection from psychologic threat. Increased learning. Increased reality perception and problem-solving ability.

Describe the breast changes expected during pregnancy
Explain that during pregnancy the breasts become enlarged; they feel stretched, full, firm, and tender. There may be tingling and throbbing. The pigmented area around the nipples widens and becomes darker and swollen. As early as the fourth month a sticky white fluid may be expressed from the nipple, and breast blood vessels become enlarged.

Rationale: An awareness of what to expect promotes comfort and safety.

Resolved Needs: Comfort. Protection from physical harm. Increased learning.

Describe the cardiac signs of physical overactivity
Explain that the signs of overexertion of a weakened heart include chest pain, labored breathing, palpitations, limited endurance, rapid pulse, pallor, and extreme weakness.

Rationale: Overexertion creates a demand for more blood for the muscles than the weakened heart can produce with its usual effort. As cardiac effort is increased, the heart's own blood supply must be increased; if it is not, as in many diseased states, chest pain, etc., will develop.

Resolved Needs: Protection from physical harm. Increased learning.

Describe the characteristics of abnormal vaginal bleeding

Explain that the use of more than four saturated sanitary napkins in an 8-hour period, or more than eight napkins in a 24-hour period, indicates excessive vaginal bleeding. Any bleeding that occurs at times other than at menstruation or any bleeding after the onset of menopause is abnormal.

Rationale: Knowledge that supports early detection of physiologic abnormalities promotes comfort.

Resolved Needs: Protection from physical harm. Increased learning.

Describe the characteristics of controlled diabetes

Explain that a feeling of well-being, maintenance of normal body weight on a well-balanced diet, negative urine tests, and normal levels of blood sugar and acetone indicate well-controlled diabetes.

Rationale: Control of diabetes is essential to the health and comfort of the diabetic.

Resolved Needs: Comfort. Protection from physical harm. Increased learning.

Describe the characteristics of edema

Explain that the characteristics of edema include swelling of subcutaneous tissue, weight gain, and shiny, tight skin.

Rationale: Edema results when fluid moves from the circulating blood into interstitial tissues. Knowledge of potentially harmful physical threats promotes safety.

Resolved Needs: Protection from physical harm. Increased learning.

Describe the characteristics of fatigue

Explain that yawning, irritability, inability to concentrate, shortness of breath, rapid pulse, and a feeling of being unable to go on are characteristics of fatigue.

Rationale: Awareness that fatigue results from depleted energy reserves and that it requires a period of restoration supports human safety.

Resolved Needs: Protection from physical harm. Increased learning.

Describe the characteristics of normal lochia

Explain that immediately after delivery the vaginal discharge should appear bloody, with small amounts of mucus. After 3 days the lochia gradually changes to a pink serous fluid. After 8 or 9 days the discharge becomes brownish. Within 3 weeks the discharge usually disappears.

Rationale: Awareness of normal physiologic processes promotes comfort and safety.

Resolved Needs: Comfort. Protection from physical harm. Increased learning.

Describe the danger signs of pregnancy Explain that during pregnancy the following signs should be reported immediately: persistent headache; nausea and vomiting; dizziness; visual disturbances; epigastric pain; edema of hands, face, or legs; decreased urinary output; constipation; vaginal bleeding; severe lower abdominal pain; shortness of breath; lumbar pain in the early months; absence of fetal movements during the fourth to ninth months; any acute illness; sudden discharge of vaginal fluid.

Rationale: Awareness of physiologic abnormalities promotes safety.

Resolved Needs: Protection from physical harm. Increased learning.

Describe the discomforts of contact lens adjustment Explain that during the period of adjustment to contact lenses, tearing, itching, burning, and light sensitivity are common.

Rationale: Awareness of what to expect promotes comfort and safety.

Resolved Needs: Comfort. Protection from physical harm. Increased learning.

Describe the early manifestations of lung cancer Explain that early signs and symptoms of lung cancer include coughing of purulent or bloody sputum, a cough that persists longer than 3 weeks, breathlessness, weight loss, wheezing, and chest or shoulder pain.

Rationale: Knowledge that supports early disease detection promotes safety.

Resolved Needs: Protection from physical harm. Increased learning.

Describe the emotional changes which normally occur during the menstrual cycle Explain that varying hormone levels during the menstrual cycle cause women to experience different emotions at different times of the month. From the 1st day to the 4th day, when hormone levels are low, a woman feels tired, blue, and depressed. From the 5th day to the 14th day, when the estrogen level is high, the woman feels quite well. This feeling gradually increases, reaching a peak on the day of ovulation. From the 14th day to the 20th day, when both estrogen and progesterone are high, she feels her best. After the 20th day, as both hormones reach low levels, she again feels tired, blue, and depressed.

Rationale: Awareness of normal physiologic processes promotes comfort and safety.

Resolved Needs: Comfort. Protection from psychologic threat. Increased learning.

Describe the factors associated with the occurrence of the problem Describe those factors that are commonly linked with a particular nonhealth episode, such as the life stage during which the problem usually occurs, its probability in certain races, its limitations to geographic areas, and its frequency in the population.

Rationale: Knowledge of the factors associated with a problem can help overcome the problem.

Resolved Needs: Protection from physical harm. Increased learning.

Describe the manifestations of a drug reaction   Explain that undesirable reactions to the drug being taken will cause specific signs and symptoms. Teach the patient exactly what to watch for and what to do if these signs and symptoms occur.

Rationale: Hypersensitivity to drugs, cumulative toxic responses, and other undesirable effects from drug therapy are always possibilities. An informed patient can recognize early evidence of such reactions and obtain medical assistance before the condition becomes critical.

Resolved Needs: Protection from physical harm. Increased learning.

Describe the manifestations of circulatory impairment
Explain that the signs indicating diminished blood flow to a body part include skin coldness, cyanosis, nonpalpable pulse, numbness and tingling, and slowed capillary filling.

Rationale: A diminished supply of oxygen to tissues resulting from impaired circulation causes tissue death.

Resolved Needs: Protection from physical harm. Increased learning.

Describe the manifestations of impending cataract   Explain that blurred vision, inability to find light bright enough to read by, double vision, spots before the eyes, and frequent need for new glasses are warning signs of impending cataract.

Rationale: Awareness of impending cataract can prevent serious visual impairment.

Resolved Needs: Protection from physical harm. Increased learning.

Describe the manifestations of impending diabetic coma
Explain that frequent copious urination, constant thirst, persistent hunger, flushed and dry skin, weakness, fatigue, and drowsiness indicate impending diabetic coma.

Rationale: Diabetic coma (ketoacidosis) indicates a lack of insulin, which causes inadequate metabolic breakdown of glucose and excess production of acetone bodies and requires immediate treatment.

Resolved Needs: Protection from physical harm. Increased learning.

Describe the manifestations of impending insulin shock   Explain that sweating, dizziness, palpitations, pale and moist

skin, shallow breathing, trembling, blurred or double vision, hunger, and confusion (if on NPH insulin) indicate impending insulin shock.

Rationale: Excessive insulin in the blood lowers the level of blood sugar to a dangerous degree and requires immediate treatment.

Resolved Needs: Protection from physical harm. Increased learning.

Describe the manifestations of impending seizure
Explain that seeing bright flashes of light, hearing unusual noises, smelling strange odors, and experiencing confusion and lightheadedness indicate an impending seizure.

Rationale: Some patients have an aura that warns of impending seizure. Early identification of such warnings and prompt action can prevent many seizure-related injuries.

Resolved Needs: Protection from physical harm. Increased learning.

Describe the manifestations of labor onset
Explain that the onset of labor is indicated by lightening, in which the infant moves down into the pelvis, thus relieving the pressure against the maternal diaphragm, as well as by a pink vaginal mucous plug discharge, uterine membrane rupture, and labor pains.

Rationale: Awareness of what to expect promotes comfort and safety.

Resolved Needs: Protection from psychologic threat. Increased learning.

Describe the manifestations of pregnancy
Explain that the early signs of pregnancy include nausea, vomiting, frequent voiding, breast tenderness, fullness, and increased pigmentation, as well as cessation of menstruation.

Rationale: Awareness of normal physiologic changes promotes comfort.

Resolved Needs: Comfort. Increased learning.

Describe the manifestations of premenstrual tension
Explain that certain discomforts are normal a few days before the onset of menstruation: nervousness, irritability, mild depression, dull backache and headache, temporary edema (especially of fingers and ankles), breast tenderness, restlessness, abdominal bloating, urinary frequency, increased thirst and appetite, fatigue, inability to concentrate, and hyperactivity or underactivity; there may be emotional outbursts or weeping without cause.

Rationale: Knowledge of normal physiologic responses promotes safety and comfort.

Resolved Needs: Comfort. Protection from psychologic threat. Increased learning.

Describe the normal behavior pattern common during labor
Explain that there is a wide range of normal emotional reactions as labor progresses: happy anticipation, fear, anxiety, frustration, discour-

agement, and overwhelming delight. Expressive reactions to pain are normal and acceptable and should not cause feelings of shame and guilt.

Rationale: Awareness that the normal emotional outlets are culturally accepted promotes comfort.

Resolved Needs: Comfort. Protection from psychologic threat. Increased learning.

Describe the normal behavior pattern common during male puberty   Explain that during male puberty the normal youth becomes increasingly interested in the opposite sex; he develops a consciousness of his own identity, but he experiences contradictory desires for independence and for peer group identity. He becomes irritable, has difficulty with emotional adjustments, and expresses inconsistent attitudes.

Rationale: Knowledge of normal behavior patterns during puberty promotes comfort.

Resolved Needs: Comfort. Protection from psychologic threat. Increased learning.

Describe the normal behavior pattern common during pregnancy   Explain that most pregnant women experience joy, but also fear of death, fear of losing the baby, fear of child abnormalities, and superstitious fears; sometimes a mother rejects her child. A woman should know that such emotions are normal and are common to most pregnant women.

Rationale: Awareness that such feelings are culturally accepted promotes comfort and helps to reduce the physiologic side effects that result from emotional tension.

Resolved Needs: Comfort. Protection from physical harm. Increased learning.

Describe the normal changes associated with male climacteric   Explain that between the ages of 50 and 60 years men can expect to experience decreased sexual desire, fatigue and muscle weakness, emotional depression or excessive emotional response, hot or cold flushes, rapid heartbeat and palpitations, dizziness, profuse perspiration, numbness and tingling of toes and fingers, nervousness, irritability, shortness of breath, spots before the eyes, tinnitus, flatulence and abdominal distention after meals, inability to sleep well, headaches at the base of the neck and top of the head, decreased physical energy, poor concentration, and feelings of inadequacy.

Rationale: Awareness of normal physiologic processes promotes comfort and safety.

Resolved Needs: Comfort. Protection from psychologic threat. Increased learning.

Describe the normal changes associated with male puberty   Explain that the developments in male secondary sex charac-

teristics between the ages of 14 and 15 years include the following: appearance of pubic, axillary, and facial hair; onset of rapid growth; ejaculation; accentuation of the Adam's apple; voice huskiness; diminished pulse rate; skin disorders; increased biologic tensions.

Rationale: Knowledge of normal physiologic processes promotes comfort.

Resolved Needs: Comfort. Protection from psychologic threat. Increased learning.

Describe the normal changes associated with menopause
Explain that permanent cessation of menstruation usually occurs between the ages of 40 and 50 years. The usual pattern involves scanty periods at first, then occasionally absent periods, and finally cessation of menstruation altogether. As the production of estrogen diminishes, one can expect facial and body flushing, sweating, chills, excitability, irritability, dyspnea, vertigo, headaches, fatigue, depression, urinary frequency, joint pain and stiffness, sparsity of scalp and pubic hair, hair growth on the upper lip and chin, loss of skin elasticity, increased wrinkling, breast sagging, skin dryness, brittle nails, perineal pruritus, vaginal discharge, painful intercourse as a result of atrophy of genital mucous membranes, palpitations with constrictive chest pressure, cold hands and feet, and numbness and tingling. Sedentary life may lead to excessive weight gain. Complacency often leads to less concern with physical appearance. Many women have feelings of worthlessness or of being unneeded because their children have become independent. Many women fear change-of-life pregnancy, but they also may find sexual activity more pleasurable because of decreased fear of pregnancy.

Rationale: Knowledge of normal physiologic processes promotes comfort.

Resolved Needs: Comfort. Protection from psychologic threat. Increased learning.

Describe the normal changes associated with premenopause
Explain that during premenopause there are bodily changes, such as weight gain around the hips, abdomen, thighs, waist, and breasts. Normal discomforts include nervousness, weakness, fatigue, depression, insomnia, palpitations, irritability, headache, numbness, and tingling; there may be excessive emotional responses and tearfulness.

Rationale: Knowledge of normal physiologic responses promotes safety and comfort.

Resolved Needs: Comfort. Protection from psychologic threat. Increased learning.

Describe the normal menstrual cycle changes during premenopause
Explain that during premenopause many normal variations in the menstrual cycle can occur: the regular menstrual cycle may continue to occur for a time and then suddenly stop; menstruation may stop for 6 or 8 months and then reappear; the cycle may remain regular in regard to date of onset, but there may be gradually decreasing flow; the cycle

may remain regular in regard to date of onset, but there may be a decrease in the number of days of flow; menstruation may occur for the same number of days and the same amount of flow, but there may be an increase in the length of time between two onsets; the cycle may be regular, but there may be longer and more profuse flow; cyclic onsets may change to become 2 to 3 weeks apart or 7 to 8 weeks apart; there may be total irregularity of onset; the cycle may occur now and then without ovulation.

Rationale: Awareness of normal physiologic responses promotes safety and comfort.

Resolved Needs: Comfort. Protection from psychologic threat. Increased learning.

Describe the normal psychic changes common during menopause   Explain that emotional instability, weeping, melancholia, insomnia, worry, fatigue, self-depreciation, and sometimes suicidal thoughts are common during menopause.

Rationale: Awareness of normal behavior reduces psychologic threat and promotes comfort.

Resolved Needs: Comfort. Protection from psychologic threat. Increased learning.

Describe the normal stages of grief   Explain that grief is a normal emotional phenomenon and that it follows certain patterns. During the initial stage of grief there exists a state of shock and disbelief. Gradually the person comes to a realization of his loss. During the period called grief work, he focuses on the lost person almost continuously and mentally relives experiences that were shared with the lost person. The period of resolving grief involves a gradual change of focus from the lost person to other interests. During this period the grieving person attempts to reestablish stable life patterns and form new relationships.

Rationale: Knowledge of normal behavior patterns reduces anxiety and threat, promotes comfort and increased reality perception, and supports mature growth.

Resolved Needs: Comfort. Protection from psychologic threat. Personal growth and maturity. Increased learning. Increased reality perception and problem-solving ability.

Describe the normal stages of tooth development   Explain that teeth appear between the ages of 6 and 9 months. At 12 months there are usually 6 teeth; at 18 months, 12 teeth; at 24 months, 16 teeth; at 2½ years, 20 teeth. Explain that teeth should come in straight.

Rationale: Knowledge of normal physiologic processes promotes comfort and safety.

Resolved Needs: Comfort. Protection from physical harm. Increased learning.

Describe the process of labor and delivery Explain to the pregnant woman the normal course of labor. During the first stage of labor, labor pains gradually increase in intensity. There is a marked increase in show, and cervix dilatation occurs. At this point, bearing down accomplishes nothing and may exhaust the mother. During the second stage of labor, pain is severe and long, occurring every 2 to 3 minutes. The membranes rupture with a gush of amniotic fluid from the vagina. By bearing down, the mother assists in the child's birth. The infant's head causes pressure against the vagina, finally becoming visible. The infant then passes through the birth canal and is born. During the third stage of labor, the placenta drops into the lower uterus and, with applied pressure, is expelled from the uterus.

Rationale: Knowledge of what to expect promotes human comfort.

Resolved Needs: Comfort. Increased learning.

Contraindications: Delay if explanation heightens anxiety.

Describe the signs of infant readiness to be weaned Explain that when a child begins to shorten the periods of time that he breast-feeds or bottle-feeds, or when he is restless because of his mother's hold on him, he is demonstrating a desire for independent feeding. At that time a gradual introduction to the cup should be started, with decreased feeding from breast or bottle.

Rationale: The joy of independent feeding replaces the pleasure of breast or bottle feeding when developmental skills allow for independence.

Resolved Needs: Comfort. Independence. Increased learning.

Describe the specific dangerous effects of poor health practices Explain that poor health practices can have potentially dangerous effects on health; e.g., excessive consumption of alcohol impairs liver function; insufficient rest inhibits adequate healing; poor nutrition impairs normal growth.

Rationale: Recognition of the potentially dangerous effects of certain health practices can minimize unhealthy practices and provide motivation toward the practice of better health.

Resolved Needs: Protection from physical harm. Increased learning. Increased reality perception.

Describe the symptoms commonly associated with tobacco withdrawal Explain that the following symptoms frequently occur when one is attempting to stop smoking: For several days or a week the person may experience occasional dizziness, headache, irritability, tremor, sweating, constipation or diarrhea, inability to sleep, inability to concentrate, impaired memory, anxiety, restlessness, craving for tobacco, gnawing stomach, and mouth soreness or blisters. At the end of 2 weeks the desire to smoke is greatly relieved, except when seeing others smoking. Gradually, over a 3-month to 6-month period, the craving decreases and subsides.

Rationale: Awareness of the normal symptoms associated with tobacco withdrawal reduces anxiety and supports completion of the withdrawal phase.

Resolved Needs: Comfort. Protection from psychologic threat. Increased learning.

Describe the undesirable effects of specific therapies

Describe the side effects of specific therapies that the patient can expect to experience. Explain that the urine turns orange when one is on Pyridium therapy, that the stools become black when one is taking iron, that hair falls out when one takes anticancer drugs or radiation therapy, that diuretics produce urinary frequency, and that thyroid drugs increase one's activity level.

Rationale: Awareness of what to expect reduces needless anxiety and promotes comfort.

Resolved Needs: Comfort. Protection from psychologic threat. Increased learning.

Describe those behaviors which usually occur in communication impairment

Explain that persons unable to communicate usually display frustration, embarrassment, irritation with the listener, depression, and agitation.

Rationale: Awareness that certain uncharacteristic behavior by a patient is to be expected reduces the sensitivity of his loved ones to behavior that would ordinarily be perceived as threatening.

Resolved Needs: Comfort. Protection from psychologic threat. Increased learning.

Describe those factors which intensify fear (or anxiety)

Explain that being alone and being in the dark tend to magnify fear and anxiety. Relatively mild, but deep-rooted, fears and anxieties may grow out of proportion when one encounters situations that require considerable emotional adaptation or change in normal living patterns, such as relocation for a new job or the occurrence of pregnancy.

Rationale: Awareness of the factors that intensify fear and anxiety supports control and prevention of the emotions.

Resolved Needs: Comfort. Protection from psychologic threat. Personal growth and maturity. Increased learning. Increased reality perception and problem-solving ability.

Describe those symptoms which should be reported

Explain the specific signs and symptoms that may be related to the patient's particular health problem and that should be reported to medical or nursing personnel without delay.

Rationale: Prompt care can minimize the harmful effects of nonhealth conditions.

Resolved Needs: Comfort. Protection from physical harm. Increased learning.

Emphasize that a car should never be started in a closed garage
Emphasize that when one is warming up the motor of a car either the garage door should be open or the car should be in the open air.

Rationale: Warming up the motor of a car in a closed garage can result in carbon monoxide poisoning.

Resolved Needs: Protection from physical harm. Increased learning.

Emphasize that bulging food cans should be discarded
Emphasize that when a food can bulges around the lid, the can and contents should be thrown away.

Rationale: A bulging can is usually the result of gas formed by the action of pathogenic microorganisms.

Resolved Needs: Protection from physical harm. Increased learning.

Emphasize that children need guidance
Emphasize that because the judgment of a child is not developed and he has no experience to fall back on, he requires guidance by those who are more experienced.

Rationale: Guidance from his elders keeps the child safe from physical and psychologic harm.

Resolved Needs: Protection from physical harm. Protection from psychologic threat. Increased learning. Increased reality perception and problem-solving ability.

Emphasize that clotheslines should be kept high to prevent strangulation
Emphasize that clotheslines should be strung high enough so that one cannot walk into them.

Rationale: Walking into clotheslines can cause strangulation, eye injury, or serious wounds.

Resolved Needs: Protection from physical harm. Increased learning.

Emphasize that contaminated clothing should be changed immediately
Emphasize that whenever dust particles, bacteria, vapors, fumes, or other harmful products come in contact with clothing, the clothing should be changed as soon as possible and properly cleaned.

Rationale: Contaminated clothing can cause skin or respiratory disorders.

Resolved Needs: Protection from physical harm. Increased learning.

Emphasize that contaminated skin should be washed immediately
Emphasize that whenever dust particles, bacteria, vapors, fumes, or other harmful products come in contact with the skin, the skin should be washed.

Rationale: Skin contamination can result in infectious or allergic conditions.

Resolved Needs: Protection from physical harm. Increased learning.

Emphasize that cracked dishware should be discarded
Emphasize that cracked or chipped glasses or dishes should be thrown away.

Rationale: Cracked or chipped glasses or dishes can result in accidental cuts, and growth of disease-causing organisms (bacteria) can occur in the cracks.

Resolved Needs: Protection from physical harm. Increased learning.

Emphasize that dangerous products should be stored out of reach   Emphasize that all dangerous household substances should be stored on high shelves, preferably in locked cabinets, out of reach of young children or irresponsible adults.

Rationale: Easy access to dangerous products increases the potential for serious accidental injury.

Resolved Needs: Protection from physical harm. Increased learning.

Emphasize that extension cords should be secured in place   Emphasize that extension cords should be securely fastened to the wall or floor and should never be allowed to lie on the floor or hang loose.

Rationale: Electrical cords loosely placed can cause injury from tripping and falling.

Resolved Needs: Protection from physical harm. Increased learning.

Emphasize that fireplaces should be screened   Emphasize that a screen should be placed in front of a fireplace whenever a fire is burning or when hot ashes remain.

Rationale: Sparks from unscreened open fires can ignite carpets, clothing, and other nearby materials and cause severe burns.

Resolved Needs: Protection from physical harm. Increased learning.

Emphasize that floors and stairways should be litter-free   Emphasize that stairways and floors should be kept free of loose objects. Small children should be taught to put toys away when they are not in use.

Rationale: Scattered objects on the floor can cause injury from tripping and falling.

Resolved Needs: Protection from physical harm. Increased learning.

Emphasize that food wastes should be burned in animal-inhabited outdoor areas   Emphasize that anyone living or camping in outdoor areas where there are bears or raccoons should burn food wastes.

Rationale: Raccoons and bears can smell buried food and dig it up; they leave what they don't eat to the flies, who in turn transmit disease.

Resolved Needs: Protection from physical harm. Increased learning.

Emphasize that fume-producing substances should be used in the open air   Emphasize that all products giving off dangerous fumes should be used only in the open air.

Rationale: If products that emit fumes are used only in the open air, toxic inhalation can be prevented.

Resolved Needs: Protection from physical harm. Increased learning.

Emphasize that garbage should be covered   Emphasize that garbage should be placed in tightly covered containers, preferably inside sealed bags.

Rationale: Tightly sealed garbage containers prevent flies and rats from transmitting infection.

Resolved Needs: Protection from physical harm. Increased learning.

Emphasize that heaters should be vented to the outside   Emphasize that oil and gas heaters should be vented to the outdoors.

Rationale: Venting heaters to the outside prevents fumes from remaining in the room and causing asphyxiation.

Resolved Needs: Protection from physical harm. Increased learning.

Emphasize that in outdoor living, human wastes should be buried   Emphasize that when people are living outdoors, human excreta and food wastes should be placed in the ground and covered with dirt.

Rationale: Uncovered human excreta and food wastes attract flies, who in turn transmit disease.

Resolved Needs: Protection from physical harm. Increased learning.

Emphasize that knife racks should be covered   Emphasize that all sharp knives should be placed in covered racks, or the knife blade should be enclosed in a heavy cardboard guard. Sharp knives should never be kept loose in a drawer.

Rationale: Exposed knife blades can cause severe injury to anyone reaching into a drawer where knives are kept.

Resolved Needs: Protection from physical harm. Increased learning.

Emphasize that large icicles should be removed   Emphasize that large icicles hanging from a roof should be broken off before they fall and cause injury.

Rationale: Large icicles can cause penetrating wounds.

Resolved Needs: Protection from physical harm. Increased learning.

Emphasize that matches should be stored in a metal container
Emphasize that matches should be stored in metal, not cardboard, containers and kept out of reach of small children and irresponsible adults.

Rationale: Fire resulting from combustion of matches within a metal container will be confined to that container. When matches are stored in cardboard containers, such fires will spread.

Resolved Needs: Protection from physical harm. Increased learning.

Emphasize that medicine cabinets should be locked
Emphasize that all medicines should be safely locked in cabinets where they are inaccessible to young children and irresponsible adults.

Rationale: Locking medicines in cabinets reduces the potential for a drug overdose.

Resolved Needs: Protection from physical harm. Increased learning.

Emphasize that open heaters should be screened
Emphasize that open gas or electric heaters should be covered with metal screening.

Rationale: Sparks from open heaters can ignite carpets, clothing, and other nearby materials and cause severe burns.

Resolved Needs: Protection from physical harm. Increased learning.

Emphasize that outdated foods (or drugs) should be discarded
Emphasize that dated foods, which spoil easily, should not be used after the expiration date. Drugs should always be discarded when outdated.

Rationale: Foods and drugs are dated for the purpose of assuring their fitness for consumption. Discarding foods after the expiration date assures safety from food poisoning. Since time, light, and moisture alter the chemical composition of drugs, discarding them after the expiration date prevents drug side effects.

Resolved Needs: Protection from physical harm. Increased learning.

Emphasize that plastic bags should be shredded and discarded
Emphasize that plastic bags should be stored out of reach and should be shredded when discarded, since small children often put them over their heads while playing.

Rationale: Because air cannot penetrate a plastic bag, suffocation occurs quickly if one is placed over the head.

Resolved Needs: Protection from physical harm. Increased learning.

Emphasize that play areas should be fenced
Emphasize that small children should play only in fenced areas.

Rationale: Small children are not sufficiently experienced to recognize many dangers, and their distraction during play further decreases their perception of danger.

Resolved Needs: Protection from physical harm. Increased learning.

Emphasize that pools should be protected against entry   Emphasize that fishponds, swimming pools, wells, and cisterns should be closed off by a covering, a rail, or a screen.

Rationale: Preventing access to pools reduces the potential for drowning.

Resolved Needs: Protection from physical harm. Increased learning.

Emphasize that potentially unsafe water should be boiled for ten minutes   Emphasize that outdoor water or water in foreign countries should be boiled for 10 minutes to make it safe for consumption. If it has a flat taste after boiling, vigorously shake it in a container to aerate it. Keep it well covered at all times.

Rationale: Boiling water drives off air and gases and destroys bacteria.

Resolved Needs: Protection from physical harm. Increased learning.

Emphasize that safety guards should be placed over electrical outlets   Emphasize that safety plugs should be attached to all electrical outlets when small children are in the crawling stage and are learning to walk.

Rationale: Electrical guards keep small children from poking fingers or other objects into electrical sockets, thus preventing electrical shock.

Resolved Needs: Protection from physical harm. Increased learning.

Emphasize that seat belts should be fastened   Emphasize that safety belts on passenger vehicles should be fastened before the vehicle is set in motion.

Rationale: Safety belts maintain the body's position and prevent the injuries that can result from being thrown about or thrown out of a vehicle during a collision.

Resolved Needs: Protection from physical harm. Increased learning.

Emphasize that small children should always be attended   Emphasize that small children should never be left alone for extended periods.

Rationale: The perception and judgment of small children are not sufficiently developed for them to recognize potential danger.

Resolved Needs: Protection from physical harm. Increased learning.

Emphasize that snow should be removed from stairs   Emphasize that steps should be kept clear of ice and snow.

Rationale: Removing ice and snow from stairs reduces the potential for falling.

Resolved Needs: Protection from physical harm. Increased learning.

Emphasize that stoves should be kept free of grease

Emphasize that grease should be removed from a stove as soon as it is spilled.

Rationale: Serious fires can result if grease comes in contact with an open flame.

Resolved Needs: Protection from physical harm. Increased learning.

Emphasize that unused electrical equipment should be disconnected

Emphasize that appliances and equipment such as toasters, can openers, radios, and handsaws that are used only intermittently should be unplugged when not in use.

Rationale: Wherever there are electrical contacts, the potential for fire exists.

Resolved Needs: Protection from physical harm. Increased learning.

Emphasize that unused refrigerators should be locked or the doors removed

Emphasize that old refrigerators should be locked or should have their doors removed, since children like to play inside refrigerators and close the doors behind them.

Rationale: Refrigerators are airtight, and suffocation results when the limited oxygen supply is used up.

Resolved Needs: Protection from physical harm. Increased learning.

Emphasize that worn electrical cords should be repaired immediately

Emphasize that all electrical cords should be repaired or replaced at the first sign of wear.

Rationale: Exposed electrical cords can cause fire or electrical shock.

Resolved Needs: Protection from physical harm. Increased learning.

Emphasize the danger of breathing cold air

Explain that in very cold weather the mouth should be covered with a scarf, and breathing should be nasal rather than oral in order to prevent injury to respiratory tissue.

Rationale: Breathing cold air through the mouth burns respiratory passages, increases the chance of infection, and stimulates the cough reflex. Nasal breathing is preferable because the nasal mucous membranes warm the air as it passes through.

Resolved Needs: Comfort. Protection from physical harm. Increased learning.

Emphasize the danger of crash-dieting   Explain that attempting to lose a large amount of weight in a short time places severe stress on the body's adaptive mechanisms.

Rationale: The severe stress placed on the body by crash-dieting increases susceptibility to illness.

Resolved Needs: Protection from physical harm. Increased learning.

Emphasize the danger of cutting calloused skin   Explain that thick, hardened skin should not be cut off with scissors but should be softened with skin lubricants.

Rationale: Cutting calloused skin traumatizes underlying tissue; it can cut into vessels and cause bleeding and can introduce bacteria into the open wound.

Resolved Needs: Protection from physical harm. Increased learning.

Emphasize the danger of diving into shallow water   Explain that the potential for hitting one's head on the bottom of the pool and compressing the cervical vertebrae is great when diving into shallow water. Young children should be warned of the danger when first learning to swim.

Rationale: Cervical trauma can result in paralysis.

Resolved Needs: Protection from physical harm. Increased learning.

Emphasize the danger of excessive body weight   Explain that excessive body weight places stress on all body systems, thereby increasing the potential for a system breakdown.

Rationale: Excessive weight increases the heart's work load and the potential for impaired oxygenation of tissues. Excessive weight imposes strain on spinal disks, increases weight-bearing pressure on bones, and weakens the muscular supportive structures of the body.

Resolved Needs: Comfort. Protection from physical harm. Increased learning.

Emphasize the danger of excessive coffee consumption
Explain that drinking five or more cups of coffee a day increases blood pressure, intraocular pressure, and stomach acid. It causes arteriosclerosis and disguises fatigue.

Rationale: The caffeine in coffee has a stimulating effect; taken in excess, it is detrimental to health.

Resolved Needs: Protection from physical harm. Increased learning.

Emphasize the danger of excessive exposure to noise
Explain that loud, prolonged, and high-frequency noise can cause diminished hearing or deafness and can place stress on the nervous system.

Rationale: Sound waves more intense than 80 decibels cause auditory damage and overstimulate the nervous system.

Resolved Needs: Protection from physical harm. Increased learning.

Emphasize the danger of excessive use of nose drops   Explain that excessive use of nose drops can injure nasal tissue.

Rationale: Injury to nasal mucous membrane interferes with the olfactory and filtering functions of the membrane.

Resolved Needs: Protection from physical harm. Increased learning.

Emphasize the danger of highly waxed floors   Explain that floors should never be waxed to the point of being slippery.

Rationale: Slippery floors can cause accidental injury from falling.

Resolved Needs: Protection from physical harm. Increased learning.

Emphasize the danger of induced abortion   Explain that abortion induced by external means can cause vaginal infection and hemorrhage.

Rationale: Induced abortion that results in vaginal infection and hemorrhage can cause serious and sometimes fatal illness.

Resolved Needs: Protection from physical harm. Increased learning.

Emphasize the danger of massaging a painful calf   Explain that rubbing or kneading a painful calf poses the danger of dislodging a thrombus.

Rationale: Calf tenderness often results from blood vessel obstruction caused by blood clot formation and localization.

Resolved Needs: Protection from physical harm. Increased learning.

Emphasize the danger of mixing drugs and alcohol   Explain that simultaneous use of drugs and alcohol can cause dangerous chemical reactions that often result in death.

Rationale: Both drugs and alcohol have sedative effects, and when they are mixed the sedation can be so severe that respiratory depression and death can occur.

Resolved Needs: Protection from physical harm. Increased learning.

Emphasize the danger of self-regulation of intravenous fluids   Explain to the patient that he must not release the regulating clamp on an intravenous infusion in order to facilitate more rapid flow; doing so could overload the circulatory system with fluid. This problem is sometimes encountered with anxious patients who want to get the intravenous infusion completed and be rid of it.

Rationale: Knowledge that rapid flow of intravenous fluid can overload the heart and cause circulatory failure promotes safety.

Resolved Needs: Protection from physical harm. Increased learning.

Emphasize the danger of sharing drugs between persons
Explain that a drug that affects one person in a certain way may affect another person in another way, not in the intended therapeutic manner, but with serious side effects. Therefore drugs should never be shared.

Rationale: Chemical reactions within the body that result from the combination of incompatible elements can produce a poisoning effect.

Resolved Needs: Protection from physical harm. Increased learning.

Emphasize the danger of sleeping with an infant
Explain that the newborn infant should sleep in a separate bed, not in bed with an adult.

Rationale: An infant sleeping with an adult is in danger of suffocation; an adult could accidentally roll onto or over the child.

Resolved Needs: Protection from physical harm. Increased learning.

Emphasize the danger of smoking around oxygen
Explain that smoking is not permitted in areas where pressurized oxygen is being used because of the fire hazard.

Rationale: When oxygen-saturated materials come in contact with a spark or open flame, they burst into flame and burn rapidly.

Resolved Needs: Protection from physical harm. Increased learning.

Emphasize the danger of smoking in bed
Explain that one should never smoke in bed because of the fire hazard.

Rationale: If one falls asleep while smoking, the cigarette may be dropped onto bed linens, whereupon the mattress smolders and causes suffocation, followed by body burns.

Resolved Needs: Protection from physical harm. Increased learning.

Emphasize the danger of using excessive hair dye
Explain that excessive use of hair dye irritates the scalp and damages the hair follicles, making them coarse and brittle.

Rationale: Many hair dyes contain silver nitrate or aniline dyes, which are chemically irritating to the skin and eyes.

Resolved Needs: Protection from physical harm. Increased learning.

Emphasize the danger of X-ray exposure during early pregnancy
Explain that women in the first 3 months of pregnancy should avoid exposure to any type of X-ray therapy.

Rationale: X-ray therapy may cause injury to the fetus or may interfere with fetal development.

Resolved Needs: Protection from physical harm. Increased learning.

Emphasize the importance of planning and anticipating future activities   Emphasize the importance of planning one's activities in advance so that some pleasant event or situation can be looked forward to in the near future.

Rationale: Planned use of one's time encourages a positive attitude, allows for development of creative talents, skills, and interests, and helps to maintain social contacts. Looking forward to something offers a psychologic lift for the present and provides a predictable and orderly world.

Resolved Needs: Comfort. Protection from psychologic threat. Predictable, orderly world. Personal growth and maturity. Increased learning. Increased pleasantness.

Emphasize the importance of recognizing tension within oneself   Emphasize that reduction of tension can be accomplished only by conscious recognition of tension. Irritability, nervousness, and tight muscles indicate the presence of tension.

Rationale: Recognizing and relieving tension can promote comfort, since there is decreased demand placed on the body to respond to stimuli.

Resolved Needs: Protection from physical harm. Protection from psychologic threat. Increased learning. Increased reality perception and problem-solving ability.

Emphasize the importance of wearing safety goggles   Emphasize that safety goggles should be worn when there is potential for eye injury.

Rationale: Safety goggles prevent eye injury.

Resolved Needs: Protection from physical harm. Increased learning.

Emphasize the need to check for gas leakage and fire   Emphasize that persons who cannot distinguish odors easily should check frequently for gas leaks and fire, especially before going to sleep. Smear a small amount of diluted soap around a gas jet and its connections; if it does not bubble there is no leakage. One can also listen for a hissing sound from gas jets. A brief check of the house will determine if a fire is in progress.

Rationale: Checking for gas leakage and fire reduces the potential for injury.

Resolved Needs: Protection from physical harm. Increased learning.

Emphasize the need to develop self-reliance   Explain that each person must learn that he can rely on his internal and external resources when meeting life's challenges.

Rationale: Self-confidence is based on the conviction that one's internal and external resources are adequate for any task.

Resolved Needs: Protection from psychologic threat. Self-reliance. Personal growth and maturity. Increased learning. Increased reality perception and problem-solving ability.

Emphasize the need to fly in pressurized airplanes Emphasize that persons in poor health should fly only in airplanes that have controlled barometric pressure. Light private planes should be avoided.

Rationale: The lowered barometric pressure that is encountered at high altitudes decreases the pressure and amount of oxygen going to the lungs, which can cause anoxia, pneumothorax, or cardiac impairment. Unequal internal and external pressures may cause the ear's tympanic membrane to rupture. Unequal abdominal pressures may cause fecal contents to be expelled from a colostomy.

Resolved Needs: Protection from physical harm. Increased learning.

Emphasize the need to maintain sturdy stair rails Emphasize that stair railings should be well maintained and should never be allowed to become loose or wobbly.

Rationale: Sturdy stair railings reduce the potential for injury from falling.

Resolved Needs: Protection from physical harm. Increased learning.

Emphasize the need to use only an approved sewage facility Emphasize that drainage systems for toilets, sinks, and tubs should be approved and should meet sanitation standards.

Rationale: Safe waste disposal prevents the spread of infection.

Resolved Needs: Protection from physical harm. Increased learning.

Emphasize the need to use only an approved water supply Emphasize that only water that has been inspected and approved by government agencies should be used for drinking.

Rationale: Water that has not been decontaminated is a potential source of disease.

Resolved Needs: Protection from physical harm. Increased learning.

Emphasize the need to use safe ladders Emphasize that ladders should never be used unless they are of solid construction and have nonskid legs. One should never try to reach too far when on a ladder; it is easy to lose one's balance.

Rationale: Safe use of ladders can reduce the potential for injury.

Resolved Needs: Protection from physical harm. Increased learning.

Emphasize the need to use safety straps to prevent falling
Emphasize that a person with poor coordination or limited range of motion should be protected with safety straps when sitting in a chair. Safety straps applied around the waist and anchored to the bed can protect sleepwalkers.

Rationale: Safety straps prevent injury from falling.

Resolved Needs: Protection from physical harm. Increased learning.

Explain and offer hope that the emotional pain will decrease with time
Explain that intensely severe emotional pain that may seem unbearable at the moment will gradually decrease in intensity and be more endurable as time goes on and adjustment occurs.

Rationale: An awareness that severe emotional pain will gradually subside in the future promotes comfort and strength as the person realizes it is a temporary stress.

Resolved Needs: Comfort. Protection from psychologic threat. Endurance. Increased learning.

Explain how and where organ donations are made
Explain that organs for transplant come from two major sources: unrelated persons who have recently died and living relatives. Recommend those organizations or physicians whose prime function is to secure such donations.

Rationale: Inquiries about organ donation can result in the giving of an organ needed to preserve life or improve body function.

Resolved Needs: Increased learning.

Explain how impending insulin shock can be interrupted
Explain that when a person is going into insulin shock, he should be given one of the following: sugar, a piece of candy, a carbonated beverage, or fruit juice with sugar in it. This should be followed by a regular meal or by some high-protein food.

Rationale: Excessive insulin in the blood lowers the level of blood sugar. A normal level of blood sugar can be rapidly reestablished by giving foods or fluids containing sugar.

Resolved Needs: Protection from physical harm. Increased learning.

Explain how the equipment works
Explain as simply as possible how the specific equipment associated with the patient's care functions. If there are flashing lights, buzzer signals, etc., explain their meanings.

Rationale: Knowledge of the functioning of devices associated with one's care reduces anxiety and promotes comfort.

Resolved Needs: Comfort. Protection from psychologic threat. Increased learning.

Explain how the infant grows in utero Explain the sequence of child development in utero. At the end of the *first month*, the embryo head is very prominent, as is the backbone. It is only ¼ inch long. At the end of the *second month*, the fetus has a human face and arms and legs. It is about 1 inch long and weighs 1/30 ounce. At the end of the *third month*, sex can be distinguished and nails appear, as well as teeth buds. Kidneys develop and secrete small amounts of urine into the bladder. The fetus is 3 inches long and weighs 1 ounce. At the end of the *fourth month*, downy hair appears, and faint fetal movements are sometimes felt. The fetus is 6½ inches long and weighs 4 ounces. At the end of the *fifth month*, fetal heart tones can be heard and fetal movements felt. It is 10 inches long and weighs 6 ounces. At the end of the *sixth month*, the fetus begins to resemble an infant. It develops a skin coating called vernix caseosa. It is 12 inches long and weighs 1½ pounds. At the end of the *seventh month*, the fetus is 15 inches long and weighs 2½ pounds. At the end of the *eighth month*, the fetus is 16½ inches long and weighs 4 pounds. At the end of the *ninth month*, the infant becomes mature; it is 19 inches long and weighs about 6 pounds.

Rationale: Knowledge of physiologic processes promotes comfort.

Resolved Needs: Comfort. Increased learning.

Explain how the loss of an organ will affect the donor's future health Explain that if a living person sacrifices one of duplicate organs within his body, there is always the possibility that the remaining organ could develop impaired function. Explain that in most cases the donor enjoys a lifetime of good health.

Rationale: Knowledge of what to expect reduces anxiety and permits realistic assessment of whether to donate the organ.

Resolved Needs: Comfort. Protection from psychologic threat. Increased learning. Increased reality perception and problem-solving ability.

Explain how to adjust clothing to meet health problems Explain that some clothing is more appropriate in certain health conditions than in others. High-necked clothing, long sleeves, and scarves can cover wounds and scars. Following mastectomy, clothing worn before surgery can be filled in with soft materials, or seams can be adjusted for the current body shape. Women who breast-feed should wear nursing bras and clothes that open down the front. When one is wearing a brace, culottes, wide pants, shift dresses, and A-line dresses offer freedom of movement; loosely knit underwear should be avoided, and the inside seams of trousers should be finished off so that they are not caught in the brace. Patients with limited range of motion should use clothing one size too large when dressing themselves. Wide sleeves and pants legs should be worn over casts. Oversize clothing is needed for body casts, and clothes that button down the front are needed for body and neck casts. A heavy sock instead of a shoe is necessary on a casted foot.

Rationale: The proper use of clothing for comfort, reduction of fatigue, and safety during movement supports positive health action.

Resolved Needs: Comfort. Protection from physical harm. Independence. Increased learning.

Explain how to apply elastic stockings or an elastic bandage

Explain that elastic hose and elastic bandages should be applied in the morning before getting out of bed. A wrinkle-free application that provides an evenly distributed and moderate amount of pressure is the goal. To apply an elastic stocking, turn it inside out down to the heel, fit the foot part on snugly, and then gradually work the length of the stocking up onto the leg, making sure no tourniquet effect is created. To apply elastic bandages to the leg, begin wrapping on the foot, enclosing the foot, heel, and ankle with the figure-eight wrap. Continue with a smooth spiral wrap to midthigh, making sure that the second or third bandage is not placed over or too close to the knee joint. To bandage the arm, use the same technique, beginning at the hand.

Rationale: Evenly distributed, moderate external pressure applied to the extremity diverts the venous blood from the smaller veins into the large veins that lie deeper; this increases the flow rate and decreases the chance of thrombosis. The superficial veins must be relatively empty as a result of having been in an elevated position prior to application of pressure; otherwise, blood will be trapped and thrombi will form.

Resolved Needs: Circulation. Comfort. Protection from physical harm. Mastery and competence in skills. Increased learning.

Contraindications: Circulatory thrombus or embolus.

Explain how to budget

Explain how to plan for health needs and how to judge the comparable values of health essentials such as bandages, food, etc. Teach a realistic approach from the standpoint of priorities and the available budget.

Rationale: Budgeting for health essentials supports improved health care.

Resolved Needs: Increased learning. Increased problem-solving ability.

Explain how to calculate the delivery date

Explain that the approximate date of delivery can be determined as follows: count back 3 calendar months from the first day of the last menstrual period; add 7 days; this will give the anticipated date of delivery.

Rationale: Knowledge of the anticipated birth date of a child promotes comfort.

Resolved Needs: Comfort. Increased learning.

Explain how to channel emotional energy into activity

Explain that emotional tension (involving fear, anxiety, sex drive, etc.) can be channeled into accomplishments. When such energy is diverted toward work, hobbies, sports, travel, or other activities, the emotional tension is weakened.

Rationale: Emotion stimulates energy resources; if the energy is not used, muscular tension increases. Body movements can absorb and decrease tension and at the same time channel the energy into successful endeavors.

Resolved Needs: Comfort. Protection from psychologic threat. Personal growth and maturity. Increased learning.

Explain how to clean the external part of the indwelling urinary catheter
Explain that the external portion of the urinary catheter should be kept clean with soap and water. Clean especially well where the catheter enters the meatus.

Rationale: Cleanliness minimizes the potential for urinary tract infection.

Resolved Needs: Cleanliness. Protection from physical harm. Increased learning.

Explain how to collect a specimen
Explain how to collect the specific specimens that are required for analysis.

Rationale: Employing the correct procedures in collecting and transporting specimens can contribute to the accuracy of the analysis.

Resolved Needs: Increased learning.

Explain how to control weight gain during pregnancy
Explain that during pregnancy the total weight gain should not exceed 25 pounds, although weight gain will depend on the mother's size. Weight gain should be limited to ½ pound each week from the fourth month through the sixth month and ¾ pound a week from the seventh month through the ninth month.

Rationale: Excessive weight gain enhances the potential for difficult labor and delivery. Excessive pregnancy weight places unnecessary pressure on the leg and back muscles and may cause backache, leg pain, and fatigue.

Resolved Needs: Protection from physical harm. Increased learning.

Explain how to correctly store guns and ammunition
Explain that guns and ammunition should be stored in locked cabinets or drawers, that guns should be stored unloaded, and that guns and ammunition should never be touched by persons (especially children) who have not had supervised training in handling them.

Rationale: Severe injury and death can result from gunshot wounds.

Resolved Needs: Protection from physical harm. Increased learning.

Explain how to correctly wash diapers
Explain that mild soap should be used when washing diapers. They should be rinsed thoroughly and, if possible, allowed to dry in the sunshine.

Rationale: Removal of all foreign particles from diapers decreases skin irritation.

Resolved Needs: Cleanliness. Protection from physical harm. Increased learning.

Explain how to counteract the theories of drug users   When a drug user justifies his habit by stating that he has the right of free choice, the right to destroy his body, or the right to manipulate reality, be prepared to rebut such statements. Suggest that free choice is based on the intent of man to improve himself. Free choice also implies compromise in consideration of the rights of the majority. If the drug user claims the right to destroy his body because he sees destruction of human life throughout the world, agree that destruction does exist, but emphasize that it is not acceptable behavior. If there are destructive elements significant in the user's own life, perhaps a change can be brought about. When the drug user claims the right to manipulate reality because he sees people manipulating one another for their own gain, agree that manipulation does exist, but emphasize that it diminishes human dignity.

Rationale: Recognition and discussion of social problems promote realistic solutions and release of socially imposed tensions.

Resolved Needs: Protection from psychologic threat. Increased learning.

Explain how to describe pain   Explain that there are standard terms used to express the intensity, duration, and quality of pain and that use of these terms clarifies perception of the patient's problem by other persons.

Rationale: Comfort and safety can derive from an ability to communicate one's needs.

Resolved Needs: Protection from physical harm. Protection from psychologic threat. Increased learning.

Explain how to detect pacemaker failure   Explain that the average pacemaker battery has a life of 30 to 36 months. Signs that a battery is beginning to fail may include chest pain, dizziness, pulse rate increase or decrease, and loss of consciousness.

Rationale: Since pacemakers are usually essential to maintenance of adequate cardiac output, they must be kept in optimum working order.

Resolved Needs: Protection from physical harm. Increased learning.

Explain how to determine proper cane length (97)   Explain that a cane is the proper length when the patient's arm is at a 30° angle as the cane is held a few inches in front of and to the side of his foot.

Rationale: Proper cane length is essential for safe and comfortable mobility.

Resolved Needs: Comfort. Protection from physical harm. Increased learning.

Explain how to determine proper crutch length (97)

Explain that the following measurements will determine whether crutch length is correct. For an axillary crutch, have the patient lie in bed or stand; then measure the length from the axilla to a point 6 inches out from the side of the foot. When the patient's hand is on the handbar, the elbow should be bent at a 30° angle. When a forearm (Lofstrand) crutch fits properly, the elbows will be bent at a 30° angle and the crutch tips will be 6–8 inches to the side of and in front of the foot. When crutches are too short, the head, shoulders, and body will be bent forward and downward in a stooped-shoulder crutch-walking posture. When crutches are too long, the shoulders will be bent into an arch in a hunched-shoulder crutch-walking posture, and there will be pain in the axilla from crutch pressure.

Rationale: Correct crutch length is essential for adequate body support, mobility, and comfort. Crutches that are too long can cause nerve damage under the axilla.

Resolved Needs: Comfort. Protection from physical harm. Increased learning.

Explain how to determine proper walker height (97)

Explain that if the walker height is correct, the patient's elbows will be bent at a 30° angle. When the walker is too short, the shoulders will be bent in a slumped position. When the walker is too tall, the shoulders will be bent slightly backward.

Rationale: Correct walker height is essential for adequate body support, mobility, and comfort.

Resolved Needs: Comfort. Protection from physical harm. Increased learning.

Explain how to determine the optimum time for conception

Explain that the best time to attempt conception is 7 to 10 days after menstrual bleeding stops.

Rationale: Ovulation usually occurs between the 10th day and the 16th day after menstrual bleeding begins. If pregnancy is to occur, there must be discharge of ovum and male germ cell impregnation.

Resolved Needs: Comfort. Increased learning.

Explain how to disinfect contaminated linen

Explain that linens contaminated with infectious material should be either boiled or burned.

Rationale: Disinfection or destruction of contaminated articles prevents the spread of infection.

Resolved Needs: Cleanliness. Protection from physical harm. Increased learning.

Explain how to dispose of infectious expectoration

Explain that infectious expectorated material should be burned or disposed of through the sewer system.

Rationale: Removing infectious microorganisms from locations where they might contact other people reduces the potential for transfer of disease.

Resolved Needs: Cleanliness. Protection from physical harm. Increased learning.

Explain how to dispose of soiled dressings   Explain that soiled dressings should be placed in paper or plastic sacks, tightly sealed, and then burned or placed in the container for city or institution garbage collection.

Rationale: Isolating infectious objects prevents the spread of infection.

Resolved Needs: Cleanliness. Protection from physical harm. Increased learning.

Explain how to estimate temperature by touch   Explain that when a thermometer is not available, one can estimate fever by touching the skin, especially the forehead and face. Temperature estimation is as follows:

very hot skin	dangerous fever
hot skin	high fever
very warm skin	slight fever
warm skin	normal
cool skin	slightly subnormal temperature
cold skin	moderately low temperature
very cold skin	dangerously low temperature

Rationale: Abnormal body temperature may indicate excessive heat production or loss or a poor temperature regulating mechanism.

Resolved Needs: Protection from physical harm. Increased learning.

Explain how to file the nails correctly   Explain that nails should be shaped by filing only the undesirable areas and by filing in only one direction. A metal file should be used for shaping long, hard nails. The coarse side of an emery board should be used for shaping normal nails, with the fine side being used to finish off the shaping.

Rationale: Proper nail shaping prevents nail splitting and tearing of nails.

Resolved Needs: Protection from physical harm. Increased learning.

Explain how to give medications to children   Explain that although children may be irritable and fussy when ill, medicines can be given successfully. Infants accept medicines well from a plastic dropper. Young children do better if allowed some independence, such as choosing between tablet and liquid, putting the tablet into a gelatin capsule, choosing the flavor of syrup to mix with the medicine, or drinking the medicine from a doll's teacup. Avoid restraining the child unless it is absolutely necessary. Children appreciate explanations of why the medication is necessary.

Rationale: Successful administration of medications to children increases the potential for improved health.

Resolved Needs: Comfort. Protection from physical harm. Increased learning.

Explain how to illuminate a room correctly   Explain that proper lighting involves both immediate illumination of the work area and distant illumination from a second light in the room. Explain that light should come over the left shoulder if the person is right-handed and over the right shoulder if the person is left-handed.

Rationale: Proper room illumination promotes visual acuity.

Resolved Needs: Comfort. Protection from physical harm. Increased learning.

Explain how to integrate the hemodialysis procedure into the home routine   Suggest to the patient and his family how the hemodialysis procedure might best fit into their schedule with the least interruption of daily routine.

Rationale: Fitting essential therapeutic treatments into daily living patterns with the least disruption of lifestyle provides the comfort of a nearly normal existence.

Resolved Needs: Comfort. Increased learning.

Explain how to maintain a correct sitting position   Explain that when one is sitting, the body weight should be equally distributed on the thighs and buttocks. The lower back should rest against the back of the chair, with the feet flat on the floor.

Rationale: Proper body alignment keeps organs in their correct positions and functioning well; it can favor gravity pull or support against gravity; it reduces fatigue and maintains skeletal balance, which in turn promotes effective circulation and respiration.

Resolved Needs: Comfort. Protection from physical harm. Increased learning.

Explain how to maintain a diabetic diet when away from home   Explain that diabetics can eat any time and anywhere without worry. When traveling, they can take along nonperishable foods if meals are delayed or unavailable on trains or airplanes. They should take the following precautions: Eat only clear broths and consomme soups. Eat only unglazed, unbuttered, and uncreamed meat, poultry, fish, and vegetables. Eat leafy salads containing celery, lettuce, tomatoes, cucumbers, or pickles. Eat fresh fruits for dessert. Avoid casseroles, since their contents vary. Use only lemon and vinegar for salad dressings.

Rationale: Knowing how to manage a diabetic diet away from home can support good health and allow the diabetic increased social comfort.

Resolved Needs: Comfort. Protection from physical harm. Increased learning.

Explain how to maintain body alignment Explain the various methods used to position and support the extremities and other body parts in a normal line for functioning.

Rationale: Functional body alignment promotes circulation and comfort; it helps prevent joint deformities, painful stretching or shortening of tendons, and further damage to vital tissues by fractured bones.

Resolved Needs: Circulation. Comfort. Protection from physical harm. Increased learning.

Explain how to maintain cleanliness of the ostomy appliance Explain that the ostomy bag and tubing should be cleaned daily with soap and water, rinsed in cold water, and dried.

Rationale: A clean ostomy appliance minimizes the potential for infection, promotes comfort, and supports independent self-care.

Resolved Needs: Comfort. Cleanliness. Protection from physical harm. Increased learning.

Explain how to maintain environmental cleanliness Explain that a clean environment is essential for health. Cleaning should include the following: damp-dusting of furniture, uncarpeted floors, baseboards, pictures, doors, and drapes; washing of floors, baseboards, windows, cabinets, tables, and shelves with antiseptic solutions; daily rug vacuuming; periodic vacuuming of stuffed furniture and drapes.

Rationale: Cleanliness inhibits the growth of harmful microorganisms.

Resolved Needs: Cleanliness. Protection from physical harm. Increased learning.

Explain how to maintain ileostomy (or colostomy) cleanliness Explain that the ileostomy or colostomy stoma and the surrounding skin should be kept clean with mild soap and water.

Rationale: Cleansing of an ostomy stoma prevents skin excoriation, decreases offensive odor, promotes comfort, and supports independent self-care.

Resolved Needs: Comfort. Cleanliness. Protection from physical harm. Increased learning.

Explain how to maintain maximum nutrients in food Explain that the maximum nutrient value of foods can be retained by employing slow cooking methods rather than rapid boiling, by steaming rather than cooking in water, and by broiling and baking.

Rationale: Conservation of nutrients in food promotes improved nutrition.

Resolved Needs: Food balance. Protection from physical harm. Increased learning.

Explain how to manage seizure episodes   Explain that when seizures occur, the patient's clothing should be loosened. He should not be restrained, nor should there be interference with seizure movements. All surrounding objects that might cause harm to the patient should be removed. If the patient's mouth is open, place something soft between the jaw teeth on one side only. If the teeth are tightly clenched, do not attempt to force anything between them. Allow the patient to rest once the seizure is over.

Rationale: Knowledge of the methods for safe handling of patients having seizures promotes comfort and safety.

Resolved Needs: Comfort. Protection from physical harm. Increased learning.

Explain how to massage bony prominences   Explain that bony prominences such as the heels, ankles, knees, iliac crest, scapula and clavicle, wrists, and elbows should be frequently massaged with rhythmic, stimulating strokes.

Rationale: Prolonged pressure of bone against skin can result in decreased circulation, with increased potential for irritation and necrosis. Stimulation of the bony prominences prevents tissue damage.

Resolved Needs: Protection from physical harm. Increased learning.

Explain how to measure intake and output   Explain how to measure and record the volume of fluids taken in and excreted from the body in a 24-hour period.

Rationale: Assistance from the patient and family in measuring intake and output promotes accuracy.

Resolved Needs: Protection from physical harm. Increased learning.

Explain how to minimize intraocular pressure   Explain that ways of preventing increased pressure within the eyes include avoidance of the following factors: emotional excitement, excessive fluid intake, heavy lifting, elimination straining, sudden or up-and-down head movements, and tight clothing around the head and neck. Teach moderation when using the eyes for work and reading.

Rationale: Intraocular pressure can cause hemorrhage or rupture of surgical eye incisions that have not completely healed.

Resolved Needs: Protection from physical harm. Increased learning.

Explain how to observe respirations   Explain that respiration count is the number of times a person breathes in 1 minute. Explain the need to watch for deviations from normal respiratory patterns.

Rationale: Normal oxygen and carbon dioxide exchange through respiration is essential to tissue cell life.

Resolved Needs: Protection from physical harm. Increased learning.

Explain how to obtain release from emotional stress   Explain that pent-up emotional stress can be relieved in a number of ways: strenuous physical activity such as hammering, competitive sports, running, swimming, bicycling, chopping wood, cleaning out the garage, or moving the furniture; creative activities such as painting and writing; catharses such as crying in private, laughing heartily, or simply talking things over with another person.

Rationale: Release of pent-up emotions temporarily relieves emotional distress.

Resolved Needs: Comfort. Protection from physical harm. Protection from psychologic threat. Increased learning.

Explain how to obtain therapeutic supplies   When therapeutic supplies are needed, tell the patient where and how to obtain them at minimum cost.

Rationale: Having the appropriate supplies supports continuity of health therapy.

Resolved Needs: Comfort. Protection from physical harm. Increased learning.

Explain how to pad bony prominences   Explain that all bony prominences should be padded with soft materials whenever they are subject to prolonged pressure. This is essential for persons undergoing prolonged rest, for those with paralyzed limbs, etc.

Rationale: Pressure on bony prominences causes irritation and impaired circulation, which can result in necrosis.

Resolved Needs: Comfort. Protection from physical harm. Increased learning.

Explain how to pad rough cast edges   Explain that all rough or ragged cast edges should be padded (petaled) so as to minimize pressure against the skin and prevent plaster particles from falling under the cast and causing decubitus ulcer.

Rationale: Small rough particles rubbed into the skin can cause abrasion and infection.

Resolved Needs: Comfort. Protection from physical harm. Increased learning.

Explain how to prepare for the diagnostic study   Explain what the patient needs to do to prepare himself for a particular study. This includes such preparations as limiting food and fluids for a specified time, eating special diets, taking special drugs or dyes, taking laxatives and enemas, and collecting specimens. Be sure that the patient understands when, how, and why the preparations should be carried out.

Rationale: Adequate preparation for studies facilitates accurate diagnostic findings.

Resolved Needs: Comfort. Increased learning.

Explain how to prepare the breasts during pregnancy for postdelivery breast feeding
Explain that breast care during pregnancy can bring the breasts to optimum condition for breast feeding after delivery. Instruct the woman to massage her breasts once or twice daily, apply lanolin to her breasts, gently pull on the nipples, and rub the nipples with a terrycloth towel.

Rationale: Massaging and rubbing the breasts will toughen the nipples and prevent cracking, bleeding, and pain during breast feeding. Lubricating the breasts makes them more elastic so that they will stretch and the nipple will not split.

Resolved Needs: Comfort. Cleanliness. Protection from physical harm. Increased learning.

Explain how to prevent coughing
Explain that coughing may be deferred by taking slow, gentle deep breaths when the cough reflex seems imminent.

Rationale: Coughing causes increased intrathoracic, intraocular, intraabdominal, and intracranial pressure. Unproductive coughing wastes energy.

Resolved Needs: Protection from physical harm. Freedom from pain. Increased learning.

Explain how to prevent cross infection
Explain that cross infection can be reduced by room and article decontamination, limited direct human contact, hand washing, and wearing a gown and mask.

Rationale: Removing infectious microorganisms from surfaces and preventing contact with organisms can decrease the potential for disease transfer from one person to another.

Resolved Needs: Protection from physical harm. Increased learning.

Explain how to prevent sneezing
Explain that sneezing may be prevented by exerting finger pressure above the lip and under the nose or by taking deep breaths through the mouth. The nares should not be squeezed together in an attempt to prevent sneezing.

Rationale: Since sneezing causes increased intranasal pressure and can dislodge blood clots that have sealed off bleeding, sneezing should be avoided when there has been nasal bleeding or trauma.

Resolved Needs: Protection from physical harm. Increased learning.

Explain how to prevent the common cold
Explain that good basic health practices such as adequate rest and balanced nutrition make one less susceptible to colds. In addition, other measures include wearing warm clothing to protect against chill, maintaining good room ventilation, staying away from persons with colds and persons who are sneezing or

coughing, wearing a mask when one has a cold and is caring for others, preventing the drying out of respiratory mucous membrane linings, avoiding dieting during the cold season, avoiding breathing cold air, and avoiding sudden temperature changes.

Rationale: Prevention of the common cold preserves health and reduces suffering.

Resolved Needs: Comfort. Protection from physical harm. Increased learning.

Explain how to recognize the outgrowth of a brace   Explain that brace joints should coincide with body joints. When it is noticed that brace joints do not coincide with body joints, the patient is outgrowing his brace.

Rationale: A brace that does not fit properly causes pressure on skin areas and does not provide the intended support.

Resolved Needs: Protection from physical harm. Increased learning.

Explain how to reduce muscular tension   Explain that muscular tension can be reduced by stretching the muscles, yawning, and suddenly letting the muscles go limp. It can also be accomplished by assuming a lying or sitting position and allowing all muscles to become limp.

Rationale: Stretching brings the muscles to peak contraction, and this is followed by relaxation. Muscle contraction during illness consumes energy that is vital for healing. Relief of musclar tension promotes comfort.

Resolved Needs: Sleep, rest, relaxation. Energy. Comfort. Protection from physical harm. Increased learning.

Explain how to remove earwax   Explain that earwax may be softened by placing a few drops of warmed glycerin in the ear; this is followed by gentle removal with a small piece of twisted gauze or tissue gently inserted, not packed, into the canal to absorb the solution.

Rationale: Removal of earwax promotes cleanliness and can improve impaired hearing when impacted cerumen is its cause.

Resolved Needs: Comfort. Cleanliness. Protection from physical harm. Increased learning.

Contraindications: Ear infection, inflammation, or drainage. Ruptured tympanic membrane. Presence of a myringotomy tube.

Explain how to remove hair lice   Explain that lice can be removed from the hair and scalp by moistening the hair with hot vinegar and combing the ova out with a fine-tooth comb; a mixture of kerosene and olive oil in equal amounts may also be used; there are also prescription shampoos.

Rationale: Head lice cause scalp inflammation, which has the potential for bacterial infection.

Resolved Needs: Cleanliness. Protection from physical harm. Increased learning.

Explain how to replace monitor electrodes   Explain to the patient wearing a battery-operated portable monitor how to retape or repaste external electrodes if they come loose.

Rationale: Proper adherence of electrodes to the skin is essential for correct monitor recordings.

Resolved Needs: Comfort. Increased learning.

Explain how to set behavioral limits   Explain that limits are set on another person's behavior by clearly stating what constitutes acceptable and unacceptable behavior.

Rationale: External control of behavior supports internal control when the latter cannot be maintained. Limitations protect against future shame that can result from uncontrolled behavior.

Resolved Needs: Protection from psychologic threat. Personal growth and maturity. Increased learning. Increased reality perception and problem-solving ability.

Explain how to shampoo the hair (or scalp)   Explain how to shampoo hair so that optimum cleanliness is attained. The technique may include shampooing in bed as well as out of bed.

Rationale: Cleanliness prevents infection and promotes comfort.

Resolved Needs: Comfort. Cleanliness. Protection from physical harm. Increased learning.

Explain how to splint an incision   Explain that patients who experience discomfort while coughing should splint or support the painful site with a pillow while coughing.

Rationale: Supporting a painful site during coughing decreases tension and stretching of the severed muscles.

Resolved Needs: Comfort. Protection from physical harm. Increased learning.

Explain how to sterilize contaminated dishes   Explain that contaminated dishes can be sterilized by submerging them in a large pan of disinfecting solution, by boiling them, or by placing them in a dishwasher that attains the proper temperature.

Rationale: Sterilization destroys all surface microorganisms and helps prevent infection.

Resolved Needs: Protection from physical harm. Increased learning.

Explain how to stimulate an infant during feeding   Explain that some infants fall asleep during feeding time. Changing the infant's position or moving his bottle will usually awaken him.

Rationale: Knowledge that infants may go to sleep before receiving adequate nourishment increases the parents' ability to ensure proper nourishment.

Resolved Needs: Protection from physical harm. Increased learning.

Explain how to strain urine   Explain how to filter urine output through a gauze or strainer to catch urinary stones.

Rationale: Catching urinary stones provides evidence that the stones have been passed. Analysis of urinary stones facilitates the prescription of measures to prevent future stone formation.

Resolved Needs: Protection from physical harm. Increased learning.

Explain how to take allergy precautions   Suggest that persons with allergies take the following precautions: travel in air-conditioned vehicles; do not bring cut flowers indoors; stay out of smoke-filled rooms; avoid using perfumes and scented cosmetics; do not engage in water sports that necessitate swimming under water; avoid excessive sun; get adequate rest; avoid fog, rain, and road dust as much as possible; have a short-haired dog instead of a long-haired one; do not keep birds in the house; avoid eating fish, nuts, chocolate, oranges, and tomatoes; use hypoallergenic cosmetics; avoid fuzzy blankets and wool clothing; do not use insecticides; do not apply dust-catching oils to the skin; avoid sudden temperature changes, especially becoming overheated.

Rationale: Avoidance of allergic stimuli promotes safety and comfort.

Resolved Needs: Comfort. Protection from physical harm. Increased learning.

Explain how to use a bed rope   Teach the patient to use a rope or a strong piece of sheeting that has been attached to the foot of the bed so that he can pull himself from a lying position to a sitting position.

Rationale: The ability to move about prevents stasis of secretions, stimulates circulation, restores strength, and promotes independence.

Resolved Needs: Activity, exercise. Comfort. Protection from physical harm. Independence. Increased learning.

Explain how to use a paper bag to reduce hyperventilation   Teach patients who experience dizziness because of habitual rapid breathing to breathe into a paper bag for about 5 minutes, or until the dizziness and rapid breathing cease.

Rationale: When the patient rebreathes the exhaled carbon dioxide collected in the paper bag, the level of carbon dioxide in his blood is raised to normal, reestablishing respiratory acid-base balance.

Resolved Needs: Acid-base balance. Protection from physical harm. Increased learning.

Contraindications: Elevated blood levels of carbon dioxide. Emphysema.

Explain how to use toilet tissue correctly Explain that when cleansing the perineal area with toilet tissue, wiping should begin at the anterior (front) perineum and continue to the posterior (back) perineum. Never wipe toward the front or wipe twice with the same piece of tissue.

Rationale: Bacteria-containing fecal matter can cause urinary tract infection when spread from the posterior to the anterior perineum.

Resolved Needs: Cleanliness. Protection from physical harm. Increased learning.

Explain how venereal disease is transmitted Explain that venereal diseases are transmitted primarily by sexual intercourse and that persons who frequently change sexual partners run a high risk because they do not always know the health status of these partners. Explain that venereal disease can be transmitted to the fetus through the placenta or through contact in an infected birth canal. If there are lip lesions, venereal disease can be contracted by kissing.

Rationale: Prevention of venereal disease preserves health and reduces suffering.

Resolved Needs: Protection from physical harm. Increased learning.

Explain that a child should become accustomed to dry diapers during toilet training Explain that toilet training is facilitated if the child's diaper is changed frequently so that he becomes accustomed to a dry diaper.

Rationale: Children accustomed to dry diapers find wet diapers uncomfortable and are more amenable to toilet training.

Resolved Needs: Comfort. Increased learning.

Explain that a light is needed in the television viewing room Explain that soft indirect lighting should be provided in the television viewing room and that the light should not be reflected in the screen.

Rationale: The contrast between a bright television screen and a darkened room causes eye fatigue.

Resolved Needs: Comfort. Protection from physical harm. Increased learning.

Explain that a pacifier should not be hung around an infant's neck Explain that a pacifier should never be hung on a string or ribbon around a child's neck.

Rationale: As the child moves about, the pacifier may become caught on something or twisted about the child's neck, causing strangulation.

Resolved Needs: Protection from physical harm. Increased learning.

Explain that a sugared pacifier should not be given at bedtime Explain that a child should not be allowed to suck on a pacifier coated with sugar prior to napping or sleeping.

Rationale: Carbohydrates cause tooth decay.

Resolved Needs: Protection from physical harm. Increased learning.

Explain that care should be taken to prevent scratching of the contact lenses   Explain that contact lenses should be handled gently and never placed on a rough surface where scratching can occur.

Rationale: A scratched contact lens impairs vision and causes discomfort.

Resolved Needs: Comfort. Protection from physical harm. Increased learning.

Explain that childbirth is a normal process   Explain that childbirth is not a disease, but a natural physiologic process, just as are the processes of breathing and digestion.

Rationale: Awareness that physiologic processes are normal promotes comfort.

Resolved Needs: Comfort. Protection from psychologic threat. Increased learning.

Explain that clear, correct product labeling is essential   Explain that household products, drugs, etc., should be labeled clearly and accurately so that there can be no error in determining the contents of any container. Avoid putting poisonous substances in the same types of containers that are used for products for internal consumption.

Rationale: Clear, correct labeling of containers promotes safety.

Resolved Needs: Protection from physical harm. Increased learning.

Explain that clothes should be laid out in the order of dressing for persons with impaired cerebral function   Explain that confused or retarded persons should have their clothes laid out in the proper order of dressing when attempting to dress themselves.

Rationale: Orderliness reduces confusion and supports the development of skill and self-reliance.

Resolved Needs: Comfort. Self-reliance. Mastery and competence in skills. Independence. Increased learning.

Explain that commode sittings should be scheduled during toilet training   Explain that during toilet training the child should be placed on the commode every day at the same time.

Rationale: Placing the child on the commode at the same time every day facilitates adaptation to routine physiologic functioning.

Resolved Needs: Comfort. Increased learning.

Explain that communication should be encouraged despite impairment   Teach the family to assist the patient to communicate in

any way possible, whether it be by speech, writing, or symbols, and to select the method that causes the least frustration and self-depreciation.

Rationale: Comfort is promoted by a sense of effective communication with others.

Resolved Needs: Comfort. Warm, communicating relationships. Increased learning.

Contraindications: When a patient is relearning to speak, he should not be encouraged to use short-cut methods to communicate.

Explain that controlled elimination should be praised during toilet training   Explain that toilet training is facilitated by words of approval and appreciation when elimination control is successful.

Rationale: Praise gives the child a sense of satisfaction and a desire to master the behavior that precipitates praise.

Resolved Needs: Comfort. Increased learning.

Explain that corrective eye lenses require periodic adjustment   Explain that persons wearing glasses or contact lenses should have their eyes checked for visual changes at least every 2 years and should have their glasses or contact lenses adjusted to meet these changes.

Rationale: Periodic readjustment of eye lenses supports improved vision.

Resolved Needs: Protection from physical harm. Increased learning.

Explain that daily bowel elimination is not essential   Explain that as long as feces are not hard and dry, daily elimination is not necessary; elimination is dependent on body routine and food consumption.

Rationale: Awareness that daily bowel elimination is not essential can prevent the use of poor health practices to stimulate elimination.

Resolved Needs: Comfort. Protection from physical harm. Increased learning.

Explain that drug dependence is an illness   Explain that the excessive use of drugs or alcohol indicates a basic psychologic disorder that must be dealt with in order to overcome the problem. Although addicts may commit criminal acts to obtain drugs, addiction itself is not a crime. Addiction is an illness.

Rationale: Recognizing that drug dependence is an illness supports a realistic approach to solution of the problem.

Resolved Needs: Comfort. Protection from physical harm. Protection from psychologic threat. Increased learning. Increased reality perception and problem-solving ability.

Explain that drug use is not socially essential   Explain that one does not have to use drugs or alcohol to be accepted within a peer group. Those who prefer not to use drugs are generally held in equal, if not higher, esteem than those who do.

Rationale: The mistaken notion that one must conform to every peer pressure in order to be accepted frequently overrides intelligent recognition of the inadvisability of an activity.

Resolved Needs: Comfort. Protection from physical harm. Protection from psychologic threat. Personal growth and maturity. Increased learning. Increased reality perception and problem-solving ability.

Explain that extreme cold cracks contact lenses   Explain that if a contact lens is stored in solution and left in an extremely cold environment, the lens will crack.

Rationale: Proper care of contact lenses assures their availability as a visual aid.

Resolved Needs: Protection from physical harm. Increased learning.

Explain that fatigue should be recognized as a stress factor   Help families recognize that high percentages of disagreements occur when family members are fatigued. This is especially true in the evening, when the father comes home from a hard day's work, the children are tired from school, and the mother, who has been housekeeping or working at outside employment, has the additional stress of meal preparation.

Rationale: Understanding stress factors promotes preventive behavior and acceptance of the behavior of others.

Resolved Needs: Protection from physical harm. Protection from psychologic threat. Increased learning. Increased reality perception and problem-solving ability.

Explain that fear (or anxiety) often disguises itself   Explain that an expressed fear or anxiety is often a substitute for another fear or anxiety that is not socially acceptable. Disguising fear or anxiety can convert the original fear or anxiety into a form that is socially approved.

Rationale: Facing fear or anxiety in its original form reduces the complexity of the fear situation.

Resolved Needs: Comfort. Protection from psychologic threat. Personal growth and maturity. Increased learning. Increased reality perception and problem-solving ability.

Explain that fluid intake and output should be balanced   Explain that maintenance of balance in body fluids requires daily consumption of approximately 2000 cc (six to eight 240-cc glasses of liquid), with about equal output.

Rationale: Water balance is essential for normal cell function, production of secretions, elimination of urine and feces, maintenance of electrolyte balance, and other important physiologic functions.

Resolved Needs: Water-salt balance. Protection from physical harm. Increased learning.

Explain that fluids should not be given to persons unable to swallow   Explain that nothing should be given by mouth to patients who are unable to swallow. This includes those who are unconscious or stuporous, those with throat paralysis, and those who cough and spit up when attempting to swallow.

Rationale: Difficulty in swallowing or inability to swallow poses the threat of food or liquid aspiration into the lungs and consequent airway obstruction.

Resolved Needs: Protection from physical harm. Increased learning.

Explain that hair lost during illness usually returns   Explain that hair loss resulting from high fever or drug reactions is temporary and that hair will return when body processes are restored to normal.

Rationale: Awareness that lost hair will return to normal promotes comfort.

Resolved Needs: Comfort. Increased learning.

Explain that heat warps contact lenses   Explain that a contact lens should never be placed near a stove or heater because it will change shape.

Rationale: Proper care of contact lenses assures their availability as a visual aid.

Resolved Needs: Protection from physical harm. Increased learning.

Explain that ill persons are often hypersensitive   Explain that most ill persons are highly susceptible to emotional upsets inadvertently caused by others. The patient is keenly aware of others' responses regarding the acceptability of his illness, and he often prefers that his illness not be discussed outside the family. Ill persons are also sensitive to environmental confusion and noise.

Rationale: Awareness of the hypersensitivity of ill persons supports behavior modification on the part of well persons to meet the needs of the sick.

Resolved Needs: Comfort. Protection from psychologic threat. Personal growth and maturity. Increased learning. Increased reality perception and problem-solving ability.

Explain that immobility related to pain causes further pain   Explain that despite the pain involved, noninflamed arthritic and age-stiffened joints should be moved as much as possible; otherwise, greater pain and stiffness will be experienced.

Rationale: Maintenance of joint mobility promotes comfort.

Resolved Needs: Comfort. Protection from physical harm. Freedom from pain. Increased learning.

Explain that it is acceptable to admit the existence of pain
Explain that admitting the existence of pain is culturally acceptable and that when it is reported relief measures can be taken.

Rationale: Psychologic safety requires that the person experience acceptance by others.

Resolved Needs: Comfort. Protection from psychologic threat. Increased learning.

Explain that it is essential to foster healthy drinking attitudes
Explain that it is the family's responsibility to their children to communicate moderate and positive attitudes toward alcohol consumption.

Rationale: Moderate and positive attitudes taught during early childhood support healthy behavior in adult life.

Resolved Needs: Protection from physical harm. Protection from psychologic threat. Personal growth and maturity. Increased learning. Increased reality perception and problem-solving ability.

Explain that long-term drug abuse reduces the pleasures derived from drug abuse
Explain to persons taking drugs for their pleasurable effects that the experience becomes less and less pleasurable with time. Even as drug dosage is increased to stimulate ecstasy, the quality of the experience gradually deteriorates.

Rationale: Awareness that drugs cannot indefinitely maintain a heightened pleasurable experience supports recognition that drug abuse for the sake of pleasure is futile.

Resolved Needs: Protection from psychologic threat. Personal growth and maturity. Increased learning. Increased reality perception and problem-solving ability.

Explain that monitors are safe
Explain that the application of a monitor is harmless.

Rationale: Assurance that monitors are safe reduces anxiety.

Resolved Needs: Comfort. Protection from psychologic threat. Increased learning.

Explain that mothers have a choice of single or double breast feeding
Explain that once lactation is well established, the mother may alternate breasts with each feeding or may use both breasts for each feeding. The decision depends on the milk flow, on infant demand for feeding, and on the mother's comfort.

Rationale: Proper breast feeding supports maternal and infant health.

Resolved Needs: Comfort. Protection from physical harm. Increased learning.

Explain that nails should be soaked before trimming   Explain that nails should be soaked in warm soapy water before being cut.

Rationale: Soaking softens the nail, making trimming easier and reducing the potential for nail injury.

Resolved Needs: Protection from physical harm. Increased learning.

Explain that nursing the infant on alternate breasts reduces tenderness   Explain that during the first few days of breast feeding, if the mother experiences breast tenderness or soreness, she may prefer to alternate breasts with each feeding.

Rationale: Alternating breasts with each feeding decreases irritation from infant sucking and promotes comfort.

Resolved Needs: Comfort. Protection from physical harm. Increased learning.

Explain that objects should be consistently placed in the same location for the visually impaired   Explain that when persons have difficulty in seeing, objects should always be kept in their accustomed places according to individual needs.

Rationale: Consistently keeping objects in their usual places reduces the stress of adapting to an unfamiliar situation; it promotes comfort, meets dependency needs, supports independent mobility, and reduces the potential for injury.

Resolved Needs: Comfort. Protection from physical harm. Dependence. Predictable, orderly world. Independence. Increased learning.

Explain that one's face should be kept visible when speaking to a deaf person   Explain that in speaking to a deaf person, the speaker should directly face the deaf person and maintain a position such that light falls on the face of the speaker.

Rationale: Deaf persons depend on facial expressions to clarify messages.

Resolved Needs: Comfort. Warm, communicating relationships. Increased learning.

Explain that pacemakers are safe   Explain that the electrical current in a pacemaker is not sufficient to do harm, only to stimulate the heart.

Rationale: Assurance that pacemakers are safe reduces anxiety.

Resolved Needs: Comfort. Protection from psychologic threat. Increased learning.

Explain that parental attitudes affect child development
Explain that the attitudes parents communicate to children, both verbally and nonverbally, affect the child's perception of himself and his world and results in child behavior that reflects that perception.

Rationale: Awareness of the effect that one's attitudes have on others supports favorable behavior toward others.

Resolved Needs: Protection from physical harm. Protection from psychologic threat. Personal growth and maturity. Increased learning. Increased reality perception and problem-solving ability.

Explain that persons making emotional adjustments prefer doing so at their own pace   Explain that persons who are making emotional adjustments should not be forced into activities and contacts with other people, but should be allowed to participate as they desire.

Rationale: Forcing rapid adaptation and adjustment increases the threat of internal tension, especially when the person feels inadequate to cope with the situation.

Resolved Needs: Comfort. Protection from psychologic threat. Increased learning. Increased reality perception and problem-solving ability.

Explain that persons wearing leg braces should avoid contact sports   Explain that persons wearing braces should not participate in sports that bring them into physical contact with others, such as football, basketball, and soccer. Tennis, volleyball, baseball, and swimming are safer.

Rationale: Severe injury can result from impact with the steel brace frame.

Resolved Needs: Protection from physical harm. Increased learning.

Explain that persons with impaired cerebral function require close observation   Explain that persons whose cerebral functioning is impaired are often not responsible and should not be left alone; they require constant and close supervision.

Rationale: Persons with impaired cerebral function require close supervision because of their increased potential for accidental injury.

Resolved Needs: Protection from physical harm. Increased learning. Increased reality perception and problem-solving ability.

Explain that persons with limited attention span require message repetition   Explain that messages should be repeated to a person whose attention span is limited.

Rationale: Repetition enhances communication by reinforcing perception of the intended ideas and thoughts.

Resolved Needs: Warm, communicating relationships. Increased learning.

Explain that poor speech is not outgrown   Explain that a child's poor speech habits will not correct themselves as the child matures; correct speech habits must be taught and practiced.

Rationale: If a child learns to speak incorrectly, he must relearn the speech process in order to correct the problem.

Resolved Needs: Increased learning. Increased reality perception and problem-solving ability.

Explain that positive retirement goals are essential to health
Explain that as retirement approaches, a person should have some specific activity he can step into that he perceives as pleasant and worthwhile. Retirement should be a positive step, not a loss.

Rationale: Loss evokes grief and depression. Anticipation of pleasantness promotes positive feelings and stimulation.

Resolved Needs: Comfort. Stimulation. Protection from physical harm. Protection from psychologic threat. Personal growth and maturity. Increased learning.

Explain that powder should be applied between the diabetic's toes after bathing
Explain that after diabetics bathe, they should apply a light, smooth layer of dusting powder between the toes.

Rationale: Diabetics are prone to hardening and narrowing of the arteries, which cause poor circulation to the skin. Maintaining dry skin with absorbent dusting powder minimizes irritation to their easily traumatized skin and promotes comfort.

Resolved Needs: Comfort. Protection from physical harm. Increased learning.

Explain that pregnancy results from sexual activity
Explain that sexual intercourse, when occurring at ovulation, results in pregnancy.

Rationale: Knowledge of physiologic processes promotes comfort.

Resolved Needs: Comfort. Increased learning.

Explain that premature infants require at-home supervision
Explain that premature infants discharged from the hospital cannot be taken to nurseries or left in the care of babysitters. They must be kept at home and supervised by family members specifically instructed in their care.

Rationale: Since the health status of the premature infant is more fragile than that of the full-term baby, early care must be carefully supervised to assure health maintenance.

Resolved Needs: Protection from physical harm. Increased learning. Increased reality perception and problem-solving ability.

Explain that premature infants require prescribed foods
Explain that premature infants at home must have specifically prescribed foods for proper growth and development.

Rationale: Since premature infants are not as well developed physiologically as full-term infants, they cannot digest the same foods at the same age.

Resolved Needs: Protection from physical harm. Increased learning.

Explain that questions need to be phrased for yes and no answers when there is impaired speech delivery   Explain that when a person has difficulty in speaking, he is most comfortable when he is able to give a yes or no answer to a question, rather than having to respond in detail to conversation.

Rationale: Simple and direct communication reduces frustration and anxiety and promotes comfort.

Resolved Needs: Comfort. Protection from psychologic threat. Warm, communicating relationships. Increased learning.

Explain that recreation aids total health   Explain that recreation provides a balance to the working world and supports health.

Rationale: The movement and motor coordination experienced in recreational activities stimulate physical and mental processes.

Resolved Needs: Protection from physical harm. Protection from psychologic threat. Increased learning. Increased reality perception and problem-solving ability.

Explain that recreation and relaxation differ   Explain that recreation is voluntary play performed during leisure time and requiring physical, mental, and emotional activity, while relaxation is the reduction of muscle tension that occurs with the cessation of all body activity.

Rationale: Since recreation and relaxation are commonly thought of as synonymous, one or the other is often omitted. An awareness that they differ can facilitate the use of both for improved health.

Resolved Needs: Protection from physical harm. Protection from psychologic threat. Increased learning. Increased reality perception and problem-solving ability.

Explain that recreation should fit individual interests   Explain that any activity that holds a person's attention is good recreation for that person, regardless of the preferred activity in his peer group. Recreation should be considered in relation to the person's health.

Rationale: One's interests derive from past pleasurable experiences and support positive attitudes toward future pleasant experiences.

Resolved Needs: Comfort. Increased learning. Increased reality perception and problem-solving ability. Increased pleasantness.

Explain that recreation supports personal growth and is not an escape mechanism   Explain that recreation should not be considered an escape, but rather a growth factor that gives personal satisfaction.

Rationale: Negative feelings lead to escape activity. Growth results from positive attitudes that enrich and develop the personality, often by recreational means.

Resolved Needs: Comfort. Personal growth and maturity. Increased learning. Increased reality perception and problem-solving ability. Increased pleasantness.

Explain that relaxation is essential for successful sexual response
Explain that an important aspect of successful sexual activity involves relaxing and allowing natural responses to occur.

Rationale: The body performs best when relaxed.

Resolved Needs: Relaxation. Sexuality. Increased learning. Increased reality perception and problem-solving ability.

Explain that sexual activity should be temporarily limited
Explain that when recovering from cardiac disease, the patient should refrain from sexual activity for several months. During pregnancy, sexual activity should be avoided if the membrane has ruptured or if there is vaginal bleeding. Intercourse should be avoided when a vaginal infection exists.

Rationale: Sexual intercourse increases the heart rate, respirations, blood pressure, and cardiac output and can result in cardiac overload. Sexual activity after the membrane has ruptured can cause vaginal infection, placenta previa, or perforation of the placenta. When vaginal infection exists, sexual activity can extend the infection in the female and cause infection of the male's genitourinary tract.

Resolved Needs: Protection from physical harm. Increased learning.

Explain that sexual response normally varies
Explain that the degree of sexual satisfaction varies from day to day and is dependent on fatigue level, mood, current life problems, muscular tension caused by anxiety, and other such factors.

Rationale: Awareness that sexual response varies promotes comfort and reality perception.

Resolved Needs: Comfort. Sexuality. Protection from psychologic threat. Increased learning. Increased reality perception and problem-solving ability.

Explain that socialization depletes the ill person's energy
Explain that socializing with visitors fatigues sick persons and therefore should be limited.

Rationale: Socializing consumes energy that ill persons need for healing and recovery.

Resolved Needs: Protection from physical harm. Protection from psychologic threat. Increased learning.

Explain that some tension is normal Explain that one normally experiences a certain amount of tension and should not expect to feel tension-free.

Rationale: Normal tension gives pleasure and stimulates activity.

Resolved Needs: Comfort. Protection from psychologic threat. Increased learning. Increased reality perception and problem-solving ability.

Explain that the behavior of one family member is not a reflection on other family members Explain that the abnormal behavior of a family member does not reflect negatively on other family members. Despite family ties, each person is independently responsible for his behavior.

Rationale: Awareness that each person is solely responsible for his behavior reduces the anxiety commonly experienced when the values and behavior of one family member are in conflict with the basic values of the family.

Resolved Needs: Comfort. Protection from psychologic threat. Increased learning. Increased reality perception and problem-solving ability.

Explain that the common cold is contagious for 48 hours after symptom onset Explain that the common cold can be given or contracted from others during the first 48 hours after symptoms (heightened sneezing) appear.

Rationale: Reduced contact with those who have colds for the first 48 hours after their symptoms appear can prevent the spread of infection.

Resolved Needs: Protection from physical harm. Increased learning.

Explain that the diabetic's feet should be washed gently Explain that diabetics should wash their feet gently with mild soap and a soft cloth.

Rationale: Diabetics are prone to hardening and narrowing of the arteries, which cause poor circulation to the skin. Washing the feet gently is more comfortable, and it decreases the trauma caused by excess friction.

Resolved Needs: Comfort. Protection from physical harm. Increased learning.

Explain that the person's emotional response is appropriate and commonly experienced Explain that the emotion the person is experiencing is considered a normal response in the particular situation and that other persons often experience the same emotion in similar situations.

Rationale: Feelings of adequacy and comfort evolve from an awareness that one's emotions are normal and are similarly experienced by others.

Resolved Needs: Comfort. Protection from psychologic threat. Adequacy. Increased learning. Increased reality perception and problem-solving ability.

Explain that the teeth should not be brushed with potentially unsafe water
Explain that the teeth should not be brushed with contaminated water. Boiled, chlorinated or carbonated water can be used.

Rationale: Brushing the teeth with contaminated water introduces bacteria into the mouth that eventually can enter the intestinal tract.

Resolved Needs: Protection from physical harm. Increased learning.

Explain that the urinary catheter should be taped to the abdomen
Explain that a male patient having an indwelling catheter for a prolonged period should tape the end of the catheter to his abdomen.

Rationale: Taping the urinary catheter to the abdomen prevents ulceration at the penile-scrotal junction by keeping pressure off the glans and urethra.

Resolved Needs: Protection from physical harm. Increased learning.

Contraindications: An unhealed abdominal surgical incision.

Explain that the use of drugs to solve problems is dangerous
Explain that drugs and alcohol should not be taken in an effort to resolve problems. Not only does drug use fail to resolve problems, it also creates new ones.

Rationale: Drugs and alcohol have damaging effects on the body; they deaden one's perception of any solution to the problem that is causing the drug use.

Resolved Needs: Protection from physical harm. Protection from psychologic threat. Increased learning.

Explain that there are nondrug methods available for pain relief
Explain that pain relief methods other than drugs can be used: heat or cold therapy, positioning, tension reduction, therapeutic soaks, elastic bandage support, body alignment, supportive garments. Discuss which of these is applicable to the patient's specific situation.

Rationale: Relieving pain without using drugs reduces the potential for drug habituation and drug side effects.

Resolved Needs: Comfort. Protection from physical harm. Freedom from pain. Increased learning.

Explain that undesirable thoughts and feelings are normal
Explain that every person occasionally has thoughts, feelings, and impulses whose consequences he would consider wrong if he were to act upon them.

Rationale: Awareness that undesirable thoughts and feelings are normal promotes comfort in persons who have difficulty accepting such thoughts and feelings within themselves.

Resolved Needs: Comfort. Protection from psychologic threat. Personal growth and maturity. Increased learning. Increased reality perception and problem-solving ability.

Explain that unpleasant conversation increases stress   Explain to visitors that the stress of unpleasant conversation depletes the energy that the patient needs for healing purposes. Therefore conversation should be pleasant.

Rationale: Awareness that unpleasant conversation increases stress encourages behavior that can reduce stress.

Resolved Needs: Protection from physical harm. Protection from psychologic threat. Increased learning.

Explain that wet face masks are ineffective   Explain that once a face mask becomes wet, it should be replaced immediately with a dry one.

Rationale: Moisture accumulation on a mask decreases the shielding property of the mask and allows infectious microorganisms to be transmitted through the material.

Resolved Needs: Protection from physical harm. Increased learning.

Explain that yawning and swallowing will equalize ear pressure   Explain that if pressure, pain, or hearing loss occurs as an airplane descends for a landing, one should yawn or swallow several times. Chewing gum will promote swallowing.

Rationale: As an airplane descends, the air pressure in the passenger's middle ear is less than the increasing atmospheric pressure. Yawning or swallowing opens the eustachian tube and allows the outside air at higher pressure to enter the ear, with resulting equalization of pressures.

Resolved Needs: Comfort. Protection from physical harm. Increased learning.

Explain the advantages and disadvantages of breast feeding   Explain that breast feeding has several advantages. Breast milk contains the best nutritional composition known for infants; it is the correct temperature, it is free from bacteria, and it seldom causes allergic reactions. Breast feeding reduces formula preparation, and fewer women who breast-feed their infants have breast cancer.

There are also disadvantages to breast feeding: being committed to a rigid home schedule in order to be available for infant feeding; breast discomforts associated with lactation.

Rationale: Awareness of the advantages and disadvantages of breast feeding assists in making the proper choice of whether to breast-feed.

Resolved Needs: Comfort. Increased learning. Increased reality perception and problem-solving ability.

Contraindications: Insufficient lactation. Breast infection or irritation.

Explain the causes of fear of death Explain that man fears death because it is an unknown, because no one has returned from death to explain what lies ahead. We fear death because we fear losing the pleasures of life, time, and the self.

Rationale: Awareness of the causes of fear tends to reduce the degree of fear.

Resolved Needs: Comfort. Protection from psychologic threat. Increased learning. Increased reality perception and problem-solving ability.

Explain the causes of fear of pain Explain that fear of pain results from past unpleasant experiences and that pain is associated with threat to life, destruction by disease, or impending disaster.

Rationale: Awareness of the causes of fear tends to reduce the degree of fear.

Resolved Needs: Comfort. Protection from psychologic threat. Increased learning. Increased reality perception and problem-solving ability.

Explain the causes of pain Discuss with the patient what he considers to be the cause of his pain. If his interpretation is correct, verify it. If further clarification is needed, provide it.

Rationale: Awareness of causes promotes comfort and reduces the internal tension and anxiety that result from fear of the unknown.

Resolved Needs: Comfort. Protection from psychologic threat. Increased learning. Increased reality perception and problem-solving ability.

Contraindications: Avoid the explanation if it appears to severely heighten anxiety.

Explain the causes of the health problem Explain the significant factors that brought about the patient's health problem.

Rationale: Awareness of the causes of problems reduces the anxiety that is associated with the unknown and decreases the potential for recurrence of the problem.

Resolved Needs: Comfort. Protection from physical harm. Protection from psychologic threat. Increased learning. Increased reality perception and problem-solving ability.

Contraindications: Delay explanation if it appears to heighten anxiety.

Explain the criteria for acceptance of an organ donor Explain that close relatives, especially identical twins, are usually the most compatible kidney donors. The process of determining compatibility is as follows: Blood types are determined; they must be compatible. When the blood types are cross-matched, agglutination (clumping) of the cells must not occur. Tissue typing is performed; if any one of the 11 known antigens is present in the donor but not in the recipient, the tissues are incompatible. If an antigen is present in the recipient but not in the donor, there is only minor incompatibility. It is preferable that the donor be living and well and that he have no history of urinary tract disease. Pyelography, renal function studies, and renal arteriograms are performed. Corneal donations are acceptable so long as the cornea is healthy.

Rationale: Knowledge of what to expect promotes feelings of comfort and safety.

Resolved Needs: Comfort. Protection from psychologic threat. Increased learning.

Explain the difference between a mature and a rigid conscience   Explain that a rigid conscience is shaped by fear of punishment learned in childhood. The mature adult conscience is based on what one perceives as his personal value system and is not shaped by blind adherence to society's standards.

Rationale: A mature conscience is essential to growth and development and personal inner peace.

Resolved Needs: Protection from psychologic threat. Personal growth and maturity. Increased learning. Increased reality perception and problem-solving ability.

Explain the difference between freedom from fear and freedom from problems   Explain that when a person is free of fear, there are no feelings of dread or doubt as he attempts to solve a problem; instead, he approaches the problem with positive solutions. As long as we live we will never be free of problems.

Rationale: Some persons perceive fears and problems as being the same, because the challenge of a problem evokes fear in them. Awareness that the two are different and that problems can be solved by a sound, fearless approach supports good mental health.

Resolved Needs: Protection from psychologic threat. Personal growth and maturity. Increased learning. Increased reality perception and problem-solving ability.

Explain the difference between guilt and shame   Explain that guilt consists in self-imposed internal judgment, criticism of oneself, that results from fear of punishment or a desire for self-punishment. Shame is a feeling of humiliation or disgrace that is externally imposed by the disapproval of others because of one's nonconformity to cultural norms.

Rationale: Awareness of the sources and meanings of guilt and shame supports increased insight into healthy behavioral responses to these emotions.

Resolved Needs: Protection from psychologic threat. Personal growth and maturity. Increased learning. Increased reality perception and problem-solving ability.

Explain the difference between pain and discomfort Explain that pain and discomfort differ: discomfort may include hunger, nausea, thirst, dizziness, distention, fullness, and congestion; pain is distressful hurting.

Rationale: Awareness of the difference between pain and discomfort reduces anxiety and threat and supports verbal clarification when reporting symptoms.

Resolved Needs: Protection from physical harm. Protection from psychologic threat. Increased learning.

Explain the difference between real and neurotic guilt Explain that real guilt occurs after some wrongdoing as one repents of his misdeed. In neurotic guilt one recognizes within himself an unacceptable intent or wish and reacts as if he had actually performed the misdeed.

Rationale: Awareness of normal and abnormal responses supports increased insight into healthy behavioral responses.

Resolved Needs: Protection from psychologic threat. Personal growth and maturity. Increased learning. Increased reality perception and problem-solving ability.

Explain the difference between salt and sodium diet restriction Explain that common table salt is sodium chloride and that dietary restriction of salt limits only the intake of sodium chloride. But sodium is not found only in salt (sodium chloride); it occurs in a variety of chemical compounds: sodium bicarbonate, sodium phosphate, sodium bromide, sodium carbonate, sodium citrate, sodium sulfate. A sodium-restricted diet restricts all these forms of sodium, and it necessitates very careful reading of product labels.

Rationale: In the presence of certain circulatory and renal disorders, excess sodium is not excreted effectively; this results in edema, excess vascular fluid, and electrolyte imbalance.

Resolved Needs: Water-salt balance. Protection from physical harm. Increased learning.

Explain the difference between true and false labor pains Explain that true labor pains occur at regular intervals that gradually become shorter; the pains increase in intensity, they are intensified by walking, they are located mainly in the back, and they are accompanied by bloody show. Explain that false labor pains occur at irregular, long intervals; they do not increase in intensity, they are located mainly in the abdomen, they are either relieved or unaffected by walking, and they are not accompanied by bloody show.

Rationale: Knowledge that helps to differentiate one problem from another promotes comfort.

Resolved Needs: Comfort. Increased learning.

Explain the effects of the specific type pacemaker   Explain the specific effects of the type of pacemaker being used. An asynchronous pacemaker stimulates the ventricle at a preset rate regardless of the patient's activity. A synchronous pacemaker stimulates the ventricle at a specific rate according to the patient's activity and is often used by young persons. A demand pacemaker stimulates the ventricle if there is delayed natural stimulation.

Rationale: Awareness of the effects of therapeutic devices supports effective use of the devices.

Resolved Needs: Comfort. Increased learning.

Explain the emotional causes of reduced sexual response   Explain that the emotional causes of reduced sexual response are: fear of motherhood; fear of venereal disease; fear of organic damage; fear that one's own passionate appetite will cause self-degradation and loss of love; perception of sex as disgusting; inability to give oneself to another; homosexual tendencies; feeling dominated by one's partner; feeling that it is wrong to enjoy sexual activity because of its procreative purpose; feeling inadequate as a person; feeling guilty because of extramarital relations; feeling that the sexual relationship with the husband indicates disloyalty to one's father.

Rationale: Awareness of causes of a situation frequently resolves the problem.

Resolved Needs: Comfort. Sexuality. Protection from psychologic threat. Personal growth and maturity. Increased learning. Increased reality perception and problem-solving ability.

Explain the genetic factors involved in the disease   Explain that certain diseases are passed from parents to children by transmission of genes in chromosomes. Explain to the parents the degree of probability that their child will inherit their disease. Make it clear to the parents that transmission of genes has not yet been brought under scientific control. Keep them informed of any medical breakthrough involving their particular disease.

Rationale: Knowledge of the genetic factors involved in disease transmission promotes understanding and offers some degree of comfort.

Resolved Needs: Comfort. Protection from psychologic threat. Increased learning.

Explain the importance of blood replacement after transfusion   Explain that in order for health facilities to have adequate blood supplies, blood should be replaced by donations of family or friends when a transfusion is administered.

Rationale: Blood is available only through human donations, and a standby supply is essential to community health.

Resolved Needs: Protection from physical harm. Increased learning.

Explain the importance of correct message interpretation

Explain that the person communicating a message must be certain that the receiver has interpreted the message correctly. If the interpretation is inconsistent with the message, the misinterpretation must be corrected immediately.

Rationale: Correct message interpretation is essential to human understanding and good interpersonal relationships.

Resolved Needs: Protection from psychologic threat. Warm, communicating relationships. Increased learning.

Explain the importance of individual use of a comb and brush

Explain that each person should use only his own comb and brush.

Rationale: Individual use of a comb and brush prevents the transfer of scalp bacteria, parasites, dirt particles, and dandruff to other persons.

Resolved Needs: Cleanliness. Protection from physical harm. Increased learning.

Explain the importance of learning and practicing health principles

Explain that by learning and practicing health principles, the potential for good health will be increased.

Rationale: Awareness of the importance of health information supports improved health.

Resolved Needs: Protection from physical harm. Increased learning. Increased reality perception and problem-solving ability.

Explain the importance of maintaining a positive self-attitude

Explain that each person must have a consistent, positive attitude toward himself. At some time in each day, he should briefly consider that which is good about himself.

Rationale: Positive attitudes toward oneself promote positive behavior.

Resolved Needs: Comfort. Protection from psychologic threat. High evaluation of self. Personal growth and maturity. Increased learning.

Explain the importance of offering emotional support to one another

Explain that every person needs to feel that family and friends will support him during times of stress or crisis. This support should be freely offered between significant persons.

Rationale: Psychologic comfort and safety are promoted by support from significant persons who help meet physical and psychologic needs in times of stress.

Resolved Needs: Protection from psychologic threat. Unity with loved ones. Warm, communicating relationships. Personal growth and maturity. Increased learning. Increased reality perception.

Explain the importance of periodic breast inspection   Explain that breast inspection for tumors should be done once a month, 1–2 days after completion of menstruation. After menopause occurs, the examination should be done once a month, at the same time each month. Assist the patient to develop skill in performing the breast examination, and provide her with appropriate literature.

Rationale: Early detection of breast abnormalities reduces the potential for severe breast disease.

Resolved Needs: Protection from physical harm. Increased learning.

Explain the importance of remaining calm   Explain that the ability to control one's emotions in a stressful situation is extremely important for oneself and for others.

Rationale: Calmness reduces internal tension, conserves the energy needed for action, supports realistic problem solving, and sets an example for others less likely to remain calm. If one person seeks self-gratification by attempting to cause another person emotional upset, only to find that the second person remains calm, he receives the communication that his attempt has served no purpose. This usually leads to calm, favorable behavior on the part of the instigator.

Resolved Needs: Energy. Protection from psychologic threat. Personal growth and maturity. Increased learning. Increased reality perception and problem-solving ability.

Explain the importance of setting an example through abstinence from drug use   Explain that if the family does not want its children to use drugs, alcohol, or tobacco, then the family must set an example by not using them. This also applies to those in the presence of anyone struggling to curtail habituation.

Rationale: Children who grow up in families where drugs, alcohol, and tobacco are not used are less likely to indulge in them. Seeing others use drugs for pain relief can cause an automatic expectation of relief of distress through drugs. Alcoholics frequently resent seeing others drink when they are struggling not to, and this often precipitates a drinking episode.

Resolved Needs: Protection from psychologic threat. Increased learning.

Explain the importance of standing on dry surfaces and wearing insulated rubber gloves and rubber-soled shoes when working with electricity   Explain that when working with electrical equipment or outlets, one should be absolutely sure that his hands and the earth or floor beneath him are perfectly dry. Rubber gloves and rubber-soled shoes should always be worn.

Rationale: Water conducts electricity, and it will cause the electrical current to go into and stay within the body, causing severe shock or death. Rubber gloves and rubber-soled shoes are protective nonconductors; thus if a current accidentally passes to the body it will flow through the body and into the earth in a relatively harmless manner.

Resolved Needs: Protection from physical harm. Increased learning.

Explain the importance of staying well informed on drug abuse
Advise parents of teenage children to keep up with the latest scientific information on drug abuse.

Rationale: Well-informed parents can give accurate information to their children and make realistic decisions if drug problems arise.

Resolved Needs: Comfort. Increased learning. Increased reality perception and problem-solving ability.

Explain the importance of testing cosmetics for skin irritation
Explain that before new cosmetics are applied to the face, they should be tested on other skin areas such as the inner arm. If no irritation occurs, then it is probably safe to use them on the face.

Rationale: Early detection of potential skin irritants reduces the possibility of severe skin disorders.

Resolved Needs: Protection from physical harm. Increased learning.

Explain the importance of testing the water temperature
Explain that before getting into a tub of water, one should test the water temperature by placing a wrist in the water. If the degree of heat feels comfortable to the wrist, then the water temperature is safe.

Rationale: Testing water before exposing the body to its heat can prevent skin burns.

Resolved Needs: Protection from physical harm. Increased learning.

Explain the importance of using grounded electrical equipment and appliances
Explain that one should only use equipment or appliances that have built-in grounding.

Rationale: Grounded equipment prevents accidental passage of electric current into the body.

Resolved Needs: Protection from physical harm. Increased learning.

Explain the importance of washing combs and brushes with each shampoo
Explain that each time the hair is cleansed by shampooing, the person's comb and brush should be cleaned with soap and water.

Rationale: Cleanliness prevents infection.

Resolved Needs: Cleanliness. Protection from physical harm. Increased learning.

Explain the importance of wearing a Medic Alert tag
Explain that persons with chronic illnesses or diseases should wear Medic Alert tags

in case they are in accidents or other situations in which they are unable to communicate.

Rationale: A Medic Alert tag assures the person of prompt and accurate treatment for his chronic illness, and it minimizes the potential for adverse reactions to treatments used for his other injuries.

Resolved Needs: Protection from physical harm. Increased learning.

Explain the limitations imposed by isolation   Explain that quarantine patients are limited to a designated area and should not leave that area or invite unexposed persons to visit them.

Rationale: Limiting human contact minimizes pathogen transfer from one person to another.

Resolved Needs: Protection from physical harm. Increased learning.

Explain the meaning of premature birth   Explain that an infant is considered premature if he weighs less than 5½ pounds and is born sooner than 37 weeks after conception.

Rationale: Knowing the factors associated with prematurity clarifies perception of the special needs of the infant.

Resolved Needs: Increased learning. Increased reality perception.

Explain the meaning of the diagnostic report(s)   Explain to the patient what X-ray reports, laboratory findings, and other studies mean in relation to his specific problem.

Rationale: An understanding of one's health problem promotes comfort, safety, and confidence in handling the problem.

Resolved Needs: Comfort. Protection from physical harm. Warm, communicating relationships. Increased learning.

Contraindications: Delay explanation if it appears to heighten anxiety.

Explain the need for maintaining a firm surface under the hip of an amputated leg   Explain that a firm mattress should be placed under the hips of a patient who has had a leg amputated; this prevents hip sagging.

Rationale: Hip sagging will cause flexion contracture of the amputation stump, which will impair the effective use of a prosthesis.

Resolved Needs: Protection from physical harm. Increased learning.

Explain the need for nail cleanliness   Explain that fingernails and toenails should be cleaned daily by brushing or soaking in soap and water.

Rationale: Cleanliness prevents infection in body areas that come in contact with the fingers.

Resolved Needs: Cleanliness. Protection from physical harm. Increased learning.

Explain the need for pleasant mealtimes   Explain that mealtime conversation should revolve around pleasant subjects. The atmosphere should be unhurried and relaxed.

Rationale: Unpleasant conversation causes muscular tension, reduces appetite, and impairs digestion.

Resolved Needs: Protection from physical harm. Increased learning.

Explain the need for properly fitting dentures   Explain that dentures that do not fit properly should be readjusted.

Rationale: Dentures that do not fit properly irritate the mouth and prevent effective chewing of food.

Resolved Needs: Protection from physical harm. Increased learning.

Explain the need for realistic expectations of others   Explain that in most cases in which a person feels he is not being treated with the consideration he deserves, he is expecting more from others than he should realistically expect.

Rationale: Some persons perceive the normal self-concerns of others to be threatening to their own self-concerns. Realizing that most people are normally preoccupied with their own problems supports realistic perception that this normal concern is not an expression of rejection of others.

Resolved Needs: Comfort. Protection from psychologic threat. Personal growth and maturity. Increased learning. Increased reality perception and problem-solving ability.

Explain the need for scheduled bowel elimination   Explain that it is advisable to set a time for daily bowel elimination, preferably at an unhurried hour of the day.

Rationale: Body systems function best when a regular schedule is followed.

Resolved Needs: Waste elimination. Comfort. Protection from physical harm. Increased learning.

Explain the need for weekly hair shampoo   Explain that the hair should be shampooed once a week.

Rationale: Cleanliness prevents infection of hair and scalp.

Resolved Needs: Cleanliness. Protection from physical harm. Increased learning.

Contraindications: Severe head trauma.

Explain the need to associate pleasant experiences with feared objects   Explain that fear can be alleviated or reduced by associating pleasure with the feared object. When a child who fears dogs experiences the pleasure of cuddling a soft puppy, his fear is reduced.

Rationale: By consistently associating pleasure with feared objects, the previous fear response can gradually be replaced with a positive response.

Resolved Needs: Comfort. Protection from psychologic threat. Personal growth and maturity. Increased learning. Increased reality perception and problem-solving ability.

Explain the need to avoid contaminated soil

Explain that soil contaminated with parasites or worms should be kept away from the hands and face.

Rationale: Parasites and worms promote disease.

Resolved Needs: Protection from physical harm. Increased learning.

Explain the need to avoid lip licking

Explain that licking the lips should be avoided, especially during cold weather.

Rationale: Lip licking dries out lip tissue, promotes cracking and bleeding, and irritates lip blisters and pustules.

Resolved Needs: Comfort. Protection from physical harm. Increased learning.

Explain the need to avoid mechanical trauma

Explain that forceful body contact with other objects should be avoided. This includes dropping heavy objects on oneself, accidentally cutting oneself, and running into doors, chairs, table corners, or other potentially harmful objects.

Rationale: Avoiding mechanical trauma prevents injury.

Resolved Needs: Protection from physical harm. Increased learning.

Explain the need to avoid overexertion

Explain that exercising beyond normal limits, or exercising strenuously when unaccustomed to doing so, places excessive stress on the body. If the body cannot accommodate the stress, one or more systems may fail to function.

Rationale: Strenuous exercise increases tissue requirements for oxygen and rate and amount of blood that must be pumped through the heart to the muscles. This causes elevated arterial and venous pressures and may result in inadequate tissue oxygenation. Overexertion taxes the body's energy supply.

Resolved Needs: Oxygen, circulation. Energy. Protection from physical harm. Increased learning.

Explain the need to avoid sudden movements of an extremity having an arteriovenous shunt

Explain that an extremity containing an arteriovenous shunt should not be moved suddenly and forcefully, especially not in a twisting motion. It should be moved slowly and smoothly.

Rationale: Sudden extremity movements can pull an arteriovenous shunt joint apart and cause hemorrhage.

Resolved Needs: Protection from physical harm. Increased learning.

Explain the need to maintain balanced brace-shoe heels
Explain that brace-shoe heels should be kept even and should not be allowed to wear more on one side than on the other.

Rationale: Good body balance depends on an even walking surface.

Resolved Needs: Protection from physical harm. Increased learning.

Explain the need to predict and plan for change
Explain that anxiety can be reduced by admitting that certain changes probably will occur and by making definite plans to meet those changes. For instance, we are reasonably sure of growing old and can realistically plan for it.

Rationale: Anxiety results from a sense of helplessness. Helplessness can be overcome through prediction and planning.

Resolved Needs: Comfort. Protection from psychologic threat. Predictable, orderly world. Personal growth and maturity. Increased learning. Increased reality perception and problem-solving ability.

Explain the need to recognize highly stressful situations
Explain the importance of being aware of situations that place one under intense stress. Each person should learn to recognize which situations cause him stress. Significant others should avoid causing situations that place undue stress on a person.

Rationale: Recognition of highly stressful situations gives the person and his significant others an opportunity to avoid such situations or modify the degree of stress.

Resolved Needs: Comfort. Protection from physical harm. Protection from psychologic stress. Increased learning.

Explain the physical causes of reduced sexual response
Explain that the physical causes of reduced sexual response include pathology of sex organs or nearby organs, external genital lesions, endocrine disorders, drug- or alcohol-induced anesthesia, and fatigue.

Rationale: Awareness of the causes of sexual problems reduces anxiety and supports solution of the problem.

Resolved Needs: Comfort. Sexuality. Protection from psychologic threat. Increased learning. Increased reality perception and problem-solving ability.

Explain the psychologic cause of organic pain
Explain that organic pain can result from muscle tension and nerve stimulation caused by stress situations.

Rationale: Awareness that stress can produce organic pain should support attempts at reducing stress situations, with emphasis on relaxation.

Resolved Needs: Protection from physical harm. Protection from psychologic threat. Personal growth and maturity. Increased learning. Increased reality perception and problem-solving ability.

Contraindications: Delay explanation if it appears to heighten anxiety.

Explain the reason for and intended effect of the therapy, (study, or examination)   Explain why certain specific treatments, studies, and examinations are recommended or are being incorporated into the patient's plan of care. Let him know what effects they will have on his health condition.

Rationale: Knowledge of why treatments, studies, and examinations are performed and their intended effects reduces anxiety and promotes comfort.

Resolved Needs: Comfort. Protection from psychologic threat. Increased learning.

Explain the reason for delaying the prosthesis application   Explain that applying a stump prosthesis is often delayed to allow for deep tissue healing, which takes about 6 weeks. If pressure is applied to the tissue before healing is complete, tissue injury and excessively long inactivity may result.

Rationale: Knowledge of why treatments are delayed reduces anxiety and promotes comfort.

Resolved Needs: Comfort. Protection from psychologic threat. Increased learning.

Explain the reason for the delay in giving a pain relief drug   Explain that the administration of pain relief drugs is often delayed because of the possibility of side effects occurring from frequent drug dosage. Be sure that the patient understands that staff apathy is not the reason for the delay.

Rationale: Knowledge of why treatments are delayed reduces anxiety and promotes comfort.

Resolved Needs: Comfort. Protection from psychologic threat. Increased learning.

Explain the relationship between conflict and psychogenic pain   Explain that psychogenic pain is a symbolic means of attempting to solve emotional conflict and that it occurs at the subconscious level.

Rationale: Awareness of behavioral mechanisms supports healthy behavioral responses.

Resolved Needs: Protection from psychologic threat. Personal growth and maturity. Increased learning. Increased reality perception and problem-solving ability.

Explain the reproductive process   Explain that pregnancy results from union of a female egg with a male spermatozoon. One egg is discharged from the ovary each month; it then works its way into the fallopian tube. If intercourse occurs at the right time, the spermatozoon penetrates the egg in the fallopian tube and fertilization takes place. The fertilized egg then moves itself into the uterus and embeds itself in the uterine lining, where fetal development begins.

Rationale: Knowledge of physiologic processes promotes comfort and safety.

Resolved Needs: Comfort. Protection from physical harm. Increased learning.

Explain the significance of premature membrane rupture and that it does not indicate difficult labor   Explain that once the uterine membrane ruptures, labor onset will follow within 24–46 hours. Reassure the patient that early rupture of the membrane does not mean that labor will be difficult. Even though the bulk of amniotic fluid is lost at membrane rupture, the fluid is continuously being produced until delivery occurs. Its lubricating quality facilitates ease of birth.

Rationale: Knowledge of normal physiologic responses promotes comfort.

Resolved Needs: Comfort. Increased learning.

Explain the significance of regressive behavior in illness   Explain that return to an earlier behavior pattern is the patient's way of coping with the anxiety and insecurity of illness or hospitalization. When a child displays regressive behavior, the parents may need help in accepting his behavior until he is ready to resume behavior appropriate for his developmental stage. Adults often display regressive behavior by desiring more attention and wanting to be waited on.

Rationale: Significant others are often embarrassed by the regressive behavior of a loved one. If such behavior occurs in a child, they may scold or punish the child, increasing his feelings of insecurity and inadequacy. Loving acceptance during the stressful period will help the person adjust more quickly.

Resolved Needs: Protection from psychologic threat. Dependence. Increased learning.

Explain those menstrual variations which indicate abnormality   Explain that menstruation is considered abnormal if it occurs more frequently than every 21 days, if it occurs less frequently than every 35 days, if its duration is less than 3 days or more than 7 days, or if more than 12 perineal pads are used in a 24-hour period.

Rationale: Knowledge of normal physiologic processes promotes safety.

Resolved Needs: Protection from physical harm. Increased learning.

Explain what is considered justifiable aggression Explain that in most cultures aggression is justified when self-defense is necessary.

Rationale: Healthy adjustment maintains a balance between appropriate assertiveness and antisocial aggressive impulses.

Resolved Needs: Protection from psychologic threat. Personal growth and maturity. Increased learning. Increased reality perception and problem-solving ability.

Explain when showering should be substituted for tub bathing during pregnancy Explain that pregnant women may bathe in a tub until such time as the membrane ruptures, the mucus plug is passed, or bleeding occurs. Showering is recommended after any one of these occurs.

Rationale: After the membrane ruptures or the mucus plug is passed or bleeding occurs, tub bathing heightens the potential for vaginal infection because of vaginal exposure to unclean water. Showering provides constantly running clean water, which reduces the chance of vaginal infection.

Resolved Needs: Comfort. Cleanliness. Protection from physical harm. Increased learning.

Explain when the postpartum flow normally resumes Explain that when a mother is not breast feeding her infant, menstruation usually resumes about 8 weeks after delivery. Mothers who are breast feeding usually do not resume menstruation until breast feeding has stopped. However, both menstruation and pregnancy have been known to occur during the period of breast feeding.

Rationale: Knowledge of normal physiologic processes promotes comfort.

Resolved Needs: Comfort. Increased learning.

Explain why persons resort to drug abuse Explain that persons take drugs for group acceptance, for kicks, to cope with emotional problems, as a means of rejecting and shaming parents by whom they feel rejected, and as a stimulant to increase efficiency.

Rationale: Knowledge of the causes of drug abuse facilitates understanding the problem as an illness.

Resolved Needs: Increased learning. Increased reality perception and problem-solving ability.

Explain why persons should maintain self-control Explain that self-control is maintained out of respect for other persons and to obtain social approval.

Rationale: Awareness of the reasons for behavior supports healthy behavioral responses.

Resolved Needs: Personal growth and maturity. Increased learning. Increased reality perception and problem-solving ability.

Inform about careers available to diabetics   Inform diabetics that various careers are open to them: medicine, nursing, dentistry, law, business administration, engineering, scientific research, architecture, photography, teaching, radio and television, skilled crafts, secretarial work, etc. Careers closed to diabetics include military service, law enforcement and firefighting, driving and piloting taxis, busses, trains, airplanes, and ships, and similar hazardous occupations.

Rationale: Diabetics can lead normal lives provided that they choose nonhazardous careers compatible with their disease. Involvement in a productive occupation supports independence.

Resolved Needs: Protection from physical harm. Independence. Increased learning.

Inform as to the correct terminology used for elimination   Explain that the proper terms to describe defecation are stool, feces, and bowel movement. Explain that the proper terms for passing urine are voiding and urinating.

Rationale: Small children being toilet trained should be taught the proper terminology for elimination.

Resolved Needs: Increased learning.

Inform of the recommended length of infant nursing periods   Explain that the length of the infant nursing period varies with each baby and mother. Much depends on the comfort or discomfort the mother experiences. When infants are first fed by the breast, the usual time is from 1 to 10 minutes, with gradual daily increases up to 20 minutes. If the mother's breasts are cracked, nursing should be limited to short periods.

Rationale: Adequate nursing periods are essential for the comfort and safety of the mother and infant.

Resolved Needs: Comfort. Protection from physical harm. Increased learning.

Inform of the recommended minimum hours of sleep (325)   Explain that it is recommended that average healthy persons obtain these amounts of sleep each day, although sleep requirements are individualized somewhat:

Infants	10–20 hours
Children	10–14 hours
Adults	7–9 hours
Aging persons	5–7 hours

Ill persons require more sleep than healthy persons.

Rationale: Adequate daily sleep is essential to the replacement of energy within tissue cells.

Resolved Needs: Sleep, rest. Energy. Protection from physical harm. Increased learning

Inform of the resources available for health care
Make known to the patient the health agencies and institutions that are available to assist in solving his particular health problem, such as rehabilitation, financial resources, etc.

Rationale: Knowledge and use of available health resources promote improved health status and independent self-care.

Resolved Needs: Protection from physical harm. Independence. Increased learning.

Inform of the therapies available for the specific condition
Provide information on the different therapeutic approaches that can be used to improve the patient's specific condition.

Rationale: Awareness of the therapies available for improving health reduces anxiety and provides factual information that can support optimum decision-making.

Resolved Needs: Comfort. Protection from psychologic threat. Increased learning. Increased reality perception and problem-solving ability.

Inform of those conditions which precipitate seizures
Explain that certain conditions should be avoided because they tend to stimulate epileptic seizures. They include excessive food or liquid intake, excitement, overexertion, inadequate rest, fever, infection, an irregular daily schedule, and flashing light patterns.

Rationale: Avoiding conditions that precipitate seizures reduces the potential for seizures.

Resolved Needs: Protection from physical harm. Increased learning.

Inform that a brown vaginal discharge often indicates uterine carcinoma
Explain that a foul-smelling, watery, dark brown vaginal discharge is indicative of a cancerous lesion and should be reported immediately.

Rationale: Malignant cells within an organ cause tissue damage.

Resolved Needs: Protection from physical harm. Increased learning.

Inform that a child should be diapered only at night during toilet training
Explain that during toilet training, a child should be diapered only at night and should wear pants during the day.

Rationale: Diapers imply elimination without heed to time or place. Gradually discontinuing the use of diapers supports accommodation to more acceptable patterns of elimination and introduces the child to greater feelings of comfort.

Resolved Needs: Comfort. Increased learning.

Inform that a child should be dressed in easily removable clothes for toileting Explain that toilet training can be facilitated if the child is dressed in pants that slip down easily, in trousers with a few large buttons, and in easily removed playsuits.

Rationale: Hard-to-remove clothing results in frustration and rebellion, which retard learning.

Resolved Needs: Comfort. Increased learning.

Inform that a child should be fully awakened during nighttime toileting Explain that when a child is taken to the bathroom at night, he should be fully awakened so that he knows that toileting is taking place.

Rationale: To learn conscious sphincter control, full awareness is necessary.

Resolved Needs: Comfort. Increased learning.

Inform that a clear, mucoid vaginal discharge occurs with ovulation Explain that a clear, stringy vaginal discharge indicates that ovulation is occurring.

Rationale: Knowledge of normal physiologic processes promotes comfort.

Resolved Needs: Comfort. Increased learning.

Inform that a predisposition to the illness exists Inform the patient that inherited factors passed from parents to children make the children susceptible to certain diseases. Explain that frequent physical examinations should be scheduled as a precautionary measure when a certain disease is prevalent in a family.

Rationale: Recognition of a predisposition to specific diseases should support early detection and treatment of the disease.

Resolved Needs: Protection from physical harm. Increased learning.

Inform that a yellow, purulent vaginal discharge indicates inflammation Explain that a yellow, puslike vaginal discharge is indicative of inflammation and infection in the reproductive system. It should be reported immediately.

Rationale: Infection or inflammation of organs causes tissue damage.

Resolved Needs: Protection from physical harm. Increased learning.

Inform that after-birth pains following delivery are normal Explain that for 24 to 48 hours after delivery, spasm-type abdominal pains will normally be felt.

Rationale: Awareness that after-birth pains are normal involuntary uterine contractions produced to expel lochia and return the uterus to normal size promotes comfort.

Resolved Needs: Comfort. Increased learning.

Inform that airway noise indicates obstruction   Explain that snoring or wheezing breath sounds indicate that an obstruction is preventing optimal ventilation of the lungs.

Rationale: A patent airway is essential for respiratory exchange of oxygen and carbon dioxide.

Resolved Needs: Protection from physical harm. Increased learning.

Inform that an unused leg brace should be stored in an aligned position   Explain that braces not in use should be placed on a flat surface in order to maintain alignment. Explain that braces should never be hung up.

Rationale: Hanging a brace can distort its alignment and diminish its effectiveness in body support.

Resolved Needs: Protection from physical harm. Increased learning.

Inform that artificial larynxes are available   Explain to the person who has had a laryngectomy that several kinds of electronic and mechanical larynx devices are available.

Rationale: The use of an artificial larynx device supports verbal communication.

Resolved Needs: Comfort. Warm, communicating relationships. Increased learning.

Inform that bathing is permitted when wearing a pacemaker   Teach the patient wearing a pacemaker that he may bathe so long as he keeps the wires and generator box dry.

Rationale: Knowledge of how to use therapeutic equipment promotes safety.

Resolved Needs: Protection from physical harm. Increased learning.

Inform that bathrooms require daily cleaning   Explain that since most hygienic care occurs in the bathroom, sinks, commodes, showers, and tubs should be cleaned daily.

Rationale: Cleanliness minimizes the potential for infection.

Resolved Needs: Cleanliness. Protection from physical harm. Increased learning.

Inform that bathtubs require cleaning after each use   Explain that the bathtub should be cleaned with soap or scouring powder and thoroughly rinsed after each use.

Rationale: Cleanliness minimizes the potential for infection.

Resolved Needs: Cleanliness. Protection from physical harm. Increased learning.

Inform that battery monitors should be disconnected during tub bathing or showering   Teach the patient who has a battery-operated monitor to disconnect the monitor from the leads when taking a tub bath or shower and reconnect them later. Disconnecting the monitor is not necessary for sponge bathing.

Rationale: If a battery-operated monitor becomes wet, it can damage the monitoring equipment. Knowledge that there is no danger of electrocution from a wet monitor promotes comfort.

Resolved Needs: Comfort. Increased learning.

Inform that battery-operated objects should be used when wearing a pacemaker   For patients who have pacemakers, suggest that battery-operated appliances be used rather than plug-in appliances. This includes razors, radios, television remote controls, call buttons, tape recorders, and automatic toothbrushes.

Rationale: The electrical pacemaker wires that pierce the skin and are inserted into the heart increase the body's conductance to external electrical current; this requires additional precautionary measures.

Resolved Needs: Protection from physical harm. Increased learning.

Inform that bearing down aids the progress of second stage labor   Teach the patient to strain, as if to force a bowel movement, during the second stage of labor.

Rationale: Bearing down assists in pushing the infant through the vaginal canal.

Resolved Needs: Protection from physical harm. Increased learning.

Contraindications: First stage of labor.

Inform that bilateral hand activity should be avoided   Explain that stuttering children should be discouraged from activities that require two hands, such as playing a piano or drum and making model airplanes.

Rationale: Bilateral hand activities tend to inhibit the development of a dominant hemisphere, which is necessary for normal speech.

Resolved Needs: Protection from physical harm. Increased learning.

Inform that brace locks and joints need to be oiled   Explain that brace locks and joints should be oiled once a week with one drop of machine oil.

Rationale: A therapeutic brace kept in good repair effectively supports weakened muscles, joints, and bones and facilitates motion or temporarily reduces motion while healing occurs.

Resolved Needs: Protection from physical harm. Increased learning.

Inform that brace straps require cleanliness and repair   Explain that the leather straps on braces should be washed periodically with soap and water. When signs of wear appear, the straps should be replaced.

Rationale: A therapeutic brace kept in good repair effectively supports weakened muscles, joints, and bones and facilitates motion or temporarily reduces motion while healing occurs.

Resolved Needs: Protection from physical harm. Increased learning.

Inform that bribing and threatening are ineffective child discipline methods
Explain that in disciplining children, the use of material rewards and gifts leads the child to believe that favorable behavior earns him a reward, whereas it should be seen as merely a part of social interaction. Expressed intentions to inflict injury do not gain the child's cooperation; they result in hostility. The child begins to perceive the adult-child relationship with resentment, and he comes to feel threatened because his previously secure relationship has been weakened.

Rationale: Effective methods of discipline support child socialization while maintaining a secure child-parent relationship and a sense of adequacy.

Resolved Needs: Protection from psychologic threat. Adequacy. Personal growth and maturity. Increased learning. Increased reality perception and problem-solving ability.

Inform that carbonated beverages are safe to drink in foreign countries
Explain that it is safe to drink carbonated soft drinks, mineral water, and beer in foreign countries.

Rationale: The carbonation process makes liquids safe from contamination.

Resolved Needs: Protection from physical harm. Increased learning.

Inform that children are receptive to stages of toilet training at different ages

Bladder control: Explain that the infant's bladder has minimal urine retention capacity until the age of 12 to 18 months.

At 15 to 16 months the bladder is sufficiently developed that the child will stay dry for about 2 hours at a time.

At 18 to 24 months the child is aware of his full bladder. He notifies adults when he is wet, he may want to go to the bathroom frequently because of pride of accomplishment, and he needs assistance with dressing and getting on the seat. He wears training pants.

At age 2 to 2½ years the child goes alone to the bathroom; he stays dry most of the day, but he still has occasional accidents.

At age 3 to 3½ years the child usually stays dry at night but has occasional accidents.

Bowel control: Beginning at 7 or 8 months of age, the child has no voluntary control, but he may have bowel movements at the same time every day.

At age 12 to 18 months the child is irregular. He can verbally identify the bowel movement, he is proud of his accomplishment, and he may have a movement immediately after getting off the commode. If he fusses about being placed on the commode, this indicates, that training should be delayed.

At age 18 to 24 months the child will notify adults that his diaper is soiled. Dirtiness bothers him, and he may show aversion to the stool. He likes to flush the commode, but he may have the fear that he will be flushed down the commode. He wears training pants.

At age 2 years the child has developed control, with only occasional accidents.

At age 2½ years the child uses the toilet alone.

Rationale: Knowledge of what to expect in the way of normal behavior promotes comfort.

Resolved Needs: Comfort. Increased learning.

Inform that clean linens are essential   Explain that bed linens should be washed at least once a week, and towels and washcloths should be washed several times a week. If possible, a clean towel and washcloth should be used for each bath, especially when bathing infants.

Rationale: Cleanliness reduces the potential for infection.

Resolved Needs: Cleanliness. Protection from physical harm. Increased learning.

Inform that cleanliness is basic to health   Explain that cleanliness inhibits the growth of bacteria and therefore reduces the potential for disease.

Rationale: Cleanliness prevents infection.

Resolved Needs: Cleanliness. Protection from physical harm. Increased learning.

Inform that clothing should be worn between the brace and the skin   Explain that socks or stockings should be worn under a leg brace. A T-shirt should be worn under a body brace. Long lightweight sleeves should be worn under an arm brace.

Rationale: Clothing between a brace and the skin prevents skin irritation by the steel brace frame.

Resolved Needs: Comfort. Protection from physical harm. Increased learning.

Inform that coughing should be avoided   Explain that it is important that the patient avoid coughing as much as possible.

Rationale: Coughing should be avoided in situations where increased pressure within the body can lead to tissue damage, bleeding, or pain. This is especially true when intravascular, intraocular, intracranial, intraabdominal, and intrathoracic pressures need to be kept to a minimum.

Resolved Needs: Protection from physical harm. Freedom from pain. Increased learning.

Inform that deep carpeting should be avoided by persons in a wheelchair   Explain to persons in wheelchairs that they should not have deep pile carpeting on their floors. Instead, they should use outdoor carpeting.

Rationale: The friction from a deep carpet makes it difficult to move a wheelchair. Smooth outdoor carpeting permits easier wheelchair manipulation and will provide sufficient cushioning if the patient falls.

Resolved Needs: Comfort. Protection from physical harm. Independence. Increased learning. Increased reality perception and problem-solving ability.

Inform that elimination is advisable before abdominal examinations and procedures   Explain that physical examinations and procedures are more successful if the patient has a bowel elimination and voids shortly before the procedure.

Rationale: Bowel and bladder elimination before an examination or procedure makes for easier palpation and reduces the potential for organ rupture.

Resolved Needs: Protection from physical harm. Increased learning.

Inform that elimination straining should be avoided   Explain that it is important that the patient avoid straining when attempting to eliminate stool.

Rationale: Elimination straining should be avoided, because increased pressure within the body can lead to tissue damage, bleeding, or pain. This is especially true when intravascular, intraocular, intracranial, intraabdominal, and intrathoracic pressures need to be kept to a minimum.

Resolved Needs: Protection from physical harm. Freedom from pain. Increased learning.

Inform that esophageal speech therapy is available   Explain to the patient who has had a laryngectomy that esophageal speech can be learned. It is basically a method of speaking by regurgitating swallowed air.

Rationale: Knowledge of available methods for improved communications promotes comfort.

Resolved Needs: Comfort. Warm, communicating relationships. Increased learning.

Inform that extended breast sucking indicates hunger   Explain that when an infant sucks at the breast 30 to 45 minutes or longer, this may be an indication that he is still hungry.

Rationale: Awareness that the breast milk may not be sufficient to satisfy the infant can facilitate use of a supplementary formula.

Resolved Needs: Protection from physical harm. Increased learning.

Inform that eyeglasses should be kept clean, rested on their rims to prevent lens scratching, and placed in a case when unused   Explain that eyeglasses should be kept clean at all times, that they should be set to rest on their rims and not on their lens, and that they should be put in a cushioned case.

Rationale: Eyeglass cleanliness promotes visual acuity, which is essential to safety and comfort. Resting eyeglasses on their rims prevents lens scratching, which can result in distorted vision. Undamaged eyeglasses are essential for optimum vision.

Resolved Needs: Comfort. Protection from physical harm. Increased learning.

Inform that foods causing allergies fall into specific categories (11)   Explain that foods that cause allergic reactions fall into specific groupings: chicken, turkey, duck, and fowl; chocolate and cola drinks; radishes, cabbage, Brussels sprouts, turnips, cauliflower, broccoli, and lettuce; strawberries and raspberries; peanuts, peas, soybeans, and lima beans; cantaloupe, cucumbers, and watermelons; shrimp and oysters; potatoes and sweet potatoes; ginger and cinnamon; buckwheat and wheat; corn, salad oils, and cottonseed; apricots, peaches, plums, and nectarines. Other foods that cause allergic reactions are milk, eggs, pork, spicy foods, shellfish, and tomatoes.

Rationale: Knowledge of the specific items to avoid when one has an allergic condition promotes comfort and safety.

Resolved Needs: Comfort. Protection from physical harm. Increased learning.

Inform that Halazone tablets should be added to potentially unsafe water   Explain that Halazone tablets, which are found in most first-aid kits, may be used to chlorinate potentially contaminated water. Allow the treated water to stand 30 minutes before drinking.

Rationale: Knowledge that chlorination of water destroys bacteria promotes safety.

Resolved Needs: Protection from physical harm. Increased learning.

Inform that handwashing is essential before touching the laryngectomy stoma   Teach the patient who has had a laryngectomy to avoid touching the stoma until he has first washed his hands.

Rationale: Cleanliness prevents infection of the laryngectomy stoma and respiratory tract.

Resolved Needs: Cleanliness. Protection from physical harm. Increased learning.

Inform that heavy lifting should be avoided Explain that one should not lift heavy objects. If objects must be moved, it is preferable to slide them across the floor.

Rationale: Lifting heavy weights strains muscles, increases cardiac load, and uses large quantities of energy reserves. Heavy lifting causes increased intravascular, intraocular, intrathoracic, intracranial, and intraabdominal pressures.

Resolved Needs: Energy. Comfort. Protection from physical harm. Increased learning.

Inform that high-frequency signals should be avoided when wearing a pacemaker   Teach persons wearing pacemakers to stay way from equipment that transmits high-frequency electromagnetic signals. This includes machines for diathermy and electrocautery, dielectric welders, radar installations, UHF radio transmitters, and microwave ovens.

Rationale: High-frequency electromagnetic signals may cause the pacemaker to malfunction, and it may fail to stimulate adequate cardiac output.

Resolved Needs: Protection from physical harm. Increased learning.

Inform that immunity does not occur with venereal infection Explain that having a venereal disease does not confer immunity from future contagion.

Rationale: Persons who believe that having had a disease makes them immune tend to neglect precautions against future contagion.

Resolved Needs: Protection from physical harm. Increased learning.

Inform that isolation, loss of treat, and restitution are effective child discipline methods   Explain that the most effective forms of child discipline include the following: temporary removal of the child from the pleasure of social contacts, so long as the isolation does not include the threat of or the actual loss of parent or parental love; depriving the child of special treats, especially if peers are receiving the treats; requiring that the child make up for his misbehavior. For instance, if he breaks another child's toy, he must give up one of his toys, or he must be required to apologize.

Rationale: Isolation from others forces the child to realize that it is his own fault that he is missing the pleasure of human relationships. Loss of treats forces the child to realize the advantages of being good. When compensating for misbehavior requires more time and effort than behaving, the child realizes that good behavior is easier than bad. Discipline should put emphasis on the misbehavior, not on the child.

Resolved Needs: Adequacy. Personal growth and maturity. Increased learning.

Inform that large-print reading material is available
Explain that popular reading material can be obtained in very large print from public libraries.

Rationale: Large-print reading material supports ease of reading for persons with impaired vision.

Resolved Needs: Comfort. Protection from physical harm. Increased learning.

Inform that lint should be removed from brace locks and joints
Explain that lint should be removed from locks and joints of braces at least once a week.

Rationale: A therapeutic brace kept in good repair effectively supports weakened muscles, joints, and bones and facilitates motion or temporarily reduces motion while healing occurs.

Resolved Needs: Protection from physical harm. Increased learning.

Inform that menopause does not interfere with sex life
Explain that one's sex life is not affected by menopause, since sexual desire and response are of psychologic, emotional, and sensory origin.

Rationale: An awareness that menopause does not interfere with sex life supports comfort.

Resolved Needs: Comfort. Increased learning.

Inform that new foods should be introduced to children at the beginning of the meal
Explain that when new foods are to be introduced to a child, they should be presented at the beginning of the meal.

Rationale: Since the appetite is greatest at the beginning of a meal, the child is more likely to accept the food at that time.

Resolved Needs: Food balance. Increased learning.

Inform that participation in cultural rituals enhances security feelings
Explain that anxiety can be reduced by participating in ritualistic holidays, games, and pageants important to one's culture and locale.

Rationale: Rituals provide for continuity in everyday life. They integrate the society and forestall the threat of fragmentation and anxiety.

Resolved Needs: Comfort. Protection from psychologic threat. Stability. Personal growth and maturity. Increased learning. Increased reality perception and problem-solving ability.

Inform that powered wheelchairs are available
Explain that battery-powered wheelchairs are available.

Rationale: Battery-powered wheelchairs minimize energy depletion and provide independence for persons with severely impaired mobility.

Resolved Needs: Energy. Protection from physical harm. Independence. Increased learning.

Inform that precautions should be taken when using sprays
Explain that when using any type of spray, care should be taken not to spray the contents in or near the eyes and not to inhale the fumes.

Rationale: Chemicals in commercial sprays will burn the eyes, which can result in diminished vision or blindness. Inhaling fumes can impair respiratory function.

Resolved Needs: Protection from physical harm. Increased learning.

Inform that seizures are noncontagious
Explain that epilepsy is not a contagious disease and that it indicates a neurologic lesion or disorder. Explain that touching the froth on the mouth of seizuring epileptics does not transfer the disease.

Rationale: Awareness that seizures are not contagious can reduce the fear that is commonly associated with the disorder.

Resolved Needs: Comfort. Protection from psychologic threat. Increased learning.

Inform that spinal injury often impairs sexual potency
Explain that sexual potency after spinal cord injury depends on the level and the amount of cord injury. Future sexual capacity cannot be predicted early. If the reflex arcs are intact, there will be contraction of the external sphincter when a rectal examination is done. Sensation in the penile skin, scrotal skin, and saddle area is also a favorable sign. Reflex erections are not indicative of sexual potency. If there has been complete transection of the cord, both voluntary and reflex impulses are abolished. When the lumbar and sacral regions are affected, erection is not possible, except occasionally by psychic stimulation. When the upper lumbar region or a region below that is affected, ejection of seminal fluid from the urethra (ejaculation) is rare. When the third or fourth sacral region or a region above that is affected, male discharge of semen (or female orgasm) cannot occur. If there is incomplete transection of the cord, some reflex impulses may be possible. When the lumbar and sacral regions are affected, erection occurs from both organic and psychic stimulation most of the time, but not necessarily with every stimulation. When the upper lumbar region or a region below that is affected, ejection of seminal fluid from the urethra (ejaculation) is possible 30%–70% of the time. When the third or fourth sacral region or a region above that is affected, male discharge of semen (or female orgasm) may, but seldom does, occur.

Rationale: Factual information about physical limitations promotes reality perception and supports adaptation to the affected phase of life.

Resolved Needs: Sexuality. Increased learning. Increased reality perception and problem-solving ability.

Inform that stooping and lowering the head should be avoided
Explain that it is inadvisable to bend forward and downward or to lower the head.

Rationale: Stooping and lowering the head should be avoided when intraocular and intracranial pressures need to be kept to a minimum. This precaution will help to prevent tissue damage, bleeding, and pain.

Resolved Needs: Comfort. Protection from physical harm. Freedom from pain. Increased learning.

Inform that television should be viewed from a moderate distance
Explain that one should sit a moderate distance from a television set. The correct distance for viewing television depends on the size of the screen and the size of the room.

Rationale: Viewing television from too close or too far away causes eyestrain.

Resolved Needs: Comfort. Protection from physical harm. Increased learning.

Inform that the color and taste of outdoor water do not indicate its safety
Explain that although water coming from springs and rivers may be clear and may taste fresh and cool, it may be contaminated.

Rationale: Since people use outdoor water for bathing, wading, dumping wastes, etc., there is always the possibility of contamination.

Resolved Needs: Protection from physical harm. Increased learning.

Inform that the extremities should be kept warm when the circulation is impaired
Explain that when there is poor circulation in the extremities, loosely fitting soft wool socks or gloves and lightweight blankets can be used to maintain natural warmth. Heavy blankets should be avoided because their pressure on the extremities may further reduce circulation. Heat applications should also be avoided, since they increase metabolism, which in turn reduces the blood supply to the extremities.

Rationale: Natural body warmth helps maintain circulation in the extremities through vasodilatation.

Resolved Needs: Protection from physical harm. Increased learning.

Inform that the laryngectomy stoma should be protected against sunburning
Teach the patient who has had a laryngectomy to be careful that the stoma does not become sunburned. The area should be covered in strong sunlight.

Rationale: If a laryngectomy stoma becomes sunburned, it will swell and decrease the airway size.

Resolved Needs: Protection from physical harm. Increased learning.

Inform that the skin should be protected from windburn Explain that the skin should be covered with a protective scarf when the wind is either cold or hot and dry.

Rationale: Wind at high velocity and extremes of temperature dries the skin and results in tissue irritation.

Resolved Needs: Comfort. Protection from physical harm. Increased learning.

Inform that the tracheostomy must be covered in order to speak Teach the patient who has had a tracheostomy to cover the tracheostomy opening for a few moments, with sterile mesh, if he wants to speak.

Rationale: The ability to communicate by speech reduces anxiety and promotes comfort.

Resolved Needs: Comfort. Protection from psychologic threat. Warm, communicating relationships. Increased learning.

Contraindications: Severe respiratory distress. Following laryngectomy.

Inform that the use of a lightweight wheelchair is preferable Explain that it is wise to purchase a lightweight wheelchair.

Rationale: Lightweight wheelchairs are easily handled independently, and they minimize fatigue in patients whose muscle strength is limited.

Resolved Needs: Energy. Comfort. Protection from physical harm. Independence. Increased learning.

Inform that the use of a walker without wheels is preferable Explain that it is best to use a walker that does not have wheels.

Rationale: Wheels on a walker make it less stable for supporting body weight.

Resolved Needs: Protection from physical harm. Increased learning.

Inform that the use of a wheelchair with good brakes is preferable Explain that a wheelchair should always have a good brake system.

Rationale: Good brakes provide the safety inherent in being able to stop quickly.

Resolved Needs: Protection from physical harm. Increased learning.

Inform that the use of unadjustable crutches for heavyweight persons is preferable Explain that a patient who weighs a great deal should use crutches that are not adjustable and are made of a solid piece of wood.

Rationale: Weight puts stress on the bolts, nuts, and holes in adjustable crutches, whereas a solid piece of wood has greater strength and is thus safer.

Resolved Needs: Protection from physical harm. Increased learning.

Inform that toilet training should be delayed until the child can sit up   Explain that toilet training should be delayed until a child can sit up comfortably.

Rationale: If sitting is beyond the child's physiologic capability, he will experience anxiety and discomfort when placed in a sitting position.

Resolved Needs: Comfort. Protection from psychologic threat. Increased learning.

Inform that toilet training should be limited to short periods daily   Explain that the child should be placed on the commode seat for only a short period each day.

Rationale: If prolonged sitting results in discomfort, the child will develop antagonism toward the training situation.

Resolved Needs: Comfort. Protection from psychologic threat. Increased learning.

Inform that toys should be small enough to hold   Teach parents to provide children with toys that are compatible with the size of the child's hands.

Rationale: Small toys help the child develop fine motor skills.

Resolved Needs: Comfort. Protection from physical harm. Increased learning.

Inform that underweight persons require additional sleep   Explain that persons who weigh less than normal usually require more sleep than those of normal weight. This is especially true of children who are failing to thrive satisfactorily.

Rationale: Underweight persons have less energy reserve than those of normal weight, and they require more energy restoration through sleep.

Resolved Needs: Sleep, rest. Energy. Protection from physical harm. Increased learning.

Inform that vegetables should be introduced to children before fruits at the meal   Explain that when new foods are to be introduced to a child, the vegetables should be presented before the fruits.

Rationale: Eating sweet foods first deadens the appetite for less sweet foods that follow.

Resolved Needs: Food balance. Increased learning.

Inform that water should be kept out of infected ears Explain that water must be kept out of the ears when one has a fungus infection or is susceptible to fungus infections or when there has been rupture of the tympanic membrane.

Rationale: Water, when mixed with hard earwax, promotes fungal and bacterial growth. The force of water rushing into the ears may push earwax farther into the ear.

Resolved Needs: Protection from physical harm. Increased learning.

Inform that when there is limited movement, the affected body side should be dressed first Teach patients with impaired mobility to put their affected limb into an armhole or pant leg first and then dress the unaffected limb.

Rationale: Since the unaffected limb has the greatest mobility, moving it into the strained positions often associated with the final stages of dressing is easier than moving the affected limb.

Resolved Needs: Comfort. Mastery and competence in skills. Independence. Increased learning.

Instruct in the use of projections on wheelchair wheel rims Explain that small wooden or plastic squares can be placed around the rim of a wheelchair wheel for persons who find it difficult to grasp the narrow rim when manipulating the wheelchair.

Rationale: Wooden or plastic projections on wheelchair wheel rims make them easier to grasp and facilitate independent manipulation of the wheelchair.

Resolved Needs: Energy. Independence. Increased learning.

Instruct not to blow the nose Explain that whenever there is nasal bleeding or trauma, nose blowing should be avoided until healing occurs.

Rationale: Nose blowing increases intranasal pressure, thus traumatizing sensitive tissue and dislodging blood clots.

Resolved Needs: Protection from physical harm. Increased learning.

Instruct not to dangle the legs Instruct the patient not to sit with his feet and legs hanging off the side of the bed. Advise that pressure not be placed under the back of the knee.

Rationale: The force of gravity on the dangling leg causes fluid to be pulled into the interstitial tissue spaces, which causes edema; it also decreases venous return from the extremities to the heart. Pressure behind the knees impairs arterial and venous circulation.

Resolved Needs: Circulation. Protection from physical harm. Increased learning.

Instruct not to insert foreign objects into body orifices
Explain that all objects other than food and fluids should be kept out of the mouth. Beads, pins, and buttons should never be put in the mouth, nose, or ears; such objects should be kept away from small children.

Rationale:　Foreign objects irritate internal mucosa, and they can cause fatal airway obstruction.

Resolved Needs:　Protection from physical harm. Increased learning.

Instruct not to kill animals suspected of being infected
Explain that when an animal has injured a person, the animal should not be destroyed; it should be captured and held for observation. An exception is that snakes should be killed and brought to medical authorities.

Rationale:　A diseased animal that is alive will develop evidence of disease; such evidence will not be observable if the animal is killed.

Resolved Needs:　Protection from physical harm. Increased learning.

Instruct not to massage the breast
Explain that when one is attempting to dry up lactating breasts one should avoid rubbing, stroking, or kneading the breasts.

Rationale:　Breast massage stimulates the mammary glands and promotes lactation. If a tumor is present, massaging the breast can spread tumor cells.

Resolved Needs:　Protection from physical harm. Increased learning.

Instruct not to pick the nose
Explain that picking the nose should be avoided because it traumatizes nasal tissue and causes bleeding.

Rationale:　Injury to nasal mucous membranes interferes with the olfactory and filtering functions of the membrane.

Resolved Needs:　Protection from physical harm. Increased learning.

Instruct not to swallow blood during epistaxis
Tell the patient with a bleeding nose not to swallow the blood but to lean forward and allow the blood to drain from the nose.

Rationale:　Swallowing blood leads to vomiting.

Resolved Needs:　Comfort. Protection from physical harm. Increased learning.

Instruct not to use a drinking straw
Explain that the patient should not use a drinking straw for transporting liquids to the mouth.

Rationale:　Sucking on a straw creates a vacuum within the oral cavity and can cause bleeding by disrupting clots formed around healing tissue. Sucking on a straw increases air swallowing, which can increase the discomfort of flatulence.

Resolved Needs: Comfort. Protection from physical harm. Increased learning.

Instruct not to use rubber rings and doughnuts   Explain that inflated rubber rings or doughnuts should not be used in the treatment of existing or potential decubitus ulcer.

Rationale: Pressure from rubber rings impairs circulation, thus increasing the potential for decubitus ulcer.

Resolved Needs: Protection from physical harm. Increased learning.

Instruct not to use ungrounded electrical equipment when wearing a pacemaker   Teach patients wearing pacemakers to stay away from electrical equipment that is ungrounded. This includes two-prong electrical plugs, electric tools such as drills and saws, ungrounded television sets and radios, and motors of automobiles, boats, and lawnmowers.

Rationale: Ungrounded electrical equipment could cause the pacemaker to malfunction so that it would fail to stimulate adequate cardiac output.

Resolved Needs: Protection from physical harm. Increased learning.

Instruct not to vigorously rinse the mouth   Instruct the patient who has had oral surgery or who has suffered trauma to oral mucous membranes not to rinse out his mouth unless he does so very gently.

Rationale: Pressure applied to the oral mucous membrane when rinsing out the mouth may cause bleeding.

Resolved Needs: Protection from physical harm. Increased learning.

Instruct that a soft towel should be used to dry the diabetic's feet   Teach the diabetic to dry his feet with a towel made of very soft material.

Rationale: Diabetics are prone to poor circulation in the skin. Using a soft towel reduces friction, thus decreasing the potential for irritation of easily traumatized tissue.

Resolved Needs: Protection from physical harm. Increased learning.

Instruct that contact lenses should not be worn beyond the prescribed time, during an eye disorder, or while sleeping   Explain that contact lenses should not be worn any longer than 10 to 16 hours a day and should not be worn when the eyes are infected or traumatized. Contact lenses should be removed during sleep or naps because of the danger of eye injury.

Rationale: Improper use of contact lenses can cause corneal irritation, laceration, and ulceration.

Resolved Needs: Protection from physical harm. Increased learning.

Instruct that diabetics should not fry foods　Teach the diabetic that unless he uses the amount of fat allowed in his diet for cooking instead of eating, he cannot have fried foods. Meats, fish, potatoes, etc., should be baked, boiled, or broiled. It is preferable to use the fat allowance for salad dressings and spreads on bread.

Rationale:　The stability of diabetic metabolism is dependent on a limited caloric intake.

Resolved Needs:　Protection from physical harm. Increased learning.

Instruct that douching be avoided　Explain that douching should be avoided during pregnancy, before a vaginal examination, during puerperium healing, when abortion is habitual, and during a vaginal infection, unless it is ordered for therapeutic reasons.

Rationale:　Vaginal irrigations disrupt the natural vaginal flora and pH, which increases susceptibility to infection in the vagina and can further spread existing infection. The pressure of vaginal irrigations can precipitate abortion. Douching before a vaginal examination may remove bacteria and cells that have diagnostic value.

Resolved Needs:　Protection from physical harm. Increased learning.

Instruct that it is essential to carry an arteriovenous shunt clamp　Explain that arteriovenous shunt clamps must be carried by the patient at all times in case the shunt comes apart.

Rationale:　Hemorrhage from a disconnected arteriovenous shunt can result in death.

Resolved Needs:　Protection from physical harm. Increased learning.

Instruct that only water, not milk or juice, be given in the infant's bottle at bedtime　Explain that when a child prefers a bottle before going to sleep, the bottle should be filled with nothing but plain water.

Rationale:　Carbohydrates that are allowed to remain in the mouth will cause tooth decay. Water, a noncarbohydrate, will not cause tooth decay.

Resolved Needs:　Protection from physical harm. Increased learning.

Instruct that pillows (blankets or trochanter rolls) not be placed under the knee　Explain that pillows, blankets, and trochanter rolls should not be placed under the knee, especially after a below-knee amputation. If a pillow must be placed under the knee to prevent hemorrhage, it should be removed as soon as possible.

Rationale:　The flexion position of an amputation stump causes contractures. Pressure behind the knee (popliteal area) can impair circulation in the lower legs.

Resolved Needs:　Circulation. Protection from physical harm. Increased learning.

Instruct that premature infants require a moderate environmental temperature   Explain that premature infants at home require a consistently moderate environmental temperature and should not be exposed to extreme heat or cold.

Rationale: Premature infants require a moderate environmental temperature because their poorly developed internal temperature control system cannot protect them from temperature extremes.

Resolved Needs: Normal temperature. Protection from physical harm. Increased learning.

Instruct that premature infants require protection against infection   Explain that the premature infant at home must be protected from infection by a clean, uncrowded environment. Stress the necessity for handwashing before touching the infant.

Rationale: The premature infant has poor resources for fighting infection. Cleanliness minimizes the potential for infection.

Resolved Needs: Cleanliness. Protection from physical harm. Increased learning.

Instruct that several stump socks should not be worn simultaneously   Teach amputees that it is unwise to wear several stump socks in order to obtain a snug prosthesis fit. Suggest that the prosthesis be adjusted to fit properly.

Rationale: An improperly fitting prosthesis impairs mobility and irritates the skin.

Resolved Needs: Protection from physical harm. Increased learning.

Instruct that soap should not be used on the laryngectomy stoma   Teach the patient who has had a laryngectomy not to use soap for cleaning the stoma.

Rationale: Soap will damage the mucosa and stimulate coughing if it gets into the stoma.

Resolved Needs: Protection from physical harm. Increased learning.

Instruct that sun gazing be avoided even when wearing sunglasses   Explain that one should never gaze at the sun and that sunglasses do not protect the eyes from the direct rays of the sun.

Rationale: Sunglasses do not filter out infrared rays, and these can damage the retina.

Resolved Needs: Protection from physical harm. Increased learning.

Instruct that the amputation stump should not be rested on the crutch handrail   Teach the amputee to avoid resting his amputation stump on the handrail of his crutch.

Rationale: The flexion position of an amputation stump causes contractures, which make the use of a prosthesis impossible. Pressure from resting the stump on the hard handrail will impair circulation to the stump.

Resolved Needs: Protection from physical harm. Increased learning.

Instruct that the drainage container should be held below the bladder (kidney, stomach, or chest) level   Explain that any drainage container should be kept below the level of the insertion site of the tube that is draining.

Rationale: A drainage apparatus kept below the level of its drain tube prevents backflow of the drainage into the tubing insertion site. This reduces the potential for infection and promotes better drainage.

Resolved Needs: Protection from physical harm. Increased learning.

Instruct that the eyes should not be wiped with soiled towels   Explain that soiled towels should not be rubbed in or near the eyes.

Rationale: Dirt and bacteria transferred into the eye from towels can cause tissue trauma and infection.

Resolved Needs: Cleanliness. Protection from physical harm. Increased learning.

Instruct that the flexion stump position be avoided   Teach the amputee not to let his amputation stump hang over the edge of a bed, wheelchair, or chair.

Rationale: The flexion position of an amputation stump results in contractures.

Resolved Needs: Protection from physical harm. Increased learning.

Instruct that the nonhemiplegic leg be placed down first when getting out of bed   Teach the patient with one-sided paralysis to put his strong foot down first when getting out of bed.

Rationale: The strong side of the body can support body weight, but the affected side cannot.

Resolved Needs: Comfort. Protection from physical harm. Mastery and competence in skills. Independence. Increased learning.

Instruct to align brace joints with body joints when applying a brace   Explain that when applying a brace, the joints of the brace should not be allowed to twist; they should be aligned with the body joints.

Rationale: A properly applied therapeutic brace will effectively support weakened muscles, joints, and bones and facilitate motion.

Resolved Needs: Protection from physical harm. Increased learning.

Instruct to anchor the urinary catheter   Explain that the urinary catheter should be taped to the inner thigh. The extended tubing should then be pinned to the sheet or mattress.

Rationale: Anchoring the urinary catheter will prevent tension on the catheter and minimize the potential for pulling it out.

Resolved Needs: Comfort. Protection from physical harm. Increased learning.

Instruct to apply a warm, moist compress to the laryngectomy stoma for dyspnea   If the patient who has had a laryngectomy becomes short of breath, teach him to place a warm moist compress over the stoma and breathe quietly. This will ease those breathing difficulties caused by dried secretions.

Rationale: Warm moist air liquefies secretions and promotes comfortable breathing.

Resolved Needs: Waste elimination. Comfort. Protection from physical harm. Increased learning.

Instruct to avoid artificial leg abduction   Teach the patient wearing a lower limb prosthesis to avoid moving his leg to the side and outward from his body when walking.

Rationale: Poor body alignment impairs body balance and mobility.

Resolved Needs: Protection from physical harm. Increased learning.

Instruct to avoid foods having strong odors   Explain that foods with strong odors should not be eaten. This includes onions, cauliflower, Brussels sprouts, garlic, strong cheese, sausage, corned beef, and fish.

Rationale: Foods with strong odors tend to increase the odor from a colostomy, ileostomy, ureterostomy, or ureteroileostomy stoma. When intake of such foods is reduced, the odor decreases.

Resolved Needs: Comfort. Increased learning.

Instruct to avoid hiking the shoulder when walking with a leg prosthesis   Teach the patient wearing a lower limb prosthesis to avoid raising one shoulder higher than the other when walking.

Rationale: Poor body alignment impairs body balance and mobility.

Resolved Needs: Protection from physical harm. Increased learning.

Instruct to avoid pushing and pulling activities   Explain that fatigue can be reduced by abstaining from pushing or pulling heavy objects.

Rationale: Fatigue results from energy-depleting activity.

Resolved Needs: Energy. Comfort. Protection from physical harm. Increased learning.

Instruct to avoid rubbing the eyes Explain that eye rubbing should be avoided because foreign and infectious material can be transferred to the eyes from the fingers and because rubbing causes friction and pressure against the eyelids and eye tissue.

Rationale: Foreign objects in the eyes or pressure on the eyes can cause tissue infection or trauma.

Resolved Needs: Comfort. Cleanliness. Protection from physical harm. Increased learning.

Instruct to carefully move the injured body part Explain that an injured body area, if movable, may be moved slowly and gently with extreme care during mobility or position change.

Rationale: Carefully moving injured body parts can reduce pain and prevent further injury.

Resolved Needs: Comfort. Protection from physical harm. Increased learning.

Instruct to change position frequently Explain that a patient who is bedridden should be moved from one position to another, from side to side, and from back to abdomen at least every 2 hours day and night.

Rationale: Changing body positions prevents congestion of respiratory secretions, facilitates expectoration, promotes circulation, provides comfort by preventing prolonged pressure on body areas, reduces fatigue, and prevents contractures.

Resolved Needs: Comfort. Protection from physical harm. Increased learning.

Instruct to change position gradually Explain that when the body position is changed from lying to sitting or from sitting to standing, it should be done slowly. The head should be gradually elevated upward, and there should be a rest period between each position change. This is especially true when there are blood pressure abnormalities, when there is bleeding or when there could be bleeding, when there are injured bones, and when an arteriovenous cannula is in place.

Rationale: Changing position gradually minimizes blood pressure adaptations in arteries and veins, promotes good circulation, and decreases the pressure placed on one body part by another.

Resolved Needs: Comfort. Protection from physical harm. Increased learning.

Instruct to check the pulse daily when wearing a pacemaker Teach the patient who has a pacemaker to check his pulse rate twice a day and to report any increase or decrease of more than five beats per minute.

Rationale: In one who is wearing a pacemaker, an increase or decrease in pulse rate usually indicates battery failure or a weakening battery.

Resolved Needs: Protection from physical harm. Increased learning.

Instruct to clean the nails with a cotton-tipped stick   Explain that a soft cotton-tipped orange stick should be used to clean the nails and that sharp objects should be avoided.

Rationale: Use of sharp objects increases the chance of tissue puncture and resulting infection.

Resolved Needs: Comfort. Cleanliness. Protection from physical harm. Increased learning.

Instruct to comb dandruff up from the scalp   Explain that dandruff can be removed by gently pressing the comb against the scalp and pushing the dandruff up and away from the hair roots.

Rationale: Dandruff causes hair dullness and itching.

Resolved Needs: Comfort. Cleanliness. Protection from physical harm. Increased learning.

Instruct to cover the mouth when coughing   Explain that the mouth should be covered with a handkerchief, a tissue, or a hand when coughing.

Rationale: Covering the mouth when coughing minimizes the spread of droplets that can carry infection.

Resolved Needs: Cleanliness. Protection from physical harm. Increased learning.

Instruct to cover the nose when sneezing   Explain that the nose should be covered with a handkerchief or tissue when sneezing.

Rationale: Covering the nose when sneezing minimizes the spread of droplets that can carry infection.

Resolved Needs: Cleanliness. Protection from physical harm. Increased learning.

Instruct to cut the toenails straight across   Explain that nails should be cut straight across; they should never be cut shorter than the tips of the toes and should be rounded gently with an emery board.

Rationale: Cutting the nails straight across prevents ingrown nails, which can become infected.

Resolved Needs: Protection from physical harm. Increased learning.

Instruct to do wheelchair pushups   Teach the patient who is confined to a wheelchair to place the palms of his hands against the chair seat or chair arms and push himself off the wheelchair cushion every 30 minutes.

Rationale: Wheelchair pushups relieve pressure on areas of diminished circulation and reduce the potential for decubitus ulcers.

Resolved Needs: Protection from physical harm. Increased learning.

Instruct to eat only at mealtime   Teach the patient to eat only at mealtimes. One should refrain from snacking between meals and at bedtime.

Rationale: When diabetics eat unprescribed foods between meals, they disrupt carbohydrate metabolism and heighten the potential for diabetic coma. When patients with gastric ulcers eat between meals, they stimulate gastric acidity, thus increasing the potential for further ulceration and reducing the potential for healing.

Resolved Needs: Protection from physical harm. Increased learning.

Contraindications: If between-meal or bedtime snacks are prescribed as in diabetic diets.

Instruct to eat only prescribed foods and amounts of foods   Explain that it is not advisable to substitute unprescribed foods and amounts of foods in a therapeutic diet.

Rationale: Indiscriminate experimentation with one's prescribed therapeutic diet can have adverse effects and can cause recurrence or complication of the nonhealth condition.

Resolved Needs: Protection from physical harm. Increased learning.

Instruct to elevate the body part   Explain that an injured, inflamed, or inflicted body part should be positioned above other adjacent body parts.

Rationale: Elevation of a body part reduces edema and promotes circulation.

Resolved Needs: Circulation. Comfort. Protection from physical harm. Increased learning.

Instruct to frequently wash the stump sock   Explain that the stump sock should be washed thoroughly with soap and water daily.

Rationale: Unclean perspiration residue on the stump sock causes skin irritation.

Resolved Needs: Comfort. Cleanliness. Protection from physical harm. Increased learning.

Instruct to gradually increase the wearing time of the prosthesis   Explain that the length of time the prosthesis is worn should gradually be increased each day.

Rationale: Gradually increasing the prosthesis wearing time allows for slow, comfortable adjustment of the stump to pressure.

Resolved Needs: Comfort. Protection from physical harm. Increased learning.

Instruct to immediately change wet diapers

Explain that as soon as an infant's diaper is wet, it should be changed and replaced with a dry diaper. Explain that the child should be checked frequently to determine whether the diaper is wet.

Rationale: Acidic urine in contact with the skin causes skin irritation.

Resolved Needs: Comfort. Cleanliness. Protection from physical harm. Increased learning.

Instruct to immediately report serious symptoms

Explain that certain symptoms should be reported as soon as they occur, with no delay.

Rationale: Certain symptoms indicate serious threats to health, and any lapse of time before treatment is begun can greatly affect outcome.

Resolved Needs: Protection from physical harm. Increased learning.

Instruct to immediately respond to the elimination reflex

Explain that it is advisable to respond to the bladder and bowel elimination reflexes as soon as they occur.

Rationale: Prolonged retention of feces in the lower colon causes pressure and discomfort. Water continues to be absorbed from the feces, making them harder and more difficult to expel. Prolonged retention of urine in the bladder causes discomfort because of distention and promotes urinary tract infection.

Resolved Needs: Waste elimination. Comfort. Protection from physical harm. Increased learning.

Instruct to increase fluid intake

Explain that the amount of fluid taken each day should be increased by whatever amount is appropriate to the situation.

Rationale: Increased fluid intake in certain situations assures adequate hydration of body tissues. During jet travel, increased fluid intake offsets the potential for dehydration caused by atmospheric pressure changes.

Resolved Needs: Water-salt balance. Protection from physical harm. Increased learning.

Instruct to inspect the skin (scalp or hair)

Explain that patients, especially diabetics and patients confined to bed or wheelchair, should inspect the skin for redness, irritation, duskiness, and intactness. The back, buttocks, and soles of the feet can be inspected with a hand mirror. Explain that where there is the possibility of lice, etc., the scalp should be inspected periodically.

Rationale: Skin inspection facilitates early detection and treatment of skin disorders. Infestation can cause scalp inflammation and facilitates bacterial infection.

Resolved Needs: Protection from physical harm. Increased learning.

Instruct to lanolinize the diabetic's feet, but not the toes
Teach diabetics that they should lubricate their feet with lanolin cream or lotion but should not moisturize between their toes.

Rationale: Lanolin is a nonabsorbable oil. When applied to body creases such as between the toes, it can trap perspiration, and the consequent wetness can cause fungal infection.

Resolved Needs: Comfort. Protection from physical harm. Increased learning.

Instruct to lean forward for improved ventilation
Teach the orthopneic patient to lean forward and rest his arms on a table for easier breathing.

Rationale: Good positioning facilitates lung ventilation and improved oxygenation and promotes comfort.

Resolved Needs: Oxygen. Comfort. Increased learning.

Instruct to lie in the prone position
Teach the patient with an amputated lower extremity to lie on his abdomen several times a day and place the stump in a straightened (extended) position. Teach the mother to sleep and lie on her abdomen after child delivery.

Rationale: Using the prone position to extend the hip after amputation will reduce flexion contractures. Abdominal positioning helps the uterus resume its normal position.

Resolved Needs: Comfort. Protection from physical harm. Increased learning.

Contraindications: Delay until C-section incision is well healed.

Instruct to lightly rub the diabetic's feet with alcohol
Teach diabetics to rub their feet lightly with alcohol one or two times a day, especially when perspiring heavily.

Rationale: Alcohol has a drying effect on the skin. It prevents the perspiration wetness that can irritate easily traumatized skin and promotes comfort.

Resolved Needs: Comfort. Protection from physical harm. Increased learning.

Instruct to limit direct contact with infected persons
Limit direct physical contacts of the infected patient to those persons responsible for his care.

Rationale: Pathogen transfer from person to person is decreased by limiting human contact.

Resolved Needs: Cleanliness. Protection from physical harm. Increased learning.

Instruct to lock the wheelchair before transferring Explain that the wheelchair brake should be locked before the patient attempts to get in or out of the chair.

Rationale: Locking the wheelchair brake provides a stable base for weight-bearing when getting in and out of the chair and prevents accidental injury.

Resolved Needs: Protection from physical harm. Increased learning.

Instruct to lower the head Teach the patient to sit and place his head down between his knees when feeling faint.

Rationale: Placing the head between the knees increases circulation to the brain.

Resolved Needs: Protection from physical harm. Increased learning.

Contraindications: Increased intracranial or intraocular pressure. Hypertension.

Instruct to lubricate the skin (scalp or nails) Explain that dry skin should be moistened daily with a soothing, lubricating solution or cream. Recommend oil treatments for a dry, scaling scalp.

Rationale: Lubrication prevents skin and scalp drying.

Resolved Needs: Comfort. Protection from physical harm. Increased learning.

Contraindications: Excessively oily skin or hair. Acned skin.

Instruct to maintain a moist laryngectomy bib Teach the patient who has had a laryngectomy to keep the bib moist at all times.

Rationale: Maintaining a moist laryngectomy bib prevents crusting around the stoma and promotes comfort.

Resolved Needs: Comfort. Protection from physical harm. Increased learning.

Instruct to maintain skin dryness Explain that as soon as the skin becomes wet from any body discharge, the excretion should be removed with mild soap and water and the skin thoroughly dried. Persons who are incontinent or who experience profuse perspiration or drainage should be checked frequently to determine skin wetness.

Rationale: Prolonged wetness irritates the skin.

Resolved Needs: Comfort. Protection from physical harm. Increased learning.

Instruct to maintain skin (or scalp) cleanliness   Explain that the skin should be thoroughly cleaned periodically with soap and water, and the scalp with shampoo, so that dirt and bacteria are removed.

Rationale: Removal of dirt and bacteria from the skin and scalp promotes comfort and reduces the potential for infection.

Resolved Needs: Comfort. Cleanliness. Protection from physical harm. Increased learning.

Instruct to measure foods after cooking   Explain that food should be weighed or measured after it has been cooked in order to assure accuracy of allowable amounts.

Rationale: Cooking alters the fluid content and weight of food. Exact diet measurements are essential to maintaining many health states, especially stable diabetic metabolism.

Resolved Needs: Protection from physical harm. Increased learning.

Instruct to place a pillow between the thighs in below-knee amputation   Teach the patient who has had a below-knee amputation to place a pillow between his thighs when lying in bed.

Rationale: Placing a pillow between the thighs promotes extension and alignment of the amputation stump.

Resolved Needs: Protection from physical harm. Increased learning.

Instruct to place the infant in a pillow-free crib   Explain that when a small child is placed in a crib, pillows should not be placed in the crib with the child.

Rationale: Since infants and small children are unable to handle pillows, they can suffocate if pillows fall on them.

Resolved Needs: Protection from physical harm. Increased learning.

Instruct to protect the laryngectomy (or tracheostomy) from water   Explain that the patient who has had a laryngectomy or tracheostomy should not swim. When he takes a shower, he should shield the opening from the water.

Rationale: The potential for drowning is high if water enters a laryngectomy or tracheostomy stoma.

Resolved Needs: Protection from physical harm. Increased learning.

Instruct to remove dentures   Explain that dentures should be removed from persons who are unconscious, those who are having seizures, and those who have obstructed airways.

Rationale: Removing dentures when a person is unable to control their movement prevents airway obstruction and injury to the oral mucosa.

Resolved Needs: Protection from physical harm. Increased learning.

Instruct to take medications immediately after meals
Recommend that medications be taken immediately after the meal is finished.

Rationale: Drugs taken after a meal are less likely to cause gastric irritation because of the fullness of the intestinal tract.

Resolved Needs: Comfort. Protection from physical harm. Increased learning.

Contraindications: Drugs such as penicillin G should be taken on an empty stomach because food interferes with their absorption.

Instruct to thoroughly dry the skin between the diabetic's toes   Teach diabetics that they should dry their skin thoroughly after bathing.

Rationale: Keeping the skin dry between the toes minimizes the chance of fungal infection.

Resolved Needs: Comfort. Protection from physical harm. Increased learning.

Instruct to toilet frequently   Recommend that the patient go to the bathroom at frequent intervals. This is especially important for patients who have bladder infections or who are recovering from bladder infections.

Rationale: Frequent toileting reduces the amount of urine that the bladder must handle at one time, minimizes the chance of accidental or uncontrolled voiding, and helps to prevent prolongation or recurrence of infection.

Resolved Needs: Comfort. Increased learning.

Instruct to use a footboard   Explain that a board should be placed at the foot of the bed, with the feet positioned against the board at a right angle to the legs with the patient in the prone position.

Rationale: Placing the feet against a footboard prevents footdrop and keeps pressure from covers off the feet; it can promote circulation when pressing exercises are performed against the board.

Resolved Needs: Protection from physical harm. Increased learning.

Instruct to use a soft, new toothbrush and to apply only mild toothbrush pressure   Explain that a new (not old or bent) soft toothbrush should be used when gums are easily injured, degenerating, or bleeding. The pressure applied should be gentle but firm, never excessive.

Rationale: Bent toothbrush bristles cannot be controlled; they can puncture soft gum tissue. Excessive toothbrush pressure causes gum surface irritation. A new soft toothbrush minimizes trauma to gums and oral mucosa but provides gum stimulation and the comfort of clean teeth.

Resolved Needs: Comfort. Cleanliness. Protection from physical harm. Increased learning.

Instruct to use a water-base lubricant around the laryngectomy stoma   Instruct the patient to use a lubricant (K-Y jelly or Lubafax) that has a water base rather than an oil base around the laryngectomy stoma. Instruct the patient to apply small amounts of lubricant twice a day; it should be allowed to soak in for 2 minutes and then removed. Caution against applying lubricant into the stoma.

Rationale: Lubricating a stoma can prevent crusting and promote comfort. A water-base lubricant is preferred, since oil-base lubricants can be inhaled into the lungs and cause pneumonia.

Resolved Needs: Comfort. Protection from physical harm. Increased learning.

Instruct to use a wide supportive stance for good body balance   Explain that when the body is erect, the feet should be placed at equal distances from the body midline.

Rationale: Equal support on both sides of the body promotes balanced movement.

Resolved Needs: Protection from physical harm. Increased learning.

Instruct to use ice applications to control bleeding   Explain that applying ice or an ice bag or pack to a bleeding site will stop bleeding and prevent or minimize the formation of hematomas.

Rationale: Cold applications cause vasoconstriction, which reduces blood supply to the area.

Resolved Needs: Protection from physical harm. Increased learning.

Contraindications: Decubitus ulcers. Gangrenous tissue. Recent skin graft. Varicose veins. Areas of paralysis or sensation loss.

Instruct to use pressure applications to control bleeding   Explain that bleeding can be stopped by applying finger pressure or a tight bandage to the bleeding area.

Rationale: Pressure obstructs blood flow.

Resolved Needs: Protection from physical harm. Increased learning.

Instruct to use simple words when speaking with persons having impaired communication reception   Explain that short, simple statements are best for communicating with persons who have impaired communication reception.

Rationale: Short, simple statements are most easily understood and promote effective communication.

Resolved Needs: Comfort. Warm, communicating relationships. Increased learning.

Instruct to use vagal stimulation methods to terminate dysrhythmias (290)   Explain that the following methods can be used to stimulate the vagus nerve:

Hold a deep breath for 6–8 seconds after inspiration
Bend the body at the waist and hold the chest parallel to the floor for a few seconds
Hold the breath after inspiration, and press the right or left carotid artery
Stimulate the gagging reflex by inserting a finger down the throat
Drink ice water

Rationale: Heart rate is regulated by an inhibiting nervous system and an accelerating nervous system, each working against the other. When the vagus nerve, which is part of the inhibiting nervous system, is stimulated, it slows the heart rate.

Resolved Needs: Circulation. Comfort. Protection from physical harm. Increased learning.

Instruct to use wide crutch tips   Explain that the tips on crutches should be as wide as is comfortable for the user.

Rationale: A firm, stable base is essential to safe ambulation. The larger the crutch tip, the greater the friction and stability.

Resolved Needs: Protection from physical harm. Increased learning.

Instruct to wear well-fitting shoes   Explain that one should wear shoes that are not tight, do not rub against the skin, give good support, and are comfortable.

Rationale: Friction causes skin pressure and irritation, which can result in tissue injury. A firm supportive base promotes stability of body movement and comfort.

Resolved Needs: Comfort. Protection from physical harm. Increased learning.

Recommend a daily change of clean clothing   Suggest that clean clothing be worn each day.

Rationale: Clean clothing promotes comfort and reduces the potential for infection.

Resolved Needs: Comfort. Cleanliness. Protection from physical harm. Increased learning.

Recommend a habitual, positive mental attitude   Suggest that the patient avoid dwelling on possible failure and unpleasantness. Suggest

that he develop positive approaches to problems, plan for the success he hopes to attain, and have a definite alternative plan in case failure does occur. If negative thinking has been his approach in the past, he will encounter considerable difficulty in developing a positive approach.

Rationale: A positive mental attitude supports self-confidence, which overcomes fear and anxiety and leads to success.

Resolved Needs: Comfort. Protection from psychologic threat. Personal growth and maturity. Increased learning. Increased reality perception and problem-solving ability.

Recommend a periodic chest X-ray Suggest that a chest X-ray be taken periodically. Advise use of mobile units if other facilities are not practical. This is especially important for persons who smoke.

Rationale: Periodic chest X-rays can permit early detection of lung disorders, many of which can be cured if found in the early stages.

Resolved Needs: Protection from physical harm. Increased learning.

Recommend a regular meal schedule Suggest that meals be served at approximately the same time each day so that a regular eating pattern is established.

Rationale: Body systems adapt more readily to routine functioning than to unrelated phenomena and activity. Scheduled feeding reduces the visceral hunger sensation and promotes comfort.

Resolved Needs: Food balance. Comfort. Protection from physical harm. Increased learning.

Recommend a regular sleeping schedule Suggest that one make it a habit to go to bed at the same time each night.

Rationale: Stable sleep habits promote physical and emotional health.

Resolved Needs: Sleep, rest. Protection from physical harm. Protection from psychologic threat. Increased learning.

Recommend activities which improve circulation Teach the patient to perform exercises, to walk briskly, or to rock in a chair.

Rationale: Activities that alternately cause vasodilatation and vasoconstriction improve circulation.

Resolved Needs: Oxygen, circulation. Activity, exercise. Protection from physical harm. Increased learning.

Recommend adequate food refrigeration Suggest that perishable foods and foods labeled as requiring refrigeration be kept cold in a tightly closed refrigerator.

Rationale: Adequate refrigeration prevents bacterial growth in food.

Resolved Needs: Protection from physical harm. Increased learning.

Recommend adherence to a moderate pace of living Explain that it is essential to control one's pace of living so that stress is kept to a minimum but productivity is satisfactory. This can be done by starting the day unhurriedly, by allowing extra time for activities, and by not becoming involved in more activities than one can comfortably perform.

Rationale: Living at a rapid pace consumes the energy that is vital to healing. Prolonged stress caused by a rapid pace breaks down the health of vital body organs and diminishes the capacity for healthy emotional adaptation.

Resolved Needs: Energy. Comfort. Protection from physical harm. Protection from psychologic threat. Increased learning.

Recommend an appropriate breast prosthesis Depending on the stage of recovery, give advice regarding a breast prosthesis. Shortly after surgery the patient will not be able to tolerate a commercial prosthesis. Suggest that she fill her regular brassiere with cotton or a sanitary pad as a temporary measure. Later recommend a professional prosthesis fitter for a prosthesis that is filled with air, fluid, or sponge and is designed to order.

Rationale: A breast prosthesis provides a feeling of body balance and a symmetric appearance.

Resolved Needs: Comfort. Increased learning.

Recommend communication by gesture Teach the patient who is unable to communicate by speech to convey messages by using hand movements, such as pointing, signs, and drawing in the air.

Rationale: Effective communication promotes comfort.

Resolved Needs: Comfort. Warm, communicating relationships. Increased learning.

Recommend consideration of occupation change When a patient is experiencing health impairment because of the nature of his job, advise him of the advantages of seeking other employment.

Rationale: Changing from an occupation that is impairing one's health can result in improved health.

Resolved Needs: Protection from physical harm. Increased learning.

Recommend distributing heavy tasks throughout the week Explain that tasks that consume a lot of energy should be planned so that they are spread out over the entire week, with about the same work load each day. A heavy wash load can be split, with half being done on one day and half on another. A large closet can be cleaned by doing one shelf each day. Task distribution is also suggested for light tasks that will require a great deal of time.

Rationale: When energy resources are limited, tasks that require a large expenditure of energy can be accomplished by distributing them over a period of time.

Resolved Needs: Energy. Comfort. Protection from physical harm. Independence. Increased learning.

Recommend eating and drinking in moderation
Suggest that the patient eat and drink moderately and not indulge in excessive food or drink.

Rationale: Overconsumption distends the stomach wall and causes pain and discomfort. It accelerates the digestive process, which increases heart rate and makes sleeping difficult. Excessive intake of food (calories) causes obesity.

Rationale: Comfort. Protection from physical harm. Increased learning.

Recommend eating only well-cooked meat in foreign countries
Explain that meat should be ordered well done, not rare, when one is visiting a foreign country.

Rationale: Thorough cooking decreases the potential for infection from bacteria or infestation (blood flukes, trichina).

Resolved Needs: Protection from physical harm. Increased learning.

Recommend energy-conserving methods for lifting and moving objects
Explain that the entire body weight should be employed in pushing or pulling, rather than just the arms or legs. Objects should be lifted with the arms close to the body, rather than extended outward from the body, and the weight of an object should be borne equally by both arms.

Rationale: Fatigue results from energy-consuming activity. The use of efficient methods conserves strength, promotes comfort, and supports independent activity.

Resolved Needs: Energy. Comfort. Protection from physical harm. Independence. Increased learning.

Recommend financial nonsupport of the drug user's habit
Explain that money should not be given to drug users to buy drugs. But it should be made known that love and emotional support are always available to the drug user.

Rationale: Financial support of a drug habit perpetuates drug use. Giving love and emotional support makes the person feel significant and may help overcome the drug abuse.

Resolved Needs: Comfort. Protection from psychologic threat. Increased learning.

Recommend housing with few doors and hallways for persons in a wheelchair
Suggest that physically disabled persons obtain living quarters where the doors and hallways are few in number and at least 48 inches wide.

Rationale: Housing of appropriate construction for the disabled promotes independent mobility.

Resolved Needs: Comfort. Independence. Increased learning.

Recommend limiting jet flying time to five consecutive hours when possible   Suggest that persons engaging in jet travel plan stop-overs after 4 or 5 hours of flight whenever possible.

Rationale: Interrupting lengthy jet flights can reduce fatigue and the stress imposed by time-zone changes.

Resolved Needs: Energy. Protection from physical harm. Increased learning.

Recommend limiting one's involvement in monotonous tasks   Explain that reduction of muscle tension can be facilitated by avoiding boring, unstimulating, and repetitive tasks.

Rationale: Having to perform unpleasant tasks increases tension, which consumes energy. Relief of muscular tension promotes comfort because of the decreased demands placed on the body.

Resolved Needs: Relaxation. Comfort. Protection from physical harm. Increased learning.

Recommend living in a single level, ground floor dwelling   Recommend that disabled patients live in ground level residences that have no stairs, basements, or attics.

Rationale: Single level dwellings support independent mobility for disabled persons. The absence of stairs can alleviate stress on the cardiac and respiratory systems.

Resolved Needs: Comfort. Protection from physical harm. Independence. Increased learning.

Recommend low window sills for persons in a wheelchair   Suggest that physically disabled persons obtain living quarters where at least one window sill is no higher than 36 inches.

Rationale: Window sills no higher than 36 inches allow the person in a wheelchair to look out without having to rely on assistance from others.

Resolved Needs: Comfort. Independence. Increased learning.

Recommend methods for achieving total relaxation   Suggest that total relaxation can be accomplished by setting aside some time each day when one is totally free from all mental and physical activity. Explain that one should not feel that doing nothing is a waste of time, since relaxation is essential to health. Controlled breathing, involving a conscious and gradual decrease in respirations below 10 times a minute, promotes relaxation. Quietly listening to soft music is also recommended. These methods should be practiced daily.

Rationale: Sitting and relaxing can reduce the muscular contraction and tension associated with activity. Soothing music aids relaxation because of its calming effect on the nervous system and because it distracts the mind from other mental activity. Slow, rhythmic breathing lowers oxygen intake, which slows the nervous system and general body function, quiets the emotions, and reduces muscular contraction.

Resolved Needs: Relaxation. Energy. Comfort. Protection from physical harm. Protection from psychologic threat. Increased learning.

Contraindications: Respiratory distress.

Recommend methods for eating suggested for the visually impaired   Explain that by gently touching food, the blind person can learn to distinguish food differences. The liquid level in a glass can be found by bending the forefinger into the glass and determining the distance between the liquid and the top of the glass. A piece of bread can be used to scoop food onto an eating utensil. Food for the blind person can be placed on the plate according to a system similar to the hours on a clock face: the meat can be at 5 o'clock, the salad at 9 o'clock, the potatoes at 1 o'clock.

Rationale: Special techniques for eating support independence for the blind person.

Resolved Needs: Adequacy. Independence. Mastery and competence in skills. Increased learning.

Recommend methods for increasing sensory stimulation   Suggest that there are many ways in which sensory stimulation can be increased: avoid monotonous tasks; increase room lighting; use bright room colors; add background sound by turning on a radio, television, or tape recorder; open windows to admit street noises; use unfamiliar routes to and from places; find employment in a large organization; mingle with crowds; attend exciting entertainments such as disaster movies, horse races, and competitive sports; use many nonpermanent articles; travel; seek out a variety of friends; live in a big city.

Rationale: Adequate sensory stimulation is essential for sound physical and mental health. Sensory stimulation increases motivation and encourages creativity.

Resolved Needs: Comfort. Stimulation. Protection from physical harm. Protection from psychologic threat. Increased learning. Increased creativity.

Recommend methods for noise reduction   Suggest that noise can be reduced by closing doors and windows, using heavy drapes, turning radios, recorders, or televisions off or to low volume, wearing earplugs or mufflers, and carpeting areas where noisy equipment is used.

Rationale: Sound waves at intensities above 80 decibels irritate the human ear. The noise level inside the home should be limited to 35 or 40 decibels. Excessive environmental stimuli increase stress.

Resolved Needs: Comfort. Protection from physical harm. Protection from psychologic threat. Increased learning.

Recommend methods for preparing a sick room at home
Suggest ways in which the sick room can be prepared or improved: room location, equipment needed, furniture placement, and the like.

Rationale: A properly located and equipped sick room meets the patient's needs and facilitates ease in caring for the patient.

Resolved Needs: Comfort. Protection from physical harm. Increased learning.

Recommend methods for reducing sensory stimulation
Suggest ways in which sensory stimulation can be limited: use subdued room light; decrease the noise level by turning off radios and televisions; close windows to reduce street noises; avoid offensive environmental odors; use familiar routes to and from places; find employment in a small, quiet office; remain away from crowds; attend light entertainment that does not involve tension and excitement; participate in noncompetitive games; dismiss unimportant matters so that the mind is not overstressed; delegate decision-making to other capable persons; reduce change by using permanent articles instead of throwaway articles; minimize travel or limit travel to only familiar places; keep the same job, the same car, and several very close friends; limit change to one change at a time whenever possible; live in a small or moderate-size community; become involved only up to a comfortable level, not to a higher level that might please others.

Rationale: Reduction of sensory stimulation decreases the amount of physical and psychologic adaptation that one must make to deal with stress, which in turn supports good health.

Resolved Needs: Comfort. Protection from physical harm. Protection from psychologic threat. Increased learning. Increased pleasantness.

Recommend methods used to stop smoking
Explain that there are many different methods used to stop smoking: withdrawing gradually by cutting one's smoking in half each day; stopping suddenly; keeping cigarettes in one's pocket or purse so that they are available if one feels desperate; delaying each smoke by an hour; quitting while on vacation, when normal pressures are decreased; promising to stop smoking, but keeping it to oneself so as to reduce the social pressures; puffing on an empty cigarette holder; chewing on a pipe; chewing on root ginger, which will cause a bad taste if one resumes smoking; letting a cigarette burn unsmoked; smoking only part of a cigarette; smoking bad-tasting cigarettes; chewing gum or eating candy; treating oneself each time one avoids smoking; changing the habits of living associated with smoking, such as going for a walk after meals instead of having a cigarette.

Rationale: Smoking increases the carbon monoxide content in hemoglobin and reduces its capacity to carry oxygen; it contracts airway muscles, thus narrowing respiratory passages and reducing air flow; it constricts and thickens blood vessels, which decreases circulation, especially to the extremities; it increases the catecholamine level, which increases the heart's need for oxygen; it irritates the intestines, causing ulceration; it retards healing of peptic ulcers because of vasoconstriction; it causes paralysis of respiratory cilia, which prevents the cilia from expelling foreign particles from the respiratory system; it thickens the respiratory mucous membranes and obstructs them with secretions; it causes growth of abnormal lung cells and produces tissue inflammation.

Resolved Needs: Protection from physical harm. Increased learning.

Recommend more effective methods of coping   If the patient is not coping in the most effective manner, suggest coping mechanisms that will lead to greater success in the struggle. For instance, if a person is angrily venting his frustration on loved ones, suggest that these frustrations can better be vented on the tennis court.

Rationale: Effective coping methods are essential to good mental health and happiness.

Resolved Needs: Comfort. Protection from psychologic threat. Increased learning.

Recommend napping whenever possible   Suggest that one nap on buses, airplanes, and trains or during work breaks, if possible.

Rationale: Fatigue results from energy-consuming activity. Sleep and rest restore energy.

Resolved Needs: Sleep, rest. Energy. Comfort. Protection from physical harm. Increased learning.

Recommend polyethylene doorsills for persons in a wheelchair   Suggest that the person in a wheelchair either have metal doorsills removed or use compressible polyethylene doorsills.

Rationale: Removing doorsills or using polyethylene doorsills facilitates independent mobility for the disabled.

Resolved Needs: Comfort. Independence. Increased learning.

Recommend strict adherence to safety rules   Explain that safety rules should be followed without exception.

Rationale: Safety rules are devised to protect one from accidental injury or disease.

Resolved Needs: Protection from physical harm. Increased learning.

Recommend that a high glucose source be carried at all times   Teach the person who is prone to develop low blood sugar to carry a ready source of glucose, such as sugar packets or candy.

Rationale: Ingestion of glucose will raise a low blood sugar to normal and maintain body cell activity and energy production. Prolonged and severe low blood sugar can result in brain damage.

Resolved Needs: Protection from physical harm. Increased learning.

Recommend that alkalis be used conservatively
Explain that when alkalis are taken in large doses, they disturb acid-base balance. Foods such as milk, cream, and buttermilk and antacid and alkali medications should be taken in moderation.

Rationale: Normal body function is dependent on acid-base balance.

Resolved Needs: Acid-base balance. Protection from physical harm. Increased learning.

Contraindications: When large doses of alkali are prescribed as an ulcer regimen.

Recommend that behavioral limits be set
Suggest that there are times when one must set limits on how far one will go to meet the demands of another person. It should be made clear that excessive demands cannot be met, and an explanation or a reason should be given.

Rationale: Setting limits gives the demanding person a guideline by which to control behavior. Giving a reason for not meeting a person's demand reduces the possibility that the refusal will be perceived as rejection.

Resolved Needs: Protection from psychologic threat. Personal growth and maturity. Increased learning. Increased reality perception and problem-solving ability.

Recommend that bones be removed from food before eating
Explain that bones should be removed before food is placed in the mouth, not after.

Rationale: Once bones are in the mouth, they can easily be aspirated, which can cause lung or tracheal injury.

Resolved Needs: Protection from physical harm. Increased learning.

Recommend that children be introduced to a wide variety of food
Suggest that a child taste as many different foods as possible at the earliest appropriate time.

Rationale: Exposing children to a wide variety of food supports taste development and good nutrition.

Resolved Needs: Food balance. Comfort. Protection from physical harm. Increased learning.

Recommend that doorknobs and switches be placed 36 inches above the floor
Suggest that physically disabled persons have their doorknobs and light switches placed 36 inches above the floor.

Rationale: Doorknobs and light switches placed 36 inches above the floor can be reached easily from a sitting or standing position.

Resolved Needs: Comfort. Independence. Increased learning.

Recommend that electrical outlets be placed 18 inches above the floor
Suggest that physically disabled persons have their electrical outlets placed 18 inches above the floor.

Rationale: Electrical outlets placed 18 inches above the floor can be reached easily by a person in a wheelchair and by anyone who cannot stoop down.

Resolved Needs: Comfort. Independence. Increased learning.

Recommend that extra therapeutic supplies be carried
Suggest that the patient wearing a drainage collection appliance or absorbent dressings carry extra supplies.

Rationale: Extra supplies provide the comfort of being ready for accidents.

Resolved Needs: Comfort. Increased learning.

Recommend that food be cut in small bite sizes
Suggest that food be cut into small bite-size portions rather than into large chunks.

Rationale: If small bites of food are aspirated, they are less likely to cause fatal airway obstruction than large bites.

Resolved Needs: Protection from physical harm. Increased learning.

Recommend that food servings be in proportion to the appetite
Suggest that the size of the food serving be appropriate to the person's appetite. Never serve more food than a person wants and can eat.

Rationale: Serving large portions of food to the person with a poor appetite has a discouraging effect and further diminishes his desire to eat.

Resolved Needs: Comfort. Increased learning.

Recommend that high altitudes be avoided after cardiac damage
Explain that patients with heart disease should avoid traveling to areas high above sea level.

Rationale: The partial pressure of oxygen in the blood is decreased at high altitudes, thus placing extra stress on the heart.

Resolved Needs: Oxygen. Protection from physical harm. Increased learning.

Recommend that independence be encouraged
Explain that every person needs freedom from control by others and should have the opportunity to try new things.

Rationale: Balancing dependence-independence needs is essential to growth, maturity, adequacy, and self-reliance. Independence supports the development of one's potential.

Resolved Needs: Protection from psychologic threat. Adequacy. Self-reliance. Independence. Personal growth and maturity. Awareness of potential. Increased learning. Full development of potential. Increased reality perception and problem-solving ability.

Recommend that infants be fed on a self-demand schedule
Suggest that infants be fed when they indicate hunger through crying. Most babies will put themselves on a regular schedule.

Rationale: An infant fed on a self-demand schedule is most likely to obtain adequate nutrition, since his food demand is based on physiologic needs.

Resolved Needs: Food balance. Comfort. Protection from physical harm. Increased learning.

Recommend that jet travelers reduce stress by arriving 24 hours before scheduled activity
Suggest that the person engaged in extensive jet travel arrive at his destination 24 hours before planned meetings or sightseeing activities.

Rationale: Arriving 24 hours before scheduled activity allows time for rest and adjustment to time-zone changes. This is particularly important if one is working and major decisions have to be made.

Resolved Needs: Energy. Protection from physical harm. Protection from psychologic threat. Increased learning.

Recommend that passive activities be avoided
Explain that passive activities such as sleeping, reading, watching television, and listening to radio should be avoided as much as possible by healthy persons. Explain that active activities are preferable.

Rationale: Passive activities lead to boredom and frustration and reduce involvement in healthy activity and exercise.

Resolved Needs: Protection from physical harm. Protection from psychologic threat. Increased learning.

Recommend that self-medication be avoided
Explain that prescribing drugs for oneself or one's children can result in serious side effects, because faulty determination of the cause of the problem will result in taking the wrong drug.

Rationale: Chemical reactions within the body resulting from combination of incompatible elements can produce poisoning effects. Drugs taken during pregnancy can cause birth defects or impair fetal development.

Resolved Needs: Protection from physical harm. Increased learning.

Recommend that the approximate eating schedule be maintained despite long jet trips   Suggest that the person engaged in extensive jet travel eat three times a day at 5- to 6-hour intervals, or as near to his normal schedule as possible.

Rationale: Adequate nutrition reduces the fatigue associated with travel.

Resolved Needs: Food balance. Protection from physical harm. Increased learning.

Recommend that the tongue be brushed   Suggest using a toothbrush to brush the tongue gently.

Rationale: Brushing the tongue cleans its surface and removes food particles from cracks in the tongue.

Resolved Needs: Comfort. Cleanliness. Protection from physical harm. Increased learning.

Contraindications: Tongue inflammation or pain.

Recommend that time be divided between energy- and nonenergy-consuming activities   Suggest that stress be reduced by balancing activities between those that require much energy and those that require little energy.

Rationale: Equally distributing one's efforts between high- and low-energy-consuming activities reduces stress and conserves energy.

Resolved Needs: Energy. Comfort. Protection from physical harm. Protection from psychologic threat. Increased learning.

Recommend that toys be washable   Suggest that parents provide children with toys that can be washed or cleaned. Plush unwashable toys can be cleaned by sprinkling them with corn meal, letting them stand awhile, and then brushing out the corn meal.

Rationale: Unclean toys can carry bacteria and lead to infection.

Resolved Needs: Cleanliness. Protection from physical harm. Increased learning.

Recommend that two ostomy appliances be alternately used   Suggest that the patient have two ostomy appliances so that one can be used while the other is being prepared for use.

Rationale: Having two ostomy appliances allows for one to be thoroughly cleaned and dried while the other is in use.

Resolved Needs: Comfort. Cleanliness. Increased learning.

Recommend that windows be screened   Suggest that screens be put on windows to keep insects out.

Rationale: Insects carry microorganisms from one person to another and transmit disease.

Resolved Needs: Protection from physical harm. Increased learning.

Recommend that work activities be combined   Suggest that work be simplified, possibly by doubling the amount of work done at one time and limiting how often work is done. This might include washing dishes only once a day, thorough housecleaning only once a week, making two cakes at one time and freezing one, and buying groceries in larger quantities.

Rationale: Work simplification reduces energy consumption and supports independent activity.

Resolved Needs: Energy. Comfort. Protection from physical harm. Independence. Increased learning.

Recommend the duplication of equipment in work areas   Suggest that work can be simplified by having several frequently used equipment items in different work areas. This might include dust mops upstairs and downstairs, scouring powder in each bathroom, hot pads on the stove and the table, etc.

Rationale: Work simplification minimizes energy consumption and supports independent activity.

Resolved Needs: Energy. Comfort. Protection from physical harm. Independence. Increased learning.

Recommend the elimination of unnecessary work   Suggest that work can be simplified by determining which details can be eliminated. This might include the following: not ironing sheets, towels, and underwear; buying drip-dry clothing; using paper dishes whenever possible; using partially prepared food; using the same dish to cook, serve, and store food; planning simple meals.

Rationale: Work simplification minimizes energy consumption and supports independent activity.

Resolved Needs: Energy. Comfort. Protection from physical harm. Independence. Increased learning.

Recommend the installation of a smoke alarm   Suggest that one install an alarm that signals when a fire is still in the smoldering stage.

Rationale: If a person is unable to detect odors easily, a smoke alarm can warn him that a fire is in its early stages. Smoke alarms will wake a sleeping person in time to escape a fire.

Resolved Needs: Protection from physical harm. Increased learning.

Recommend the preferable age for introducing specific foods to children (400)   Explain that certain solid foods should be introduced to young children at certain ages. At age 1–4 months the child should begin to eat cereals; age 2–4 months, stewed or strained fruits and very ripe

bananas; age 3–5 months, strained vegetables; age 2–6 months, pureed egg yolk; age 6 months and older, puddings, potatoes, and finger foods such as toast and zwieback; age 7–12 months, lumpy foods; age 9 months, soft-boiled eggs or scrambled whole eggs and mashed foods; age 10–12 months, boiled or broiled fish that has been boned.

Rationale: Sound nutrition is essential to healthy growth and development.

Resolved Needs: Comfort. Food balance. Protection from physical harm. Increased learning.

Recommend the pursuit of only one activity at a time
Explain that muscular tension can be reduced by engaging in only one activity at a time. When that activity is completed, then one can move on to the next task.

Rationale: Performing only one activity at a time reduces the number of stimuli to which the body must respond, thus promoting relaxation and decreasing energy consumption.

Resolved Needs: Relaxation. Energy. Comfort. Protection from physical harm. Protection from psychologic threat. Increased learning.

Recommend the sitting position for improved ventilation
Suggest that when a person has difficulty breathing, he should take a sitting position.

Rationale: The sitting position promotes free passage of air through the respiratory tract.

Resolved Needs: Oxygen. Comfort. Protection from physical harm. Increased learning.

Recommend the use of a back-support garment
Suggest that snugly fitting garments be worn to give back support.

Rationale: Back-support garments reduce muscle strain and promote body alignment and comfort.

Resolved Needs: Comfort. Freedom from pain. Increased learning.

Recommend the use of a brassiere for breast support
Suggest that during pregnancy and lactation, or after a mastectomy, a comfortable supportive brassiere be worn. The brassiere should have a sufficiently large cup; it should cover all breast tissue in the underarm area and should have wide supportive straps.

Rationale: Use of a supportive brassiere during pregnancy, lactation, or breast engorgement can relieve discomfort from breast weight, shield the breast for cleanliness, and minimize fluid congestion. Breast support prevents overstretching and tearing of muscle fibers, thus forestalling premature breast sagging. Since the absence of one breast tends to pull the body to one side, breast support following mastectomy brings the body into normal alignment.

Resolved Needs: Comfort. Cleanliness. Protection from physical harm. Increased learning.

Recommend the use of a canister vacuum for energy conservation
Suggest that the physically disabled person use a canister vacuum cleaner with a swivel top.

Rationale: Canister vacuums are more easily manipulated than upright vacuums; they help conserve energy and reduce fatigue.

Resolved Needs: Energy. Comfort. Protection from physical harm. Independence. Increased learning.

Recommend the use of a car backrest
Suggest that the person with back problems use a backrest, especially designed for automobiles, when driving.

Rationale: A car backrest offers firm support, which promotes comfort.

Resolved Needs: Comfort. Freedom from pain. Increased learning.

Recommend the use of a face mask
Suggest that whenever dust, bacteria, vapor, or fumes come in contact with the face, a mask should be worn.

Rationale: A face mask protects the skin and respiratory system against injurious foreign objects.

Resolved Needs: Protection from physical harm. Increased learning.

Recommend the use of a fluoride toothpaste
Suggest that a toothpaste containing fluoride be used every day.

Rationale: Trace amounts of the element fluorine in water or toothpaste help prevent tooth decay.

Resolved Needs: Protection from physical harm. Increased learning.

Recommend the use of a foot pedal on appliance doors when hand dexterity is impaired
For a person who has limited hand movement, suggest the use of a foot pedal instead of a handle on appliance doors.

Rationale: A foot pedal makes it easier to use an appliance for one whose hand dexterity is impaired.

Resolved Needs: Comfort. Independence. Increased learning. Increased reality perception and problem-solving ability.

Recommend the use of a hernia support
Suggest that the patient apply a hernia support to the inguinal area.

Rationale: Supportive garments decrease stress on abdominal muscles and organs, promote comfort, and reduce pain.

Resolved Needs: Comfort. Protection from physical harm. Freedom from pain. Increased learning.

Recommend the use of a laryngectomy bib   Suggest that the patient who has had a laryngectomy wear a cotton or crocheted bib to keep clothing clean.

Rationale: Expulsion of mucus from the laryngectomy stoma will stain clothing. A bib helps maintain cleanliness and offers protection from irritants.

Resolved Needs: Comfort. Cleanliness. Increased learning.

Recommend the use of a night light   Suggest that a night light be kept on when a patient has visual or mobility impairment.

Rationale: Use of a night light prevents accidents; it keeps sleep disturbance to a minimum when one must get up during the night, and it prevents distorted perception.

Resolved Needs: Protection from physical harm. Increased learning.

Recommend the use of a nipple shield   Suggest that when a breast nipple is cracked or irritated, a soft protective shield be placed over the nipple, especially while the infant is nursing.

Rationale: A nipple shield prevents irritation of breast nipple tissue, facilitates healing, promotes cleanliness, and permits continued breast feeding.

Resolved Needs: Comfort. Cleanliness. Protection from physical harm. Increased learning.

Recommend the use of a pacemaker shirt   Suggest that an undershirt with a pocket large enough to hold a pacemaker be worn.

Rationale: An undershirt can hold a pacemaker in place and prevent skin irritation from the pacemaker.

Resolved Needs: Comfort. Protection from physical harm. Increased learning.

Recommend the use of a pegboard for ease in storing utensils   Suggest that the physically disabled person hang utensils on a pegboard instead of placing them in drawers or cabinets.

Rationale: Removing utensils from a pegboard requires less energy than pulling out drawers and opening cabinets.

Resolved Needs: Energy. Comfort. Independence. Increased learning.

Recommend the use of a scrotal support

Suggest that the male patient apply a supportive garment to the scrotum.

Rationale: A scrotal support can protect the reproductive organ from injury and reduce postsurgical edema.

Resolved Needs: Comfort. Protection from physical harm. Increased learning.

Contraindications: Skin irritation.

Recommend the use of a sheepskin

Suggest that sheep's wool be placed under a patient who must lie or sit for prolonged periods.

Rationale: The air spaces in a sheepskin help to keep the patient's skin dry; its softness eases pressure on the skin and helps prevent decubitus ulcer.

Resolved Needs: Comfort. Protection from physical harm. Increased learning.

Recommend the use of a shower chair

Suggest that the weak patient sit on a waterproof chair or stool in the shower.

Rationale: Using a chair or stool in the shower can reduce the potential for falling and can conserve energy.

Resolved Needs: Energy. Comfort. Protection from physical harm. Increased learning.

Recommend the use of a typewriter when unable to write

Suggest that the person who is unable to write but who still has coarse finger movements use a typewriter.

Rationale: Use of a typewriter can facilitate communication with others.

Resolved Needs: Warm, communicating relationships. Increased learning.

Recommend the use of absorbent padding

Suggest that padding made of a material that will soak up liquid excretions and drainage be placed under the patient and around draining wounds.

Rationale: Many materials can absorb wetness that otherwise would remain in contact with the skin and cause skin irritation.

Resolved Needs: Comfort. Cleanliness. Protection from physical harm. Increased learning.

Recommend the use of an abdominal-support garment

Suggest that a girdle or binder be worn when the patient is out of bed.

Rationale: Supportive garments prevent muscle sagging.

Resolved Needs: Comfort. Protection from physical harm. Increased learning.

Contraindications: Impaired circulation.

Recommend the use of an antiperspirant
Suggest the use of commercial antiperspirants on the axilla after bathing for control of sweating and skin odor.

Rationale: Body odor may be controlled by oxidizing odoriferous material or by inhibiting bacterial growth.

Resolved Needs: Comfort. Cleanliness. Increased learning.

Contraindications: Axillary skin irritation or inflammation. Allergy.

Recommend the use of an antiperspirant foot powder
Explain that foot odor can be controlled by a thin application of a commercial foot powder that prevents sweat secretion.

Rationale: Inhibiting sweat secretion reduces skin odor and promotes cleanliness and comfort.

Resolved Needs: Comfort. Cleanliness. Increased learning.

Contraindications: Skin irritation or inflammation. Allergy.

Recommend the use of an electric garage door for energy conservation
Suggest that the physically disabled person have electric garage doors installed.

Rationale: Electric garage doors support independent activity and minimize the number of times one must get in and out of a car.

Resolved Needs: Comfort. Independence. Increased learning.

Recommend the use of bedrails
Suggest that young children, old persons, and irresponsible persons be protected with siderails on their beds.

Rationale: Siderails minimize the potential for falling.

Resolved Needs: Protection from physical harm. Increased learning.

Recommend the use of closed shoes for foot protection
Suggest that shoes closed at the toes and heels be worn to protect against foot injury.

Rationale: A protective shoe can prevent trauma to an injured foot or to the stump of an amputated toe.

Resolved Needs: Comfort. Protection from physical harm. Increased learning.

Recommend the use of dental floss
Suggest that dental floss be used to clean between the teeth at least once a day.

Rationale: Dental floss removes food particles and plaque from between the teeth and reduces the potential for decay.

Resolved Needs: Protection from physical harm. Increased learning.

Recommend the use of denture adherent   Suggest that an adherent be used to assure snug-fitting dentures.

Rationale: Properly fitting dentures are necessary for comfort, for normal chewing, and for prevention of oral mucosa injury.

Resolved Needs: Comfort. Protection from physical harm. Increased learning.

Contraindications: Oral mucosal infection, inflammation, or irritation. Allergy.

Recommend the use of disposable dishes for contagious diseases   Suggest that paper or plastic disposable dishes and utensils be used when caring for the patient with a communicable disease.

Rationale: Disposable dishes minimize the possibility of transmitting infection.

Resolved Needs: Cleanliness. Protection from physical harm. Increased learning.

Recommend the use of double thickness tissue for infectious sputum   Suggest that when infective sputum is expectorated, double thickness tissue should be used.

Rationale: It is difficult for microorganisms to penetrate double thickness tissue. This reduces the potential for transmitting infection.

Resolved Needs: Protection from physical harm. Increased learning.

Recommend the use of dry shampoo   Suggest that dry shampoo may be used to clean and freshen the hair when it cannot be washed.

Rationale: Dry shampoo cleans superficial dirt and oil from the hair by absorbing greasy materials that hold dirt.

Resolved Needs: Comfort. Cleanliness. Protection from physical harm. Increased learning.

Contraindications: Scalp infection, abrasions, or bleeding.

Recommend the use of ear mufflers   Suggest that mufflers be placed over the ears when working in noisy environments, such as in manufacturing plants, at airports, and around loud music.

Rationale: Ear mufflers reduce the potential for hearing loss from exposure to intense sound.

Resolved Needs: Protection from physical harm. Increased learning.

Recommend the use of eye shields for sleeping
Suggest that persons traveling by airplane use eye shields for sleeping, especially when flying all night and into the dawn.

Rationale: Eye shields provide darkness, which is conducive to sleep.

Resolved Needs: Sleep, rest. Protection from physical harm. Increased learning.

Recommend the use of eyeglass safety lens
Suggest that eyeglasses with shatterproof lenses be purchased.

Rationale: Shatterproof eyeglasses reduce the potential for eye injury.

Resolved Needs: Protection from physical harm. Increased learning.

Recommend the use of front stove controls for persons in a wheelchair
Suggest that the person in a wheelchair be provided with a stove that has front controls and that the oven and broiler be placed at a low level.

Rationale: Front controls on stoves and low-level ovens are easiest to use when one is in a wheelchair; they support independent activity.

Resolved Needs: Comfort. Independence. Increased learning.

Recommend the use of front-loading washers and dryers for persons in a wheelchair
Suggest that the person in a wheelchair be provided with a front-loading dishwasher, washing machine, and dryer with front panel controls.

Rationale: Front-loading machines are easiest to use when one is in a wheelchair; they support independent activity.

Resolved Needs: Comfort. Independence. Increased learning.

Recommend the use of handrails
Suggest that handrails be provided when the patient has impaired coordination or limited range of motion. Handrails are useful in bathtubs and showers, on bedside commodes, and in long hallways.

Rationale: Handrails assist body balance and coordination of movement and help prevent accidental injury.

Resolved Needs: Protection from physical harm. Increased learning.

Recommend the use of high storage cabinets for persons unable to stoop
Suggest that persons who are unable to stoop store things in upper cabinets.

Rationale: There is easier access to high cabinets for persons who are unable to stoop; their use can support independent activity.

Resolved Needs: Comfort. Independence. Increased learning.

Recommend the use of individual dishes, utensils, and drinking glasses Suggest that each person have his own dishes, utensils, and glasses and that dishes not be shared between persons.

Rationale: Use of separate dishes minimizes the potential for transfer of infectious microorganisms.

Resolved Needs: Cleanliness. Protection from physical harm. Increased learning.

Recommend the use of individual towels and washcloths Suggest that each person have his own towel and washcloth and not use linens used by others.

Rationale: Using individual towels and washcloths promotes cleanliness and minimizes the spread of disease.

Resolved Needs: Cleanliness. Protection from physical harm. Increased learning.

Recommend the use of iodized salt Suggest that salt containing sodium iodide or potassium iodide be used to season food.

Rationale: Use of iodized salt will prevent iodine deficiency, and its use during early iodine deficiency will usually correct the problem. Iodine is essential to the production of thyroxine, which is necessary for normal metabolism.

Resolved Needs: Protection from physical harm. Increased learning.

Recommend the use of knots to distinguish clothing color for the visually impaired Suggest that different numbers of embroidery knots placed inside of clothing can designate the color: two knots might indicate brown, three knots green, etc.

Rationale: Coding clothes by knots enables persons with impaired vision to know the colors of their clothing and to dress independently.

Resolved Needs: Comfort. Mastery and competence in skills. Independence. Increased learning.

Recommend the use of lightweight clothing Suggest that the patient wear clothing made of cool material, such as cottons instead of polyesters. Also, recommend clothing that weighs as little as possible.

Rationale: Lightweight clothing can help maintain a cool body temperature, decrease pressure on irritating lesions, and reduce the weight a weakened body must carry.

Resolved Needs: Normal temperature. Energy. Comfort. Protection from physical harm. Increased learning.

Recommend the use of lightweight utensils Suggest the use of small utensils that are lightweight, versatile, easily stored, and easily gripped.

Rationale: Lightweight utensils are easily used by small children or weak persons.

Resolved Needs: Comfort. Protection from physical harm. Independence. Increased learning.

Recommend the use of long, even strokes to propel the wheelchair
Suggest that the best method of propelling a wheelchair is to push both wheels forward simultaneously, using long, even, intermittent strokes.

Rationale: Use of efficient means to propel a wheelchair reduces energy consumption, which minimizes fatigue.

Resolved Needs: Energy. Comfort. Protection from physical harm. Increased learning.

Recommend the use of low clothes racks for persons in a wheelchair
Suggest that the person in a wheelchair use clothes racks about half the height of standard racks.

Rationale: Low clothing racks are easily reached by persons in wheelchairs, which supports independent activity.

Resolved Needs: Comfort. Independence. Increased learning.

Recommend the use of low storage cabinets for persons in a wheelchair
Suggest that the person in a wheelchair store products in low cabinets.

Rationale: For someone in a wheelchair, low cabinets are easy to reach; they facilitate ease in handling items.

Resolved Needs: Comfort. Independence. Increased learning.

Recommend the use of low-heeled shoes
Suggest that shoes having no heels or slight heels be worn in preference to high-heeled shoes.

Rationale: Low-heeled shoes maintain correct body alignment. High-heeled shoes throw the skeleton and abdominal organs forward and increase the potential for falling.

Resolved Needs: Protection from physical harm. Increased learning.

Recommend the use of mouthwash
Suggest the use of salt solution or commercial mouthwash to rinse the mouth. When oral bleeding occurs, mouthwash should be used gently, or a padded tongue blade may be soaked in mouthwash and swabbed around the mouth.

Rationale: Use of a mouthwash removes food particles from the teeth, refreshes the breath, and provides a pleasant taste.

Resolved Needs: Comfort. Cleanliness. Protection from physical harm. Increased learning.

Contraindications: Avoid using mouthwash when there are blood clots in the mouth or when the oral mucosa is inflamed or irritated.

Recommend the use of nipple padding Suggest that pads be placed over the breast nipple or inserted into the brassiere when lactation secretions threaten to soil clothes.

Rationale: Nipple padding promotes comfort and cleanliness by preventing seepage of breast secretions onto clothes.

Resolved Needs: Comfort. Cleanliness. Protection from physical harm. Increased learning.

Recommend the use of nonskid throw rugs Explain that it is inadvisable to place small rugs throughout a home. If rugs are used, they should have nonskid backing.

Rationale: The use of nonskid rugs decreases the potential for injury from falling.

Resolved Needs: Protection from physical harm. Increased learning.

Recommend the use of push-bar windows for energy conservation Suggest that disabled persons be provided with windows that open and close by use of a push-bar at the windowsill level.

Rationale: Use of a push-bar for opening a window conserves energy and encourages independent activity.

Resolved Needs: Comfort. Independence. Increased learning.

Recommend the use of revolving cabinet shelves Suggest that physically disabled persons be provided with revolving shelves in deep cabinets.

Rationale: Revolving shelves make it easy to reach items in cabinets, which supports independent activity.

Resolved Needs: Comfort. Independence. Increased learning.

Recommend the use of rolling tables to ease work Suggest the use of sturdy tables with wheels for moving many items at a time and for support in walking.

Rationale: Work simplification reduces energy consumption and supports independent activity.

Resolved Needs: Energy. Comfort. Protection from physical harm. Independence. Increased learning.

Recommend the use of rubber gloves Suggest that rubber gloves be worn whenever the hands are placed in harsh detergents.

Rationale: Harsh detergents irritate the skin and cause chapping, cracking, and allergic responses.

Resolved Needs: Comfort. Cleanliness. Protection from physical harm. Increased learning.

Recommend the use of slow, distinct speech with persons having impaired communication reception
Suggest that slow, clear speech be used when talking to persons who have difficulty receiving messages.

Rationale: Slow, distinct speech enhances communication perception.

Resolved Needs: Comfort. Protection from psychologic threat. Warm, communicating relationships. Increased learning.

Recommend the use of stair gates
Suggest that safety gates be placed at the tops and bottoms of stairways when small children are learning to walk.

Rationale: Safety gates on stairways help prevent the severe injury or death that can result from falls.

Resolved Needs: Protection from physical harm. Increased learning.

Recommend the use of suction tub mats
Suggest that suction-type rubber mats be used in bathtubs.

Rationale: A suction-type rubber mat provides a firm base for standing and helps prevent injury from falling.

Resolved Needs: Protection from physical harm. Increased learning.

Recommend the use of top stove controls for persons unable to stoop
Suggest that persons who are unable to stoop be provided with stoves with controls on the top and with oven and broiler at or above waist level.

Rationale: Top controls on stoves and high ovens are easiest to use when one is unable to stoop; they support independent activity.

Resolved Needs: Comfort. Independence. Increased learning.

Recommend the use of top-loading washers and dryers for persons unable to stoop
Suggest that persons who are unable to stoop be provided with top-loading dishwashers, washing machines, and dryers.

Rationale: Top-loading machines are easiest to use when one is unable to stoop; they support independent activity.

Resolved Needs: Comfort. Independence. Increased learning.

Recommend the use of warm clothing
Suggest that adequately warm clothing be worn in cold weather, including hats and gloves.

Rationale: Warm clothing protects the body from the harmful effects of cold weather. Warm clothing in bed prevents chilling, which stimulates bed-wetting.

Resolved Needs: Comfort. Protection from physical harm. Increased learning.

Recommend the use of well-padded pot holders Suggest that pot holders and kitchen mits be well padded and that they not be used after they have worn thin.

Rationale: Well-padded pot holders prevent burns.

Resolved Needs: Protection from physical harm. Increased learning.

Recommend thorough food chewing Suggest that food be chewed slowly and thoroughly before swallowing.

Rationale: The first step toward adequate digestion is chewing one's food into small particles. Thorough chewing helps offset deficient digestive secretion if saliva production is diminished, and it enhances digestive enzyme activity when food reaches the stomach and intestines.

Resolved Needs: Comfort. Protection from physical harm. Increased learning.

Recommend throat gargling Suggest the use of a salt gargle or medicated gargle whenever the throat feels scratchy or painful.

Rationale: Warm isotonic saline gargles are cleansing and soothing. Antiseptic gargles are astringent and cleansing. Anesthetic gargles have analgesic effects.

Resolved Needs: Comfort. Cleanliness. Protection from physical harm. Increased learning.

Contraindications: Impaired swallowing.

Recommend wearing a hard hat for head protection Suggest that a hard hat be worn when a person is standing or working where objects might fall on the head.

Rationale: Hard hats protect against head injury.

Resolved Needs: Protection from physical harm. Increased learning.

Relate the accepted criteria for commitment of drug users Explain that confinement of persons on drugs to health institutions is a matter of conscience. If the person is a minor, is unable to function normally, or breaks with reality, it is generally accepted that commitment is needed.

Rationale: Legal action for confinement taken by one person against another should be instigated for the well-being of the sick person and should be based on sound reasoning so as to reduce the potential for guilt.

Resolved Needs: Protection from psychologic threat. Increased learning.

Relate the accepted criteria for commitment of the mentally ill
Explain that if a person appears to be in danger of harming himself or others, he is considered a candidate for enforced hospitalization.

Rationale: Legal action for confinement taken by one person against another should be instigated for the well-being of the sick person and should be based on sound reasoning so as to reduce the potential for guilt.

Resolved Needs: Protection from psychologic threat. Increased learning.

Relate the accepted criteria for notifying authorities of drug abuse
Explain that notifying legal authorities of drug abuse is basically a matter of conscience. It is generally accepted that if a person is a minor or is a drug pusher, then he should be reported to the authorities.

Rationale: Law-enforcement action taken by one person against another should be for the well-being of the sick person and should be based on sound reasoning so as to reduce the potential for guilt.

Resolved Needs: Protection from psychologic threat. Increased learning.

Relate the criteria for determining mental illness
Explain that some of the signs indicating mental illness are severe behavioral changes, periodic confusion or memory loss, feelings of persecution or grandiose feelings, talking to oneself, hearing voices, seeing visions, complaints of strange odors or tastes, bodily complaints that are physically not possible, severe depression, and physical abuse of others.

Rationale: Awareness of the manifestations of mental illness can support early and effective treatment.

Resolved Needs: Protection from physical harm. Protection from psychologic threat. Increased learning. Increased reality perception and problem-solving ability.

Relate the criteria for successful sexual response
Explain that if one experiences satisfaction, completeness, euphoria, or contentment, then the sexual relationship is successful.

Rationale: Awareness that one has successful sexual relationships supports comfort and feelings of adequacy.

Resolved Needs: Comfort. Sexuality. Protection from psychologic threat. Adequacy. Increased learning.

Teach correct weight-bearing on the crutch handbar
Teach the patient to bear his weight on the crutch handbar; he should not lean on the crutches or suspend his weight from the point where his axillae meet the tops of the crutches.

Rationale: The pressure of one's weight against the crutches at the axillae can cause nerve damage, with resulting paralysis of the hand or arm.

Resolved Needs: Protection from physical harm. Increased learning.

Teach decubitus ulcer care
Explain how to take care of a decubitus ulcer. Include skin cleansing, use of toughening and healing agents, frequent turning, and use of sheepskin.

Rationale: Decubitus ulcer care promotes healing of pressure-damaged tissue.

Resolved Needs: Protection from physical harm. Mastery and competence in skills. Increased learning.

Teach good body mechanics
Explain that lifting an object from the ground should be accomplished with both the back muscles and leg muscles. In carrying a heavy object, one should use the muscles of the shoulders, back, legs, and arms. Stooping should be avoided; one should squat by bending the knees and keeping the back straight.

Rationale: Good body mechanics can prevent injury to the skeletal system.

Resolved Needs: Comfort. Protection from physical harm. Increased learning.

Teach good crutch-walking posture
Teach the patient walking with crutches to stand with his chest high, to fully extend (straighten) his hips and knees, and to look forward rather than down at his feet.

Rationale: Proper use of crutches is essential for correct body alignment, weight-bearing, and mobility.

Resolved Needs: Comfort. Protection from physical harm. Mastery and competence in skills. Increased learning.

Teach good prosthesis-walking posture
Teach the patient wearing a lower-extremity prosthesis to avoid taking longer steps with the prosthesis foot than with the natural foot, to avoid walking with his feet far apart, and to avoid hip and shoulder hiking with each prosthetic step. The body should be held in good alignment.

Rationale: Proper use of a prosthesis is essential for maximum weight-bearing and mobility.

Resolved Needs: Comfort. Protection from physical harm. Mastery and competence in skills. Increased learning.

Teach how to administer medications
Explain the proper dosage and method for administering prescribed drugs. Include information about the purpose of the drug and the potential side effects.

Rationale: Knowledge of correct drug administration increases the potential for effectiveness of therapy, reduces the potential for drug side effects, and supports independence.

Resolved Needs: Protection from physical harm. Independence. Increased learning.

Teach how to administer tube feeding Explain how to determine whether the tube is correctly placed in the stomach; explain that the prescribed tube feeding formula should be of moderate temperature and should be given by slow drip followed by a small amount of water. Explain proper attachment, adjustment, and cleaning of the tube feeding set.

Rationale: Adequate nutritional intake is essential to cellular activity and energy production from food.

Resolved Needs: Food balance. Protection from physical harm. Mastery and competence in skills. Independence. Increased learning.

Teach how to apply a breast binder Explain how a wide binder (8-inch Ace bandage or muslin binder) is encircled around the breasts; the breasts should be held in normal position while the binder is being applied snugly, but not too tightly; it is best to pin the binder from the bottom up.

Rationale: The application of a breast binder to an engorged or lactating breast aids in preventing fluid congestion. It shields the breast for cleanliness, relieves discomfort from breast weight by offering support, and prevents backache by enhancing good posture.

Resolved Needs: Comfort. Protection from physical harm. Mastery and competence in skills. Increased learning.

Teach how to apply a stump sock Explain that a clean stump sock should be applied smoothly over the stump without any wrinkles.

Rationale: Wrinkles or creases in a stump sock can cause skin irritation, with resulting decubitus ulcers.

Resolved Needs: Protection from physical harm. Mastery and competence in skills. Increased learning.

Teach how to apply a urinary-collection container Explain how to connect a plastic or waterproof bag and tubing to the urinary drainage tubing for collecting urinary output.

Rationale: A collection apparatus for urine assures accurate output measurement, maintains dryness and thus prevents skin irritation, and provides the comfort of cleanliness.

Resolved Needs: Comfort. Cleanliness. Protection from physical harm. Mastery and competence in skills. Increased learning.

Teach how to apply an arm sling Explain how a triangular bandage is laid flat across the chest with one tail over the shoulder opposite the injury and the pointed end across the elbow of the injured arm. Position the forearm a little higher than at a right angle. Lift the hanging tail up under the arm and around the neck. Tie the two tails behind the unaffected shoulder. Support the hand and wrist in the sling. Fold the point of the sling smoothly around the elbow and pin it in the front.

Rationale: Support of a traumatized body part prevents further injury and promotes comfort.

Resolved Needs: Comfort. Protection from physical harm. Mastery and competence in skills. Increased learning.

Teach how to apply an external urinary catheter   Explain how to apply a balloon-type catheter to the external male genitalia. Caution against anchoring the catheter too tightly, and explain how to attach it to a drainage container.

Rationale: An external urinary catheter assures accurate output measurement, maintains dryness and thus prevents skin irritation, and provides the comfort of cleanliness.

Resolved Needs: Comfort. Cleanliness. Protection from physical harm. Mastery and competence in skills. Increased learning.

Teach how to apply and remove a leg brace   Explain the procedure for putting on a leg brace: Sit in a chair and place the unaffected leg midline in front of the body. Cross the affected leg over the unaffected leg. Pull up the tongue of the shoe. Hold the brace at the top, swinging the shoe far enough forward so the toes can be inserted into the shoe. Turn the shoe slightly inward so that the toes can be inserted at a slight angle. Pull the brace up as far as possible onto the leg. If a shoehorn is needed, hold the brace between the two legs. Move the shoehorn back and forth until the foot fits into the shoe. Fasten the laces and straps. Also explain the procedure for removing a leg brace: Cross the affected leg over the unaffected leg. Unfasten the laces and straps on the brace. Push downward until the shoe is off the foot.

Rationale: Proper application and removal of a leg brace assure correct use of the device.

Resolved Needs: Protection from physical harm. Mastery and competence in skills. Increased learning.

Contraindications: Delay brace application if severe skin irritation exists.

Teach how to apply cold therapy   Explain how and when to administer cold applications to body areas. This includes ice collars, cold packs, ice bags, and soaks in cold water. Explain that extremities should not be immersed in ice water or kept in ice packs for long periods because of the danger of frostbite.

Rationale: Cold applications decrease circulation by means of mild vasoconstriction; they relieve pain and congestion and reduce pus formation, swelling, and bleeding. Correct application of therapeutic measures assures their effectiveness and promotes safety.

Resolved Needs: Protection from physical harm. Increased learning.

Contraindications: Do not apply cold applications to decubitus ulcers, gangrenous tissue, skin graft areas, varicose veins, areas of paralysis or sensation loss, or aged or debilitated skin.

Teach how to apply disinfecting solutions
Explain how to use cleansing products to disinfect household surfaces.

Rationale: Cleanliness inhibits bacterial and viral growth and minimizes infection.

Resolved Needs: Cleanliness. Protection from physical harm. Increased learning.

Teach how to apply heat therapy
Explain how and when to apply heating pads, hot-water bottles, and warm, moist compresses. Explain that whenever heat, wet or dry, is applied to the body surface, it should first be tested against the inner wrist to determine if the degree of heat is comfortable to the skin. If not, the application should be allowed to cool.

Rationale: Heat applications cause mild vasodilatation, which increases skin circulation; they relieve pain and congestion, promote muscle relaxation, and bring the pus of an abscess to the skin surface. Correct application of therapeutic measures assures their effectiveness and promotes safety.

Resolved Needs: Comfort. Protection from physical harm. Increased learning.

Contraindications: Do not apply heat to areas of paralysis, sensation loss, edema, vasodilatation, or allergic response. Do not apply heat to any body part after heart surgery or to areas of hemorrhage or trauma. Do not apply heat following head injury.

Teach how to apply preventive splints
Explain that preventive splints should be put on with the body part in the functional position and should fit securely.

Rationale: Proper use of preventive splints will hold affected body parts in functional positions so that muscles can be used after healing; their use can also prevent contractures.

Resolved Needs: Protection from physical harm. Mastery and competence in skills. Increased learning.

Teach how to apply the ostomy appliance
Explain the methods for applying an ostomy collection apparatus. This applies to the appliances used following colostomy, ileostomy, and ureteroileostomy. Emphasize skin care and cleanliness of the immediate and surrounding areas. Acquaint the patient with the disposable bags, which are not reused, and the reusable permanent bags, which require daily soap and water cleaning and exposure to fresh air.

Rationale: Proper application of a collection apparatus assures accurate output measurement, maintains dryness and thus prevents skin irritation, and provides the comfort of cleanliness.

Resolved Needs: Comfort. Cleanliness. Protection from physical harm. Mastery and competence in skills. Increased learning.

Teach how to bathe an infant

Explain that infants should be bathed at the same time each day. Clean bathing equipment and clean hands are essential. The infant should never be left alone during a bath. Sponge baths are usually given before the umbilical cord is shed. Bath water should be checked for moderate temperature. One should avoid splashing water because it tends to startle the infant. Once undressed, the infant should be kept warm with a towel. It is easier to hold and bathe a baby if one wears clean white cotton gloves. This prevents the baby from slipping out of one's grasp, and one glove can serve as a washcloth. Cleansing proceeds as follows: The nose, outer ear, and face are washed with plain water. Hair and scalp are washed with soap and water, followed by body and limbs, uncovering only one area at a time and giving special attention to creases and areas between toes and fingers. The genital area is washed last. The infant is wrapped in an absorbent towel and thoroughly dried. Since the towel will become wet, the child should be placed in a cotton receiving blanket until dressed. Lotion can be applied around fingernails, toenails, and genitals. Powder should be used sparingly, if at all.

Rationale: Bathing cleans the skin, promotes comfort, and stimulates circulation.

Resolved Needs: Circulation. Comfort. Cleanliness. Protection from physical harm. Mastery and competence in skills. Increased learning.

Teach how to blow the nose correctly

Explain that one side of the nose should be blown at a time and that the mouth should be kept open while blowing.

Rationale: Proper nose blowing prevents excessive pressure in the middle ear and facilitates removal of secretions.

Resolved Needs: Comfort. Cleanliness. Protection from physical harm. Increased learning.

Teach how to bottle-feed an infant

Explain that infants should be fed at reasonable intervals and that the amount of feeding depends on the child's needs during different growth stages. Bottle feedings should be at room temperature or warm—never cold. The infant should be held with his head supported and turned slightly to one side. The neck of the bottle should be full at all times.

Rationale: Proper bottle feeding increases comfort, provides adequate nutrition, and reduces the potential for aspiration.

Resolved Needs: Food balance. Comfort. Protection from physical harm. Mastery and competence in skills. Increased learning.

Contraindications: Vomiting. High fever. Diarrhea.

Teach how to breast-feed an infant   Explain how to feed an infant
with milk from the mother's breast. After the mother has rested from the
delivery, the infant is usually breast fed. If the mother prefers to lie down,
she should lie on her side with the arm on that side raised and a pillow
under her head. The baby should be placed on his side, either flat or supported with pillows. If the mother prefers to sit up, she should sit in a comfortable chair and support the infant with her arm or a pillow. The infant
should be fed at a moderate pace and should be bubbled every 5 minutes.
The breasts should be washed with warm water before feeding.

Rationale: Proper breast-feeding supports maternal and infant comfort
and provides adequate infant nutrition.

Resolved Needs: Food balance. Comfort. Protection from physical harm.
Mastery and competence in skills. Increased learning.

Contraindications: Breast infection or inflammation.

Teach how to brush the teeth correctly   Explain that the tooth-
brush bristles should be pointed toward the roots of the teeth. The brush
should be rotated so that the bristles sweep over the gums and teeth in the
direction of the biting surface. The teeth should be brushed in the following
sequence: the chewing surfaces of the upper and lower teeth, the outside
surfaces of the upper and lower back teeth, the inside surfaces of the upper
and lower back teeth, the front teeth, the outer surfaces of the upper and
lower front teeth. The teeth should be brushed after every meal.

Rationale: Brushing the teeth properly reduces bacterial action and decay
through cleansing and provides the comfort of a clean mouth.

Resolved Needs: Comfort. Cleanliness. Protection from physical harm.
Mastery and competence in skills. Increased learning.

Teach how to calculate a diet   Explain that special diets are based
on daily need for the four basic food groups. Help the patient or family to
select foods from the exchange lists and to interchange them in quantities
specified so that the special diet needs are met along with the essential food
requirements.

Rationale: Proper calculation of a therapeutic diet is essential if the diet is
to be effective for improved health.

Resolved Needs: Protection from physical harm. Mastery and competence in skills. Increased learning.

Teach how to care for a hearing aid   Explain that when a hearing
aid is not in use, it should be placed where it will not be damaged, and the
batteries should be removed. The hearing aid should be checked for efficiency at least every 2 years.

Rationale: A properly functioning hearing aid is essential for optimum
hearing.

Resolved Needs: Comfort. Protection from physical harm. Increased learning.

Teach how to care for an arteriovenous shunt

Teach the patient to clean the shunt connection sites and the skin of the entire extremity, to change the dressing daily, and to observe for kinks in the joint and slipping of the rings that hold the joint together.

Rationale: Cleaning an arteriovenous shunt prevents infection. Proper care of the shunt assures its availability for hemodialysis.

Resolved Needs: Cleanliness. Protection from physical harm. Mastery and competence in skills. Increased learning.

Teach how to care for an artificial eye

Explain that normal saline solution or tap water may be used to soak and clean an artificial eye.

Rationale: A clean artificial eye minimizes the potential for eye socket infection and promotes comfort.

Resolved Needs: Comfort. Cleanliness. Protection from physical harm. Increased learning.

Teach how to clean a thermometer

Explain that soap, cool water, and friction are used to clean a thermometer. The soap and water should be brought from the top of the thermometer down to the bulb with rotating friction on the glass. Caution against cleaning with boiling water.

Rationale: Thermometer cleanliness helps prevent the spread of infection to others and reduces the potential for reinfection of the patient.

Resolved Needs: Cleanliness. Protection from physical harm. Increased learning.

Teach how to clean a tracheostomy (or laryngectomy) tube

Explain that the tracheostomy or laryngectomy tube outer cannula is cleaned by suctioning. The inner cannula is soaked in hydrogen peroxide. Pipe cleaners or sterile gauze may be inserted in the center hole of the inner cannula for further cleaning and to assure patency. After the cannula is clean, it should be soaked for a few minutes in sterile water to remove any cleansing agent that might irritate tracheal tissue. The skin around the tracheostomy or laryngectomy stoma should be cleaned with hydrogen peroxide or saline, and the dressing should be changed frequently.

Rationale: A clean tracheostomy or laryngectomy tube is essential to provide adequate respiratory gas exchange and to prevent infection.

Resolved Needs: Oxygen. Comfort. Cleanliness. Protection from physical harm. Increased learning.

Teach how to clean an elastic bandage or stockings

Explain that elastic bandages and stockings should be washed daily with mild soap and warm (not hot) water, laid flat for drying, and rolled loosely when dry.

Rationale: Cleaning removes perspiration residue on stockings and bandages that might irritate the skin. Hanging elastic bandages and stockings when they are wet or rolling them tightly after they dry decreases their elasticity.

Resolved Needs: Comfort. Cleanliness. Protection from physical harm. Increased learning.

Teach how to clean an infant's ears   Explain that extreme care must be exercised when cleaning an infant's ear. The head must be held still. The creases of the auricle should be cleaned with a washcloth, and a few drops of mineral oil may be put into the ear before cleaning in order to soften earwax.

Rationale: Cleaning the ear promotes comfort and minimizes the potential for infection and impaired hearing from wax accumulation.

Resolved Needs: Comfort. Cleanliness. Protection from physical harm. Increased learning.

Teach how to clean an infant's nose   Explain that an infant's nose should be cleaned gently with a washcloth, with flexible cotton-tipped sticks moistened with warm water, or by suctioning with a bulb syringe.

Rationale: Cleanliness of the nares assures a patent airway.

Resolved Needs: Comfort. Cleanliness. Protection from physical harm. Increased learning.

Teach how to clean and dress a wound   Teach the patient how to clean a wound and how to use sterile technique when doing so. The specific method of cleaning and bandaging will depend on the particular condition.

Rationale: Cleaning and covering a wound with a sterile dressing help to minimize infection, prevent trauma, restrict motion, and absorb secretions.

Resolved Needs: Comfort. Protection from physical harm. Mastery and competence in skills. Increased learning.

Teach how to clean contact lenses   Explain that contact lens should be cleaned frequently with a noncaustic, sterile solution.

Rationale: Keeping contact lenses clean promotes visual acuity and minimizes the potential for eye infection. A caustic, nonsterile solution on a contact lens could cause ulceration or abrasion of the cornea.

Resolved Needs: Comfort. Cleanliness. Protection from physical harm. Increased learning.

Teach how to clean dentures   Explain that dentures should be cleaned with denture powder or solution at least twice a day.

Rationale: Denture cleaning provides a clean breath and refreshing mouth and prevents gum tissue injury from hardened food particles on dentures.

Resolved Needs: Comfort. Cleanliness. Protection from physical harm. Increased learning.

Teach how to clean respiratory equipment
Explain the procedure for cleaning the respiratory equipment the patient is using. Explain how to disassemble the equipment for maximum cleanliness, which cleaning solutions to use, and how often the cleaning procedure should be done. Emphasize that respiratory equipment should not be shared between patients.

Rationale: Clean respiratory equipment is essential to minimize the spread of respiratory infection.

Resolved Needs: Cleanliness. Protection from physical harm. Increased learning.

Teach how to control breathing to aid the labor process (357)
Explain that breathing during uterine contractions should consist of slow, deep breathing at the beginning of the contraction, shallow breathing during the peak of the contraction, and renewed slow, deep breathing as the contraction subsides. Be certain that the patient does not hyperventilate.

Rationale: By tensing abdominal muscles and relaxing the perineum, controlled breathing helps the progress of labor.

Resolved Needs: Relaxation. Comfort. Increased learning.

Teach how to count a pulse
Explain that when one is taking a pulse, the patient should be sitting or lying down. One's forefingers should be placed on the thumb side of the patient's wrist, and the pulse beats should be counted for one minute using a watch with a second hand. One should not use one's thumb for counting the patient's pulse, because it is possible to feel one's own pulse in the thumb.

Rationale: Pulse abnormalities may indicate cardiac or circulatory pathology.

Resolved Needs: Protection from physical harm. Mastery and competence in skills. Increased learning.

Teach how to dilate the stoma with a sterile catheter
In the patient who has an ileal conduit, it is possible for the orifice to become obstructed; teach the patient how to insert a sterile catheter gently into the orifice.

Rationale: The ileal conduit orifice can become plugged with mucus produced by mucosa of the ileum. Insertion of a sterile catheter into the orifice removes the mucus and allows for adequate urine drainage.

Resolved Needs: Waste elimination. Increased learning.

Teach how to do a catheterization
Explain how to insert an indwelling catheter. Explain correct positioning, how to maintain sterile

technique, cleaning of the genitalia, catheter insertion into the meatus, and how to attach the catheter to a drainage system.

Rationale: Self-catheterization facilitates urine flow, assures accurate output measurement, maintains dryness and thus prevents skin irritation, and provides the comfort of cleanliness.

Resolved Needs: Comfort. Cleanliness. Waste elimination. Protection from physical harm. Mastery and competence in skills. Increased learning.

Teach how to do abdominal breathing   Instruct the patient to place one hand on his abdomen and the other on his chest. As he takes a deep breath, have him watch his abdomen rise. As he exhales, have him contract the abdominal muscles. During abdominal breathing, the chest will remain still.

Rationale: When lung elasticity is lost or lung alveoli become distended (as in emphysema), breathing puts stress on the thoracic muscles. Abdominal breathing can reduce the stress placed on the thorax.

Resolved Needs: Oxygen. Protection from physical harm. Increased learning.

Teach how to do abdominal postpartum exercises   Instruct the patient to lie on her back and do these exercises: With feet braced against the wall and arms crossed over the chest, raise the head and shoulders to a 15° angle and then return to a flat position. Stretch the arms straight out from the sides and raise the arms above the head until the hands touch. With legs together and arms extended at the sides of the body, breathe slowly and deeply with the diaphragm. Without using pillows, raise and lower the head without moving the rest of the body. Raise one leg without bending the knee, allowing it to return slowly to the bed and using the abdominal muscles to control its descent; then alternate legs. With the bed covers well tucked in at the foot, try to raise first one foot and then the other.

Rationale: Abdominal exercises strengthen abdominal muscles.

Resolved Needs: Exercise. Protection from physical harm. Mastery and competence in skills. Increased learning.

Contraindications: Delay until C-section incision is well healed.

Teach how to do above-knee stump exercises   Instruct the patient who has had an above-knee amputation to move the stump inward (adduction) toward the body centerline and then outward (abduction) or away from the body and to straighten the stump (extension) in alignment with the hip.

Rationale: Stump exercises prepare the stump for a prosthesis and for future mobility.

Resolved Needs: Activity, exercise. Protection from physical harm. Mastery and competence in skills. Increased learning.

Teach how to do below-knee stump exercises Instruct the patient who has had a below-knee amputation to move the straightened leg upward as much as possible and then return the leg to the neutral position (hip extension). Have him move the stump outward (abduction) or away from the body by contracting the large muscles on the anterior thigh (quadriceps setting).

Rationale: Stump exercises prepare the stump for a prosthesis and for future mobility.

Resolved Needs: Activity, exercise. Protection from physical harm. Mastery and competence in skills. Increased learning.

Teach how to do breath-holding Teach the patient who is hyperventilating or experiencing atrial tachycardia to take a deep breath and hold it for a few seconds.

Rationale: Holding the breath prevents carbon dioxide exhalation and increases the level of carbon dioxide in the blood to normal. Holding the breath causes vagal stimulation, which reduces cardiac rate and interrupts tachycardia.

Resolved Needs: Comfort. Protection from physical harm. Increased learning.

Contraindications: Elevated blood level of carbon dioxide. Emphysema.

Teach how to do home dialysis Explain how to assemble an artificial kidney, how to mix hemodialysis fluid, and how to run and clean the machine. Explain what to do in case of power failure, how to measure hematocrit, how to operate a portable centrifuge for blood sampling, and how to store blood plasma in the freezer.

Rationale: Competence in hemodialysis therapy is essential to maintaining life in a patient experiencing renal failure.

Resolved Needs: Water-salt balance. Waste elimination. Comfort. Protection from physical harm. Mastery and competence in skills. Increased learning.

Teach how to do isometric exercises Teach the patient how to exercise his muscles without moving the injured body part. If his leg is in a cast, the nurse's hand may be placed under his knee while he pushes downward. If his arm is in a cast, he may open and close his hand for several minutes each hour. He also may be taught to move his fingers and toes for several minutes every half hour. Teach the cardiac patient to perform mild leg exercises while in bed by bending his foot up (dorsiflexion) and down (extension) ten times each hour.

Rationale: Exercises stimulate circulation and prevent muscle atrophy.

Resolved Needs: Circulation. Activity, exercise. Protection from physical harm. Increased learning.

Contraindications: Circulatory thrombus.

Teach how to do nipple eversion exercises   Teach the patient to rub her breast nipple gently with a towel and roll it between her finger and thumb in order to evert it.

Rationale: An everted breast nipple facilitates breast feeding.

Resolved Needs: Comfort. Protection from physical harm. Increased learning.

Contraindications: Suspicion of breast malignancy.

Teach how to do perineal care   Teach the patient with perineal stitches that after voiding one should pour a moderate amount of warm water over the sutured area and gently pat the area dry.

Rationale: Perineal care cleans the area of urine and reduces the potential for infection. Warm water provides comfort to the healing area.

Resolved Needs: Comfort. Cleanliness. Protection from physical harm. Increased learning.

Teach how to do perineal exercises   Teach the patient that in order to do the Kegal perineal exercises, she should tighten the vaginal, urethra, rectal, and abdominal musculature to the count of four and then relax. This exercise should be repeated 50 to 100 times a day during the postpartum period.

Rationale: Perineal exercises promote good elasticity of the tissues around the vagina and support good circulation, which increase healing of the epiosotomy.

Resolved Needs: Exercise. Protection from physical harm. Increased learning.

Teach how to do postmastectomy exercises (583)   Explain that after removal of a breast, the affected arm must be exercised.

The *hair brushing exercise* involves brushing the hair with the affected arm while keeping the head erect. One should start brushing at one side of the head and slowly work around to the other side.

For the *jump rope exercise*, a rope ½ yard long is attached to a doorknob or dresser knob. The patient stands with her affected side toward the rope, keeping her feet apart, and places her unaffected hand on her hip. She then swings the rope from the affected shoulder as one would swing a jump rope, alternating directions, without bending her waist or arm.

For the *rod rope exercise*, a rope 5 feet long is tossed over a shower rod. A knot is tied at each end of the rope. Sitting in a chair under the rod, with a knot held between the second and third fingers of each hand, the patient pulls down on the rope, alternating the unaffected and affected sides. Pulling down on the rope with the unaffected arm pulls the affected arm up. This should be done five times in the morning and evening, with gradual increases to 25 times.

For the *rubber ball exercise*, a rubber ball with a string is needed. The ball is held in the hand of the affected arm; the hand is alternately squeezed and relaxed. The ball can also be thrown against a wall with the affected arm from gradually increasing distances.

For the *shoulder rotating exercise*, the patient bends her elbows to shoulder level and then rolls her shoulders as far back and around as possible. The rotation should occur in both directions, five times on each side. Then, with elbows bent, the patient rolls both arms back and around until the shoulder blades almost meet.

For the *wall climbing exercise*, the patient faces a wall with the palms and forearms resting against the wall. Slowly the fingers of the affected arm climb the wall, reaching higher and higher each time. This exercise should be done several times a day, keeping the climbing arm as close to the head as possible.

For the *window shade exercise*, the patient raises or lowers window shades or blinds many times each day, reaching the top and bottom of the window.

Rationale: Postmastectomy exercises prevent muscle shortening, preserve muscle tone, extend the range of motion, and promote lymphatic drainage from the arm.

Resolved Needs: Activity, exercise. Protection from physical harm. Increased learning.

Contraindications: Incisional bleeding or infection.

Teach how to do postpartum exercises (460)
Explain how to do the various postpartum exercises. For the *back and pelvis strengthening exercise*, the patient lies on her back, places her feet slightly apart, and draws her knees up until her legs almost form a right angle. Then she raises her buttocks so that her body rests only on the soles of her feet and on her shoulders. Next she presses her knees together, contracting the gluteal muscles, and then relaxes. For the *gluteal and pelvic strengthening exercise*, the patient lies on her back, bends one knee sharply toward her abdomen, brings her head down toward her buttocks, then straightens her leg and lies flat. She then alternates legs. For the *knee-chest postpartum exercise*, the patient takes a kneeling position with knees widely separated and head turned to one side. She bends her body forward until her shoulders and chest touch a bed or the floor as close to her knees as possible, all the while keeping her back straight. For the *monkey-trot postpartum exercise*, the patient walks along on her feet and hands simultaneously.

Rationale: Postpartum exercises strengthen the lower back muscles and the gluteal and pelvic muscles and assist the uterus to resume the prepregnant pelvic position.

Resolved Needs: Exercise. Protection from physical harm. Mastery and competence in skills. Increased learning.

Contraindications: Delay until C-section incision is well healed.

Teach how to do pre-crutch-walking exercises
In anticipation of using crutches, teach the patient to do pushups while lying on his abdomen, to do pushups on the palms of his hands while in a sitting position, to

lift weights or sandbags while lying on his back, and to do straight elbow pushups in bed with crutches sawed off just below the handbars.

Rationale: Pre-crutch-walking exercises strengthen the arm and shoulder muscles for crutch-walking.

Resolved Needs: Activity, exercise. Protection from physical harm. Increased learning.

Teach how to do range-of-motion exercises
Teach the patient exercises that move the joints through the functional range so that function will not be lost. Cover active-assistance, active, passive, and resistive range of motion.

Rationale: Range-of-motion exercises promote joint mobility, strengthen muscle tone, develop coordination, prevent nonfunctional contractures, and increase blood circulation.

Resolved Needs: Circulation. Activity, exercise. Comfort. Protection from physical harm. Mastery and competence in skills. Increased learning.

Teach how to do resistive breathing exercises (181)
Instruct the patient to lie on his back without a pillow and with his legs elevated. Then have him place a book or some other object weighing about 1 pound on his abdomen. Have him breathe and try to push with his abdomen against the weight. This should be done five to ten times twice a day. Every third day, ½ pound of weight should be added until the weight reaches 5 pounds and the patient can comfortably do the exercise for 30 minutes. Another resistive exercise involves having the patient blow out a candle at gradually increasing distances or blow a pencil or pen to various spots on the top of a table.

Rationale: When the patient has emphysema, there is a tendency to let the chest muscles do most of the breathing work, with the diaphragm doing less and less. Resistive breathing exercises help restore the normal breathing function of the diaphragmatic and abdominal muscles.

Resolved Needs: Oxygen. Waste elimination. Protection from physical harm. Increased learning.

Teach how to do therapeutic soaks
Explain how to apply a warm, moist compress or immerse a particular body part in warm water.

Rationale: Moist heat applications cleanse, relieve the edema and pain of inflammation, and remove necrotic tissue.

Resolved Needs: Comfort. Cleanliness. Protection from physical harm. Mastery and competence in skills. Increased learning.

Teach how to do umbilical care
Explain how to clean the newborn's umbilical area by wiping it gently with alcohol.

Rationale: Proper umbilical care promotes comfort and reduces the potential for infection; alcohol dries the cord.

Resolved Needs: Comfort. Cleanliness. Protection from physical harm. Increased learning.

Teach how to dress an infant
Explain that when dressing an infant, the garment should be gathered from the bottom to the neck so that the infant's head can be slipped easily into the opening before his arms are dressed. Explain that clothing on children should not be restrictive.

Rationale: Proper infant dressing promotes comfort and safety.

Resolved Needs: Comfort. Protection from physical harm. Mastery and competence in skills. Increased learning.

Teach how to elevate from a sitting to a standing position with crutches (97)
Teach the patient who must use crutches to rise: He should back his chair against a stable surface, then move his body to the chair's edge and place his unaffected leg against the chair's edge. Then he should hold both crutches together at the handpiece with one hand and place the other hand on the chair armrest. Pushing upward with both hands, he should straighten his strong leg and stand up. Balancing on the crutches and his strong leg, he should then transfer one crutch at a time to the underarm position.

Rationale: Safe mobility is essential to carrying out daily activities and maintaining independence.

Resolved Needs: Activity, exercise. Comfort. Protection from physical harm. Mastery and competence in skills. Independence. Increased learning.

Teach how to elevate from a sitting to a standing position with leg braces (97)
Teach the patient with a brace to rise: He should back his chair against a stable surface, move his body to the chair's edge, and lock one brace at the knee. Then he should cross the locked and braced leg over the foot of the other leg and turn his body at the waist toward the unlocked and braced leg until his head and shoulders face the back of the chair. Then he should grasp the chair armrests with both hands and push the body upward until the leg with the locked brace is supporting the body. After locking the brace of the other leg at the knee, he should place the crutches, one at a time, under his arms, bearing weight on the crutches while coming to a standing position. He should back a few steps away from the chair before turning to move forward.

Rationale: Safe mobility is essential to carrying out daily activities and maintaining independence.

Resolved Needs: Activity, exercise. Comfort. Protection from physical harm. Mastery and competence in skills. Independence. Increased learning.

Teach how to get into a bathtub when hemiplegic (97)
Teach the person with one-sided paralysis to get into the bathtub so that his weak side is next to the wall. This will allow him to emerge from the tub putting his strong leg out first.

Rationale: Safe mobility is essential to carrying out daily activities and maintaining independence.

Resolved Needs: Activity, exercise. Comfort. Protection from physical harm. Mastery and competence in skills. Independence. Increased learning.

Teach how to give a bed bath Explain how to bathe the patient confined to bed. Include draping the patient, washing with soap and water, drying, and maintaining a warm environment during the bath.

Rationale: A bed bath cleans the skin, promotes comfort, stimulates circulation, and reduces energy consumption.

Resolved Needs: Circulation. Energy. Comfort. Cleanliness. Protection from physical harm. Increased learning.

Teach how to give a douche Explain that a douche is given in the reclining position with the knees flexed and thighs separated. The external genitalia are cleaned with soap and water. The irrigating nozzle is gently inserted into the vagina. An irrigating solution at approximately 105°F is allowed to flow slowly in and out of the vagina by careful nozzle rotation. The perineum is then wiped dry.

Rationale: Vaginal irrigations discourage bacterial growth, remove foul and irritating discharges, and provide heat therapy.

Resolved Needs: Comfort. Cleanliness. Protection from physical harm. Mastery and competence in skills. Increased learning.

Contraindications: Vaginal bleeding.

Teach how to give an enema Explain that before giving an enema, the bladder should be emptied. The patient should lie on his left side with his right leg flexed. He should be properly draped and have adequate privacy. After preparation of the appropriate solution at 105°F, the enema tubing should be lubricated and inserted 2–3 inches into the rectum. The enema container should be held no more than 2 feet above the patient, and the patient should take several deep breaths while the fluid flows into his colon. If the patient complains of abdominal cramping, the tubing should be clamped for a few minutes and then unclamped until all the solution is given. The tube should be removed slowly. The patient should retain the solution as long as possible. Then he should be placed on a bedpan or commode. The results of the enema should be checked, and it should be determined that the patient is dry.

Rationale: Proper administration of an enema promotes elimination of food residue and gases from the intestinal tract.

Resolved Needs: Waste elimination. Comfort. Stimulation. Cleanliness. Protection from physical harm. Increased learning.

Teach how to give insulin Explain the different types and strengths of insulin and the supplies needed for its administration. Explain how to

obtain and store insulin, how to draw up the prescribed dose, how to administer it, and how to rotate injection sites.

Rationale: Correct insulin dosage is essential to regulation of diabetes.

Resolved Needs: Acid-base balance. Comfort. Protection from physical harm. Mastery and competence in skills. Increased learning.

Teach how to give oxygen therapy   Teach the patient who has been prescribed oxygen therapy how and when to use the equipment and how to make regulatory adjustments specific to his problem.

Rationale: Oxygen therapy provides a higher intake of oxygen than normal, which can ease difficult breathing. Oxygen toxicity is less likely to occur if the patient knows the correct use of oxygen equipment.

Resolved Needs: Oxygen. Comfort. Protection from physical harm. Mastery and competence in skills. Independence. Increased learning.

Contraindications: Oxygen toxicity.

Teach how to give positive pressure breathing   Teach the patient who has been prescribed positive pressure breathing how and when to use the equipment and how to make regulatory adjustments specific to his problem.

Rationale: Intermittent positive pressure breathing inflates the lungs, pushes pressurized air past mucus secretions, and stimulates coughing for secretion elimination.

Resolved Needs: Waste elimination. Protection from physical harm. Mastery and competence in skills. Independence. Increased learning.

Contraindications: Cardiac insufficiency. Pulmonary hemorrhage.

Teach how to give vaporized air inhalation   Explain how to use a vaporizing apparatus for breathing moistened air. Explain that many household objects can be used for inhalation of humidified air, such as an electric percolator, a teakettle, or a funnel made from a newspaper or a paper bag and attached to a kettle.

Rationale: Inhalation of heated humidified air decreases respiratory tissue dryness, prevents tissue friction during respirations, and loosens and thins mucus secretions.

Resolved Needs: Comfort. Protection from physical harm. Increased learning.

Teach how to handle an infant   Explain that infants should be handled in a gentle but firm manner. They require good body support, especially of the head and neck, and they should be made to feel safe at all times.

Rationale: Proper infant handling is essential to infant safety, comfort, and security.

Resolved Needs: Comfort. Protection from physical harm. Mastery and competence in skills. Increased learning.

Teach how to inflate and deflate an airway cuff   Explain how to insert air into and remove air from an airway cuff. Emphasize the importance of suctioning the trachea during cuff deflation to remove secretions. Explain that the cuff should be inflated while the patient is eating or taking inhalation therapy and then deflated.

Rationale: Deflating an airway cuff relieves pressure from the tracheal and laryngeal mucosa, which decreases the potential for tissue necrosis. Inflation of an airway cuff provides a tight seal between the tube and the trachea. It prevents air leakage during ventilation procedures and food aspiration during meals.

Resolved Needs: Comfort. Protection from physical harm. Increased learning.

Teach how to insert a vaginal suppository   Explain that insertion of a vaginal suppository involves the following: handwashing prior to insertion; douching, when ordered, prior to insertion; positioning oneself lying down with the hips elevated on a pillow; use of the longest finger to insert the suppository gently upward and back, or use of a suppository applicator; remaining in the same position for 10 to 15 minutes after insertion. The same procedure is used for vaginal cream applications.

Rationale: Vaginal suppositories and creams reduce vaginal irritation, inflammation, and infection.

Resolved Needs: Comfort. Protection from physical harm. Mastery and competence in skills. Increased learning.

Contraindications: Abnormal vaginal bleeding.

Teach how to insert and remove an artificial eye   For insertion of an artificial eye, have the patient pull down on his lower eyelid and gently slip the eye into position. For removal, have him place gentle pressure below the eye with the index finger until the prosthesis slips out of the socket. A suction cup may be used instead of the fingers to hold the artificial eye for insertion and removal.

Rationale: Artificial eye replacement promotes comfort and prevents eye socket shrinkage. Removal of the artificial eye permits prosthesis cleansing, prevents orbit irritation, and promotes comfort.

Resolved Needs: Comfort. Cleanliness. Protection from physical harm. Mastery and competence in skills. Increased learning.

Contraindications: Eye socket irritation, inflammation, or infection.

Teach how to insert and remove contact lenses   Explain that the proper way to insert a contact lens is as follows: Pull the upper lid up and the lower lid down with the index finger and thumb of one hand. Place

wetting solution on the inner side of the lens. With the index finger of one hand, gently place the lens over the cornea of the opposite eye. Be careful to place the left lens on the left cornea and the right lens on the right cornea. The right contact lens is identified by a black dot. Explain that the proper way to remove a contact lens is as follows: Pull the side of the eye (near the ear) outward with one hand. With the other hand, gently pull the lids together; the lens should then pop out. Place the lens, with fluid, safely in its container. Be sure to place the right lens in its receptacle and vice versa.

Rationale: Proper contact lens insertion promotes visual acuity; proper contact lens removal prevents corneal injury.

Resolved Needs: Comfort. Protection from physical harm. Mastery and competence in skills. Increased learning.

Contraindications: Delay insertion during eye irritation, inflammation, or infection.

Teach how to instill ear drops   Explain that when ear drops are to be instilled, the patient should lie so that the ear to be medicated is facing upward. The person instilling the drops should straighten the adult auditory canal by gently pulling the ear auricle (lobe) upward, backward, and outward. The ears of children should be gently pulled down and back. When drainage is present, it should be wiped clean; warm drops should then be placed into the ear. The patient should remain on his side for approximately 5 minutes. Cotton may be gently inserted into the ear if desired.

Rationale: Correct instillation of ear drops supports effective drug therapy.

Resolved Needs: Comfort. Protection from physical harm. Mastery and competence in skills. Increased learning.

Teach how to instill eye drops   Explain that when instilling eye drops, the patient should tilt his head back, look up, gently pull down his lower eyelid, place the drops just inside his lower lid, and close his eyes. Explain that the eyedropper should never come in contact with tissue.

Rationale: Correct instillation of eye drops supports effective drug therapy.

Resolved Needs: Comfort. Protection from physical harm. Mastery and competence in skills. Increased learning.

Teach how to irrigate a colostomy   Teach the person who has had a colostomy to irrigate the stoma while sitting up in bed or on a commode. Explain that a 500–1500-cc solution of soap, plain water, or saline at about 105°F is used. A catheter is inserted 2–3 inches into the colostomy stoma, and the irrigating can is placed about 2 feet above the colostomy opening to allow for solution flow. Explain that colostomy irrigations should be done daily or on alternate days.

Rationale: Colostomy irrigations empty the colon of fecal material and gases and provide the comfort of cleanliness.

Resolved Needs: Waste elimination. Cleanliness. Mastery and competence in skills. Increased learning.

Contraindications: Delay if the patient is not psychologically ready.

Teach how to irrigate a urinary catheter   Explain how to introduce sterile normal saline, 0.25% acetic acid, or another prescribed solution into the urinary catheter at periodic intervals. Explain how to use sterile technique and how to use gravity flow for return of the solution.

Rationale: A patent catheter facilitates urine output. Irrigation with an acetic acid solution destroys microorganisms and dissolves calcium precipitates.

Resolved Needs: Protection from physical harm. Mastery and competence in skills. Increased learning.

Teach how to irrigate a wound   Explain how to flush a wound with sterile solution until the injured tissue appears clean and free of debris.

Rationale: Flushing a wound with a sterile solution promotes comfort and healing by cleaning the tissue and removing foreign particles.

Resolved Needs: Comfort. Cleanliness. Protection from physical harm. Mastery and competence in skills. Increased learning.

Teach how to make an occupied bed   Explain that changing the bed linen of a person confined to bed involves the following: loosening all linen tucked under the mattress; rolling the patient to one side of the bed; rolling the soiled linen up to the patient's back; placing the fresh sheet, folded in half lengthwise, on the mattress at the patient's back; tucking in half the sheet and rolling the other half up to the patient's back; turning the patient onto the clean sheet; going to the other side of the bed and pulling off the soiled sheets; pulling the clean sheets over the mattress and tucking them in; turning the patient on his back.

Rationale: Changing the bed linen of the patient who cannot get out of bed promotes cleanliness and comfort.

Resolved Needs: Comfort. Cleanliness. Increased learning.

Teach how to manually express breast milk   Explain that when breast milk is expressed by hand, the breast should be gently massaged for a few moments. One hand is placed on top of the other above the breast. The hands are then brought down over the breast and the fingers turned downward as the hands are drawn apart to encircle the breast. Three fingers should cup and support under the breast as well as bring the breast forward and upward. The forefinger is then placed below the alveoli and the thumb above the alveoli with gentle pressure until the milk flows in a stream. The fingers should be gently rotated around the alveoli until all milk is expressed. The opposite hand is used for holding a sterile collecting container. Handwashing is essential before breast milk expression.

Rationale: When breast feeding is temporarily curtailed, breast milk must be removed manually so that lactation will not cease.

Resolved Needs: Comfort. Protection from physical harm. Mastery and competence in skills. Increased learning.

Contraindications: Intentional suppression of lactation.

Teach how to massage the uterine fundus   Teach the patient to place her hand on her abdomen, grasp the body of the uterus, and externally massage by applying moderate pressure.

Rationale: Uterine fundus massage reduces hemorrhage.

Resolved Needs: Protection from physical harm. Mastery and competence in skills. Increased learning.

Teach how to mechanically express breast milk   Explain that breast milk may be expressed by use of a hand pump or an electric pump. When using a hand pump, the suction cup is applied to the nipple, and the suction bulb is alternately squeezed and released. When using an electric pump, the suction cup is applied to the nipple, and a low degree of vacuum is applied. Breast suctioning should be gradual and intermittent; it should be continued for no more than 15 minutes and should be stopped earlier if the breast is empty. The milk should be measured and saved in a sterile container for later infant feeding. Handwashing is essential before milk expression.

Rationale: When breast feeding is temporarily curtailed, breast milk must be removed manually so that lactation will not cease.

Resolved Needs: Comfort. Protection from physical harm. Mastery and competence in skills. Increased learning.

Contraindications: Intentional suppression of lactation.

Teach how to move from a bed to a chair when hemiplegic (97)   Teach the patient with one-sided paralysis to place a chair on the same side of the bed as his unaffected (strong) side. He should move into a dangling position and place his strong hand on the far armrest of the chair. Then, bearing most of his weight on the strong hand and leg, he can pivot and lift his body into the chair.

Rationale: Safe mobility is essential for carrying out daily activities and maintaining independence.

Resolved Needs: Activity, exercise. Comfort. Protection from physical harm. Mastery and competence in skills. Independence. Increased learning.

Teach how to move from a chair to a bed when hemiplegic (97)   Teach the patient with one-sided paralysis to place his chair so that his unaffected (strong) body side is nearest the bed. He then moves to the edge of the chair and places his strong hand on the bed. Then, bearing most of his weight on his strong hand and leg, he can pivot and lift his body onto the bed.

Rationale: Safe mobility is essential for carrying out daily activities and maintaining independence.

Resolved Needs: Activity, exercise. Comfort. Protection from physical harm. Mastery and competence in skills. Independence. Increased learning.

Teach how to move from a sitting to a standing position when hemiplegic (97)   Teach the patient with one-sided paralysis to sit on a bed or chair edge with his feet flat on the floor. The person assisting him should face the hemiplegic and grasp him under the arms. The patient leans forward and supports his affected (weak) leg by bracing his foot and knee against the foot and knee of the assisting person. When the assisting person pulls the patient to a standing position, the patient should bear most of his weight on the unaffected (strong) leg and as much weight as possible on the affected (weak) leg.

Rationale: Safe mobility is essential for carrying out daily activities and maintaining independence.

Resolved Needs: Activity, exercise. Comfort. Protection from physical harm. Mastery and competence in skills. Independence. Increased learning.

Teach how to percuss the amputation stump   Teach the amputee to gently tap his stump against a soft pillow or his hand; he should gradually increase the pressure by tapping on firmer surfaces until a hard surface can be used. Percussion must be done in proportion to the gradual decrease in stump pain.

Rationale: Stump percussion toughens the skin, gradually decreases nerve sensitivity, and prepares the stump for the pressure of a prosthesis.

Resolved Needs: Comfort. Protection from physical harm. Increased learning.

Contraindications: Nonhealing of the stump wound. Stump hemorrhage.

Teach how to prepare a formula   Explain the several methods for preparing a formula. For the presterilized method, clean and sterilize the bottles, nipples, and formula equipment; add formula to the bottles and store them in a refrigerator. For the thermal heat method, clean the bottles, nipples, and formula equipment; pour the formula into the bottles, sterilize them, cool them, and store them in the refrigerator. Explain what is available in the prepackaged formulas. Explain how to prepare various tube feeding formulas.

Rationale: Correctly prepared and stored formulas are less likely to cause problems of digestion, absorption, or infection and are more likely to provide the essentials for food and fluid balance.

Resolved Needs: Water-salt balance. Food balance. Comfort. Protection from physical harm. Mastery and competence in skills. Increased learning.

Teach how to prepare balanced meals   Assist the patient in planning a series of meals, each of which provides good nutrition. Plan a variety of foods, even where there are dietary limitations.

Rationale: Well-balanced meals contribute to better health and good nutritional habits and increase one's appetite.

Resolved Needs: Food balance. Protection from physical harm. Increased learning.

Teach how to spoon feed an infant   Explain how to hold or sit an infant for feeding and how to put the spoon well back into his mouth; one should give moderate, not large, food portions with each spoonful.

Rationale: Proper feeding methods promote infant comfort and protect against aspiration.

Resolved Needs: Comfort. Protection from physical harm. Mastery and competence in skills. Increased learning.

Contraindications: Delay spoon feeding if he is prone to vomiting.

Teach how to stimulate the gums   Explain that gums can be stimulated by eating fibrous foods or by using a water jet.

Rationale: Gum stimulation strengthens the gum tissue so that it can hold the teeth firmly in the mouth.

Resolved Needs: Protection from physical harm. Increased learning.

Teach how to suction an airway   Explain the proper method for suctioning the nose, mouth, tracheostomy stoma, endotracheal tube, etc. Explain how to insert catheters and prevent tissue trauma, as well as appropriate suctioning techniques.

Rationale: Removal of secretions maintains a patent airway.

Resolved Needs: Oxygen. Protection from physical harm. Mastery and competence in skills. Increased learning.

Teach how to take a blood pressure   Explain the method for reading blood pressure; include proper cuff application, differentiation of systolic and diastolic blood pressures, undelayed cuff release, and accepted norms.

Rationale: Knowledge of blood pressure status is necessary for patients with hypertension and for those who are receiving home hemodialysis therapy.

Resolved Needs: Protection from physical harm. Mastery and competence in skills. Increased learning.

Teach how to take a sitz bath   Teach the patient to sit in a tub of hot water (96–106°F) with the tub filled so that the water comes up to the umbilicus. Caution the patient to rise slowly when getting out of a hot sitz bath because of the potential for hypotension.

Rationale: Moist heat promotes relaxation and healing by cleansing and increases circulation to the pelvic area through vasodilatation.

Resolved Needs: Circulation. Relaxation. Comfort. Cleanliness. Protection from physical harm. Increased learning.

Contraindications: New abdominal surgical incision.

Teach how to take a temperature   Explain that before taking a temperature, the thermometer should read 95°F or below. For oral temperature, the thermometer bulb should be placed well under the tongue with the lips kept closed for at least 3 minutes. For rectal temperature, the thermometer bulb should be inserted about 1½ inches into the rectum for 3–5 minutes. For axillary temperature, the thermometer bulb should be placed in the axilla, with the arm pressed against the body for 5 minutes. When the thermometer is removed, the temperature should be read and recorded and the thermometer wiped clean.

Rationale: Knowledge of temperature status is necessary to determine excessive body heat production or loss or poor temperature control.

Resolved Needs: Protection from physical harm. Mastery and competence in skills. Increased learning.

Teach how to test the blood for glucose using the finger-stick method   Explain how to use Dextrostix to determine the glucose level in blood.

Rationale: Knowledge of the glucose level in blood promotes safety for diabetics and persons with hypoglycemia.

Resolved Needs: Protection from physical harm. Mastery and competence in skills. Increased learning.

Teach how to test the urine for pH   Explain how to check the urine acid level with litmus or Nitrazine paper or other appropriate chemical agents.

Rationale: Urinary pH (acidity or alkalinity) affects urinary stone formation.

Resolved Needs: Protection from physical harm. Mastery and competence in skills. Increased learning.

Teach how to test the urine for protein   Explain how to use Combistix or Urostix to determine the protein level in urine.

Rationale: Protein in the urine indicates impaired renal function, prostatitis, epididymitis, or impending pregnancy toxemia, or kidney transplant rejection.

Resolved Needs: Protection from physical harm. Mastery and competence in skills. Increased learning.

Teach how to test the urine for sugar-acetone   Explain how to use Clinitest, Diastix, or Tes-Tape to determine the level of urine sugar (glucose) and how to use Acetest or Ketostix to determine the level of acetone (ketone bodies) in the urine.

Rationale: Sugar in the before-meal urine of a diabetic indicates inadequate insulin or excess carbohydrate intake. Acetone in the urine indicates abnormal metabolism of body fat.

Resolved Needs: Acid-base balance. Protection from physical harm. Mastery and competence in skills. Increased learning.

Teach how to transfer from a bathtub to a wheelchair (97)   When a patient who is in a bathtub wants to get into a wheelchair, he should place the front of the wheelchair toward the side of the bathtub as close to the bathtub as possible and lock the wheelchair. Making sure that his hands are dry, he places one hand on each side of the tub and carefully raises his body to sit on the edge of the tub. Then he moves his body backward into the wheelchair.

Rationale: Safe mobility is essential for carrying out daily activities and maintaining independence.

Resolved Needs: Activity, exercise. Comfort. Protection from physical harm. Mastery and competence in skills. Independence. Increased learning.

Teach how to transfer from a bed to a wheelchair (97)   When a patient who is in bed wants to get into a wheelchair, he should place the front of the wheelchair toward the side of the bed as close to the bed as possible and lock the brakes. In a sitting position, with his back facing the chair, he should move his body to the edge of the bed. He should place his hands on the arms of the chair and slide his body backward off the bed into the wheelchair. Then he should lift his legs off the bed into the chair.

Rationale: Safe mobility is essential for carrying out daily activities and maintaining independence.

Resolved Needs: Activity, exercise. Comfort. Protection from physical harm. Mastery and competence in skills. Independence. Increased learning.

Teach how to transfer from a chair to a wheelchair (97)   When a patient who is in a regular chair wants to move into a wheelchair, he should place the regular chair and the wheelchair so that they face each other as close together as possible. Then he should lock the wheelchair brakes. He should move his body to the edge of the chair, place one hand on the chair seat and the other on the wheelchair arm, and pivot his body into the wheelchair.

Rationale: Safe mobility is essential for carrying out daily activities and maintaining independence.

Resolved Needs: Activity, exercise. Comfort. Protection from physical harm. Mastery and competence in skills. Independence. Increased learning.

Teach how to transfer from a wheelchair to a bathtub
(97)   When a patient who is in a wheelchair wants to get into a bathtub, he should place the front of the wheelchair toward the side of the bathtub as close to the bathtub as possible and lock the wheelchair. He should lift his feet and legs into the tub, place each hand on an arm of the wheelchair, and move his body forward off the wheelchair to a sitting position on the edge of the tub. Then he should place one hand on the near side of the tub and the other hand on the far side and carefully lower his body into the water.

Rationale: Safe mobility is essential for carrying out daily activities and maintaining independence.

Resolved Needs: Activity, exercise. Comfort. Protection from physical harm. Mastery and competence in skills. Independence. Increased learning.

Teach how to transfer from a wheelchair to a bed (97)   When a
patient who is in a wheelchair wants to get into bed, he should place the front of the wheelchair toward the bed as close to the bed as possible and lock the wheelchair brakes. He should put his feet on the floor, place one hand firmly on the mattress and the other on the nearest wheelchair arm, and then pivot his body onto the bed.

Rationale: Safe mobility is essential for carrying out daily activities and maintaining independence.

Resolved Needs: Activity, exercise. Comfort. Protection from physical harm. Mastery and competence in skills. Independence. Increased learning.

Teach how to transfer from a wheelchair to a chair (97)   When
a patient who is in a wheelchair wants to get into a regular chair, he should place the wheelchair and the regular chair so that they face each other as close together as possible and lock the wheelchair brakes. He should move his body to the edge of the wheelchair, place one hand on the wheelchair arm and the other on the seat of the regular chair, and pivot his body onto the chair.

Rationale: Safe mobility is essential for carrying out daily activities and maintaining independence.

Resolved Needs: Activity, exercise. Comfort. Protection from physical harm. Mastery and competence in skills. Independence. Increased learning.

Teach how to transfer from a wheelchair to an automobile
(97)   When a patient who is in a wheelchair wants to move into a car, he should open the car door as far as possible and move the wheelchair close to the side of the car facing the car. Then he should lock the wheelchair brakes. He should move his body to the edge of the wheelchair, turning it in the direction of the front of the car, and place one hand on the window ledge of the car door and the other on the wheelchair arm. Then he should lift his body onto the car seat and lift his legs and feet into the car.

Rationale: Safe mobility is essential for carrying out daily activities and maintaining independence.

Resolved Needs: Activity, exercise. Comfort. Protection from physical harm. Mastery and competence in skills. Independence. Increased learning.

Teach how to transfer from an automobile to a wheelchair (97)   When a patient who is in a car wants to get into a wheelchair, he should open the car door as far as possible and place the wheelchair close to the car facing the side of the car. He should lock the wheelchair brakes and then move to the edge of the car seat. Then he can swing his legs out of the car, place one hand on the car window ledge and the other on the farthest wheelchair arm, and lift his body into the wheelchair.

Rationale: Safe mobility is essential for carrying out daily activities and maintaining independence.

Resolved Needs: Activity, exercise. Comfort. Protection from physical harm. Mastery and competence in skills. Independence. Increased learning.

Teach how to turn over when hemiplegic (97)   When a patient with one-sided paralysis wants to turn on his affected (weak) side, he should bend the unaffected (strong) leg and pull on the bedrail with his strong arm. This will turn his body onto the affected side. If he wants to turn on his unaffected (strong) side, he should grasp the pajama leg of the affected (weak) side and pull the paralyzed leg across the strong leg. Then, placing his paralyzed arm on his chest, he can grasp the bedrail and pull his body onto his strong side.

Rationale: Frequent turning prevents fluid congestion in the lungs, stimulates circulation, and promotes comfort. Safe mobility encourages independence.

Resolved Needs: Activity, exercise. Comfort. Protection from physical harm. Mastery and competence in skills. Independence. Increased learning.

Teach how to use a cane for balancing (97)   Explain that body balance can be maintained by holding a cane in the hand opposite the weak leg and moving the cane forward at the same time the weak leg moves forward.

Rationale: A cane can provide the body support and stability necessary for active locomotion.

Resolved Needs: Activity. Comfort. Protection from physical harm. Mastery and competence in skills. Increased learning.

Teach how to use a cane for weight-bearing (97)   Explain that weight-bearing can be accomplished by holding a cane in the hand on the side of the weak leg and bearing weight on the cane as one steps forward with the good leg.

Rationale: A cane can provide the body support and stability necessary for active locomotion.

Resolved Needs: Activity. Comfort. Protection from physical harm. Mastery and competence in skills. Increased learning.

Teach how to use a hand nebulizer   Explain how to use a hand nebulizer: keep the mouth open and simultaneously breathe in and squeeze the nebulizer so that the medication is inhaled.

Rationale: Medication by hand nebulizer can reduce respiratory spasm or loosen secretions.

Resolved Needs: Protection from physical harm. Increased learning.

Teach how to use a hydraulic hoist   Explain the use of a hoist to make lifting the body easier.

Rationale: Use of a hydraulic hoist can provide even weight distribution and limit skin pressure when the body is moved, and it supports independent activity.

Resolved Needs: Protection from physical harm. Mastery and competence in skills. Independence. Increased learning.

Teach how to use a temporary prosthesis   Explain that when a temporary prosthesis is used shortly after amputation surgery, only 10% of the body weight should be borne on the prosthesis; a stump wrap should be applied at night to prevent swelling.

Rationale: Use of a temporary prosthesis supports early ambulation.

Resolved Needs: Activity. Comfort. Protection from physical harm. Mastery and competence in skills. Increased learning.

Teach how to use assistive dressing devices   Explain how to use self-help devices for dressing, such as buttonhooks, Velcroe clothing closures, and long-handled shoehorns.

Rationale: Use of assistive dressing devices promotes independence.

Resolved Needs: Comfort. Mastery and competence in skills. Independence. Increased learning.

Teach how to use assistive eating devices   Explain how to use self-help devices for eating, such as a feeder cuff for spoon and fork, long straws, removable handles to make a cup from a glass, one-handed rocking knives for easy cutting, plate guards, extension forks, swivel spoons, and suction plates.

Rationale: Use of assistive eating devices promotes independence.

Resolved Needs: Comfort. Mastery and competence in skills. Independence. Increased learning.

Teach how to use assistive grooming devices Explain how to use self-help devices for grooming, such as a suction nailbrush, a suction brush for cleaning dentures, a long-handled bath brush, soap mits, a feeder cuff to hold the toothbrush, and a long-handled hairbrush.

Rationale: Use of assistive grooming devices promotes the comfort of being refreshed and having a pleasant appearance and encourages independence.

Resolved Needs: Comfort. Cleanliness. Protection from physical harm. Independence. Increased learning.

Teach how to use assistive holding-reaching devices Explain how to use self-help devices for holding things or reaching for things, such as a cigarette holder, a telephone holder, a pencil holder, reaching tongs, handrails on bathtubs, bedside commodes, and rails used for walking.

Rationale: Use of assistive holding-reaching devices promotes independence.

Resolved Needs: Comfort. Mastery and competence in skills. Independence. Increased learning.

Teach how to use the forearm to push up from a lying position when hemiplegic (97) Teach the patient with one-sided paralysis to use his unaffected (strong) arm to lift his body from the bed and then push up with his forearm and hand to move his body to a sitting position.

Rationale: Safe mobility is essential for carrying out daily activities and maintaining independence.

Resolved Needs: Activity, exercise. Comfort. Protection from physical harm. Mastery and competence in skills. Independence. Increased learning.

Teach how to use the problem-solving method Explain that a systematic method for solving problems should include defining the problem, gathering and analyzing data related to the problem, examining the possible solutions, and evaluating the effectiveness of the chosen solution.

Rationale: Successful problem solving is essential to mental health.

Resolved Needs: Comfort. Protection from psychologic threat. Mastery and competence in skills. Personal growth and maturity. Increased learning. Increased reality perception and problem-solving ability.

Teach how to use the unaffected leg to move the hemiplegic leg (97) Teach the patient with one-sided paralysis to place his unaffected (strong) leg under his affected (weak) leg and lift his affected (weak) leg to the edge of the bed and over the side.

Rationale: Safe mobility is essential for carrying out daily activities and maintaining independence.

Resolved Needs: Activity, exercise. Comfort. Protection from physical harm. Mastery and competence in skills. Independence. Increased learning.

Teach how to weigh   Explain how to measure and record body weight.

Rationale: Changes in body weight may indicate loss or retention of fluid, changes in appetite, abnormalities of food absorption or metabolism, or poor nutrition.

Resolved Needs: Protection from physical harm. Increased learning.

Teach how to wrap an amputation stump   Teach the amputee that a stump wrapping is applied by beginning at the mid-anterior thigh and bringing one length of bandage down to the stump end, under the stump, and over the anterior stump and thigh. A crisscross or figure-eight pattern is used, never a circular pattern. The bandage must be applied with even pressure, and it should be changed in the morning, in the afternoon, and before bedtime.

Rationale: Wrapping shrinks and shapes the stump in preparation for the prosthesis, supports soft tissue, and decreases edema.

Resolved Needs: Comfort. Protection from physical harm. Mastery and competence in skills. Increased learning.

Teach menstrual cycle physiology   Explain that menstruation is the monthly discharge of uterine blood, mucus, and epithelial cells. It occurs at intervals of approximately 28 days between the ages of 12 and 45 years. The menstrual cycle begins on the 1st day of menstruation, when the discharge of blood, mucus, and epithelial cells occurs. At the end of this period, or approximately 5 days later, the uterine membrane becomes very thin. From the 5th day to about the 10th or 12th day, estrogen secretion causes the uterus lining to become thick and cushiony. Around the 12th or 14th day ovulation occurs, during which a small body in the ovaries (the graafian follicle) ruptures, releasing an egg and then forming the corpus luteum, which secretes progesterone. The egg moves into the fallopian tube and down into the uterus. The progesterone stimulates increased blood supply to the uterine lining, making it even thicker in preparation for a fertilized egg. If fertilization does not occur by about the 25th day, the corpus luteum stops its activity and the uterine lining degenerates and is shed. Bleeding occurs because of the rupture of the small blood vessels in the uterine lining.

Rationale: Knowledge of physiologic body processes promotes comfort and safety.

Resolved Needs: Comfort. Protection from physical harm. Increased learning.

Teach menstrual hygiene   Explain that during menstrual flow, bathing, shampooing, exercise, and other normal activities are important to good health. Answer questions specific to the person's needs.

Rationale: Good menstrual hygiene promotes comfort and health.

Resolved Needs: Comfort. Cleanliness. Increased learning.

Teach mobility down a curb with crutches (97)   Teach the patient to approach the curb, stand still, move his crutches down off the curb, and then move his affected (weak) leg down, followed by his unaffected (strong) leg.

Rationale: Safe mobility is essential for carrying out daily activities and maintaining independence.

Resolved Needs: Activity, exercise. Comfort. Protection from physical harm. Mastery and competence in skills. Independence. Increased learning.

Teach mobility down stairs and curbs with leg braces (97)   Teach the patient to place one hand on the stair rail and both crutches under his opposite arm. He should move the crutches down to the next step, place as much weight as possible on his hands, and swing both braced legs down to that step. He should repeat the procedure for each step.

Rationale: Safe mobility is essential for carrying out daily activities and maintaining independence.

Resolved Needs: Activity, exercise. Comfort. Protection from physical harm. Mastery and competence in skills. Independence. Increased learning.

Teach mobility down stairs with crutches (97)   Teach the patient to place one hand on the stair rail and both crutches under his opposite arm. He should place as much weight as possible on his hands and arms, move the crutches to the step below, and then move his affected (weak) leg down, followed by his unaffected (strong) leg. He should repeat the procedure at each step.

Rationale: Safe mobility is essential for carrying out daily activities and maintaining independence.

Resolved Needs: Activity, exercise. Comfort. Protection from physical harm. Mastery and competence in skills. Independence. Increased learning.

Teach mobility from a standing to a sitting position with crutches (97)   Teach the patient to back a chair against a stable surface. He should move as close to the chair as possible, hold both crutches together at the handpiece with one hand, and place his other hand on the chair arm. Then he can slide into the chair.

Rationale: Safe mobility is essential for carrying out daily activities and maintaining independence.

Resolved Needs: Activity, exercise. Comfort. Protection from physical harm. Mastery and competence in skills. Independence. Increased learning.

Teach mobility from a standing to a sitting position with leg braces (97)   Teach the patient to back a chair against a stable surface. He should move as close to the chair as possible, unlock one brace at the

knee, grasp the chair arms with both hands, and slide into the chair. Then he should unlock the other leg brace.

Rationale: Safe mobility is essential for carrying out daily activities and maintaining independence.

Resolved Needs: Activity, exercise. Comfort. Protection from physical harm. Mastery and competence in skills. Independence. Increased learning.

Teach mobility up a curb with crutches (97)   Teach the patient to use his crutches to maintain balance as he approaches a curb. Then he should step up on the curb with his strong leg, straighten that leg, and lift his weak leg and his crutches onto the curb.

Rationale: Safe mobility is essential for carrying out daily activities and maintaining independence.

Resolved Needs: Activity, exercise. Comfort. Protection from physical harm. Mastery and competence in skills. Independence. Increased learning.

Teach mobility up a curb with leg braces (97)   Teach the patient to use his crutches to maintain balance as he backs up to the curb. He should swing one leg back and up onto the curb while leaning on both crutches. Then he should shift his weight to the leg on the curb and swing the other leg back and up onto the curb. He should balance his body on one crutch and both legs and bring first one crutch and then the other up onto the curb.

Rationale: Safe mobility is essential for carrying out daily activities and maintaining independence.

Resolved Needs: Activity, exercise. Comfort. Protection from physical harm. Mastery and competence in skills. Independence. Increased learning.

Teach mobility up stairs with crutches (97)   Teach the patient to place one hand on the stair rail and both crutches under his opposite arm. He should place as much weight as possible on his hands and arms and then step up with his strong leg, straighten that leg, and lift his weak leg and crutches. He should repeat the procedure at each step.

Rationale: Safe mobility is essential for carrying out daily activities and maintaining independence.

Resolved Needs: Activity, exercise. Comfort. Protection from physical harm. Mastery and competence in skills. Independence. Increased learning.

Teach mobility up stairs with leg braces (97)   Teach the patient to place one hand on the stair rail and both crutches under his opposite arm. He should place as much weight as possible on his hands and arms and step up by lifting his legs and then bringing the crutches up to that step. He should repeat the procedure at each step.

Rationale: Safe mobility is essential for carrying out daily activities and maintaining independence.

Resolved Needs: Activity, exercise. Comfort. Protection from physical harm. Mastery and competence in skills. Independence. Increased learning.

Teach postural drainage   After determining which lobe of the lung needs draining, teach the patient proper positioning for drainage.

Rationale: Postural drainage removes secretions from the lung by utilizing the force of gravity.

Resolved Needs: Protection from physical harm. Increased learning.

Contraindications: Do not place the patient in the head-down position if he has increased intracranial or intraocular pressure or hypertension.

Teach prenursing nipple hygiene   Explain that immediately before breast feeding, the nipples should be washed with warm water.

Rationale: Cleanliness helps prevent infection and promotes comfort.

Resolved Needs: Comfort. Cleanliness. Protection from physical harm. Increased learning.

Teach reverse isolation   Explain that persons who are highly susceptible to infection can be protected somewhat if those with whom they come in contact wash their hands and wear gowns and masks.

Rationale: Wearing gowns and masks and washing the hands help to protect the susceptible person from infectious organisms carried by others.

Resolved Needs: Protection from physical harm. Increased learning.

Teach that weight-bearing should be done on the unaffected side   Explain that in almost any injury, weight should be borne by the unaffected side of the body.

Rationale: Use of the body's strongest side helps prevent further injury to the weak side; it promotes healing and provides support for the total body.

Resolved Needs: Protection from physical harm. Increased learning.

Teach the principles of good nutrition   Explain the daily need for the basic foods in every diet: one or more servings of leafy green or yellow vegetables; one or more servings of citrus fruit, tomatoes, or raw cabbage; two or more servings of potatoes and other vegetables and fruits; 2–4 cups of milk, or the equivalent in cheese or ice cream; one or more servings of meat, poultry, fish, eggs, or dried peas or beans; one or more servings of bread, flour, or cereals; some butter or margarine.

Rationale: A balanced nutritional intake is essential to cellular activity and energy production from food.

Resolved Needs: Food balance. Energy. Protection from physical harm. Increased learning.

Teach the proper gait to use with a walker (97)   Explain that the standard gait pattern used with a walker involves moving the walker forward first, followed by the right foot and then the left foot.

Rationale: Proper use of a walker promotes safe mobility.

Resolved Needs: Protection from physical harm. Increased learning.

Teach the proper gait to use with crutches (97)   Teach the patient the crutch-walking gait appropriate for his condition. For *two-point crutch-walking*, the patient should move forward by advancing the right crutch and left foot together and the left crutch and right foot together at a reasonable pace. In *three-point crutch walking*, the patient should stand on his good leg and place both crutches the same distance ahead of him. He should swing himself forward ahead of the crutches, then place his body weight on his good leg, and regain his balance before advancing the crutches again. For *four-point crutch-walking*, the patient should employ the pattern of right crutch, left foot, left crutch, right foot. In *swing-through crutch-walking*, the patient should place the crutches ahead of him and then raise his entire body off the floor and up to and through the crutches. For *tripod crutch-walking*, the patient should place the crutches slightly ahead of him and drag his body up to the crutches, then repeat the process.

Rationale: The ability to move about is essential to daily living activities. Three-point crutch-walking facilitates walking following an amputation or a fractured hip. Four-point crutch-walking is best for patients who can manipulate both lower extremities. Swing-through crutch-walking facilitates movement where there is severe lower-extremity involvement, such as in paraplegia. Tripod crutch-walking facilitates movement for the person who cannot lift his body off the floor.

Resolved Needs: Protection from physical harm. Mastery and competence in new skills. Increased learning.

Teach the specific procedure   When a patient needs to perform a certain health procedure, teach him which supplies he will need and how to perform the procedure. After the explanation, have him give a return demonstration.

Rationale: Correct performance of health procedures increases the potential for effectiveness of the procedure.

Resolved Needs: Protection from physical harm. Mastery and competence in skills. Increased learning.

Teach weight-bearing on the entire foot   Explain that one should walk on the entire foot, not primarily on the ball of the foot.

Rationale: Proper walking promotes correct body alignment and mobility.

Resolved Needs: Protection from physical harm. Increased learning.

Teach which drugs and chemicals have the potential for habituation   Explain that the following drugs can lead to drug habituation: hallucinogenic drugs (LSD, DMT, mescaline), sleeping pills and barbiturates (Amytal, Nembutal, phenobarbital), amphetamine pep pills and diet pills (Benzedrine, Dexedrine, Methedrine), opiates and narcotics (morphine, heroin, codeline, paregoric), tranquilizers (Valium, Meprobamate, Librium), marijuana, and deliriants such as airplane glue, gasoline, lighter fluid, paint thinner, varnish, shellac, and Freon.

Rationale: Accurate knowledge about drugs that can lead to habituation can result in abstinence or cautious use of such drugs.

Resolved Needs: Protection from physical harm. Increased learning.

34.
Medical Treatments
Performed by Nurses

Administer a bladder instillation Instill a prescribed solution into the bladder at periodic intervals using sterile technique.

Rationale: Instilling medicated solutions into the bladder can help prevent or alleviate bladder infection.

Resolved Needs: Protection from physical harm.

Administer a blood transfusion Infuse typed and cross-matched blood into the vein.

Rationale: A blood infusion increases circulating blood volume, red cell volume, and hemoglobin content, and these facilitate oxygen transport to cells. It provides protein and essential nutrient elements. Freshly drawn blood also restores platelets and white blood cells.

Resolved Needs: Oxygen, circulation. Water-salt balance. Protection from physical harm.

Contraindications: Known allergies. Polycythemia vera. Circulatory overload.

Administer a medicated enema Dispense a medicated solution into the colon. Encourage the patient to retain the solution for 30 minutes to 1 hour.

Rationale: In the presence of liver damage, the intestinal flora increases ammonia production. Cleaning the bowel with neomycin or lactulose decreases intestinal bacteria and reduces the ammonia level.

Resolved Needs: Protection from physical harm.

Administer aerosol mist by nebulizer Dispense a fine mist of liquid particles suspended in air by running oxygen or compressed air through a nebulizer to produce a spray.

Rationale: Aerosol mist can liquefy mucus secretions and promote their elimination from the respiratory tract.

Resolved Needs: Waste elimination. Comfort. Protection from physical harm.

Administer carbon dioxide whiffs
Dispense inhalation therapy of 5% carbon dioxide in oxygen for very short intermittent periods.

Rationale: Carbon dioxide stimulates failing respirations.

Resolved Needs: Oxygen. Stimulation. Protection from physical harm.

Contraindications: Elevated blood level of carbon dioxide. Emphysema.

Administer continuous positive pressure breathing
Administer continuous pressurized air into the lungs by using positive pressure equipment.

Rationale: Continuous positive pressure breathing treatments promote inhalation and exhalation of air that is at a pressure higher than the local atmospheric pressure. Mechanical ventilation can maintain normal respirations despite irregular respiratory patterns set by the body.

Resolved Needs: Oxygen. Waste elimination. Comfort. Protection from physical harm.

Contraindications: Impaired cardiac output. Decreased blood volume from fluid or blood loss (hemorrhage). Pulmonary embolus.

Administer continuous positive pressure breathing by expiratory positive pressure mask
Administer continuous positive pressure breathing with an expiratory positive pressure mask attached to the ventilator.

Rationale: The expiratory positive pressure mask has a multihole valve with varying diameters. The smaller the disk hole, the greater the alveolar and airway pressures. The greater the pressure, the less venous return to the thorax. This reduces pulmonary capillary pressure and decreases pulmonary edema. Continuous positive pressure breathing provides forced air flow on inspiration and expiration.

Resolved Needs: Oxygen. Protection from physical harm.

Contraindications: Pulmonary embolus. Pulmonary hemorrhage.

Administer controlled positive pressure breathing
Dispense intermittent positive pressure breathing, which completely controls the breathing pattern.

Rationale: When normal respirations cannot be maintained, controlled positive pressure breathing supports respirations at normal rate, depth, and rhythm; it prevents respiratory failure, promotes carbon dioxide elimination, and supports acid-base balance.

Resolved Needs: Oxygen. Acid-base balance. Waste elimination. Protection from physical harm.

Contraindications: Pulmonary hemorrhage.

Administer fluids by hypodermoclysis   Insert two small-gauge needles into the appropriate subcutaneous tissue, and administer through sterile tubing a bottle of physiologic sodium chloride solution. Regulate the flow rate in accordance with the absorption rate.

Rationale: Balance of fluid intake and output is essential to cell functioning. Improper fluid balance damages and impairs cell activity. Hypodermoclysis replaces the normal salt solution that is a basic component of blood; it is used when the intravenous route is not feasible.

Resolved Needs: Water-salt balance. Protection from physical harm.

Contraindications: Never give solutions containing glucose or electrolytes other than sodium and chloride by hypodermoclysis. Do not give during circulatory overload, which is evidenced by vein distention, etc.

Administer heated humidified oxygen (ET) (listed under Nursing Treatments, p. 1243)

Administer humidified oxygen (ET) (listed under Nursing Treatments, p. 1243)

Administer intermittent positive pressure breathing (ET) (listed under Nursing Treatments, p. 1244)

Administer intermittent positive pressure by expiratory positive pressure mask   When giving IPPB for pulmonary edema, use an expiratory positive pressure mask that has a multihole valve with disks of varying diameters.

Rationale: The expiratory positive pressure mask maintains positive pressure in the alveoli and airway. The smaller the disk hole, the greater the positive pressure. It retards blood flow back to the heart during exhalation, which decreases blood flow to the lungs.

Resolved Needs: Oxygen. Protection from physical harm.

Contraindications: Pulmonary embolus. Pulmonary hemorrhage.

Administer intermittent positive pressure with 100% oxygen   Give positive pressure treatments with 100% oxygen at regular intervals.

Rationale: Intermittent positive pressure with 100% oxygen increases pressure within the alveoli and diminishes venous return to the thorax. This reduces pulmonary capillary pressure and reduces edema.

Resolved Needs: Oxygen. Protection from physical harm.

Contraindications:　Pulmonary hemorrhage. Oxygen toxicity.

Administer intravenous fluids (ET) (listed under Nursing Treatments, p. 1244)

Administer oxygen by nasal cannula　Give humidified oxygen with a double-prong nasal cannula.

Rationale:　The nasal cannula provides high oxygen concentrations and the comfort of freedom of movement.

Resolved Needs:　Oxygen. Comfort. Protection from physical harm.

Administer oxygen by nasal catheter　Give oxygen by a small plastic tube inserted through the nose to the oropharynx at a flow rate of 2 to 4 liters per minute.

Rationale:　A nasal catheter provides highly concentrated oxygen.

Resolved Needs:　Oxygen. Protection from physical harm.

Administer oxygen by nonrebreathing mask　Give oxygen therapy with a mask having a safety inlet valve between the mask and oxygen reservoir bag.

Rationale:　A nonrebreathing mask prevents rebreathing of the same air, thus providing fresh oxygen concentration.

Resolved Needs:　Oxygen. Protection from physical harm.

Administer oxygen by partial rebreathing mask　Give oxygen therapy with a mask having no valve between the mask and oxygen reservoir bag.

Rationale:　A partial rebreathing mask allows for one-third of the exhaled air to be rebreathed. In severe oxygen deficiency, a very high therapeutic oxygen concentration elevates the body's oxygen level to normal.

Resolved Needs:　Oxygen. Comfort. Protection from physical harm.

Administer oxygen by tent, croupette, or incubator　When giving oxygen to a patient who requires environmental control, use an oxygen tent, croupette, or incubator in which oxygen and humidified air are circulated.

Rationale:　An oxygen tent, croupette, or incubator provides high oxygen concentrations and controls environmental humidity and temperature. Humidified air prevents tissue friction during respirations, loosens secretions, and promotes comfort.

Resolved Needs:　Oxygen. Comfort. Protection from physical harm.

Administer oxygen by Venturi mask　Give oxygen with a mask that delivers precise oxygen concentrations.

Rationale: When respirations have been depressed by oxygen excess or carbon dioxide retention, it is essential that precise amounts of oxygen be given for maintenance of normal blood levels and prevention of further respiratory depression.

Resolved Needs: Oxygen. Waste elimination. Protection from physical harm.

Administer phototherapy treatment   Expose jaundiced skin to ultraviolet rays (bili light), and protect the patient's eyes with bandages during exposure to the light.

Rationale: Exposure of jaundiced skin to ultraviolet rays reduces the yellow skin color.

Resolved Needs: Comfort. Protection from physical harm.

Contraindications: Sensitivity of skin or eyes to light.

Administer the hemodialysis treatment   Give the hemodialysis treatment according to the physician's prescribed order.

Rationale: Hemodialysis removes those body wastes that are not being removed because of renal failure. Hemodialysis is essential to maintenance of life when renal failure occurs.

Resolved Needs: Waste elimination. Protection from physical harm.

Advance the intestinal tube as ordered   Gently push the intestinal tube farther into the intestinal tract. Insert as frequently as ordered and the number of inches ordered for each insertion.

Rationale: Slow advancement of an intestinal tube opens blocked areas of the intestinal tract.

Resolved Needs: Protection from physical harm.

Apply a biologic dressing (47)   Apply skin from another human (homograft) or pig skin (heterograft) to the burned area. This skin is available from skin banks.

Rationale: Biologic dressings are applied to burned skin because they provide a barrier to reduce water vaporization, decrease protein and exudate loss, protect against infection, relieve pain, support joint movement, help in debridement, and support the growth of epithelium and granulation tissue.

Resolved Needs: Water-salt balance. Activity. Comfort. Protection from physical harm.

Apply a medicated dressing   Apply a sterile dressing dampened with medicinal solution. Most medication solutions are not heated because heat destroys the active properties of most drugs.

Rationale: A wet medicated wound dressing soothes and cools by moisture evaporation from the dressing; it allows for slow medication penetration into the wound; it softens wound discharges, promotes drainage, localizes the area of infection, and has a bacteriostatic-bactericidal effect.

Resolved Needs: Comfort. Cleanliness. Protection from physical harm.

Contraindications: Known medication allergy.

Apply the prescribed preventive splint Apply to the limb a prescribed supportive splint. Such splints are applied primarily at night, but occasionally during the day.

Rationale: Preventive splints hold limbs in functional positions, thus preventing contractures, and supporting future muscle use after healing.

Resolved Needs: Protection from physical harm.

Apply the prescribed prosthesis Put the artificial body part that the physician has prescribed on the patient.

Rationale: A prescribed prosthesis provides the patient with a means of functioning and substitutes for the loss of a body part that has impaired normal function.

Resolved Needs: Activity. Independence.

Apply the prescribed topical agent (47) Apply to the skin the prescribed drug usually in salve or ointment form. In burn therapy, topical agents include Sulfadiazine, Silver Nitrate, Sulfamylon cream, Betadine, Cerium Nitrate.

Rationale: Topical agents applied to the skin reduce pain, infection, promote comfort and support healing.

Resolved Needs: Comfort. Protection from physical harm.

Apply the prescribed traction Exert weighted pulling pressure against designated bones and establish their alignment, as prescribed by the physician.

Rationale: Skeletal traction helps to disengage bone fragments, position and immobilize bones for healing, decrease muscle spasms, prevent deformities, and increase future mobility of currently injured and immobile bones.

Resolved Needs: Protection from physical harm.

Attach the gastric tube to suction Remove gastric contents from the stomach or duodenum by attaching the gastric tube to a suction device.

Rationale: Removal of gastric fluids and gas decreases gastric activity and pressure and promotes healing and comfort.

Resolved Needs: Waste elimination. Comfort. Protection from physical harm.

Bivalve and spread the cast to relieve pressure (ET) (listed under Nursing Treatments, p. 1268)

Clamp the suprapubic catheter and have the patient attempt to void   Clamp the suprapubic catheter (usually for 4 hours), and then release it for the ordered time (usually 15–30 minutes). Suggest that the patient attempt to void during the period that the catheter is clamped.

Rationale: Clamping the suprapubic catheter is a method used to reestablish normal voiding patterns.

Resolved Needs: Waste elimination. Comfort.

Defibrillate the heart muscle (ET) (listed under Nursing Treatments, pp. 1281–1282)

Give the prescribed diet   Give diets explicitly calculated for a specific disease.

Rationale: Certain nutritional elements, when given in proper amounts, can correct certain diseases and imbalances.

Resolved Needs: Food balance. Water-salt balance. Acid-base balance. Protection from physical harm.

Give the prescribed drugs   Give medicinal substances that require a physician's prescription in specified doses at specified times.

Rationale: Drugs consist of chemicals that combine with body processes to alter or improve body function, promote comfort, or balance body fluid, salts, and acid-base levels. They promote elimination, stimulate body functions, regulate body temperature, and protect from inflammatory or infectious conditions.

Resolved Needs: Water-salt balance. Acid-base balance. Waste elimination. Normal temperature. Sleep, rest, relaxation. Comfort. Stimulation. Protection from physical harm. Freedom from pain.

Contraindications: Drug intolerance. Drug allergy.

Give the prescribed exercise(s)   Exercise the patient as prescribed by the physician. Prescribed exercises include those specific to cardiac conditions and Buerger-Allen exercises. The Buerger-Allen exercise involves placing the patient in the flat position and elevating the legs above the heart level for two minutes. Then have the patient dangle his legs, exercise his feet for three minutes, and lie flat for 5 minutes.

Rationale: Prescribed exercises improve arterial blood flow which supports better circulation.

Resolved Needs: Circulation. Exercise. Stimulation. Protection from physical harm.

Give the prescribed fluids   Give the specific amounts and kinds of fluids prescribed by the physician.

Rationale: Prescribed fluids assist in the maintenance of fluid and electrolyte balance, especially in such conditions as edema, ascites, renal insufficiency, and congestive heart failure.

Resolved Needs: Water-salt balance. Comfort. Protection from physical harm.

Give the prescribed hyperalimentation feeding   Administer the hyperalimentation feedings as prescribed by the physician.

Rationale: Hyperalimentation feedings provide additional nutrients essential to health and healing that cannot be ingested or absorbed.

Resolved Needs: Water-salt balance. Food balance. Energy. Protection from physical harm.

Give the prescribed number of peritoneal dialysis exchanges   Give the number of dialysis treatments the physician has ordered. This includes instillation, leaving the fluid in the abdomen, and drainage. Most treatments are given every hour for 24–36 hours.

Rationale: The numbers of peritoneal dialysis exchanges are ordered according to blood levels of electrolytes and urea.

Resolved Needs: Waste elimination. Protection from physical harm.

Give the prescribed tube feeding   Administer food and fluids through a gastric, gastrostomy, or jejunostomy (enterostomy) tube.

Rationale: Balanced nutritional intake is essential to cellular activity and energy production from food products. Relief of the visceral hunger sensation promotes comfort.

Resolved Needs: Water-salt balance. Food balance. Comfort. Protection from physical harm.

Instill dialysate into the peritoneum, allow it to remain in the abdomen, then drain the dialysate   Instill the dialysate fluid, leave it in the peritoneal cavity, and drain according to the physician's prescription for amount and length of each stage of treatment.

Rationale: The effectiveness of removal of waste material by the dialysate fluid depends on the amount of fluid and the length of time it is left in the peritoneum.

Resolved Needs: Waste elimination. Protection from physical harm.

Irrigate the bladder by tidal drainage   Gradually fill the bladder with irrigating solution and periodically empty the solution from the bladder.

Rationale: Gradual bladder distention increases muscle tone. Periodic bladder filling stimulates bladder emptying and conditions the bladder for activity not controlled by the central nervous system. The flow of irrigating fluid into the catheter prevents obstruction by clots, facilitates the application of warmth to the mucous lining, and allows for medication instillations.

Resolved Needs: Waste elimination. Protection from physical harm.

Irrigate the nephrostomy tube   Using sterile technique, irrigate the nephrostomy tube with sterile saline or distilled water. Never irrigate a nephrostomy tube without a physician's order, which includes the exact amount of solution to use. Be sure that the irrigating solution returns.

Rationale: Nephrostomy tube irrigation maintains tube patency.

Resolved Needs: Waste elimination. Comfort. Protection from physical harm.

Irrigate the ostomy   Dispense a water solution into the colon through an artificial anus or stoma surgically placed in the anterior abdominal wall and stimulate the defecation reflex.

Rationale: Distention and irritation of the colon stimulate fecal elimination. Colostomy irrigation maintains cleanliness by preventing defecation at socially inappropriate times.

Resolved Needs: Waste elimination. Comfort. Cleanliness.

Irrigate the transtracheal catheter   Inject sterile saline onto the tracheal mucous membrane through a nasal, pharyngeal, or transtracheal catheter.

Rationale: A transtracheal catheter irrigation liquefies secretions and irrigates the tracheal mucous membrane, thus stimulating the cough reflex.

Resolved Needs: Waste elimination.

Lavage the stomach (ET) (listed under Nursing Treatments, p. 1363)

Maintain the decompression drainage Y-tube at the ordered level   When the patient is undergoing decompression drainage of the bladder, periodically lower the Y-tube the number of inches prescribed (usually 1 inch every hour).

Rationale: The Y-tube level is gradually lowered so that the bladder will be slowly decompressed and bladder muscle tone will be maintained.

Resolved Needs: Stimulation. Protection from physical harm.

Mobilize with the prescribed brace   Apply to the limb the prescribed supportive brace.

Rationale: A therapeutic brace supports weakened muscles, joints, and bones; it facilitates motion or temporarily reduces motion during healing.

Resolved Needs: Activity, exercise. Protection from physical harm.

Contraindications: Delay if severe skin irritation exists.

Mobilize with the prescribed crutches Help the patient move about with crutches specifically ordered and fitted to him.

Rationale: Crutches facilitate good body balance and independent mobility.

Resolved Needs: Activity, exercise. Comfort. Protection from physical harm. Independence.

Contraindications: Severe energy depletion.

Place on a hypothermia blanket Maintain a low body temperature by placing the patient on a cooling blanket.

Rationale: Lowering the body temperature decreases metabolic demand for oxygen, reduces blood pressure, and decreases fever.

Resolved Needs: Normal temperature. Comfort. Protection from physical harm.

Place on the prescribed bed rest Encourage the patient to adhere to the amount of bed rest the physician has prescribed. The amount of rest needed each day will be determined by the nature of the disease or injury being treated.

Rationale: Rest is essential to maintenance of body function; it replenishes the cell energy that the body uses for maintenance of life and activity and promotes healing and comfort.

Resolved Needs: Sleep, rest. Energy. Comfort. Protection from physical harm.

Resuscitate breathing (ET) (listed under Nursing Treatments, p. 1434)

Resuscitate mouth-to-neck when the patient has a laryngectomy (ET) (listed under Nursing Treatments, p. 1435)

Soak in a medicated bath Apply medication to the skin by placing the medication in a tub of water and soaking the patient's body in it.

Rationale: Use of a tub provides for overall and equal body coverage of medications.

Resolved Needs: Comfort. Cleanliness. Protection from physical harm.

Contraindications: Known allergy to the medication.

Soak in a medicated solution Immerse the arm, hand, fingers, leg, foot, or toes in a warm medicated solution for approximately 20–30 minutes three to four times a day.

Rationale: Local application of a warm medicated solution promotes comfort by relieving inflammation; it removes necrotic tissue and has cleansing or bacteriostatic-bactericidal effects.

Resolved Needs: Comfort. Cleanliness. Protection from physical harm.

Contraindications: Known allergy to the medication.

Part 4.

References and Indexes

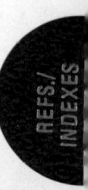

References

BOOKS

1. Abbott Laboratories. *Fluid and Electrolytes*. Chicago: Abbott Laboratories, 1969.
2. Abdellah, Faye, and Eugene Levine. *Better Patient Care Through Nursing Research*. London: Macmillan & Co., 1965.
3. Abdellah, Faye, Irene Beland, Almeda Martin, and Ruth Matheney. *Patient Centered Approaches to Nursing*. New York: Macmillan Co., 1964.
4. Abrahamsen, David. *The Road to Emotional Maturity*. Englewood Cliffs, N.J.: Prentice-Hall, Inc., 1966.
5. Abrahamson, E. M., and A. W. Pezet. *Body, Mind and Sugar*. New York: Holt, Rinehart and Winston, 1972.
6. Ackerman, Lloyd. *Health and Hygiene*. Tempe, Ariz.: Jaques Cattell Press, 1943.
7. Adams, John. *Viruses and Colds*. New York: American Elsevier Publishing Co., 1967.
8. Ainsworth, Stanley. *Speech Correction Methods*. New York: Prentice-Hall, Inc., 1948.
9. Aldrich, C. Knight. *An Introduction to Dynamic Psychiatry*. New York: McGraw-Hill Book Co., 1966.
10. Allen, James H. *May's Diseases of the Eye*. Baltimore: Williams & Wilkins Co., 1963.
11. Allergy Foundation of America. *Allergy—Its Mysterious Causes and Modern Treatment*. New York: Grosset & Dunlap, 1967.
12. Allport, Gordon W. *Pattern and Growth in Personality*. New York: Henry Holt & Co., 1937.
13. Allport, Gordon W. *Personality—A Psychological Interpretation*. New York: Henry Holt & Co., 1937.
14. Alpers, Bernard, and Elliott Mancall. *Clinical Neurology*. Philadelphia: F. A. Davis Co., 1971.
15. Alvarez, Walter. *Live at Peace With Your Nerves*. Englewood Cliffs, N.J.: Prentice-Hall, Inc., 1961.
16. American Medical Association. *Current Medical Terminology*. Chicago: American Medical Association, 1966.
17. American Medical Association. *Drug Dependence—A Guide for Physicians*. Chicago: American Medical Association, 1961.
18. American Red Cross. *Advanced First Aid and Emergency Care*. Garden City, N.Y.: Doubleday & Co., Inc., 1973.
19. American Red Cross. *Standard First Aid and Personal Safety*. Garden City, N.Y.: Doubleday & Co., Inc., 1973.
20. Anderson, W.A., and Thomas Scotti. *Synopsis of Pathology*. St. Louis: C.V. Mosby Co., 1968.
21. Armed Forces Information Service—Dept. of Defense. *Drug Abuse—Game Without Winners*. Washington, D.C.: U.S. Gov-

22. Arnold, Magda. *Feelings and Emotions*. New York: Academic Press, 1960.

23. Arieti, Silvano. *American Handbook of Psychiatry*. Volumes I, II, III. New York: Basic Books, 1966.

24. Artz, Curtis, and John Moncrief. *The Treatment of Burns*. Philadelphia: W. B. Saunders Co., 1969.

25. Backus, Ollie, and Jane Beasley. *Speech Therapy With Children*. Boston: Houghton Mifflin Co., 1951.

26. Bacon, Edgar. *Your Child's Teeth*. New York: E. P. Dutton & Co., 1957.

27. Bailey, June, and Karen Claus. *Decision Making in Nursing*. St. Louis: C. V. Mosby Co., 1975.

28. Baker, Charles. *Physician's Desk Reference*. Oradell, N.J.: Medical Economics, Inc., 1976.

29. Barbata, Jean, Deborah Jensen, and William Patterson. *A Textbook of Medical-Surgical Nursing*. New York: G. P. Putnam's Sons, 1964.

30. Barber, Janet, Lillian Stokes, Diane Billings. *Adult and Child Care—A Client Approach to Nursing*. St. Louis: C. V. Mosby Co., 1973.

31. Beintema, David, and Heinz Prechtl. *A Neurological Study of Newborn Infants*. London: Lanvenham Press, Ltd., 1968.

32. Beland, Irene. *Clinical Nursing—Pathophysiological and Psychosocial Approaches*. New York: Macmillan Co., 1970.

33. Belgum, David. *Guilt: Where Religion and Psychology Meet*. Englewood Cliffs, N.J. Prentice-Hall, Inc., 1963.

34. Bellet, Samuel. *Clinical Disorders of the Heart Beat*. Philadelphia: Lea & Febiger Co., 1971.

35. Benedek, Therese. *Insight and Personality Adjustment*. New York: Ronald Press, 1946.

36. Bergersen, Betty, Edith Anderson, Morgant Duffy, Mary Lohr, and Rose Marion. *Current Concepts in Clinical Nursing*. St. Louis: C. V. Mosby Co. 1967.

37. Bergman, B. Abraham, J. Bruce Beckwith, and C. George Ray. *Sudden Infant Death Syndrome*. Seattle: University of Washington Press, 1970.

38. Bergstrom, Doris. *Care of Patients With Bowel and Bladder Problems: A Nursing Guide*. Minneapolis, Minn.: American Rehabilitation Foundation, 1968.

39. Berland, Theodore, and Mitchell Spellberg. *Living With Your Ulcer*. New York: St. Martin's Press, 1971.

40. Berland, Theodore, and Alfred Seyler. *Your Children's Teeth*. New York: Meredith Press, 1968.

41. Bernard, Jessie, and Deborah Jensen. *Sociology*. St. Louis: C. V. Mosby Co., 1962.

42. Bernard, Jessie, and Lida Thompson. *Sociology—Nurses and Their Patients in a Modern Society*. St. Louis: C. V. Mosby Co., 1970.

43. Berne, Eric. *A Layman's Guide to Psychiatry and Psychoanalysis*. New York: Simon and Schuster, 1968.

44. Bernhardt, Karl. *Practical Psychology*. New York: McGraw-Hill Book Co., 1953.

45. Berry, Mildred Freburg. *Language Disorders of Children: The Bases and Diagnosis*. New York: Appleton-Century-Crofts, 1969.

46. Beutner, Karl, and Nathan Hale. *Emotional Illness—How Families Can Help*. New York: G. P. Putnam's Sons, 1957.

47. Beyers, Marjorie, and Susan Dudas. *Medical Surgical Nursing*. Chapter: Nursing Care Delivery for the Thermally Injured Patient. Boston: Little, Brown & Co., 1977.

48. Blake, Florence, F. Howell Wright, and Eugenia Waechter. *Nursing Care of Children*. Philadelphia: J. B. Lippincott Co., 1970.

49. Block, Marvin. *Alcohol and Alcoholism*. Belmont, Calif.: Wadsworth Publishing Co., 1970.

50. Boas, Ernst. *Treatment of the Patient Past Fifty*. Chicago: Year Book Medical Publishers, Inc., 1947.

51. Bogert, L. Jean, George Briggs, and Doris Callaway. *Nutrition and Physical Fitness*. Philadelphia:

W. B. Saunders Co., 1966.

52. Bonney, Merl. *Mental Health in Education.* Rockleigh, N.J.: Allyn and Bacon, Inc., 1960.

53. Bookmiller, Mae, George Bowen, and Dolores Carpenter. *Textbook of Obstetrics and Obstetric Nursing.* Philadelphia: W. B. Saunders Co., 1967.

54. Bordicks, Katherine. *Patterns of Shock.* New York: Macmillan Co., 1965.

55. Boucheron, Pierre. *How to Enjoy Life After Sixty.* New York: Archer House, Inc., 1959.

56. Bragg, Shirley, and Olive Rees. *Scientific Principles in Nursing.* St. Louis: C. V. Mosby Co., 1970.

57. Brain, Lord, and John N. Walton. *Brain Diseases of the Nervous System.* New York: Oxford University Press, 1969.

58. Brams, William. *Managing Your Coronary.* Philadelphia: J. B. Lippincott Co., 1966.

59. Brams, William. *Your Blood Pressure.* Philadelphia: J. B. Lippincott Co., 1956.

60. Brauer, Earle. *Your Skin and Hair.* London: Macmillan & Co., 1969.

61. Braun, M. D., and Gerald Diettert. *Coronary Care Unit Nursing—Part I.* Missoula, Mont,: Montana Clinic Foundation, 1968.

62. Braverman, Irvin, M.D. *Skin Signs of Systemic Disease.* Philadelphia: W. B. Saunders Co., 1970.

63. Bray, Patrick. *Neurology in Pediatrics.* Chicago: Year Book Medical Publishers, Inc., 1969.

64. Breckenridge, Marina E., and Margaret N. Murphy. *Growth and Development of the Young Child.* Philadelphia: W. B. Saunders Co., 1969.

65. Brichall, Ellen, and Noll Gerson. *Sex and the Adult Woman.* New York: Gilbert Press, 1965.

66. Brighthill, Charles. *Man and Leisure.* Englewood Cliffs, N.J.: Prentice-Hall, Inc., 1961.

67. Brown, Jason W. *Aphasia, Apraxia and Agnosia.* Springfield, Ill.: Charles C Thomas Publisher, 1972.

68. Brown, Martha, and Grace Fawler. *Psychodynamic Nursing—A Biosocial Orientation.* Philadelphia: W. B. Saunders Co., 1966.

69. Brughera-Jones, Antonella. *Manual of Laboratory Medicine.* New York: Harper & Row, Publishers, Inc., 1970.

70. Brunner, Lillian, Charles Emerson, L. Kraeer Ferguson, and Doris Suddarth. *Textbook of Medical-Surgical Nursing.* Philadelphia: J. B. Lippincott Co., 1970.

71. Brunner, Lillian, and Doris Suddarth. *The Lippincott Manual of Nursing Practice.* Philadelphia: J. B. Lippincott Co., 1974.

72. Bryant, Richard, and Anna Overland. *Obstetric Management and Nursing.* Philadelphia: F. A. Davis Co., 1964.

73. Buckley, Joseph. *The Retirement Handbook.* New York: Harper & Row, Publishers, Inc., 1967.

74. Buffum, Herbert, A. T. Lovering, Ira Warren, A. E. Small, William Thorndike, Herbert Smith, and Charles Lyman. *The Household Physician.* Boston: Woodruff Publishing Co., Inc., 1905.

75. Burd, Shirley, and Margaret Marshall. *Some Clinical Approaches to Psychiatric Nursing.* New York: Macmillan Co., 1963.

76. Burgess, Ann, and Aaron Lazare. *Psychiatric Nursing in the Hospital and the Community.* Englewood Cliffs, N.J.: Prentice-Hall, Inc., 1973.

77. Burrell, Zeb, Jr., and Lenette Owens Burrell. *Intensive Nursing Care.* St. Louis: C. V. Mosby Co., 1969.

78. Byers, Virginia. *Nursing Observation.* Dubuque, Iowa: William C. Brown Co., 1971.

79. Byrd, Oliver. *Health.* Philadelphia: W. B. Saunders Co., 1971.

80. Cammer, Leonard. *Up From Depression.* New York: Simon and Schuster, 1971.

81. Canfield, Norton. *Hearing—A Handbook for Laymen.* Garden City, N.Y.: Doubleday & Co., Inc., 1959.

82. Cannon Walter. *The Wisdom of the Body.* New York: W. W. Norton & Co., Inc., 1939.

83. Caprio, Frank. *Helping Yourself With Psychiatry.* Englewood Cliffs, N.J.: Prentice-Hall, Inc., 1957.

84. Carini, Esta, and Guy Owens. *Neurological and Neurosurgical*

Nursing. St. Louis: C. V. Mosby Co., 1970.

85. Carlson, Carolyn. *Behavioral Concepts and Nursing Intervention.* Philadelphia: J. B. Lippincott Co., 1970.

86. Chapman, Frederick. *Recreation Activities for the Handicapped.* New York: Ronald Press, 1960.

87. Chess, Stella, Alexander Thomas, and Herbert Berch. *Your Child Is a Person.* New York: Viking Press, 1965.

88. Child Study Association of America, Inc. *You, Your Child and Drugs.* New York: Child Study Press, 1971.

89. Clark, Marguerita. *Why So Tired? The Ways of Fatigue and the Ways of Energy.* New York: Duell, Sloan and Pearce, 1962.

90. Clements, H. *What to Do About a Bad Back and Disc Trouble.* New York: Drake Publishers, 1972.

91. Coffin, Margaret. *Nursing Observations of the Young Patient.* Dubuque, Iowa: William C. Brown Co., 1970.

92. Cohen, Sidney. *The Drug Dilemma.* New York: McGraw-Hill Book Co., 1969.

93. Cohen, Yehudi. *Social Structure and Personality.* New York: Holt, Rinehart and Winston, 1961.

94. Coleman, James. *Psychology and Effective Behavior.* Glenview, Ill.: Scott, Foresman & Co., 1969.

95. Coleman, Lester. *Freedom From Fear.* New York: Hawthorn Books, Inc., 1959.

96. Collins, Daniel. *Your Teeth.* Garden City, N.Y.: Doubleday & Co., Inc., 1967.

97. Colorado State Department of Public Health. *Elementary Rehabilitation Nursing Care.* Washington, D.C.: U.S. Dept. of Health, Education and Welfare, 1967.

98. Combs, Arthur. *Perceiving, Behaving, Becoming.* Washington, D.C.: National Education Association, 1962.

99. Combs, Arthur, and Donald Snygg. *Individual Behavior.* New York: Harper & Brothers, 1959.

100. Confield, Norton. *Hearing—A Handbook for Laymen.* Garden City, N.Y.: Doubleday & Co., Inc., 1959.

101. Cooper, Signe Skott. *Contemporary Nursing Practice.* New York: McGraw-Hill Book Co., 1970.

102. Cowdry, E. V. *The Care of the Geriatric Patient.* St. Louis: C. V. Mosby Co., 1968.

103. Craig, W. S. *Care of the Newly Born Infant.* Baltimore: Williams & Wilkins Co., 1969.

104. Creighton, Helen, *Law Every Nurse Should Know.* Philadelphia: W. B. Saunders Co., 1970.

105. Crews, Eli Rush. *A Practical Manual for the Treatment of Burns.* Springfield, Ill.: Charles C Thomas Publisher, 1967.

106. Crohn, Burrell. *Understand Your Ulcer.* New York: Sheridan House Publishers, 1969.

107. Culver, Vivian. *Modern Bedside Nursing.* Philadelphia: W. B. Saunders Co., 1969.

108. Danforth, David. *Textbook of Obstetrics and Gynecology.* New York: Harper & Row Publishers, Inc., 1966.

109. Danowski, T. S. *Diabetes as a Way of Life.* New York: Coward-McCann Inc., 1957.

110. Davis, Keith. *Human Behavior at Work.* New York: McGraw-Hill Book Co., 1972.

111. Davis, Maxine. *Every Woman's Book of Health.* New York: McGraw-Hill Book Co., 1969.

112. Davis, M. Edward, and Reva Rubin. *Obstetrics for Nurses.* Philadelphia: W. B. Saunders Co., 1966.

113. DeGowin, Elmer, and Richard DeGowin. *Bedside Diagnostic Examination.* New York: Macmillan Co., 1969.

114. Delacato, Carl H. *The Diagnosis and Treatment of Speech and Reading Problems.* Springfield, Ill.: Charles C Thomas Publisher, 1965.

115. De Levita, David. *The Concept of Identity.* Paris: Mouton and Company, 1965.

116. Delp, Mahlon, and Robert Manning. *Major's Physical Diagnosis.* Philadelphia: W. B. Saunders Co., 1968.

117. De Myer, William. *Technique of the Neurological Examination.* New

York: McGraw-Hill Book Co., 1969.

118. Dennis, Lorraine. *Psychology of Human Behavior for Nurses.* Philadelphia: W. B. Saunders Co., 1967.

119. De Ropp, Robert. *Drugs and the Mind.* New York: Grove Press Inc., 1961.

120. Diamond, Solomon. *Personality and Temperament.* New York: Harper & Brothers, 1957.

121. Diehl, Harold, and Stewart Thompson. *Textbook of Healthful Living.* New York: McGraw-Hill Book Co., 1960.

122. Diehl, Harold S., and Willard Dalrymple. *Healthful Living.* New York: McGraw-Hill Book Co., 1968.

123. Dolger, Henry, and Bernard Seeman. *How to Live With Diabetes.* New York: Pyramid Publications, Inc., 1970.

124. Dollard, John, and Neal Miller. *Personality and Psychotherapy.* New York: McGraw-Hill Book Co., 1950.

125. Dorland, W. A. Newman. *American Pocket Medical Dictionary.* Philadelphia: W. B. Saunders Co., 1946.

126. Duke-Elder, Sir Stewart. *Parson's Diseases of the Eye.* London: J. & A. Churchill Co., 1970.

127. Dushkin, David. *Psychology Today—An Introduction.* Del Mar, Calif.: CRM Books, 1970.

128. Eckelberry, Grace. *Administration of Comprehensive Nursing.* New York: Appleton-Century-Crofts, 1971.

129. Eliason, Eldridge, M.D., L. Kraeer Ferguson, M.D., and Lillian Sholtis, R.N. *Surgical Nursing.* Philadelphia: J. B. Lippincott Co., 1950.

130. Elliott, Frank. *Clinical Neurology.* Philadelphia: W. B. Saunders Co., 1964.

131. Emerson, Charles, and Jane Taylor. *Essentials of Medicine.* Philadelphia: J. B. Lippincott Co., 1950.

132. Engeelberg, Hyman, and Henry F. Greenberg. *The Doctor's Modern Heart Attack Prevention Program.* New York: Funk and Wagnalls, 1974.

133. English, Horace. *Child Psychology.* New York: Henry Holt & Co., 1951.

134. Epp, Theodore. *Why Do Christians Suffer?* Lincoln, Neb.: Good News Broadcasting Assn., Inc., 1970.

135. Erikson, Erik. *Childhood and Society.* New York: W. W. Norton & Co., Inc., 1963.

136. Erven, Lawrence W. *First Aid and Emergency Rescue.* Beverly Hills, Calif.: Glencoe Press, 1970.

137. Fabricant, Noah D., and Groff Conklin. *The Dangerous Cold.* New York: Macmillan Co., 1965.

138. Farley, John, and Howard Mold. *The Teaching Role.* St. Paul, Minn.: College of St. Thomas, 1968.

139. Fast, Julius. *Body Language.* Philadelphia: J. B. Lippincott Co., 1970.

140. Feifel, Herman. *The Meaning of Death.* New York: McGraw-Hill Book Co., 1965.

141. Fink, David. *For People Under Pressure.* New York: Simon and Schuster, 1956.

142. Finnerty, Frank, Jr., and Shirley Motter Linde. *High Blood Pressure.* New York: David McKay, Co., Inc., and Pavilion Publishing Co., Inc., 1975.

143. Fishbein, Anna Mantel. *Modern Woman's Medical Encyclopedia.* Garden City, N.Y.: Doubleday & Co., Inc., 1966.

144. Fishbein, Morris. *The Modern Family Health Guide.* Garden City, N.Y.: Doubleday & Co., Inc., 1967.

145. Fishbein, Morris. *Modern Home Medical Adviser.* Garden City, N.Y.: Doubleday & Co., Inc., 1969.

146. Fitzpatrick, Elise, Sharon Reeder, and Luigi Mastroianni. *Maternity Nursing.* Philadelphia: J. B. Lippincott Co., 1971.

147. Fleming, Mary, and Marion Benson. *Home Nursing Handbook.* Boston: D. C. Heath and Co., 1961.

148. Francis, Gloria, and Barbara Munjas. *Promoting Psychological Comfort.* Dubuque, Iowa: William C. Brown Co., 1968.

149. Fredericks, Carlton. *Nutrition—Your Key to Good Health*. North Hollywood, Calif.: London Press, 1964.

150. Fredericks, Carlton, and Herman Goodman. *Low Blood Sugar and You*. New York: Constellation International, 1969.

151. Freedman, Alfred, and Harold Kaplan. *Comprehensive Textbook of Psychiatry*. Baltimore: Williams & Wilkins Co., 1967.

152. Freeman, Ruth. *Community Health Nursing Practice*. Philadelphia: W. B. Saunders Co., 1970.

153. Freeman, Ruth. *Public Health Nursing Practice*. Philadelphia: W. B. Saunders Co., 1957.

154. French, Ruth. *The Nurse's Guide to Diagnostic Procedures*. New York: McGraw-Hill Book Co., 1971.

155. Frohlich, Edward. *Pathophysiology—Altered Regulatory Mechanism in Disease*. Philadelphia: J. B. Lippincott Co., 1972.

156. Fromm, Erich. *The Art of Loving*. New York: Bantam Books, Inc., 1963.

157. Fromme, Allan. *The Ability to Love*. New York: Farrar, Straus and Giroux, 1963.

158. Fuerst, Elinor, and Lu Verne Wolff. *Fundamentals of Nursing*. Philadelphia: J. B. Lippincott Co., 1969.

159. Galton, Lawrence. *The Silent Disease—Hypertension*. New York: Crown Publishers, Inc., 1973.

160. Ganong, William. *Review of Medical Physiology*. Los Altos, Calif.: Lange Medical Publishers, 1969.

161. Garb, Solomon. *Laboratory Tests in Common Use*. New York: Springer Publishing Co., Inc., 1966, 1971.

162. Gardner, A. Ward, and Peter Roylance. *New Essential First Aid*. Boston: Little, Brown & Co., 1971.

163. Gebbie, Kristine, and Mary Ann Lavin. *Classification of Nursing Diagnosis: Proceedings of the First National Conference*. St. Louis: C. V. Mosby Co., 1975.

164. Gesell, Arnold, and Frances Ilg. *Child Development*. New York: Harper & Brothers, 1949.

165. Gibson, James. *The Perception of the Visual World*. Dallas: Houghton Mifflin Co., 1950.

166. Gifford-Jones. *Hysterectomy*. Toronto: University of Toronto Press, 1961.

167. Gilmer, B. von Haller. *Applied Psychology—Problems in Living and Work*. New York: McGraw-Hill Book Co., 1967.

168. Ginott, Haim. *Between Parent and Child*. New York: Macmillan Co., 1955.

169. Given, Barbara, and Sandra Simmons. *Nursing Care of the Patient With Gastrointestinal Disorders*. St. Louis: C. V. Mosby Co., 1971.

170. Goodale, Raymond. *Clinical Interpretation of Laboratory Tests*. Philadelphia: F. A. Davis Co., 1964, 1969.

171. Goode, William. *The Dynamics of Modern Society*. New York: Atherton Press, 1968.

172. Goodrich, Frederick. *Infant Care*. Englewood Cliffs, N.J.: Prentice-Hall, Inc., 1968.

173. Gordon, David. *Overcoming the Fear of Death*. New York: Macmillan Co., 1970.

174. Gray, J. Stanley. *Psychology Applied to Human Affairs*. New York: McGraw-Hill Book Co., 1954.

175. Gray, Madeline. *The Normal Woman*. New York: Charles Scribner's Sons, 1967.

176. Greenhill, J. P., and Emanuel Friedman. *Biological Principles and Modern Practice of Obstetrics*. Philadelphia: W. B. Saunders Co., 1974.

177. Grenard, Steve, Gustav Beck, and George Rich. *Introduction to Respiratory Therapy—Workbook Study Guide*. New York: Glenn Educational Medical Services, Inc., 1971.

178. Gross, Harry, and Abraham Gezer. *Treatment of Heart Disease*. Philadelphia: W. B. Saunders, 1956.

179. Gruenberg, Sidonie Matsner. *The Encyclopedia of Child Care and Guidance*. New York: Doubleday & Co., Inc., 1954.

180. Guyton, Arthur. *Textbook of Medical Physiology*. Philadelphia: W. B. Saunders Co., 1976.

181. Haas, Albert. *Essentials of Living*

With Pulmonary Emphysema. New York: The Institute of Physical Medicine and Rehabilitation, 1963.

182. Hall, Robert. *Nine Months' Reading.* Garden City, N.Y.: Doubleday & Co., Inc., 1960.

183. Hamilton, James Alexander. *Post Partum Psychiatric Problems.* St. Louis: C. V. Mosby Co., 1962.

184. Hampers, Constatine L., and Eugene Schupak. *Long-Term Hemodialysis.* New York: Grune and Stratton, 1967.

185. Harmer, Bertha. *Textbook of the Principles and Practice of Nursing.* New York: Macmillan Co., 1960.

186. Harvey, A. McGehee, and James Bardley. *Differential Diagnosis.* Philadelphia: W. B. Saunders Co., 1970.

187. Hays, Samhammer Joyce, and Kenneth Larson. *Interacting With Patients.* New York: Macmillan Co., 1965.

188. Head, Henry. *Aphasia and Kindred Disorders of Speech.* London: Hafner Publishing Co., 1963.

189. Heather, Arthur. *Manual of Care for the Disabled Patient.* New York: Macmillan Co., 1960.

190. Heidgerken, Loretta. *Teaching and Learning in Schools of Nursing.* Philadelphia: J. B. Lippincott Co., 1965.

191. Hellman, Louis, and Jack Pritchard. *Williams Obstetrics.* New York: Appleton-Century-Crofts, 1971.

192. Henderson, John. *Emergency Medical Guide.* St Louis: McGraw-Hill Book Co., 1973.

193. Henderson, Virginia. *The Nature of Nursing.* London: Macmillan & Co., 1970.

194. Hess, George. *Living at Your Best With Multiple Sclerosis.* Springfield, Ill.: Charles C Thomas, Publisher, 1962.

195. Hilgard, Ernest. *Introduction to Psychology.* New York: Harcourt, Brace and Co., 1953.

196. Hiltner, Seward, and Karl Menninger. *Constructive Aspects of Anxiety.* New York: Abingdon Press, 1963.

197. Hinsie, Leland, and Robert Campbell. *Psychiatric Dictionary.* New York: Oxford University Press, 1970.

198. Hoff, Ebbe Curtis. *Aspects of Alcoholism.* Philadelphia: J. B. Lippincott Co., 1963.

199. Hofling, Charles, and Madelune Leininger. *Basic Psychiatric Concepts in Nursing.* Philadelphia: J. B. Lippincott Co., 1960, 1967.

200. Holtgrew, Marian. *A Guide for Public Health Nurses Working With Mentally Retarded Children.* Washington, D.C.: U.S. Government Printing Office, 1964.

201. Holvey, David. *The Merck Manual.* Rahway, N.J.: Merck & Co., Inc., 1972.

202. Horney, Karen. *Neurosis and Human Growth.* New York: W. W. Norton & Co., Inc., 1950.

203. Horracks, John. *The Psychology of Adolescence.* Boston: Houghton Mifflin Co., 1962.

204. Hughes, James. *Synopsis of Pediatrics.* St. Louis: C. V. Mosby Co., 1967.

205. Hull, Edgar, and Cecilia Perrodin. *Medical Nursing.* Philadelphia: F. A. Davis Co., 1960.

206. Hunt, Robert. *Personalities and Culture.* New York: Natural History Press, 1967.

207. Hurlock, Elizabeth. *Adolescent Development.* New York: McGraw-Hill Book Co., 1967.

208. Hurlock, Elizabeth. *Child Growth and Development.* New York: McGraw-Hill Book Co., 1970.

209. Hurst, J. Willis, M.D., and R. Bruce Logue. *The Heart.* New York: McGraw-Hill Book Co., 1970.

210. Hurst, J. Willis, M.D., and Robert Schlant, M.D. *Examination of the Heart—Inspection and Palpitation of the Anterior Chest.* New York: American Heart Association, 1967.

211. Illingworth, R. S. *Common Symptoms of Disease in Children.* Philadelphia: F. A. Davis Co., 1969.

212. Illingworth, Ronald and Illingworth, Cynthia. *Babies and Young Children.* London: Churchill Livingston, 1972.

213. Immerman, Harold, and T. Blanchard Dewey. *What Women Want to Know.* New York: Crown Publishers, 1959.

214. Ingalls, A. Jay, and M. Constance Salerno. *Maternal and Child Health Nursing.* St. Louis: C. V. Mosby Co., 1971.

215. Ingram, Madeline. *Principles and Techniques of Psychiatric Nursing.* Philadelphia: W. B. Saunders Co., 1960.

216. Irving, Susan. *Basic Psychiatric Nursing.* Philadelphia: W. B. Saunders Co., 1973.

217. Israel, S. Leon. *Menstrual Disorders and Sterility.* New York: Harper & Row, Publishers, Inc., 1967.

218. Jacob, Stanley, and Clarice Francone. *Laboratory Manual of Structure and Function in Man.* Philadelphia: W. B. Saunders Co., 1970.

219. Jacobson, Edmond. *You Must Relax.* New York: McGraw-Hill Book Co., 1948.

220. Jeans, Philip, Winifred Rand, and Florence Blake. *Essentials of Pediatrics.* London: J. B. Lippincott Co., 1946.

221. Jensen, Deborah. *Sociology and Social Problems.* St. Louis: C. V. Mosby Co., 1947.

222. Johnson, Mae, Mary David, and Mary Bilitch. *Problem Solving in Nursing Practice.* Dubuque, Iowa: William C. Brown Co., 1970.

223. Johnson, Wendell. *Stuttering and What You Can Do About It.* Danville, Ill: The Interstate Printers and Publishers, Inc., 1961.

224. Jones, W. Gifford. *On Being a Woman—The Modern Woman's Guide to Gynecology.* New York: Macmillan Co., 1969.

225. Judge, Richard D., and George D. Zuidema. *Physical Diagnosis: A Physiologic Approach to the Clinical Examination.* Boston: Little, Brown & Co., 1963.

226. Kalmer, John. *Clinical Diagnosis by Laboratory Examination.* New York: Appleton-Century-Crofts, 1961.

227. Kark, Robert, and James Lawrence. *A Primer of Urinalysis.* New York: Harper & Row, Publishers Inc., 1964.

228. Kelly, Lucie Young. *Dimensions of Professional Nursing.* New York: Macmillan Co., 1975.

229. Kempe, C. Henry, Henry K. Silver, and Donough O'Brien. *Current Pediatric Diagnosis and Treatment.* Los Altos, Calif.: Lange Medical Publications, 1970.

230. Kendig, Edwin. *Disorders of the Respiratory Tract in Children.* Philadelphia: W. B. Saunders, 1967.

231. Kendler, Howard. *Basic Psychology.* New York: Appleton-Century-Crofts, 1968.

232. Kennedy, Joseph. *Relax and Live.* Englewood Cliffs, N.J.: Prentice-Hall, Inc., 1961.

233. Kenyon, Herbert. *The Prostate Gland.* New York: Random House, 1970.

234. Kernicki, Jeanette, Barbara Bullock, and Joan Matthews. *Cardiovascular Nursing— Rationale for Therapy and Nursing Approach.* New York: G. P. Putnam's Sons, 1970.

235. Keuhnelian, John, and Virginia Sanders. *Urologic Nursing.* New York: Macmillan Co., 1970.

236. Kilander, H. Fredrick. *Health for Modern Living.* Englewood Cliffs, N.J.: Prentice-Hall, Inc., 1957.

237. Kirk, Samuel, Merle Karnes, and Winifred Kirk. *You and Your Retarded Child.* Palo Alto, Calif.: Pacific Books Publishers, 1965.

238. Klee, James. *Problems of Selective Behavior.* Lincoln, Neb.: University of Nebraska, 1951.

239. Knight, James. *Conscience and Guilt.* New York: Appleton-Century-Crofts, 1969.

240. Koas, Earl. *The Sociology of the Patient.* New York: McGraw-Hill Book Co., 1959.

241. Kordels, Lelord. *Natural Folk Remedies.* New York: G. P. Putnam's Sons, 1974.

242. Kozier, Barbara, and Beverly DuGas. *Fundamentals of Patient Care.* Philadelphia: W. B. Saunders Co., 1968.

243. Kraus, Hans. *Backache—Stress and Tension.* New York: Simon and Schuster, 1965.

244. Krause, Marie. *Food, Nutrition and Diet Therapy.* Philadelphia: W. B. Saunders Co., 1966.

245. Kroger, William. *Psychosomatic Obstetrics, Gynecology and Endocrinology.* Springfield, Ill.:

Charles C Thomas Publisher, 1962.

246. Krug, Elsie, and Hugh McGuigan. *An Introduction to Materia Medica and Pharmacology*. St. Louis: C. V. Mosby Co., 1951.

247. Krupp, Marcus, and Milton Chatton. *Current Diagnosis and Treatment*. Los Altos, Calif.: Lange Medical Publications, 1973.

248. Kubler-Ross, Elizabeth. *On Death and Dying*. New York: Macmillan Co., 1970.

249. Laing, J. Ellsworth, and Joyce Harvey. *The Management and Nursing of Burns*. London: English Universities Press, 1967.

250. Lally, James. *The Over 50 Health Manual*. Englewood Cliffs, N.J.: Prentice-Hall, Inc., 1961.

251. Lamb, Lawrence. *Your Heart and How to Live With It*. New York: Viking Press, 1969.

252. Lara, Dorothy, and Lucille Gidseg. *The Home Nurse's Handbook*. New York: Wilfred Funk Inc., 1951.

253. Larson, Carroll, and Marjorie Gould. *Orthopedic Nursing*. St. Louis: C. V. Mosby Co., 1970.

254. Lascelles, P. T., and D. Donaldson. *Diagnostic Tests*. New York: G. P. Putnam's Sons, 1971.

255. Lehner, George, and Ella Kube. *The Dynamics of Personal Adjustment*. New York: Prentice-Hall Inc., 1955.

256. Lekoff, William, Bernard Segal, and Lawrence Galton. *Your Heart*. Philadelphia: J. B. Lippincott Co., 1972.

257. Lennard, Henry, Leon Epstein, Arnold Bernstein, and Donald Ransom. *Mystification and Drug Abuse*. San Francisco: Jossey-Bass Inc., 1971.

258. Lerch, Constance. *Maternity Nursing*. St. Louis: C. V. Mosby Co., 1974.

259. Lesnik, Milton, and Bernice Anderson. *Nursing Practice and the Law*. Philadelphia: J. B. Lippincott Co., 1955, 1969.

260. Levitt, Eugene, and Karl Meninger. *The Psychology of Anxiety*. New York: Bobbs-Merril Co., Inc., 1967.

261. Lewis, Lucile. *Planning Patient Care*. Dubuque, Iowa: William C. Brown Co., 1970.

262. Lidz, Theodore. *The Person—His Development Throughout the Life Cycle*. New York: Basic Books, 1968.

263. Lindgren, Henry Clay. *Meaning: Antidote to Anxiety*. New York: Thomas Nelson and Sons, 1956.

264. Lipkin, Gladys, and Robert Cohen. *Effective Approaches to Patient's Behavior*. New York: Springer Publishing Co., Inc., 1973.

265. Little, Dolores, and Doris Carnevali. *Nursing Care Planning*. Philadelphia: J. B. Lippincott Co., 1969.

266. Louria, Donald. *Overcoming Drugs*. New York: McGraw-Hill Book Co., 1971.

267. Louria, Donald. *The Drug Scene*. New York: McGraw-Hill Book Co., 1968.

268. Lowsley, Oswald, and Thomas Kirwin. *Clinical Urology*. Vol. II. Baltimore: Williams & Wilkins Co., 1956.

269. Luce, Gay Gaer, and Julius Segal. *Insomnia—The Guide for Troubled Sleepers*. Garden City, N.Y.: Doubleday & Co., Inc., 1969.

270. Luce, Gay Gaer, and Julius Segal. *Sleep*. New York: Coward-McCann, Inc., 1966.

271. Lyght, Charles. *The Merck Manual of Diagnosis and Therapy*. Rahway, N.J.: Merck & Co., Inc., 1956.

272. Lynch, Matthew, Stanley Raphael, Leslie Mellon, Peter Sparc, and Martin Inwood. *Medical Laboratory Technology and Clinical Pathology*. Philadelphia: W. B. Saunders Co., 1969.

273. Lysaught, Jerome P. *An Abstract for Action*. St. Louis: McGraw-Hill Book Co., 1970.

274. MacBryde, Cyril M. *Signs and Symptoms—Applied Pathologic Physiology and Clinical Interpretation*. Philadelphia: J. B. Lippincott Co., 1964.

275. McCary, J. L. *Psychology of Personality*. New York: Logas Press, 1956.

276. McClain, M. Esther, and Shirley Gragg. *Scientific Principles in Nursing*. St. Louis: C. V. Mosby Co., 1962.

277. McDonald, Linda. *Contact Lenses: How to Wear Them Successfully.* Garden City, N.Y.: Doubleday & Co., Inc., 1972.

278. McKinney, Fred. *Psychology of Personal Adjustment.* New York: John Wiley & Sons, Inc., 1941.

279. Magda, Arnold. *Emotion and Personality.* Volume I. New York: Columbia University Press, 1960.

280. Mager, Robert F. *Preparing Instructional Objectives.* Palo Alto, Calif.: Fearon Publishers, 1962.

281. Maier, Norman. *Frustration—The Study of Behavior Without a Goal.* New York: McGraw-Hill Book Co., 1949.

282. Maloney, Elizabeth. *Interpersonal Relations.* Dubuque, Iowa: William C. Brown Co., 1966.

283. Maltz, Maxwell. *Creative Living for Today.* New York: Pocket Books, 1970.

284. Maltz, Maxwell. *Psycho-Cybernetics.* Englewood Cliffs, N.J.: Prentice-Hall Inc., 1960.

285. Manfreda, Marguerite. *Psychiatric Nursing.* Philadelphia: F. A. Davis Co., 1968.

286. Marlow, Dorothy. *Textbook of Pediatric Nursing.* Philadelphia: W. B. Saunders Co., 1973.

287. Marlow, Dorothy, and Gladys Sellew. *Textbook of Pediatric Nursing.* Philadelphia: W. B. Saunders Co., 1961.

288. Maroon, Joseph. *What You Can Do About Cancer.* Garden City, N.Y.: Doubleday & Co., Inc., 1969.

289. Marriner, Ann. *The Nursing Process.* St. Louis: C. V. Mosby Co., 1975.

290. Marvin, H. M. *Your Heart.* Garden City, N.Y.: Doubleday & Co., Inc., 1960.

291. Mash, Jean Bulger, and Margaret Dickens. *Armstrong and Browder's Nursing Care of Children.* Philadelphia: F. A. Davis Co., 1970.

292. Maslow, Abraham. *Motivation and Personality.* New York: Harper & Brothers, 1954.

293. Matheney, Ruth, Breda Nolan, Alice Hogan, and Gerald Griffin. *Fundamentals of Patient-Centered Nursing.* St. Louis: C. V. Mosby Co., 1972.

294. May, Rollo. *Psychology and the Human Dilemma.* Princeton, N.J.: D. Van Nostrand Co., Inc., 1966.

295. May, Rollo. *The Meaning of Anxiety.* New York: Ronald Press, 1950.

296. Mayers, Marlene Glover. *A Systematic Approach to the Nursing Care Plan.* New York: Appleton-Century-Crofts, 1972.

297. Meares, Ainslie. *Relief Without Drugs.* Garden City, N.Y.: Doubleday & Co., Inc., 1967.

298. Meares, Ainslie. *The Management of the Anxious Patient.* Philadelphia: W. B. Saunders Co., 1963.

299. Megargie, Edwin, and Jack Hokanson. *The Dynamics of Aggression.* New York: Harper & Row, Publishers, Inc., 1970.

300. Meltzer, Lawrence, Faye Abdellah, and Roderick Kitchell. *Concepts and Practices of Intensive Care for Nurse Specialists.* Philadelphia: Charles Press, 1970.

301. Meltzer, Lawrence, Rose Pinneo, and Roderick Kitchell. *Intensive Coronary Care—A Manual for Nurses.* Philadelphia: Charles Press, 1968.

302. Menard, Richard. *Introduction to Arrhythmia Recognition.* San Francisco: California Heart Association, 1968.

303. Meng, H. C., and David Law. *Parenteral Nutrition.* Springfield, Ill.: Charles C Thomas, Publisher, 1970.

304. Miller, Ashton, W. Slade, and H. M. Leather. *A Synopsis of Renal Diseases and Urology.* Great Britain: John Wright and Sons, 1966.

305. Miller, Benjamin, and Lawrence Galton. *The Family Book of Preventive Medicine.* New York: Simon and Schuster, 1971.

306. Miller, Benjamin, Lawrence Galton, and Daniel Brunner. *Freedom From Heart Attacks.* New York: Simon and Schuster, 1972.

307. Miller, Robert. *How to Live With a Heart Attack.* Radnor, Pa.: Chilton Book Company, 1971.

308. Mitchell, J. B. *Urology for Nurses.* Great Britain: John Wright and Sons, 1965, 1969.

309. Mitchell, Helen, Henderika Ryn-

bergen, Linnea Anderson, and Marjorie Dibble. *Cooper's Nutrition in Health and Disease*. Philadelphia: J. B. Lippincott Co., 1968.

310. Mitford, Jessica. *The American Way of Death*. New York: Simon and Schuster, 1963.

311. Modell, Walter, and Doris Schwartz. *Handbook of Cardiology for Nurses*. New York: Springer Publishing Co., Inc., 1958.

312. Moidel, Harriet, Gladys Sorensen, Elizabeth Giblin, and Margaret Kaufmann. *Nursing Care of the Patient With Medical-Surgical Disorders*. New York: McGraw-Hill Book Co., 1971.

313. Molloy, Julia. *Teaching the Retarded Child to Talk*. New York: John Day Company, 1961.

314. Moncrieff, R. W. *The Chemical Senses*. New York: John Wiley & Sons, Inc., 1944.

315. Montag, Mildred, and Ruth Swenson. *Fundamentals in Nursing Care*. Philadelphia: W. B. Saunders Co., 1959.

316. Morgan, William, and George Engel. *The Clinical Approach to the Patient*. Philadelphia: W. B. Saunders Co., 1969.

317. Morressey, Alice. *Rehabilitation Nursing*. New York: G. P. Putnam's Sons, 1951.

318. Mosby, C. V. Company. *Mosby's Comprehensive Review of Nursing*. St. Louis: C. V. Mosby Co., 1951.

318a. Mowbray, A. Q. *The Transplant*. New York: David McKay Co., Inc., 1974.

319. Mullan, Sean. *Essentials of Neurosurgery*. New York: Springer Publishing Co., Inc., 1961.

320. Mullen, Robert. *The Latter-Day Saints: The Mormons Yesterday and Today*. Garden City N.Y.: Doubleday & Co., Inc., 1966.

321. Murchison, Irene, and Thomas Nichols. *Legal Foundations of Nursing Practice*. London: Macmillan & Co., 1970.

322. Murray, Ruth, and Judith Zenter. *Nursing Concepts for Health Promotion*. Englewood Cliffs, N.J.: Prentice-Hall, Inc., 1975.

323. Neilson, William. *Webster's New International Dictionary*. Springfield, Mass.: G. & C. Merriam Co., 1950.

324. Nelson, Waldo, Victor Vaughn, and R. James McKay. *Textbook of Pediatrics*. Philadelphia: W. B. Saunders Co., 1969.

325. Nordmark, Madelyn, and Anne Rohweder. *Scientific Foundations of Nursing*. Philadelphia: J. B. Lippincott Co., 1967.

326. Nordmark, Madelyn, and Anne Rohweder. *Scientific Principles Applied to Nursing*. Philadelphia: J. B. Lippincott Co., 1959.

327. Northrup, Eric. *Science Looks at Smoking*. New York: Coward-McCann Inc., 1957.

328. Nose, Yukihiko. *The Artificial Kidney*. Volume I. St. Louis: C. V. Mosby Co., 1969.

329. Nosow, Sigmund, and William Form. *Man, Work and Society*. New York: Basic Books, 1962.

330. Novak, Edmund, and J. Donald Woodruff. *Gynecologic and Obstetric Pathology*. Philadelphia: W. B. Saunders Co., 1962.

331. Noyes, Arthur P., William P. Camp, and Mildred Van Sickel. *Psychiatric Nursing*. New York: Macmillan Co., 1964.

332. Nurenberg, Gerard, and Henry Calero. *How to Read a Person Like a Book*. New York: Hawthorn Books Inc., 1971.

333. Ochsner, Alton. *Smoking—Your Choice Between Life and Death*. New York: Simon and Schuster, 1970.

334. Odlum, Doris. *Mental Health, the Nurse and the Patient*. Philadelphia: J. B. Lippincott Co., 1960.

335. O'Hara, Frank, and Herman Reith. *Psychology and the Nurse*. Philadelphia: W. B. Saunders Co., 1966.

336. Olson-Dorland, W. A. *A Reference Handbook and Dictionary of Nursing*. Philadelphia: W. B. Saunders, 1960.

337. Orton, Samuel Torrey. *Reading, Writing and Speech Problems in Children*. New York: W. W. Norton & Co., Inc., 1964.

338. Page, Irvine H. *Strokes*. New York: E. P. Dutton & Co., Inc., 1961.

339. Papper, Solomon. *Clinical Nephrol-*

ogy. Boston: Little, Brown & Co., 1971.

340. Parker, Elizabeth. *The Seven Ages of Woman.* Baltimore: Johns Hopkins Press, 1967.

341. Patton, Edwin. *Pediatric Index.* St. Louis: C. V. Mosby Co., 1958.

342. Peale, Norman Vincent. *A Guide to Confident Living.* Greenwich, Conn.: Fawcett Publications, Inc., 1948.

343. Peale, Norman Vincent. *Stay Alive All Your Life.* Greenwich, Conn.: Fawcett Publications, Inc., 1957.

344. Peplau, Hildegard. *Aspects of Psychiatric Nursing: Therapeutic Concepts.* New York: National League for Nursing, 1957.

345. Peyton, Alice. *Practical Nutrition.* Philadelphia: J. B. Lippincott Co., 1957.

346. Phillips, Raymond, and Mary Feeney. *The Cardiac Rhythms.* Philadelphia: W. B. Saunders Co., 1973.

347. Pirenne, M. H. *Vision and the Eye.* London: Chapman and Hall, Ltd., 1967.

348. Pitorak, Elizabeth, Carolyn Hudak, Joan O'Gureck, and Patricia Hanusz. *Nurses Guide to Cardiac Surgery and Nursing Care.* New York: McGraw-Hill Book Co., 1971.

349. Porter, Joseph. *Stamford Curriculum Guide for Drug Abuse Education.* Chicago: J. G. Ferguson Publishing Co., 1971.

350. Price, Alice. *The Art, Science and Spirit of Nursing.* Philadelphia: W. B. Saunders Co., 1965.

351. Prior, John, and Jack Silberstein. *Physical Diagnosis.* St. Louis: C. V. Mosby Co., 1959.

352. Race, George. *Laboratory Medicine.* Volume I. New York: Harper & Row, Publishers, Inc., 1973.

353. Rapaport, Howard G., and Shirley Motter Linde. *The Complete Allergy Guide.* New York: Simon and Schuster, 1970.

354. Ratner, Herbert. *The Womanly Art of Breastfeeding.* Franklin Park, Ill.: La Leche League International, 1969.

355. Ravin, Abe. *Cardiac Auscultation—An Audio Presentation.*

Philadelphia: Merck, Sharp, and Dohme, 1969.

356. Redman, Barbara Klug. *The Process of Patient Teaching in Nursing.* St. Louis: C. V. Mosby Co., 1968.

357. Reeder, Sharon, Luis Mastroianni, Jr., Leonide L. Martin, and Elsie Fitzpatrick. *Maternity Nursing.* Philadelphia: J. B. Lippincott, 1976.

358. Regnier, Edme. *There Is a Cure for the Common Cold.* New York: Parker Publishing Co., Inc., 1971.

359. Reich, Nathaniel, and Rudolph Fremont. *Chest Pain—Systematic Differentiation and Treatment.* New York: Macmillan Co., 1961.

360. Render, Helena, and M. Olga Weiss. *Nurse Patient Relationships in Psychiatry.* New York: McGraw-Hill Book Co., 1959.

361. Robinson, Corinne. *Proudfit-Robinson's Normal and Therapeutic Nutrition.* New York: Macmillan Co., 1967.

362. Rodman, Morton J., and Dorothy Smith. *Pharmacology and Drug Therapy in Nursing.* Philadelphia: J. B. Lippincott Co., 1968.

363. Roeske, Nancy, Clare Assue, Richard French, and Toner Overley. *Examination of the Personality.* Philadelphia: Lea and Febiger, 1972.

364. Rogers, Carl. *Client-Centered Therapy.* Boston: Houghton Mifflin Co., 1951.

365. Rothweiler, Ella L., and Jean Martin White. *The Art and Science of Nursing.* Philadelphia: F. A. Davis Co., 1950.

366. Rothweiler, Ella, Jean White, and Doris Geitgey. *The Art and Science of Nursing.* Philadelphia: F. A. Davis Co., 1959.

367. Rubinstein, Max. *You and Your Hormones.* New York: Twayne Publishers, 1960.

368. Ruslink, Doris. *Family Health and Home Nursing.* New York: Macmillan Co., 1963.

369. Sammis, Florence Eastly. *The Allergic Patient and His World.* Springfield, Ill.: Charles C Thomas, Publishers, 1953.

370. Sanford, Nevitt. *Self and Society.*

New York: Atherton Press, 1966.

371. Sarason, Irwin. *Personality An Objective Approach.* New York: John Wiley & Sons, Inc., 1967.

372. Sartain, A. O., A. J. North, J. R. Strange, and H. M. Chapman. *Understanding Human Behavior.* Dallas: Southern Methodist University Press, 1955.

373. Saxton, Dolores F., and Phyllis W. Haring. *Care of Patients With Emotional Problems.* St. Louis: C. V. Mosby Co., 1971.

374. Sawyer, Janet. *Nursing Care of Patients With Urologic Diseases.* St. Louis: C. V. Mosby Co., 1963.

375. Schindler, John. *How to Live 365 Days a Year.* Englewood Cliffs, N.J.: Prentice-Hall, Inc., 1956.

376. Schmidt, Jacob. *Attorneys' Dictionary of Medicine and Word Finder.* New York: Matthew Bender & Co., Inc., 1962. Cumulative Supplement and Revision, May 1975.

377. Scholz, Ray. *Sight—A Handbook for Laymen.* Garden City, N.Y.: Doubleday & Co., Inc., 1960.

378. Schultz, Duane. *Sensory Restriction.* New York: Academic Press, 1965.

379. Schwartz, Herman. *The Art of Relaxation.* New York: Thomas Crowell Co., 1954.

380. Seyle, Hans. *The Stress of Life.* New York: McGraw-Hill Book Co., 1956.

381. Shafer, Kathleen, Janet Sawyer, Audrey McCluskey, and Edna Lifgren. *Medical Surgical Nursing.* St. Louis: C. V. Mosby Co., 1958.

382. Sharp, LaVaughn, and Beatrice Rabin. *Nursing in the Coronary Care Unit.* Philadelphia: J. B. Lippincott Co., 1970.

383. Sheen, Fulton. *Peace of Soul.* New York: Image Books, 1949.

384. Sherman, Henry, and Caroline Lanford. *Essentials of Nutrition.* New York: Macmillan Co., 1957.

385. Shipp, Thomas. *Helping the Alcoholic and His Family.* Englewood Cliffs, N.J.: Prentice Hall, Inc., 1963.

386. Shires, G. Tom, and Charles R. Baxter. *Care of the Trauma Patient.* New York: McGraw-Hill Book Co., 1966, Chapter 13.

387. Shires, G. Tom, and Robert McClelland. *Care of the Trauma Patient.* New York: McGraw-Hill Book Co., 1966, Chapter 38.

388. Simonson, Josephine. *According to the Aphasic Adult.* Dallas: University of Texas Medical School, 1971.

389. Slavson, S. R. *An Introduction to Group Therapy.* New York: Oxford University Press, 1943.

390. Smith, Christine. *Maternal-Child Nursing.* Philadelphia: W. B. Saunders Co., 1963.

391. Smith, Dorothy, Carol Germain, and Claudia Gips. *Care of the Adult Patient—Medical-Surgical Nursing.* Philadelphia: J. B. Lippincott Co., 1971.

392. Smith, Henry Clay. *Sensitivity to People.* New York: McGraw-Hill Book Co., 1966.

393. Smith, Henry Clay. *Personality Development.* New York: McGraw-Hill Book Co., 1968.

394. Smithers, R. Brinkley. *Biochemical and Nutritional Aspects of Alcoholism.* New York: Clayton Foundation Biochemical Institute, 1964.

395. Sodeman, William. *Pathologic Physiology.* Philadelphia: W. B. Saunders Co., 1950.

396. Southard, Samuel. *Religion and Nursing.* Nashville, Tenn.: Broadman Press, 1959.

397. Spencer, Marietta. *Blind Children—In Family and Community.* Minneapolis: University of Minnesota Press, 1960.

398. Spencer, Roberta T. *Patient Care in Endocrine Problems.* Philadelphia: W. B. Saunders, 1973.

399. Spielberger, Charles. *Anxiety and Behavior.* New York: Academic Press, 1966.

400. Spock, Benjamin, Dr. *Baby and Child Care.* New York: Meredith Press, 1968.

401. Stagner, Ross. *Psychology of Personality.* New York: McGraw-Hill Book Co., 1937.

402. Steele, Harold, and Charles Crow. *High Blood Pressure—Cholesterol and You.* Huntsville, Ala.: Strode Publishers, 1969.

403. Stein, Edward. *Guilt: Theory and Therapy.* Philadelphia: Westminister Press, 1969.

404. Steincrohn, Peter. *How to Get a Good Night's Sleep*. Chicago: Henry Regnery Company, 1968.

405. Stevenson, George. *Mental Health Planning for Social Action*. New York: McGraw-Hill Book Co., 1956.

406. Stevenson, Ian. *The Psychiatric Examination*. Boston: Little, Brown & Co., 1969.

407. Stone, Joseph L., and Joseph Church. *Childhood and Adolescence*. New York: Random House, 1957.

408. Storlie, Francis. *Principles of Intensive Nursing Care*. New York: Appleton-Century-Crofts, 1969.

409. Strang, Ruth. *Helping Your Child Develop His Potentialities*. New York: E. P. Dutton & Co., Inc., 1965.

410. Sutton, Audrey. *Bedside Nursing Technique*. Philadelphia: W. B. Saunders Co., 1969.

411. Sutton, Audrey. *Bedside Nursing Techniques in Medicine and Surgery*. Philadelphia: W. B. Saunders Co., 1964.

412. Sutton, Maurice. *Cancer Explained*. New York: Hart Publishing Co., Inc., 1966.

413. Swartz, Harry. *The Allergy Guide Book*. New York: Frederick Unger Publishing Co., 1961.

414. Taber, Clarence. *Taber's Cyclopedic Medical Dictionary*. Worchester, Mass.: F. A. Davis Publications, Inc., 1975.

415. Terman, Lewis, and Catharine Cox Miles. *Sex and Personality*. New York: McGraw-Hill Book Co., 1936.

416. Terry, Florence, Gladys Benz, Dorothy Mereness, and Frank Kleffner. *Principles and Technics of Rehabilitation Nursing*. St. Louis: C. V. Mosby Co., 1961.

417. Thompson, Edward, and Adaline Hayden. *Standard Nomenclature of Diseases and Operations*. New York: McGraw-Hill Book Co., 1969.

418. Thompson, George. *Child Psychology*. Boston: Houghton Mifflin Co., 1952.

419. Thompson, Lloyd. *Reading Disability—Developmental Dyslexia*. Springfield, Ill.: Charles C Thomas, Publisher, 1966.

420. Toch, Hans. *Violent Men—An Inquiry Into the Psychology of Violence*. Chicago: Aldine Publishing Co., 1969.

421. Toole, James. *Diagnosis and Management of Stroke*. New York: American Heart Association, 1968.

422. Townsend, Carolynn. *Nutrition and Diet Modification for the Nurse*. New York: Delmar Publishers, Inc., 1966.

423. Travelbee, Joyce. *Interpersonal Aspects of Nursing*. Philadelphia: F. A. Davis Co., 1966.

424. United States Department of Health, Education and Welfare. *International Classification of Diseases*. Eighth Revision. Volume I. National Center for Health Statistics.

425. U.S. Department of Health, Education and Welfare. *Nursing Problem Classification for Children and Youth*. Rockville, Md., 1976.

426. Vail, Derrick. *The Truth About Your Eyes*. New York: Farrar, Straus and Cudahy, 1959.

427. Van Riper, Charles. *Your Child's Speech Problems*. New York: Harper & Row, Publishers, Inc., 1961.

428. Vaughn, Daniel, Robert Cook, and Asbury Taylor. *General Ophthalmology*. Los Altos, Calif.: Lange Medical Publications, 1965.

429. Victor, Diana. *Care of the Maternity Patient*. New York: McGraw-Hill Book Co., 1971.

430. Wagman, Richard and J. G. Ferguson. *The New Concise Family Health and Medical Guide*. Chicago: J. G. Ferguson Publishing Co. Distributed by Doubleday & Co., Inc., 1972.

431. Wallace, Margaret Ann Jaeger. *Handbook of Child Nursing Care*. New York: John Wiley & Sons, Inc., 1971.

432. Watson, Jeannette. *Medical-Surgical Nursing and Related Physiology*. Philadelphia: W. B. Saunders Co., 1972.

433. Watson, Robert. *Psychology of the Child*. New York: John Wiley & Sons, Inc., 1965.

434. Wayler, Thelma, and Rose Klein. *Applied Nutrition*. New York: Macmillan Co., 1965.

435. Weed, Lawrence. *Medical Records, Medical Education, and Patient Care.* Chicago: Case Western Reserve University Press, 1971.

436. Weinberg, George. *The Action Approach.* New York: World Publishing Co., 1969.

437. Weisenburg, Theodore, and Katherine McBride. *Aphasia.* New York: Oxford University Press, 1935.

438. Weller, Charles, and Brian Boylan. *How to Live With Hypoglycemia.* Garden City, N.Y.: Doubleday & Co., 1968.

439. Weller, Charles, and Brian Boylan. *The New Way to Live With Diabetes.* Garden City, N.Y.: Doubleday and Co., 1966.

440. Wells, H. G. *The Anatomy of Frustration.* New York: Macmillan Co., 1936.

441. Wenar, Charles. *Personality Development.* Boston: Houghton Mifflin Co., 1971.

442. Wepman, Joseph M. *Asphasia and the Family.* New York: American Heart Association, 1969.

443. Wepman, Joseph M. *Recovery From Aphasia.* New York: Ronald Press, 1951.

444. White, Dorothy, Edith Rubino, and Philip DeLorey. *Fundamentals: The Foundation of Nursing.* Englewood Cliffs, N.J.: Prentice-Hall, Inc., 1972.

445. Whitehead, Sylvia. *Nursing Care of the Adult Urology Patient.* New York: Appleton-Century-Crofts, 1970.

446. Widenbach, Ernestine. *Family-Centered Maternity Nursing.* New York: G. P. Putnam's Sons, 1958.

447. Wiebe, Anne. *Orthopedics in Nursing.* Philadelphia: W. B. Saunders Co., 1961.

448. Wiggins, Jerry, Edward Renner, Gerald Clare, and Richard Rose. *The Psychology of Personality.* Reading, Mass.: Addison-Wesley Publishing Co., 1971.

449. Wilson, Eva, Katherine Fisher, and Mary Fuqua. *Principles of Nutrition.* New York: John Wiley & Sons, Inc., 1966.

450. Wilson, J. Robert, Clayton Beechan, and Elsie Reid Carrington. *Obstetrics and Gynecology.* St. Louis: C. V. Mosby Co., 1971.

451. Winter, Chester, and Marilyn Roehm. *Sawyer's Nursing Care of Patients With Urologic Diseases.* St. Louis: C. V. Mosby Co., 1968.

452. Winter, Ruth. *Do You Have Sinus Trouble?* New York: Grosset & Dunlap, 1973.

453. Wintrobe, M. M., George Thorn, Raymond Adams, Ivan Bennett, Eugene Braunwald, Kurt Isselbacher, and Robert Petersdorf. *Harrison's Principles of Internal Medicine.* New York: McGraw-Hill Book Co., 1971.

454. Wood, Lucile A. *Nursing Skills for Allied Health Services.* Volumes 1–3. Philadelphia: W. B. Saunders Co., 1975.

455. Wretlind, A. *Complete Intravenous Nutrition.* Switzerland: Ludin, Liestel, A. G., 1972.

456. Wright, Milton. *The Art of Conversation.* New York: McGraw-Hill Book Co., 1936.

457. Yacorzynski, George. *Medical Psychology.* New York: Ronald Press, 1951.

458. Young, Kimball. *Personality and Problems of Adjustment.* New York: F. S. Crofts and Co., 1941.

459. Yura, Helen, and Mary Walsh. *The Nursing Process.* Washington, D.C.: Catholic University of America Press, Inc., 1971.

460. Zabriskie, Louise, and N. J. Eastman. *Nurses' Handbook of Obstetrics.* Philadelphia: J. B. Lippincott Co., 1952.

461. Ziegel, Erna, and Carolyn Van Blarcom. *Obstetric Nursing.* New York: Macmillan Co., 1972.

462. Zubek, John P. *Sensory Deprivation: Fifteen Years of Research.* New York: Appleton-Century-Crofts, 1969.

ARTICLES

463. Alexander, Leo, M. D. "Differential Diagnosis Between Psychogenic and Physical Pain." *Journal of American Medical Association* (September 8, 1962), 149–155.

464. Anderson, Bernice. "Legal Aspects of Nursing Care for Cardiac Patients." *Cardiovascular Nursing,* Vol. 5, No. 2 (March–April 1969), 5–7.

465. Baer, Eva, Lois Jean Davitz, and

Renee Lieb. "Inferences of Physical Pain." *Nursing Research*, Vol., 19, No. 5 (September–October 1970), 388–401.

466. Baker, J. B., and H. Merskey. "Pain in General Practice." *Journal of Psychosomatic Residence*, Vol. 10 (1967), 383–387.

467. Barnard, Jan. "Understanding and Treating the Patient in Pain." *R.N. Magazine* (May 1967), 73–75.

468. Baxter, Charles, R. P. William Curreri, and Janet A. Marvin. "The Control of Burn Wound Sepsis by the Use of Quantitative Bacteriologic Studies and Sebeschar Clysis With Antibiotics." *Surgical Clinics of North America*, Vol. 53 (December 1973), 1509–1517.

469. Bayless, Colin E., et al. "The Pacemaker—Twiddler's Syndrome: A New Complication of Implantable Transvenous Pacemakers." *Canadian Medical Association Journal* (August 24, 1968), 371–373.

470. Beecher, Henry, M.D. "The Powerful Placebo." *Journal of American Medical Association* (December 24, 1955), 1602–1606.

471. Benjamin, Harry, and Charles Ihlenfeld. "Transsexualism." *American Journal of Nursing* (March 1973), 457–461.

472. Berry, Margaret, and Colette Kerlin. "The Drops of Life: Fluids and Electrolytes." *R. N. Magazine*, Vol., 33, No. 9. (September 1970), 35–67.

473. Betson, Carol. "Blood Gases." *American Journal of Nursing* (May 1968), 1010–1012.

474. Billars, Karen. "You Have Pain? I Think This Will Help." *American Journal of Nursing*, Vol. 70, No, 10 (October 1970), 2143–2145.

475. Billing, Dorothy. "Nursing Care of Patients With Mechanical Cardiac Pacemakers." *Nursing Clinics of North America*, Vol. 7, No. 3 (September 1972), 509–515.

476. Blaylock, Jerry. "Nursing Functions and the Tradition of Nursing." *The Bulletin—Texas Nurses Association* (October 1970), 8–11.

477. Blaylock, Jerry. "The Psychological and Cultural Influences on the Reaction to Pain." *Nursing Forum*, Vol. 7, No. 3 (1968), 263–274.

478. Bloom, Judith. "Problem Oriented Charting." *American Journal of Nursing*, Vol. 19 (November 1971), 2144–2148.

479. Bonkowsky, Marilyn. "Adapting the POMR to Community Child Health Care." *Nursing Outlook* (August 1972), 515–518.

480. Brabenstetter, Joan. "Synthetic Fat Helps Prevent Pressure Sores." *American Journal of Nursing* (July 1968), 1521.

481. Bruegel, Mary Ann. "Relationship of Preoperative Anxiety to Perception of Post Operative Pain." *Nursing Research*, Vol. 20, No. 1 (January–February 1971), 26–31.

482. Burnell, A. W. "Bedsore Control and a Multipurpose Mattress." *The American Journal of Australia* (November 1969), 958–960.

483. Busse, Ewald. "How to Handle Problems of Aging." *Today's Health* (July 1969), 28–31, 58.

484. Campbell, Margaret. "Identifying Nursing Problems." *Canadian Nurse* (February 1965), 96–99.

485. Carbeil, Madeline. "Nursing Process for a Patient With a Body Image Disturbance." *Nursing Clinics of North America*, Vol. 6, No. 1 (March 1971), 155–163.

486. Chambers, Wilda. "Nursing Diagnosis." *American Journal of Nursing* (November 1962), 102–104.

487. Chernov, Merrill, Harry Hale, and MacDonald Wood. "Prevention of Stress Ulcers." *The American Journal of Surgery*, Vol. 122 (November 1971), 674–677.

488. Clark, Nancy Fairchild. "Pump Failure." *Nursing Clinics of North America*, Vol. 7, No. 3 (September 1972), 529–539.

489. Dallas Times Herald. "Doctor Offers These Tips on Conquering Jet Lag." *Dallas Times Herald*, Section J7 (August 22, 1976), 1.

490. Davis, Anne. "The Skills of Communication." *American Journal of Nursing* (January 1963), 66–70.

491. Davis, Barbara. "Until Death Ensues." *Nursing Clinics of North America*, Vol. 7, No. 2 (June 1972), 303–309.

492. Drew, Frances, Richard Moriarity, and Alvin Shapiro. "An Approach to the Measurement of the Pain and Anxiety Response of Surgical Patients." *Psychosomatic Medicine*, Vol. 30, No. 6 (1948), 826–836.

493. Durand, Mary, and Rosemary Prince. "Nursing Diagnosis: Process and Decision." *Nursing Forum*, Vol. 5, No. 4 (1966), 50 64.

494. Engel, George. "Grief and Grieving." *American Journal of Nursing* (September 1964), 93–98.

495. Farnsworth, Dana L. "Pain and the Individual." *The New England Journal of Medicine*, Vol. 254, No. 12 (March 22, 1956), 559–562.

496. Fellows, Barbara. "Hemodialysis at Home." *American Journal of Nursing*, Vol. 66 (August 1966), 1775–1778.

497. Foley, Mary F. "Air Travel for Patients." *American Journal of Nursing* (June 1973), 1020–1023.

498. Gadboys, H. L., et al. "Long-Term Follow-up of Patients With Cardiac Pacemakers." *American Journal of Cardiology* (January 1968), 55–59.

499. Garrison, Webb. "Pain: Your Body's Early Warning System." *Today's Health* (October 1969), 29–66.

500. Gebbie, Kristine, and Mary Ann Lavin. "Classifying Nursing Diagnosis." *American Journal of Nursing*, Vol. 74 (February 1974), 250–253.

501. Golub, Sharon. "Recognizing the Drug Abuser." *R. N. Magazine* (July 1969), 44–45.

502. Graffam, Shirley R. "Nurse Response to the Patient in Distress—Development of an Instrument." *Nursing Research*, Vol. 19, No. 4 (July–August 1970), 331–336.

503. Grant, Jo Ann Nallinger. "Patient Care in Parenteral Hyperalimentation." *Nursing Clinics of North America*, Vol. 8, No. 1 (March 1973), 165–181.

504. Gregg, Dorothy. "Reassurance." *American Journal of Nursing* (February 1955), 171–173.

505. Haferkorn, Virginia. "Assessing Individual Learning Needs as a Basis for Patient Teaching." *Nursing Clinics of North America*, Vol. 6, No. 1 (March 1971), 199–209.

506. Hamdi, Mary, and Carol Hutelmyer. "A Study of the Effectiveness of an Assessment Tool in the Identification of Nursing Care Problems." *Nursing Research*, Vol. 19 (July–August 1970), 354–358.

507. Harnug, Gertrude. "The Nursing Diagnosis—An Exercise in Judgment." *Nursing Outlook* (January 1956), 29–30.

508. Hart, Betty, and Anne Rohweder. "Support in Nursing." *American Journal of Nursing* (October 1959), 1398–1401.

509. Hubert, Sister Mary. "Spiritual Care for Every Patient." *The Journal of Nursing Education*, Vol. 2, No. 2 (May–June 1963), 9–11.

510. Hunter, John. "The Mark of Pain." *American Journal of Nursing*, Vol. 61, No. 10 (October 1961), 96–99.

511. Jensen, Hellene N., and Gene Tillotson. "Dependency in Nurse-Patient Relationships." *American Journal of Nursing* (February 1961), 81–84.

512. Johnson, JoAnn Rao. "Discharge Planning." *Texas Nursing* (November 1976), 9–10.

513. Kanner, Leo. "Judging Emotions From Facial Expressions." *Psychological Review*, Vol. 61, No. 3 (1931), 16–20.

514. Kaufmann, Margaret, and Dorothy Brown. "Pain Wears Many Faces." *American Journal of Nursing*, Vol. 61, No. 1 (January 1961), 48–51.

515. Keats, Arthur S. "Postoperative Pain—Research and Treatment." *Journal of Chronic Diseases*, Vol. 4, No. 1 (July 1956), 72–83.

516. Kelly, Katherine. "Clinical Inference in Nursing." *Nursing Research* (Winter 1966), 23–26.

517. Komarita, Nori. "Nursing Diagnosis." *American Journal of*

Nursing (December 1963), 83–86.

518. Langford, Teddy. "The Evaluation of Nursing: Necessary and Possible." *Supervisor Nurse* (November 1971), 65–75.

519. Larson, Duane, and Rita Gaston. "Current Trends in the Care of Burned Patients." *American Journal of Nursing*, Vol. 67, No. 2 (February 1967), 319–327.

520. Lasagna, Louis, Fredrick Mosteller, John M. Von Felsinger, and Henry Beecher. "A Study of Placebo Response." *American Journal of Medicine* (June 1954), 770–779.

521. Lawson, Betty. "Clinical Assessment of Cardiac Patients in Acute Care Facilities." *Nursing Clinics of North America*, Vol. 7, No. 3 (September 1972), 431–444.

522. Lehmann, Sister Janet. "Auscultation of Heart Sounds." *American Journal of Nursing* (July 1972), 1242–1246.

523. Levin, Nathaniel, John E. McClear, Vitus F. Pekarek, and James Shanks. "Rehabilitation—Sound the Way for Laryngectomees." *Patient Care* (August 15, 1972), 58–8.

524. Levine, Rhoda. "Disengagement in the Elderly—Its Causes and Effects." *Nursing Outlook* (October 1969), 28–30.

525. Littmann, David. "Stethoscopes and Auscultation." *American Journal of Nursing* (July 1972), 1239–1241.

526. McBride, Mary. "Additive to the Analgesic." *American Journal of Nursing* (May 1969), 974–976.

527. McBride, Mary Angela. "Nursing Approach, Pain and Relief: An Exploratory Experiment." *Nursing Research*, Vol. 16, No. 4 (Fall 1967), 337–340.

528. McCaffery, Margo, and Faye Moss. "Nursing Intervention for Bodily Pain." *American Journal of Nursing*, Vol. 67, No. 6 (June 1967), 1224–1227.

529. McCain, Faye. "Nursing by Assessment—Not Intuition." *American Journal of Nursing* (April 1965), 82–84.

530. McQuade, Anne, and Alvin I.

Goldfarb. "Coping With Feelings of Helplessness." *American Journal of Nursing* (May 1963), 77–79.

531. Martin, Harry W., and Arthur J. Prange. "The Stage of Illness—Psychosocial Approach." *Nursing Outlook* (March 1962), 169–170.

532. Maskopp, Mary Elizabeth, and Joan Sloan. "Nursing Care for the Amputee." *American Journal of Nursing*, Vol. 50, No. 9 (September 1950), 550–555.

533. Maslow, Abraham. "Deficiency Motivation and Growth Motivation." *Personality Dynamics and Effective Behavior*. Edited by James Coleman. Glenview, Ill.: Scott, Foresman & Co., 1960, 475–485.

534. Mazzara, James, and Stephen Ayres. "Fluid, Electrolytes, and Acid-Base Disturbances in the Coronary Care Unit." *Nursing Clinics of North America*, Vol. 7, No. 3 (September 1972), 549–562.

535. Moss, Faye, and Burton Meyer. "The Effects of Nursing Interaction Upon Pain Relief in Patients." *Nursing Research*, Vol. 15, No. 4 (Fall 1966), 303–306.

536. Mundinger, Mary O'Neil, and Grace Dotterer Jauron. "Developing a Nursing Diagnosis." *Nursing Outlook* (February 1975), 94–98.

537. Nalls, Sandra. "Developing a Therapeutic Relationship." *American Journal of Nursing* (December 1965), 114–118.

538. Nehren, Jeanette, and Naomi Gilliam. "Separation Anxiety." *American Journal of Nursing* (January 1965), 109–112.

539. Neylan, Margaret. "The Nurse in a Healing Milieu." *American Journal of Nursing* (April 1964), 72–74.

540. Norris, Catherine. "The Professional Nurse and Body Image." *Behavioral Concepts and Nursing Intervention*. Philadelphia: J. B. Lippincott Co., 1970, 39–60.

541. Norris, Catherine. "Toward a Science of Nursing." *Nursing Forum*, Vol. 3, No. 3 (1964), 10–45.

542. O'Donnell, D. R. "The Internal Clock of the International Jet Traveler." *The Medical Journal of Australia* (June 5, 1971), 1227–1230.

543. Patterson, Edith, and Frances Stence. "Thinking Together to Solve Care Problems." *American Journal of Nursing* (August 1970), 1703–1706.

544. Peplau, Hildegard E. "Talking With Patients." *American Journal of Nursing* (July 1960), 964–966.

545. Plorde, James J. "Advice to Foreign Travelers." *Postgraduate Medicine*, Vol. 51 (January 1972), 179–183.

546. Pohl, Margaret. "Teaching Activities of the Nurse Practitioner." *Nursing Research*, Vol. 14 (1965), 4–11.

547. Puder, Barbara. "What You Should Know About Nursing Diagnosis." *Medical Records News* (August 1975), 87–90.

548. Ripley, Herbert. "Psychological Factors in Pain." *Nebraska State Medical Journal*, Vol. 9, No. 4 (April 1964), 166–169.

549. Rothberg, June. "Why Nursing Diagnosis?" *American Journal of Nursing* (May 1967), 1040–1042.

550. Rowan, Noel M. "New Systems for Supporting the Patient in the Management of Decubitus Ulcer: Preliminary Report." *Journal of the American Geriatrics Society* (May 1970), 422–424.

551. Roy, Sister Callista. "A Diagnostic Classification System for Nursing." *Nursing Outlook*, Vol. 23, No. 2 (February 1975), 90–92.

552. Rubin, Reva. "Body Image and Self Esteem." *Nursing Outlook* (June 1968), 20–23.

553. Schell, Pamela L., and Alla T. Campbell. "POMR—Not Just Another Way to Chart." *Nursing Outlook*, Vol. 20 (August 1972), 510–514.

554. Searcy, Laurel. "Nursing Care of the Laryngectomy Patient." *R. N. Magazine* (October 1972), 35–41.

555. Skalka, Patricia. "Solving the Mystery of the Decaying Teeth." *Today's Health* (January 1974), 27–28, 70.

556. Skipper, James, Daisy Tagliacazzo, and Hans Mauksch. "What Communication Means to Patients." *American Journal of Nursing* (April 1964), 101–103.

557. Traver, Gayle. "Assessment of Thorax and Lungs." *American Journal of Nursing* (March 1973), 466–471.

558. Ullman, Montague. "Disorders of Body Image After Stroke." *American Journal of Nursing* (October 1964), 89–91.

559. Van Meter, Margaret, and Romaine Hart. "Chest Tubes —Basic Techniques for Better Care." *Nursing '74.* (December 1974), 48–55.

560. Varvaro, Filomena Fanelli. "Teaching the Patient About Open Heart Surgery." *American Journal of Nursing* (October 1965), 111–115.

561. Verwoerdt, Ardian, M.D. "Communications With the Fatally Ill." *A Cancer Journal for Clinicians*, Vol. 15 (1965), 105–111.

562. Washington State Board of Nursing. "Statement on Advanced Registered Nurse/Specialized Registered Nurse Rules and Regulations." *Washington State Journal of Nursing* (Winter 1975), 15–16.

563. Weaver, Barbara, and Elsie Williams. "Teaching the Tuberculosis Patient." *American Journal of Nursing*, Vol. 63 (December 1963), 80–82.

564. Weed, L. L. "Medical Records That Guide and Teach." Part 1. *New England Journal of Medicine* (March 14, 1968), 593–600.

565. Weed, L. L. "Medical Records That Guide and Teach." Part 2. *New England Journal of Medicine* (March 21, 1968), 652–657.

566. Wenkler, Gerald,· and Robert Young. "Efficacy of Chronic Propranolol Therapy in Action Tremors of the Familial, Senile or Essential Varieties." *The New England Journal of Medicine*, Vol. 290 (May 2, 1974), 984–988.

567. Western Pennslyvania Regional Medical Program. "The Nursing Process." University of Pittsburg School of Nursing, 1973.

568. William, Mary. "The Patient

Profile." *Nursing Research*, Vol. 9, No. 3 (Summer 1960), 122–124.

569. Wilson, W. P., and B. S. Nashold. "Pain and Emotion." *Postgraduate Medicine* (May 1970), 182–187.

570. Wolf, Stewart, and Ruth Pinsky. "Effects of Placebo Administration and Occurrence of Toxic Reactions." *Journal of American Medical Association* (May 22, 1954), 339–341.

571. Wu, Ruth. "Explaining Treatments to Young Children." *American Journal of Nursing*, Vol. 65 (July 1965), 71–73.

572. Zimmerman, Dorothy, and Carol Gohrke. "The Goal Directed Nursing Approach—It Does Work." *American Journal of Nursing* (February 1970), 306–310.

PAMPHLETS, BOOKLETS, AND MANUALS

573. American Cancer Society. "First Aid for Laryngectomees." New York: American Cancer Society, 1973.

574. American Cancer Society. "Helping Words for the Laryngectomee." New York: American Cancer Society, 1972.

575. American Cancer Society. "Rehabilitating Laryngectomees." New York: American Cancer Society, 1971.

576. American Diabetes Association. "Calorie Control for You." New York: The Upjohn Company, 1966.

577. American Diabetes Association. "Facts About Diabetes." New York: American Diabetes Association, 1966.

578. De Jong, Russell, A. L. Sahs, C. K. Aldrich, and John Milligan. "Essentials of the Neurological Examination." Philadelphia: Smith, Kline and French Laboratories, 1962.

579. Eli Lilly and Company. "A Guide for the Diabetic." Indianapolis: Eli Lilly and Company, 1971.

580. Epilepsy Foundation of America. "Epilepsy." Washington, D.C.: Epilepsy Foundation of America, 1972.

581. Epilepsy Foundation of America. "Teacher Tips." Washington, D.C.: Epilepsy Foundation of America, 1972.

582. Hurst, J. Willis, Robert Schlant, W. Dallas Hall, and H. Kenneth Walker. "The Problem-Oriented Medical System." Atlanta: Emory University School of Medicine, 1972.

583. Johnson and Johnson. "Narcotic Addiction in the Newborn." New York: Medical Programs Incorporated, 1972.

584. Lasser, Terese. "Reach to Recovery." American Cancer Society, 1953.

585. Leonard, James, M.D., and Frank Kroetz, M.D. "Examination of the Heart: Auscultation." New York: American Heart Association, 1967.

586. National Association for Mental Health. "How to Deal With Mental Problems." New York: National Association for Mental Health, Undated.

587. National Association for Mental Health. "Mental Health Is 1, 2, 3." Arlington, Va.: National Association for Mental Health, 1976.

588. National Association for Mental Health. "What Every Child Needs." New York: National Association for Mental Health, 1954.

589. National Institute of Mental Health. "Alcohol and Alcoholism." Washington D.C.: U.S. Government Printing Office, 1969.

590. National Society for the Prevention of Blindness, Inc. "Cataract: Fact and Fancy." New York: National Society for the Prevention of Blindness, Inc., 1971.

591. National Society for the Prevention of Blindness, Inc. "Television and Your Eyes." New York: National Society for the Prevention of Blindness, Inc., 1968.

592. National Society for the Prevention of Blindness, Inc. "Your Eyes for a Lifetime of Sight." New York: National Society for the Prevention of Blindness, Inc., 1968, 1971.

593. National Tuberculosis Association. "Homemaking Hints." New

York: National Tuberculosis Association, 1954

594. Normand, Hal. "A Procedure Manual for the Voluntary or Involuntary Commitment of the Mentally Ill." Dallas: Beddoe Printing Co., Undated.

595. Reynolds, William. "Home Care Programs in Arthritis." New York: The Arthritis Foundation, 1969.

596. Roche Laboratories. "Facts at Your Fingertips." Nutley, N.J.: Roche Laboraties, Undated.

597. Rosenthal, Helen, and Joseph Rosenthal. "Diabetic Care in Pictures." Philadelphia: J. B. Lippincott, 1960.

598. Sprague, Howard. "Examination of the Heart—History Taking." New York: American Heart Association, 1967.

599. Van Allen, M. W. "Pictorial Manual of Neurologic Tests." Chicago: Year Book Medical Publications, Inc., 1969.

600. Van Dolak, John. "You and Your Contented Baby." Carnation Company, 1955.

601. Vazuka, Francis. "Essentials of the Neurological Examination." Philadelphia: Smith, Kline and French Laboratories, 1962.

PAPERS

602. American Druggist. "Counterdoses for the Home." 1965.

603. American Heart Association. "High Blood Pressure Screening Clinic Instructions." Dallas County Chapter. 1976.

604. American Heart Association and National Academy of Sciences—National Research Council. "Standards for Cardiopulmonary Resuscitation (CRP) and Emergency Cardiac Care (ECC). Washington, D.C. 1973.

605. American Medical Association Committee on Nursing. "Medicine and Nursing in the 1970's, a Position Statement." Chicago: American Medical Association, June 1970, p. 2.

606. American Nurses Association. "A Position Paper." New York: American Nurses Association, 1965.

607. American Nurses Association. "H.E.W. report on Licensure and Related Health Personnel Credentialing." New York: American Nurses Association, 1972.

608. American Nurses Association. Task Force for Review and Revision of ANA's Model Practice Act of the ANA Congress for Nursing Practice. "Legal Barriers to Expanded Nursing Role Responsibilities." New York: American Nurses Association, 1973.

609. American Nurses Association. "Standards of Nursing Practice." Kansas City, Mo.: American Nurses Association, 1973.

610. American Nurses Association. "Practice of Nursing Defined in State Nursing Practice Acts." New York: American Nurses Association, 1973.

611. American Nurses Association. "The American Nurse." Kansas City, Mo.: American Nurses Association, September 1, 1976, Volume 8, Number 11, p. 9.

612. Barnett, E. Kathryn. "The Development of a Theoretical Construct of the Concepts of Touch as They Relate to Nursing." Ph.D. dissertation, North Texas State University, Denton, Texas, 1970.

613. Cross, Harold. "Teaching Methods and Patient Care with Emphasis on the Weed Method." Paper presented at the University of Medicine Symposium at Emory University, Atlanta, Ga. September 10–11, 1971.

614. Health, Education and Welfare. "Extending the Scope of Nursing Practice." Washington, D.C.: November 1971, p. 12.

615. Health, Education and Welfare. "Guidelines for the Utilization of Nurse Practioners." Public Law 94–63.

616. Health, Education and Welfare. "Report on Licensure and Related Health Personnel Credentialing." Presented at the Educational Conference Council of State Boards of Nursing, Detroit, Mich., 1972, pp. 2–3.

617. Henderson, Betty. "Physical Assessment of the Respiratory System." Texas Woman's Uni-

versity, Denton, Texas, 1973.

618. Kenner, Cornelia. "Assessment of the Thermally Injured." Texas Woman's University, Denton, Texas, 1973.

619. Kuempel, Anne. "Individual Reaction to Pain." Unpublished paper, April 1971.

620. National Foundation—March of Dimes (in collaboration with the American Medical Association and Woman's Day). "Family Medical Record." New York: Fawcett Publications, Inc., 1972.

621. Olson, Mary. "Postoperative Patients Evaluate Preoperative Teaching." Master's thesis, Texas Woman's University, December 1971.

622. Pinterich, Shirley. "Deliberate Nursing Care for the Quiet Patient." Unpublished paper, December 1970.

623. Robertson, K. Joy, M.D. "Outline of Chest Physical Diagnosis." Unpublished paper, Dallas, Texas, 1973.

624. Texas Nurses Association. "Working Draft: Professional Nursing Practice Act for Texas for Study Purposes Only." 1976.

625. Western Pennsylvania Regional Medical Program. "The Nursing Process." University of Pittsburg School of Nursing, p. 2.

Nursing Diagnoses Alphabetical Index

Nursing Diagnoses Subject Index

NURSING DIAGNOSES

A

ABSCESS

External abscess, 751–752

ACCIDENTAL INJURY

Potential accidental automobile injury, 571–572

Potential accidental burn, 572–573
Potential accidental falling, 573–574
Potential accidental poisoning, 574–575
Potential accidental suffocation, 575–576
Potential accidental wound, 577
Predisposition to accidental injury, 899–900

ACIDOSIS

Emergency phase acidosis, 108–110
Emergency phase diabetic acidosis, 110–112
Predisposition to acidosis, 105–107

ACTIVITY TOLERANCE

Mild activity tolerance, 1072–1074
Minimum activity tolerance, 1071–1072
Moderate activity tolerance, 1074–1076

ADRENAL HYPERFUNCTION

Adrenal hyperfunction, 835–837

ADRENAL HYPOFUNCTION

Emergency phase impending adrenal shock (emergency phase impending adrenal crisis), 837–838

AIR TRAVEL

Inadequate information related to air-travel fitness, 591–592
Inadequate information related to jet lag, 594–595

AIRWAY PATENCY

Dependence on airway-patency maintenance, 1119–1121

AIRWAY OBSTRUCTION

Airway obstruction, 1121–1122
Potential airway obstruction, 1123–1124

ALCOHOL ABUSE

Inadequate information related to alcohol abuse, 524–525
Inadequate information related to coping with the alcohol abuser, 525–527

ALKALOSIS

Emergency phase alkalosis, 112–114
Potential alkalosis, 107–108

ALLERGY

Cluster headache (histamine headache), 989–991
Emergency phase anaphylactic shock (emergency phase allergic shock), 452–454
Inadequate information related to drug allergy, 758–759
Inadequate information related to food allergy, 759–760
Inadequate information related to respiratory allergy, 760–761
Inadequate information related to skin allergy, 761–762

ALONENESS

Inadequate emotional support related to aloneness, 240–242

AMBULATION

Difficulty ambulating, 851–853

AMPUTATION

Dependence on amputation stump care, 902–903
Phantom pain, 1015–1016

ANESTHESIA, POST

Dependence on nursing supervision of postanesthesia recovery, 1229–1231

ANGER

Anger related to being ill, 115–116
Anger related to desertion by a departed loved one, 116–118
Inability to control anger, 118–120
Maladaptive coping related to anger, 120–123
Potential active aggression, 123–125

ANGINA

Angina, 979–981

ANIMAL BITE

Animal bite, 807–808

ANOREXIA

Anorexia, 925–927

ANOXIA

Emergency phase oxygen insufficiency

NURSING DIAGNOSES

A

ABSCESS

External abscess, 751–752

ACCIDENTAL INJURY

Potential accidental automobile injury, 571–572

H

HAIR

Cradle cap, 763–764
Dandruff, 764–765
Dependence on hair care, 719–721
Inadequate hair care, 703–704
Parasite infestation, 765–766
Potential infestation transmission, 766–767

HANDS

Limited hand dexterity, 858–860

HEADACHE

Cluster headache (histamine headache), 989–991
Eyestrain headache, 991–992
Febrile headache, 992–994
Hypertensive headache, 994–995
Meningeal headache, 995–997
Menstrual-migraine headache, 997–998
Migraine headache, 998–1000
Potential headache, 1055–1056
Sinus headache, 1000–1001
Spinal puncture headache, 1001–1003
Tension headache, 1003–1004
Toxic headache, 1004–1006
Trauma headache, 1006–1007

HEALING

Immobility requirement related to tissue healing, 806–807
Increased nutritional requirement related to tissue healing, 924–925

HEALTH CARE

Conflict related to the health care of a significant other, 145–147
Failure to seek health care, 687–689
Inability to obtain health care, 689–690

HEALTH CARE TERMINATION

Difficult adaptation to health care termination, 149–151

HEALTH MAINTENANCE

Inadequate motivation related to health maintenance, 690–691
Spiritually restricted health maintenance, 1238–1239

HEALTH PRINCIPLES

Inadequate information related to mental health principles, 359–360

HEALTH PROCEDURE

Conflict related to a high-risk procedure, 143–145

HEALTH STATUS

Dependence on nursing assessment of health status, 685–686

HEALTH TREATMENT

Inadequate emotional support related to the endurance of health treatment, 258–260
Reluctance to accept health treatment, 692–694

HEARING

Dependence on communication assistance related to impaired hearing, 474–476
Impending drug deafness, 505
Potential hearing loss related to trauma, 1192–1193
Sound sensitivity, 1191–1192

HEARING AID

Inadequate information related to hearing aid use, 1219–1220

HEARTBURN

Heartburn (pyrosis), 603–604

HEAT

Heat intolerance, 584–585

HEAT EXHAUSTION

Emergency phase heat exhaustion, 390–391

HEAT STROKE

Emergency phase heat stroke, 391–392
Inadequate information related to heat stroke, 392–393

HEMODIALYSIS

See also Dialysis
Dependence on hemodialysis management, 670–671

Dependence on nasogastric tube management, 630–631
Dependence on T-tube management, 627–628
Inadequate information related to laryngectomy management, 1185–1186
Inadequate information related to tracheostomy management, 1186–1187

TURNING

Difficulty turning self, 857–858

TWITCHING, MUSCLE

Involuntary muscle twitching, 889–890

U

ULCER

Decubitus ulcer (skin breakdown) (bedsore), 788–790
Potential decubitus ulcer (potential skin breakdown) (potential bedsore), 796–797
Predisposition to stress ulcer, 610–611
Stasis ulcer, 790–791
Threatening decubitus ulcer (threatening skin breakdown) (threatening bedsore), 791–792
Ulcerated skin tissue, 794–795

UMBILICUS

Dependence on umbilical hygiene, 727–728

UREMIC FROST

Uremic frost skin discomfort, 782–783

URETERILEOSTOMY

Dependence on ureterileostomy management (dependence on ileal conduit management) (dependence on Bricker procedure management), 663–665

URETEROSIGMOIDOSTOMY

Dependence on ureterosigmoidostomy management, 655–657

URETEROSTOMY

Dependence on ureterostomy management, 667–668

URINARY-ELIMINATION THERAPY DEPENDENCE

Dependence on decompression urinary drainage management, 655–657
Dependence on indwelling urinary catheter management, 657–658
Dependence on nephrostomy drainage management, 659–660
Dependence on suprapubic drainage management (dependence on cystostomy drainage management), 660–662
Dependence on tidal drainage management, 662–663
Dependence on ureterileostomy management (dependence on ileal conduit management) (dependence on Bricker procedure management), 663–665
Dependence on ureterosigmoidostomy management, 665–667
Dependence on ureterostomy management, 667–668

URINATION

Painful urination (dysuria), 986–987

URTICARIA

Urticaria skin discomfort, 786–787

UTERUS

Inadequate information related to uterine cancer, 1104–1105
Uterine fundus nondescent (subinvolution), 1100

V

VAGINA

Inadequate information related to abnormal vaginal bleeding, 1114–1115
Inadequate information rleated to postsurgical vaginal bleeding, 1116–1117

VARICOSE VEINS

Potential varicose veins, 404–405

VENOUS STASIS

Potential impaired peripheral circulation (potential venous stasis) (potential blood pooling) (potential thrombus formation), 405–407

VENTILATION, ARTIFICIAL

Artificial-ventilation discomfort, 1156–1157

Nursing Interventions Alphabetical Index

NURSING TREATMENTS

A

Accept and attempt to relieve unexplainable body complaints, 1241
Acknowledge dependency, 1241
Acknowledge emotional concealment, 1241
Administer a drug sensitivity test, 1242
Administer a hot foot bath, 1242
Administer a vaginal douche, 1242
Administer a warm bath, 1242
Administer an enema, 1242–1243
Administer heated humidified oxygen (ET), 1243
Administer humidified oxygen (ET), 1243–1244
Administer intermittent positive pressure breathing (ET), 1244
Administer intravenous fluids (ET), 1244
Administer isotonic saline intravenous fluid between the blood transfusion and glucose infusion, 1244–1245
Administer vaporized air, 1245
Allow time for thought comprehension, 1245
Allow unlimited visiting, 1245
Ambulate the patient, 1245–1246
Anchor the tubing securely, 1246
Anticipate needs, 1246
Apply a bandana to the unamputated breast, 1246
Apply a bed cradle, 1246
Apply a brassiere, 1246–1247
Apply a breast binder, 1247
Apply a cold, moist compress, 1247
Apply a cool, damp cloth to the face, 1247

Apply a greasy substance over the tick, 1247
Apply a heat cradle, 1247–1248
Apply a heating pad, 1248
Apply a hernia support, 1248
Apply a hot water bottle, 1248
Apply a parasiticide, 1249
Apply a precordial blow (ET), 1249
Apply a pressure dressing, 1249
Apply a safety helmet to the head, 1249
Apply a saline compress, 1249
Apply a scrotal support, 1249
Apply a sterile dressing, 1249–1250
Apply a stump sock, 1250
Apply a supportive splint, 1250
Apply a tourniquet between the extremity wound and the body, 1250
Apply a warm, moist compress, 1250
Apply after-bath powder, 1250–1251
Apply alcohol to the skin, 1251
Apply aluminum paste to the skin, 1251
Apply an abdominal support garment, 1251
Apply an analgesic ointment, 1251
Apply an antibiotic ointment (or spray), 1251–1252
Apply an antiperspirant, 1252
Apply an arm sling, 1252
Apply an elastic bandage, 1252
Apply an external urinary catheter, 1252
Apply an ice bag, 1252–1253
Apply an ice collar, 1253
Apply an occlusive dressing, 1253
Apply an ostomy appliance, 1253
Apply calamine lotion, 1253–1254
Apply corn starch to the skin, 1254
Apply elastic stockings, 1254
Apply heat by a gooseneck lamp, 1254

E

NURSING OBSERVATIONS

O

Health Teaching

MEDICAL TREATMENTS PERFORMED BY NURSES

A

B

C

D

G

Nursing Interventions
Subject Index

Explain the need to avoid overexertion, 1639

Instruct to avoid pushing and pulling activities, 1665

Observe the person's activity pattern, 1542

Recommend activities which improve circulation, 1676

ADENOIDS

Inspect the adenoids for enlargement, 1485

ADHESIVE STRIPS

Use sterile adhesive stips for wound closure, 1455

ADHESIVE TAPE

Advise not to use adhesive tape on the skin, 1572

Remove adhesive tape and adhesive debris, 1426–1427

Use paper or transparent tape instead of adhesive on the skin, 1454

AIRBORNE IRRITANTS

Advise against exposure to airborne irritants, 1562

AIRWAY

Change the catheter each time the airway is suctioned, 1270

Deflate the airway-tube cuff periodically, 1282

Hold the jaw forward to maintain an airway, 1352–1353

Inflate the airway tube cuff, 1356

Inform that airway noise indicates obstruction, 1647

Insert a nasal airway, 1357

Insert an oral airway, 1358

Observe for airway obstruction, 1522

Suction the airway, 1445

Teach how to inflate and deflate an airway cuff, 1718

Teach how to suction an airway, 1723

AIRWAY CUFF

Deflate the airway-tube cuff periodically, 1282

Inflate the airway tube cuff, 1356

Teach how to inflate and deflate an airway cuff, 1718

ALCOHOL

Apply alcohol to the skin, 1251

Clean with alcohol, 1275

Instruct to lightly rub the diabetic's feet with alcohol, 1670

Irrigate the foreign particle with alcohol, 1361

Refrain from cleansing with alcohol, 1413

ALCOHOL AND DRIVING

Advise not to drive for three hours after two alcoholic drinks, 1571

ALCOHOL RUB

Refrain from giving an alcohol rub, 1415

ALIGNMENT, BODY

Explain how to maintain body alignment, 1609

Inspect the bones for alignment, 1486

Maintain alignment of the drying cast through positioning, 1369

Maintain body alignment, 1369–1370

ALKALI

Recommend that alkalis be used conservatively, 1683

ALLERGY

Damp-dust the room of allergy-prone persons daily, 1280

Explain how to take allergy precautions, 1615

Inform that foods causing allergies fall into specific categories, 1652

Observe for a hypersensitivity response, 1521

ALTITUDES

Recommend that high altitudes be avoided after cardiac damage, 1684

ALUMINUM PASTE

Apply aluminum paste to the skin, 1251

AMBULATION

Ambulate the patient, 1245–1246

Walk with the patient, 1456

AMNIOTIC FLUID

Inspect the amniotic fluid for meconium, 1485–1486

CARBON DIOXIDE

Administer carbon dioxide whiffs (MD Rx), 1738

CARBONATED BEVERAGE

Give carbonated beverages, 1337
Inform that carbonated beverages are safe to drink in foreign countries, 1649
Refrain from giving carbonated beverages, 1415

CARDIAC DULLNESS

Percuss the chest for widened cardiac dullness, 1550–1551

CARDIAC MASSAGE

Initiate external cardiac massage (ET), 1356

CARDIOGRAM

Monitor the cardiogram, 1512

CARPETING

Inform that deep carpeting should be avoided by persons in a wheelchair, 1651
Place in a heavily draped, carpeted room to reduce noise, 1383

CAST

Bivalve and spread the cast to relieve pressure (ET), 1268
Explain how to pad rough cast edges, 1611
Expose the drying cast to air, 1332
Inspect the cast for tightness, 1486
Lay the drying cast on pillows, 1363
Lift the drying cast with the palms of the hand, 1363
Maintain alignment of the drying cast through positioning, 1369
Move the entire cast as a single unit, 1376
Observe the cast for an expanding bleeding area, 1539
Observe the cast for odor, 1539–1540
Pad the rough cast edges, 1380
Waterproof the cast surface, 1457

CATARACT

Describe the manifestations of impending cataract, 1583

CATHETER, NASAL

Change the nasal oxygen catheter every eight hours, 1270–1271

CATHETER, SUCTION

Change the catheter each time the airway is suctioned, 1270

CATHETER, TRANSTRACHEAL

Irrigate the transtracheal catheter (MD Rx), 1745

CATHETER, URINARY

Apply an external urinary catheter, 1252
Avoid disconnecting the urinary catheter, 1263
Catheterize with an indwelling urinary catheter, 1269–1270
Change the urinary catheter, 1272
Clamp the indwelling urinary catheter intermittently, 1273
Clamp the suprapubic catheter and have the patient attempt to void (MD Rx), 1743
Clean the urinary catheter externally at the meatus, 1274–1275
Explain how to clean the external part of the indwelling urinary catheter, 1604
Explain that the urinary catheter should be taped to the abdomen, 1628
Instruct to anchor the urinary catheter, 1665
Irrigate the urinary catheter, 1361
Tape the urinary catheter onto the abdomen, 1450
Teach how to apply an external urinary catheter, 1703
Teach how to dilate the stoma with a sterile catheter, 1709
Teach how to irrigate a urinary catheter, 1720

CATHETERIZATION

Catheterize one time only, 1269
Catheterize with an indwelling urinary catheter, 1269–1270
Do not withdraw by catheter more than 1000 cc of urine at one time, 1290–1291
Teach how to do a catheterization, 1709–1710

CENTRAL VENOUS PRESSURE

Monitor the central venous pressure, 1512–1513

CEREBRAL SPINAL FLUID

Inspect the ears and nose for cerebral spinal fluid leakage, 1487

CEREBRAL SPINAL FLUIDS STUDIES

See Studies, Cerebral Spinal Fluid

CERVIX

Palpate the cervix for dilatation, 1545

CHAIR

Mobilize by invalid chair, 1374
Recommend the use of a shower chair, 1691
Sit the patient in an armchair, 1439

CHAPLAIN

Encourage the chaplain's visit, 1323
Prepare the patient for the clergy's visit, 1394

CHARCOAL

Give charcoal solution orally, 1337

CHEST

Auscultate the chest for abnormal breath sounds, 1460–1461
Auscultate the chest for abnormal heart sounds, 1461–1463
Auscultate the chest for abnormal voice sounds (pectoriloquy, bronchophony, or egophony), 1463
Auscultate the chest for crepitation, 1463
Auscultate the chest for lung aeration, 1463
Auscultate the chest for pleural friction rub, 1464
Auscultate the chest for rales and/or rhonchi, 1464
Inspect the chest for precordial bulge, 1486
Inspect the chest for respiratory rate and rhythm, 1486–1487
Inspect the chest for symmetrical expansion, 1487
Palpate the chest for a precordial heave, 1545
Palpate the chest for a thrill, 1546
Palpate the chest for abnormal vocal fremitus, 1546
Palpate the chest for an abnormal precordial thrust, 1546
Percuss the chest for abnormal resonance, 1550

Percuss the chest for cracked-pot sounds, 1550
Percuss the chest for widened cardiac dullness, 1550–1551
Percuss the posterior chest for decreased diaphragmatic descent, 1551

CHEST TUBE

Attach the chest tube to a water-seal drainage, 1261–1262
Clamp the chest tube but for only a short time, 1272–1273
Strip the chest tube, 1444

CHEWING

Observe for chewing difficulty, 1522
Provide foods and toys for chewing, 1403
Recommend thorough food chewing, 1699

CHILLS

Observe for chills, 1522

CHOLESTEROL

Encourage decreased cholesterol-food intake, 1302

CHVOSTEK'S SIGN

Test for Chvostek's sign, 1552

CIRCOLECTRIC BED

Place on a CircOlectric bed, 1388

CIRCULATION

Advise that positions which impair circulation be avoided, 1576
Describe the manifestations of circulatory impairment, 1583
Inform that the extremities should be kept warm when the circulation is impaired, 1656
Inspect the extremity (or extremities) for adequate circulation, 1487
Observe for clothing which constricts circulation, 1522–1523
Recommend activities which improve circulation, 1676

CIRCULATORY OVERLOAD

Observe for water intoxication, 1538

CONSCIENCE

Explain the difference between a mature and a rigid conscience, 1631

Explore with the patient the difference between his child and adult conscience, 1331

CONSCIOUSNESS, LEVEL OF

Explain that persons with impaired cerebral function require close observation, 1623

Observe the level of consciousness, 1540–1541

Observe the preoperative and postoperative response level, 1542

CONSTIPATION

Observe for complaints of constipation, 1523

CONTACT LENS

Advise that contact lenses not be used for eye color change, 1574

Clean the contact lenses, 1273

Describe the discomforts of contact lens adjustment, 1582

Explain that care should be taken to prevent scratching of the contact lenses, 1617

Explain that extreme cold cracks contact lenses, 1619

Explain that heat warps contact lenses, 1620

Insert and remove the contact lens, 1358

Instruct that contact lenses should not be worn beyond the prescribed time, during an eye disorder, or while sleeping, 1661

Remove the contact lens, 1429

Safeguard the patient's contact lenses, 1436

Teach how to clean contact lenses, 1708

Teach how to insert and remove contact lenses, 1718–1719

CONTAMINATION

Disinfect contaminated articles, 1286

Emphasize that contaminated skin should be washed immediately, 1590–1591

Explain how to sterilize contaminated dishes, 1614

Explain the need to avoid contaminated soil, 1639

CONTRACTIONS

Palpate the uterus for contraction quality, 1549

Time the uterine contractions, 1556–1557

CONTRACTURES

Inspect the joints for impending contractures, 1490

CONVULSIONS

See Seizures

COORDINATION

Test for impaired coordination, 1552–1553

CORN STARCH

Apply corn starch to the skin, 1254

COSMETICS

Explain the importance of testing cosmetics for skin irritation, 1636

COTTON PLEDGET

Insert an oiled cotton pledget into the ear, 1357

COUGH DROPS

Give cough drops, 1338

COUGHING

Encourage coughing, 1300

Explain how to prevent coughing, 1612

Inform that coughing should be avoided, 1650–1651

Instruct to cover the mouth when coughing, 1667

Observe for coughing, 1526

Observe the characteristics of the cough, 1540

CRACKED-POT SOUNDS

Percuss the chest for cracked-pot sounds, 1550

CRACKERS

Give dry crackers, 1339

CRADLE, BED OR HEAT

Apply a bed cradle, 1246

Apply a heat cradle, 1247–1248

FLUID WAVE

FOOD

FLUID WAVE

FOOD

Explain how to maintain maximum nutrients in food, 1609
Give bland foods, 1337
Give clear liquid foods, 1338
Give flavor-intensified food, 1339
Give full-liquid foods, 1340
Give light foods before sleep, 1343
Give mechanically soft foods, 1345
Give pureed foods, 1347
Give soft foods, 1348–1349
Give strongly seasoned foods, 1349
Inform that new foods should be introduced to children at the beginning of the meal, 1654
Instruct that diabetics should not fry foods, 1662
Instruct to avoid foods having strong odors, 1665
Instruct to eat only at mealtime, 1668
Instruct to eat only prescribed foods and amounts of foods, 1668
Open packaged foods, 1379
Provide extra food helpings at mealtimes, 1402–1403
Provide finger food, 1403
Provide food selection, 1404
Provide foods and toys for chewing, 1403
Provide foods at their most appetizing temperature, 1404
Recommend adequate food refrigeration, 1676
Recommend eating only well-cooked meat in foreign countries, 1678
Recommend that children be introduced to a wide variety of food, 1683
Recommend that food be cut in small bite sizes, 1684
Recommend that food servings be in proportion to the appetite, 1684
Recommend the preferable age for introducing specific foods to children, 1687–1688
Refrain from giving crumbling, flaking foods, 1416
Remove food from the mouth, 1427
Season the food for individual taste, 1438
Withhold food until the patient requests it, 1458

FOOD PREPARATION

Instruct to measure foods after cooking, 1672
Teach how to prepare a formula, 1722
Teach how to prepare balanced meals, 1723

FOOT BATH

Administer a hot foot bath, 1242

FOOTBOARD

Instruct to use a footboard, 1673
Place a footboard at the feet, 1381

FOOTSTOOL

Place a footstool at the bedside, 1381

FOREIGN OBJECTS OR PARTICLES

Inspect for foreign bodies, 1483
Instruct not to insert foreign objects into body orifices, 1660
Irrigate the foreign particle with alcohol, 1361
Remove foreign object(s), 1427

FORESKIN

Retract and clean the foreskin, 1435

FREMITUS, VOCAL

Palpate the chest for abnormal vocal fremitus, 1546

FRICTION RUB

Auscultate the chest for pleural friction rub, 1464
Auscultate the head for cranial friction sounds, 1465

FRUITS

Give fresh fruits, 1339–1340

FUMES

Emphasize that fume-producing substances should be used in the open air, 1592
Emphasize the need to check for gas leakage and fire, 1599

G

GAIT

Observe for abnormal gait, 1521
Teach the proper gait to use with a walker, 1734
Teach the proper gait to use with crutches, 1734

GARGLE

Encourage the use of a warm, saline gargle, 1325

Instruct to inspect the skin (scalp or hair), 1669–1670

Moisten the hair with conditioning formula, 1376

Remove hair with a depilatory cream, 1427–1428

Shampoo the hair (scalp), 1438

Shave the hair surrounding the burned area, 1438

Soften the hair with a cream rinse, 1441

HAIR DYE

Emphasize the danger of using excessive hair dye, 1598

HAIR SPRAY

Advise limited use of hair spray, 1570

HALAZONE TABLETS

Inform that Halazone tablets should be added to potentially unsafe water, 1652

HALLUCINATIONS

See Behavior

HAND ROLL

Place a hand roll under the fingers, 1381

HANDLING

Advise minimal infant handling, 1570
Handle gently, 1352
Reduce infant-handling to a minimum, 1412

HANDRAILS

Recommend the use of handrails, 1694

HANDS

Assist with skilled hand activities, 1261
Cover the hands with mittens, 1279
Inform that bilateral hand activity should be avoided, 1648
Inspect the hands for impaired grasp, 1489
Inspect the hands for tremors, 1489–1490
Inspect the palms for coloration, 1492
Place only warm hands and objects on the patient, 1391
Tape implements to the bandaged hands, 1450

HANDWASHING

Advise handwashing after elimination, 1569

Advise handwashing before meals, 1569–1570

Inform that handwashing is essential before touching the laryngectomy stoma, 1652–1653

Wash the patient's hands, 1456
Wash your hands between contacts, 1457

HEAD

Apply a safety helmet to the head, 1249
Auscultate the head for cranial bruit, 1464
Auscultate the head for cranial crepitation sounds, 1464–1465
Auscultate the head for cranial friction sounds, 1465
Cover the head, 1279
Elevate the head, 1294
Inform that stooping and lowering the head should be avoided, 1656
Inspect the head for Battle's sign, 1490
Measure the head for abnormal size, 1497
Palpate the cranial suture line for separation, 1546
Palpate the fontanel for abnormality, 1547
Palpate the head for a cranial bulge, 1547
Place the head below the knees, 1392
Recommend wearing a hard hat for head protection, 1699

HEADACHE

Observe for complaints of headache, 1523

HEAD-ROLLING

Observe for infant head-rolling, 1531

HEALING

Observe for delayed healing, 1527
Observe for signs of healing, 1536

HEALTH PRACTICES

Describe the specific dangerous effects of poor health practices, 1588

HEALTH PRINCIPLES

Explain the importance of learning and practicing health principles, 1634

HEALTH RESOURCES

Inform of the resources available for health care, 1645

HEARING AID

Provide hearing-aid care, 1405
Safeguard the patient's hearing aid, 1436
Teach how to care for a hearing aid, 1706–1707

HEART FAILURE

Observe for heart failure, 1529

HEART SOUNDS

Auscultate the apical heartbeat for rate and rhythm, 1460
Auscultate the chest for abnormal heart sounds, 1461–1463
Monitor the fetal heart sounds, 1513

HEAT APPLICATIONS

Apply a heat cradle, 1247–1248
Apply a heating pad, 1248
Apply a hot water bottle, 1248
Apply a warm, moist compress, 1250
Apply heat by a gooseneck lamp, 1254
Apply hot packs to the breast before breast feeding, 1254
Refrain from giving local heat applications, 1417–1418
Teach how to apply heat therapy, 1704

HEIGHT

Measure the height, 1497

HEIMLICH MANEUVER

Apply the Heimlich maneuver, 1256

HEMODIALYSIS

Administer the hemodialysis treatment (MD Rx), 1741
Check the hemodialysis AV shunt for cleanliness and patency, 1467
Check the hemodialysis equipment for mechanical breakdown, 1467
Explain how to integrate the hemodialysis procedure into the home routine, 1608

HEMOPTOSIS

Observe for hemoptosis, 1529

HEMORRHAGE

See also Bleeding
Inspect for hemorrhage, 1483–1484

HICCOUGHS

Observe for hiccoughs, 1529

HIGH-FREQUENCY SIGNALS

Inform that high-frequency signals should be avoided when wearing a pacemaker, 1653

HOMAN'S SIGN

Test for a positive Homan's sign, 1552

HOME ADAPTATIONS

Recommend housing with few doors and hallways for persons in a wheelchair, 1678–1679
Recommend living in a single level, ground floor dwelling, 1679
Recommend low window sills for persons in a wheelchair, 1679
Recommend methods for preparing a sick room at home, 1681
Recommend polyethylene doorsills for persons in a wheelchair, 1682
Recommend that doorknobs and switches be placed 36 inches above the floor, 1683–1684
Recommend the use of a foot pedal on appliance doors when hand dexterity is impaired, 1689
Recommend the use of a pegboard for ease in storing utensils, 1690
Recommend the use of front stove controls for persons in a wheelchair, 1694
Recommend the use of front-loading washers and dryers for persons in a wheelchair, 1694
Recommend the use of high storage cabinets for persons unable to stoop, 1694
Recommend the use of top stove controls for persons unable to stoop, 1698
Recommend the use of top-loading washers and dryers for persons unable to stoop, 1698
Suggest home adaptations appropriate to the health problem, 1445–1446

HOME CARE

Suggest that volunteers might offer assistance with home care, 1447

HOME VISIT

Provide a home visit, 1397

Immunize against infectious disease (ExR), 1353
Inform that immunity does not occur with venereal infection, 1653

INACTIVITY

Avoid placing the patient on enforced inactivity, 1263

INCISION

See also Wound
Splint the incisional area, 1442

INCISION AND DRAINAGE

Incise and drain the wound (ExR), 1353

INCONTINENCE

Fold a towel between the legs during incontinence, 1335
Observe for incontinence, 1530–1531

INCUBATOR

Administer oxygen by tent, Croupette, or incubator (MD Rx), 1740
Check the environmental controls on the incubator periodically, 1467
Place the newborn in an incubator, 1392

INFANT CARE

Teach how to bathe an infant, 1705
Teach how to bottle-feed an infant, 1705
Teach how to breast-feed an infant, 1706
Teach how to clean an infant's ears, 1708
Teach how to clean an infant's nose, 1708
Teach how to handle an infant, 1717–1718

INFANT SEAT

Place in an infant seat, 1383–1384

INFECTION

Explain how to prevent cross infection, 1612
Inform that water should be kept out of infected ears, 1659
Inspect for signs of infection, 1484
Instruct that premature infants require protection against infection, 1663
Instruct to limit direct contact with infected persons, 1670–1671
Isolate infected persons, 1361–1362
Recommend the use of disposable dishes for contagious diseases, 1693
Recommend the use of double thickness

tissue for infectious sputum, 1693
Recommend the use of individual towels and washcloths, 1695

INFILTRATION

Check for infiltration of the solution, 1465

INFLAMMATION

Inspect for inflammation, 1484

INFORMATION

Determine the extent of lack of information, 1471
Provide reliable information, 1408

INJECTIONS

Refrain from giving intravenous or intramuscular injections, 1417

INSECT BITE

Remove the insect stinger, 1429

INSULIN

Refrain from giving insulin, 1417
Teach how to give insulin, 1716–1717

INSULIN SHOCK

Describe the manifestations of impending insulin shock, 1583–1584
Explain how impending insulin shock can be interrupted, 1601

INTAKE

Balance fluid intake to equal output, 1265
Balance nutritional intake, 1266
Explain how to measure intake and output, 1610
Explain that fluid intake and output should be balanced, 1619
Measure the intake, 1497–1498
Observe and record the food intake, 1520
Observe for abnormal fluid intake, 1521
Restrict the intake to nothing by mouth, 1433

INTERMITTENT POSITIVE PRESSURE

Administer continuous positive pressure breathing (MD Rx), 1738
Administer continuous positive pressure breathing by expiratory positive pressure mask (MD Rx), 1738

Use a waist safety strap during mobility, 1453

MODESTY

Drape modestly, 1291

MONITOR, CARDIAC

Check the monitor electrodes for placement periodically, 1468

Explain how to replace monitor electrodes, 1614

Explain that monitors are safe, 1621

Inform that battery monitors should be disconnected during tub bathing or showering, 1648

Unplug the electrical monitor during a bath, 1452

MOTOR FUNCTION

Observe the extremities for motor function, 1540

MOUTH

Inspect the gums for abnormalities, 1489

Inspect the mouth for abnormal salivation, 1490

Inspect the mucous membranes for abnormalities, 1490

Inspect the patient's mouth for concealed medications, 1492

Inspect the teeth for abnormalities, 1494

Inspect the throat for impaired swallowing reflex, 1494

Inspect the tongue for abnormalities, 1494–1495

Take nasal and oral secretion precautions, 1449

Test for impaired taste perception, 1553

MOUTH CARE

See also Mouthwash

Instruct not to vigorously rinse the mouth, 1661

Instruct to cover the mouth when coughing, 1667

Moisten the mouth with cracked ice, 1376

Provide cold water for mouth rinsing but not swallowing, 1401

Rinse the mouth with dilute hydrogen peroxide, 1435

Swab the mouth with diluted glycerine, 1448–1449

MOUTH FRESHENER

Refresh with a mouth freshener, 1425

MOUTHWASH

Advise mouth rinsing when brushing is inconvenient, 1571

Refresh with a mouthwash, 1426

Recommend the use of mouthwash, 1696–1697

MUCOUS MEMBRANES

Inspect the mucous membranes for abnormalities, 1490

MUSCLES

Inspect the muscles for impaired tone, 1490–1491

Test for the degree of muscle strength, 1553

N

NAILS

Advise that lanolin be applied to brittle nails, 1575

Clean the nails, 1274

Explain how to file the nails correctly, 1607

Explain that nails should be soaked before trimming, 1622

Explain the need for nail cleanliness, 1637

File the nails in one direction and only on the underside, 1335

Inspect the nails for abnormalities, 1491

Instruct to clean the nails with a cotton-tipped stick, 1667

Instruct to cut the toenails straight across, 1667

Instruct to lubricate the skin (scalp or nails), 1671

Pack sterile cotton between the ingrown nail and the skin, 1379

Soak the nails in warm oil, 1441

Trim the hangnail, 1452

NASAL FLARE

Observe for nasal flare, 1534

NAUSEA

Observe for complaints of nausea, 1524

NEBULIZATION

Administer aerosol mist by nebulizer (MD Rx), 1737–1738

Drain condensation from the nebulizer tubing periodically, 1291

Teach how to test the urine for protein, 1724

Test the urine for protein, 1556

PUBERTY

See Behavior

PULSE

Auscultate the apical and palpate the radial pulses for a pulse deficit, 1460

Instruct to check the pulse daily when wearing a pacemaker, 1666–1667

Palpate for arterial pulsations, 1543–1544

Palpate the abdominal aorta for increased pulsation, 1544–1545

Palpate the pulse for rate, rhythm, and volume, 1548

Teach how to count a pulse, 1709

PULSE PRESSURE

Monitor the pulse pressure, 1514–1515

PUPIL RESPONSE

Inspect the eyes for pupil equality and response changes, 1488

Q

QUESTIONS

Ask simple, direct questions, 1259

Encourage patient (parent or family) questions, 1318

QUIET

Provide quiet, 1407–1408

R

RADIATION

Collect radiation-contaminated linen in a special laundry bag, 1276

Collect radiation-contaminated urine in a lead-lined container, 1276

Limit the amount of time visitors are exposed to radiation, 1365

Limit the distance from which visitors approach the radiated patient, 1365–1366

Shield visitors from exposure to radiation, 1439

RALES

Auscultate the chest for rales and/or rhonchi, 1464

RANGE OF MOTION

Excercise in range of motion, 1328

READING

Advise against reading or looking out the window while in a moving vehicle, 1565

Encourage light reading before sleep, 1314

Inform that large-print reading material is available, 1654

Offer reading material with familiar content, 1378

Provide braille reading material, 1401

Provide large-print reading material, 1405

Provide religious reading material, 1408

Read to the patient, 1410

REFERRAL

Make a referral, 1372–1373

REFLEXES

Inspect the throat for an impaired swallowing reflex, 1494

Stimulate the sucking reflex through jaw or lip pressure, 1444

Test for abnormal deep-reflex responses, 1552

Test the eyes for decreased corneal reflex, 1554

Test the infant for the Moro reflex, 1555

Test the infant for the neck-righting reflex, 1555–1556

Test the infant for the rooting reflex, 1556

RELAXATION

Explain that recreation and relaxation differ, 1625

Recommend methods for achieving total relaxation, 1679–1680

RELIGION

Assist with bedside religious observances, 1260–1261

Determine the level of participation in spiritual rituals, 1472–1473

Encourage chapel-service attendance, 1299

Encourage discussion of the patient's spiritual values, 1305–1306

Encourage spiritually uplifiting conversation, 1322

Encourage the chaplain's visit, 1323

S

SAFETY, PHYSICAL

Advise against exposure to airborne irritants, 1562

Apply a safety helmet to the head, 1249

Emphasize that a car should never be started in a closed garage, 1590

Emphasize that bulging food cans should be discarded, 1590

Emphasize that clotheslines should be kept high to prevent strangulation, 1590

Emphasize that contaminated clothing should be changed immediately, 1590

Emphasize that contaminated skin should be washed immediately, 1590–1591

Emphasize that cracked dishware should be discarded, 1591

Emphasize that dangerous products should be stored out of reach, 1591

Emphasize that extension cords should be secured in place, 1591

Emphasize that fireplaces should be screened, 1591

Emphasize that floors and stairways should be litter-free, 1591

Emphasize that food wastes should be burned in animal-inhabited outdoor areas, 1591–1592

Emphasize that fume-producing substances should be used in the open air, 1592

Emphasize that garbage should be covered, 1592

Emphasize that heaters should be vented to the outside, 1592

Emphasize that, in outdoor living, human wastes should be buried, 1592

Emphasize that knife racks should be covered, 1592

Emphasize that large icicles should be removed, 1592–1593

Emphasize that matches should be stored in a metal container, 1593

Emphasize that medicine cabinets should be locked, 1593

Emphasize that open heaters should be screened, 1593

Emphasize that outdated foods (or drugs) should be discarded, 1593

Emphasize that plastic bags should be shredded and discarded, 1593

Emphasize that play areas should be fenced, 1593–1594

Emphasize that pools should be protected against entry, 1594

Emphasize that potentially unsafe water should be boiled for ten minutes, 1594

Emphasize that safety guards should be placed over electrical outlets, 1594

Emphasize that seat belts should be fastened, 1594

Emphasize that small children should always be attended, 1594

Emphasize that snow should be removed from stairs, 1594–1595

Emphasize that stoves should be kept free of grease, 1595

Emphasize that unused electrical equipment should be disconnected, 1595

Emphasize that unused refrigerators should be locked or the doors removed, 1595

Emphasize that worn electrical cords should be repaired immediately, 1595

Emphasize the danger of diving into shallow water, 1596

Emphasize the danger of highly waxed floors, 1597

Emphasize the danger of sleeping with an infant, 1598

Emphasize the danger of smoking around oxygen, 1598

Emphasize the danger of smoking in bed, 1598

Emphasize the importance of wearing safety goggles, 1599

Emphasize the need to check for gas leakage and fire, 1599

Emphasize the need to maintain sturdy stair rails, 1600

Emphasize the need to use only an approved sewage facility, 1600

Emphasize the need to use only an approved water supply, 1600

Emphasize the need to use safe ladders, 1600

Emphasize the need to use safety straps to prevent falling, 1601

Evaluate the safety of the environment, 1477

Explain how to correctly store guns and ammunition, 1604

Explain that clear, correct product labeling is essential, 1617

Explain that persons with impaired cerebral function require close observation, 1623

Provide safe play equipment for children, 1409

Recommend strict adherence to safety rules, 1682

Recommend the use of handrails, 1694

Recommend the use of nonskid throw rugs, 1697

Recommend the use of stair gates, 1698
Recommend the use of suction tub mats, 1698
Recommend the use of well-padded pot holders, 1699
Recommend wearing a hard hat for head protection, 1699
Remove harmful objects from the environment, 1428
Remove immediately to a safe area, 1428
Safeguard with siderail padding, 1437
Safeguard with siderails, 1437
Use a waist safety strap during mobility, 1453

SALINE

Apply a saline compress, 1249
Encourage the use of a warm, saline gargle, 1325
Refrain from giving saline laxatives, 1419
Soak in saline solution, 1440–1441

SALIVATION

Inspect the mouth for abnormal salivation, 1490
Stimulate salivation with sour-flavored foods, 1443

SALT

Explain the difference between salt and sodium diet restriction, 1632
Give iodized salt, 1343
Recommend the use of iodized salt, 1695
Refrain from giving table salt, 1419

SALT, ARTIFICIAL

Substitute artificial salt, 1445

SALT SOLUTION

Give salt solution orally, 1347

SALT-SODA SOLUTION

Give salt-soda solution orally, 1347

SANDBAGS

Position with sandbags, 1394
Restrict head movements with sandbags and pillows, 1432

SANITARY PADS

Advise frequent sanitary pad change, 1569

Change the sanitary pads frequently, 1271
Count the number of sanitary pads used, 1470

SCALP

Advise against prolonged skin (or scalp) exposure to the sun, 1564
Advise against prolonged skin (or scalp) exposure to water, 1565
Explain how to shampoo the hair (or scalp), 1614
Instruct to comb dandruff up from the scalp, 1667
Instruct to inspect the skin (scalp or hair), 1669–1670
Instruct to lubricate the skin (scalp or nails), 1671
Instruct to maintain skin (or scalp) cleanliness, 1672
Shampoo the hair (scalp), 1438

SCRATCHING DEVICE

Provide a scratching device, 1399

SECRETIONS

Advise against drawing secretions to the back of the throat, 1561
Clear nasal secretions, 1276

SEIZURES

Describe the manifestations of impending seizure, 1584
Explain how to manage seizure episodes, 1610
Inform of those conditions which precipitate seizures, 1645
Inform that seizures are noncontagious, 1655
Observe for convulsions, 1526
Observe the seizure characteristics, 1542

SENSORY PERCEPTIONS

Test for impaired smell perception, 1553
Test for impaired taste perception, 1553

SEWAGE

Emphasize the need to use only an approved sewage facility, 1600

SEXUAL ACTIVITY

Explain that pregnancy results from sexual activity, 1624

Soak in a medicated solution (MD Rx), 1747
Soak in cold water, 1440
Soak in saline solution, 1440–1441
Soak the nails in warm oil, 1441
Teach how to do therapeutic soaks, 1714

SOAP

Clean the skin with a drying soap, 1274
Clean with castile or lanolin soap, 1275
Clean with surgical soap, 1275
Refrain from using a cream-based soap, 1425
Refrain from using an alkaline soap on the skin, 1425

SOCIALIZATION

Encourage social activities, 1322
Explain that socialization depletes the ill person's energy, 1626
Socialize gradually, 1441

SODIUM

Encourage decreased sodium-food intake, 1304
Encourage increased sodium-food intake, 1312–1313
Explain the difference between salt and sodium diet restriction, 1632
Give high-sodium fluids orally, 1341
Give low-sodium fluids orally, 1341

SODIUM BICARBONATE

Apply sodium bicarbonate to the skin, 1256
Give sodium bicarbonate solution orally, 1348

SPASTICITY

Control excessive spasticity with firm hand pressure, 1278

SPECIAL REQUESTS

Grant special requests, 1352

SPECIMENS

Explain how to collect a specimen, 1604

SPIRITUAL

Assist with bedside religious observances, 1260–1261
Determine the level of participation in spiritual rituals, 1472–1473

Encourage chapel-service attendance, 1299
Encourage discussion of the patient's spiritual values, 1305–1306
Encourage spiritually uplifting conversation, 1322
Encourage the chaplain's visit, 1323
Encourage the use of spiritual resources, 1326
Evaluate the significance of spirituality in the patient's life, 1477
Guide the patient in simple prayer, 1352
Pray with the patient, 1394
Provide desired religious articles, 1402
Provide information about spiritual programs, 1405
Provide religious reading material, 1408

SPLEEN

Palpate the spleen for enlargement, 1548

SPLINT

Apply a supportive splint, 1250
Apply the prescribed preventive splint (MD Rx), 1742
Teach how to apply preventive splints, 1704

SPLINTING

Explain how to splint an incision, 1614
Splint the incisional area, 1442

SPUTUM

Explain how to dispose of infectious expectoration, 1606–1607
Inspect the sputum for characteristics, 1494
Monitor the laboratory findings of sputum analysis, 1513
Provide a sputum container, 1399–1400
Recommend the use of double thickness tissue for infectious sputum, 1693
Take sputum precautions, 1499

SPUTUM STUDIES

See Studies, Sputum

STANDING

Advise not to stand for prolonged periods, 1571–1572

STERILE TECHNIQUE

Use sterile technique, 1455
Wear sterile gloves, 1457

STIMULANTS

Discourage oral stimulants, 1284
Refrain from giving oral stimulants, 1418

STIMULATION

Advise that mental stimulation be maintained through variety, 1575
Explain how to stimulate an infant during feeding, 1614–1615
Offer environmental stimulation through contact with varied personnel, environmental change, and variety in daily routine, 1378
Recommend methods for increasing sensory stimulation, 1680
Recommend methods for reducing sensory stimulation, 1681
Refrain from making sudden, stimulating movements, 1420–1421
Remove the stimuli which support the misperception, 1430
Remove the stimulus for the emotion, 1430
Stimulate by movement, touch, sternal pressure, or speech, 1442
Stimulate gagging with a tongue blade, 1443
Stimulate salivation with sour-flavored foods, 1443
Stimulate the infant with a mobile, 1443
Stimulate the infant with back stroking or foot thumping, 1443
Stimulate the memory by repeating the patient's last expressed thought, 1443
Stimulate the reflex bladder by applying cold to the abdomen, stroking the inner thigh, or running water, 1443–1444
Stimulate the reflex bowel by abdominal stroking and anal stimulation, 1444
Stimulate the sucking reflex through jaw or lip pressure, 1444
Teach now to stimulate the gums, 1723

STOOL

Inspect for stool abnormalities, 1484
Take stool precautions, 1449

STOVES

Emphasize that stoves should be kept free of grease, 1595
Recommend the use of front stove controls for persons in a wheelchair, 1694
Recommend the use of top stove controls for persons unable to stoop, 1698

STRANGULATION

Emphasize that clotheslines should be kept high to prevent strangulation, 1590

STRAW

Instruct not to use a drinking straw, 1660–1661
Provide a drinking straw, 1397
Provide a short drinking straw, 1399

STRESS

See Behavior

STRETCHER

Mobilize by stretcher, 1375

STRYKER FRAME

Place on a Stryker frame, 1389

STUDIES, BLOOD

Monitor blood studies for abnormal acid-base, 1499
Monitor blood studies for abnormal adrenal function, 1499–1500
Monitor blood studies for abnormal carbohydrate metabolism, 1500
Monitor blood studies for abnormal cardiac enzymes, 1500
Monitor blood studies for abnormal cholesterol, 1500
Monitor blood studies for abnormal clotting mechanism, 1500–1501
Monitor blood studies for abnormal electrolytes, 1501–1502
Monitor blood studies for abnormal gas exchange, 1502–1503
Monitor blood studies for abnormal glucose, 1503
Monitor blood studies for abnormal hematology, 1503–1505
Monitor blood studies for abnormal liver function, 1505–1506
Monitor blood studies for abnormal pancreatic function, 1506
Monitor blood studies for abnormal parathyroid function, 1506
Monitor blood studies for abnormal pituitary function, 1506
Monitor blood studies for abnormal renal function, 1506–1507
Monitor blood studies for abnormal thyroid function, 1507
Monitor blood studies for biliary obstruction, 1507

STUDIES, CEREBRAL SPINAL FLUID

STUDIES, GASTRIC ANALYSIS

STUDIES, LABORATORY

STUDIES, SPUTUM

STUDIES, TIDAL VOLUME

STUDIES, URINE

STUMP SOCK

SUBCLAVIAN INTRACATH

SUCTION

SUFFOCATION